Clayton's Basic Pharmacology for Nurses

EDITION
18

Clayton's Basic Pharmacology for Nurses

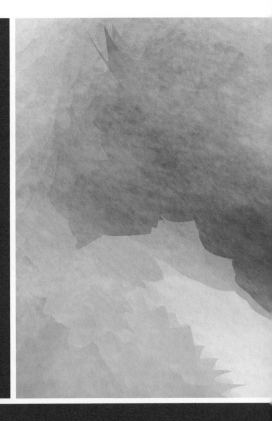

Michelle J. Willihnganz, MS, RN, CNE
RCTC Nursing Instructor
Rochester Community and Technical College
Rochester, Minnesota

Samuel L. Gurevitz, PharmD, CGP
Associate Professor
College of Pharmacy and Health Sciences
Butler University
Indianapolis, Indiana

Bruce D. Clayton, BS Pharm, PharmD, RPh
Professor of Pharmacy Practice
College of Pharmacy and Health Sciences
Butler University
Indianapolis, Indiana

ELSEVIER

Notices

Knowledge and best practice in this field are constantly changing. As new research and experience broaden our understanding, changes in research methods, professional practices, or medical treatment may become necessary.

Practitioners and researchers must always rely on their own experience and knowledge in evaluating and using any information, methods, compounds, or experiments described herein. In using such information or methods they should be mindful of their own safety and the safety of others, including parties for whom they have a professional responsibility.

With respect to any drug or pharmaceutical products identified, readers are advised to check the most current information provided (i) on procedures featured or (ii) by the manufacturer of each product to be administered, to verify the recommended dose or formula, the method and duration of administration, and contraindications. It is the responsibility of practitioners, relying on their own experience and knowledge of their patients, to make diagnoses, to determine dosages and the best treatment for each individual patient, and to take all appropriate safety precautions.

To the fullest extent of the law, neither the Publisher nor the authors, contributors, or editors, assume any liability for any injury and/or damage to persons or property as a matter of products liability, negligence or otherwise, or from any use or operation of any methods, products, instructions, or ideas contained in the material herein.

Previous editions copyrighted 2017, 2013, 2010, 2007, 2004, 2001, 1997, 1993, 1989, 1985, 1981, 1977, 1973, 1969, 1965, 1961, and 1957.

International Standard Book Number: 978-0-323-55061-1

Senior Content Manager: Ellen Wurm-Cutter
Senior Content Strategist: Nancy O'Brien
Senior Content Development Specialist: Rebecca Leenhouts
Publishing Services Manager: Catherine Albright Jackson
Senior Project Manager: Claire Kramer
Design Direction: Renee Duenow

Printed in Canada.

Last digit is the print number: 9   8   7   6   5   4   3   2   1

ELSEVIER

3251 Riverport Lane
St. Louis, Missouri 63043

Working together
to grow libraries in
developing countries

www.elsevier.com • www.bookaid.org

Reviewers and Ancillary Contributors

REVIEWERS

Kimberly Ann Amos, PhD, MSN, RN, CNE
Interim Director
Practical Nursing Education
Isothermal Community College
Spindale, North Carolina

Virginia L. Christensen, RN, BSN
Practical Nursing/Health Education Coordinator
Tennessee College of Applied Technology–Livingston
Livingston, Tennessee

Patricia Donovan, MSN, RN
Director of the Practical Nursing Program and
    Curriculum Chair
Nursing Education
The Porter and Chester Institute
Rocky Hill, Connecticut

Linda Gambill, MSN/Ed, RN, ENPC
Instructor and Clinical Coordinator
Practical Nursing
Southwest Virginia Community College
Cedar Bluff, Virginia

Lorraine Kelley, MSN, BSHA, RN
Nursing Department Faculty
Practical Nursing Program Coordinator
Department of Nursing
Pensacola State College
Pensacola, Florida

Nora MacLeod-Glover, BSc (Pharm), PharmD
Associate Professor, Health Systems
University of Toronto
Toronto, Ontario, Canada

Mary Ruiz-Nuve, RN, MSN
Director of Nursing
Licensed Practical Nursing
St. Louis College of Health Careers
Fenton, Missouri

Travis E. Sonnett, PharmD
Clinical Pharmacy Specialist/Adjunct Clinical Professor
Mann-Grandstaff VA Medical Center
College of Pharmacy
Washington State University
Spokane, Washington

Ashley Williams, MSN, RN, CEN
Assistant Professor of Nursing
Capito Department of Nursing
University of Charleston
Charleston, West Virginia

ANCILLARY CONTRIBUTOR

Laura Bevlock Kanavy, RN, BSN, MSN
Director, Practical Nursing Program
Career Technology Center of Lackawanna County
Scranton, Pennsylvania
Test Bank, NCLEX Review Questions

LPN/LVN Advisory Board

Preface

The eighteenth edition of *Clayton's Basic Pharmacology for Nurses*, in the tradition of the book's standards first established in 1957, advocates the administration of medication with safety and precision while focusing on medication safety through medication monitoring and patient education. In the practice setting, the nurse not only must demonstrate knowledge of the underlying disease process but also must be able to perform an accurate assessment to identify individualized nursing diagnoses. The nurse must also plan and implement care in a manner that involves the patient as an active participant in decisions affecting care. Therefore, a primary concern throughout this book is the integration of patient teaching about drug therapy to enable the patient to reach therapeutic goals and attain an optimum level of health. The nurse must also validate patient understanding to ensure that the individual has the ability to provide safe self-care and monitoring of the prescribed treatment plan. User friendly in content, structure, and layout, the text is concise and easy to read. With its emphasis on the seven Rights of Drug Administration (right drug, right time, right indication, right dosage, right patient, right route, and right documentation), *Clayton's Basic Pharmacology for Nurses* provides students with the information needed to provide safe, effective nursing care for patients receiving drug therapy.

ORGANIZATION AND SPECIAL FEATURES

CONTENT THREADS

Clayton's Basic Pharmacology for Nurses, eighteenth edition, shares some features and design elements with other Elsevier books that you may be using. The purpose of these Content Threads is to make it easier for students and instructors to use the variety of books required by a fast-paced and demanding curriculum.

The shared features in *Basic Pharmacology for Nurses*, eighteenth edition, include the following:
- Cover and internal design similarities; the colorful, student-friendly design encourages reading and learning of this core content
- Numbered lists of Objectives that begin each chapter
- Key Terms with pronunciations at the beginning of each chapter; the key terms are in color when they are defined in the chapter
- Bulleted lists of Key Points at the end of each chapter

- Multiple-choice and multiple-response Review Questions for the NCLEX® Examination at the end of each chapter; answers are provided on the Evolve student website.

In addition to content and design threads, these textbooks benefit from the advice and input of the Elsevier Advisory Board.

CONTENTS

Unit I explores pharmacology foundations, principles, life span considerations, the nursing process with pharmacology, and patient education. Unit II contains the unique Illustrated Atlas of Medication Administration that provides extensive step-by-step instructions and illustrations that show primary routes of administration and proper administration techniques for all forms of medications.

Units III through X provide an overview of each drug class, followed by narrative discussions of the most common individual drugs. The units and chapters are organized by body system.

CHAPTER ORGANIZATION

- Each drug chapter in Units III through X begins with an overview of a clinical problem and its management.
- The general nursing implications section includes clearly identified headings for Assessment, Implementation, and Patient Education. The Patient Education section helps the nurse incorporate patient education designed to promote health into the overall treatment plan.
- Drug monographs are provided for each major drug class. These monographs describe Actions, Uses, and Therapeutic Outcomes for each class.
- A drug class–specific nursing implications section for each drug monograph highlights Premedication Assessment, Product Availability, Dosing Instructions, Common Adverse Effects, Serious Adverse Effects, and Drug Interactions.

SPECIAL FEATURES

Clayton's Basic Pharmacology for Nurses includes special features designed to foster effective learning and comprehension.
- Chapter opening features include lists of Objectives and Key Terms with pronunciations.

- Clinical Pitfall and Medication Safety Alert boxes highlight critically important clinical considerations to help students practice safety and reduce medication errors.
- Clinical Goldmine boxes put a spotlight on tips and best practices for clinical procedures.
- Life Span Considerations boxes focus on the implications of drug therapy for children, pregnant and breastfeeding women, and older adults.
- Herbal Interactions boxes discuss well-documented interactions among drugs, herbal therapies, and dietary supplements.
- A handy bulleted list of Key Points at the end of most chapters facilitates review of essential chapter content.

NEW TO THIS EDITION

- This edition includes the latest FDA approvals and withdrawals, including up-to-date clinical drug indications and new drugs.
- Increased emphasis on medication safety stresses imperative information for patient protection.
- Additional information on genetics, pharmacogenomics, and racial/gender factors in drug actions is included to highlight the most up-to-date research.
- Several chapters have been renamed to incorporate medications that previously were only under the miscellaneous chapter, and this change allows for expansion of new medications as they are produced and used for common conditions such as Alzheimer's and osteoporosis.

TEACHING AND LEARNING PACKAGE

FOR STUDENTS

- The Evolve Website provides free student resources, including answers and rationales for in-text Review Questions for the NCLEX® Examination, a math review, animations, video clips, a collection of Patient Teaching handouts, fully customizable Patient Self-Assessment Forms provided as "completable" PDF documents, and a collection of 500 NCLEX®-style Review Questions.
- The revised Study Guide provides additional learning resources that complement those in the textbook. Questions for each chapter follow the objectives in the book for additional focus on these key concepts. A new section on matching starts each chapter, and a patient scenario is included with the chapters that detail the medications. Each question has a page number identified to help the student find the answer in the textbook. Answers to the Study Guide questions are available from instructors.

FOR INSTRUCTORS

The comprehensive *Evolve Resources with TEACH Instructor Resource* provides a rich array of resources that includes the following:

- Updated TEACH Lesson Plans, based on textbook learning objectives, provide ready-to-use lesson plans that tie together all of the text and ancillary components provided for *Clayton's Basic Pharmacology for Nurses.*
- The collection of PowerPoint Lecture Slides is specific to the text.
- A Test Bank, delivered in ExamView, now provides an expanded collection of approximately 900 multiple-choice and alternate-format NCLEX®-style questions. Each question includes the Correct Answer, Rationale, Step of the Nursing Process, and NCLEX® Patient Needs Category, as well as corresponding text page numbers.
- The Image Collection contains every reproducible image from the text. Images are suitable for incorporation into classroom lectures, PowerPoint presentations, or distance-learning applications.
- Answer keys are provided for the Study Guide.

Special Features

Clayton's Basic Pharmacology for Nurses focuses on medication safety through medication monitoring and patient education. Full-color art and design features accompany detailed, understandable discussions of drugs organized by body system.

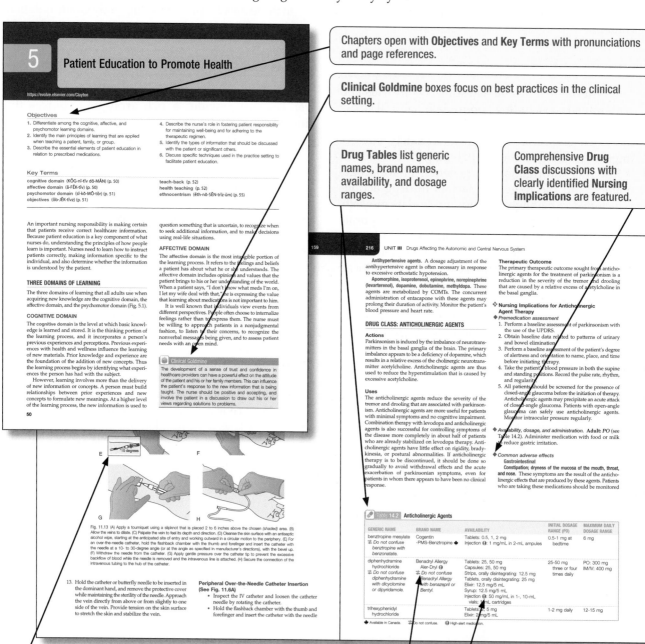

Chapters open with **Objectives** and **Key Terms** with pronunciations and page references.

Clinical Goldmine boxes focus on best practices in the clinical setting.

Drug Tables list generic names, brand names, availability, and dosage ranges.

Comprehensive **Drug Class** discussions with clearly identified **Nursing Implications** are featured.

Step-by-step **full color art** shows proper medication administration techniques.

Do-Not-Confuse icons highlight look-alike/sound-alike drugs.

High-Alert Medication icons identify drugs that require special safeguards to reduce the risk of administration errors.

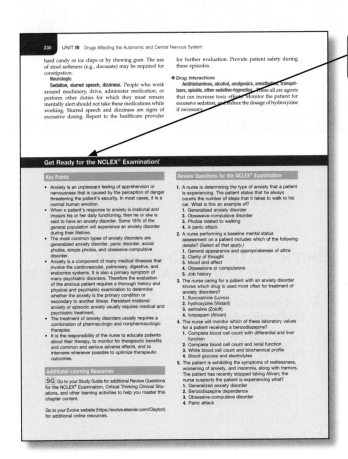

Get Ready for the NCLEX® Examination! sections include Key Points, Additional Learning Resources, and Review Questions for the NCLEX® Examination.

- **Patient Education and Health Promotion** is emphasized in the overall treatment plan.
- **Life Span Considerations** boxes focus on implications of drug therapy for children, pregnant and breastfeeding women, and older adults.
- **Clinical Pitfall and Medication Safety Alert** boxes highlight critically important clinical considerations.
- **Herbal Interactions** boxes describe possible adverse effects of alternative therapies.

Chapters open with **Objectives** and **Key Terms** with pronunciations and page references.

STUDY GUIDE

Includes *Practice Questions for the NCLEX® Examination* for each textbook chapter. Answers to the revised study guide are available from your instructor.

Contents

Clayton's
Basic Pharmacology
for Nurses

Drug Definitions, Standards, and Information Sources

Objectives

1. Differentiate between the chemical, generic, and brand names of drugs.
2. Identify the various methods used to classify drugs.
3. Identify sources of drug information available for healthcare providers.
4. Cite sources of credible drug information on the Internet.
5. Discuss the difference between prescription and nonprescription drugs.
6. Describe the process of developing and bringing new drugs to market.
7. Differentiate between the Canadian *chemical* names and the *proper* name of a drug.

Key Terms

Pharmacology (făr-mă-KŎL-ŏ-jē) (p. 1)
therapeutic methods (thĕr-ă-PYŪ-tĭk MĚTH-ĕdz) (p. 1)
drugs (p. 1)
biologic therapies (p. 1)
chemical name (KĔM-ĭ-kŭl) (p. 2)
generic name (jĕ-NĀR-ĭk) (p. 2)
brand name (p. 2)
prescription drugs (p. 2)
nonprescription drugs (p. 2)

over-the-counter (OTC) drugs (p. 2)
illegal drugs (ĭl-LĒ-gŭl) (p. 2)
biosimilar (p. 2)
schedules (SKĔD-jūlz) (p. 5)
black box warnings (p. 8)
orphan drugs (ŌR-făn) (p. 9)
Food and Drugs Act and Regulations (p. 10)
Controlled Drugs and Substances Act (p. 10)

Pharmacology (from the Greek *pharmakon,* meaning "drugs," and *logos,* meaning "science") deals with the study of drugs and their actions on living organisms. Diseases that cause illness may be treated in several different ways, which are referred to as *therapies.* The various approaches to therapy are called ***therapeutic methods.*** Examples of therapeutic methods include the following:

- **Drug therapy:** Treatment with drugs
- **Diet therapy:** Treatment with diet (e.g., a low-salt diet for patients with cardiovascular disease)
- **Physiotherapy:** Treatment with natural physical forces (e.g., water, light, heat)
- **Psychological therapy:** The identification of stressors and methods that can be used to reduce or eliminate stress

Most illnesses caused by diseases require a combination of therapeutic methods for successful treatment.

Drugs (from the Dutch *droog,* meaning "dry") are chemical substances that have an effect on living organisms. Therapeutic drugs, which are often called *medicines,* are those drugs that are used for the prevention or treatment of diseases. Up until the early to mid-20th century, dried plants were the most abundant source of medicines, thus the word *drug* was applied to them.

Whereas most drugs are individual chemicals that cause a response in living tissues, a new class known as **biologic therapies** have been discovered that have transformed treatment of patients with disorders that attack the body's own organs, tissues, and cells (autoimmune disorders), blood (hematologic disorders), and cancers. Biologic agents are large, complex proteins manufactured in a living system such as a microorganism, or within plant or animal cells. Biologics have added major therapeutic choices for the treatment of many diseases for which no effective therapies were available or previously existing therapies were clearly inadequate.

DRUG NAMES, STANDARDS, LEGISLATION, AND DEVELOPMENT IN THE UNITED STATES

DRUG NAMES

All drugs have several names, which may cause confusion. When administering the prescribed drug, the spelling on the drug package must correspond exactly with the spelling of the drug ordered to ensure that the proper medicine is administered.

Each drug has three names: (1) a *chemical* name, (2) a *generic* name, and (3) a *brand* name. The **chemical name** is most meaningful to the chemist. By means of the chemical name, the chemist understands the exact chemical constitution of the drug and the exact placement of its atoms or molecular groupings.

Before a drug becomes official, it is given a **generic name** or common name. The generic name is simpler than the chemical name. It may be used in any country and by any manufacturer. The first letter of the generic name is not capitalized. Students are strongly encouraged to learn and refer to drugs by their generic names because formularies (i.e., lists of medicines available through a pharmacy) are maintained by generic names. When a therapeutically equivalent drug becomes available in generic form, the generic medicine is routinely substituted for the brand-name medicine.

Generic names are provided by the United States Adopted Names Council, which is an organization sponsored by the United States Pharmacopeial Convention, the American Medical Association, and the American Pharmacists Association. The official name, which is virtually always the generic name in the United States, is the name under which the drug is listed by the US Food and Drug Administration (FDA). The FDA is empowered by federal law to generically name the drugs for human use in the United States.

A trademark or **brand name** is followed by the symbol ®. This symbol indicates that the name is registered and that the use of the name is restricted to the owner of the drug, which is usually the manufacturer. Most drug companies place their products on the market under brand names rather than generic names. The brand names are deliberately made easier to pronounce, spell, and remember. The first letter of the brand name is capitalized.

Example of Chemical, Generic, and Brand Names for Drugs

Chemical name: [2-[4-[(4-Chlorophenyl) phenylmethyl]-1-piperazinyl]ethoxy]acetic acid dihydrochloride (see Fig. 1.1)
Generic name: Cetirizine
Brand name: Zyrtec Allergy

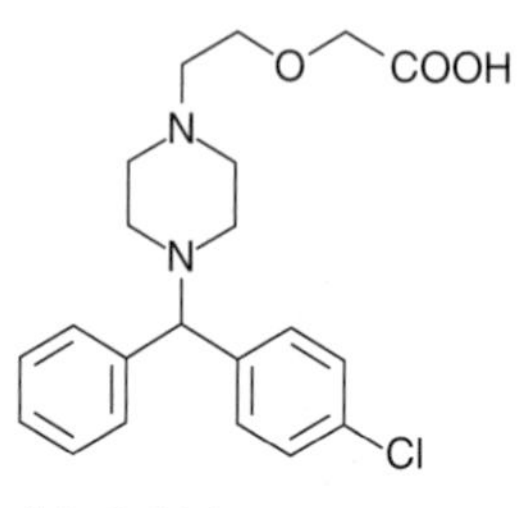

Fig. 1.1 Cetirizine, an antihistamine.

DRUG CLASSIFICATIONS

Drugs may be classified by a variety of methods according to the *body system* that they affect (e.g., the central nervous system, the cardiovascular system, the gastrointestinal system); their *therapeutic use* or *clinical indications* (e.g., antacids, antibiotics, antihypertensives, diuretics, laxatives); and their *physiologic* or *chemical action* (e.g., anticholinergics, beta-adrenergic blockers, calcium channel blockers, cholinergics).

Drugs may be further classified as prescription or nonprescription. **Prescription drugs** require an order by a health professional who is licensed to prescribe drugs, such as a physician, a nurse practitioner, a physician assistant, a pharmacist, or a dentist. **Nonprescription drugs**, or **over-the-counter (OTC) drugs**, are sold without a prescription in a pharmacy or in the health section of department or grocery stores. **Illegal drugs**, sometimes referred to as *recreational drugs*, are drugs or chemical substances used for nontherapeutic purposes. These substances either are obtained illegally or have not received approval for use by the FDA. See Chapter 48 for further information about substance abuse.

A **biosimilar** is a biologic product that is close in structure and function to an existing approved biologic product, known as a *reference product*. For example, infliximab-dyyb (Inflectra) and infliximab-abda (Renflexis) are biosimilars for the reference product infliximab (Remicade) used to treat rheumatoid arthritis. With many patents for biologics expiring, biosimilar agents will become available. In 2010, legislation created an abbreviated licensure pathway for biologic products that are demonstrated to be biosimilar. Biosimilars offer an opportunity to increase access to biologics while lowering the cost of therapy. However, unlike generic medicines in which the active ingredients are identical to the reference small-molecule drugs, biosimilars will not be identical to the reference biologics. This is due to the inherent complexity of biologic proteins. Biosimilars made by different manufacturers will differ from the reference product and from each other, making each biosimilar a unique therapeutic option for patients (Table 1.1).

SOURCES OF DRUG STANDARDS AND DRUG INFORMATION

Drug products made by different manufacturers or in different batches by the same manufacturer must be uniformly pure and potent. The United States Pharmacopeial Convention is a nongovernment organization that promotes public health by establishing state-of-the-art standards to ensure the quality of medicines and other healthcare technologies. These standards are developed by a unique process of public involvement, and they are accepted worldwide. The Convention publishes a single-volume text, the *United States Pharmacopeia (USP)/National Formulary (NF)*, which is revised annually. The primary purpose of this volume is to

Table 1.1	Comparing and Contrasting Biosimilar and Generic Products	
PROPERTIES	**BIOSIMILARS (BIOLOGICS)**	**GENERICS (SMALL-MOLECULE DRUGS)**
Size	Large	Small
Structure	Complex with potential structural variations	Simple and well defined
Manufacturing	Unique bank of living cells Unlikely to achieve identical copy	Predictable chemical reaction Identical copy can be made
Complexity	Difficult to fully characterize	Easy to fully characterize
Stability	More sensitive to storage and handling conditions	Less sensitive to storage and handling conditions
Immunogenicity (promotes immune response; potential for allergy)	Higher potential	Lower potential
Approval requirements	Large clinical trials in patients	Small clinical trials for safety in healthy volunteers

provide standards for the identity, quality, strength, and purity of substances used in the practice of healthcare. The standards described in the *USP/NF* are enforced by the FDA as the official standards for the manufacture and quality control of medicines and nutritional supplements produced in the United States. The *USP/NF* is also recognized by the Canadian Food and Drugs Act as an authoritative source of drug standards in Canada.

Table 1.2 lists and describes the common sources of drug information available for the professional healthcare provider; additional resources are described in the following sections.

PACKAGE INSERTS

Manufacturers of drugs are required to develop a comprehensive but concise description of the drug, indications and precautions for clinical use, recommendations for dosage, known adverse reactions, contraindications, and other pharmacologic information relating to the drug. Federal law mandates that this material be approved by the FDA before the product is released for marketing and that it be presented on an insert that accompanies each package of the product.

The FDA adopted a format for package inserts to help reduce medication errors and to improve patient education. The labeling reduces practitioners' time looking for information, decreases the number of preventable medication errors, and improves treatment effectiveness and patient education. Because this labeling represents considerable effort and is most critical for newer and less familiar drugs, the formatting applies only to relatively new prescription drug products, developed since 2006.

Clinical Goldmine

 DailyMed (see Online Resources), which is sponsored by the US National Library of Medicine, provides a database for new package inserts that is searchable by product name, indications, dosage and administration, warnings, description of drug product, active and inactive ingredients, and how the drug is supplied. See the section Electronic Databases.

NURSING JOURNALS

Many specialty journals have articles about drug therapy as it relates to a specific field of interest (e.g., *Geriatric Nursing, American Journal of Critical Care*). Nursing journals such as *RN* and *American Journal of Nursing* provide drug updates and articles that discuss nursing considerations related to drug therapy and drugs. Nurses must keep in mind that the purpose of using resources such as journals is to obtain professional knowledge of current evidence-based practice changes and they should not be used as a primary source for drug information. Nurses must be mindful of the accuracy of the information contained and should check the dates on articles to validate the currency of the information.

ELECTRONIC DATABASES

With the exponential growth of information about medicines and health, it is almost impossible to make the information available without the use of electronic databases. The National Library of Medicine provides Medline and other searchable databases at no cost. Most of the drug information sources listed in Table 1.2 are also available via electronic retrieval from libraries. Many college libraries subscribe to the Cumulative Index to Nursing and Allied Health Literature (CINAHL). These databases give nurses access to a wealth of information from sources published in the United States and other countries.

Databases for practitioners are also available by subscription. UpToDate, Lexicomp, and ePocrates are three vendors with several different packages of regularly updated information (see Online Resources). Lexicomp has a particularly strong database because the American Hospital Formulary Service is available through its portal.

The DailyMed system (see Online Resources) was developed in collaboration with federal agencies— including the FDA, the National Library of Medicine, the Agency for Healthcare Research and Quality, the National Cancer Institute in the US Department of Health and Human Services, and the US Department of Veterans

Table 1.2   Sources of Drug Information for Healthcare Providers

SOURCES OF DRUG INFORMATION	DESCRIPTION
USP Dictionary of United States Adopted Names (USAN) and International Drug Names	Published annually Compilation of more than 10,000 drug names Describes the criteria by which drugs are named Online version available
American Drug Index	Index of medicines available in the United States Useful for quickly comparing brand names and generic names and for checking available strengths and dosage forms
AHFS Drug Information	Contains monographs about virtually every single-entity drug available in the United States Describes therapeutic uses of drugs, including approved and unapproved uses Online version available
Drug Interaction Facts	Currently considered the most comprehensive book available about drug interactions
Drug Facts and Comparisons	Contains drug monographs that describe all drugs in a therapeutic class Monographs are formatted as tables to allow comparison of similar products, brand names, manufacturers, cost indices, and available dosage forms Online version available
ASHP's *Handbook on Injectable Drugs: IV Decision Support*	Collection of monographs about 332 injectable drugs with sections on available concentrations, compatibility with other drugs, dosage and rate of administration, stability, pH, and other useful information Interactive version available
Handbook of Nonprescription Drugs: An Interactive Approach to Self-Care	Most comprehensive text available about over-the-counter medications that can be purchased in the United States Online version available
Martindale: The Complete Drug Reference	Considered one of the most comprehensive texts available for information about drugs in current use throughout the world Contains extensive referenced monographs about the international names, pharmacologic activity, and side effects of more than 5500 drugs Online subscription available
Physicians' Desk Reference (PDR)	Discusses more than 3000 therapeutic agents Divided into six sections: (1) manufacturers' index; (2) brand and generic name index; (3) product category index; (4) product identification guide; (5) product information section; and (6) dietary supplements Includes a tear-out form for the MedWatch program for use by health professionals to voluntarily report adverse effects of drugs
Natural Medicines Comprehensive Database	Scientific gold standard for evidence-based information about herbal medicines and combination products involving herbal medicines Only available in an online database by subscription or at libraries
LactMed (Drugs and Lactation Database)	Contains information on drugs and other chemicals to which breastfeeding mothers may be exposed Includes information on the levels of such substances in breast milk and infant blood, and the possible adverse effects in the nursing infant Provides suggested therapeutic alternatives to those drugs, where appropriate All data are derived from the scientific literature and are fully referenced A peer-review panel evaluates the data to ensure scientific validity and currency Database is updated monthly *https://toxnet.nlm.nih.gov/newtoxnet/lactmed.htm*
Developmental and Reproductive Toxicology Database (DART)	Provides more than 200,000 journal references covering teratology and other aspects of developmental and reproductive toxicology Funded by several federal agencies Contains references from the early 1900s to the present *https://toxnet.nlm.nih.gov/newtoxnet/dart.htm*

Table 1.2	Sources of Drug Information for Healthcare Providers—cont'd
SOURCES OF DRUG INFORMATION	**DESCRIPTION**
Canadian Drug Standards	
European Pharmacopoeia *Pharmacopée Française* *The International Pharmacopoeia* (Ph. Int.) *British Pharmacopoeia* *Canadian Formulary* *The National Formulary* *Pharmaceutical Codex* *United States Pharmacopeia*	All recognized by the Canadian Food and Drugs Act as authoritative sources of drug standards
Canadian Drug Information	
Compendium of Pharmaceuticals and Specialties (CPS)	Published annually by the Canadian Pharmacists Association Comprehensive list of the pharmaceutical products distributed in Canada, as well as other practical information e-CPS available
Patient Self-Care: Helping Patients Make Therapeutic Choices	Published by the Canadian Pharmacists Association Provides comprehensive information for health professionals and consumers about nonprescription drug products available in Canada e-Therapeutics available
Compendium of Self-Care Products (CSCP)	Nonprescription companion to CPS and Patient Self-Care Offers at-a-glance comparative tables for thousands of products and monographs about hundreds of commonly used nonprescription products

AHFS, American Hospital Formulary Service; *ASHP,* American Society of Health-System Pharmacists; *USP,* United States Pharmacopeia.

Affairs—to provide high-quality information about marketed drugs. DailyMed makes available to healthcare providers and the public a standard, comprehensive, up-to-date resource about medicines.

UNITED STATES DRUG LEGISLATION

Drug legislation provides a legal basis for drug treatments and protects the consumer from false claims made by the drug manufacturer. The need for such protection is great because manufacturers and advertisers may make unfounded claims about the benefits of their products.

FEDERAL FOOD, DRUG, AND COSMETIC ACT

The Federal Food, Drug, and Cosmetic Act of 1938 requires the FDA to determine the safety of drugs before marketing and to ensure that certain labeling specifications and standards in advertising are met in the marketing of products. Manufacturers are required to submit new drug applications to the FDA for the review of safety studies before the products can be released for sale.

There are two key amendments to the 1938 act. The Durham Humphrey Amendment of 1951 divides medicines into prescription and nonprescription (OTC) categories based on safety. Prescription medicine labels are required to contain the statement "Caution: Federal Law prohibits dispensing without a prescription" or "Prescription only." The Kefauver-Harris Drug Amendment was brought about in 1962 as a result of

the thalidomide tragedy. Thalidomide was an incompletely tested drug that had been approved for use as a sedative-hypnotic during pregnancy. Fetuses exposed to thalidomide were born with serious birth defects. This amendment provides greater control and surveillance of the distribution and clinical testing of investigational drugs and requires that a product be proven both safe and effective before release for sale.

CONTROLLED SUBSTANCES ACT

The Comprehensive Drug Abuse Prevention and Control Act, which is commonly referred to as the *Controlled Substances Act,* was passed by Congress in 1970. This statute repealed almost 50 other laws written between 1914 and 1970 that related to the control of drugs. The new composite law was designed to improve the administration and regulation of the manufacturing, distribution, and dispensing of drugs that require control by the government because of their high incidence of abuse. The basic structure of the Controlled Substances Act consists of five classifications, or **schedules,** of controlled substances. The degree of control, the conditions of record keeping, the particular order forms required, and other regulations depend on these classifications (Box 1.1).

Drug Enforcement Administration

The US Drug Enforcement Administration (DEA) was organized to enforce the Controlled Substances Act, to gather intelligence, to train its officers, and to conduct research in the area of dangerous drugs and drug abuse.

| Box 1.1 | Controlled Substance Drug Schedules[a] |

SCHEDULE I DRUGS
1. Very high potential for abuse
2. Not currently accepted for medical use in the United States
3. Lack of accepted safety for use under medical supervision
   Examples: lysergic acid diethylamide (LSD), peyote, heroin, hashish

SCHEDULE II DRUGS
1. High potential for abuse
2. Currently accepted for medical use in the United States
3. Abuse potential that may lead to severe psychological or physical dependence
4. Requires new prescription; no refills
   Examples: amphetamines, morphine, hydrocodone/acetaminophen (Vicodin), hydrocodone/acetaminophen (Lortab), hydrocodone/acetaminophen (Norco), methadone, oxycodone/aspirin (Percodan), methylphenidate (Ritalin), amphetamine/dextroamphetamine (Adderall)

SCHEDULE III DRUGS
1. High potential for abuse but less so than drugs in Schedules I and II
2. Currently accepted for medical use in the United States
3. Abuse potential that may lead to moderate or low physical dependence or high psychological dependence

4. Prescription outdates in 6 months; no more than five refills in that 6 months
   Examples: aspirin/codeine (Empirin with codeine), aspirin/butalbital/caffeine (Fiorinal), acetaminophen/codeine (Tylenol with codeine)

SCHEDULE IV DRUGS
1. Low potential for abuse compared with drugs in Schedule III
2. Currently accepted for medical use in the United States
3. Abuse potential that may lead to limited physical or psychological dependence compared with drugs in Schedule III
4. Prescription outdates in 6 months; no more than five refills in that 6 months
   Examples: phenobarbital, chlordiazepoxide, diazepam, flurazepam, temazepam

SCHEDULE V DRUGS
1. Low potential for abuse compared with drugs in Schedule IV
2. Currently accepted for medical use in the United States
3. Abuse potential of limited physical or psychological dependence liability compared with drugs in Schedule IV; because abuse potential is low, a prescription may not be required
4. Prescription outdates in 6 months, no more than five refills in that 6 months
   Example: atropine/diphenoxylate (Lomotil, Virtussin AC)

[a]Drugs that are listed in Schedule I are not available for other than highly controlled research purposes. Drugs in Schedule II are available by prescription only in limited quantities, usually no more than a 30-day supply. The prescription cannot be refilled; a new prescription must be issued for continued use. Drugs categorized as Schedule III, IV, or V may be ordered by prescription with a maximum supply of 30 days of medicine. The prescription may be refilled up to five times but outdates at 6 months, at which time a new prescription is required if the medicine is to be continued. Prescription medicines that are not classified as controlled substances may be refilled for up to 1 year, if approved by the prescriber. Most state laws mandate that a prescription outdates in 1 year.

The DEA is a bureau of the Department of Justice, and the director of the DEA reports to the Attorney General of the United States. The US Attorney General, after public hearings, has the authority to reschedule a drug, to bring an unscheduled drug under control, or to remove controls on scheduled drugs.

Every manufacturer, physician, nurse practitioner, physician assistant, dentist, pharmacy, and hospital that manufactures, prescribes, or dispenses any of the drugs listed in the five schedules must register biannually with the DEA. A healthcare provider's prescription for substances named in this law must contain the healthcare provider's name, address, DEA registration number, and signature; the patient's name and address; and the date of issue. The pharmacist cannot refill such prescriptions without the approval of the healthcare provider.

Controlled Substances in Hospitals
The use of controlled substances in hospitals is discussed in Chapter 6.

Possession of Controlled Substances by Individuals
Federal and state laws make the possession of controlled substances without a valid prescription a crime, except

in specifically exempted cases. The law makes no distinction between professional and practical nurses with regard to the possession of controlled drugs. Nurses may give controlled substances only under the direction of a healthcare provider who has been licensed to prescribe or dispense these agents. Nurses may not have controlled substances in their possession unless the following conditions are met: (1) the nurse is giving them to a patient under an order from a healthcare provider, (2) the nurse is a patient for whom a healthcare provider has prescribed scheduled drugs, or (3) the nurse is the official custodian of a limited supply of controlled substances on a unit or for a department of the hospital. Controlled substances that are ordered for patients but not used must be returned to the source from which they were obtained (i.e., the physician or pharmacy). Violation of or failure to comply with the Controlled Substances Act is punishable by fine, imprisonment, or both and by the possible loss of professional licensing.

EFFECTIVENESS OF DRUG LEGISLATION
Enforcing the laws regarding the proper distribution and use of drugs is dependent on many organizations working together to ensure the understanding of the

reasons for the drug legislation. The National Council on Patient Information and Education (NCPIE) is a driving force behind the effort to educate healthcare professionals and the public with regard to the possible consequences of indiscriminate use of drugs. Other organizations involved in this very important effort are the American Medical Association, the American Dental Association, the American Pharmacists Association, the American Society of Health-System Pharmacists, and local, county, and state health departments.

NEW DRUG DEVELOPMENT

It currently takes an average of 8 to 15 years and more than $2 billion in research and development costs to bring a single new drug to market; healthcare professionals and consumers alike often have a lack of understanding about this process. The Pharmaceutical Research and Manufacturers of America estimates that only 1 of 10,000 chemicals investigated is actually found to be "safe and effective" and ultimately brought to the pharmacist's shelf.

The Food, Drug, and Cosmetic Act of 1938 charged the FDA with the responsibility of regulating new drugs. Rules and regulations evolved by the FDA divide new drug development into four stages: (1) preclinical research and development; (2) clinical research and development; (3) New Drug Application (NDA) review; and (4) postmarketing surveillance (Fig. 1.2).

PRECLINICAL RESEARCH AND DEVELOPMENT STAGE

The preclinical research phase of new drug development begins with the discovery, synthesis, and purification of the drug. The goal at this stage is to use laboratory studies to determine whether the experimental drug has therapeutic value and whether the drug appears to be safe in animals. Enough data must be gained to justify testing the experimental drug in humans.

The preclinical phase of data collection may require 1 to 3 years, although the average length of time is 18 months. Near the end of this phase, the investigator (often a pharmaceutical manufacturer) submits an Investigational New Drug (IND) application to the FDA; this application describes all of the studies completed to date, discusses the expected safety of the drug, and explains the testing that is planned for human subjects. Within 30 days, the FDA must make a decision on the basis of safety considerations about whether to allow the human study to proceed. Only about 20% of the chemicals tested in the preclinical phase advance to the clinical testing phase.

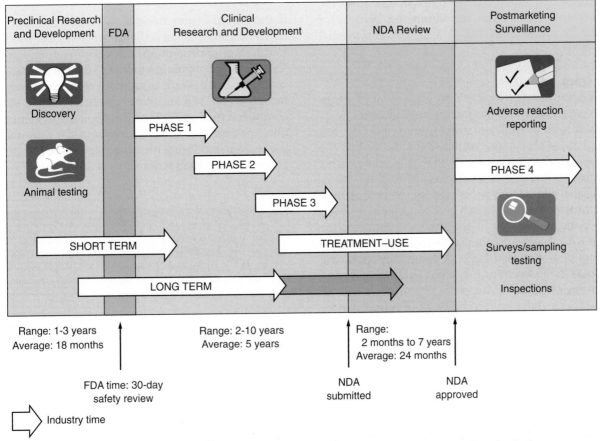

Fig. 1.2 The new drug review process. *FDA*, US Food and Drug Administration; *NDA*, New Drug Application.

CLINICAL RESEARCH AND DEVELOPMENT STAGE

The stage in which humans are first tested (i.e., the clinical research or IND stage) is usually subdivided into three phases. Phase 1 studies determine an experimental drug's pharmacologic properties, such as its pharmacokinetics, metabolism, safe dosage range, potential for toxicity at a certain dosage, and safe routes of administration. The study population is composed of normal volunteers or the intended treatment population, such as those patients for whom the standard treatments of certain cancers or dysrhythmias have been ineffective. Phase 1 studies usually require 20 to 100 subjects who are treated for 4 to 6 weeks.

If phase 1 trials are successful, the drug is moved to phase 2 trials, which involve a smaller population of patients who have the condition that the drug is designed to treat. Studies at various dosages are conducted to determine the success rate and safety of a drug for its intended use. If successful, the drug is advanced to phase 3 trials, in which larger patient populations are used to ensure the statistical significance of the results. Phase 3 studies also provide additional information about proper dosing and safety.

The entire clinical research phase may require 2 to 10 years, with the average experimental drug requiring 5 years. Each study completed is reviewed by the FDA to help ensure patient safety and efficacy. Only one of five drugs that enter clinical trials makes it to the marketplace. The others are eliminated because of efficacy or safety problems or a lack of commercial interest.

Fast Tracking

To expedite the development and approval of drugs for the treatment of life-threatening illnesses (e.g., acquired immunodeficiency syndrome), the FDA has drafted rules that allow certain INDs to receive the highest priority for review within the agency. This procedure is sometimes known as *fast tracking*. Additional rules allow INDs to be used for the treatment of a life-threatening disease in a particular patient—even if the patient does not fit the study protocol for the drug—when there is no alternative therapy. These cases are known as *treatment INDs*. A potentially lifesaving drug may be allowed for treatment IND status during late phase 2 studies, during phase 3 studies, or after all clinical studies have been completed but before marketing approval.

Parallel Tracking

Another mechanism to make INDs available to patients with life-threatening illnesses is known as *parallel tracking*. With this procedure, an IND may be used for patients who cannot participate in controlled clinical trials and when there is no satisfactory standard therapeutic alternative. Parallel track studies are conducted along with the principal controlled clinical trials; however, unlike a controlled study, the parallel track study does not involve a concurrent control group.

Investigators and patients must realize that there may be greater uncertainty regarding the risks and benefits of therapy with agents that are in relatively early stages of testing and development. Parallel tracking is similar to the treatment IND process but allows for access to investigational agents when there is less accumulated evidence of efficacy than required for a treatment IND. A drug may be released through the parallel track mechanism when phase 2 trials have been given approval to proceed but have not necessarily been started.

NEW DRUG APPLICATION REVIEW

When sufficient data have been collected to demonstrate that the experimental drug is both safe and effective, the investigator submits an NDA to the FDA to formally request approval to market a new drug for human use. Thousands of pages of NDA data are reviewed by a team of pharmacologists, toxicologists, chemists, physicians, and others (as appropriate), who then make a recommendation to the FDA about whether the drug should be approved for use. The average NDA review takes 24 months. After a drug is approved by the FDA, it is the manufacturer's decision as to when to bring a product to the marketplace.

POSTMARKETING SURVEILLANCE STAGE

If the manufacturer decides to market the medicine, the postmarketing surveillance stage begins; this is the fourth stage of drug product development. This process consists of an ongoing review of adverse effects of the new drug and periodic inspections of the manufacturing facilities and the resulting products. Other studies completed during the fourth stage include identifying other patient populations for whom the drug may be useful, refining dosing recommendations, and exploring potential drug interactions.

 Clinical Goldmine

Healthcare providers make a significant contribution to the knowledge of drug safety by reporting adverse effects to the FDA using the MedWatch program for the voluntary reporting of adverse events and product problems (see Online Resources).

BLACK BOX WARNING

Although the FDA's drug approval process is one of the most stringent in the world, the value of ongoing safety review of medicines has been demonstrated through the use of the MedWatch program. If safety concerns are identified after a drug is approved for marketing, the FDA can issue **black box warnings** to the package insert of the product. When a medication's risks and known dangers outweigh its benefits, the FDA and/or the manufacturer may decide that the product should be withdrawn from the market.

The probability of a drug acquiring a new black box warning or being withdrawn from the market within 25 years of being released is estimated at 20%. Consequently, it is the responsibility of all healthcare professionals to constantly monitor their patients for adverse effects of drugs and to complete a MedWatch form when adverse effects are suspected. More than 200,000 MedWatch forms are filed with the FDA annually.

From a safety standpoint, prescribers and patients should be aware that recently marketed medicines carry a risk of causing unsuspected serious adverse effects. Even with the high probability that there will be no serious complications, the devastating—and sometimes fatal—consequences cannot be ignored. When choosing medicines for treatment, it becomes important to consider whether an equally effective alternative drug is already available. At a minimum, this reduces the risk of an undiscovered adverse drug reaction, and it is often less expensive. At a maximum, the patient, the family, and the prescriber are saved the anguish of an avoidable adverse drug reaction.

RARE DISEASES AND THE DEVELOPMENT OF ORPHAN DRUGS

The National Organization for Rare Disorders, which is a coalition of 140 rare-disease groups, estimates that more than 6000 rare health conditions exist in about 20 million Americans. Examples of these rare diseases are cystic fibrosis, Hansen's disease (leprosy), sickle cell anemia, blepharospasm, infant botulism, and *Pneumocystis jiroveci* pneumonia (see Online Resources). Historically, pharmaceutical manufacturers have been reluctant to develop products that could be used to treat these illnesses. The medicines that are developed for these conditions are known as **orphan drugs** because the manufacturers have been unable to recover the costs of the research on account of the very limited use of the final product. Because no companies were willing to "adopt" the diseases to complete extensive research to develop products for treatment, the diseases became known as *health orphans*.

In 1983, Congress passed the Orphan Drug Act to stimulate the development and market availability of products that are used for the treatment of rare diseases. The act defines the term *rare disease* as a condition that affects fewer than 200,000 people in the United States. The FDA's Office of Orphan Products Development (OOPD) promotes the development of products that demonstrate promise for the diagnosis or treatment of rare diseases or conditions. The OOPD interacts with medical and research communities, professional organizations, academia, and the pharmaceutical industry, as well as with rare-disease groups. The OOPD administers the major provisions of the Orphan Drug Act,

which provide incentives for sponsors to develop products for rare diseases.

The law provides research grants, protocol development assistance by the FDA, special tax credits for the cost of clinical trials, and 7 years of exclusive marketing rights after the product has been approved. On average, an orphan drug receives FDA approval 10 to 11 months sooner than a nonorphan drug. The act has been quite successful: more than 200 new drugs have been approved by the FDA for rare diseases, benefiting several million people. Examples include pentamidine and atovaquone for *Pneumocystis jiroveci* pneumonia, thalidomide for Hansen's disease, zidovudine for the human immunodeficiency virus, dornase alfa (Pulmozyme) for cystic fibrosis, and cladribine (Leustatin) for hairy cell leukemia.

DRUG NAMES, STANDARDS, AND LEGISLATION IN CANADA

CANADIAN DRUG NAMES

OFFICIAL DRUG

The term *official drug* pertains to any drug for which a standard is described specifically in the Food and Drug Regulations or in any publication named in the Food and Drugs Act as being satisfactory for officially meeting the standards for drugs in Canada.

CHEMICAL NAME

The *chemical name* is most meaningful to the chemist. By means of the chemical name the chemist understands the exact chemical constitution of the drug and exact placing of its atoms or molecular groupings. The chemical name is the same in both Canada and the United States.

PROPER NAME OR GENERIC NAME

The *proper name* is the nonproprietary (generic) name, which is used to identify an official drug in Canada. The *generic name* is the same in both Canada and the United States.

BRAND NAME

The *brand name* (or proprietary name) is the name assigned to the drug by its manufacturer to distinguish the drug for advertisement and sale. Brand names for the same generic drug product are frequently different between Canada and the United States. The following example and Fig. 1.3 depict the application of terminology to drug nomenclature.

Example of Canadian Drug Names

Chemical name: 4-dimethylamino-1,4,4a,5,5a,6,11,12a-octahydro-3,6,10,12,12a-pentahydroxy-6-methyl-1, 11,dioxo-2-napthacene carboxamide (see Fig. 1.3)

Proper name: tetracycline

Official name: Tetracycline, USP

Brand names: Apo-Tetra; Nu-Tetra

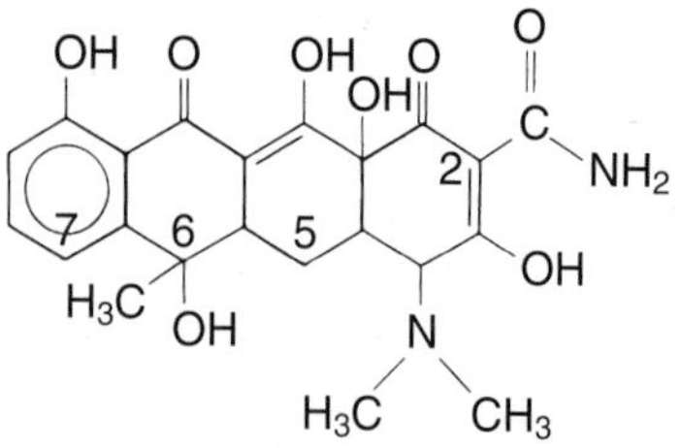

Fig. 1.3 Tetracycline, an antibiotic.

SOURCES OF CANADIAN DRUG STANDARDS

The Food and Drugs Act recognizes the standards described by international authoritative books as being acceptable for official drugs in Canada (see Table 1.2).

CANADIAN DRUG LEGISLATION

FOOD AND DRUGS ACT AND REGULATIONS

The **Food and Drugs Act** (1927) and **Regulations** (1953, 1954, 1979) empower Health Canada to protect the public from foreseeable risks related to the manufacture and sale of drugs, cosmetics, food, and therapeutic devices. The legislation provides for a review of the safety and efficacy of drugs before their clearance for marketing in Canada and determines whether the medicine is *prescription* or *nonprescription*. Also included in this legislation are requirements for good manufacturing practices, adequate labeling, and fair advertising.

In Canada (as in the United States), an effort has been made to align the provincial drug schedules so that the conditions for the sale of medicines are consistent across Canada. The National Association of Pharmacy Regulatory Authorities (NAPRA) proposed a new national drug scheduling model. This model is in various stages of implementation across the provinces and territories of Canada. With the use of this model, all medicines in Canada are assigned to one of four categories:

Schedule I: All prescription drugs, including narcotics
Schedule II: Restricted-access nonprescription drugs
Schedule III: Pharmacy-only nonprescription drugs
Unscheduled: Drugs that are not assigned to the previous categories

Schedule II drugs are available for sale directly from the pharmacist and are kept "behind the counter." Examples include insulin, pseudoephedrine, glucagon, loperamide (for children younger than age 12 years), and nitroglycerin sublingual spray and tablets (other dosage forms are Schedule I). These medications are in two categories: (1) those that patients may require urgently and cannot delay taking until after an appointment with a prescriber (insulin, nitroglycerin, glucagon); and (2) those that require appropriate counseling to avoid improper use (loperamide, pseudoephedrine). Placement with a pharmacist does not allow for patient self-selection and allows for pharmacist intervention for these medications. This restriction is meant to ensure the following: (1) that patients are not self-diagnosing

medically serious diseases (e.g., diabetes mellitus, angina); and (2) that patients are educated about the proper use of these drugs through appropriate counseling from the pharmacist.

Schedule III drugs are pharmacy-only nonprescription drugs. These medicines can be sold only through pharmacies and include levonorgestrel emergency contraception, diphenhydramine, child preparations of antihistamines, and the low-dose histamine-2 antagonists. It is expected that if patients have questions, they could easily consult with a pharmacist.

Medicines that are not categorized in Schedule I, II, or III are considered to be "unscheduled" (e.g., nicotine gum and patches, acetylsalicylic acid, lower-dose ibuprofen, some lower-dosage "cough and cold" preparations) and can be sold at any retail outlet. Adequate information is available for the patient to make a safe and effective choice, and labeling is sufficient to ensure the appropriate use of the drug without professional supervision.

Drugs requiring a prescription—except for controlled drugs—are listed on Schedule F of the Food and Drug Regulations. Schedule F drugs may be prescribed only by qualified healthcare providers because they would normally be used most safely under supervision. Most antibiotics, antineoplastics, corticosteroids, cardiovascular drugs, and antipsychotics are Schedule F drugs.

CONTROLLED DRUGS AND SUBSTANCES ACT

The **Controlled Drugs and Substances Act** (1997) established the requirements for the import, production, export, distribution, and possession of substances classified as narcotics and substances of abuse in Canada. The Controlled Drugs and Substances Act describes eight schedules of controlled substances. Assignment to a schedule is based on the potential for abuse and the ease with which illicit substances can be manufactured in illegal laboratories. The degree of control; the conditions of record keeping; assignment of penalties for possession, trafficking, and manufacturing; and other regulations depend on these classifications. (Note that Schedules I, II, and III under the US Food and Drugs Act as described earlier are different from Schedules I through VIII of the Canadian Controlled Drugs and Substances Act). Examples of controlled substances schedule assignment are as follows:

Schedule I: Opium poppy and its derivatives (e.g., heroin, morphine); coca and its derivatives (e.g., cocaine), pethidine (meperidine), methadone, fentanyl
Schedule II: Cannabis
Schedule III: Amphetamines, methylphenidate, lysergic acid diethylamide (LSD), methaqualone, psilocybin, mescaline
Schedule IV: Sedative-hypnotic agents (e.g., barbiturates, benzodiazepines); butorphanol, anabolic steroids
Schedule V: Propylhexedrine, phenylpropanolamine, pyrovalerone

Schedule VI: Part I class A precursors (e.g., ephedrine, pseudoephedrine, norephedrine [phenylpropanolamine], ergotamine) and part II precursors (e.g., acetone, ethyl ether, hydrochloric acid, sulfuric acid, toluene)

Schedule VII: Cannabis resin (3 kg); cannabis (marijuana) (3 kg) (must be read in conjunction with Schedule II)

Schedule VIII: Cannabis resin (1 g); cannabis (marijuana) (30 g) (must be read in conjunction with Schedule II)

The Controlled Drugs and Substances Act and accompanying regulations provide for the nonprescription sale of certain codeine preparations (e.g., Tylenol No. 1 with codeine, Benylin with codeine). The content must not exceed the equivalent of 8 mg of codeine phosphate per solid dosage unit or 20 mg per 30 mL of a liquid preparation, and the preparation must also contain two additional nonnarcotic medicinal ingredients. These preparations may not be advertised or displayed, and they may be sold only by pharmacists (see previous discussion of Schedule II drugs). In hospitals, the pharmacy usually requires strict inventory control of these products and other narcotics.

Requirements for the legitimate administration of drugs to patients by nurses are generally similar in Canada and the United States. Individual hospital policy determines specific record-keeping requirements on the basis of federal and provincial laws. Violations of these laws will result in fines or imprisonment in addition to the loss of professional licensing.

NONPRESCRIPTION DRUGS

The NAPRA drug schedules list three categories of nonprescription drugs: Schedule II, III, and unscheduled drugs (see discussion under Food and Drugs Act and Regulations).

Get Ready for the NCLEX® Examination!

Key Points

- In the classification system used in the United States, each drug has three names: a *chemical* name, a *generic* name, and a *brand* name. The chemical name is most meaningful to the chemist. The generic name is simpler than the chemical name. The first letter of the generic name is not capitalized. The brand names are selected by the manufacturer and deliberately made easier to pronounce, spell, and remember. A brand name is followed by the symbol ®. The first letter of the brand name is capitalized.
- Drugs may be classified by a variety of methods according to the *body system* that they affect (e.g., the central nervous system, the cardiovascular system, the gastrointestinal system); their *therapeutic use* or *clinical indications* (e.g., antacids, antibiotics, antihypertensives, diuretics, laxatives); and their *physiologic* or *chemical action* (e.g., anticholinergic agents, beta-adrenergic blockers, calcium channel blockers, cholinergic agents).
- Table 1.2 lists and describes the common sources of drug information available for the healthcare provider.
- Prescription drugs require an order by a healthcare provider who is licensed to prescribe drugs, such as a physician, a nurse practitioner, a physician assistant, a pharmacist, or a dentist. Nonprescription or over-the-counter (OTC) drugs are sold without a prescription in a pharmacy or in the health section of department or grocery stores.
- Rules and regulations evolved by the FDA divide new drug development into four stages: (1) preclinical research and development; (2) clinical research and development; (3) new drug application review; and (4) postmarketing surveillance (see Fig. 1.2).
- In Canada, the *proper name* is the nonproprietary (generic) name, which is used to identify an official drug. The *generic name* is the same in both Canada and the United States.

Additional Learning Resources

SG Go to your Study Guide for additional Review Questions for the NCLEX® Examination, Critical Thinking Clinical Situations, and other learning activities to help you master this chapter content.

Go to your Evolve website (https://evolve.elsevier.com/Clayton) for additional online resources.

🌐 Online Resources
- DailyMed: https://dailymed.nlm.nih.gov/dailymed/index.cfm
- ePocrates: http://www.epocrates.com/
- iPharmacy: https://itunes.apple.com/us/app/ipharmacy-drug-guide-pubmed-direct/id378721295
- Lexicomp: http://www.wolterskluwercdi.com/lexicomp-online/
- MedicinesComplete: https://about.medicinescomplete.com/#/
- MedWatch: https://www.fda.gov/Safety/MedWatch/default.htm
- NORD (National Organization for Rare Disorders): https://rarediseases.org/
- UpToDate: https://www.uptodate.com/home
- US National Library of Medicine: https://www.nlm.nih.gov/

🌐 Online Resources for Canadian Practitioners
- Controlled Substances and Drugs Act (Justice Laws Website): http://laws-lois.justice.gc.ca/eng/acts/c-38.8/
- Drug Product Database: https://www.canada.ca/en/health-canada/services/drugs-health-products/drug-products/drug-product-database.html
- National Association of Pharmacy Regulatory Authorities (NAPRA) proposal for drug schedule outlines: http://napra.ca/national-drug-schedules

Review Questions for the NCLEX® Examination

1. A patient has received a prescription from his primary care provider for the drug metoprolol (Lopressor). He asks the nurse why there are two names for the same drug. The nurse responds with which statements(s)? *(Select all that apply.)*
   1. "One of the names is the brand name of the drug, and the other is the generic name."
   2. "When drugs are discovered, all drugs are given a detailed chemical name and a simple generic name. If the company that discovered the drug brings it to the marketplace for sale, the manufacturer will give it a distinctive brand name."
   3. "Lopressor is the generic name, and metoprolol is the brand name."
   4. "The two names are used to determine whether the drug is a Schedule III or a Schedule IV drug."
   5. "Generally, the generic form of the drug is less expensive."

2. Antacids, antibiotics, antihypertensives, diuretics, and laxatives are examples of drugs that are classified by which method?
   1. Nonprescription status
   2. Body system
   3. Chemical action
   4. Clinical indication

3. The nurse giving a drug to a patient for the effect it will have on the cardiovascular system understands that which method is used to classify the drug?
   1. Therapeutic use
   2. Physiologic action
   3. Clinical indication
   4. Body system

4. Which electronic database(s) provide(s) drug information for healthcare providers? *(Select all that apply.)*
   1. Lexicomp
   2. CINAHL
   3. Medline
   4. DailyMed
   5. Health on the Net

5. A patient asked the nurse for an example of an appropriate source for drug information on the Internet. What would be an appropriate response by the nurse?
   1. "The Internet is not an appropriate place to look up any drug information; you need to ask your physician or pharmacist."
   2. "There are several reliable sites for drug information that are from official sources, for example, DailyMed."
   3. "The Internet is reliable for any drug information that you search for."
   4. "The only acceptable drug information sources are the package inserts."

6. The nurse knows which of these factors are the differences between prescription and nonprescription drugs? *(Select all that apply.)*
   1. Nonprescription drugs are available over-the-counter.
   2. Prescription drugs are those drugs that may be prescribed by dentists, pharmacists, nurse practitioners, and physicians.
   3. Recreational drugs are available by prescription only.
   4. Over-the-counter drugs are available at a pharmacy or health section of grocery stores.
   5. Prescription drugs have been approved for use by the FDA.

7. During which stage of the process of new drug development does testing on humans start?
   1. The preclinical research and development stage
   2. The postmarketing surveillance stage
   3. The postclinical research and development stage
   4. The clinical research and development stage

8. A nurse was teaching a patient from Canada the names of her medications and reviewed the differences between Canadian names. Which statement indicates the patient understands the instructions?
   1. "The proper name of the medication is the same as the brand name in Canada."
   2. "The proper name of the medication is the same as the generic name in Canada."
   3. "The chemical name is the one used the most when buying medications in Canada."
   4. "The chemical names and the brand names are the only names used in Canada."

Objectives

1. Identify common drug administration routes.
2. Identify the meaning and significance of the term *half-life* when used in relation to drug therapy.
3. Describe the process of how a drug is metabolized in the body.
4. Compare and contrast the following terms that are used in relationship to medications: *desired action, common adverse effects, serious adverse effects, allergic reactions,* and *idiosyncratic reactions.*
5. Identify what is meant by a drug interaction.
6. Differentiate among the terms *additive effect, synergistic effect, antagonistic effect, displacement, interference,* and *incompatibility.*
7. Identify one way in which alternatives in metabolism create drug interactions.

Key Terms

receptors (rē-SĔP-tĕrz) (p. 13)
pharmacodynamics (făr-mă-kō-dī-NĂM-ĭks) (p. 13)
agonists (ĂG-ŏ-nĭsts) (p. 13)
antagonists (ăn-TĂG-ŏ-nĭsts) (p. 13)
partial agonists (PĂR-shŭl ĂG-ŏ-nĭsts) (p. 13)
enteral (ĔN-tĕr-ăl) (p. 14)
parenteral (pă-RĔN-tĕr-ăl) (p. 14)
percutaneous (pĕr-kū-TĀ-nē-ŭs) (p. 14)
pharmacokinetics (făr-mă-kō-kĭ-NĔT-ĭks) (p. 14)
absorption (ăb-SŎRP-shŭn) (p. 14)
distribution (dĭs-trĭ-BŪ-shŭn) (p. 15)
drug blood level (p. 15)
metabolism (mĕ-TĂB-ō-lĭz-ĕm) (p. 15)
excretion (ĕks-KRĒ-shŭn) (p. 15)
half-life (p. 15)
onset of action (p. 16)

peak action (p. 16)
duration of action (p. 17)
desired action (p. 17)
side effects (p. 17)
common adverse effects (ĂD-vŭrs ĕ-FĔKTS) (p. 17)
serious adverse effects (p. 17)
idiosyncratic reaction (ĭd-ē-ō-sĭn-KRĂT-ĭk rē-ĂK-shŭn) (p. 18)
allergic reactions (ă-LŬR-jĭk) (p. 18)
drug interaction (p. 18)
unbound drug (ŭn-BŌWND) (p. 18)
additive effect (ĂD-ĭ-tĭv) (p. 19)
synergistic effect (sĭn-ĕr-JĬS-tĭk) (p. 19)
antagonistic effect (ăn-tăg-ŏ-NĬST-ĭk) (p. 19)
displacement (dĭs-PLĀS-mĕnt) (p. 19)
interference (ĭn-tŭr-FĒR-ĕns) (p. 19)
incompatibility (ĭn-kŏm-păt-ĭ-BĬL-ĭ-tē) (p. 19)

BASIC PRINCIPLES RELATED TO DRUG THERAPY

DRUG RESPONSES IN THE BODY

When administered to the body, drugs do not create new responses but rather alter existing physiologic activity in several different ways. Usually the drug forms chemical bonds with specific sites, called *receptors*, within the body. This bond forms only if the drug and its receptor have similar shapes and if the drug has a chemical affinity for the receptor. The relationship between a drug and a receptor is similar to that seen between a key and lock (Fig. 2.1A). The study of the interactions between drugs and their receptors and the series of events that result in a pharmacologic response is called *pharmacodynamics*. Most drugs have several

different atoms within each molecule that interlock into various locations on a receptor. The better the fit between the receptor and the drug molecule, the better the response from the drug. The intensity of a drug response is related to how well the drug molecule fits into the receptor and to the number of receptor sites that are occupied. Drugs that interact with a receptor to stimulate a response are known as *agonists* (Fig. 2.1B). Drugs that attach to a receptor but do not stimulate a response are called *antagonists* (Fig. 2.1C). Drugs that interact with a receptor to stimulate a response but inhibit other responses are called *partial agonists* (Fig. 2.1D).

Drug response must be stated in relation to the physiologic activity expected in response to the drug therapy (e.g., an antihypertensive agent is successful if

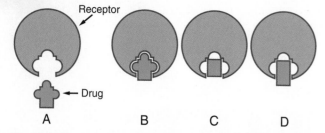

Fig. 2.1 (A) Drugs act by forming chemical bonds with specific receptor sites, similar to a key and lock. The better the fit, the better the response. (B) Drugs with complete attachment and response are called *agonists*. (C) Drugs that attach but do not elicit a response are called *antagonists*. (D) Drugs that attach and elicit a small response but also block other responses are called *partial agonists*.

the patient's blood pressure is lower after receiving the drug than it was before the drug was started). Therefore it is important to perform a thorough nursing assessment to identify the baseline data. After that is done, results from regular assessments can be compared with the baseline data by the physician, the nurse, and the pharmacist to evaluate the effectiveness of the drug therapy.

ROUTES OF DRUG ADMINISTRATION

The most common routes of drug administration are the enteral, parenteral, and percutaneous routes. When using the **enteral** route, the drug is administered directly into the gastrointestinal (GI) tract by the oral, rectal, or nasogastric route. The **parenteral** route bypasses the GI tract with the use of subcutaneous (subcut), intramuscular (IM), or intravenous (IV) injection. The **percutaneous** route involves drugs being absorbed through the skin and mucous membranes. Methods of the percutaneous route include inhalation, sublingual (under the tongue), and topical (on the skin) administration.

LIBERATION, ABSORPTION, DISTRIBUTION, METABOLISM, AND EXCRETION

After they have been administered, all drugs go through five stages: *l*iberation, *a*bsorption, *d*istribution, *m*etabolism, and *e*xcretion (LADME). After liberation from the dosage form, each drug has its own unique ADME characteristics. The study of the mathematical relationships among the ADME features of individual medicines over time is called **pharmacokinetics**.

Liberation

Regardless of the route of administration, a drug must be released from the dosage form (i.e., liberated) and dissolved in body fluids before it can be absorbed into body tissues. For example, before a solid drug that is taken orally can be absorbed into the bloodstream for transport to the site of action, the dosage form (usually a capsule or tablet) must disintegrate and the active drug must dissolve in the GI fluids so that it can be transported across the stomach or intestinal lining into

the blood. The process of converting the drug into a form that will activate a response can be partially controlled by the pharmaceutical dosage form used (e.g., solution, suspension, capsule, tablet [with various coatings]). This conversion process can also be influenced by administering the drug with or without water or food in the patient's stomach.

Absorption

Absorption is the process whereby a drug is transferred from its site of entry into the body to the circulating fluids of the body (i.e., blood and lymph) for distribution around the body. The rate at which this occurs depends on the route of administration, the blood flow through the tissue where the drug is administered, and the solubility of the drug. It is therefore important to do the following: (1) administer oral drugs with an adequate amount of fluid (usually a large [8-oz] glass of water); (2) give parenteral forms properly so that they are deposited in the correct tissue for enhanced absorption; and (3) reconstitute and dilute drugs only with the diluent recommended by the manufacturer in the package literature so that drug solubility is not impaired. Equally important are nursing assessments that reveal poor absorption (e.g., if insulin is administered subcutaneously and a lump remains at the site of injection 2 to 3 hours later, absorption from that site may be impaired).

The rate of absorption when a drug is administered by a parenteral route depends on the rate of blood flow through the tissues. Circulation or blood flow must be determined before the administration of drugs by the parenteral route to identify any circulatory insufficiency. If any such insufficiency is noted, injections will not be absorbed properly, and the drug will not be effective. Subcutaneous injections have the slowest absorption rate, especially if peripheral circulation is impaired. Intramuscular injections are more rapidly absorbed because of greater blood flow per unit weight of muscle compared with subcutaneous tissue. Cooling the area of injection slows the rate of absorption, whereas heat or massage hastens the rate of absorption. Drugs are dispersed throughout the body most rapidly when they are administered by IV injection. The nurse must be thoroughly educated regarding the responsibilities and techniques associated with administering IV medications. It is important to remember that after a drug enters the patient's bloodstream, it cannot be retrieved.

The absorption of topical drugs that have been applied to the skin can be influenced by the drug concentration, the length of contact time, the size of the affected area, the thickness of the skin surface, the hydration of the tissue, and the degree of skin disruption. Percutaneous (i.e., across-the-skin) absorption is greatly increased in newborns and young infants, who have thin, well-hydrated skin. When drugs are inhaled, their absorption can be influenced by the depth of the patient's respirations, the fineness of the droplet particles, the available surface area of the patient's mucous membranes, the contact time, the hydration state, the blood supply to the area, and the concentration of the drug itself.

Distribution

The term *distribution* refers to the ways in which a drug is transported throughout the body by the circulating body fluids to the sites of action or to the receptors that the drug affects. *Drug distribution* refers to the transport of the drug throughout the entire body by the blood and lymphatic systems and the transport from the circulating fluids into and out of the fluids that bathe the receptor sites. Organs with the most extensive blood supplies (e.g., heart, liver, kidneys, brain) receive the distributed drug most rapidly. Areas with less extensive blood supplies (e.g., muscle, skin, fat) receive the drug more slowly.

After a drug has been dissolved and absorbed into the circulating blood, its distribution is determined by the chemical properties of the drug and how it is affected by the blood and tissues that it contacts. Two factors that influence drug distribution are protein binding and lipid (fat) solubility. Most drugs are transported in combination with plasma proteins (especially albumin), which act as carriers for relatively insoluble drugs. Drugs that are bound to plasma proteins are pharmacologically inactive because the large size of the complex keeps them in the bloodstream and prevents them from reaching the sites of action, metabolism, and excretion. Only the free, or *unbound*, portion of a drug is able to diffuse into tissues, interact with receptors, and produce physiologic effects; it is also only this portion that can be metabolized and excreted. The same proportions of bound and free drug are maintained in the blood at all times. Thus as the free drug acts on receptor sites or is metabolized, the decrease in the serum drug level causes some of the bound drug to be released from protein to maintain the ratio between bound and free drug.

When a drug leaves the bloodstream, it may become bound to tissues other than those with active receptor sites. The more lipid-soluble drugs have a high affinity for adipose tissue, which serves as a repository site for these agents. Because there is a relatively low level of blood circulation to fat tissues, the more lipid-soluble drugs tend to stay in the body much longer. Equilibrium is established between the repository site (i.e., lipid tissue) and the circulation so that as the **drug blood level** drops as a result of binding at the sites of physiologic activity, metabolism, or excretion, more drug is released from the lipid tissue. By contrast, if more drug is given, a new equilibrium is established among the blood, the receptor sites, the lipid tissue repository sites, and the metabolic and excretory sites.

Distribution may be general or selective. Some drugs cannot pass through certain types of cell membranes, such as the blood-brain barrier (i.e., the central nervous system) or the placental barrier (i.e., the placenta), whereas other types of drugs readily pass into these tissues. The distribution process is very important because the amount of drug that actually gets to the receptor sites determines the extent of pharmacologic activity. If little of the drug actually reaches and binds to the receptor sites, the response will be minimal.

Metabolism

Metabolism is the process whereby the body inactivates drugs. The enzyme systems of the liver are the primary sites for the metabolism of drugs, but other tissues and organs (e.g., white blood cells, GI tract, lungs) metabolize certain drugs to a minor extent. Genetic, environmental, and physiologic factors are involved in the regulation of drug metabolism reactions. The most important factors for the conversion of drugs to their metabolites are genetic variations of enzyme systems, the concurrent use of other drugs, exposure to environmental pollutants, concurrent illnesses, and age. (For more information, see Chapter 3.)

Excretion

The elimination of drug metabolites and, in some cases, of the active drug itself from the body is called *excretion*. The two primary routes of excretion are through the GI tract into the feces and through the renal tubules into the urine. Other routes of excretion include evaporation through the skin, exhalation from the lungs, and secretion into saliva and breast milk.

Because the kidneys are major organs of drug excretion, the nurse should review the patient's chart for the results of urinalysis and renal function tests. A patient with renal failure often has an increase in the action and duration of a drug if the dosage and frequency of administration are not adjusted to allow for the patient's reduced renal function.

Fig. 2.2 shows a schematic review of the ADME process of an oral medication. It is important to note how little of the active ingredient actually reaches the receptor sites for action.

HALF-LIFE

Drugs are eliminated from the body by means of metabolism and excretion. A measure of the time required for elimination is the half-life. The **half-life** is defined as the amount of time required for 50% of the drug to be eliminated from the body. For example, if a patient is given 100 mg of a drug that has a half-life of 12 hours, the following would be observed:

TIME (HOURS)	HALF-LIFE	DRUG REMAINING IN BODY (%)
0	—	100 mg (100)
12	1	50 mg (50)
24	2	25 mg (25)
36	3	12.5 mg (12.5)
48	4	6.25 mg (6.25)
60	5	3.12 mg (3.12)

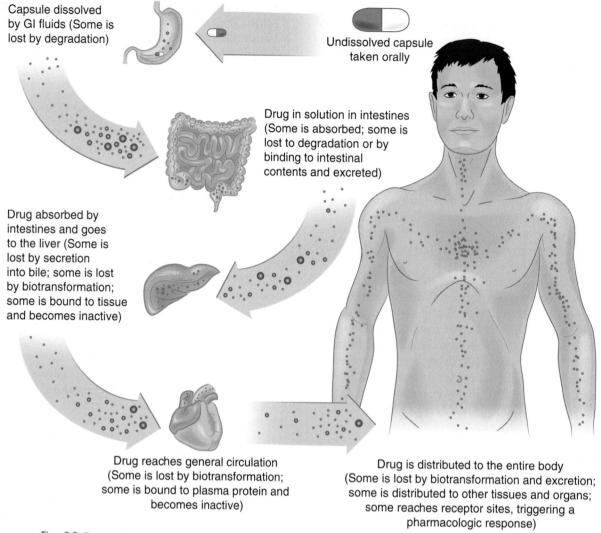

Capsule dissolved by GI fluids (Some is lost by degradation)

Undissolved capsule taken orally

Drug in solution in intestines (Some is absorbed; some is lost to degradation or by binding to intestinal contents and excreted)

Drug absorbed by intestines and goes to the liver (Some is lost by secretion into bile; some is lost by biotransformation; some is bound to tissue and becomes inactive)

Drug reaches general circulation (Some is lost by biotransformation; some is bound to plasma protein and becomes inactive)

Drug is distributed to the entire body (Some is lost by biotransformation and excretion; some is distributed to other tissues and organs; some reaches receptor sites, triggering a pharmacologic response)

Fig. 2.2 Factors that modify the quantity of drug that reaches a site of action after a single oral dose. *GI*, Gastrointestinal.

Note that as each 12-hour period (i.e., one half-life) passes, the amount remaining is 50% of what was there 12 hours earlier. After six half-lives, more than 98% of the drug has been eliminated from the body.

The half-life is determined by an individual's ability to metabolize and excrete a particular drug. Because most patients metabolize and excrete a particular drug at approximately the same rate, the approximate half-lives of most drugs are now known. When the half-life of a drug is known, dosages and frequency of administration can be calculated. Drugs with long half-lives (e.g., digoxin, with a half-life of 36 hours) need to be administered only once daily, whereas drugs with short half-lives (e.g., aspirin, with a half-life of 5 hours) need to be administered every 4 to 6 hours to maintain therapeutic activity. For patients who have impaired hepatic or renal function, the half-life may become considerably longer because of their reduced ability to metabolize or excrete the drug. For example, digoxin has a half-life of about 36 hours in a patient with normal renal function; however, it has a half-life of about 105 hours in a patient with complete renal failure. Monitoring diagnostic tests that measure renal or hepatic function is important. Whenever laboratory data reflect impairment of either function, the nurse should notify the healthcare provider.

DRUG ACTIONS

All drug actions have an onset, peak, and duration of action. The **onset of action** is when the concentration of a drug at the site of action is sufficient to start a physiologic (pharmacologic) response. Many factors—such as the route of administration and the rates of absorption, distribution, and binding to receptor sites—affect the onset of action. In general, increasing the dose of the drug hastens the onset of action by shortening the time required to achieve the necessary concentration of drug at the target site. **Peak action** is the time at which the drug reaches the highest concentrations on the target receptor sites, thereby inducing the maximal pharmacologic response for the dose given.

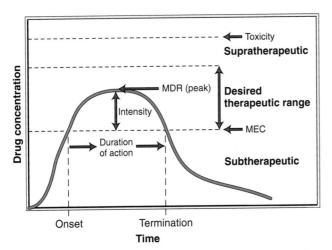

Fig. 2.3 A time-response curve, which is also known as a *drug concentration–time profile*, demonstrates the relationship between the administration of a drug and the patient's response. If the drug level does not reach the minimum effective concentration *(MEC)*, there will be no pharmacologic effect. If the peak level exceeds the toxicity threshold, toxic effects will result. The optimal drug concentration is in the middle of the therapeutic range. *MDR*, Maximum drug response (peak effect).

The **duration of action** is how long the drug has a pharmacologic effect. The onset, peak, and duration of action of a drug are often illustrated by a time-response curve, which is also known as a drug concentration–time profile (Fig. 2.3). A time-response curve demonstrates the relationship between the administration of a drug and the associated response. If the drug level does not reach the minimum effective concentration, there will be no pharmacologic effect. If the peak level exceeds the toxicity threshold, toxic effects will result. Generally, the drug concentration is targeted to be in the middle of this range, between the minimum effective response and the toxic response; this is referred to as the *therapeutic range.*

DRUG BLOOD LEVEL

When a drug is circulating in the blood, a blood sample may be drawn and assayed to determine the amount of drug present. This is known as a *drug blood level.* It is important for certain drugs (e.g., anticonvulsants, aminoglycoside antibiotics) to be measured to ensure that the drug blood level is within the therapeutic range. If the drug blood level is low, the dosage must be increased, or the medicine must be administered more frequently. If the drug blood level is too high, the patient may develop signs of toxicity; in this case, the dosage must be reduced or the medicine administered less frequently.

ADVERSE EFFECTS OF DRUGS

No drug has a single action. When a drug enters a patient and is then absorbed and distributed, the **desired action** (i.e., the expected response) usually occurs. However, all drugs have the potential to affect more than one body system simultaneously, thereby producing responses that are known as **side effects** or *common adverse effects*, which are mild, or *serious adverse effects*, which can lead to toxicity. The World Health Organization's definition of an adverse drug reaction (ADR) is "any noxious, unintended, and undesired effect of a drug, which occurs at dosages used in humans for prophylaxis, diagnosis, or therapy." A more common definition is as follows: "Right drug, right dose, right patient, bad effect." ADRs should not be confused with medication errors or adverse drug events (ADEs), which are defined as "an injury resulting from medical intervention related to a drug." (For more information, see Chapter 6.)

Recent studies have indicated the following:

- ADRs may be responsible for more than 100,000 deaths among hospitalized patients per year, which makes them one of the top six leading causes of death in the United States.
- An average of 6% of hospitalized patients experience a significant ADR at some point during their hospitalizations.
- Between 5% and 9% of hospitalization costs are attributable to ADRs.
- The most commonly seen ADRs are rash, nausea, itching, thrombocytopenia, vomiting, hyperglycemia, and diarrhea.
- The classes of medicines that account for the largest number of ADRs are antibiotics, cardiovascular medicines, cancer chemotherapy agents, analgesics, and antiinflammatory agents.

Most ADEs are predictable because of the pharmacologic effects of a drug, and patients should be monitored so that dosages can be adjusted to allow for the maximum therapeutic benefits with a minimum of adverse effects. As described in Units III through X of this text, each drug has a series of parameters (e.g., therapeutic actions to expect, adverse effects, probable drug interactions) that should be monitored by the nurse, physician, pharmacist, and patient to optimize therapy while reducing the possibility of serious adverse effects.

Accurate and appropriate drug-drug interaction information must be available to prescribers, and continual attention is currently focused on this issue. Further population-based studies still need to be conducted to meet federal initiatives to promote the meaningful use of information technologies and to integrate knowledge databases with clinical decision systems. Ideally, clinical decision systems and the databases of drug interactions that interface with them help the prescriber to identify and avoid potential medication interactions.

All hospitals have internal mechanisms for reporting suspected ADRs, and healthcare providers should not hesitate to report possible reactions. By monitoring and tracking the occurrences of ADRs, clinical protocols and improved patient screening will reduce the frequency of recurrence. The US Food and Drug Administration's

MedWatch program is also available for the voluntary reporting of adverse events. (For more information, see MedWatch on Evolve.)

Idiosyncratic Reaction

Two other types of drug actions are much more unpredictable: idiosyncratic reactions and allergic reactions. An idiosyncratic reaction occurs when something unusual or abnormal happens when a drug is first administered. The patient usually demonstrates an unexpectedly strong response to the action of the drug. This type of reaction is generally the result of a patient's inability to metabolize a drug because of a genetic deficiency of certain enzymes. Fortunately, this type of reaction is rare.

Allergic Reaction

Allergic reactions, which are also known as *hypersensitivity reactions*, occur in about 6% to 10% of patients who are taking medications. Allergic reactions occur among patients who have previously been exposed to a drug and whose immune systems have developed antibodies to the drug. On reexposure to the drug, the antibodies cause a reaction; this reaction is most commonly seen as raised, irregularly shaped patches on the skin known as *hives*, which cause severe itching, known as *urticaria.*

Occasionally, a patient has a severe, life-threatening reaction that causes respiratory distress and cardiovascular collapse; this is known as an *anaphylactic reaction.* This condition is a medical emergency, and it must be treated immediately. Fortunately, anaphylactic reactions occur much less often than the more mild urticarial reactions.

If a patient has a mild reaction, it should be understood as a warning to not take the medication again. The patient is much more likely to have an anaphylactic reaction during his or her next exposure to the drug. Patients should receive information about the drug name and be instructed to tell healthcare providers that they have had such reactions and that they must not receive the drug again. In addition, patients should wear a medical alert bracelet or necklace that explains the allergy.

DRUG INTERACTIONS

A drug interaction is said to occur when the action of one drug is altered or changed by the action of another drug. Drug interactions are elicited in two ways: (1) by agents that, when combined, *increase* the actions of one or both drugs; and (2) by agents that, when combined, *decrease* the effectiveness of one or both drugs. Some drug interactions are beneficial, such as the use of caffeine, a central nervous system stimulant, with an antihistamine, a central nervous system depressant. The stimulatory effects of the caffeine counteract the drowsiness caused by the antihistamine without eliminating the antihistaminic effects. The mechanisms of drug interactions can be categorized as those that change the absorption, distribution, metabolism, or excretion of a drug and those that enhance the pharmacologic effect of a drug.

CHANGES IN ABSORPTION

Most drug interactions that change absorption take place in the GI tract, usually the stomach. Examples of this type of interaction include the following:

- Antacids inhibit the dissolution of ketoconazole tablets by increasing the gastric pH. The interaction is managed by giving the antacid at least 2 hours after ketoconazole administration.
- Aluminum-containing antacids inhibit the absorption of tetracycline. Aluminum salts form an insoluble chemical complex with tetracycline. The interaction is managed by separating the administration of tetracycline and antacids by 3 to 4 hours.

CHANGES IN DISTRIBUTION

Drug interactions that cause a change in distribution usually affect the binding of a drug to an inactive site (e.g., circulating plasma albumin, muscle protein). When a drug is absorbed into the blood, it is usually transported throughout the body bound to plasma proteins. It often binds to other proteins, such as those in muscle. A drug that is highly bound (e.g., >90% bound) to a protein-binding site may be displaced by another drug that has a higher affinity for that binding site. Significant interactions can take place this way because little displacement is required to have a major impact. Remember, only the unbound drug is pharmacologically active. If a drug is 90% bound to a protein, then 10% of the drug is providing the physiologic effect. If another drug is administered with a stronger affinity for the protein-binding site and it displaces just 5% of the bound drug, there is now 15% unbound for physiologic activity; this is the equivalent of a 50% increase in dosage (i.e., from 10% to 15% active drug). For example, the anticoagulant action of warfarin is increased by administration with furosemide, which is a loop diuretic. Furosemide displaces warfarin from albumin-binding sites, thereby increasing the amount of unbound anticoagulant. This interaction is managed by decreasing the warfarin dosage.

CHANGES IN METABOLISM

Drug interactions usually result from a change in metabolism that involves inhibiting or inducing (stimulating) the enzymes that metabolize a drug. Medicines known to bind to enzymes and to slow the metabolism of other drugs include verapamil, chloramphenicol, ketoconazole, amiodarone, cimetidine, and erythromycin. Serum drug levels usually increase as a result of inhibited metabolism when these drugs are given concurrently, and the dosages of the inhibited drugs usually must be reduced to prevent toxicity. For example, erythromycin inhibits the metabolism of theophylline; therefore the dose of theophylline must be reduced on the basis of theophylline serum levels and signs of toxicity. Because erythromycin (an antibiotic) is usually administered only in short courses, the theophylline dosage usually needs to be increased when the erythromycin is discontinued.

Common drugs that bind to enzymes and increase the metabolism of other drugs (enzyme inducers) are phenobarbital, carbamazepine, rifampin, and phenytoin. Rapidly metabolized drugs include doxycycline, warfarin, metronidazole, theophylline, and verapamil. When administered with enzyme inducers, the dosages of the more rapidly metabolized drugs should generally be increased to provide therapeutic activity. The patient must be monitored closely for adverse effects. For example, if a woman who is taking oral contraceptives (see Chapter 40) requires a course of rifampin antimicrobial therapy, the rifampin will induce the enzymes that metabolize both the progesterone and estrogen components of the contraceptive, thereby causing an increased incidence of menstrual abnormalities and reduced effectiveness of conception control. This interaction is managed by advising the patient to use an additional form of contraception while she is receiving rifampin therapy. Adverse effects may also occur if an enzyme inducer is discontinued. The metabolism of the induced drug then decelerates, leading to accumulation and toxicity if the dosage is not reduced.

CHANGES IN EXCRETION

Drug interactions that cause a change in excretion usually act in the kidney tubules by changing the pH to enhance or inhibit excretion. The classic example of altered urine pH is the combination of acetazolamide (which elevates urine pH) and quinidine. The alkaline urine produced by acetazolamide causes quinidine to be reabsorbed in the renal tubules, which potentially increases the physiologic and toxic effects of quinidine. The frequent monitoring of quinidine serum levels and assessments for signs of quinidine toxicity are used as guides for reducing quinidine dosage.

DRUGS THAT ENHANCE THE PHARMACOLOGIC EFFECTS OF OTHER DRUGS

Major drug interactions also occur between drugs. This may occur when one drug enhances the physiologic effects of another drug. Alcohol and sedative-hypnotic agents both cause sedation, but when used together can cause significant central nervous system depression. Another drug interaction that can have serious consequences is the interaction between aminoglycoside antibiotics (gentamicin, tobramycin) and a neuromuscular blocking agent such as pancuronium. When used together, the antibiotic increases the neuromuscular blockade, prolonging return to normal respirations and recovery time. Table 2.1 defines the terminology related to drug-drug interactions.

Because it is impossible to memorize all possible drug interactions, the nurse must check for drug interactions when they are suspected. The nurse must take the time to consult drug resource books and pharmacists to ensure that a patient who is receiving multiple medications does not experience unanticipated drug interactions.

Table 2.1 Terminology Related to Drug-Drug Interactions

TERM	DEFINITION	EXAMPLE
Additive effect	Two drugs with similar actions are taken for an increased effect.	hydrocodone + acetaminophen = added analgesic effect
Synergistic effect	The combined effect of two drugs is greater than the sum of the effect of each drug given together.	aspirin + codeine = much greater analgesic effect
Antagonistic effect	One drug interferes with the action of another.	tetracycline + antacid = decreased absorption of the tetracycline
Displacement	The displacement of the first drug from protein-binding sites (i.e., bound drugs are inactive) by a second drug increases the activity of the first drug because more unbound drug is available.	warfarin + valproic acid = increased anticoagulant effect
Interference	The first drug inhibits the metabolism or excretion of the second drug, thereby causing increased activity of the second drug.	probenecid + ampicillin = prolonged antibacterial activity of ampicillin because probenecid blocks the renal excretion of ampicillin
Incompatibility	The first drug is chemically incompatible with the second drug, thereby causing deterioration when the drugs are mixed in the same syringe or solution or are administered together at the same site. Signs include haziness, formation of a precipitate, or a change in the color of the solution when the drugs are mixed.	ampicillin + gentamicin = ampicillin inactivates gentamicin

Get Ready for the NCLEX® Examination!

Key Points

- The most common routes of drug administration are the enteral, parenteral, and percutaneous routes.
- The half-life of a drug is defined as the amount of time required for 50% of the drug to be eliminated from the body.
- After administration, all drugs go through five stages: *l*iberation, *a*bsorption, *d*istribution, *m*etabolism, and *e*xcretion (LADME). The enzyme systems of the liver are the primary sites for the metabolism of drugs, but other tissues and organs (e.g., white blood cells, GI tract, lungs) metabolize certain drugs to a minor extent.
- When a drug enters a patient and is absorbed and distributed, the desired action usually occurs. However, all drugs have the potential to affect more than one body system simultaneously, causing common adverse effects, which are generally mild, or serious adverse effects, which can be more severe and lead to toxicity.
- Drug interactions are elicited in two ways: (1) by agents that, when combined, *increase* the actions of one or both drugs; and (2) by agents that, when combined, *decrease* the effectiveness of one or both of the drugs.

Additional Learning Resources

SG Go to your Study Guide for additional Review Questions for the NCLEX® Examination, Critical Thinking Clinical Situations, and other learning activities to help you master this chapter content.

Go to your Evolve website (https://evolve.elsevier.com/Clayton) for additional online resources.

Review Questions for the NCLEX® Examination

1. A nurse was reviewing the drug route for an order written to be given via nasogastric tube and understood that this meant the drug would be administered by which route?
   1. Enteral
   2. Parenteral
   3. Percutaneous
   4. Intramuscular

2. A patient takes 50 mg of a drug that has a half-life of 12 hours. What percentage of the dose remains in the body 36 hours after the drug is administered?
   1. 50 mg (100%)
   2. 25 mg (50%)
   3. 12.5 mg (25%)
   4. 6.25 mg (12.5%)

3. What is the portion of a drug that is pharmacologically active called?
   1. Protein-bound drug
   2. Unbound drug
   3. Drug tolerance level
   4. Incompatibility factor

4. When an antihypertensive drug causes a drop in blood pressure to the normal range, what is this effect called?
   1. Antagonistic effect
   2. Desired effect
   3. Side effect
   4. Additive effect

5. After the nurse injects the patient with the morning insulin dose, when will the action of the drug reach its highest physiologic effect?
   1. During peak action
   2. During displacement
   3. During the half-life
   4. During onset of action

6. When a patient has taken a drug and a rash appears along with severe itching, what is this reaction called?
   1. Idiosyncratic reaction
   2. Antagonistic effect
   3. Allergic reaction
   4. Displacement effect

7. When a patient who was prescribed warfarin and valproic acid begins experiencing an increased effect of warfarin, what is this known as?
   1. Synergistic effect
   2. Antagonistic effect
   3. Idiosyncratic effect
   4. Displacement effect

8. A person who has an increased metabolic rate (e.g., hyperthyroidism) generally requires what type of dosage?
   1. Normal dosage
   2. Lower-than-normal dosage
   3. Higher-than-normal dosage
   4. A dosage that is based on his or her thyroid function levels

9. The drug interaction between furosemide (Lasix) and warfarin (Coumadin) in which the interaction is managed by decreasing the warfarin dose is caused by which action?
   1. Changes in distribution
   2. Changes in absorption
   3. Changes in metabolism
   4. Changes in excretion

10. Drugs known to bind to an enzyme that cause the metabolism of the drug to be increased are called what?
    1. Enzyme inhibitors
    2. Enzyme inducers
    3. Enzyme enhancers
    4. Enzyme metabolizers

Drug Action Across the Life Span

Objectives

1. Explain the impact of the placebo effect and nocebo effect.
2. Identify the importance of drug dependence and drug accumulation.
3. Discuss the effects of age on drug absorption, distribution, metabolism, and excretion.
4. Explain the gender-specific considerations of drug absorption, distribution, metabolism, and excretion.
5. Describe where a nurse will find new information about the use of drugs during pregnancy and lactation.
6. Discuss the impact of pregnancy and breastfeeding on drug absorption, distribution, metabolism, and excretion.
7. Discuss the role of genetics and its influence on drug action.

Key Terms

gender-specific medicine (JĔN-dŭr spĕ-SĬ-fĭk) (p. 22)
placebo effect (plă-SĒ-bō ĕf-FĔKT) (p. 23)
nocebo effect (nō-SĒ-bō) (p. 23)
placebo (plă-SĒ-bō) (p. 23)
tolerance (TŎL-ŭr-ŭns) (p. 23)
drug dependence (dē-PĔN-dĕns) (p. 23)
drug accumulation (ă-kyū-mū-LĀ-shŭn) (p. 23)
carcinogenicity (kăr-sĭn-ō-jĕn-ĬS-ĭ-tē) (p. 23)
passive diffusion (PĂ-sĭv dĭ-FYŪ-shŭn) (p. 24)
hydrolysis (hī-DRŎ-lĭ-sĭs) (p. 24)
intestinal transit (ĭn-TĔS-tĭ-năl TRĂN-sĭt) (p. 24)

protein binding (PRŌ-tēn BĬN-dĭng) (p. 25)
drug metabolism (mĕ-TĂB-ō-lĭz-ĕm) (p. 25)
metabolites (mĕ-TĂB-ŏ-līts) (p. 26)
therapeutic drug monitoring (thĕr-ă-PYŪ-tĭk) (p. 27)
polypharmacy (pŏl-ē-FĂR-mă-sē) (p. 29)
teratogens (TĔR-ă-tō-jĕnz) (p. 31)
genetics (jĭ-NĔT-ĭks) (p. 33)
genome (JĒ-nōm) (p. 33)
polymorphisms (pŏl-ē-MŎR-fíz-ĭmz) (p. 33)
pharmacogenetics (făr-mă-kō-jĭ-NĔT-ĭks) (p. 33)

FACTORS THAT AFFECT DRUG THERAPY

Patients often say "That drug really knocked me out!" or "That drug didn't touch the pain!" The effects of drugs are unexpectedly potent in some patients, whereas other patients show little response at the same dosage. In addition, some patients react differently to the same dosage of a drug that is administered at different times. Because of individual patient variation, exact responses to drug therapy are difficult to predict. The following factors have been identified as contributors to the variable response to drugs.

AGE

Infants and the very old tend to be the most sensitive to the effects of drugs. There are important differences with regard to the absorption, distribution, metabolism, and excretion of drugs in premature neonates, full-term newborns, and children. The aging process brings about changes in body composition and organ function that can affect the older patient's response to drug therapy.

Thus the age of the patient can have a significant impact on drug therapy. When discussing the effect of age on drug therapy, it is helpful to subdivide the population into the following categories:

AGE	STAGE
<38 wk gestation	Premature
0-1 mo	Newborn, neonate
1-24 mo	Infant, toddler
3-5 yr	Young child
6-12 yr	Older child
13-18 yr	Adolescent
19-54 yr	Adult
55-64 yr	Older adult
65-74 yr	Elderly
75-84 yr	The aged
85 yr or older	The very old

BODY WEIGHT

Compared with the general population, considerably overweight patients may require an increase in drug dosage to attain the same therapeutic response.

Conversely, patients who are underweight, compared with the general population, tend to require lower dosages for the same therapeutic response. It is important to obtain an accurate height and weight on patients because dosages of medicines are often calculated with these parameters.

Most pediatric dosages are calculated by milligrams of drug per kilogram of body weight (mg/kg) to adjust for growth rate. The dosages of other medicines, particularly chemotherapeutic agents, are ordered on the basis of the body surface area (see Appendix A); this calculation requires both height and weight. For accurate measurements, the patient's weight should be taken at the same time of day and while the patient is wearing similar-weight clothing.

GENDER

Gender-specific medicine is a developing science that studies differences in the normal function of men and women and addresses how people of each gender perceive and experience disease. In almost every body system, men and women function differently, as well as perceive and experience disease differently. In the case of angina (heart pain), women will present with nausea, indigestion, and upper back and jaw pain, whereas men will generally present with left-sided chest pain or pressure. Unfortunately, few scientific data exist to document differences in the pharmacokinetics of most drugs in men compared with women. In 1993, the US Food and Drug Administration (FDA) issued guidelines stating that drug development must evaluate the effects on both genders. Testing is also needed to assess differences in pharmacokinetic parameters between men and women. In the women's studies, the research must distinguish between premenopausal and postmenopausal women and among women in different phases of the menstrual cycle.

METABOLIC RATE

Patients with a higher-than-average metabolic rate (e.g., patients with hyperthyroidism) tend to metabolize drugs more rapidly, thus requiring larger doses or more frequent administration. The converse is true for those patients with lower-than-average metabolic rates (e.g., patients with hypothyroidism). Chronic smoking enhances the metabolism of some drugs (e.g., clozapine, olanzapine), thereby requiring larger doses to be administered more frequently for a therapeutic effect.

ILLNESS

Pathologic conditions may alter the rate of absorption, distribution, metabolism, and excretion of a drug. For example, patients who are in shock have reduced peripheral vascular circulation and will absorb intramuscularly or subcutaneously injected drugs more slowly. Patients who are vomiting may not be able to retain a medication in the stomach long enough for dissolution and absorption. Patients with conditions such as nephrotic syndrome or malnutrition may have reduced amounts of serum proteins in the blood that are necessary for adequate distribution of drugs. Patients with kidney failure generally will excrete drugs at a slower rate and must have significant reductions in dosages of medications that are excreted by the kidneys (Table 3.1).

PSYCHOLOGY

Attitudes and expectations play a major role in a patient's response to therapy and in his or her willingness to take the medication as prescribed. When the disease

Table 3.1 **Selected Medications That Require Dosage Adjustment for Renal Failure[a]**

THERAPEUTIC CATEGORY	DRUG CLASS	EXAMPLES
Antibiotics	Aminoglycosides	amikacin, gentamicin, tobramycin
	Cephalosporins	cefotaxime, cefotetan, ceftazidime, ceftriaxone, cefuroxime, cefpodoxime
	Penicillins	ampicillin, piperacillin, ticarcillin
	Quinolones	ciprofloxacin, norfloxacin
	Others	vancomycin, minocycline, aztreonam, imipenem, co-trimoxazole, ethambutol
Antifungal agents	—	amphotericin B, fluconazole
Antiviral agents	—	acyclovir, ganciclovir, stavudine
Cardiovascular agents	Angiotensin-converting enzyme inhibitors	benazepril, captopril, ramipril
	Antiarrhythmic agents	dofetilide
	Beta-adrenergic blocking agents	atenolol, labetalol, pindolol, metoprolol, nadolol, propranolol
	Digitalis glycoside	digoxin
Gastrointestinal agents	Histamine-2 antagonists	cimetidine, ranitidine
Other	—	lithium, allopurinol, meperidine, methotrexate

[a]Medicines are representative examples only. See the *Physicians' Desk Reference.* 71st ed. Montvale, NJ: PDR Network LLC; 2017, or the *AHFS Drug Information 2018.* Bethesda, MD: American Society of Health-System Pharmacists; 2018, for appropriate dosing and monitoring parameters.

state physically affects the patient's ability to function, the treatment protocol is generally followed, as in a patient with insulin-dependent diabetes who needs insulin or a patient with arthritis who needs pain medication. When the disease has few symptoms (e.g., hypertension, dyslipidemia), it becomes harder to follow the treatment protocol because body cues are not present to remind patients. Patients frequently voluntarily discontinue treatment because their current lifestyle is not affected by the hypertension or dyslipidemia.

Other psychological considerations are the placebo effect and the nocebo effect. It is well documented that a patient's positive expectations about treatment and the care received can positively affect the outcome of therapy; this is a phenomenon known as the *placebo effect* (from Latin, meaning "I will please"). Although more difficult to prove because of ethical considerations, it is also believed that negative expectations about therapy and the care received can have a **nocebo effect** (from Latin, meaning "I will harm"), which results in less-than-optimal outcomes of therapy. It is thought that the nocebo effect plays a major role in psychogenic illness, especially in stress-related problems, because the patient may worry about his or her condition or treatment. A **placebo** is a drug dosage form (e.g., tablet, capsule) that has no pharmacologic activity because the dosage form has no active ingredients. However, when the placebo is taken, the patient may report a therapeutic response. Placebos are frequently used in studies of new medicines to measure the pharmacologic effects of a new medicine compared with the inert placebo. The American Pain Society and the Agency for Healthcare Research and Quality recommend the avoidance of the deceitful use of placebos in current clinical practice guidelines for pain management. It is thought that the deceitful use of placebos in pain management violates a patient's right to receive the highest quality of care possible.

TOLERANCE

Tolerance occurs when a person begins to require a higher dosage of a medication to produce the same effects that a lower dosage once provided. An example is the person who is addicted to heroin. After a few weeks of use, larger doses are required to provide the same "high." Tolerance can be caused by psychological dependence, or the body may metabolize a particular drug more rapidly than before, thereby causing the effects of the drug to diminish more rapidly.

DEPENDENCE

Drug dependence, which is also known as *addiction* or *habituation,* occurs when a person is unable to control his or her desire for ingestion of drugs. The dependence may be *physiologic,* in which the person develops withdrawal symptoms if the drug is withdrawn for a certain period, or *psychological,* in which the patient is emotionally attached to the drug. Drug dependence

occurs most commonly with the use of the scheduled or controlled medications listed in Chapter 1 (e.g., opiates, benzodiazepines). Many people, especially older adults, worry about becoming addicted to pain medication and therefore may not take their pain medication, even when it is needed. The nurse needs to assure these individuals that studies have shown that less than 1% of patients using opioids for acute pain relief become addicted and that it is important for their overall well-being to be as free of pain as possible. (See Chapter 48 for more information.)

CUMULATIVE EFFECT

A drug may accumulate in the body if the next dose is administered before the previously administered dose has been metabolized or excreted. Excessive **drug accumulation** may result in drug toxicity. An example of drug accumulation is the excessive ingestion of alcoholic beverages. A person becomes "drunk" or "inebriated" when the rate of consumption exceeds the rate of metabolism and excretion of the alcohol.

Carcinogenicity is the ability of a drug to induce living cells to mutate and become cancerous. Many drugs have this potential, so all drugs are tested in several animal species before human investigation to eliminate this potential.

FACTORS THAT INFLUENCE DRUG ACTIONS

ABSORPTION

Drug absorption refers to the process by which drugs are absorbed in the body. This occurs by way of different routes through which the drugs are administered. For example, the most common way to administer a drug is orally (by mouth), and then the drug is absorbed by the gastrointestinal (GI) tract (enterally). Other routes include intramuscularly (in the muscle) or intravenously (in the vein). The rate of absorption is dependent on various factors such as blood flow to the area in which the drug has been administered.

Age

Pediatric and geriatric patients each require special considerations for medication administration. Medicines given intramuscularly are usually erratically absorbed in neonates and older adults. Differences in muscle mass, blood flow to muscles, and muscle inactivity in patients who are bedridden make absorption unpredictable.

Topical administration with percutaneous absorption is usually effective for infants because their outer layer of skin (the stratum corneum) is not fully developed. Because the skin is more fully hydrated at this age, water-soluble drugs are absorbed more readily. Infants who wear plastic-coated diapers are also more susceptible to skin absorption because the plastic acts as an occlusive dressing that increases the hydration of the skin. Inflammation (e.g., diaper rash) also increases the amount of drug that is absorbed.

Transdermal administration in geriatric patients is often difficult to predict. Although dermal thickness decreases with aging and may enhance absorption, factors that may diminish absorption can be seen, including drying, wrinkling, and a decrease in the number of hair follicles. With aging, decreased cardiac output and diminishing tissue perfusion may also affect transdermal drug absorption.

In most cases, medicines are administered orally. Infants and older adults often lack a sufficient number of teeth for chewable medicines. Chewable tablets should not be given to children or to any patient with loose teeth. Geriatric patients often have reduced salivary flow, which makes chewing and swallowing more difficult. However, tablet and capsule forms are often too large for pediatric or geriatric patients to swallow safely. It is often necessary to crush a tablet for administration with food or to use a liquid formulation for easier and safer administration. Taste also becomes a factor when administering oral liquids because the liquid comes into contact with the taste buds. Timed-release tablets, enteric-coated tablets, and sublingual tablets should not be crushed because this will increase their absorption rate and thus the potential for toxicity.

The GI absorption of medicines is influenced by various factors, including gastric pH, gastric emptying time, the motility of the GI tract, enzymatic activity, the blood flow of the mucous lining of the stomach and intestines, the permeability and maturation of the mucosal membrane, and concurrent disease processes. Absorption by **passive diffusion** across the membranes and gastric emptying time depend on the pH of the environment.

Newborns and geriatric patients have reduced gastric acidity and prolonged transit time compared with adults. Premature infants have a high gastric pH (6 to 8) as a result of the immature acid-secreting cells in their stomachs. In a full-term newborn, the gastric pH is also 6 to 8, but within 24 hours the pH decreases to 2 to 4 in response to gastric acid secretion. At 1 year old, the child's stomach pH approximates that of an adult (i.e., pH of 1 to 2 when empty, up to 5 when full).

Geriatric patients often have a higher gastric pH because of the loss of acid-secreting cells. Drugs that are destroyed by gastric acid (e.g., ampicillin, penicillin) are more readily absorbed in older adults because of the decrease in acid production, which results in higher serum concentrations. By contrast, drugs that depend on an acidic environment for absorption (e.g., phenobarbital, acetaminophen, phenytoin, aspirin) are more poorly absorbed, thereby resulting in lower serum concentrations in older adults.

Premature infants and geriatric patients also have a slower gastric emptying time, partly because of their reduced acid secretion. A slower gastric emptying time may allow the drug to stay in contact with the absorptive tissue longer, thereby allowing for increased absorption with a higher serum concentration. There is also the potential for toxicity caused by extended contact time in the stomach for drugs that have the potential to cause gastric ulcers (e.g., nonsteroidal antiinflammatory drugs).

Another factor that affects drug absorption in the newborn is the absence of the enzymes needed for **hydrolysis**. Hydrolysis is the process that uses water to initiate a chemical reaction. Infants cannot metabolize palmitic acid from chloramphenicol palmitate (an antibiotic), thereby preventing the absorption of the chloramphenicol. Oral phenytoin dosages are also greater in infants who are less than 6 months old because of poor absorption (i.e., in neonates, the dosage is 15 to 20 mg/kg/24 hr compared with infants and children, in whom the dosage is 4 to 7 mg/kg/24 hr).

The **intestinal transit** refers to the speed at which the intestine moves foods, secretions, and other ingested matter along, and this rate varies with age. Premature and full-term newborns have a slower transit time. As the healthy newborn matures into infancy, the GI transit rate increases to a relatively standard rate by about 4 months of age. Older adults develop decreased GI motility and intestinal blood flow. This has the potential for altering the absorption of medicines and for causing constipation or diarrhea, depending on the medicine.

Gender

Generally, a woman's stomach empties solids more slowly than a man's does, and it may have greater gastric acidity, thus slowing the absorption of certain types of medicines (e.g., aspirin). A slower gastric emptying time may allow the drug to stay in contact with the absorptive tissue longer, thereby allowing for more absorption and a higher serum concentration. Women also have lower gastric levels of the enzyme alcohol dehydrogenase, which is needed to metabolize ingested alcohol. Thus larger amounts of ingested alcohol may be absorbed instead of metabolized in the stomach, thereby leading to a higher blood alcohol level in a woman than in a man for equal amounts of ingested alcohol. Other factors, such as body weight and drug distribution (see the next section of this chapter), may aggravate the higher blood alcohol level and state of intoxication in women compared with men.

DISTRIBUTION

The term *distribution* refers to the ways in which drugs are transported by the circulating body fluids to the sites of action (receptors), metabolism, and excretion. Distribution is dependent on pH, body water concentrations (i.e., intracellular, extracellular, and total body water), the presence and quantity of fat tissue, protein binding, cardiac output, and regional blood flow.

Age and Gender

Most medicines are transported either dissolved in the circulating water (i.e., in blood) of the body or bound to plasma proteins within the blood. Total body water content of a preterm infant is 83%, whereas that of an

Table 3.2 Proportions of Body Water[a]			
AGE (WEIGHT)	EXTRACELLULAR WATER (%)	INTRACELLULAR WATER (%)	TOTAL BODY WATER (%)
Premature (1.5 kg)	60	40	83
Full term (3.5 kg)	56	44	74
5 months (7 kg)	50	50	60
1 year (10 kg)	40	60	59
Adult male	40	60	60

[a]Developmental changes from birth to adulthood. Extracellular and intracellular water values are expressed as percentages of total body weight.
Data from Friis-Hansen B. Body composition during growth. *Pediatrics.* 1971;47(suppl 2):264.

adult man is 60%; this drops to 50% in older persons. The significance of this is that infants have a larger volume of distribution for water-soluble drugs and thus require a higher dose on a milligram-per-kilogram basis than an older child or an adult (Table 3.2).

With aging, lean body mass and total body water decrease and total fat content increases. The body weight of a preterm infant may be composed of 1% to 2% fat, whereas a full-term newborn may have 15% fat. Adult total body fat ranges from 18% to 36% for men and 33% to 48% for women between the ages of 18 and 35 years. Drugs that are highly fat soluble (e.g., antidepressants, phenothiazines, benzodiazepines, calcium channel blockers) require a longer onset of action and accumulate in fat tissues, thereby prolonging their action and increasing the potential for toxicity. For water-soluble drugs (e.g., ethanol, aminoglycoside antibiotics), a woman's greater proportion of body fat produces a higher blood level compared with that of a man when the drug is given as an equal dose per kilogram of body weight. In the case of ethanol, this effect tends to cause a higher level of ethanol in the brain cells, which results in greater intoxication. Highly fat-soluble medicines (e.g., diazepam) must be given in smaller milligram-per-kilogram dosages to low-birth-weight infants, because there is less fat tissue to bind the drug, thereby leaving more drug to be active at receptor sites.

Drugs that are relatively insoluble are transported in the circulation by being bound to plasma proteins (albumin and globulins), especially albumin. **Protein binding** is reduced in preterm infants because of decreased plasma protein concentrations, lower binding capacity of protein, and decreased affinity of proteins for drug binding. Drugs that are known to have lower protein binding in neonates than in adults include phenobarbital, phenytoin, theophylline, propranolol, lidocaine, and penicillin. Because serum protein binding is diminished, the drugs are distributed over a wider area of the neonate's body, and a larger loading dose is required than is needed in older children to achieve therapeutic serum concentrations. Several drugs that are used to treat neonatal conditions may compete for binding sites. Little difference exists between albumin protein in men and women, although there are some differences between the globulin proteins (i.e., corticosteroid-binding and sex-hormone–binding globulins). In adults who

are more than 40 years old, the composition of body proteins begins to change. Although the total body protein concentration is unaffected, albumin concentrations gradually decrease and other protein levels (e.g., globulins) increase. As albumin levels diminish, the level of unbound active drug increases. Increased levels of naproxen and valproate have been found in older adults, presumably as a result of decreased albumin levels. Disease states such as cirrhosis, renal failure, and malnutrition can lower albumin levels. Initial doses of highly protein-bound drugs (e.g., warfarin, phenytoin, propranolol, diazepam) should be reduced and then increased slowly if there is evidence of decreased serum albumin. Lower protein binding may also lead to a greater immediate pharmacologic effect because more active drug is available; however, the duration of action may be reduced because more of the unbound drug is available for metabolism and excretion.

METABOLISM

Drug metabolism is the process whereby the body inactivates medicines. It is controlled by factors such as genetics, diet, age, health, and the maturity of enzyme systems. Enzyme systems, primarily in the liver, are the major pathways of drug metabolism.

Age

All enzyme systems are present at birth, but they mature at different rates, taking several weeks to a year to fully develop. Liver weight, the number of functioning hepatic cells, and hepatic blood flow decrease with age; this results in the slower metabolism of drugs in older adults. Reduced metabolism can be seriously aggravated by the presence of liver disease or heart failure. Drugs that are extensively metabolized by the liver (e.g., morphine, lidocaine, propranolol) can have substantially prolonged durations of action if hepatic blood flow is reduced. Dosages usually must be reduced or the time interval between doses extended to prevent the accumulation of active medicine and potential toxicity. Drug metabolism can also be affected in all age groups by genetics, smoking, diet, gender, other medicines, and diseases (e.g., hepatitis, cirrhosis). Liver enzymes are monitored to determine any elevated levels during the course of drug therapy. No specific laboratory tests are available for measuring liver function that can be used to adjust drug dosages (Table 3.3). Renal function must be assessed and dosages adjusted based on creatinine clearance.

Gender

It is now recognized that males and females differ with regard to the concentrations of enzyme systems throughout life. The CYP3A4 component of the cytochrome P450 (CYP) system of enzymes metabolizes more than 50% of all drugs, and it is 40% more active in women. Drugs such as erythromycin, prednisolone, verapamil, and diazepam are metabolized faster in women than in men.

EXCRETION

Metabolites of drugs, which are the products of metabolism—and, in some cases, the active drug itself—are eventually excreted from the body. The primary routes are through the renal tubules into the urine and through the GI tract into the feces. Other generally minor routes of excretion include evaporation through the skin, exhalation from the lungs, and secretion into the saliva and breast milk.

Age

At birth, a preterm infant has up to 15% of the renal capacity of an adult, whereas a full-term newborn has approximately 35% of that capacity. The filtration capacity of an infant increases to about 50% of adult capacity at 4 weeks of age and is equivalent to full adult function at 9 to 12 months. Drugs that are excreted primarily by the kidneys (e.g., penicillin, gentamicin, tobramycin, vancomycin) must be administered in increased dosages or given more often to maintain adequate therapeutic serum concentrations as renal function matures.

As the body ages, important physiologic changes take place in the kidneys, including decreased renal blood flow caused by atherosclerosis and reduced cardiac output, a loss of glomeruli, and decreased tubular function and urine-concentrating ability. However, there is a great degree of individual variation with regard to changes in renal function, and no prediction of renal function can be made solely on the basis of a person's age. The renal function of older adult patients should be estimated using equations that factor in the patient's age. More optimally, renal function should be calculated

Table 3.3 Medications That Require Hepatic Monitoring[a,b]

GENERIC NAME	BRAND NAME	GENERIC NAME	BRAND NAME
acetaminophen	Tylenol	methotrexate	Rheumatrex
amiodarone	Pacerone	methsuximide	Celontin
atorvastatin	Lipitor	naproxen	Naprosyn
azathioprine	Imuran	nevirapine	Viramune
carbamazepine	Tegretol	niacin	Niaspan
diclofenac	Voltaren	oxcarbazepine	Trileptal
efavirenz	Sustiva	pemoline	
ethosuximide	Zarontin	pentamidine	Pentam
ethotoin	Peganone	pioglitazone	Actos
felbamate	Felbatol	piroxicam	Feldene
fenofibrate	Tricor	pravastatin	Pravachol
fluvastatin	Lescol	rifampin	Rifadin
gemfibrozil	Lopid	ritonavir	Norvir
griseofulvin	Gris-PEG	rosiglitazone	Avandia
indinavir	Crixivan	rosuvastatin	Crestor
isoniazid	Nydrazid	simvastatin	Zocor
ketoconazole	Nizoral	tacrine	Cognex
lamivudine	Epivir	terbinafine	Lamisil
leflunomide	Arava	tizanidine	Zanaflex
lovastatin	Mevacor	tolcapone	Tasmar
meloxicam	Mobic	valproic acid	Depakote

[a]This is a list of the more common drugs that require periodic liver function tests, usually at the beginning of therapy and then every few weeks to months thereafter (see individual monographs).
[b]Enzymes that are routinely monitored for liver function are alkaline phosphatase, alanine aminotransferase, and aspartate aminotransferase. If the patient's levels become elevated, the physician should be notified for individualized treatment.
Data from Tice SA, Parry D. Medications that require hepatic monitoring. *Hosp Pharm.* 2001;36(4):456-464; Tice SA, Parry D. Medications that require hepatic monitoring. *Hosp Pharm.* 2004;39(6):595-606; Porter RS, Kaplan JL, eds. *The Merck Manual of Diagnosis and Therapy.* 19th ed. Whitehouse Station, NJ: Merck; 2012; American Geriatrics Society 2015 Beers Criteria Update Expert Panel. American Geriatrics Society 2015 Updated Beers criteria for potentially inappropriate medication use in older adults. *J Am Geriatr Soc.* 2015;63(11):2227-2246.

by measuring urine creatinine levels over time. Serum creatinine can give a general estimate of renal function, but in older adult patients these determinations tend to exaggerate actual functional capability. This happens because the production of creatinine depends on muscle mass, which is diminished in older adults. Significant elevations occur only when there has been major deterioration of renal function. Blood urea nitrogen concentration is also a poor predictor of renal function because it is significantly altered by diet, status of hydration, and blood loss.

THERAPEUTIC DRUG MONITORING

Therapeutic drug monitoring is the measurement of a drug's concentration in biologic fluids to correlate the dosage administered and the level of medicine in the body with the pharmacologic response. Assays of blood (serum) samples for drug concentrations are most commonly used, but assays that involve the use of saliva are being perfected for some medicines. Saliva samples have the advantage of the easy collection of specimens without pain or the loss of blood that may require replacement by transfusion at a later date. Therapeutic drug monitoring is essential for neonates, infants, and children to ensure that drugs are within an appropriate therapeutic range, given the major physiologic changes that affect drug absorption, distribution, metabolism, and excretion.

The dosage and the frequency of administration must often be adjusted to help maintain therapeutic serum concentrations. Therapeutic drug monitoring is routine for conditions such as epilepsy (e.g., phenytoin, carbamazepine, valproic acid, phenobarbital), stroke (e.g., warfarin), heart failure (e.g., digoxin), and antimicrobial therapy (e.g., gentamicin, tobramycin, vancomycin) to prevent toxicities and to ensure that dosages are adequate to provide appropriate therapeutic levels. Blood levels of drugs can be measured if toxicity is suspected. The extent to which a serum drug level is elevated may dictate how the toxicity should be treated (e.g., acetaminophen, digoxin). Blood and urine samples can also be obtained for legal purposes if it is suspected that drugs (e.g., ethanol, amphetamines, marijuana, benzodiazepines, cocaine) have been consumed illicitly.

The timing of the drug's administration and the collection of the specimen are crucial to the accurate interpretation of the data obtained after assay. Certain medicines (e.g., aminoglycosides, gentamicin, tobramycin) require that blood be drawn before and after the administration of the drug to assess subtherapeutic levels and the potential for toxicity. One sample is drawn immediately before the next dose is to be administered to obtain the *trough*, or lowest, blood level of medicine, and another is drawn 20 minutes after the medicine has been administered intravenously or 60 minutes after the medicine has been administered orally to obtain the *peak*, or highest, blood level. All institutions have

policies that prescribe the best approach to therapeutic drug monitoring with specific medicines to ensure the accuracy and usefulness of results. To coordinate blood draws with the timing of drug administration, institutional policies regarding the handling of laboratory requests should be checked.

NURSING IMPLICATIONS WHEN MONITORING DRUG THERAPY

Chapter 4 discusses in detail the nursing process as it applies to pharmacology. In this chapter, which discusses drug action across the life span, it is appropriate to discuss nursing actions that relate to high-risk populations, such as pediatric patients, older adult patients, pregnant patients, and breastfeeding patients.

MONITORING PARAMETERS

All medicines have a number of parameters (e.g., expected therapeutic actions, common adverse effects, serious adverse effects, and any drug interactions) that a nurse must be knowledgeable about before taking on the responsibility of administering medications to patients. When peak and trough blood levels for a medication have been ordered, it is important that the nurse check the laboratory results in a timely manner and make sure that the prescriber is notified of the laboratory results. The next dose of the medication should not be given until the dosage has been clarified on the basis of the blood levels measured.

Although many of the same monitoring parameters (e.g., vital signs, urine output, renal function tests) are used to plan dosages and to monitor the effects of drug therapy in patients of all ages, it is absolutely crucial that the normal values for these monitoring parameters and laboratory tests be related to the age of the patient being monitored. For example, neonates have higher respiratory and heart rates and lower normal blood pressures than adults. As with all medications, patient education is important. Involving the appropriate family members, caregivers, and the school nurse in the overall health teaching plan is essential (see Chapter 5).

Pediatric Patients

Children are not just smaller versions of adults; therefore the principles of drug therapy cannot be extrapolated to infants and children only on the basis of size. Infants and children are at greater risk for complications from drug therapy because their body and organ functions are in an ongoing state of development.

General principles that a nurse can apply to the care of a pediatric patient include the following:
- Although infants and young children have a higher total body water content, they are more susceptible to dehydration from fever, vomiting, or diarrhea.
- Weight variations and growth spurts are expected in pediatric patients during normal maturation. Dosage adjustments are frequently necessary for

patients who are taking medicine on a regular basis (e.g., seizure medicines, allergy medicines) because they outgrow their dosages (see Appendix A for a nomogram for estimating body surface area). Therefore it is important to obtain accurate height and weight measurements on a regular basis.

- Therapeutic drug monitoring is essential for neonates, infants, and children to ensure that drugs are within an appropriate therapeutic range. The nurse must document the precise times that blood samples are drawn and the time over which the medicine was infused for accurate interpretation of the results.

- It is often difficult to assess the therapeutic response to the medicines administered to neonates, infants, and young children because these patients are often nonverbal or cannot tell us where it hurts. The nurse must rely more on laboratory values and assessment parameters such as temperature, pulse, respirations, heart sounds, lung sounds, bowel sounds, intake and output data, appetite, general appearance, and responsiveness.

- Nurses may find it difficult to measure and administer doses of oral medicines to pediatric patients accurately. The volume delivered by a household teaspoon ranges from 2.5 to 7.5 mL and may vary when the same spoon is used by different caregivers. The American Academy of Pediatrics recommends the use of appropriate devices for liquid administration, such as a medication cup, an oral dropper, or an oral syringe. Although tablets and capsules can usually be swallowed by a child who is 5 years old or older, the nurse should evaluate each child's ability to swallow a tablet before administration. Tablets that are not sustained-release or enteric-coated formulations may be crushed. Most capsules may be opened and the contents sprinkled on small amounts of food (e.g., applesauce, jelly, pudding). Box 3.1 provides selected pediatric administration guidelines for oral administration.

- Oral and parenteral medicines available in powder form must be diluted properly in accordance with the manufacturer's directions to allow for the accurate measurement of doses and to prevent hyperosmolar solutions from being administered. When taken orally, hyperosmolar solutions may cause diarrhea and dehydration.

- Many medicines are not approved by the FDA for use in children. Physicians may still legally prescribe medicines for what is termed *off-label use,* but it is important for the nurse to question a specific dose of medicine if it is not readily available for cross-checking with reference texts or with the drug information service in the pharmacy. The nurse must document in the nurses' notes that the drug order was verified before the prescribed medicine was administered. Nurses must be well versed in the monitoring parameters of the drug, and report adverse effects to the healthcare provider.

Box 3.1   Selected Guidelines for the Administration of Oral Medicine to Pediatric Patients[a]

INFANTS
- Use a calibrated dropper or an oral syringe.
- Support the infant's head while holding the infant in the lap.
- Give small amounts of medicine to prevent choking.
- If desired, crush non–enteric-coated or slow-release tablets into a powder and then sprinkle the powder on small amounts of food.
- Provide physical comforting while administering medications to help calm the infant.

TODDLERS
- Allow the toddler to choose a position in which to take the medication.
- If necessary, disguise the taste of the medication with a small volume of flavored drink or a small amount of food; also, a rinse with a flavored drink or water will help to remove any unpleasant aftertaste.
- Use simple commands in the toddler's jargon to obtain cooperation.
- Allow the toddler to choose which medication to take first if more than one is being taken.
- Provide verbal and tactile responses to promote cooperation.
- Allow the toddler to become familiar with the oral dosing device.

PRESCHOOL CHILDREN
- If possible, place a tablet or capsule near the back of the tongue, and then provide water or a flavored liquid to help with the swallowing of the medication.
- If the child's teeth are loose, do not use chewable tablets.
- Use a straw to administer medications that could stain teeth.
- Use a follow-up rinse with a flavored drink to help minimize any unpleasant aftertaste.
- Allow the child to help make decisions about the dosage formulation, the place of administration, which medication to take first, and the type of flavored drink to use.

[a]For all age groups listed, use a liquid dosage form, if available. From Brown LM, Isetts BJ. Patient assessment and consultation. In: Krinsky DL, Berardi RR, eds. *Handbook of Nonprescription Drugs: An Interactive Approach to Self-Care.* 17th ed. Washington, DC: American Pharmacists Association; 2012:27. Reproduced with permission from the American Pharmacists Association.

- In general, salicylates (aspirin) should not be administered to pediatric patients from infancy through adolescence. These children are susceptible to a life-threatening illness known as Reye's syndrome if they ingest aspirin at the time of or shortly after viral infection with chickenpox or influenza.

- Medicines that are routinely used for analgesia and antipyresis (fever reduction) in pediatric patients are ibuprofen and acetaminophen.

- Allergic reactions can occur rapidly in children, particularly if the medicine is administered intravenously. Reactions occur most commonly to antibiotics, especially penicillins. The nurse needs to be observant for responses to medication administration; if an event should occur, prompt intervention is needed. The first symptoms may be intense anxiety, weakness, sweating, and shortness of breath. Other symptoms may include hypotension, shock, dysrhythmia, respiratory congestion, laryngeal edema, nausea, and defecation. The nurse should summon assistance (call a code if severity warrants), stay with the child to provide comfort, facilitate breathing (administer oxygen, as needed), and, if the child stops breathing, initiate cardiopulmonary resuscitation.

Geriatric Patients

Geriatric patients represent an ever-increasing portion of the population. Although people who are more than 65 years old represent about 14% of the US population, they consume more than 25% of all prescription medicines and 33% of all nonprescription medicines sold. The prevalence of prescription medication use in the ambulatory adult population increases with advancing age. A recent study of the US noninstitutionalized adult population has indicated that more than 90% of persons 65 years old or older use at least one medication per week. More than 40% use 5 or more medications and 12% use 10 or more different medications per week.

Life Span Considerations

Older Adults

It is important that healthcare professionals understand the physiologic and pathologic changes that develop with advancing age and adjust drug therapy for the individual patient accordingly. Factors that place older adults at greater risk for drug interactions or drug toxicity include reduced renal and hepatic function, chronic illnesses that require multidrug therapy (**polypharmacy**), and a greater likelihood of malnourishment.

Unfortunately, a lack of complete understanding of the effects of medicines in older adults also leads to a problem that is the opposite of overuse: underuse. Caregivers walk a fine line between polypharmacy and undertreatment because of the complexity of chronic illnesses, changes in physiology and nutrition, compliance with multidrug regimens, and the pharmacokinetic factors associated with drug therapy during the later decades of a person's life. Although medicines may impair an older patient's quality of life, medicines are also the most cost-effective treatment for preventing illness and disability in the geriatric population.

When caring for a geriatric patient, it is important to complete a thorough drug history that includes the patient's use of nonprescription and herbal medicines (especially laxatives and antacids), nutritional and herbal supplements, and alternative therapies (e.g., aromatherapy, heat therapy, cold therapy). Similarly, a thorough nutrition history should be completed for the patient. Determine whether the patient's diet is balanced with regard to carbohydrates, fats, proteins, and vitamins. Assess whether a loss of teeth or loose-fitting dentures could interfere with chewing. A functional health assessment that includes sight and fine-motor control should be completed to assess the patient's ability to self-medicate.

When evaluating a new symptom in a geriatric patient, determine first whether it was induced by medicines that the patient is taking. The adjustment of dosages or the elimination of certain medicines is often the easiest, quickest, and most cost-effective therapy available.

When discontinuing drug therapy, it is important to taper the dosage when appropriate (e.g., beta blockers, antidepressants) to prevent symptoms that could occur as a result of sudden discontinuation.

When initiating therapy with a geriatric patient, remember the following:

- Start at one-third to one-half of the normal adult recommended dosage, and then gradually increase the dosage at appropriate intervals to assess for the therapeutic effect and the development of adverse effects.
- Keep multidrug regimens simple; use aids such as a calendar or a pillbox with time slots to prevent confusion.
- Use therapeutic drug monitoring when serum drug level data are available for a particular medicine.
- Offer assistance with destroying expired prescriptions to minimize confusion with the current medication regimen.
- Periodically review the regimen to see whether any medications can be discontinued (e.g., allergy medicines outside of allergy season). Ask whether new prescriptions from other healthcare providers or nonprescription or herbal medicines have been started.
- Be alert to prescriptions for the medications listed in Table 3.4. This list of medicines is part of the Beers Criteria, which are used to evaluate prescription quality and safety in nursing homes. These medicines are considered to be potentially inappropriate (but not contraindicated) for older patients. Their use should be documented as the best alternative for a patient's particular needs. The Centers for Medicare and Medicaid Services has incorporated the Beers Criteria into federal safety regulations for long-term care facilities.
- Geriatric patients may have difficulty with swallowing large tablets or capsules. Tablets may need to be broken in half or crushed if there is a score mark on the tablet. Remember that timed-release tablets, enteric-coated tablets, and sublingual tablets should never be crushed because of the effect on the absorption rate and the potential for toxicity. Applesauce, ice cream, pudding, and jelly are good foods to use to administer crushed medications.

Table 3.4 **Potentially Inappropriate Drugs for Older Adult Patients**[a]

GENERIC NAME	BRAND NAME	RATIONALE
Medications to Avoid		
Antidepressants		
amitriptyline	Elavil	Highly anticholinergic
doxepin greater than 6 mg		Sedating and cause orthostatic hypotension
paroxetine	Paxil	
Antihistamines		
chlorpheniramine	Chlor-Trimeton	Highly anticholinergic
cyproheptadine		Risk of confusion, dry mouth, and constipation
diphenhydramine	Benadryl	Diphenhydramine used for acute treatment of severe allergic reactions may
hydroxyzine	Vistaril	be appropriate
Antiinfective		
nitrofurantoin	Macrobid	Avoid in individuals with creatinine clearance of less than 30 mL/min or for long-term suppression of bacteria
Antispasmodics		
dicyclomine	Bentyl	Highly anticholinergic
hyoscyamine	Levsin	
Antipsychotics		
First Generation (Typical)		All increase risk of cerebrovascular accident and greater cognitive decline
fluphenazine		and mortality in patients with dementia
haloperidol	Haldol	Do not use for behavior problems of dementia
Second Generation (Atypical)		Avoid, except for schizophrenia, bipolar disorder, or as antiemetic during chemotherapy
aripiprazole	Abilify	
quetiapine	Seroquel	
Barbiturates		
butalbital		Risk of physical dependence, greater risk of overdose
phenobarbital		Butalbital is used in combination with acetaminophen and caffeine (e.g., Fioricet) for tension or muscle contraction headache
Benzodiazepines		
Short and Intermediate Acting		Older patients are very sensitive to benzodiazepines and have decreased
alprazolam	Xanax	ability to metabolize long-acting benzodiazepines
lorazepam	Ativan	All benzodiazepines increase risk of cognitive impairment, delirium, falls, and
temazepam	Restoril	fractures
Long Acting		Long-acting benzodiazepines may be appropriate for seizure disorders,
clonazepam	Klonopin	ethanol withdrawal, severe generalized anxiety disorder
diazepam	Valium	
flurazepam		
Cardiovascular Drugs		
Antiarrhythmics		
amiodarone	Pacerone	Amiodarone is effective for maintaining sinus rhythm but has greater toxicities than other antiarrhythmics; avoid as first line unless patient has heart failure
disopyramide	Norpace	Disopyramide is highly anticholinergic; may induce heart failure
digoxin	Lanoxin	Digoxin may be associated with increased mortality in atrial fibrillation and heart failure; do not use first line and limit dose to less than 0.125 mg/day
Peripheral Alpha-1 Blockers		High risk of orthostatic hypotension
doxazosin	Cardura	
terazosin	Hytrin	
Central Alpha Blockers		High risk of central nervous system effects; may cause bradycardia and orthostatic hypotension
clonidine	Catapres	

Table 3.4 Potentially Inappropriate Drugs for Older Adult Patients—cont'd

GENERIC NAME	BRAND NAME	RATIONALE
Nonsteroidal Antiinflammatory Drugs		
aspirin greater than 325 mg		Increased gastrointestinal bleeding Avoid chronic use
ibuprofen	Motrin	
naproxen	Naprosyn	
Nonbenzodiazepines		
eszopiclone	Lunesta	Have adverse effects similar to benzodiazepines
zolpidem	Ambien	

aThese medicines are still approved for use; however, it is believed that the adverse effects are generally more common, and thus the medicines should be avoided in older adult patients unless treatment has failed with other medicines.

Data from American Geriatrics Society 2015 Beers Criteria Update Expert Panel. American Geriatrics Society 2015 Updated Beers Criteria for potentially inappropriate medication use in older adults. *J Am Geriatr Soc.* 2015;63(11):2227-2246.

- It is extremely important that patients understand the purposes of the medications that they are taking and any complications that could occur if they discontinue their drugs.
- When handing a patient a new prescription to be filled, inquire about his or her ability to pay for the new medicine. Do not let an inability to pay be a barrier to therapy; refer the patient to social services, as needed.

Pregnant Patients

During pregnancy, the fetus is exposed to most medicines and foreign substances that are circulating in the mother's blood. Fetuses are particularly sensitive to toxic substances while in utero for the following reasons: (1) they have few circulating proteins that can bind drugs; (2) their enzyme systems, which will later metabolize drugs, are not yet developed or are immature; and (3) their excretory systems are only minimally functioning. Some drugs known as *teratogens* will cause the abnormal development of key tissues (i.e., birth defects) if they are taken at a certain time during pregnancy (Table 3.5).

Because of the potential for injury to the developing fetus, drug therapy during pregnancy should be avoided if at all possible. However, studies indicate that about two-thirds of women take at least one drug while pregnant and that about two-thirds of the medicines are nonprescription self-care remedies. The medicines that are most commonly taken include acetaminophen, antacids, and cold and allergy products. Because few data are available for determining the safety of medicines in humans during pregnancy, very few medicines can be considered completely safe for use during pregnancy.

In 1975, the FDA started requiring that all medicines be assigned to a use-in-pregnancy category: A, B, C, D, or X. These categories weigh the degree to which available information has ruled out the risk to the fetus for birth defects (teratogenicity) balanced against the drug's potential benefit to the patient. However, in 2015 the FDA instituted new rules for drug labels that replace the lettered categories with new categories on pregnancy, lactation, and reproductive potential. In addition to

Table 3.5 Drugs Known to Be Teratogens

DRUG CLASS	EXAMPLE(S)
Androgenic and estrogenic hormones	oral contraceptives, diethylstilbestrol, conjugated estrogens, clomiphene, exemestane
Angiotensin-converting enzyme inhibitors	benazepril, captopril, enalapril, fosinopril, lisinopril, moexipril, perindopril, ramipril, trandolapril
Angiotensin II receptor antagonists	azilsartan, candesartan, eprosartan, irbesartan, losartan, olmesartan, telmisartan, valsartan
Anticonvulsants	carbamazepine, phenytoin, trimethadione, valproic acid
Antimanic agents	lithium
Antithyroid drugs	propylthiouracil, methimazole
Chemotherapeutic agents	busulfan, cyclophosphamide, methotrexate
Hydroxymethylglutaryl coenzyme A reductase inhibitors (statins)	atorvastatin, fluvastatin, lovastatin, pravastatin, rosuvastatin, simvastatin
Other teratogens	ambrisentan, anastrozole, azathioprine, cocaine, dronedarone, dutasteride, ethanol (high dose, frequent use), isotretinoin, alitretinoin, ribavirin, tetracycline, thalidomide, vitamin A (>18,000 units/day), warfarin

including information that summarizes the risks of using a drug during pregnancy and lactation, labeling must now include relevant information about contraception, pregnancy testing, and infertility to inform the healthcare provider prescribing drugs for females and males of reproductive potential (and for the consumer). It will be several years before the older system is completely phased out, but the new format will allow for consistency of information regarding risks and benefits of prescription drugs used during pregnancy and lactation and by females and males of reproductive potential. Information regarding drug use in pregnancy, in lactation, and in females and males of reproductive potential is found in section 8 of the package insert and in other online drug information resources such as ePocrates and Lexicomp. Two excellent resources—LactMed and DART—are available on the National Library of Medicine's Toxnet website. These resources include information on nonprescription medications, whereas the new labeling requirements do not provide information on these drugs. (See Online Resources for links.)

General principles that a nurse can apply to the care of a pregnant patient include the following (see also Chapter 39):

- When taking a history, be alert to the possibility of pregnancy in any woman of childbearing age, especially in those showing symptoms of early pregnancy, including nausea, vomiting (especially in the morning), and frequent urination.
- Complete a thorough drug history, including the use of nonprescription and herbal medicines and nutritional supplements.
- Complete a thorough nutrition history; assess for a diet that is balanced with regard to carbohydrates, fats, proteins, and vitamins. Good nutrition with the appropriate ingestion of vitamins (especially folic acid) and minerals (calcium and phosphorus) is particularly important for preventing birth defects.
- Instruct the patient to avoid drugs in general at any stage of pregnancy, unless such use is recommended by the patient's physician.
- Advise against the consumption of alcohol during pregnancy. Excessive use may cause the child to be born with fetal alcohol syndrome, which is a lifelong condition that can be avoided by eliminating alcohol during pregnancy. If the woman is planning to become pregnant, it is recommended that she stop using alcohol 2 to 3 months before the planned conception.
- Advise against the use of tobacco. Mothers who smoke have a higher frequency of miscarriage, stillbirths, premature births, and low-birth-weight infants.
- Before they use medicines, advise pregnant women to try nonpharmacologic treatments. For morning sickness, the patient can try lying down when she feels nauseated; ingesting crackers or sipping small quantities of liquids before arising; eating small, frequent meals that are high in carbohydrates; and lowering fat content of meals. Pregnant women with morning sickness should avoid spicy foods, dairy products, and smells or situations that might cause vomiting.
- Herbal medicines that have not been scientifically tested in women during pregnancy should be avoided.

Breastfeeding Infants

Many drugs are known to enter the breast milk of nursing mothers and have the potential to harm the infant. The American Academy of Pediatrics provides a list of medicines and their potential effects on nursing infants (Table 3.6).

Nurses should keep in mind when caring for patients who are breastfeeding that although drug levels in breast milk may be safe, it is always best for the mother to discuss all medicines she uses—including prescription, nonprescription, and herbal products—with a healthcare provider before taking them. If medicine is being taken, encourage the mother to take it immediately after the infant finishes breastfeeding or just before the infant's

Table 3.6 Drugs and Nursing Infants	
DRUGS' POTENTIAL ADVERSE EFFECTS	**EXAMPLES**
Drugs that may interfere with the metabolism of a nursing infant	cyclophosphamide, cyclosporine, doxorubicin, methotrexate, capecitabine, cytarabine, gemcitabine, pemetrexed
Drugs of abuse reported to have adverse effects on nursing infants	amphetamine, cocaine, heroin, marijuana, phencyclidine, ethanol
Drugs for which effect on nursing infants is unknown but may be of concern Antianxiety medications Antidepressants Others	Benzodiazepines: alprazolam, diazepam, quazepam Cyclic antidepressants: amitriptyline, clomipramine, nortriptyline, desipramine, imipramine, doxepin, bupropion, trazodone Serotonin reuptake inhibitors: fluoxetine, fluvoxamine, paroxetine, sertraline Antipsychotic drugs: chlorpromazine, clozapine, haloperidol, mesoridazine, trifluoperazine amiodarone, lamotrigine, metronidazole
Drugs associated with significant effects on nursing infants[a]	aspirin, beta-adrenergic blocking agents (acebutolol, atenolol), clemastine, lithium, phenobarbital, primidone

[a]Drugs for which the effect on nursing infants is unknown but may be of concern. Give to nursing mothers with caution.

longer sleep periods. Educate the mother about what adverse effects of the drug might occur in the infant so that other therapy can be considered.

GENETICS AND DRUG METABOLISM

Genetic composition serves as the basic foundation for all drug responses and their duration of action in the body throughout the person's lifetime. Many other factors have an impact on drug action and duration, but the foundation starts with the genetic blueprint. **Genetics** is the study of how living organisms inherit the characteristics or traits of their ancestors, such as hair color, eye color, and skin pigmentation. Other much less obvious—but extremely important—traits of inheritance include the function of the metabolic pathways and susceptibility to illnesses (e.g., heart disease or cancer).

A **genome** is the complete package of genetic coding of an organism. The human genome is composed of 23 chromosome pairs, 22 of which are known as autosomal (i.e., not gender related) pairs; the remaining pair is the X or Y chromosome that determines the presence of male or female sex characteristics. Twenty-three chromosomes each are donated by the biologic mother and father. Genetic information is carried on the chromosomes by a large molecule called *deoxyribonucleic acid* (DNA), which is copied and passed on to future generations. Traits are carried in DNA as instructions for building and operating an organism. These instructions are contained in segments of DNA called *genes*. The sequence of the DNA linkages in a gene determines what traits the gene controls. The sequence of DNA is similar to a sequence of words that are linked together to form a meaningful sentence. Several genes are frequently responsible for a specific trait or function. The sequence of genes is known as the *genetic code*. The organism reads the sequence of these units and decodes the instructions. **Polymorphisms** are naturally occurring variations in the structures of genes and the instructions that they give to the organism.

In 1989, the National Center for Human Genome Research was created to lead the US contribution to the Human Genome Project, an international public effort to sequence all 3 billion DNA base pairs of the human genetic blueprint. The Human Genome Project was completed in April 2003, and the database is now available for worldwide biomedical research.

An unfolding science based on genetics is **pharmacogenetics**, which is the study of how drug response may vary in accordance with inherited differences. As described in Chapter 2, drug action depends on five factors: liberation, absorption, distribution, metabolism, and excretion. Each of these factors is greatly influenced by genetic polymorphisms, but each also varies on the basis of such factors as age, gender, organ function, other drug therapy, and drug interactions. Research has shown significant differences among racial and ethnic groups with regard to the metabolism, clinical effectiveness, and side effect profiles of different medications.

Most studies to date have concentrated on cardiovascular and psychiatric drugs, analgesics, antihistamines, and ethanol. The research so far primarily applies to African Americans, whites, and Asians, but more research is now focusing on Hispanic Americans because they represent the largest racial or ethnic group after whites in the United States. It is anticipated that discoveries in pharmacogenetics will allow a blood sample to be analyzed for specific gene characteristics (genotyped) that are important determinants of drug pharmacokinetics and pharmacodynamics, thereby allowing drug selection to be tailored to the individual patient's genetic makeup.

Monoclonal antibodies are early examples of medicines that were synthesized to attack certain types of cancers on the basis of the presence of genetically determined types of cells in some cancers. Laboratory tests are used to determine the presence of these proteins in a patient's cancer cells and whether the cancer cells will be susceptible to the monoclonal antibody. Another recent discovery is the potential for fatal skin reactions (i.e., Stevens-Johnson syndrome, toxic epidermal necrolysis) that can be caused by carbamazepine therapy in patients with the human leukocyte antigen allele HLA-B*1502. This allele is most common in persons of Asian and South Asian Indian ancestry (see the discussion of carbamazepine in Chapter 18). The FDA maintains a website that lists genomic biomarkers that have been identified (see Online Resources). These can be tested for before the initiation of drug therapy to target therapy or prevent potentially fatal drug reactions.

Get Ready for the NCLEX® Examination!

Key Points

- The placebo effect occurs when a patient believes he or she had a positive response to a drug, even though the patient did not have any chemically active drug. The nocebo effect occurs when the patient has negative expectations about therapy and the patient believes that a drug is not working.
- Drug dependence occurs when a patient develops physical withdrawal symptoms if the drug is withdrawn for a certain period, or when a patient is emotionally attached to a drug.
- The age of the patient has significant effects on the absorption, distribution, metabolism, and excretion of the drug. Pediatric patients and elderly patients are more susceptible to the effects of drugs than adult patients. Physical changes that occur during the aging process impact the effect drugs will have on the elderly patient.
- Men and women often do not respond to drugs or physical disease states in the same way, and gender differences impact the effect of drugs.
- Pregnant and breastfeeding women need to be aware that any drug they take will have an effect on their unborn fetus and/or infant.
- Pharmacogenetics currently focuses on determining the appropriate drug to use based on the individual's genetic composition.

Additional Learning Resources

SG Go to your Study Guide for additional Review Questions for the NCLEX® Examination, Critical Thinking Clinical Situations, and other learning activities to help you master this chapter content.

Go to your Evolve website (https://evolve.elsevier.com/Clayton) for additional online resources.

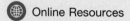 Online Resources
- DART: https://toxnet.nlm.nih.gov/newtoxnet/dart.htm
- LactMed: https://toxnet.nlm.nih.gov/newtoxnet/lactmed.htm
- Pharmacogenomic biomarkers: https://www.fda.gov/Drugs/ScienceResearch/ucm572698.htm

Review Questions for the NCLEX® Examination

1. A patient who has been asked to participate in a study asks the nurse what the term *placebo* means. What would be an appropriate response by the nurse?
   1. "The word *placebo* refers to the type of abnormal response that may occur when taking medications."
   2. "That term means the body has built up a resistance to a drug and that more of the drug is needed to get the same response."
   3. "The term *placebo* refers to a dosage form that has no active ingredients; these are frequently used in studies to determine the effect of a new medication."
   4. "The word *placebo* comes from Latin and means 'I will harm.'"

2. What is the reason it is important to understand the difference between drug dependence and drug accumulation?
   1. Drug accumulation can be detected more easily than drug dependence.
   2. Drug accumulation may result in drug toxicity, and drug dependence can result in cell mutation.
   3. Drug dependence can be prevented, and drug accumulation is inevitable.
   4. Drug dependence can be the result of taking addictive substances for a prolonged time, and drug accumulation can result in drug overdose.

3. When drugs are circulating in the bloodstream and reach the sites of action, what is this process known as?
   1. Absorption
   2. Metabolism
   3. Distribution
   4. Excretion

4. Which nursing action(s) would be essential when monitoring drug therapy in the geriatric patient? *(Select all that apply.)*
   1. Monitoring renal and liver function
   2. Monitoring for drug interactions
   3. Completing a thorough drug history, including over-the-counter and alternative therapies
   4. Inquiring about the ability to pay for medications
   5. Educating the patient and caregivers about all drugs and potential complications

5. Drug absorption in the elderly is affected by which of these physiologic factors? *(Select all that apply.)*
   1. Changes in albumin levels
   2. Increased filtration capacity of the kidneys
   3. Reduced cardiac output
   4. Higher gastric pH
   5. Decreased GI motility

6. While discussing with a mother the importance of administering furosemide orally to an infant with a cardiac abnormality, the nurse would recognize the need for further explanation if the mother makes which statement?
   1. "I know that my baby needs this drug every day at approximately the same time."
   2. "My baby will have no problem taking this tablet."
   3. "I will check to make sure that the furosemide is working by monitoring the number of wet diapers."
   4. "I understand that my baby will continue to grow even while taking this drug."

7. A pregnant woman asked a nurse at the obstetrician's clinic how she could determine which drug was safe to take during pregnancy. What would be an appropriate response by the nurse?
   1. "Because there are few studies done to determine the safe use of drugs during pregnancy, it is okay to keep taking what was previously prescribed by your physician."
   2. "Because there are few studies done to determine the safe use of drugs during pregnancy, it is advisable to ask your physician or pharmacist regarding taking prescription and over-the-counter drugs."
   3. "You are not to take any drugs during pregnancy."
   4. "It would be fine to take over-the-counter drugs, since they never cause any issues."

8. An expecting mother asks the nurse if it would be okay for her to take some cold medicine. What would be an appropriate response by the nurse?
   1. "There are not a lot of studies done with regard to how safe medications are to take during pregnancy."
   2. "I am sure it is safe to take, no problem."
   3. "I believe the cold medication is contraindicated for pregnant women."
   4. "Animal studies have revealed no evidence of harm to the fetus using these drugs."

9. A patient was discussing with the nurse the idea that in the future we will be able to determine which drug will be effective depending upon a person's genetic makeup. Which term does this refer to?
   1. Polymorphisms
   2. Pharmacogenetics
   3. Genome coding
   4. Pharmacokinetics

10. Why is it important for nurses to know about drug actions and current developments in drug therapy?
    1. Patients who are hospitalized need drug monitoring.
    2. Drug actions detail how effective the drug will be for everyone.
    3. The elderly population has a greater likelihood of polypharmacy.
    4. Prescription medication use decreases as a person ages.

4   The Nursing Process and Pharmacology

Objectives

1. Discuss the components and purpose of the nursing process.
2. Explain what the nurse does to collect patient information during an assessment.
3. Discuss how nursing diagnosis statements are written.
4. Differentiate between a nursing diagnosis and a medical diagnosis.
5. Discuss how evidence-based practice is used in planning nursing care.
6. Differentiate between nursing interventions and expected outcome statements.
7. Explain how Maslow's hierarchy of needs is used to prioritize patient needs.
8. Compare and contrast the differences between dependent, interdependent, and independent nursing actions.
9. Discuss how the nursing process applies to pharmacology.

Key Terms

nursing process (NŬR-sĭng PRŎ-sĕs) (p. 36)
nursing classification systems (klă-sĭ-fĭ-KĀ-shŭn SĬS-tĕmz) (p. 37)
assessment (ă-SĔS-mĕnt) (p. 39)
nursing diagnosis (NŬR-sĭng dī-ăg-NŌ-sĭs) (p. 39)
defining characteristics (dĕ-FĪN-ĭng kăr-ăk-tĕr-ĬS-tĭks) (p. 40)
medical diagnosis (p. 40)
collaborative problem (kŏ-LĂB-ĕr-ă-tĭv) (p. 41)
focused assessment (FŌ-kŭst ă-SĔS-mĕnt) (p. 41)
planning (p. 41)
nursing care plan (p. 41)
critical pathways (KRĬ-tĭ-kŭl PĂTH-wāz) (p. 41)
evidence-based practice (ĔV-ĭ-dĕns BĀSD PRĂK-tĭs) (p. 41)
core measures (p. 42)
priority setting (prī-ŌR-ĭ-tē SĔT-tĭng) (p. 42)
measurable goal statement (MĔ-zhŭr-ĕ-bŭl GŌL STĀT-mĕnt) (p. 42)

patient goals (p. 43)
implementation (ĭm-plĕ-mĕn-TĀ-shŭn) (p. 43)
nursing interventions (p. 43)
nursing actions (p. 43)
dependent actions (dē-PĔN-dĕnt) (p. 43)
interdependent actions (ĭn-tŭr-dē-PĔN-dĕnt) (p. 43)
independent actions (ĭn-dē-PĔN-dĕnt) (p. 43)
nursing orders (p. 44)
anticipated therapeutic statements (p. 44)
expected outcome statements (p. 44)
drug history (HĬS-tō-rē) (p. 44)
primary source (PRĪ-măr-ē SŌRS) (p. 44)
subjective data (sŭb-JĔK-tĭv DĀ-tă) (p. 44)
objective data (ŏb-JĔK-tĭv DĀ-tă) (p. 44)
secondary sources (SĔK-ŏn-dār-ē SŌR-sĕz) (p. 45)
tertiary sources (TĔR-shē-ăr-ē) (p. 45)
drug monographs (MŎN-ō-grăfs) (p. 45)
therapeutic intent (thĕr-ă-PYŪ-tĭk) (p. 45)

THE NURSING PROCESS

The practice of nursing is an art and science that uses a systematic approach to identify and solve the potential problems that individuals may experience as they strive to maintain basic human function along the wellness-illness continuum. The focus of all nursing care is to help individuals maximize their potential for maintaining the highest possible level of independence for the meeting of self-care needs. Conceptual frameworks for the basis of nursing practice—such as Henderson's Complementary-Supplement Model (1980), Roger's Life Process Theory (1979, 1980), Roy's Adaptation Model (1976), and the Canadian Nurses Association Testing Service (1980)—are examples of the models that are used today.

The **nursing process** is the foundation for the clinical practice of nursing. It provides the framework for consistent nursing actions and involves the use of a problem-solving approach rather than an intuitive approach. When implemented properly, the nursing process also provides a method for evaluating the outcomes of the therapy delivered. In addition to quality of care, the nursing process provides a scientific, transferable method for healthcare planners to assign nursing staff to patients and to determine and justify the cost of providing nursing care in this age of soaring healthcare costs.

Nursing classification systems such as the Nursing Minimum Data Set, the Nursing Interventions Classification (NIC), and the Nursing Outcomes Classification (NOC) are designed to provide a standardized language for reporting and analyzing nursing care delivery that has been individualized for the patient. These information systems promote input from *multidisciplinary team* members who provide valuable clinical expertise, a holistic approach, and collaboration for the healthcare of individual patients. These systems can measure and validate the impact of actual nursing diagnoses and interventions on outcomes for patients, families, and communities.

Many nursing education programs and healthcare facilities use a five-step nursing process model: (1) assessment, (2) nursing diagnosis, (3) planning, (4) implementation, and (5) evaluation. These five steps are actually an overlapping process (Fig. 4.1). Information from each step is used to formulate and develop the next step in the process. Box 4.1 illustrates the process that is used to assemble data and organize information into categories that help the learner to identify the patient's strengths and problem areas. Thereafter, nursing diagnosis statements can be developed and focused nursing assessments can be initiated. Planning can be individualized, and measurable goals and anticipated therapeutic outcomes can be identified. Concurrently, individualized nursing interventions can be developed to coincide with the individual's abilities and resources as well as the disease processes being treated. During the implementation process, the individual's physical, psychosocial, and cultural needs must be considered. The assessment process should continue to focus not only on the evolving changes in the presenting symptoms and problems but also on the detection of potential complications that may occur.

Nurses should familiarize themselves with the nurse practice act in the state in which they practice to identify the educational and experiential qualifications that are necessary for the performing of assessments and the

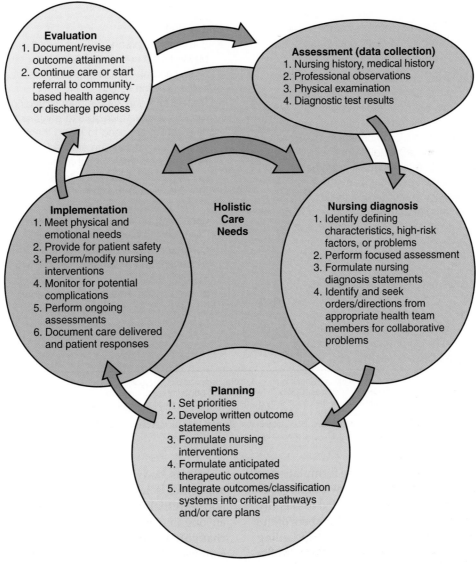

Fig. 4.1 The nursing process and the holistic needs of the patient.

Box 4.1 Principles of the Nursing Process and Their Application to Pharmacologic Needs

ASSESSMENT
- Collect all relevant data associated with the individual patient's symptoms; his or her history and physical, laboratory, and diagnostic data; and medical diagnosis to detect actual and risk/high-risk problems that require intervention.
- Data sources can be primary, secondary, or tertiary.
- Specific assessments related to the patient's pharmacologic needs include collecting the drug history; allergies; height and weight; age and disease process; hepatic function results (AST, ALT, alkaline phosphatase, LDH, bilirubin [total and direct]); and renal function results (serum creatinine, creatinine clearance, BUN, urinalysis, protein [total and 24-hour urine]), as well as discussing the patient's understanding of drug therapy and the treatment plan and determining his or her readiness to learn.

NURSING DIAGNOSIS
- On the basis of the data collected, formulate a statement about the behaviors or problems of concern and their cause.
- Formulate nursing diagnosis statements for problems that are amenable to nursing actions (see Table 4.1).
- Identify and seek orders or direction from appropriate healthcare team members for collaborative problems.[a]

PLANNING
- Prioritize the problems identified from the assessment data, with the most severe or life threatening addressed first. Other problems are arranged in descending order of importance. (Maslow's hierarchy of needs is frequently used as a basis for prioritizing; other approaches may be equally valid.)
- Develop short- and long-term patient goals and outcomes in measurable statements that are appropriate to the clinical setting and the length of stay.
- Identify the monitoring parameters to be used to detect possible complications of the disease process or the treatments being used.
- Plan nursing approaches to correlate with each identified patient goal or outcome.
- Integrate outcomes and classification systems into critical pathways or standardized care plans to be used in clinical settings.
- Specific planning related to the patient's pharmacologic needs includes examining drug monographs and developing an individualized teaching plan.

IMPLEMENTATION
- Perform the nursing intervention planned to achieve the established goals or outcomes.
- Monitor the patient's response to treatments, and monitor for complications related to existing pathophysiology.
- Provide for patient safety.
- Perform ongoing assessments on a continuum.
- Document the care given and any additional findings on the patient's chart.[b]
- Specific interventions related to the patient's pharmacologic needs include administering the prescribed drug using the seven rights: verifying the right patient, the right drug, the right dose, the right route, the right time, the right indication, and the right documentation. The nurse also will be monitoring the patient using diagnostic parameters; monitoring for adverse effects of medications; and performing and documenting health teaching, which includes having the patient understand the drug name, the dose, the route of administration, the anticipated therapeutic response, the adverse effects, what to do if a dose is missed, and how to fill a prescription.

EVALUATION
- Evaluation is an ongoing process that occurs at every phase of the nursing process. Establish target data to review and analyze at intervals prescribed by guidelines in the practice setting.
- Review and analyze the data regarding the patient, and modify the care plan so that goals and outcomes of care, which are used to return the patient to the highest level of functioning, are attained.
- Evaluate outcomes with the use of the classification systems, critical pathways, or standardized care plans that are used in the clinical setting.
- Follow a systematic approach to recording progress, depending on the setting and charting methodology.
- Continue the nursing process, initiate referral to a community-based health agency, or execute discharge procedures as ordered by the healthcare provider.
- Specific evaluation criteria related to the patient's pharmacologic needs include evaluating the patient's tolerance of drug therapy and his or her understanding of the treatment regimen.

[a]Because not all patient problems are amenable to resolution by nursing actions, those complications or problems associated with medical diagnosis or that result from treatment-related issues are placed in a category known as "Collaborative Problems," which the nurse monitors.
[b]Integrate the classification system that is currently in use in the clinical setting when charting (e.g., Nursing Minimum Data Set, Nursing Interventions Classification, Nursing Outcomes Classification, Omaha System, Home Health Care Classification System).
ALT, Alanine aminotransferase; *AST,* aspartate aminotransferase; *BUN,* blood urea nitrogen; *LDH,* lactate dehydrogenase.

development of nursing diagnoses. The formulation of nursing diagnoses requires a broad knowledge base to make the discriminating judgments needed to identify the individual patient's care needs. All members of the healthcare team need to contribute data regarding the patient's care needs and his or her response to the prescribed treatment regimen.

Just as body functions are constantly undergoing adjustments to maintain homeostasis in the internal and external environments, the nursing process is an ongoing cyclic process that must respond to the changing requirements of the patient. The nurse must continually interact with people in a variety of settings to establish and execute nursing functions creatively and cooperatively to meet the holistic care needs of patients (see Fig. 4.1).

ASSESSMENT

Assessment is the first phase of the five-step nursing process. Assessment starts when the patient is admitted and continues until the patient is discharged from care. It is the problem-identifying phase of the nursing process. The initial assessment must be performed by a registered nurse with the necessary skills to complete the physical examination and the knowledge base to analyze the data, and who can identify patient problems based on defining characteristics (i.e., signs, symptoms, and clinical evidence). In addition, the nurse should identify risk factors that make an individual or group of people more vulnerable to developing certain problems in response to a disease process or to its prescribed therapy (e.g., adverse effects of drugs that may require modification of the regimen).

During the assessment, the nurse collects a comprehensive information base about the patient from the physical examination, the nursing history, the medication history, and professional observations. Formats commonly used for data collection, organization, and analysis are the head-to-toe assessment, body systems assessment, and Gordon's Functional Health Patterns Model. The head-to-toe and body systems approaches focus on the patient's physiology, whereas the Gordon's Functional Health Patterns Model (Box 4.2) includes sociocultural, psychological, spiritual, and developmental factors that affect the individual's needs.

NURSING DIAGNOSIS

Nursing diagnosis is the second phase of the five-step nursing process. NANDA International (NANDA-I, formerly the North American Nursing Diagnosis Association) approved the following official definition of the term *nursing diagnosis:* "[a] clinical judgment about individual, family, or community responses to actual or potential health problems/life processes." Nursing diagnoses provide the basis for the selection of nursing interventions to achieve outcomes for which the nurse is accountable (Fig. 4.2).

A systematic method of working with patients is used to identify four types of nursing diagnoses: (1) actual, (2) risk/high-risk, (3) health promotion and wellness, and (4) syndrome (Table 4.1). This text will focus on actual and risk/high-risk nursing diagnoses (particularly those related to drug therapy) that influence the actions that the nurse must initiate to correct the problems that are encountered.

Box 4.2	Gordon's Functional Health Patterns Model

Health Perception–Health Management Pattern
Nutrition-Metabolic Pattern
Elimination Pattern
Activity-Exercise Pattern
Cognitive-Perceptual Pattern
Sleep-Rest Pattern
Self-Perception–Self-Concept Pattern
Role-Relationship Pattern
Sexuality-Reproductive Pattern
Coping–Stress Tolerance Pattern
Value-Belief Pattern

Adapted from Gordon M. *Manual of Nursing Diagnosis.* 11th ed. Sudbury, MA: Jones & Bartlett; 2007.

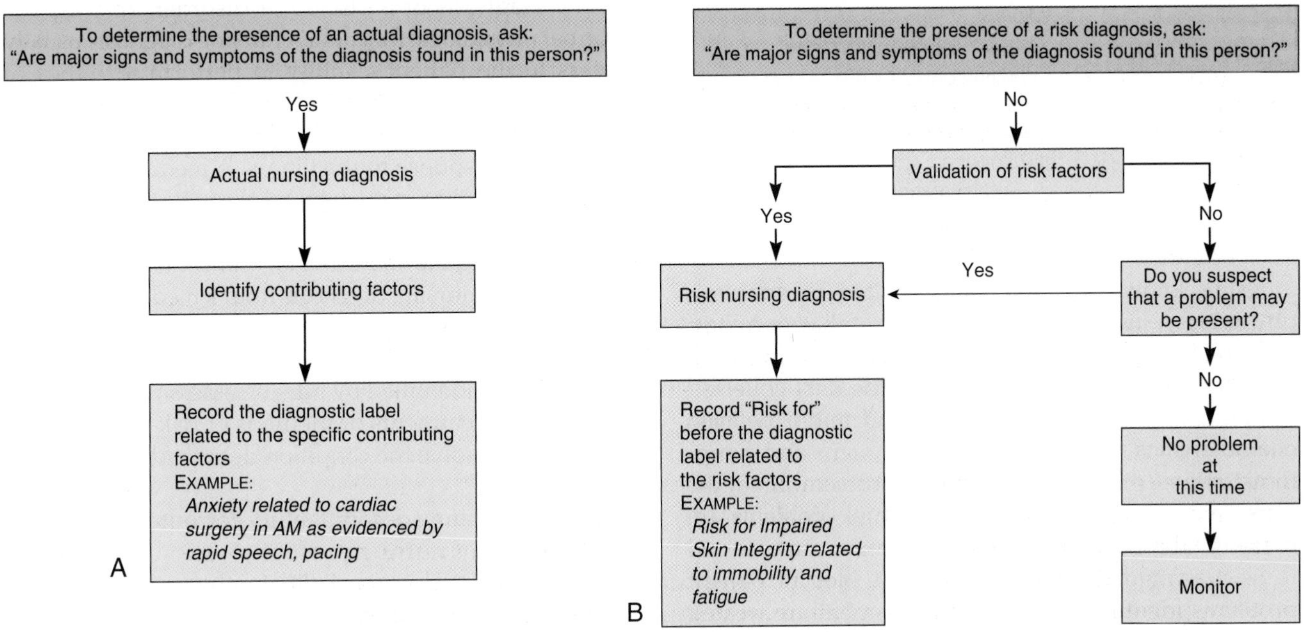

Fig. 4.2 Decision tree for actual (A) and risk (B) nursing diagnoses. (From Carpenito-Moyet LJ: *Nursing Diagnosis: Application to Clinical Practice.* 15th ed. Philadelphia: Lippincott; 2016.)

Table 4.1   Types of Nursing Diagnoses

NURSING DIAGNOSIS TYPE	DESCRIPTION
Actual	Based on human responses to health conditions and life processes that exist in an individual, a family, or a community Supported by defining characteristics (i.e., manifestations or signs and symptoms) that cluster in patterns of related cues or inferences
Risk/high-risk	A clinical judgment that an individual, a family, or a community is more susceptible to the problem than others in the same or a similar situation Supported by risk factors that contribute to increased vulnerability In some cases, when an individual is more likely to develop a particular problem, the term *high risk for* is added
Health promotion and wellness	A clinical judgment about an individual, a group, or a community in transition from a specific level of wellness to a higher level of wellness
Syndrome	These nursing diagnoses cluster actual or high-risk signs and symptoms that are predictive of certain circumstances or events The causative or contributing actors for the diagnosis are contained in the diagnostic label The five currently approved syndrome diagnoses are as follows: (1) rape-trauma syndrome (2) disuse syndrome (3) posttrauma syndrome (4) relocation stress syndrome (5) impaired environmental interpretation syndrome

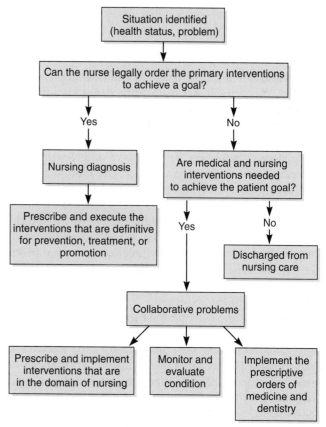

Fig. 4.3 The differentiation of nursing diagnoses from collaborative problems. (From Carpenito-Moyet LJ: *Nursing Diagnosis: Application to Clinical Practice.* 15th ed. Philadelphia: Lippincott; 2016.)

Using knowledge and skills related to anatomy, physiology, nutrition, psychology, pharmacology, microbiology, nursing practice skills, and communication techniques, the nurse analyzes the data collected to identify whether certain major and minor **defining characteristics** (i.e., manifestations or signs and symptoms) relate to a particular patient problem. If so, the nurse may conclude that certain actual problems are present. These patient-related problems are referred to as *nursing diagnoses* (see Fig. 4.2). Not all patient problems identified during an assessment are treated by the nurse alone. Many of these problems require a multidisciplinary approach. When the nurse cannot legally order the definitive interventions required under the presenting circumstances, a collaborative problem exists (Fig. 4.3).

A **medical diagnosis** is a statement of the patient's alterations in structure and function, and this results in the diagnosis of a disease or disorder that impairs normal physiologic function. A nursing diagnosis usually refers to the patient's ability to perform activities of daily living (ADLs) in relation to the impairment induced by the medical diagnosis; it identifies the individual's or group's response to the illness. A medical diagnosis also tends to remain unchanged throughout the illness, whereas nursing diagnoses may vary, depending on the patient's state of recovery. Concepts that help to distinguish a nursing diagnosis from a medical diagnosis include the following:

1. Conditions described by nursing diagnoses can be accurately identified by nursing assessment methods.
2. Nursing treatments or methods of risk-factor reduction can resolve the condition described by a nursing diagnosis.
3. Nurses assume accountability for outcomes within the scope of nursing practice.
4. Nurses assume responsibility for the research required to clearly identify the defining characteristics and causative factors of conditions described by nursing diagnoses.

5. Nurses engage in improving methods of treatment and treatment outcomes for conditions described by nursing diagnoses.

The wording of an actual nursing diagnosis takes the form of a three-part statement. These statements consist of the following: (1) a patient problem summarizing the issue; (2) the contributing factors or cause, which may include deficits in ADLs or the medical diagnosis; and (3) the defining characteristics (i.e., manifestations or signs and symptoms). An example related to pharmacology would state: *Insufficient knowledge related to polypharmacy as evidenced by inability to state what prescribed medications are used for.*

The risk/high-risk nursing diagnosis statement consists of two parts: (1) the diagnostic label from the NANDA-I–approved list and (2) the risk factors that make the individual or group more susceptible to the development of the problem. A risk diagnosis is validated by the presence of risk factors that would contribute to the individual or group developing the stated problem (see Fig. 4.2). High-risk diagnoses are used for patients who are particularly vulnerable to a problem.

A health promotion or wellness nursing diagnosis statement only has a one-part label. This label is initiated by the words "readiness for enhanced" followed by the nursing diagnosis being applied to the situation or group. The individual or group must understand that the higher level of functioning is feasible. This diagnosis can be applied only to individuals or groups when the potential for a higher level of wellness is realistic.

Further discussion of the philosophy and clinical use of nursing diagnoses—including the specifics regarding the wording of actual and risk/high-risk diagnoses, as well as the new categories of health promotion and wellness and syndrome nursing diagnoses—can be found in other primary texts and references, especially in those developed solely for the purpose of explaining nursing diagnoses.

Collaborative Problems

Not all patient problems identified by the nurse can be resolved by nursing actions; many care plans include multidisciplinary input and planning to maximize patient outcomes. However, the nurse is responsible for monitoring the patient on a continuum for potential complications that are associated with the medical diagnosis, the diagnostic procedures, or the treatments prescribed. To differentiate between a problem that requires a nursing diagnosis and a **collaborative problem**, the nurse must decide whether definitive interventions can be ordered to prevent or treat the problem to maintain the health status of the patient (Carpenito, 2013). A collaborative problem statement is worded as a potential complication, which is abbreviated as *PC*. An example would be "PC: Hypokalemia." Outcome criteria for collaborative problems are found on critical pathways or multidisciplinary plans.

Focused Assessment

A **focused assessment** is the process of collecting additional data specific to a patient or family that validates a suggested problem or nursing diagnosis. The questions asked or the data collected are used to confirm or rule out the defining characteristics associated with a specific nursing diagnosis statement. During the focused assessment, collaborative problems that require prescriptive orders can be identified and differentiated from solutions that the nurse can implement and that are within the nurse's scope of practice.

PLANNING

Planning is the third phase of the five-step nursing process. After the patient has been assessed and problems have been diagnosed, plans should be formulated to meet the patient's needs. Planning usually encompasses four phases: (1) priority setting, (2) the development of measurable goal and outcome statements, (3) the formulation of nursing interventions, and (4) the formulation of anticipated therapeutic outcomes that can be used to evaluate the patient's status. The written or computer-generated document that evolves from this planning process is called the *nursing care plan*. Handwritten care plans are being replaced by **critical pathways**, which are standardized, automated care plans that integrate standards, interventions, goals, and outcomes into the patient's electronic medical record.

Critical pathways are also referred to as *integrated care plans*, *care maps*, or *clinical maps*. These documents are comprehensive standardized plans of care that are individualized on admission by the healthcare provider and the nurse case manager. A critical pathway describes a multidisciplinary plan that is used by all caregivers to track the patient's progress toward expected outcomes within a specified period. Standardized outcomes and timetables require healthcare providers to make assessments regarding the patient's progress toward the goals of discharge while maintaining quality care. Revisions are made as necessary and communicated to all healthcare team members so that patient care continues uninterrupted toward the discharge goals. Critical pathway programs are developed to monitor the care delivered at a specific clinical setting, but they are based on data that are gathered from many clinical sites. The use of standardized outcomes is designed to improve the quality of care provided, to reduce the cost of care, and to document the effect of the nursing care on patient outcomes.

Evidence-Based Practice

Evidence-based practice is the application of data from scientific research to make clinical decisions about the care of individual patients. Past medical and nursing practice relied largely on the clinical intuition of practitioners. The shift to evidence-based decision making is possible because of the vast array of clinical studies that have been completed and the existence of large databases, which can be quickly accessed and searched for the best scientific evidence when making healthcare decisions. An example of this concept that is seen in today's healthcare institutions is the quality measures known as *core measures*. Core measures are measures of care that are tracked to show how often hospitals and healthcare providers use the care recommendations identified by evidence-based practice standards for patients who are being treated for conditions such as heart attack, heart failure, and pneumonia or for patients who are undergoing surgery. Hospitals voluntarily submit data from the medical records of adults who have been treated for these conditions to help track standards of care and clinical outcomes.

Priority Setting

After the nursing diagnoses and collaborative problems have been identified, they must be prioritized. Maslow's hierarchy of needs is a model that is often used for establishing priorities. Maslow identified five levels of needs, beginning with physiologic needs at the lowest point on the hierarchy and ending with self-actualization needs at the highest point. Nurses can use Maslow's hierarchy to perform the **priority setting** of an individual patient's needs, determining which care aspect needs to be addressed first. These care delivery options are often organized in relation to their direct effects on the maintenance of homeostasis. Thus after determining that the patient is oxygenating appropriately by pulse oximetry (first priority), the nurse can then increase the patient's activity (second priority). Box 4.3 lists the priority ranking of subcategories of Maslow's hierarchy of human needs.

Measurable Goal and Outcome Statements

After the patient's needs have been prioritized, goals must be established and statements written. Goals are usually divided into short-term and long-term plans, depending on the length of stay and the clinical site. The **measurable goal statement** starts with an action word (i.e., a verb) that is followed by the behavior or behaviors to be performed by the patient or the patient's family within a specific amount of time.

All goal and outcome statements must be individualized and based on the patient's abilities. An example of a goal statement that follows the nursing diagnosis of knowledge deficit would be: *The patient will create a list of all the medications that are currently prescribed along with the reasons for taking them, by the end of the day.* The nurse must also refer to critical pathways when establishing the parameters. Statements must take into consideration the degree of rehabilitation that is realistic for the patient to expect for the amount of time during which care will be delivered. It is sometimes difficult to accept that not everyone can return to their preillness health status; therefore the nurse must be realistic when setting a measurable goal and strive to assist the patient with obtaining an optimal degree of functioning that is consistent with that patient's abilities.

Box 4.3 Priority Ranking of Subcategories of Maslow's Hierarchy of Human Needs

PHYSIOLOGIC NEEDS
- Oxygen, circulation
- Water-salt balance
- Food balance
- Acid-base balance
- Waste elimination
- Normal temperature
- Sleep, rest, relaxation
- Activity, exercise
- Energy
- Comfort
- Stimulation
- Cleanliness
- Sexuality

SAFETY NEEDS
- Protection from physical harm
- Protection from psychological threat
- Freedom from pain
- Stability
- Dependence
- Predictable, orderly world

BELONGING NEEDS
- Love, affection
- Acceptance
- Warm, communicating relationship
- Approval from others
- Unity with loved ones
- Group companionship

SELF-ESTEEM NEEDS
- Recognition
- Dignity
- Appreciation from others
- Importance, influence
- Reputation of good character
- Attention
- Status
- Dominance over others

SELF-ACTUALIZATION NEEDS
- Personal growth and maturity
- Awareness of potential
- Increased learning
- Full development of potential
- Improved values
- Religious, philosophic satisfaction
- Increased creativity
- Increased reality perception and problem-solving abilities
- Less rigid conventionality
- Less of the familiar, more of the novel
- Greater satisfaction in beauty
- Increased pleasantness
- Less of the simple, more of the complex

From Campbell C. *Nursing Diagnosis and Intervention in Nursing Practice.* New York: John Wiley & Sons; 1978. This material is reproduced with permission of John Wiley & Sons.

When goals are being established, it is important to include the patient and appropriate significant others in decision making because the patient and his or her support systems will be responsible for accomplishing the goals. Involvement of the patient is essential to promote cooperation and compliance with the therapeutic regimen and to provide the patient with a sense of control over the disease process and the course of treatment. The goals that are established should be **patient goals** rather than nursing goals for the patient.

With the advent of shorter hospital stays, most of the goal statements will involve short-term goals. The nurse must keep in mind the usual length of hospitalization and be realistic about the number and types of goals and outcomes being established. Short-term goals should serve as a bridge to meet the long-term goals established in a care plan. Long-term goals can be established with assistance from referral agencies in accordance with the individual's needs and circumstances. Long-term goals are then implemented in long-term care settings, rehabilitation centers, mental health facilities, and community-based home healthcare delivery settings.

Most goal statements are based on the patient's need to do the following:
1. Reduce or resolve the symptoms (usually the chief complaint) of the disease that caused the person to seek medical attention.
2. Understand the disease process and its effect on lifestyle and ADLs.
3. Gain knowledge and skills associated with the treatment procedures in an effort to attain the highest level of functioning possible (e.g., nutrition, comfort measures, medication regimen, physical therapy).
4. Have reasonable expectations of the therapy, including understanding signs and symptoms of improvement versus complications that require consultation with a healthcare provider.
5. Identify monitoring parameters that should be maintained on a written record that reflects the response to the prescribed therapy.
6. Establish a schedule for follow-up evaluation.

Nursing outcomes classification. The NOC is a comprehensive standardized classification system of patient outcomes that was developed to evaluate the effect of nursing interventions on patient care. These outcomes have been linked to NANDA-I diagnoses, Gordon's Functional Health Patterns Model, the Taxonomy of Nursing Practice, Omaha System problems, resident admission protocols used in nursing homes, the Outcome and Assessment Information Set system used in home care, and NIC interventions, which are discussed later in this chapter. Each outcome has a definition, a list of indicators that is used to evaluate patient status in relation to the outcome, a target outcome rating, a place to identify the source of the data, a five-point Likert scale to measure patient status, and a short list of references used in the development of the outcome. Standardized outcomes are necessary for documentation

in electronic records, use in clinical information systems, the development of nursing knowledge, and the education of professional nurses. The NOC is one of the standardized languages recognized by the American Nurses Association.

IMPLEMENTATION

Implementation of **nursing interventions** is the fourth phase of the nursing process, and it consists of carrying out the established plan of care. Nursing care is directed at meeting the physical and emotional needs of the patient, providing for patient safety, monitoring for potential complications, and performing ongoing assessments as part of the continual process of data collection and evaluation to identify changes in the patient's care needs.

Nursing actions are suggested by the etiology of the problems identified in the nursing diagnoses, and they are used to implement plans. They may include activities such as counseling, teaching, providing comfort measures, coordinating, referring, using communication skills, and performing the actions listed in a healthcare provider's orders. Documentation of all care given, including patient education and the patient's apparent response, should be performed regularly—both to assist with evaluation and reassessment and to make other healthcare professionals aware of the patient's changing needs.

Within the nursing process are three types of nursing actions: (1) dependent, (2) interdependent, and (3) independent. **Dependent actions** are those performed by the nurse on the basis of the healthcare provider's orders, such as the administration of prescribed medications and treatments. It is important to note that even though these are dependent functions, the nurse is still responsible for exercising professional judgment when performing these actions. **Interdependent actions** are those nursing actions that the nurse implements cooperatively with other members of the healthcare team for restoring or maintaining the patient's health. This allows the nurse to coordinate his or her interventions with those of other healthcare professionals to maximize knowledge and skills from various disciplines for the well-being of the patient. Collaborative communication among multidisciplinary team members is essential for maximizing patient outcomes in today's healthcare environment. **Independent actions** are those nursing actions that are not prescribed by a healthcare provider that a nurse can provide by virtue of the education and licensure that he or she has attained. These actions are usually written in the nursing care plan and originate from the nursing diagnosis.

Nursing Action or Intervention Statements
Nursing action or intervention statements list in a concise format exactly what the nurse will do to achieve each goal that has been developed for each nursing diagnosis. A nursing action is a statement that describes nursing interventions that are applicable to any patient (e.g.,

promote adequate respiratory ventilation). **Nursing orders** describe how specific actions, including time intervals, will be implemented for an individual patient.

Example of Nursing Interventions for Patient With Respiratory Issues

(date): Cough, turn, deep breathe: 0800, 1000, 1200, 1400, 1600, 1800, 2000, 2200

(date): Educate patient re: abdominal breathing, splinting the abdomen, pursed-lip breathing, and assuming correct position to facilitate breathing

(date): Auscultate breath sounds: 0800, 1200, 1600, 2000

(date): Increase patient's fluid intake to at least 2000 mL/ 24 hr:

0700-1500: 1000 mL

1500-2300: 800 mL

2300-0700: 200 mL

(date): Assess respiratory depth and rate: 0800, 1200, 1600, 2000, 2400

Nursing interventions classification. The NIC is a comprehensive, research-based, standardized classification of interventions that nurses perform. This is useful for clinical documentation, the communication about care across settings, the integration of data across systems and settings, effectiveness research, productivity measurement, competency evaluation, reimbursement, and curriculum design. This system includes the interventions that are carried out by nurses on behalf of patients or clients: these include independent and collaborative interventions that guide direct and indirect care. The NIC can be used in all settings and for all specialties.

Anticipated Therapeutic and Expected Outcome Statements

Outcome statements are measured along the continuum of care and include **anticipated therapeutic statements** and **expected outcome statements** that are developed to document the effectiveness of the care delivered. In the previous example, the patient would do the following:

- Improve the ability to perform coughing technique.
- Maintain an adequate fluid intake as evidenced by achieving a mutually set goal of 2000 mL within 24 hours.
- Attain a respiratory rate between 18 and 24 breaths/ min.
- Perform ADLs without feeling fatigued.

Therapeutic outcomes have been identified throughout this book for each drug classification. These can be used by the student to identify the outcomes that are anticipated from the use of the drugs listed in a particular classification.

Example of a Therapeutic Outcome

Using the nursing diagnosis "Anxiousness related to hospitalization and unknown prognosis," the *primary therapeutic outcome* expected from the benzodiazepine antianxiety agents is a decrease in the level of anxiety to a manageable level for the patient. This decreased anxiety may be manifested by a reduction in physical signs of anxiety, such as a worried look or pacing, and an improvement in coping.

EVALUATION

Evaluation is the fifth and final phase of the five-step nursing process. Evaluation involves the nurse determining whether the expected outcomes were met. All care is evaluated by comparison with the established nursing diagnoses (goal statements), the planned nursing actions, and the anticipated therapeutic outcomes. For the evaluation process to be successful, the participants (i.e., the patient, the patient's family and significant others, and the nurse) must be willing to receive feedback. Therefore plans for evaluation must involve the patient, the family, and significant others from the beginning and should recognize the needs of a culturally diverse population with varying beliefs about healthcare.

Although the evaluation phase is the last step in the nursing process, it is not an end in itself. Evaluation recognizes the successful completion of previously established goals, but it also provides a means for the input of new significant data that indicate the development of additional problems or a lack of therapeutic responsiveness, which may require additional nursing diagnoses or collaboration with the healthcare provider or other professionals on the healthcare team as plans for therapy are revised.

RELATING THE NURSING PROCESS TO PHARMACOLOGY

ASSESSMENT

Assessment is an ongoing process that starts with the admission of the patient and is completed at the time of discharge. With regard to relating the nursing process to the nursing functions associated with medications, assessment includes taking a **drug history** for three reasons: (1) to evaluate the patient's need for medication; (2) to obtain his or her current and past use of over-the-counter medications, prescription medications, herbal products, and street drugs; and (3) to identify problems related to drug therapy. Nurses will also want to identify risk factors such as allergies to certain medications (e.g., penicillins) or the presence of other diseases that may limit the use of certain types of drugs (e.g., sympathomimetic agents in patients with hypertension).

The nurse draws on three sources to build the medication-related information base. Whenever the patient is able to provide reliable information, the patient should be used as the **primary source** of information. Subjective and objective data serve as the baseline for the formulation of drug-related nursing diagnoses. **Subjective data** are pieces of information provided by the patient (e.g., "Whenever I take this medicine, I feel sick to my stomach"). **Objective data** are gained from observations that the nurse makes with the use of physiologic parameters (e.g., "skin pale, cold, and moist; temperature, 99.2°F orally"). Other required objective information is the patient's height and weight, which may be needed to select drug regimens and to use as a monitoring parameter for drug therapy later during the patient's treatment.

In some cases, it is necessary to obtain information from **secondary sources** (e.g., relatives, significant others, medical records, laboratory reports, nurses' notes, other healthcare professionals). Secondary sources of information are subject to interpretation by someone other than the patient. Data collected from secondary sources should be analyzed with the use of other portions of the database to validate the conclusions that are reached.

Tertiary sources of information (e.g., a literature search) provide an accurate depiction of the characteristics of a disease, the nursing interventions and diagnostic tests used, the pharmacologic treatment prescribed, the dietary interventions and physical therapy undertaken, and other factors pertinent to the patient's care requirements. When using these sources, the nurse should be aware that the patient has individual needs and that the plan of care must be adapted to fit the patient's identified needs.

Assessment related to drug therapy continues throughout the hospitalization period. Examples of ongoing assessment activities include visiting with the patient, determining the need for and administering as-needed (PRN) medications, monitoring vital signs, and observing for therapeutic effects in addition to common and adverse effects and potential drug interactions.

In preparation for the patient's eventual discharge and his or her need for education about new health-related responsibilities, the assessment process should include the collection of data related to the patient's health beliefs, existing health problems, prior compliance with prescribed regimens, readiness for learning (both emotionally and experientially), and ability to learn and execute the skills required for self-care.

NURSING DIAGNOSES

To deal effectively with identified problems (i.e., diagnoses), the nurse must recognize both the causative and contributing factors. The etiology and contributing factors are those clinical and personal situations that can cause the problem or influence its development. Situations can be organized into five categories: (1) pathophysiologic, (2) treatment related, (3) personal, (4) environmental, and (5) maturational (Carpenito, 2013).

When identifying problems related to medication therapy, the nurse should review the **drug monographs** starting in Chapter 12. These are detailed explanations of the purpose for which a drug is intended, and assist the nurse to identify common and adverse effects and drug interactions for patient monitoring. Several nursing diagnoses can be formulated on the basis of the patient's drug therapy. Although the most commonly observed problems are those associated with the drug treatment of a disease or the adverse effects of drug therapy, nursing diagnoses can also originate from pathophysiology caused by drug interactions.

Example of a Nursing Diagnosis

Drugs prescribed for Parkinson's disease are administered to provide relief of symptoms (e.g., muscle tremors, slowness of movement, muscle weakness with rigidity, alterations in posture and equilibrium). An actual nursing diagnosis of *Compromised mobility related to neuromuscular impairment* (Parkinson's disease) would be formulated on the basis of the defining characteristics established for this nursing diagnosis. The evaluation of the therapeutic and expected outcomes from the prescribed medications is based on the degree of improvement noted in the symptoms that are present.

A second nursing diagnosis would be *Potential for injury related to amantadine adverse effects* (confusion, disorientation, dizziness, lightheadedness).

In this example, common adverse effects of the drug amantadine, which is prescribed for treatment of the symptoms of Parkinson's disease, are also the basis of the second nursing diagnosis. The second nursing diagnosis is a collaborative problem that requires the nurse to monitor the patient for the development of these adverse effects. In other words, a patient with Parkinson's disease is at risk for developing the defining characteristics. When the defining characteristics are observed, notification of these to the healthcare provider is required, and the nurse would need to intervene to provide for the patient's safety.

Two nursing diagnoses that apply to all types of medications prescribed are as follows:
- Insufficient knowledge (actual, risk) related to the medication regimen (patient education)
- Noncooperation (actual, risk) related to the patient's value system, cognitive ability, cultural factors, or economic resources

PLANNING

Planning, with reference to the prescribed medications, must include the following steps:
1. The identification of the **therapeutic intent** of each prescribed medication. Determine why the drug was prescribed and what symptoms will be relieved.
2. Review of the drug monographs provided in this text, starting in Chapter 12, to identify the common and adverse effects that can be alleviated or prevented by actions of the nurse or patient and that will require immediate planning for patient education. The nurse should continuously monitor the patient for adverse effects of drug therapy and report these suspected adverse effects to the prescriber.
3. The identification of the recommended dosage and route of administration. The nurse should compare the recommended dosage with the dosage ordered and confirm that the route of administration is correct and that the dosage form ordered can be tolerated by the patient.

4. The scheduling of the administration of the medication on the basis of the prescriber's orders and the policies of the healthcare facility. Medications prescribed must be reviewed for drug-drug interactions and drug-food interactions; laboratory tests may also need to be scheduled if serum levels of the drug have been ordered.

5. Teaching the patient to keep written records of his or her responses to the prescribed medications using the Patient Self-Assessment Form (see Appendix B for more information).

6. Providing additional education as needed about techniques of self-administration (e.g., injection, the use of topical patches, the instillation of drops), as well as information as needed about proper storage and how to refill a medication. Priority ranking in preparation for health education may encompass several factors: (1) the patient's concerns, his or her health belief system, and the patient's priorities; (2) the urgency or time available for the learning to take place; (3) a sequence that allows the patient to move from simple to more complex concepts; and (4) a review of the overall needs of the individual. The content taught to the patient should be well planned and delivered in increments that the patient is capable of mastering. The complete teaching plan should be in the patient's Kardex, on the patient's chart, or in the patient's electronic medical record.

Example of Planning Medication Education

Mr. Jones will be able to state the following for each prescribed medication by (date) and will show retention of this information by repeating it on (date):
1. Drug name
2. Dosage
3. Route and administration times
4. Anticipated therapeutic response
5. Common adverse effects
6. Serious adverse effects
7. What to do if a dose is missed
8. When, how, or whether to refill the medication

To attain this goal, the patient's ability to name all of these factors would need to be checked at the initial time of exposure and on subsequent meetings to validate retention. After the goals have been formulated, they should not be considered final but rather should be reevaluated as needed throughout the course of treatment.

Possible NOC labels that could be used for the previously mentioned nursing diagnoses that apply to all types of medications are as follows:
- Insufficient knowledge (actual, risk) related to the medication regimen (patient education)
  - NOC—Knowledge: Medication
- Noncooperation (actual, risk) related to the patient's value system, cognitive ability, cultural factors, or economic resources
  - NOC—Compliance Behavior

IMPLEMENTATION

Nursing actions applied to pharmacology may be categorized as dependent, interdependent, or independent.

Dependent Nursing Actions

Dependent nursing actions are directly related to the orders that are written by the healthcare provider. These orders include diagnostic procedures and medications for the immediate well-being of the patient. The healthcare provider reviews data on a continuing basis to determine the risks and benefits of maintaining or modifying the medication orders. The maintenance or modification of the medication orders is the healthcare provider's responsibility. The nursing action of carrying out the medication orders is considered dependent because the nurse must follow the order written.

Interdependent Nursing Actions

The nurse performs baseline and subsequent focused assessments that are valuable for establishing therapeutic goals, the duration of therapy, the detection of drug toxicity, and the frequency of reevaluation.

The nurse should approach any problems related to the medication prescribed collaboratively with appropriate members of the healthcare team. Whenever the nurse is in doubt about medication calculations, monitoring for therapeutic efficacy and adverse effects, or the establishment of nursing interventions or patient education, another qualified professional should be consulted.

The pharmacist reviews all aspects of the drug order, prepares the medications, and then sends them to the unit for storage in a medication room or on a unit-dose medication cart. If any portion of the drug order or the rationale for therapy is unclear, the nurse and the pharmacist should consult with each other or the healthcare provider for clarification.

The frequency of medication administration is defined by the healthcare provider in the original order. The nurse and the pharmacist establish the schedule of the medication on the basis of the standardized administration times used at the practice setting. The nurse (and occasionally the pharmacist) also coordinates the schedule of medication administration and the collection of blood samples with the laboratory phlebotomist to monitor drug serum levels.

As soon as laboratory and diagnostic test results are available, the nurse and the pharmacist review them to identify values that could have an influence on drug therapy. The results of the tests are conveyed to the healthcare provider. The nurse should also have current assessment data available for the collaborative discussion of signs and symptoms that may relate to the medications prescribed, the dosage, the therapeutic efficacy, or any adverse effects.

Patient education, including discharge medications, requires that an established plan be developed, written in the patient's medical record, implemented, documented, and reinforced by all those who are delivering care to the patient (see the sample teaching plan in Chapter 5, Box 5.2).

Independent Nursing Actions

The nurse visits with the patient and obtains the nursing history, which includes a medication history as described earlier in the section on Relating the Nursing Process to Pharmacology, under Assessment.

The nurse verifies the drug order and assumes responsibility for the correct transcription of the drug order to the nurse's Kardex, the medication administration record, or the electronic medical record. As part of the transcribing process, the nurse makes professional judgments about the class of the drug, the drug's therapeutic intent and usual dosage, and the patient's ability to tolerate the drug dosage form ordered. If all aspects of the verification and transcription procedure are considered correct, a copy of the original order is sent to the pharmacy.

The nurse formulates appropriate nursing diagnoses and actions to monitor for therapeutic effects and adverse effects of medications. To do this, the nurse may need to review drug monographs to formulate the diagnosis and goal statements. The criteria for therapeutic response should describe the improvements expected in the symptoms of the disease for which the medication was prescribed.

The nurse prepares the prescribed medications with the use of procedures that are meant to ensure patient safety. As part of this process, nursing professional judgments must include the following:

1. The selection of the correct supplies (e.g., needle gauge and length, type of syringe) for the administration of the medications.
2. The verification of all aspects of the medication order before preparing the medication. The order should be verified again immediately after preparation and again before actual patient administration (patients should always be identified immediately before the administration of the medication and each time that a medication is to be administered). One of the National Patient Safety Goals established by The Joint Commission is to improve the accuracy of patient identification. It is now recommended that two patient identifiers (neither of which is the room number) be used when administering medications. For example, best practice would be to look at the patient's name band for identity and to request that the patient state his or her name and birth date.
3. The collection of appropriate data, also known as *premedication assessment,* to serve as a baseline for later assessments of therapeutic effectiveness and to detect adverse effects of drugs.
4. The administration of the medication by the correct route at the correct site. The selection and rotation of sites for medication should be based on established practices for the rotation of sites and on principles of drug absorption, which in turn may be affected by the presence of pathophysiologic characteristics (e.g., poor tissue perfusion).
5. The documentation in the chart of all aspects of medication administration. Subsequent assessments to identify the drug efficacy and the development of any adverse effects should be documented.
6. The implementation of nursing actions to minimize common adverse effects and to identify serious adverse effects to be reported promptly.
7. The education of patients on medications and gaining their cooperation. When noncompliance is identified, the nurse should attempt to ascertain the patient's reasons, and the nurse and the patient should collaboratively discuss approaches to the problems viewed by the patient as hindrances. The nurse needs to be cognizant of the belief systems of a culturally diverse population regarding medications, illness, and aging among patients and their families, along with language and other barriers that may impede communication with healthcare providers.

Possible NIC labels that could be used for the previously discussed nursing diagnoses that apply to all types of medications are as follows:
- Insufficient knowledge (actual, risk) related to the medication regimen (patient education)
  - NOC—Knowledge: Medication
  - NIC—Teaching: Prescribed Medication
- Noncooperation (actual, risk) related to the patient's value system, cognitive ability, cultural factors, or economic resources
  - NOC—Cooperative Behavior
  - NIC—Learning Readiness Enhancement *or* Financial Resource Assistance

EVALUATION

Evaluation associated with drug therapy is an ongoing process that assesses the patient's response to the medications prescribed, observes for signs and symptoms of recurring illness, evaluates for therapeutic effects or the development of adverse effects of the medication, determines the patient's ability to receive patient education and to self-administer medications, and notes the potential for compliance. Box 4.1 presents examples of how the nursing process is applied to the nursing responsibilities associated with drug therapy.

Get Ready for the NCLEX® Examination!

Key Points

- The components of the nursing process are assessment, nursing diagnosis, planning, implementation, and evaluation, and they provide a framework for nursing actions.
- The nurse collects assessment data by completing the physical examination.
- Nursing diagnosis statements include a patient problem summarizing the issue; the contributing factors or cause, which may include deficits in ADLs or the medical diagnosis; and defining characteristics.
- A medical diagnosis is a statement of the patient's alterations in structure and function, and results in the diagnosis of a disease or disorder that impairs normal physiologic function.
- The goal of evidence-based practice is to improve patient outcomes by implementing best practices, which have evolved from scientific studies.
- Maslow's hierarchy of needs is a model that is often used for establishing patient care priorities.
- There are three types of nursing actions: dependent, interdependent, and independent.
- Two nursing diagnoses that apply to all types of medications prescribed are:
  - Insufficient knowledge (actual, risk) related to the medication regimen (patient education)
  - Noncooperation (actual, risk) related to the patient's value system, cognitive ability, cultural factors, or economic resources

Additional Learning Resources

SG Go to your Study Guide for additional Review Questions for the NCLEX® Examination, Critical Thinking Clinical Situations, and other learning activities to help you master this chapter content.

Go to your Evolve website (https://evolve.elsevier.com/Clayton) for additional online resources.

Review Questions for the NCLEX® Examination

1. When is the nurse supposed to use the evaluation step of the nursing process?
   1. Upon admission
   2. When the patient is ready for discharge
   3. After each intervention
   4. During the review of patient education
2. Arrange the components of the nursing process in the proper order.
   1. Implementation
   2. Assessment
   3. Diagnosis
   4. Evaluation
   5. Planning

3. The nurse applies the nursing process by gathering patient information to assess the patient using which of the following methods? (*Select all that apply.*)
   1. Body systems assessment
   2. Head-to-toe assessment
   3. Critical pathway
   4. Evidence-based practice
   5. Gordon's Functional Health Patterns Model
4. A patient develops edema as an adverse effect to a prescribed medication. A gain of 5 pounds has occurred in 24 hours, and 2+ edema is present in the legs. Which nursing diagnosis statement does the nurse allocate to this patient?
   1. Excess fluid volume related to calcium ion antagonist therapy (nifedipine), as evidenced by dependent edema (2+) and weight gain of 5 pounds in 24 hours.
   2. Excess fluid volume related to medication therapy, manifested by 5-pound weight gain and leg edema.
   3. Excess fluid volume related to adverse effects of medications, as evidenced by unknown etiology.
   4. Risk for fluid volume imbalance related to adverse effects of medications.
5. The nurse understands it is important to know the difference between a nursing diagnosis and a medical diagnosis because of which factor?
   1. The nursing diagnosis does not have any bearing on the medical diagnosis.
   2. The medical diagnosis must agree with the nursing diagnosis.
   3. The nursing diagnosis refers to how the patient is responding to an illness identified in the medical diagnosis.
   4. The medical diagnosis refers to how the patient is recovering from the illness that the nursing diagnosis has established.
6. The use of evidence-based practice to guide the formulation of nursing interventions based on research and clinical expertise is part of which component of the nursing process?
   1. Assessment
   2. Nursing diagnosis
   3. Planning
   4. Evaluation

7. What is the difference between nursing interventions and expected outcome statements?
   1. Nursing interventions are action statements, and expected outcome statements are used to identify problems.
   2. Expected outcome statements are action statements, and nursing interventions are what will be observed in the patient after specific actions.
   3. Nursing interventions are action statements, and expected outcome statements are what should be observed in the patient after specific actions.
   4. Expected outcome statements are action statements, and nursing interventions are prioritized goals.

8. When the nurse decides that the patient needs to rest before ambulating, the decision is based on what factor?
   1. The patient's wishes
   2. The family's influences
   3. The prioritization of physiologic needs
   4. The healthcare provider's orders

9. Which is an example of an independent nursing action? (Select all that apply.)
   1. Maintaining and modifying the medication orders
   2. Collaborating with qualified professionals about medication calculations
   3. Educating a patient on correct coughing and deep-breathing exercises
   4. Obtaining the patient's medication history
   5. Documenting assessments of a patient's lung sounds

10. Which type of nursing diagnosis involves the potential for a complication of drug therapy?
    1. Actual
    2. Risk/high risk
    3. Health promotion and/or wellness
    4. Syndrome

Objectives

1. Differentiate among the cognitive, affective, and psychomotor learning domains.
2. Identify the main principles of learning that are applied when teaching a patient, family, or group.
3. Describe the essential elements of patient education in relation to prescribed medications.
4. Describe the nurse's role in fostering patient responsibility for maintaining well-being and for adhering to the therapeutic regimen.
5. Identify the types of information that should be discussed with the patient or significant others.
6. Discuss specific techniques used in the practice setting to facilitate patient education.

Key Terms

cognitive domain (KŎG-nĭ-tĭv dō-MĀN) (p. 50)
affective domain (ă-FĔK-tĭv) (p. 50)
psychomotor domain (sī-kō-MŌ-tŏr) (p. 51)
objectives (ŏb-JĔK-tĭvz) (p. 51)

teach-back (p. 52)
health teaching (p. 52)
ethnocentrism (ĕth-nō-SĔN-trĭz-ŭm) (p. 55)

An important nursing responsibility is making certain that patients receive correct healthcare information. Because patient education is a key component of what nurses do, understanding the principles of how people learn is important. Nurses need to learn how to instruct patients correctly, making information specific to the individual, and also determine whether the information is understood by the patient.

THREE DOMAINS OF LEARNING

The three domains of learning that all adults use when acquiring new knowledge are the cognitive domain, the affective domain, and the psychomotor domain (Fig. 5.1).

COGNITIVE DOMAIN

The cognitive domain is the level at which basic knowledge is learned and stored. It is the thinking portion of the learning process, and it incorporates a person's previous experiences and perceptions. Previous experiences with health and wellness influence the learning of new materials. Prior knowledge and experience are the foundation of the addition of new concepts. Thus the learning process begins by identifying what experiences the person has had with the subject.

However, learning involves more than the delivery of new information or concepts. A person must build relationships between prior experiences and new concepts to formulate new meanings. At a higher level of the learning process, the new information is used to

question something that is uncertain, to recognize when to seek additional information, and to make decisions using real-life situations.

AFFECTIVE DOMAIN

The affective domain is the most intangible portion of the learning process. It refers to the feelings and beliefs a patient has about what he or she understands. The affective domain includes opinions and values that the patient brings to his or her understanding of the world. When a patient says, "I don't know what meds I'm on, I let my wife deal with that," he is expressing the value that learning about medications is not important to him.

It is well known that individuals view events from different perspectives. People often choose to internalize feelings rather than to express them. The nurse must be willing to approach patients in a nonjudgmental fashion, to listen to their concerns, to recognize the nonverbal messages being given, and to assess patient needs with an open mind.

 Clinical Goldmine

The development of a sense of trust and confidence in healthcare providers can have a powerful effect on the attitude of the patient and his or her family members. This can influence the patient's response to the new information that is being taught. The nurse should be positive and accepting, and involve the patient in a discussion to draw out his or her views regarding solutions to problems.

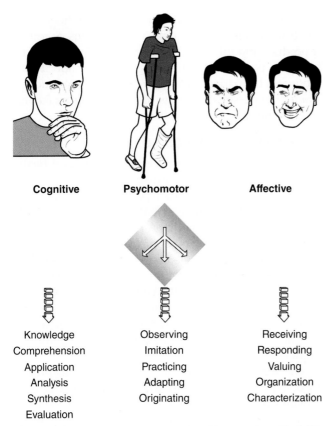

Cognitive   Psychomotor   Affective

Knowledge	Observing	Receiving
Comprehension	Imitation	Responding
Application	Practicing	Valuing
Analysis	Adapting	Organization
Synthesis	Originating	Characterization
Evaluation		

Fig. 5.1 **The Three Domains of Learning.** (Redrawn from Black BP. *Professional Nursing.* 7th ed. Philadelphia, PA: Saunders; 2014, and Washington CM, Leaver DT. *Principles and Practice of Radiation Therapy.* 4th ed. St. Louis, MO: Mosby; 2016.)

PSYCHOMOTOR DOMAIN

The **psychomotor domain** involves the learning of a new procedure or skill. It is often referred to as the *doing domain*. Teaching is usually done by demonstration of the procedure or task using a step-by-step approach. For example, the nurse can explain how to use an incentive spirometer and the patient will demonstrate his or her learning by doing it correctly.

PRINCIPLES OF TEACHING AND LEARNING

Patient education is an important nursing responsibility that carries legal implications if there is a failure to provide and document all relevant patient education. Providing information to patients so that they can understand and manage healthcare-related situations is now considered a basic patient right, and it has been mandated by The Joint Commission since 1996. Patient education involves establishing goals with the patient and family based on the healthcare needs of the patient so the patient can learn to manage his or her care at home. Principles of teaching and learning are important to keep in mind when teaching patients (Box 5.1).

Box 5.1   **Principles of Teaching and Learning**

- Focus the learning.
- Consider learning styles.
- Organize teaching sessions and materials.
- Motivate the patient to learn.
- Determine the patient's readiness to learn.
- Space the content.
- Use repetition to enhance learning.
- Consider the patient's education level.
- Incorporate cultural and ethnic diversity.
- Teach appropriate use of the Internet.
- Encourage adherence.
- Use relevant content.
- Communicate goals and expectations.

FOCUS THE LEARNING

The patient must be allowed to focus on the material or task to be learned. The environment must be conducive to learning (i.e., quiet, well lit, and equipped for a teaching session). The patient requires repetition of new information to master it. Nurses may feel obligated to teach the patient or family members everything that they know about a disease or procedure, thereby overwhelming them with information. Instead, nurses must first glean what information is essential and then consider what the patient wants to know.

When the patient starts to ask questions about any medications or procedures, this is considered a teachable moment, and it is important to recognize it as such. By beginning with what the patient brings up, the nurse is able to give the patient some control over learning and increase active participation in the process.

CONSIDER LEARNING STYLES

Learning styles vary. Some people can read and readily comprehend directions, whereas others need to see, feel, hear, touch, and think to master a task. To be effective, the nurse must fit the teaching techniques to the learner's style. Therefore a variety of materials should be made available for healthcare education, which will include all domains of learning. The nurse can select the instructional approach to be used from written materials such as pamphlets, photographs, and charts for the cognitive domain. The use of video recordings, models, and computers by the nurse to teach a task or procedure, and evaluation of a return demonstration by the patient, can correspond to the psychomotor domain.

ORGANIZE TEACHING SESSIONS AND MATERIALS

In most clinical settings, patient education materials are developed by the staff and then reviewed by a committee for adoption. Specific objectives should be formulated for patient education sessions. The **objectives** should state the purpose of the activities and the expected outcomes. Objectives may be developed in conjunction with a nursing diagnosis statement (e.g., Imbalanced nutrition: Less than body requirements), or they can be developed for common conditions that require care delivery (e.g., care of the patient who is receiving chemotherapy). Regardless of the format used, these instructional materials have established content that is given in outline form, and they are arranged so that one nurse can initiate the teaching and document the degree of understanding, and then another nurse can continue the teaching during a different shift or on a different day. The first nurse should check off what has been accomplished so that the next nurse knows where to resume the lesson.

At the start of each subsequent teaching session, it is important to review what has been covered previously and to affirm the retention of information from the previous lessons. The method known as **teach-back** refers to asking the patient to explain in his or her own words what instruction was just received. This is an important part of patient education that will identify gaps in learning and help focus the nurse on what needs to be instructed. When psychomotor skills are being taught, return demonstrations by the patient are key to helping the patient practice and gain confidence in performing the task. Giving the patient immediate feedback about the skills and then giving him or her time to practice the skills that are more difficult allows the patient time to improve on mastering the procedure. If appropriate, equipment may be left with the patient for practice before the next session.

Sometimes it is particularly useful to set up a video of skill demonstrations for the patient to view alone at a convenient time. At the next meeting, the patient can review the video together with the nurse, and important points can be discussed and clarified if the patient expresses confusion or uncertainty. This technique reinforces what has been said, reviews what has been learned, and provides the learner with repetition, which is necessary for learning.

MOTIVATE THE PATIENT TO LEARN

Before initiating a teaching plan, the nurse should be certain that the patient can focus and concentrate on the tasks and materials to be learned. The patient's basic needs (e.g., food, oxygen, pain relief) must be met before he or she can focus on learning. The nurse must recognize the individual's health beliefs when trying to motivate the patient. Because **health teaching** requires the integration of the patient's beliefs, attitudes, values, opinions, and needs, an individualized teaching plan must be developed based on the patient's beliefs and needs (Box 5.2).

Teaching does not require a formal setting. Some of the most effective teaching can be done while care is being delivered. The patient can be exposed to a skill, a treatment, or facts that must be comprehended in small increments. The nurse who explains a certain procedure and informs the patient why the procedure is being performed reinforces the need for it and motivates the patient to learn. When the patient understands the personal benefits of performing a task, his or her willingness to do it is strengthened.

DETERMINE READINESS TO LEARN

A patient's perception of his or her health and health status may differ from the nurse's judgment; therefore the values of healthcare to each patient may differ greatly. The patient may not realize that a healthy lifestyle will provide significant benefits. A person who commonly indulges in alcohol, smoking, or a high-fat diet and leads a sedentary lifestyle may not consider the consequences of these practices in relation to health. Not everyone is interested in the concept of healthy living. The nurse must respect the individuality of the patient, family, or group being treated; he or she should accept that not everyone is motivated by the possibility of a higher level of wellness.

The nurse can positively influence the learning process by being enthusiastic about the content to be taught. A patient's response to the new information will vary and depends on several factors, including the following: the need to know, the patient's life experiences and self-concept, the effect of the illness on the patient's lifestyle, the patient's experience with learning new materials, and the patient's readiness to learn. Consideration must be given to the patient's psychosocial adaptation to illness and his or her ability to focus on learning. For example, during the denial, anger, or bargaining stages of grieving, the patient usually is neither prepared nor willing to accept the limitations imposed by the disease process. During the resolution and acceptance stages of the grieving process, the patient moves toward accepting responsibility and develops a willingness to learn what is necessary to attain an optimal level of health. The nurse can use encouragement and support the patient's attempts to learn new, challenging, or difficult procedures (Fig. 5.2).

For teaching activities that are conducted with children, psychosocial, cognitive, and language abilities must be considered. Cognitive and motor development, as well as the patient's language usage and understanding, must be assessed. Age definitely influences the types and amounts of self-care activities that the child is capable of learning. The nurse should consult a text that addresses developmental theory for further information.

Adult education is usually oriented toward learning what is necessary to maintain a particular lifestyle. In general, adults need to understand why they must learn something before they undertake the effort to learn it. When planning the educational needs of the patient, the nurse must assess what the patient already knows and what additional information is desired.

Box 5.2   **Sample Teaching Plan for a Patient With Diabetes Mellitus Taking One Type of Insulin[a]**

UNDERSTANDING OF HEALTH CONDITION
- Assess the patient's and the family's understanding of diabetes mellitus.
- Clarify the meaning of the disease in terms that the patient is able to understand.
- Establish learning goals through mutual discussion. Teach the most important information first. Set dates for the teaching of content after discussion with the patient.

FOOD AND FLUIDS
- Arrange for the patient and his or her family members and significant others to attend nutrition lectures and demonstrations about food preparation.
- Reinforce knowledge of exchange lists (or other dietary methods) with the use of tactful questioning and by giving the patient a chance to practice food selections for daily meals from the menus provided.
- Explain how to manage the diabetic diet during illness (e.g., with nausea and vomiting, patient should increase fluid intake) and when to contact the healthcare provider.
- Stress the interrelationship of food with the onset, peak, and duration of the prescribed insulin.

MONITORING TESTS
- Demonstrate how to collect and test blood glucose samples and, as appropriate, urine.
- Validate understanding by having the patient collect, test, and record the results of the testing for the remainder of the hospitalization.
- Stress serum glucose testing before meals and at bedtime.
- Explain the importance of regular follow-up laboratory studies (e.g., fasting plasma glucose testing, postprandial hemoglobin A_{1c}) to monitor the patient's degree of control.

MEDICATIONS AND TREATMENTS
- Teach the name, dosage, route of administration, desired action, and storage and refilling procedures for the type of insulin prescribed.
- Explain the principles of insulin action, onset, peak, and duration (see Chapter 35).
- Demonstrate how to prepare and administer the prescribed dose of insulin.
- Teach site location and self-administration of insulin.
- Give specific instructions that address the reading of the syringe to be used at home.
- Teach the patient how to obtain supplies (e.g., disposable syringes, needles, glucometer, glucose monitoring strips, insulin pen).
- Discuss the usual timing of reactions, the signs and symptoms of hypoglycemia or hyperglycemia, and the management of each complication.
- Validate the patient's understanding of common adverse effects and serious adverse effects.
- Teach and validate family members' and significant others' understanding of the signs and symptoms of hypoglycemia and hyperglycemia and the management of each complication.

- Teach a general approach to the management of illnesses (e.g., the actions required if nausea and vomiting or fever occur; stress glucose monitoring before meals and at bedtime); discuss the situations when there is a need to call a healthcare provider.

PERSONAL HYGIENE
- Discuss the great importance of managing personal hygiene, and emphasize the need to consult a healthcare provider for guidance and discussion:
  - Regular foot care
  - Meticulous oral hygiene and dental care
  - Care of cuts, scratches, and minor and major injuries
  - Stress management and needed alterations in insulin dosage during an illness

ACTIVITIES
- Help the patient develop a detailed time schedule for usual activities of daily living. Incorporate diabetic care needs into this schedule.
- Encourage maintaining all usual activities of daily living. Discuss anticipated problems and possible interventions.
- Discuss personal care needs not only at home but also in the work setting, as appropriate. (Consider involving the industrial nurse, if available, in the work setting.)
- Discuss the effects of an increase or decrease in activity level on the management of diabetes mellitus.

HOME OR FOLLOW-UP CARE
- Arrange for outpatient or healthcare provider follow-up appointments and schedule ordered laboratory tests.
- Advise the patient to seek assistance from the healthcare provider or from the nearest emergency department service for problems that may develop.
- Arrange appropriate referrals to community health agencies, if needed.
- Complete a diabetic alert card or another means (e.g., an identification necklace or bracelet) of alerting people to the individual's needs in case of an emergency.
- Discuss an exercise program with the healthcare provider.

SPECIAL EQUIPMENT AND INSTRUCTIONAL MATERIAL
- Develop a list of equipment and supplies to be purchased; have a family member purchase and bring these to the hospital for use during teaching sessions (e.g., blood glucose monitoring supplies, syringes, insulin pen, needles, alcohol wipes).
- Show audiovisual materials that address insulin preparation, storage, and administration, as well as serum glucose testing.
- Develop a written record (see Chapter 35), and assist the patient with maintaining data during hospitalization.

OTHER
- Teach measures to make travel easier.
- Tell the patient about the American Diabetes Association and about the materials available from this resource.

[a]Each item listed must be assessed for the individual's current knowledge base and level of understanding throughout the course of teaching. The process is reassessed and the teaching continued until the patient masters all facets of self-care needs. With the advent of shorter hospitalizations, inpatient and outpatient teaching may be necessary, and it may include referral to community-based healthcare agencies, as needed. Discharge charting and referral should carefully document those facets of the teaching plan that have been mastered and those that need to be taught. The healthcare provider should be notified of deficits in the patient's learning ability or in his or her mastery of needed elements in the teaching plan.

Life Span Considerations
Older Adults

Teaching Older Adults

The older adult needs to be further assessed before the implementation of healthcare teaching; these assessments should include vision, hearing, and short- and long-term memory. If a task is to be taught, fine and gross motor abilities need to be evaluated as well. An older patient may also have major concerns regarding the cost of the proposed treatments in relation to available resources. A patient will often evaluate the benefits of planned medical interventions and their overall effect on the quality of life. Any of these situations can affect the ability of the patient to focus on the new information to be taught, thus influencing his or her response to and the overall outcome of the teaching. Older adults have often experienced losses and may be facing social isolation, physical (functional) losses, and financial constraints. Because older adults often have more chronic health problems, a new diagnosis, an exacerbation of a disease, or a new crisis may be physically and emotionally overwhelming. Therefore the timing of patient instruction is of great significance.

When teaching an older patient, it is prudent to slow the pace of the presentation and to limit the length of each session to prevent overtiring. Older adults can learn the material, but they often process things more slowly than younger people do because their short-term memory may be more limited. The nurse must work with the patient to develop ways to remember what is being taught. The more that the older person is involved in forming the associations that will be used to remember new ideas and to connect these ideas with past experiences, the better the outcome.

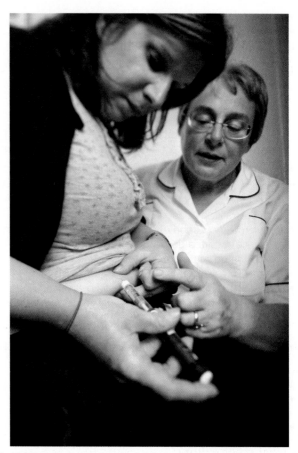

Fig. 5.2 A patient does a return demonstration of an insulin injection after being taught by the nurse. (Courtesy Jim Varney, North Yorkshire, UK.)

Many patients are embarrassed by their inability to master a task. Asking them if they understand is not going to be effective because they will not admit their embarrassment or that they do not understand. The nurse should provide information in small increments and allow for practice, review, practice, review, and practice until success is achieved. The nurse can stop at appropriate intervals and reschedule sessions to meet the patient's learning needs. *Teach-back* can be used as an important tool to help the nurse verify what information has been understood.

When the patient becomes anxious, the presentation of new information can be slowed, repeated, or stopped and the session rescheduled. Fear and anxiety often impair a person's ability to focus on the task or content being presented, so creating an environment that is conducive to learning is important.

When anxiety is high, the ability to focus on details is reduced. The nurse should anticipate periods during hospitalization when teaching can be more effective. Some teaching is most successful when it is done spontaneously, such as when the patient asks direct questions about his or her progress toward discharge. The nurse also must learn to anticipate inopportune times to initiate teaching, such as when a patient becomes withdrawn after learning about a diagnosis with a poor prognosis. With reduced hospital stays, the ability to time patient education ideally and to perform actual teaching is a challenge. It is imperative that the nurse document those aspects of healthcare teaching that have been mastered and—of equal importance—those that have not been; he or she must then request referral to an appropriate agency for follow-up teaching and assistance.

 Clinical Goldmine

Consider the lighting so that there is no glare on reading materials, face the learner for better eye contact, and speak directly and in a clear tone, without shouting. Be calm, use tact and diplomacy if frustrations develop, and try to instill confidence in the learner's ability to surmount any problems.

SPACE THE CONTENT

Spacing or staggering the amount of material given during one session should be considered, regardless of the age of the person being taught. People tend to remember what is learned first. With this principle in mind, the nurse can provide multiple short sessions rather than a few longer sessions that may overwhelm the patient.

USE REPETITION TO ENHANCE LEARNING

It is important for the nurse to recognize that patients need repetition to learn new content. The nurse needs to repeat what was previously taught to help the patient understand what is important to remember and build on it to the next level.

CONSIDER EDUCATION LEVEL

An important consideration to keep in mind when teaching adult patients is their literacy level. Just giving the patient a pamphlet to read may not be appropriate if the patient cannot read it. Instead, the nurse could review the pamphlet with the patient and then determine the level of the patient's understanding of the information.

Medical terms may not be understood, and written instructions left at the bedside may be misinterpreted or not read at all. Some patients may be illiterate, whereas others may read at a first-grade, seventh-grade, or collegiate level. Therefore if written materials are used, it is important to consider these wide variations in literacy.

INCORPORATE CULTURAL AND ETHNIC DIVERSITY

Many healthcare providers have a limited understanding of what other cultures believe and the importance of these benefits to the learning process. **Ethnocentrism** is the assumption that one's culture provides the right way, the best way, and the only way to live. Briefly, people who believe in the theory of ethnocentrism assume that their way of viewing the world is superior to that of others (Leininger, 2002). As an understanding of cultural diversity increases, healthcare providers must expand their knowledge of the basic tenets of the belief systems that they may encounter among their patients.

Because there are differing beliefs, it is important that the nurse explore the meaning of an illness with the patient. Members of other cultures do not always express themselves when their views are in conflict with those of another culture. Unless a careful assessment of psychosocial needs is performed, the true meaning of an illness or the proposed intervention may never be uncovered. Even the assessment process has obstacles attached. Patients in some cultures do not believe that family information should be shared outside of the family. For example, some Eastern European cultures prefer not to reveal any history of psychiatric illness or treatment and are usually reluctant to share any sexual history. Others, such as the Native American culture, believe that only the affected individual may reveal information.

Communication is vitally important within any cultural group. However, verbal and nonverbal types of communication mean different things to different cultures. For example, whites tend to value eye contact, whereas in other cultures (e.g., Native Americans, Asians) direct eye contact is a sign of disrespect or rudeness. As a part of communication, knowing how to address the patient is also important. African American patients often prefer to have their formal names used rather than their first names, especially older family members. Chinese people tend to be more formal than Americans, and husbands and wives do not necessarily have the same last name. The simple gesture of asking the patient how he or she prefers to be addressed is both helpful and respectful.

Working with an interpreter when a language barrier exists presents several additional challenges to understanding. The nurse should first explain the educational session to the interpreter and then discuss the types of questions that will be asked of the patient. Whenever a third person enters into the communication cycle, a lack of clarity and misinterpretation can occur. The nurse should keep questions brief and ask them one at a time to give the interpreter an opportunity to rephrase the question and obtain a response. Sometimes supplementing questions with pictures and pantomime gestures may be helpful. When using an interpreter, the nurse should look directly at the patient (not at the interpreter) while conversing.

The members of the healthcare team should always try to ascertain the patient's beliefs about illness. The following should be taken into consideration:

- Is "good health" defined as the ability to work or to fulfill family roles, or is it a reward from God or a balance with nature?
- Does the patient believe that healthcare can improve health outcomes, or does fate determine the outcome?
- Are any cultural or religious disease prevention approaches used in the household?
- Do family members wear talismans or charms for protection against illness?
- Are cultural healers important (e.g., Chinese herbalists, Native American medicine men)?

As part of the *cultural assessment*, the nurse should determine factors that relate to the cultural beliefs of the family. Inquire as to whether other family members should be included in the discussion of the patient's medical care. Be sure to include the decision makers in the teaching session so that the teaching will not be wasted. Always remain sensitive to the patient's and family's cultural beliefs and practices. Nurses can demonstrate understanding, empathy, respect, and patience for the patient's cultural values through their communication and actual delivery of healthcare. Consult assessment textbooks for more extensive coverage of ethnic and cultural issues.

As cultural mixes become more common, educational materials are being adapted to meet a variety of cultural considerations. Unfortunately, this does not solve all of the problems. Interpreting written materials still leaves room for misunderstanding because many people cannot read or do not read at the level of the provided materials.

STRATEGIES FOR HEALTHCARE TEACHING

TEACH APPROPRIATE USE OF THE INTERNET

It has become common for consumers to access the Internet for healthcare inquiries, including medical consultation from an online physician or another healthcare professional about a particular healthcare concern. Consumers can purchase medications online and research healthcare treatments. The convenience of accessing electronic healthcare information is a powerful resource for consumers, and it is one that provides anonymity and that may serve to empower the patient. Valid healthcare information can assist patients with the making of informed healthcare decisions (Table 5.1).

Today, many patients present to the healthcare provider's office with some knowledge of their disease, treatment, and medications. This has altered the nurse's role as a provider of healthcare education to resemble that of a consultant. It is the nurse's role to teach patients to use the Internet effectively, to evaluate websites for validity, and to assist patients with understanding the information that they have accessed. The nurse should also provide patients with the tools to evaluate websites for validity and to tell them about reputable sites that are specific to their healthcare needs. With the abundance of health- and disease-related information on the Internet, the quality of information varies. Therefore it is essential that the nurse maintain an educational partnership with the patient and his or her caregivers.

ENCOURAGE ADHERENCE

Healthcare providers and educators tend to think that a patient should change behaviors and adhere to a new therapeutic regimen simply because the nurse said so. However, patients do have the right to make their own life choices, and they often do. Unfortunately, there is no way to ensure adherence unless the patient recognizes its value.

Success with a healthcare regimen is enhanced when the nurse conveys an enthusiastic attitude, appears positive about the subject matter, and shows confidence in the abilities of the patient to understand the lesson. Reinforcing positive accomplishments fosters successful achievement.

The patient's response to the therapeutic regimen (including medications) and his or her degree of compliance are influenced by several variables, including the following:

- Beliefs about the seriousness of the illness
- Perceptions of the benefits of the proposed treatment plans
- Personal beliefs, values, and attitudes toward health, the provider of the medication, and the healthcare system, including prior experience with the system
- Effects of the proposed changes on personal lifestyle
- Acceptance (or denial) of the illness and its associated problems; other psychological issues, such as anger about the illness, apathy, depression, forgetfulness, and confusion
- High stress or daily stresses, such as dysfunctional families, difficult living situations, poverty, long working hours in a tense environment, and problematic parenting issues
- Comprehension and understanding of the healthcare regimen or frequent changes in the regimen; the inability to read written instructions
- Multiple physicians or healthcare providers prescribing medications
- Costs of treatment in relation to resources and possible difficulty with getting prescriptions filled
- Support of significant others or problems with assistance needed in the home
- Amount of control that the patient experiences with regard to the disease or condition

Table 5.1	Sources of Patient Information
Source	**Description**
Health on the Net Foundation (https://www.hon.ch)	Leading organization that promotes and guides the deployment of useful and reliable online medical and healthcare information and its appropriate and efficient use
Healthcare institution intranet	Data available through an institution-specific intranet Provides an online resource for drug information (e.g., Micromedex) Often includes information about diseases and diagnostic testing Information may be printed by the nurse and used for patient education
Krames Online (https://dhch.kramesonline.com/)	Patients access this site on their own Includes information about diseases, conditions, treatments, procedures, surgeries, and medications, including prescription medications and over-the-counter products
Compendium of Therapeutic Choices (CTC)	Published by the Canadian Pharmacists Association Extensive handbook that describes major diseases and their treatment Discussions of medical conditions are brief Focuses on goals of therapy, management algorithms, and the discussion of nonpharmacologic and pharmacologic therapies

- Side effects of the treatment and the degree of inconvenience, annoyance, or impairment in functioning that they produce
- Degree of positive response achieved
- Physical difficulties that limit access to or use of medication, such as difficulty swallowing tablets, difficulty with opening containers or handling small tablets, or the inability to distinguish colors or identifying markings on different medications
- Concerns about taking drugs and the fear of addiction

Evaluating the ability of a patient to comply with a proposed healthcare regimen is a complex process that involves using established criteria to reach a conclusion. The ultimate goal is to assist patients with achieving the greatest degree of control possible within the context of their beliefs, values, and needs. Healthcare professionals can offer support and encouragement, be complimentary about positive achievements, and encourage an examination of the available options and the benefits of a healthy lifestyle. It is vital to assist patients with exploring options when a problem or complication arises rather than giving up on the treatment because information about alternatives is lacking. Financial considerations may also affect the patient's decisions.

Strategies for Increasing Adherence

The challenge for nursing is to increase the adherence of patients to their healthcare regimen and to minimize hospital readmission and suffering from complications. It is estimated that poor adherence to medical therapy accounts for about $300 billion in unnecessary healthcare expenses each year. One model that has been used to induce behavioral change in patients is called the *Case Management Adherence Guidelines, version 2*. This project, developed by Pfizer and the Case Management Society of America, is a series of tools that are used by case managers (many of whom are nurses) to assess the patient's motivation level and his or her knowledge of prescribed medications and other therapies. It also assesses a patient's social support system. The tools help to identify those who are more at risk for nonadherence so that interventions can be initiated early during the care process. A key principle of this model is that the nurse must recognize that the patient will make the final decisions. The nurse must negotiate with (not dictate to) the patient to implement actions that may result in positive change. This approach gives the nurse and patient ownership of the goals to be achieved.

Another type of research technique used to study adherence is ethnography. When a patient is not meeting expected outcomes, an ethnographer may visit the patient at home to observe how the patient administers his or her healthcare regimen. Observations are made with regard to how and which procedures are accomplished and what errors are being made. Industry has used these methods for many years to help design work flow for production, and it has been discovered that this is also a valuable tool in healthcare for improving patient outcomes. It is important to remember that the patient may not be purposefully nonadherent; rather, the home environment may not be set up to allow the patient to follow care instructions.

USE RELEVANT CONTENT

Nurses tend to think that patients will do what is suggested simply because they have been told that it will be beneficial. In the hospital, the nurse and other healthcare members reinforce the basic therapeutic regimen; at discharge, however, the patient leaves the controlled environment and is free to choose to follow the prescribed treatment or to alter it as deemed appropriate on the basis of personal values and beliefs. For learning to take place, the patient must perceive the information as being relevant. Whenever possible, the nurse should start with simple and attainable goals to build the patient's confidence. It is important to correlate the teaching with the patient's perspective of the illness and his or her ability to control the signs and symptoms or the course of the disease process.

COMMUNICATE GOALS AND EXPECTATIONS OF THERAPY

Before discharge, reasonable responses to the planned therapy should be discussed. The patient should know what signs and symptoms may be altered by the prescribed medications. The precautions necessary when taking a medication must be explained by the nurse and understood by the patient (e.g., to use caution when operating power equipment or a motor vehicle, to avoid direct sunlight, to ensure that follow-up laboratory studies are carried out).

Changes in Expectations

Changes in the patient's expectations should be assessed as therapy progresses and as the patient gains understanding and skill with regard to managing the diagnosis. The expectations of therapy for patients with acute illnesses may vary widely from those of patients with chronic illnesses.

Cooperative Goal Setting

An attitude of shared input into goals and outcomes can encourage the patient to enter into a therapeutic alliance. Therefore the patient should be taught to help monitor the parameters that are used to evaluate therapy. It is imperative that the nurse nurture a cooperative environment that encourages the patient to do the following: (1) keep records of the essential data that are needed to evaluate the prescribed therapy and (2) contact the healthcare provider for advice rather than alter the medication regimen or discontinue the medication entirely. For each major class of drugs in this book, written records (located on Evolve) are provided to help the nurse identify essential data that the patient needs to understand and record. In the event that the patient and his or her family or significant others do not understand all aspects of the continuing therapy prescribed, they may be referred to a community-based agency for help with achieving long-term healthcare requirements.

Discharge Planning and Teaching

A summary statement of the patient's unmet needs must be written and placed in the medical chart. The healthcare provider should be consulted about the possibility of a referral to a community-based agency for continued monitoring or treatment. The nurse's discharge notes must identify the nursing diagnoses that have not been met and the potential collaborative problems that require continued monitoring and intervention. All counseling information should be carefully drafted in a manner that the patient can read and understand.

Get Ready for the NCLEX® Examination!

Key Points

- The three domains of learning are the cognitive, affective, and psychomotor domains.
- The main principles of learning include the patient's attitudes toward learning, readiness to learn, and individual learning style.
- Patient education in relation to medications includes understanding the benefits of the medications, the common adverse effects, and potential drug interactions.
- Nurses play an important role in teaching patients about how they can maintain and improve their own well-being by understanding the intent of the therapies prescribed.
- The types of information discussed with the patient and his or her family include the medications and treatments to be continued after discharge and activities, special equipment, and follow-up care.
- Specific techniques used to facilitate patient education include determining the patient's readiness to learn, repetition of information, motivating the patient, and understanding the patient's culture.

Additional Learning Resources

SG Go to your Study Guide for additional Review Questions for the NCLEX® Examination, Critical Thinking Clinical Situations, and other learning activities to help you master this chapter content.

Go to your Evolve website (https://evolve.elsevier.com/Clayton) for additional online resources.

Review Questions for the NCLEX® Examination

1. Which statement is an example of an objective of healthcare teaching that involves the cognitive domain of learning?
   1. The patient will demonstrate the correct way to use a peak flowmeter.
   2. The patient will verbalize an understanding of the potential side effects of digoxin.
   3. The patient will correctly place medications in the proper box when filling the drug box.
   4. The patient will discuss with his or her family how the treatment proposal will affect their lives.

2. The nurse is developing a teaching plan for a patient who will have limited activity at home after a recent fall. What principle of learning is involved when teaching this patient?
   1. The timing of the teaching is important for learning to take place.
   2. Teaching is effective when all family members are present.
   3. The affective domain is particularly useful when dealing with the grieving process.
   4. Financial considerations are not part of the issues involved in patient teaching.

3. The nurse was reviewing the discharge medication list with a patient who recently had been hospitalized for heart failure. The patient stated that the medications were not new and that everything was fine. What would be an appropriate response by the nurse?
   1. "Your medications are important to understand so that you will not have to come back to the hospital frequently."
   2. "The doctor wants you to remember all of your medications so when you go back to the clinic you will know the list."
   3. "Your medication list is not as important as remembering to take your doses every day."
   4. "I have to tell you all these medications before you can go home."

4. Which patient is most ready to begin a patient teaching session?
   1. A patient who has had nausea and vomiting for the past 24 hours
   2. A patient who has just been told that he needs to have major surgery
   3. A patient who has voiced a concern about how insulin injections will affect her lifestyle
   4. A patient who is complaining bitterly about a low-fat, low-cholesterol diet after his heart attack

5. Which of the following information about medications is important to teach patients? (Select all that apply.)
   1. The name, dosage, and route of administration of the medication
   2. The laboratory studies that need to be monitored while on the medication
   3. The common adverse effects and possible serious adverse effects to watch for
   4. The correct pharmacy to obtain the medication from
   5. The correct schedule or timing of the medication to follow

6. The patient presents with educational information about medication that has been obtained from the Internet. What does the role of the nurse as consultant include? *(Select all that apply.)*
   1. Evaluating websites for validity
   2. Assisting the patient with purchasing medications online
   3. Assisting the patient with understanding the information accessed
   4. Providing the patient with tools to evaluate websites for validity
   5. Encouraging the use of one search engine

7. Which statement is an example of an objective of healthcare teaching that involves the affective domain of learning?
   1. The patient will verbalize an understanding of the reason for taking the medication furosemide.
   2. The patient will demonstrate the correct way to use the metered-dose inhaler.
   3. The patient will discuss with the family the treatment options proposed.
   4. The patient will teach the nurse the same content just learned in the session.

6

Principles of Medication Administration and Medication Safety

https://evolve.elsevier.com/Clayton

Objectives

1. Identify the legal and ethical considerations for medication administration.
2. Compare and contrast the various systems used to dispense medications.
3. Identify what a narcotic control system entails.
4. Define the four categories of medication orders.
5. Identify common types of medication errors and actions that can be taken to prevent them.
6. Identify precautions used to ensure the right drug is prepared and given to the right patient.
7. List the seven rights of drug administration.
8. Identify the appropriate nursing documentation of medications, including the effectiveness of each medication.

Key Terms

nurse practice act (p. 61)
standards of care (p. 61)
summary section (SŬM-ă-rē SHĒT) (p. 62)
consent section (kŏn-SĔNT) (p. 62)
order section (ŌR-dŭr) (p. 62)
history and physical examination section (HĬS-tō-rē and FĬZ-ĭ-kŭl ĕgz-ăm-ĭ-NĀ-shŭn) (p. 62)
progress notes (PRŎ-grĕs) (p. 62)
nurses' notes (p. 62)
laboratory tests record (LĂB-ōr-ă-tōr-ē) (p. 62)
graphic record (GRĂ-fĭk) (p. 62)
flow sheets (FLŌ SHĒTS) (p. 63)
consultation reports (kŏn-sŭl-TĀ-shŭn) (p. 63)
medication profile (PRŌ-fīl) (p. 63)
medication administration record (MAR) (p. 64)
PRN (p. 64)
patient education record (PĀ-shĕnt ĕd-jū-KĀ-shŭn) (p. 64)
nursing care plan (p. 65)
Kardex (KĂR-dĕks) (p. 66)
floor or ward stock system (FLŌR or WŌRD STŎK SĬS-tĕm) (p. 68)
individual prescription order system (ĭn-dĭ-VĬD-jū-ăl prē-SKRĬP-shŭn) (p. 68)
unit-dose drug distribution systems (YŪ-nĭt DŌS DRŬG dĭs-trĭ-BYŪ-shŭn) (p. 69)

computer-controlled dispensing system (kŏm-PYŪ-tŭr kŏn-TRŌLD dĭ-SPĔN-sĭng) (p. 69)
bar codes (BĂR KŌDZ) (p. 70)
long-term care unit-dose system (p. 70)
narcotic control systems (năr-KŎ-tĭk kŏn-TRŌL) (p. 71)
disposal of unused medicines (dĭs-PŌ-zŭl of ŭn-YŪZD MĔD-ĭ-sĕnz) (p. 72)
stat order (STĂT ŌR-dŭr) (p. 73)
single order (SĬN-gŭl) (p. 73)
standing order (STĂN-dĭng) (p. 73)
PRN order (p. 73)
computerized provider order entry (CPOE) systems (p. 74)
medication safety (p. 74)
medication errors (ĀR-ŭrz) (p. 74)
adverse drug events (p. 74)
high-alert medications (HĪ-ă-LŬRT) (p. 74)
medication reconciliation (rĕ-kŏn-sĭl-ē-Ă-shĕn) (p. 75)
handoffs (HĂND-ŏfs) (p. 75)
verification (vĕr-ĭ-fĭ-KĀ-shĕn) (p. 75)
transcription (trăn-SKRĬP-shĕn) (p. 76)
variance (VĂR-ē-ăns) (p. 76)

Before medications are administered, the nurse must understand the professional responsibilities associated with medication administration, drug orders, medication delivery systems, and the nursing process as it relates to drug therapy. Ignorance of the nurse's overall responsibilities as part of the system may result in delays in the receiving and administering of medications and serious administration errors. In either case, care is compromised, and the patient may suffer unnecessarily.

LEGAL AND ETHICAL CONSIDERATIONS

The practice of nursing under a professional license is a privilege, not a right. When accepting this privilege, the nurse must understand that this responsibility includes accountability for one's actions and judgments during the execution of professional duties. An understanding of the **nurse practice act** and the rules and regulations established by the state boards of nursing for the various levels of entry (i.e., practical nurse, registered nurse, and nurse practitioner) is a solid foundation for beginning practice. Many state boards have developed specific guidelines for nurses to use when practicing nursing.

STANDARDS OF CARE

Standards of care are guidelines that have been developed for the practice of nursing. These guidelines are defined by the nurse practice act of each state, by state and federal laws that regulate healthcare facilities, by The Joint Commission, and by professional organizations such as the American Nurses Association and other specialty nursing organizations (e.g., the Infusion Nurses Society). Nurses must also be familiar with the established policies of the employing healthcare agency. Policies developed by the healthcare agency must adhere to the minimum standards of state regulatory authorities; however, agency policies may be more stringent than those that are recognized by the state. Employment by the agency implies the willingness of the nurse to adhere to established standards and to work within established guidelines. Examples of policy statements that are related to medication administration include the following:

1. *Educational requirements for professionals who are authorized to administer medications.* Many healthcare facilities require the passing of a written test to confirm the knowledge and skills needed for medication calculation, preparation, and administration before granting approval to an individual to administer any medications.
2. *Approved lists of intravenous solutions and medications that the nurse can start or add to an existing infusion.*
3. *Lists of restricted medications (e.g., antineoplastic agents, magnesium sulfate, allergy extracts, RhoGAM [Rh$_o$(D) immune globulin (human)], heparin) that may be administered only by certain staff members with specific credentials or training.*
4. *Lists of abbreviations that are not to be used in documentation to avoid medication errors* (see the page facing the inside back cover of this book).

Before administering any medication, the nurse must have a current license to practice, a clear policy statement that authorizes the act, and a medication order signed by a practitioner who is licensed with prescriptive privileges at that institution. The nurse must understand the individual patient's diagnosis and symptoms that correlate with the rationale for drug use. The nurse should also know why a particular medication is ordered and its expected actions, usual dosing, proper dilution, route and rate of administration, adverse effects, and the contraindications for its use. If drugs are to be administered with the use of the same syringe or at the same intravenous (IV) site, drug compatibility should be confirmed before administration. If the nurse is unsure about any of these key medication points, then he or she must consult an authoritative resource or the hospital pharmacist before administering a medication. The nurse must be accurate when calculating, preparing, and administering medications. The nurse must assess the patient to be certain that therapeutic and adverse effects associated with the medication regimen are reported. Nurses must be able to collect patient data at regularly scheduled intervals and to record observations in the patient's chart when evaluating a treatment's effectiveness. Claiming unfamiliarity with any of these nursing responsibilities when an avoidable complication arises is unacceptable; in fact, it is considered negligence of nursing responsibility.

Nurses must take an active role in educating the patient, the family, and significant others in preparation for the patient's discharge from the healthcare environment. A person's health will improve only to the extent that the patient understands how to care for himself or herself. Specific teaching goals should be developed and implemented. Nursing observations and the patient's progress toward the mastery of skills should be charted to document the patient's degree of understanding.

PATIENT CHARTS

The patient's chart or the electronic medical record is a primary source of information that is necessary for the patient assessment so that the nurse can create and implement plans for patient care. It is also where the nurse provides the documentation of the nursing assessments performed, the observations reported to the physician for further verification, the basic nursing measures implemented (e.g., daily treatments), the patient teaching performed, and the observed responses to therapy.

This record serves as the communication link among all members of the healthcare team regarding the patient's status, the care provided, and the patient's progress. The chart is a legal document that describes the patient's health, lists diagnostic and therapeutic procedures initiated, and describes the patient's response to these measures. The chart must be kept current as long as the patient is in the hospital. After the patient's discharge, this record is maintained according to policies within the institution. The patient record may be used for research to compare responses to selected therapies in a sampling of patients with similar diagnoses.

CONTENTS OF PATIENT CHARTS

Although each healthcare facility uses a slightly different format, the basic patient chart consists of the following elements.

Summary Section

The **summary section** gives the patient's name, address, date of birth, attending physician, gender, marital status, allergies, nearest relative, occupation and employer, insurance carrier and other payment information, religious preference, date and time of admission to the hospital, previous hospital admissions, and admitting problem or diagnosis. The date and time of discharge are added when appropriate.

Consent Section

The admission **consent section** grants permission to the healthcare facility and the healthcare provider to provide treatment. Other types of consent forms are used during the course of a hospitalization, such as an operative procedure permit or consent, an invasive procedure consent, a blood-product consent, and a consent to bill the patient's insurance carrier.

Order Section

All procedures and treatments are ordered by the healthcare provider in the **order section**. These orders include general care (e.g., activity, diet, frequency of recording vital signs), laboratory tests to be completed, other diagnostic procedures (e.g., radiography, electrocardiography, computed tomography), and all medications and treatments (e.g., physical or occupational therapy).

History and Physical Examination Section

During admission to the hospital, the patient is interviewed by a healthcare provider and given a physical examination. The healthcare provider records the findings on the **history and physical examination section** and lists the problems to be corrected (e.g., the diagnoses). The history and physical examination form is often referred to as "the H&P."

Progress Notes

The attending healthcare provider records frequent observations of the patient's health status in the **progress notes**. In most hospitals, other health professionals (e.g., pharmacists, dietitians, physical and respiratory therapists) may record observations and suggestions.

Nurses' Notes

Although the format varies among institutions, the **nurses' notes** generally start with the nursing history. On admission, the nurse performs a complete health assessment of the patient. This process includes a head-to-toe physical assessment, and it also incorporates a patient and family history that provides insights into individual and family needs, life patterns, psychosocial and cultural data, and spiritual needs. This assessment will serve as the basis for the development of the individualized care plan and as a baseline for comparison when ongoing assessment data are gathered.

Nurses record the following in their notes: ongoing assessments of the patient's condition; responses to nursing interventions ordered by the physician (e.g., treatments or medications) or to those initiated by the nurse (e.g., skin care, patient education); evaluations of the effectiveness of nursing interventions; procedures completed by other healthcare professionals (e.g., wound cleaning by a physician, fitting for a prosthesis by a prosthetist); and other pertinent information (e.g., physician or family visits, patient's responses after these visits). Entries may be made on the nurses' notes or flow sheets throughout a shift, but general guidelines include the following: (1) completing records, including vital signs, immediately after assessing the patient, whether when he or she is first admitted or after he or she returns from a diagnostic procedure or therapy; (2) recording all "as needed" (PRN) medications immediately after administration and addressing the effectiveness of the medication; (3) recording change in the patient's status and who was notified (e.g., healthcare provider, manager, patient's family); (4) discussing the treatment of a sudden change in the patient's status; and (5) recording information about the transfer, discharge, or death of a patient. In addition to the accurate charting of the observations in a clear and concise form, the nurse should report significant changes in a patient's status to the charge nurse. The charge nurse then makes a nursing judgment regarding the notification of the attending healthcare provider. Written nurses' notes are quickly being replaced by computerized charting methods that allow the nurse to document findings and basic care delivered using multiple screens of data and checklist-type formats.

Laboratory Tests Record

The **laboratory tests record** has all the laboratory test results in one section of the chart. Hospitals that use computerized reports may list consecutive values of the same test if that test has been repeated several times (e.g., electrolytes). Computerized laboratory data access provides online laboratory results as soon as the tests are completed. Other hospitals may attach small report forms to a full-sized backing sheet as each report returns from the laboratory. Because some medication doses are based on daily blood studies, it is important to be able to locate these data within the patient's chart.

Graphic Record

The **graphic record** (Fig. 6.1A) is an example of the manual recording of temperature, pulse, respiration, and blood pressure. Fig. 6.1B is an electronic database–generated example of the vital signs, fluid intake and output, glucose, dietary intake, and other information to be used for the ongoing assessment of the patient's status.

Pain assessment, which is now considered the fifth vital sign, can also be recorded in a graphic form. In addition to the graphic recording of pain, assessments of pain can be found on other flow sheets in the chart that will record the details of the pain events.

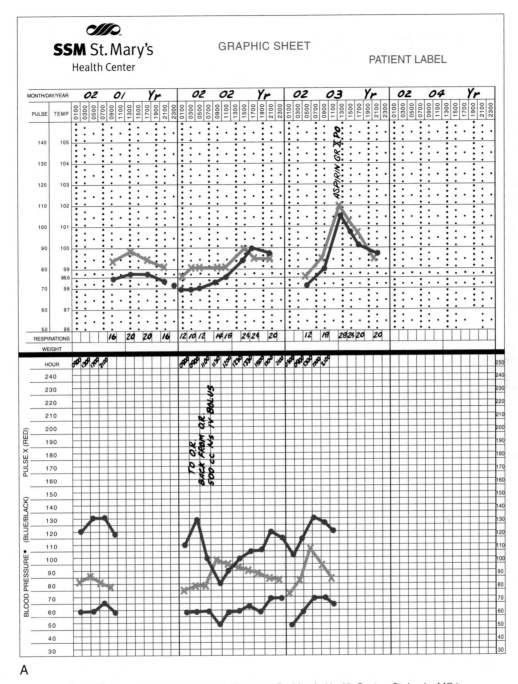

Fig. 6.1A Manual vital signs record. (Courtesy St. Mary's Health Center, St. Louis, MO.)

Flow Sheets

Flow sheets are a condensed form for recording information for the quick comparison of data. Examples of flow sheets in common use are diabetic, pain, and neurologic flow sheets. The graphic record that is used for recording vital signs is another type of flow sheet (see Fig. 6.1A).

Consultation Reports

When other physicians or healthcare professionals are asked to consult about a patient, the specialist's summary of findings, diagnoses, and recommendations for treatment are recorded in the consultation reports section of the chart.

Other Diagnostic Reports

Reports of surgery, electroencephalography, electrocardiography, pulmonary function tests, radioactive scans, and radiography are usually recorded in the other diagnostic reports section of the patient's chart.

Medication Profile and Medication Administration Record

The medication profile, also called the medication worklist when in an electronic format, lists all medications to be administered and is printed from the computerized patient database, thereby ensuring that the pharmacist and the nurse have identical medication

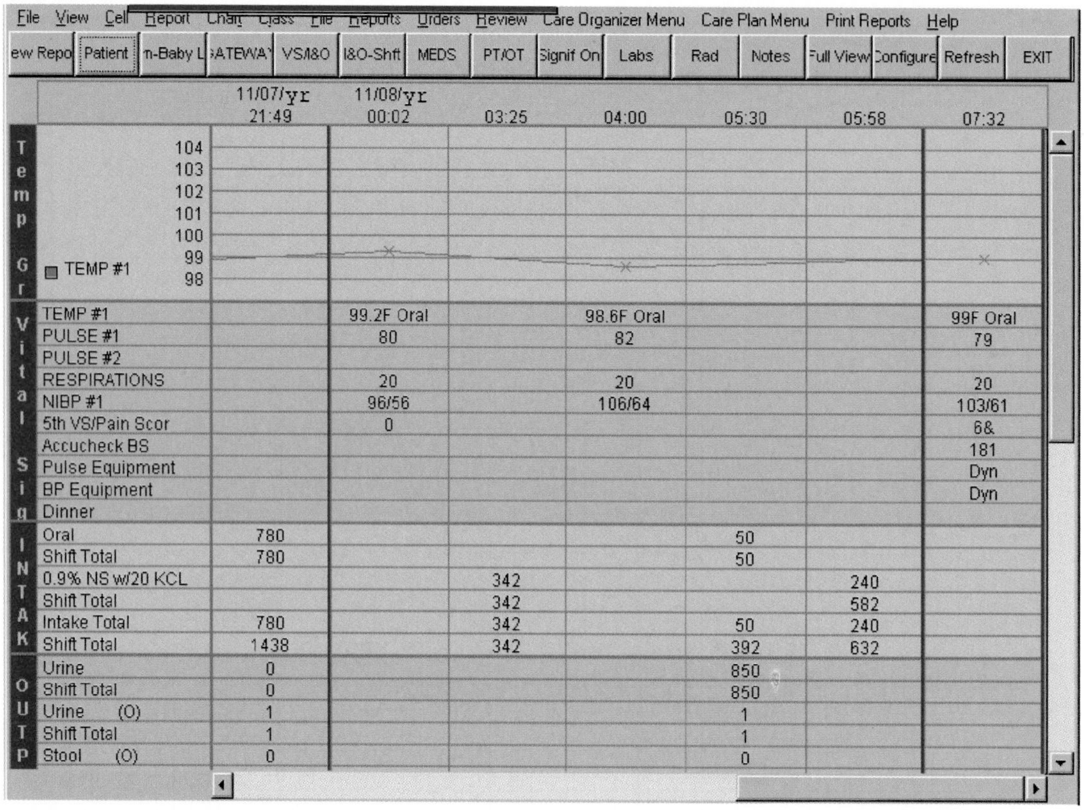

B

Fig. 6.1B Electronic charting of vital signs and intake and output. (Courtesy Creighton University Medical Center, Omaha, NE.)

profiles for the patient. The medications are usually grouped according to the following categories: medications scheduled to be given on a regular basis (e.g., every 6 hours, twice daily), parenteral medications, stat medications (from the Latin *statim*, meaning "immediately"), and preoperative orders. PRN medications (from the Latin *pro re nata*, meaning "as circumstances require") are those medications that are given on an "as needed" basis and are usually listed at the bottom of the profile, or they may be found on a separate page as unscheduled medication orders.

The medication administration record (MAR) is a record of the time that the medication was administered and identifies who gave it (Fig. 6.2A). Generally, the nurse records and initials the time that the medication was given. Medication profiles are kept in a notebook or clipboard file on the medication cart for the 24-hour period that they are in use; they then become a permanent part of the patient's chart. In the acute care setting, a new profile is generated every 24 hours at the same time that the unit-dose cart is refilled. Fig. 6.2B is an example of an electronic database–generated MAR that lists all scheduled medications for an 8-hour shift. By clicking the cursor on the highlighted area (i.e., scheduled regular insulin in this illustration), a window opens to reveal details of the order.

In the long-term care setting the MAR uses the same principles; however, it generally provides a space for medications to be recorded for up to 1 month. The MAR also includes the name of the pharmacy that dispensed the prescribed medications and the assigned prescription number. Medications that are prescribed for residents in the long-term care setting must be reviewed on a scheduled basis; therefore the MAR identifies the reviewer and the date of review.

PRN or Unscheduled Medication Record

PRN medications, or those that are given as needed, may be recorded on a separate medication record rather than the MAR to record the date, the time, the PRN medication administered, the dose, the reason for administering the PRN medication, and the patient's response to the drug given. However, in most clinical settings that involve the use of electronic forms of charting, the PRN medications are recorded on the same MAR.

Patient Education Record

The patient education record provides a means of documenting the health teaching provided to the patient, the family, or significant others, and it includes statements about the patient's mastery of the content presented.

Additional Patient Chart Records

Additional records in a patient's chart may include the following: separate MARs; operative and anesthesiology

MARTINDALE HOMETOWN HOSPITAL

MEDICATION ADMINISTRATION RECORD

NAME:	Joseph Lorenzo	RM-BD: 621-2	Init	Signature	Title
ID NO:	016-28-3978	AGE: 62			
DIAGNOSIS:	Myocardial Infarction SEX: M				
PHYSICIAN:	M. Martin, M.D. Ht: 6' Wt: 200 lb				

DATES:	**SCHEDULED MEDICATIONS** MEDICATION—STRENGTH—FORM—ROUTE	0030-0729	0730-1529	1530-0029
1/25/yr	RANITIDINE ZANTAC 150 MG TABLET ORAL TWICE A DAY		0900	1800
1/25/yr	DILTIAZEM HYDROCHLORIDE CARDIZEM 90 MG TABLET ORAL 4 TIMES DAILY		0900 1300	1800 2100
1/25/yr	WARFARIN SODIUM COUMADIN 1 MG TABLET ORAL EVERY OTHER DAY	NOT GIVEN	TODAY	
	IV AND PIGGYBACK ORDERS			
1/25/yr	CEFTAZIDIME (FORTAZ) 1 G IV SODIUM CHLORIDE 0.9% 50 ML EVERY 8 HOURS INFUSE: 20 MIN	0200	1000	1800
1/25/yr	GENTAMICIN PREMIX 80 MG IV ISO-OSMOTIC SOLN 100 ML BY IV PUMP EVERY 12 HOURS INFUSE: 30 MIN	0200	1400	
1/25/yr	BY IV PUMP 1 IV DSW-5/0.2 NACI 1000 ML RATE: 100 ML/HR			
	PRN MEDICATIONS			
1/25/yr	ACETAMINOPHEN TYLENOL 650 MG (23325) TABLET ORAL EVERY 4 HOURS AS NEEDED PRN			
1/25/yr	MAGNESIUM HYDROXIDE MILK OF MAGNESIA 60 ML (CONC) ORAL CONC AS NEEDED PRN			
1/25/yr	ALBUTEROL PROVENTIL INHALER 90 MCG/INH AEROSOL INH AS NEEDED PRN SEE RESPIRATORY THERAPY NOTES AT BEDSIDE			

Age/Sex HT WT Date	ALLERGIES: CODEINE
62/ M 6'0" 200 lb 1/25/yr	
Room-Bd Name	
621 2 Joseph Lorenzo	

A

Fig. 6.2A Medication profile. Note the separation of scheduled orders, intravenous (IV), and as-needed (PRN) medications. (Courtesy Creighton University Medical Center, Omaha, NE.)

records; recovery room records; physical, occupational, or speech therapy records; inhalation therapy reports; and a diabetic's daily record of insulin dosage and blood glucose (sugar) test results. Each page that is placed in the patient's chart is imprinted with the patient's name, registration number, and unit or room number. Nurses often use data from all of the chart sections to formulate a nursing care plan.

Nursing Care Plans

After the initial data collection, the nurse develops an individualized nursing care plan. Care plans incorporate nursing diagnoses, critical pathway information, and physician-ordered and nursing-ordered care (see Nursing Care Plan). Most acute care facilities require the nurse to chart against each identified nursing diagnosis stated in the care plan every 8 hours. Care plans are evaluated and modified on a continuum throughout the course of treatment. The plan should be shared with the healthcare team to ensure an interdisciplinary approach to care. Many institutions have developed standardized care plans for the various nursing diagnoses. It is the nurse's responsibility to identify those diagnoses, interventions, and outcomes that are appropriate for the patient.

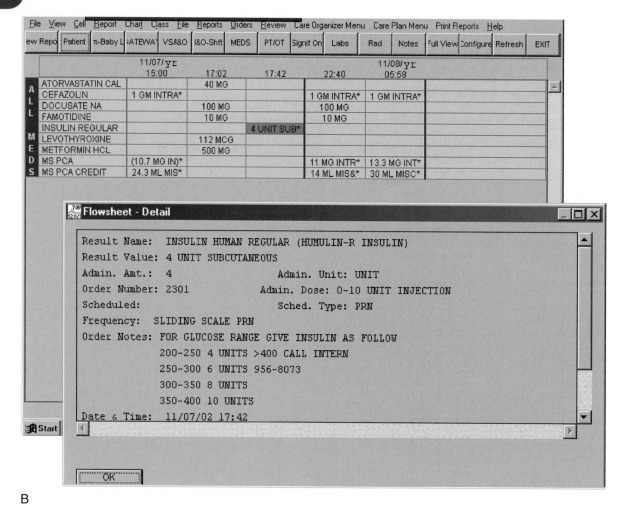

B

Fig. 6.2B Electronically generated medication sheet listing all scheduled medications for an 8-hour shift. By clicking the cursor on the highlighted area ("4 UNIT SUB" in this illustration), a window opens to reveal details of the order. (Courtesy Creighton University Medical Center, Omaha, NE.)

KARDEX RECORDS

The **Kardex** is a large index-type card that is usually kept in a flip file or a separate holder that contains pertinent information such as the patient's name, diagnosis, allergies, treatments, and the nursing care plan. When the unit-dose system is used, medications are not listed on the Kardex; rather, they are listed separately on the medication profile. Although the Kardex is used primarily by nurses, patient data can be quickly accessed by all members of the healthcare team. The Kardex is often completed in pencil and updated regularly. Because it is not a legal document, it is destroyed when the patient is discharged from the institution. Traditional Kardex information is evolving into an electronic database format that is continually updated throughout each shift.

EVOLVING CHARTING METHODOLOGIES

Regardless of the method of charting used, the documentation process needs to adhere to The Joint Commission standards that incorporate established standards of care. The Joint Commission requires that all charting methodologies incorporate nursing process criteria and evidence of teaching and discharge planning. When more than one healthcare discipline is providing patient care, a multidisciplinary care plan must be completed. This facilitates communication among interdisciplinary team members and healthcare providers. Improving patient safety at the point of care has become standard in every healthcare institution.

The format and extent of use of electronic database charting vary widely among institutions, but each method incorporates the standards of care and The Joint Commission requirements. Some clinical sites have extensive online electronic charting developed, whereas others have little or none. For example, one hospital may elect to combine all of the elements formerly found in the Kardex, the care plan, the MAR, and the critical pathways into one document known as a *patient profile* that the nurse can access during each shift. Regardless of the methodology used, the adage "If you didn't chart it, it didn't happen" still holds true.

★ Nursing Care Plan | Risk for Infection

ASSESSMENT

Mrs. Spicer was admitted to the medical nursing unit 3 days ago with a diagnosis of lymphoma. She received her first dose of multiagent chemotherapy yesterday. Jess Ralston is the student nurse who is caring for Mrs. Spicer. He begins his shift by conducting a focused assessment.

Assessment Activities	Findings/Defining Characteristics
Review the patient's chart for laboratory data that reflect immune function.	The data show a reduction in the number of white blood cells (i.e., leukopenia).
Ask the patient to describe her appetite and to review her food intake for the last 24 hr. Weigh the patient and measure her height.	The patient reports that she has not had an interest in eating for a couple of weeks. She has lost approximately 6 lb. Her current weight is 125 lb, and her height is 5'7". Her food intake yesterday consisted of a small cup of applesauce, half of a bowl of soup, some crackers, and two glasses of juice. The patient states, "I get full easily and lose interest in food."
Palpate the patient's cervical and clavicular lymph nodes.	Her lymph nodes are enlarged and painless.
Review the effects of chemotherapy in a drug reference.	Multiagent chemotherapy causes drug-induced pancytopenia.

NURSING DIAGNOSIS

Risk for infection related to chemotherapy and reduced food intake

PLANNING

Goal	Expected Outcomes[a]
RISK CONTROL: INFECTIOUS PROCESS, IMMUNE STATUS	
Patient will remain free from symptoms of infection.	Patient will observe and report signs of infection (i.e., fever, shaking, chills).
KNOWLEDGE: INFECTION CONTROL	
Patient will become knowledgeable about infection risks.	Patient will identify routines to follow in the home to reduce the transmission of microorganisms.
	Patient will identify signs and symptoms that indicate infection needing to be reported to the healthcare provider.
	Patient will demonstrate appropriate hand hygiene, and verbalize oral care and perineal care.

INTERVENTIONS

Nursing Actions	Rationale
INFECTION PROTECTION AND CONTROL	
Monitor the patient's body temperature routinely, inspect her oral cavity for lesions, inspect her IV access site for drainage, and observe her for evidence of cough; ask her about any unusual discharge or burning on urination.	Interventions are designed to prevent infection and ensure the early detection of infection in a patient who is at risk.
Teach the patient how to perform hand hygiene by handwashing or the use of alcohol-based hand rubs.	Rigorous hand hygiene reduces bacterial counts on the hands. The patient can easily come in contact with infectious agents that can cause infection.
Consult with a dietitian about providing a high-calorie, high-protein, low-bacteria diet. Minimize the patient's intake of salads, raw fruits and vegetables, undercooked meat, pepper, and paprika. Offer the patient small, frequent meals.	Maintaining calorie and protein intake will prevent weight loss. Foods high in bacteria should be avoided because they increase the risk for gastrointestinal infection.
Instruct the patient to report any of the following to the healthcare provider:	Signs of infection are indicative of local or systemic infection.
• A temperature of >100°F (38°C)	
• A persistent cough with or without sputum; pus or foul-smelling drainage from a body site	
• The presence of an abscess	
• Urine that is cloudy or foul smelling	
• Burning during urination	

[a]Outcome classification labels and interventions from Moorhead S, Johnson M, Maas M, Swanson E. *Nursing Outcomes Classification (NOC).* 5th ed. St. Louis: Elsevier; 2013.

✳ **Nursing Care Plan** | **Risk for Infection—cont'd**

Nursing Actions	Rationale
Teach the patient to do the following activities at home: • Avoid crowds and large gatherings of people. • Bathe daily. • Do not share personal toiletry items (e.g., toothbrush, washcloth, deodorant stick) with family members. • Practice hand hygiene. • Do not drink water that has been standing for >15 min. • Do not reuse cups or glasses without washing them first.	These measures are designed to prevent infection in those patients with impaired immune function.

EVALUATION

Nursing Actions	Patient Response/Finding	Achievement of Outcome
Compare the patient's body temperature and other physical findings with baseline data.	The patient remains afebrile and denies having a cough or burning during urination. There are no signs of drainage or discharge from body sites.	The patient has no active infection at this time.
Ask the patient to describe the signs and symptoms that should be reported to a healthcare provider.	The patient is able to identify the temperature range to report. She was able to describe a cough but unable to identify signs of urinary infection or local discharge.	The patient has a partial understanding of the signs and symptoms to report. She will require additional instruction and should be offered an information sheet.
Ask patient to explain the measures to take at home to reduce exposure to infectious agents.	The patient is able to discuss the need to avoid sharing personal hygiene articles. She asked for a listing of other precautions and requested that her husband be included in the discussion.	The patient has a partial understanding of restrictions. The nurse will obtain printed guidelines to give to the patient and include the patient's husband in a discussion this evening.

Adapted from Ackley BJ, Ladwig GB, Makic MB. *Nursing Diagnosis Handbook: An Evidence-Based Guide to Planning Care.* 11th ed. St. Louis: Mosby; 2017.

DRUG DISTRIBUTION SYSTEMS

Before administering medications, it is important that the nurse understand the overall medication delivery system that is used at the employing healthcare agency. Although no two drug distribution systems function in exactly the same way, the following general types are used.

FLOOR OR WARD STOCK SYSTEM

In the **floor or ward stock system**, all but the most dangerous or rarely used medications are stocked at the nursing station in stock containers. This system has generally been used in very small hospitals and hospitals in which there are no direct charges to the patient for medications (e.g., in some government hospitals). Some advantages of this system are the ready availability of most drugs, fewer inpatient prescription orders, and the minimal return of medications. The disadvantages are as follows:

• Increased potential for medication errors because of the large array of stock medications from which to choose and the lack of review by the pharmacist of a patient's medication order

• Increased danger of the unnoticed passing of expiration dates and drug deterioration, as well as increased quantities of expired drugs to be discarded

• Economic loss caused by misplaced or forgotten charges and the misappropriation of medication by hospital personnel

• Need for larger stocks and frequent total drug inventories

• Storage problems on the nursing units of many hospitals

INDIVIDUAL PRESCRIPTION ORDER SYSTEM

With the **individual prescription order system**, medications are dispensed from the pharmacy with the receipt of a prescription or drug order for an individual patient.

The pharmacist usually sends a 3- to 5-day supply of medication in a bottle that is labeled for a specific patient. After the prescriptions are received at the nurses' station, medications are placed in the medication cabinet in accordance with institutional practices. Generally, the medication containers are arranged alphabetically by the patient's name, but they may be arranged numerically by the patient's room or bed number. This system provides greater patient safety because of the review of prescription orders by the pharmacist and nurse before administration; it also involves less danger of drug deterioration, easier inventory control, smaller total inventories, and reduced revenue loss because of improved charging systems and less pilferage. Although dispensing medication to individual patients is better than the floor or ward stock system, the major disadvantages of this system are the time-consuming procedures that are used to schedule, prepare, administer, control, and record the drug distribution and administration process.

UNIT-DOSE SYSTEM

Unit-dose drug distribution systems use single-unit packages of drugs that are dispensed to fill each dose requirement as it is ordered. Each package is labeled with the drug's generic and brand names, the manufacturer, the lot number, and the expiration date. When they are dispensed by the pharmacy, the individual packages are placed in labeled drawers that are assigned to individual patients. The drawers are kept in a large unit-dose cabinet (Fig. 6.3) that is kept at the nurses' station; in some institutions, individualized containers or envelopes may be locked in a cabinet in the patient's room. With most unit-dose systems, a pharmacist refills the drawers every 24 hours. In long-term care facilities, these drawers are usually exchanged on a 3- or 7-day schedule.

Advantages of the system include the following:
- The time that is normally spent by nursing personnel preparing drugs for administration is drastically reduced.
- The pharmacist has a profile of all medications for each patient and is therefore able to analyze the prescribed medications for drug interactions or contraindications. This method increases the pharmacist's involvement and makes better use of his or her extensive drug knowledge.
- Counting drugs from multidose packets is no longer necessary as a result of unit-dose packaging, thereby reducing errors.
- It is the nurse's responsibility to check drugs and calculate dosages (see the information under Right Dose later in this chapter), thereby reducing errors.
- There is less waste and misappropriation because single units are dispensed.
- Credit is given to the patient for unused medications because each dose is individually packaged. (Under the individual prescription order system, returned bottles of unused medications are destroyed out of fear of contamination.)

The unit-dose medication is prepared under rigid controls, and it is dispensed only after pharmacists have completed quality control procedures. Nurses should always check medications before administration. If there is a discrepancy between the Kardex (i.e., the medication profile) and the medication in the cart, then the pharmacist and the original prescriber's order should be consulted.

At the time of administration, the nurse should check all aspects of the medication order as stated on the medication profile against the medication container removed from the patient's drawer for administration. The number of doses remaining in the drawer for the shift should also be checked. If the number of remaining doses is incorrect, the medication order should be checked before continuing with the drug administration. It is always possible that the drug has been discontinued or that someone else has given the dose, omitted a dose, or given the wrong patient the wrong medication. If an error has been made, it should be reported in accordance with hospital policies.

COMPUTER-CONTROLLED DISPENSING SYSTEM

A common system for medication ordering and administration is a **computer-controlled dispensing system**, such as Pyxis (Fig. 6.4), that uses the unit-dose system described earlier. It is resupplied by the pharmacy daily and is stocked with single-unit packages of medicines. When a drug order is received in the pharmacy for a patient, it is entered into the computerized system. The nurse—who is using a security code and password and, with newer systems, a fingerprint—accesses the system and selects the patient's name, the medication profile, and the drugs that are due for administration. The drug order appears on the screen, and a specific section of the cart opens so that the nurse can take a single dose of medicine out of the cart (Fig. 6.5A). This process continues until all drugs ordered for a specific time of administration are retrieved. During the actual administration process at the bedside, the nurse uses a

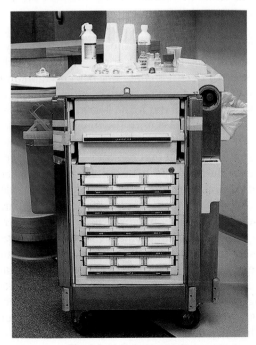

Fig. 6.3 Unit-dose cabinet.

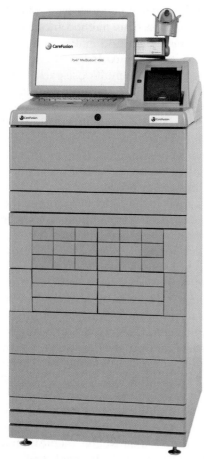

Fig. 6.4 Electronic dispensing system: the Pyxis system. (Courtesy and © Becton, Dickinson and Company, Franklin Lakes, NJ.)

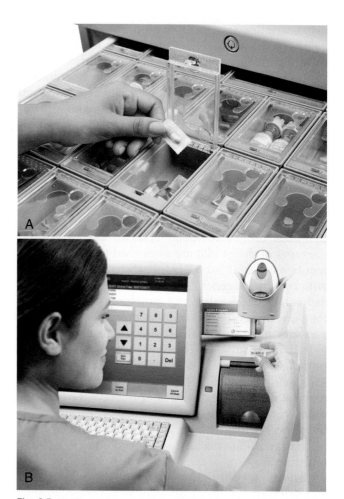

Fig. 6.5 (A) The nurse removes a single dose of medicine from the electronic dispensing system. (B) A single-dose, bar-coded medication package is scanned by the nurse before it is administered. (Courtesy and © Becton, Dickinson and Company, Franklin Lakes, NJ.)

handheld scanner that reads the **bar codes** on the nurse's identification badge, the patient's wristband, and the unit-dose medication packet, thereby linking this information with the patient database (Fig. 6.5B). If there is an error (e.g., wrong dose, wrong time of administration, wrong patient), an alert pops up on the computer and the user is unable to continue until the error is corrected. If the process is correct and the medicine is administered, there is automatic documentation in the patient's MAR of the administration.

Controlled drugs are also kept in this automated dispensing cart. The system provides a detailed record of the controlled substance dispensed, including the date, the time, and by whom it was accessed. A second qualified nurse must witness the disposal of a portion of a dose of a controlled substance or the return to the automated dispensing cart of any controlled substance that is not used. The automated dispensing system is currently the safest and most economical method of drug distribution in hospitals and long-term care facilities.

Long-Term Care Unit-Dose System

The **long-term care unit-dose system** is an adaptation of the system that is used in the acute care setting. The unit-dose cart is designed with individual drawers to

hold one resident's medication containers for 1 week. The drawer is labeled with the resident's name and room number, the pharmacy's name and telephone number, and the name of the healthcare facility. The pharmacist fills the medication container with the prescribed drug. Each container has enough compartments to contain the prescribed number of doses of the drug for each day of the week. The individual compartments may be labeled with the days of the week. The medication cart has other compartments for storing bottles of medication that cannot be placed in patients' drawers. The cart has a storage area for medication cups, a medicine crusher, drinking cups, straws, alcohol wipes, syringes, and other necessities for the preparation and administration of the medications prescribed. The entire cart has a locking system that should be secured when the medication cart is not in use or when it is unattended while medications are being dispensed.

The unit-dose system may involve the use of a color-coding system to simplify finding the medication holder for a specific time of day—for example, purple = 6 AM (0600); pink = 8 AM (0800); yellow = noon (1200); green = 2 PM (1400) or 4 PM (1600); orange = early evening;

and red = PRN. Using this method to organize the medications allows the nurse or medication aide to remove all of the pink holders for administering the prescribed 8 AM (0800) tablets or capsules. Each medication holder is also labeled with the resident's name, the physician's name, the prescription number, the generic or brand name of the drug (or both), the dose, the frequency of the drug order (e.g., four times daily), and the actual time that the drug in this holder is to be administered (e.g., 8 AM, or 0800). This system is easy to use unless the user is color blind. By using military time (e.g., 0800) to mark the individual containers, the individual who is color blind can use the military time as a guideline.

At the time of administration, the nurse or medication aide checks all aspects of the medication order (as stated on the medication profile) against the medication container that has been removed from one of the drawers. The number of doses remaining in the holder is checked against the days of the week that remain for the medication to be administered. If the resident refuses the medication, it must be charted on the record with the reason that the medication was refused. In a long-term care setting, a resident seldom wears an identification band; therefore third-party identification of the resident must be relied on until the nurse or medication aide is able to identify the resident. If pictures of the residents are used as identifiers, the institution should have a policy in place to update the photos on a regular basis. Medications should be charted as soon as they are administered. The medication aide has specific limitations on the types of medications that he or she can administer; therefore nurses should be thoroughly familiar with the laws and guidelines of their state. The nurse is ultimately responsible for verifying the qualifications of the individual who is being supervised in the medication-aide capacity and for the medications that the medication aide is administering.

NARCOTIC CONTROL SYSTEMS

As described in Chapter 1, laws regulating the use of controlled substances have been enacted in the United States and Canada and are rigidly enforced in hospitals and long-term care facilities with the use of narcotic control systems. It is a standard policy that controlled substances are issued in single-unit packages and kept in a locked cabinet. If an automated dispensing system is not available, a designated individual is responsible for the key to the cabinet. When controlled substances are issued to a nursing unit, they are accompanied by an inventory control record (Fig. 6.6) that lists each type of controlled substance being supplied. This record is used to account for the disposition of each type of medication issued. When the controlled substance supply is dispensed to the nursing unit by the pharmacist, the nurse receiving the drug supply is responsible for counting and verifying the number and types of controlled substances received. The nurse then signs a record

attesting to the accuracy and receipt of the controlled substances and locks them in the controlled substances (narcotic) cabinet.

When a controlled substance is ordered for a particular patient, the nurse caring for the patient uses a key to the cabinet to obtain and prepare the medication for administration. At the time of removal from the cabinet, the inventory control record (see Fig. 6.6) must be completed; it must indicate the time, the patient's name, the drug, and the dose, and it must include the signature of the nurse who is responsible for checking out the controlled substance. If a portion of the medication is to be discarded because of a smaller prescribed dose, two nurses must check the dose, the preparation, and the portion discarded. Both nurses must then cosign the inventory control record to verify the transaction. The cabinet is relocked, the medicine is administered, and the documentation is completed.

Before the administration of any controlled substance, the patient's chart should be checked to verify that the time interval since the last use of the drug has elapsed as specified in the healthcare provider's orders (see Chapter 19 for details about the monitoring of pain and the use of analgesics). Immediately after the administration of a controlled substance, the nurse who is administering the medication should complete the charting. At appropriate intervals after the administration of a controlled substance, the degree and duration of effectiveness should be recorded in the nurses' notes or the pain flow sheet.

At the end of each shift, the contents of the controlled substances cabinet or the controlled substances cart are counted (inventoried) by two nurses: one from the shift that is about to end and the other from the oncoming shift. Each container is counted, and the remaining numbers of tablets, ampules, and prefilled syringes are added to the amount used in accordance with the inventory control record. The amount of each drug remaining plus the amount recorded as being administered to individual patients should equal the total number issued. During the counting procedure, packages of unopened prefilled syringes are visually inspected to verify that the seal and cellophane coverings are intact. If the package seal is broken, closer scrutiny of the package is required. These observations should include tilting a package of prefilled syringes to observe the rate of air bubble movement inside the barrel, the uniformity of color of the solutions in each of the barrels, and the similarity in fluid levels in each of the barrels. The same medication in the same type of syringe should be the same color and travel through the barrel at the same rate, and all fluid levels should be similar.

Discrepancies in the number of remaining doses are checked with nursing personnel on the unit to see if all controlled substances used have been charted. If this does not reveal the source of the inaccuracy, each patient's chart is checked to be certain that all controlled substances recorded on the individual patient's chart for

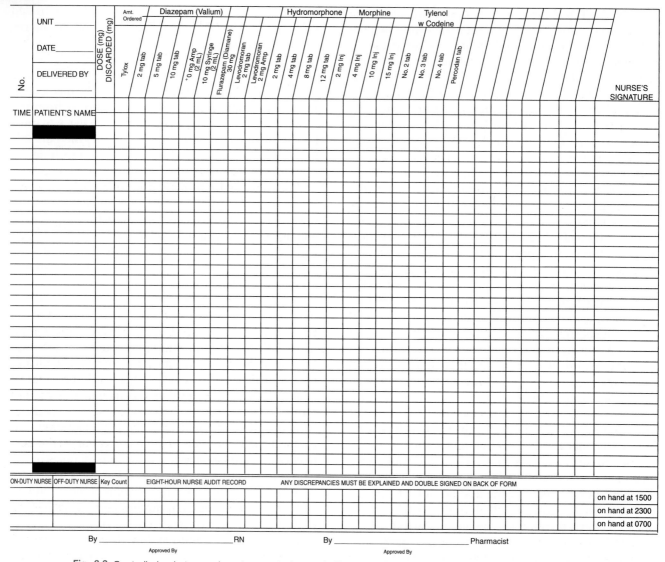

Fig. 6.6 Controlled substances inventory control record. (Courtesy University Hospital, The University of Nebraska Medical Center; © Board of Regents of the University of Nebraska, Lincoln, NE.)

the shift coincide with the controlled substances inventory record. If the error is still not found, the pharmacy and the nursing service office should be contacted in accordance with institution policy. If the count appears to be accurate but tampering with the contents of the containers is suspected, a report should be made to the pharmacy and the nursing service office. When the controlled substances inventory is complete, the two nurses who are counting sign the inventory control shift record to verify that the records and inventory are accurate at that time. With the controlled substance cart, the computer generates an end-of-shift report that also identifies discrepancies so that the staff involved can account for the use of controlled substances.

When an automated dispensing cart such as Pyxis (see Fig. 6.4) is used, the shift change narcotic check is not done. At the time of administration, the nurse will verify the correct count of the drug desired before removing the drug from the cart. At that time, the system will be activated if a discrepancy occurs. Discrepancies

are tracked by nursing and pharmacy, and they are resolved as soon as they are discovered. The pharmacy also checks for discrepancies when controlled substances are restocked in the automated dispensing system. Reconciliation sheets must be completed if there are inaccuracies in the count.

DISPOSAL OF UNUSED MEDICINES

In recent years, environmental concerns have arisen about the proper **disposal of unused medicines**, because trace levels of medicines have been found in rivers, lakes, and community water supplies. Concerns have been expressed about the appropriateness of the common practice of flushing unused medicines down the toilet, because many people assume that this is the primary source of water contamination. However, the US Food and Drug Administration's Center for Drug Evaluation and Research has stated that drugs found in ground water are primarily drugs that have been incompletely absorbed and metabolized by the body after human consumption and that have entered the environment after passing through waste-water treatment plants. Scientists from the Environmental Protection Agency have found no evidence of adverse human health effects from unmetabolized drugs in the environment.

The US Food and Drug Administration, working in conjunction with the White House Office of National Drug Control Policy, issued the following guidelines addressing prescription and nonprescription medication disposal:

- Follow specific disposal instructions on the drug label or in the patient information leaflet that accompanies the medication. Do not flush prescription drugs down the toilet unless specifically instructed to do so by the manufacturer.
- If no instructions are given, throw the drugs in the household trash, but first:
  - Empty the drugs from the container, and then mix them with an undesirable substance, such as used coffee grounds or kitty litter. This makes the product considerably less appealing to children and pets and less recognizable to people who may intentionally go through trash (e.g., dumpster divers).
  - Put this mixture in a sealable bag, an empty can, or another container to prevent the medication from leaking out of the garbage bag.
- Use community drug take-back programs that allow the public to bring unused drugs to a central location for proper disposal. The drugs are often destroyed using a biohazard-controlled incinerator.
- Before throwing out an empty prescription bottle, scratch out all identifying information on the label to make it unreadable. This will help to protect patient identity and health information.
- Controlled substances (e.g., opiate analgesics) should be flushed down the toilet to reduce the danger of unintentional use or overdose and illegal abuse. An example is the fentanyl patch, which, even after it has been used by the patient for 3 days, can still contain enough medicine to cause severe respiratory depression in babies, children, and pets.

Additional guidelines for the disposal of drugs that are classified as hazardous medications (e.g., chemotherapeutic agents) have also been defined. Refer to agency policies for proper disposal.

MEDICATION ORDERS

Medications for patient use must be ordered by licensed physicians, dentists, nurse practitioners, and physician assistants acting within their areas of professional training. Placing an order for a medication or treatment is known as *issuing a prescription*. Initially, a prescription may be issued verbally or in written form. Prescriptions that are issued for nonhospitalized patients use a form that is similar to that shown in Fig. 6.7, whereas

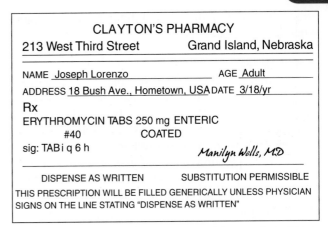

Fig. 6.7 Prescription showing patient name and age, patient address, date, drug and strength, number of tablets, directions for use, and the healthcare provider's signature.

prescriptions for hospitalized patients are written on the institution's medication order form. All prescriptions must contain the following elements: the patient's full name, the date, the drug name, the route of administration, the dose, the duration of the order, and the signature of the prescriber. Additional information may be required for certain types of medications (e.g., for IV administration, the concentration, dilution, and rate of flow should be specified in addition to the method [i.e., "IV push" or "continuous infusion"]).

TYPES OF MEDICATION ORDERS

Medication orders fall into four categories: stat, single, standing, and PRN orders. The **stat order** is generally used on an emergency basis. It means that the drug is to be administered as soon as possible, but only once. For example, if a patient is having a seizure, the physician may order "diazepam 10 mg IV stat," which means that the drug is to be given immediately and one time only.

The **single order** means administration at a certain time but only one time. For example, a one-time order may be written for "furosemide 20 mg IV to be given one time at 7 AM." Furosemide would then be administered at that time, but once only.

The **standing order** indicates that a medication is to be given for a specified number of doses: for example, "cefazolin 1 g q6h × 4 doses." A standing order may also indicate that a drug is to be administered until it is discontinued at a later date: for example, "ampicillin 500 mg PO q6h." In the interest of patient safety, however, all accredited healthcare agencies have policies that automatically cancel an order after a certain number of doses are administered or after a certain number of days of therapy have passed (e.g., surgery, after 72 hours for narcotics, after one dose only for anticoagulants, after 7 days for antibiotics).

A **PRN order** means "administer if needed." This order allows a nurse to judge when a medication should be administered on the basis of the patient's need and when it can be safely administered.

Verbal Orders

Healthcare agencies have policies regarding who may accept verbal orders and under what circumstances they should be accepted. The practice is strongly discouraged and should be avoided whenever possible to prevent medication errors. However, when a verbal order is accepted, the person who took the order is responsible for accurately entering it on the order sheet and signing it. The prescriber must cosign and date the order, usually within 24 hours.

Electronic Transmission of Patient Orders

Many physicians' offices fax new orders to the area where the patient is admitted or transferred. These fax transmissions must have an original signature within a specified time, often 24 hours. Hospital units also find it useful to fax orders to the nursing home where the individual is being transferred. This allows the receiving agency to prepare for the patient or resident, and the original orders, which have been signed by the physician, then accompany the individual at the time of transfer.

Computerized provider order entry (CPOE) systems are used to transmit orders electronically. Software has been developed that allows for the use of CPOE and clinical decision-making support systems (CDSSs). The computerized system integrates the ordering system with the pharmacy, the laboratory, and the nurses' station, thereby providing access instantly to online information that may affect a patient's care needs.

MEDICATION SAFETY

Medication safety is freedom from accidental injury from medications. The nurse should be aware of how to properly handle certain medications (e.g., chemotherapy drugs, topical hormones), which can cause a reaction when they come in contact with the skin. The nurse also needs to be aware of how to correctly prepare and administer medications to prevent injury (e.g., a needlestick).

Medication errors can be defined as the failure of a planned action to be completed as intended or the use of a wrong plan to achieve a goal. Medication errors include prescribing errors, transcription or order communication errors, dispensing errors, administration errors, and errors of monitoring or education for proper use (Box 6.1). Medication errors can result in serious complications known as *adverse drug events*. In 2005, the number of deaths from medication errors as reported to the US Food and Drug Administration was 15,107 (Moore, 2007). The National Academy of Medicine, formerly called the Institute of Medicine, has been working on initiatives to reduce these events and manage the outcomes by exploring how they occur and determining ways to prevent them.

Box 6.1	Examples of Medication Errors

PRESCRIBING ERRORS
- Suboptimal drug therapy decisions
- Drug prescribed for patient with known allergy or intolerance
- Incorrect dose for diagnosis
- Unauthorized drug prescribed

TRANSCRIPTION ERRORS
- Misinterpretation or misunderstanding of drug ordered or any directions listed
- Illegible handwriting
- Unapproved abbreviations
- Omission of orders

DISPENSING
- Wrong drug or dose sent to nursing unit
- Wrong formulation or dosage form

ADMINISTRATION
- Incorrect strength (dose) given
- Extra dose given or missed dose
- Wrong administration time
- Incorrect administration technique

MONITORING
- Suboptimal monitoring
- Suboptimal assessment of drug response or revision of regimen
- Suboptimal patient education

TECHNOLOGY AND PREVENTION OF ADVERSE DRUG EVENTS

Adverse drug events occur most commonly during ordering and at the administration stage. Therefore preventive measures are being implemented that include substantial changes in the ordering system used for medications and laboratory studies. The use of the CPOE technology checks for potential drug interactions and the appropriateness of drug dosages ordered, as well as for laboratory findings (e.g., therapeutic drug levels at the time of order entry).

Automated ordering and dispensing systems have been developed to minimize medication errors. Automated systems use robotics and bar-coding technology to fill the orders entered by the physician. Robotics in the pharmacy can free some of the pharmacists for deployment to clinical units, where they can make patient rounds, check for medication response, review current laboratory data, and work with the prescriber to select, dose, and monitor drug therapy.

HIGH-ALERT MEDICATIONS

The Institute for Safe Medication Practices (ISMP) has conducted a survey of several acute care hospitals to determine which medications cause serious patient harm or death. As a result of this study, medications and classifications that pose significant risk in the acute clinical setting were identified. These are now known as *high-alert medications*, and they include insulin, heparin, opioids, injectable potassium or potassium phosphate concentrate, neuromuscular blocking agents, and chemotherapeutic agents. Although mistakes may or may not be more common with these medicines, the consequences of an error are much more devastating to patients. The ISMP continues to monitor the frequency of drug errors in the clinical literature to update the list of high-alert medications.

High-alert medications, the role they play in medication errors, and recommended practices to aid in prevention include the following: (1) standardizing processes within the institution; (2) developing processes to make errors stand out (i.e., making staff more alert and aware to catch errors before they reach the patient); and (3) developing methods to minimize the consequences of errors that reach the patient. Cohen also discussed several practices to promote medication safety, including the following: (1) the use of technology, including CPOE, bar-coded drug administration, and smart pumps for controlled administration; (2) the restriction of high-alert medications during the dispensing process (e.g., removing neuromuscular blocking agents from readily available floor stock); (3) the avoidance of verbal orders for high-alert medicines; (4) the use of checklists for high-alert drugs; (5) the use of generic and brand names on the MAR to avoid errors with sound-alike drugs; (6) the standardizing of drug concentrations and dosing infusion charts; and (7) the performance of double-checking before administration and patient education. The Institute for Healthcare Improvement also makes recommendations for high-alert medication safety practices (http://www.ihi.org/topics/highalertmedicationsafety/pages/default.aspx).

MEDICATION RECONCILIATION

Another process that involves the goal of eliminating medication errors is **medication reconciliation**, which involves comparing a patient's current medication orders with all of the medications that the patient is actually taking. This process makes use of a single, shared, and updated medication and allergy list for patients across the continuum of inpatient and outpatient care that is to be used during **handoffs**, or the transition of patients during care. Reconciliation aims to prevent omissions, duplications, differences in dosing, and drug interactions. It should be completed as part of every transition of care during which new medications are ordered or existing orders are rewritten. Transitions in care include changes in setting, service, practitioner, or level of care (e.g., critical care to general care to rehabilitation services).

Medication reconciliation is a five-step process: (1) develop a list of current medications being administered, (2) develop a list of medications that were prescribed, (3) compare the medications on the two lists, (4) make clinical decisions on the basis of this comparison, and (5) communicate the new list to appropriate caregivers and to the patient. Accurate and complete medication reconciliation can prevent many prescribing and administration errors. Failure to reconcile medications may be compounded by the practice of writing blanket orders (e.g., "resume preop medications"), which are known to result in adverse drug events. Such orders are explicitly prohibited by The Joint Commission's medication management standards.

SOUND-ALIKE MEDICATIONS

The ISMP regularly reports medication errors that are the result of the similarity of sound-alike names (e.g., Mucomyst and Mucinex; Evista and Avinza). Manufacturers have a responsibility to avoid using brand names that are similar to those of other medicines to help avoid errors. As recommended by the ISMP, both the generic name and the brand name should be included on the CPOE screen.

Most products with sound-alike names are used for different purposes. It is important for the nurse to be familiar with patients' diagnoses and to know what medicines are used for these conditions so that they are able to question why a particular medicine may have been prescribed when a patient does not have a diagnosis that requires that medicine. For example, the generic name for Evista is raloxifene, which is used to prevent osteoporosis in postmenopausal women; alternatively, Avinza is an extended-release form of morphine sulfate that is used for severe pain. Seeing Evista dispensed for a person who requires opioid analgesia should raise a question of medication error; it should not be administered until the need for the medicine has been clarified. (Note the "do not confuse" icon ⇄ throughout this text in the appropriate drug monographs and tables.)

NURSE'S RESPONSIBILITIES

The importance of accuracy at every step during ordering, transcribing, administering, and monitoring drug therapy cannot be overemphasized.

Verification

With the nonautomated order and distribution systems, after a prescription order has been written for a hospitalized patient, the nurse interprets it and makes a professional judgment about its acceptability. Judgments must be made regarding the type of drug, the therapeutic intent, the usual dose, the associated mathematical calculations, and the physical preparation of the dose. The nurse must also evaluate the method of administration in relation to the patient's physical condition, as well as any patient allergies and the patient's ability to tolerate the dose form. If any part of an order is vague, the prescriber who wrote the order should be consulted for clarification.

Patient safety is of primary importance, and the nurse assumes responsibility for the **verification** and safety of the medication order. If, after gathering all possible information, the nurse concludes that it is inappropriate to administer the medication as ordered, the prescriber should be notified immediately. An explanation should be given as to why the order should not be executed. If the prescriber cannot be contacted or does not change the order, the nurse should notify the director of nurses, the nursing supervisor on duty, or both. The reasons for the refusal to administer the drug should be recorded in accordance with the policies of the employing institution.

Transcription

The transcription of the prescriber's order is necessary to put that order into action. After the verification of an order, a nurse or another designated person transcribes the order from the physician's order sheet onto the Kardex or medication profile. These data may also be entered into a computerized patient database that produces a Kardex or medication profile. When this process is delegated to a ward clerk or unit secretary, the nurse is still responsible for verifying all aspects of the medication order. The nurse must sign the original medication order to indicate that the order has been received, interpreted, and verified. The nurse then sends a copy of the original order to the pharmacy, often by fax. A small supply is issued, either in a unit-dose form or in a container that holds a daily supply. The container is labeled with the date, the patient's name and room number, and the drug name and strength or dose. When the supply arrives from the pharmacy, it is stored in the medication room or in the patient's medication drawer of the medication cart.

In the long-term care setting, carbon copies of new medication orders are sent to the local pharmacy to be filled. If a stat dose is needed or if the medication must be started very soon, the pharmacy is notified via telephone or fax and written verification of the medicines ordered is also supplied to the pharmacy. Because the local pharmacy generates the medication administration record only on a monthly basis, new orders must be added to the current medication record by the nurse who is transcribing the order. Nurses also send requests to the pharmacy via fax for drug reorders (e.g., PRN orders).

Using standard drug administration methodology, the nurse prepares and administers a drug by following the order on the medication profile in accordance with the seven rights of drug administration. With the new CPOE that is supported by CDSSs, both the verification and transcription of the medication orders are built into the system. It should be emphasized that bar coding and handheld devices do not eliminate the need for the nurse to use standard administration procedures for medications (e.g., checking all aspects of the drug order).

Reporting Variance

When a medication error or variance does occur, an incident report—which includes the date, the time that the drug was ordered, the drug name and dose, the route of administration, and the therapeutic response or adverse clinical observations—should be submitted. The date and time that the prescriber is notified of the error and any prescriber's orders given should also be recorded. It is important to be factual and not to state opinions on the incident report. Current practices for reporting medication errors have evolved into a process whereby facilities are being encouraged to adopt nonpunitive actions when a medication error occurs. It is much more important to determine why the error occurred and to educate all personnel regarding how to prevent repeat errors.

SEVEN RIGHTS OF DRUG ADMINISTRATION

The seven rights of drug administration are as follows: right drug, right indication, right time, right dose, right patient, right route, and right documentation.

RIGHT DRUG

The nurse needs to verify that the drug given is the one ordered. Triple-checking the drug name is one of the important steps that the nurse takes to prevent medication errors.

 Clinical Pitfall

Many drugs have similarly spelled names and variable concentrations. A significant number of medication errors occur as a result of look-alike packaging and similar drug names. Therefore before administering a medication, it is imperative to compare the exact spelling and concentration of the prescribed drug with the medication profile and the medication container. Regardless of the drug distribution system used, the drug label should be read at least three times: (1) before removing the drug from the shelf or unit-dose cart; (2) before preparing or measuring the actual prescribed dose; and (3) before replacing the drug on the shelf or before opening a unit-dose container (i.e., just before administering the drug to the patient).

RIGHT INDICATION

The nurse has the responsibility to verify the reason that the patient is receiving the medication. It is important to understand the indication, which is related to the medical diagnosis. If in doubt about the reason for the order, the nurse must verify the medication order with the prescriber before administration.

RIGHT TIME

When scheduling the administration time of a medication, factors such as timing abbreviations, standardized times, consistency of blood levels, absorption, diagnostic testing, and the use of PRN medications must be considered.

Standard Timing Abbreviations

The drug order specifies the frequency of drug administration. Standard abbreviations that are used as part of the drug order specify the times of administration. The nurse should also check institutional policy concerning medication administration. Hospitals often have standardized interpretations for abbreviations (e.g., "q6h" may mean 0600, 1200, 1800, and 2400; "qid" may mean 0800, 1200, 1600, and 2000). The nurse must memorize and use standard abbreviations to interpret, transcribe, and administer medications accurately.

Standardized Administration Times

For patient safety, certain medications are administered at specific times. This allows laboratory work or electrocardiography to be completed first so that any adjustment to the next dose can be determined. For example, warfarin or digoxin may be administered at 1300 if ordered by the prescriber. The medication administration times need to be standardized throughout a clinical facility, with all units using the same time schedule to help prevent medication errors.

Maintenance of Consistent Blood Levels

The schedule for the administration of a drug should be planned to maintain consistent blood levels of the drug to maximize the drug's therapeutic effectiveness. If blood draws to establish the current serum blood level of a specific drug are ordered, then the nurse should follow the guidelines stated in the drug monograph for the specific time at which the blood sample should be drawn in relation to the drug dose administration schedule.

Maximum Drug Absorption

The schedule for the oral administration of drugs must be planned to prevent incompatibilities and to maximize absorption. Certain drugs require administration on an empty stomach and thus are given 1 hour before or 2 hours after a meal. Other medications should be given with food to enhance absorption or reduce irritation, and still other drugs are not given with dairy products or antacids. It is important to maintain the recommended schedule of administration for maximum therapeutic effectiveness.

Diagnostic Testing

It is necessary to determine whether any diagnostic tests have been ordered for completion before initiating or continuing therapy. Before beginning antimicrobial therapy, all culture specimens (e.g., blood, urine, wound) need to be collected. If a healthcare provider has ordered serum levels of a certain drug to be obtained, then the administration time of the medication should be coordinated with the time at which the phlebotomist is going to draw the blood sample. When completing the requisition for a serum level of a medication, a notation should be made regarding the date and time that the drug was last administered. Timing is important; if tests are not conducted at the same time intervals for the same patient, then the data gained are of little value.

PRN Medications

Before the administration of any PRN medication, the patient's chart should be checked to ensure that someone else has not administered the drug and that the specified time interval has passed since the medication was last administered. When a PRN medication is given, it should be charted immediately, including the reason for administration (e.g., nausea, pain). The patient's response to the medication should also be recorded.

RIGHT DOSE

Check the drug dosage ordered against the range specified in the reference books available at the nurses' station or the institutionally accepted websites, and complete drug calculations as indicated.

Abnormal Hepatic or Renal Function

The hepatic and renal function of the specific patient who will receive the drug should always be considered. Depending on the rate of drug metabolism and the route of excretion from the body, certain drugs require a reduction in dose to prevent toxicity. Conversely, patients who are being dialyzed may require higher-than-normal doses. Whenever a dosage is outside of the normal range for that drug, it should be verified *before* administration. After verification has been obtained, a brief explanation should be recorded in the nurses' notes and on the Kardex or medication profile so that others administering the medication will have the information and the healthcare provider will not be repeatedly contacted with the same questions. The following laboratory tests are used to monitor liver function: aspartate aminotransferase (AST), alanine aminotransferase (ALT), gamma-glutamyltransferase (GGT), alkaline phosphatase, and lactate dehydrogenase (LDH). The blood urea nitrogen (BUN), serum creatinine (Cr_s), and creatinine clearance (C_{cr}) are used to monitor renal function.

Pediatric and Older Patients

Specific dosages for some drugs have not yet been firmly established for the older adult or pediatric patient. The nurse should question any order outside of the normal range *before* administration. For pediatric patients, the most reliable method is by proportional amount of body surface area or body weight (see Appendix A).

Nausea and Vomiting

If a patient is vomiting, oral medications should be held and the prescriber should be contacted for alternative medication orders, because the parenteral or rectal route may be preferred. Investigate the onset of the nausea and vomiting. If it began after the start of the medication regimen, consideration should be given to rescheduling the oral medication. Administration with food usually decreases gastric irritation.

Accurate Dose Forms

Do not break a tablet. Consult with the pharmacist about the need for scoring any tablets and have the pharmacy prepare the medication, or ask for other available dosage forms.

Accurate Calculations

When calculating drug dosages, accuracy is essential to maintain medication safety. Do not hesitate to have any calculations checked by another healthcare professional.

Clinical Pitfall

Whenever a dosage is questionable or when fractional doses are calculated, check the dose with another qualified individual. Most hospital policies require that certain medications (e.g., insulin, heparin, IV digoxin) be checked by two qualified nurses before they are administered.

Correct Measuring Devices

The accurate measurement of the volume of medication prescribed is essential. Fractional doses require the use of a tuberculin syringe, whereas insulin is generally measured in an insulin syringe that corresponds with the number of units in 1 mL (i.e., U-100 insulin is measured in a U-100 syringe).

There are numerous types of infusion pumps available, and the nurse needs to be familiar with the operation of the type used in the clinical setting. If in doubt, have another care provider with expertise in the device's use check all settings before administering a medication.

RIGHT PATIENT

When using a unit-dose system, the name on the medication profile should be compared with the individual's identification bracelet. Always check the bracelet for allergies. Some institutional policies require that the individual be called by name as a means of identification. This practice must take into consideration the patient's mental alertness and orientation. It is *always* much safer to check the identification bracelet. The Joint Commission recommends that at least two patient identifiers be used (e.g., the patient stating both his or her name and his or her birth date).

Pediatric Patients

Children should never be asked their name as a means of positive identification. They may change beds, try to avoid the staff, or seek attention by identifying themselves as someone else. Identification bracelets should be checked *every time.*

Older Patients

It is important not only to check identification bracelets, but also to confirm names verbally. In a long-term care setting, residents usually do not wear identification bracelets. In these cases, only a person who is familiar

with a specific resident should confirm his or her identity for the purpose of administering medication.

Clinical Pitfall

It is important to check the patient's identification bracelet every time that a medication is administered. The adverse effects of the administration of the wrong medication to the wrong patient and the potential for a lawsuit can thus be avoided. Although automated technology will help to reduce the frequency of medication errors, this technology does not eliminate the nurse's responsibility for checking the patient's identity and other aspects of the drug order.

RIGHT ROUTE

The drug order should specify the route to be used for the administration of the medication. One dosage form of medication should never be substituted for another unless the prescriber is specifically consulted and an order for the change is obtained. There can be a great variation in the absorption rate of the medication through different routes of administration. The IV route delivers the drug directly into the bloodstream. This route provides not only the fastest onset, but also the greatest danger of potential adverse effects (e.g., tachycardia, hypotension). The intramuscular (IM) route provides the next fastest absorption rate, which is based on the availability of the blood supply. This route can be painful, as is the case with many antibiotics. The subcutaneous (subcut) route is the next fastest, and it is also based on blood supply. In some cases, the oral route may be as fast as the IM route, depending on the medication being given, the dose form (liquids are absorbed faster than tablets), and whether there is food in the stomach. The oral route is usually safe if the patient is conscious and able to swallow. The rectal route should be avoided, if possible, because of the resultant irritation of mucosal tissues and erratic absorption rates. In case of error, the oral and rectal routes have the advantage of recoverability for a short time after administration. The drug can be removed by gastric lavage or by inducing vomiting if taken orally. If administered rectally, a drug can be diluted and rinsed out by an enema.

Clinical Pitfall

To ensure that the right drug is prepared at the right time for the right patient using the right route, it is important to maintain the highest standards of drug preparation and administration. Attention should be focused on the calculation, preparation, and administration of the ordered medication. A drug that is reconstituted by a nurse should be clearly labeled with the patient's name, the dose or strength per unit of volume, the date and time that the drug was reconstituted, the amount and type of diluent used, the expiration date or time, and the initials or name of the nurse who prepared it. Once a drug has been reconstituted, it should be administered as soon as possible; if not given right away, it should be stored in accordance with the manufacturer's recommendations.

RIGHT DOCUMENTATION

The documentation of nursing actions and patient observations has always been an important ethical responsibility, but now it is becoming a major medicolegal consideration as well. The chart should always have the following information: the date and time of medication administration; the name of the medication; and the dose, route, and site of administration. The documentation of drug action should be recorded as part of the regularly scheduled assessments for changes in the disease symptoms that the patient is exhibiting. Adverse symptoms observed should be promptly recorded and reported. Health teaching performed should be documented, and the degree of understanding exhibited by the patient should be evaluated and recorded.

- DO record when and why a drug is *not* administered.
- Under some circumstances, a patient may refuse a medication. If this occurs, DO try to obtain information about the reason for the refusal and to integrate these reasons into the care plan. In some cases, it may be because of drug side effects and a lack of understanding about how to alleviate them. Other causes could include the cost of the medicine, an inability to self-administer a drug, or the belief that the drug is ineffective. Healthcare providers must be sensitive to situations when the cause may involve a cultural belief.
- When a drug is refused, DO record all information pertaining to the incident in the nurses' notes, and notify the prescriber of the facts involved.
- DO NOT record a medication until after it has been given.

- DO NOT record in the nurses' notes that an incident report has been completed when a medication error has occurred. However, data regarding clinical observations of the patient related to the occurrence should be charted to serve as a baseline for future comparisons.

Clinical Goldmine

DO approach the patient in a firm but kind manner that conveys the feeling that cooperation is expected.

DO adjust the patient to the most appropriate position for the route of administration. For example, for oral medications, sit the patient upright to facilitate swallowing. Have appropriate fluids ready before administration.

DO remain with the patient to be certain that all medications have been swallowed.

DO use every opportunity to teach the patient and family about the drug being administered.

DO give simple and honest answers or explanations to the patient regarding the medication and the treatment plan.

DO use a plastic container, a medicine cup, a medicine dropper, an oral syringe, or a nipple to administer oral medications to an infant or small child.

DO reward the child who has been cooperative by giving praise; comfort and hold the uncooperative child after completing the medication administration.

Clinical Goldmine

CHECK the label of the container for the drug name, the concentration, and the appropriate route of administration.

CHECK the patient's chart, Kardex, medication profile, or identification bracelet for allergies. If no information is found, ask the patient, before administering the medication, if he or she has any allergies.

CHECK the patient's chart, Kardex, or medication profile for rotation schedules of injectable or topically applied medications.

CHECK medications to be mixed in one syringe with a list approved by the hospital or the pharmacy for compatibility. Normally, all drugs mixed in a single syringe should be administered within 15 minutes after mixing. Immediately before administration, always check the contents of the syringe for clarity and the absence of any precipitate; if the solution is not clear or if a precipitate is present, do not administer the contents of the syringe.

CHECK the patient's identity using two identifiers every time a medication is administered.

Clinical Pitfall

DO NOT prepare or administer a drug from a container that is not properly labeled or from a container on which the label is not fully legible.

DO NOT give any medication that has been prepared by an individual other than the pharmacist. Always check the drug name, dose, frequency, and route of administration against the order. Student nurses must know the practice limitations instituted by the hospital or school and which medications can be administered under what level of supervision.

DO NOT return an unused portion or dose of medication to a stock supply bottle.

DO NOT attempt to orally administer any drug to a comatose patient.

DO NOT leave a medication at the patient's bedside to be taken "later"; remain with the individual until the drug is taken and swallowed. (NOTE: A few exceptions to this rule are available. One is that nitroglycerin may be left at the bedside for the patient's use. Second, in a long-term care setting, certain patients are allowed to take their own medications. In both cases, a specific physician's order is required for self-medication, and the nurse must still chart the medications taken and the therapeutic response achieved.)

DO NOT dilute a liquid medication form unless there are specific written orders to do so.

Discharge Medication Teaching

1. Explain the proper method of taking prescribed medications to the patient (e.g., do not crush or chew enteric-coated tablets or any capsules; sublingual medication is placed under the tongue and is not taken with water).
2. Stress the need for punctuality with regard to the administration of medications and what to do if a dose is missed.
3. Teach the patient to store medications separately from other containers and personal hygiene items.
4. Provide the patient with written instructions that reiterate medication names, schedules, and how to obtain refills. Write the instructions in language that is understood by the patient, and use **LARGE, BOLD LETTERS** when necessary.
5. Identify the anticipated therapeutic response.
6. Instruct the patient, the family members, or significant others regarding how to collect and record data to monitor the response to drugs and other treatment modalities.
7. Give the patient (or another responsible individual) a list of signs and symptoms that should be reported to the healthcare provider.
8. Stress measures that can be initiated to minimize or prevent anticipated adverse effects to the prescribed medication. It is important to do this to further encourage the patient to be compliant with the medications prescribed.

Get Ready for the NCLEX® Examination!

Key Points

- The nurse should know why a medication is ordered and its expected actions, usual dosing, proper dilution, route and rate of administration, adverse effects, and the contraindications for the use of a particular drug.
- Medications can be dispensed by use of a floor or ward stock system, an individual prescription order system, a unit-dose system, or a computer-controlled dispensing system, which uses the unit-dose system.
- Narcotic control systems include the inventory control record, a means to keep the narcotic locked separately, and ways of verifying the correct count of the drug.
- The four categories of medication orders are stat, single, standing, and PRN orders.
- Medication errors include prescribing errors, transcription or order communication errors, dispensing errors, administration errors, and errors of monitoring or education for proper use.
- The name on the medication profile should be compared with the individual's identification bracelet using two patient identifiers to ensure the right drug is given to the right patient.
- The seven rights of drug administration are as follows: right drug, right indication, right time, right dose, right patient, right route, and right documentation.
- Appropriate documentation should always have the following information: the date and time of medication administration; the name of the medication; and the dose, route, and site of administration.

Additional Learning Resources

SG Go to your Study Guide for additional Review Questions for the NCLEX® Examination, Critical Thinking Clinical Situations, and other learning activities to help you master this chapter content.

Go to your Evolve website (https://evolve.elsevier.com/Clayton) for additional online resources.

 Online Resources

- Centers for Medicare & Medicaid Services: https://www.cms.gov
- ISMP List of High-Alert Medications in Acute Care Settings: https://www.ismp.org/recommendations/high-alert-medications-acute-list
- ISMP List of High-Alert Medications in Long-Term Care (LTC) Settings: https://www.ismp.org/recommendations/high-alert-medications-long-term-care-list
- ISMP List of High-Alert Medications in Community/Ambulatory Settings: https://www.ismp.org/recommendations/high-alert-medications-community-ambulatory-list
- The Joint Commission National Patient Safety Goals: https://www.jointcommission.org/standards_information/npsgs.aspx

2354

Review Questions for the NCLEX® Examination

1. What are the legal responsibilities for correctly preparing and administering medications to patients? (*Select all that apply.*)
   1. The nurse must ensure that the patient fully understands all the effects of the medication.
   2. The nurse must understand the patient's diagnosis and symptoms correlating to the medication.
   3. The nurse must assess the patient for adverse effects of the medication.
   4. The nurse must be accurate in calculating and preparing medications.
   5. The nurse must administer all medication orders without question.

2. What are the benefits of using CPOE technology for healthcare providers? (*Select all that apply.*)
   1. It verifies the patient has received appropriate patient education.
   2. It checks for potential drug interactions.
   3. It checks associated laboratory values.
   4. It checks for the appropriateness of the drug dosages.
   5. It frees pharmacists from filling orders.

3. The nurse preparing the narcotic hydromorphone (Dilaudid) needs to get assistance from another licensed healthcare provider when what occurs?
   1. The patient takes all the medication and then becomes nauseated and vomits the drug.
   2. The medication is delivered in a dose that is more than the amount ordered.
   3. The patient states that the drug will not work and refuses to take it.
   4. The medication ordered is locked in the narcotic drawer.

4. A nurse is having difficulty reading a physician's order for a medication. The nurse knows that the physician is very busy and does not like to be called. What does the nurse do next?
   1. Calls a pharmacist to interpret the order
   2. Calls the physician to have the order clarified
   3. Consults the unit manager to help interpret the order
   4. Asks the unit secretary to interpret the physician's handwriting

5. What nursing action causes most medication errors to occur?
   1. Failing to follow routine procedures
   2. Administering numerous medications
   3. Caring for too many patients
   4. Administering unfamiliar medications

6. List in order what steps the nurse takes when preparing and administering a patient's morning medications.
   1. Document the administration of the medications.
   2. Check the order to verify the medication is correct.
   3. Obtain the medications for administration from the medication room.
   4. Identify the patient using two patient identifiers before administration.
   5. Triple-check that the correct medication was prepared.

7. What process is used to eliminate medication errors in the healthcare environment as patients transition from one clinical setting to another?
   1. Case management
   2. Transcription
   3. Verification
   4. Medication reconciliation

8. A patient complains to his nurse about heartburn. The nurse notes in the medication profile that an antacid has been ordered PRN. What will the nurse need to do next?
   1. Give the antacid immediately.
   2. Verify the last time that the drug was given and determine whether it is appropriate to give the dose now.
   3. Inform the patient that the next scheduled medications will be given in a few hours and that the drug will be given at that time.
   4. Call the physician and ask if the antacid can be given.

9. A patient refuses an essential heart medication that has been prescribed. What does the nurse do next?
   1. Calls the physician
   2. Reports it to the head nurse
   3. Seeks patient reasons
   4. Documents refusal on the MAR

10. Immediately after administering morning medications for a patient, the nurse is expected to perform which action next?
   1. Document the medications administered.
   2. Evaluate the effectiveness of the medications.
   3. Educate the patient on the adverse effects to expect.
   4. Complete the nursing care plan for the day.

7 Percutaneous Administration

Objectives

1. Identify the equipment needed and the techniques used to apply each of the topical forms of medications to the skin.
2. Describe the purpose of and the procedure used for performing patch testing.
3. Identify the equipment needed, the sites and techniques used, and the patient education required when nitroglycerin ointment is prescribed.
4. Identify the equipment needed, the sites and techniques used, and the patient education required when transdermal patch medication systems are prescribed.
5. Describe the dose forms, the sites and equipment used, and the techniques for the administration of medications to the mucous membranes.

6. Compare the techniques that are used to administer eardrops to patients who are less than 3 years old with those that are used for patients who are 3 years and older.
7. Describe the purpose, the precautions necessary, and the patient education required for those patients who require medications via inhalation.
8. Identify the equipment needed, the site, and the specific techniques required to administer vaginal medications or douches.

Key Terms

creams (KRĒMZ) (p. 82)
lotions (LŌ-shŭnz) (p. 82)
aqueous (Ā-kwē-ŭs) (p. 82)
ointments (ŌYNT-mĕnts) (p. 83)
dressings (DRĔS-ĭngz) (p. 83)
patch testing (PĂCH) (p. 84)
allergens (ĂL-ĕr-jĕnz) (p. 84)
transdermal patch (p. 87)

buccal (BŬK-ăl) (p. 89)
ophthalmic (ŏf-THĂL-mĭk) (p. 90)
otic (Ō-tĭk) (p. 91)
aerosols (ĂR-ō-sŏlz) (p. 95)
metered-dose inhaler (MDI) (MĒ-tŭrd DŌS ĭn-HĀL-ŭr) (p. 96)
dry powder inhaler (DPI) (DRĪ PŎW-dŭr ĭn-HĀL-ŭr) (p. 96)

The routes of drug administration can be classified into three categories: enteral, parenteral, and percutaneous. The term *percutaneous administration* refers to the application of medications to the skin or mucous membranes for absorption. The absorption of topical medications can be influenced by the drug's concentration, how long the medication is in contact with the skin, the size of the affected area, the thickness of the skin, the hydration of the tissues, and the degree of skin disruption. Methods of percutaneous administration include the following: the topical application of ointments, creams, powders, or lotions to the skin; the instillation of solutions onto the mucous membranes of the mouth, eye, ear, nose, or vagina; and the inhalation of aerosolized liquids or gases for absorption through the lungs. The primary advantage of the percutaneous route is that the action of the drug, in general, is localized to the site of application, which reduces the incidence of systemic side effects.

Unfortunately, the medications are sometimes messy and difficult to apply. In addition, they usually have a short duration of action and thus require frequent reapplication.

ADMINISTRATION OF TOPICAL MEDICATIONS TO THE SKIN

DOSE FORMS

Creams

Creams are semisolid emulsions that contain medicinal agents for external application. The cream base is generally nongreasy, and it can be removed with water. Many over-the-counter creams are used as moisturizing agents.

Lotions

Lotions are aqueous (water-based) preparations that contain suspended materials. Lotions are commonly used as soothing agents to protect the skin and to relieve rashes and itching. Some lotions have a cleansing action, whereas others have an astringent or drawing effect. Lotions should be gently but firmly patted on the skin rather than rubbed into the skin to prevent increased circulation and itching. Shake all lotions thoroughly immediately before application, and use them sparingly to avoid waste.

Ointments

Ointments are semisolid preparations of medicinal substances in an oily base, such as lanolin or petrolatum. This type of preparation can be applied directly to the skin or mucous membrane, and it generally cannot be removed easily with water. The base helps to keep the medicinal substance in prolonged contact with the skin.

DRESSINGS

Several types of dressings are used to treat wounds, such as dry gauze sponges, nonadherent gauze dressings (e.g., Telfa), self-adhesive transparent films that act as a second skin (e.g., Tegaderm), and hydrocolloid dressings (e.g., DuoDERM). Hydrogel dressings are used on partial-thickness and full-thickness wounds and on skin that has been damaged by burns. There are also exudate absorbers such as calcium alginate dressings (e.g., AlgiDERM, Kaltostat, Sorbsan) manufactured from seaweed that can be used on infected wounds.

Wound care products and wound care have become a complex science. (Refer to fundamentals of nursing, medical-surgical nursing, and geriatric nursing textbooks for discussions of the principles of wound care.) Dressing recommendations for treating pressure ulcers are available from the Agency for Healthcare Research and Quality, the US Public Health Service, and the US Department of Health and Human Services.

 Clinical Goldmine

A major principle of wound healing is the need for a moist environment to promote the epithelialization of the wound, which is further enhanced by a diet that is high in protein, vitamin A, vitamin C, and zinc.

PROCEDURE PROTOCOL

The term *procedure protocol* will be used as part of the medication administration technique for the sections in this chapter. This term includes the following nursing interventions:

1. Assemble the appropriate equipment and then perform hand hygiene.
2. Use the *seven rights* of drug preparation and administration throughout the procedure: right patient, right drug, right indication, right route, right dose, right time, and right documentation.
3. Provide privacy for the patient and give a thorough explanation of the procedure and what to expect.

4. Perform a premedication assessment before applying any topical preparation. See individual drug monographs for more information.

ADMINISTRATION OF CREAMS, LOTIONS, AND OINTMENTS

Topical preparations can be used to do the following:
- Cleanse and debride a wound
- Rehydrate the skin
- Reduce inflammation
- Relieve localized signs and symptoms, such as itching and rash
- Provide a protective barrier
- Reduce a thickening of the skin, such as that involved with callus formation

EQUIPMENT

- Prescribed cream, lotion, or ointment
- 2 × 2-inch gauze sponges
- Cotton-tipped applicators
- Tongue blade
- Gloves
- Medication administration record (MAR) and medication profile

SITES

Skin surfaces affected by the disorder being treated.

TECHNIQUES

1. Follow the procedure protocol described earlier.
2. Position the patient so that the surface where the topical materials are to be applied is exposed. Assess the current status of the patient's symptoms. Provide for patient comfort before starting therapy.
3. *Cleansing:* Follow the specific orders of the healthcare provider or clinical site policies for cleansing the site of application. After the area is exposed and cleansed, perform a wound assessment.
4. *Application:* Wear gloves during the application process. Many of the agents used may be absorbed through the skin of both the patient and the person who is applying the medication.
   - *Lotions:* Shake well until a uniform appearance of the suspension is obtained. Apply lotion firmly but gently by dabbing the surface. Use gloves with medicated lotions.
   - *Ointments or creams:* Use a tongue blade to remove the desired amount from a wide-mouthed container. Alternatively, squeeze the amount needed onto a tongue blade or cotton-tipped applicator from a tube-type container. Apply ointments and creams with a gloved hand using firm but gentle strokes. Creams are to be gently rubbed into the area.
5. *Dressings:* Check specific orders regarding the type of dressing to be used. If a dressing is to be applied, spread the prescribed amount of ointment directly

onto the dressing material with a tongue blade; the impregnated dressing material can then be applied to the affected skin surface. Secure the dressing in place.

6. *Wet dressings:* Always completely remove the previous dressing. Wring out wet dressings to prevent dripping, and apply the gauze in a single layer directly to the wound surface. For deeper wounds, pack the wound loosely with moist gauze sponges so that all surfaces are in contact with the moisture. Apply a layer of dry gauze sponges and an absorbent pad to the area. To secure a dressing that requires repeated changes, apply a binder or use Montgomery tapes.

7. Clean the area and the equipment used, and make sure that the patient is comfortable after the application procedure. (NOTE: Sterile supplies, gloves, and equipment are used for some wounds; however, clean rather than sterile items [e.g., gauze, gloves] may be used when applying most types of dressings [e.g., to a pressure ulcer]. Always check institutional policies and use clinical judgment.)

8. Remove gloves and dispose of them in accordance with institutional policy.

9. Perform hand hygiene.

PATIENT TEACHING

1. If appropriate, teach the patient how to apply the medication and dressings.

2. Teach personal hygiene measures that are appropriate to the underlying cause of the skin condition (e.g., acne, contact dermatitis, infection).

3. When dressings are ordered, suggest the purchase of gauze and other necessary supplies.

4. Stress gentleness and moderation with regard to the amount of medication to be applied.

5. Emphasize that the patient must avoid touching or scratching the affected area.

6. Tell the patient to wash his or her hands before and after touching the affected area or applying the medication. Stress the prevention of the spread of infection.

DOCUMENTATION

Provide the right documentation of the medication administered and the patient's response to drug therapy.

1. Chart the date, time, drug name, dosage, and route of administration.

2. Perform and record regular patient assessments for the evaluation of the treatment's therapeutic effectiveness (e.g., change in size of affected area, reduced drainage, decreased itching, lowered temperature with an infection).

3. On the patient's record, document any signs and symptoms of adverse drug effects, and provide a narrative description of the area being treated.

4. Develop a written record for the patient to use when charting progress for the evaluation of the effectiveness of the treatments being used. List the patient's symptoms (e.g., rash on the lower leg with redness and vesicles present, decubitus ulcer on the sacrum). List the data to be collected regarding the medication prescribed and its effectiveness (e.g., vesicles now crusted, weeping, or appear to be drying; redness in lower leg is lessening; measure the area of decubitus in centimeters [cm] and indicate if the wound is extending, remaining the same, or shrinking).

5. Educate the patient on what to expect and what to do if adverse symptoms develop.

PATCH TESTING FOR ALLERGENS

Patch testing is a method that is used to identify a patient's sensitivity to contact materials (e.g., soaps, pollens, dyes). The suspected **allergens** (antigens) are placed in direct contact with the skin surface and covered with nonsensitizing, nonabsorbent tape. Unless pronounced irritation appears, the patch is usually left in place for 48 hours and then removed. The site is left open to air for 15 minutes and then "read." A positive reaction is noted by the presence of redness and swelling, called a *wheal,* which indicates an allergy to the specific allergen. It may be necessary to read the areas after 3 days and again after 7 days to detect delayed reactions.

Intradermal tests may also be used to determine the patient's allergy to specific antigens. See Chapter 10 for more information about the intradermal administration of allergens.

Perform pretesting assessments (see information provided with supplied allergen solutions).

EQUIPMENT

- Alcohol for cleansing the area
- Solutions of suspected antigens
- 1 × 1-inch gauze pads
- Droppers
- Mineral or olive oil
- Water
- Clippers
- Hypoallergenic tape
- Record for charting data about the substances applied and the patient's responses
- MAR, computer profile, or order sheet

SITES

The back, arms, or thighs are commonly used. (*Do not* apply to the face or areas that are susceptible to friction from clothing.) Selected areas are spaced 2 to 3 inches apart. The type of allergen applied and the site of application are documented on the patient's chart (Fig. 7.1). Hair is clipped from sites to ensure that the allergen is kept in close contact with the skin surface, thereby preventing a false-negative reaction.

TECHNIQUE

CAUTION: Do not start any type of allergy testing unless emergency equipment (including epinephrine) is

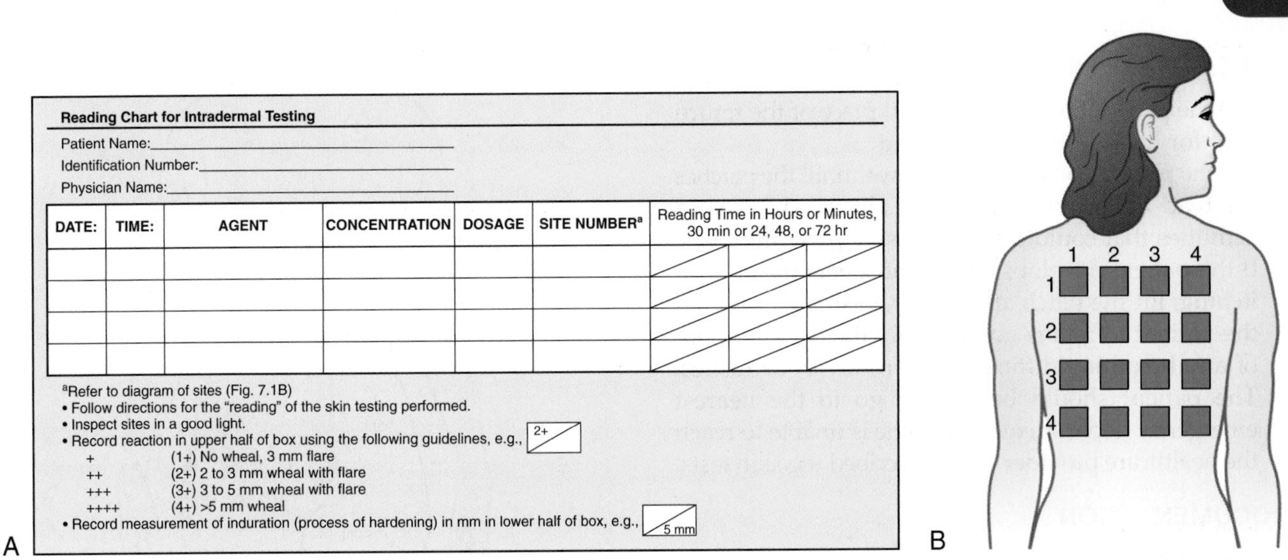

Reading Chart for Intradermal Testing

Patient Name:_____

Identification Number:_____

Physician Name:_____

DATE:	TIME:	AGENT	CONCENTRATION	DOSAGE	SITE NUMBER[a]	Reading Time in Hours or Minutes, 30 min or 24, 48, or 72 hr		

[a]Refer to diagram of sites (Fig. 7.1B)
- Follow directions for the "reading" of the skin testing performed.
- Inspect sites in a good light.
- Record reaction in upper half of box using the following guidelines, e.g.,
  - +   (1+) No wheal, 3 mm flare
  - ++   (2+) 2 to 3 mm wheal with flare
  - +++   (3+) 3 to 5 mm wheal with flare
  - ++++   (4+) >5 mm wheal
- Record measurement of induration (process of hardening) in mm in lower half of box, e.g.,

Fig. 7.1 Patch test for contact dermatitis. (A) Reading chart for patch testing. (B) Patch testing sites.

available in the immediate area in case of an anaphylactic response. Nurses should be familiar with the procedure to follow if an emergency does arise.

1. Follow the procedure protocol described earlier.
2. Check with the patient before starting the testing to ensure that no antihistamines or antiinflammatory agents (e.g., aspirin, ibuprofen, diphenhydramine, corticosteroids) have been taken for 24 to 48 hours before the test. If the patient has taken an antihistamine or an antiinflammatory agent, consult the healthcare provider before proceeding with the testing. Review the chart to ensure that the patient is not in an immunocompromised state as a result of disease or treatments such as chemotherapy or radiation therapy.
3. Position the patient so that the surface on which the test materials are to be applied is horizontal. Provide for the patient's comfort before beginning the testing.
4. Cleanse the selected testing area thoroughly with the use of an alcohol wipe. Use circular motions, starting at the planned site of application and continuing outward to the periphery. Allow the area to air-dry.
5. Prepare the designated solutions using aseptic technique (this refers to being mindful about preventing contamination of the solution by using only clean or sterile application methods).
6. Follow the specific directions of the employing healthcare agency regarding the application of liquid and solid forms of suspected allergens. A dropper is usually used to apply suspected liquid contact–type materials; solid materials are applied directly to the skin surface and then moistened with mineral or olive oil. The following methods may be used:
   - Designated amounts of standardized-strength chemical solutions are arranged in metal receptacles that are backed with hypoallergenic adhesive. These solutions are then applied to the selected sites. It is important to identify the contents of each receptacle correctly.
   - Patches that are impregnated with designated allergens are available for direct application to the prepared sites.
   - A patch test series kit is available that contains nonirritating concentrations of allergens that are packaged in syringes for dispersal. Although the kit contains 20 allergens, any number of them may be applied to individual patches or holding devices, which are then applied to the patient's skin.
   - After application, follow institutional policy for covering the test site.
7. Chart the times, agents, concentrations, and amounts applied. Make a diagram in the patient's chart, and number each location (see Fig. 7.1B). Record which agent and concentration were placed at each site (see Fig. 7.1A). Subsequent readings of each area are then performed and charted on this record.
8. Follow directions regarding the time of the reading of the skin testing being performed. The testing sites should be inspected in good light. Generally, a positive reaction (i.e., the development of a wheal) to a diluted strength of a suspected allergen is considered clinically significant. Measure the diameter of the wheal and any erythema (i.e., redness at the site of injection) in millimeters, and palpate and measure the size of any induration (i.e., the hardening of an area of the body in response inflammation). The control site should have no reaction, which should be noted.
9. Record the information from the skin test reading in the patient's chart. The following is a list of commonly used readings of reactions and their appropriate symbols:

+	(1+)	No wheal, 3-mm flare
++	(2+)	2- to 3-mm wheal with flare
+++	(3+)	3- to 5-mm wheal with flare
++++	(4+)	>5-mm wheal

PATIENT TEACHING

1. Tell the patient the time, date, and place of the return visit for having the test sites read.
2. Tell the patient not to bathe or shower until the patches are read and removed. Explain the need to avoid activities that could cause excessive perspiration.
3. If the patient develops an area of severe burning or itching, lift the patch and gently wash the area. Tell the patient to report immediately the development of any breathing difficulty, severe hives, or rashes. The patient should be told to go to the nearest emergency department if he or she is unable to reach the healthcare provider who prescribed the skin tests.

DOCUMENTATION

Provide the right documentation of the allergen testing sites and the patient's responses to the allergens that were applied.

1. Chart the date, time, allergens (including agent, concentration, and dosage), and site of administration (see Fig. 7.1A).
2. Read each site at 24, 48, and 72 hours after application as directed by the healthcare provider or the policy of the healthcare agency. Additional readings may be required for up to 7 days after application.
3. Chart and report any signs and symptoms of adverse allergen effects.
4. Perform and validate essential patient education regarding the testing and other essential aspects of intervention for the allergy that is affecting the individual.

ADMINISTRATION OF NITROGLYCERIN OINTMENT

DOSE FORM

Nitroglycerin ointment (Nitro-Bid) provides relief of anginal pain for several hours longer than sublingual preparations. When properly applied, nitroglycerin ointment is particularly effective against nocturnal attacks of anginal pain. Specific instructions for nitroglycerin ointment are reviewed in this text because it is the only ointment that is currently available for which dosage is critical to the success of use (see Chapter 24).

Perform premedication assessment; see individual drug monograph for details.

EQUIPMENT

- Clean gloves
- Nitroglycerin ointment
- Applicator paper
- Nonallergenic adhesive tape
- MAR and medication profile

SITES

Any area without hair may be used. Most people prefer the chest, flank, or upper arm area. Develop a rotation schedule for use of the ointment (Fig. 7.2). *Do not* shave

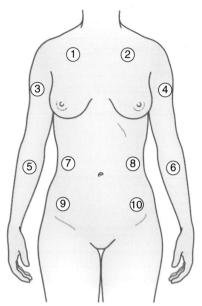

Fig. 7.2 Sites for nitroglycerin application; numbering indicates rotation schedule.

an area to apply the ointment; shaving may cause skin irritation.

TECHNIQUE

1. Follow the procedure protocol described earlier.
2. Apply clean gloves.
3. Position the patient so that the surface to which the topical material is to be applied is exposed. Provide for the patient's comfort before starting therapy. (NOTE: When reapplying ointment, first remove the plastic wrap and dose-measuring applicator paper from the previous dose, and cleanse the area of remaining ointment on the skin surface. Select a new site for the application of the medication, and then proceed with steps 4 through 7.)
4. Lay the dose-measuring applicator paper with the print side *down* on a flat surface (Fig. 7.3A). The ointment will smear the print.
5. Squeeze a ribbon of ointment of the proper length onto the applicator paper.
6. Place the measuring applicator paper on the skin surface at the site chosen on the rotation schedule, ointment side *down*. Spread in a thin, uniform layer under the applicator. DO NOT RUB IN. Leave the paper in place. NOTE: Use of the applicator paper allows you to measure the prescribed dose and prevents absorption through the fingertips as you apply the medication (see Fig. 7.3B).
7. Cover the area where the paper is placed in accordance with institutional policy (this may include covering the paper with plastic wrap), and then tape the paper in place.
8. Remove gloves and dispose of them in accordance with institutional policy.
9. Perform hand hygiene.

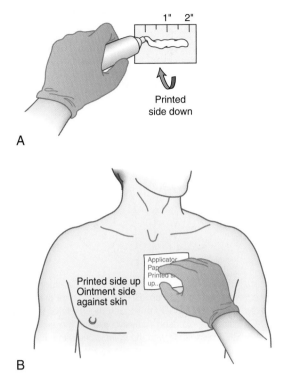

Fig. 7.3 Administering nitroglycerin topical ointment. (A) Lay the applicator paper print-side down on a hard surface and measure the ribbon of ointment. (B) Apply the applicator to the skin site, ointment-side down. Spread the ointment in a uniform layer under the applicator, and leave the paper in place.

Clinical Pitfall

Applying Nitroglycerin Ointment

To promote personal safety, the nurse should always wear gloves, whether applying nitroglycerin ointment paper or handling transdermal patches. When nitroglycerin transdermal patches are applied, chart the specific site of the application. Occasionally, patients may move the transdermal patch themselves because of convenience, skin irritation, or confusion. If the patch is not found at the original location at the scheduled time of removal, examine other areas of the body to find it; do not assume that the patch fell off or was removed. Tolerance and loss of antianginal response could develop if another patch is placed on the patient while the first patch is still on. Always dispose of used nitroglycerin paper or transdermal patches in a receptacle in which the patient, children, and pets will not have access. A substantial amount of nitroglycerin remains on the patch and can be toxic.

PATIENT TEACHING

1. Help the patient learn how to apply the ointment and ensure that the patient understands the site rotation schedule.
2. Tell the patient that the medication may discolor clothing. The use of clear plastic wrap protects clothing.
3. When the dosage is regulated properly, the ointment may be used every 3 to 4 hours and at bedtime. Remind the patient that there should be a drug-free period (usually 10 to 12 hours) every 24 hours as recommended by the healthcare provider.

4. Tell the patient to wash her or his hands after application to remove any nitroglycerin that came into contact with the fingers.
5. When terminating the use of this topical ointment, the dosage and frequency of application should be gradually reduced over a 4- to 6-week period. Tell the patient to contact the healthcare provider if adjustment is thought to be necessary. Encourage the patient not to discontinue the medication abruptly (see Chapter 24).

DOCUMENTATION

Provide the right documentation of the medication administration and the patient's responses to drug therapy.

1. Chart the date, time, drug name, dosage, site, and route of administration.
2. Perform and record regular patient assessments for the evaluation of therapeutic effectiveness (e.g., blood pressure, pulse, output, degree and duration of pain relief on a scale of 0 to 10).
3. Chart and report any signs and symptoms of adverse drug effects.
4. Perform and validate essential patient education about the drug therapy and other important aspects of intervention for the disease process that is affecting the individual.

ADMINISTRATION OF TRANSDERMAL DRUG DELIVERY SYSTEMS

DOSE FORM

The **transdermal patch** (also called a transdermal disk) provides for the controlled release of a prescribed medication (e.g., nitroglycerin, clonidine, estrogen, nicotine, scopolamine, fentanyl) through a semipermeable membrane for several hours to 3 weeks when applied to intact skin. The dose released depends on the surface area of the patch in contact with the skin surface and the individual drug. See specific drug monographs for the onset and duration of action of drugs that use this delivery system.

Perform premedication assessment; see individual drug monographs for details.

EQUIPMENT

- Clean gloves
- Transdermal patch
- Clipping equipment as appropriate for the site and the patient's skin condition
- MAR and medication profile

SITES

Any area without hair may be used. Most people prefer the chest, flank, or upper arm. Develop a rotation schedule for use of the patch (see Fig. 7.2 for an example of a nitroglycerin rotation schedule). See manufacturer's recommendations for location and frequency of application of patches other than nitroglycerin.

TECHNIQUE

1. Follow the procedure protocol described earlier.
2. Label the patch with the date, the time, and the nurse's initials. If the dosage of the medication is not printed on the patch applied, it is useful to include the dosage as part of the labeling process.
3. Apply clean gloves.
4. Position the patient so that the surface on which the topical materials are to be applied is exposed. Provide for the patient's comfort. (NOTE: When reapplying a transdermal patch, remove the old patch and cleanse the skin thoroughly. Select a new site for application. It is especially important in the older adult or the confused patient to look for the old patch if it is not where the prior application is charted. The confused patient may have moved it elsewhere on the body or removed it. The old patch can be encased in the glove as the nurse removes it; this should then be disposed of according to institutional policy.)
5. Apply the small adhesive topical patch. Fig. 7.4 illustrates nitroglycerin being applied to one of the sites recommended by the rotation schedule. The frequency of application depends on the specific medication being applied via the transdermal patch and the duration of action of the prescribed medication. Nitroglycerin is applied once daily, whereas fentanyl is reapplied every 3 days; clonidine and ethinyl estradiol/norelgestromin (Ortho Evra) are reapplied once every 7 days. Hormone replacement therapies may be applied every 4 to 7 days.
6. Remove gloves and dispose of them in accordance with institutional policy.
7. Perform hand hygiene.

PATIENT TEACHING

1. Teach the patient how and when to apply the patches. NOTE: Certain products may be worn while showering; others should be replaced after bathing or showering. Refer to the patient education instructions for specific application directions. Scopolamine, which is used for motion sickness, must be applied at least 4 hours before travel; clonidine transdermal systems are applied once every 7 days. Ortho Evra is a contraceptive patch that is reapplied weekly for 3 weeks, with the fourth week being patch free; a new patch as the first in another cycle of three patches starts the following week.
2. If a patch becomes partially dislodged, the recommendations for the product should be followed. A nitroglycerin patch is removed, and a new one is applied. Alternatively, clonidine transdermal patches come with a protective adhesive overlay to be applied over the patch to ensure skin contact with the transdermal system if the patch becomes loosened. See

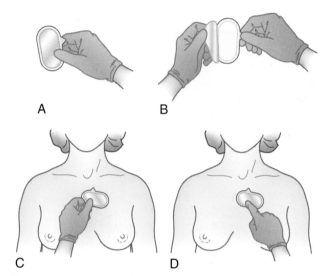

Fig. 7.4 Applying a nitroglycerin topical patch. (A) Carefully pick up the system lengthwise, with the tab up. (B) Remove the clear plastic backing from the system at the tab. Do not touch the inside of the exposed system. (C) Place the exposed adhesive side of the system on the chosen skin site. Press firmly with the palm of the hand. (D) Circle the outside edge of the system with one or two fingers.

Chapter 40 for further information about the Ortho Evra patch.
3. Patients who are receiving nitroglycerin transdermally may require sublingual nitroglycerin for anginal attacks, especially while the dose is being adjusted. In general, nitroglycerin patches are worn for 10 to 14 hours; this is followed by a drug-free period of 10 to 12 hours so that the nitroglycerin will maintain its effectiveness.
4. Fentanyl (Duragesic) may take up to 12 hours after application to be effective for the management of stable, chronic pain. Therefore it should be combined with a short-acting pain medication until a sufficient blood level of the fentanyl is achieved. Fentanyl patches are changed every 3 days. Breakthrough pain should be promptly reported to the healthcare provider. It may be necessary to increase the dosage to achieve a satisfactory level of pain relief.

DOCUMENTATION

Provide the right documentation of the medication administration and the patient's responses to the drug therapy.

1. Chart the date, time, drug name, dosage, route of administration, and location of patch.
2. Perform and record regular patient assessments for the evaluation of therapeutic effectiveness (e.g., blood pressure, pulse, degree and duration of pain relief on a scale of 0 to 10).
3. Chart and report any signs and symptoms of adverse drug effects.
4. Perform and validate essential patient education regarding the drug therapy and other essential aspects of intervention for the disease process that is affecting the individual.

ADMINISTRATION OF TOPICAL POWDERS

DOSE FORM

Powders are finely ground particles of medication that are contained in a talc base. They generally produce a cooling, drying, or protective effect where applied.

Perform premedication assessment; see individual drug monographs for details.

EQUIPMENT

- Clean gloves
- Prescribed powder
- MAR and medication profile

SITE

Apply to the skin surface of the body as prescribed.

TECHNIQUE

1. Follow the procedure protocol described earlier.
2. Apply clean gloves.
3. Position the patient so that the surface on which the topical materials are to be applied is exposed. Provide for the patient's comfort before starting therapy.
4. Wash and thoroughly dry the affected area before applying the powder.
5. Apply powder by gently shaking the container to distribute the powder evenly over the area. Gently smooth over the area for even coverage.
6. Remove gloves and dispose of them in accordance with institutional policy.
7. Perform hand hygiene.

PATIENT TEACHING

Tell the patient to cleanse the area of administration and then reapply the powder to the external surface as directed by the healthcare provider. The patient should avoid inhaling the powder during application.

DOCUMENTATION

Provide the right documentation of the medication administration and of the patient's responses to drug therapy.
1. Chart the date, time, drug name, dosage, site, and route of administration.
2. Perform and record regular patient assessments for the evaluation of therapeutic effectiveness.
3. Chart and report any signs and symptoms of adverse drug effects.
4. Perform and validate essential patient education regarding the drug therapy and other essential aspects of intervention for the disease process that is affecting the individual.

ADMINISTRATION OF MEDICATIONS TO MUCOUS MEMBRANES

Drugs are well absorbed across mucosal surfaces, and therapeutic effects are easily obtained. However, mucous membranes are highly selective with regard to absorptive activity, and they differ in sensitivity. In general, aqueous solutions are quickly absorbed from mucous membranes, whereas oily liquids are not. Drugs in suppository form can be used for local or systemic effects on the mucous membranes of the vagina, the urethra, or the rectum. A drug may be inhaled and absorbed through the mucous membranes of the nose and lungs. It may be dissolved and absorbed by the mucous membranes of the mouth or applied to the eyes or ears for local action. It may be painted, swabbed, or irrigated on a mucosal surface.

ADMINISTRATION OF SUBLINGUAL AND BUCCAL TABLETS

DOSE FORMS

Sublingual tablets are designed to be placed under the tongue for dissolution and absorption through the vast network of blood vessels in this area. Buccal tablets are designed to be held in the buccal cavity (i.e., between the cheek and the lower molar teeth) for absorption from the blood vessels of the cheek. The primary advantages of these routes of administration are the associated rapid absorption and onset of action: the drug passes directly into the systemic circulation, with no immediate pass through to the liver, where extensive metabolism usually takes place. As opposed to most other forms of administration to the mucous membranes, the action from these dose forms is usually systemic rather than localized to the mouth.

Perform premedication assessment; see individual drug monographs for details.

EQUIPMENT

- Prescribed medication (NOTE: The medications available to be administered by this route are forms of nitroglycerin. After the self-administration technique is taught, the patient should carry the medication or keep it readily available at the bedside for use as needed.)
- MAR and medication profile

SITE

Administer at the sublingual area (i.e., under the tongue; Fig. 7.5A) or the buccal pouch (i.e., between the lower molar teeth and the cheek; Fig. 7.5B).

TECHNIQUE

1. Follow the procedure protocol described earlier.
2. Put on a clean glove, and place the medication under the patient's tongue (i.e., sublingual; see Fig. 7.5A) or between the patient's lower molar teeth and his or her cheek (i.e., buccal; see Fig. 7.5B). The tablet is meant to dissolve in these locations. *Do not* administer the medication with water. Encourage the patient to allow the drug to dissolve where placed and to hold saliva in the mouth until the tablet is dissolved.

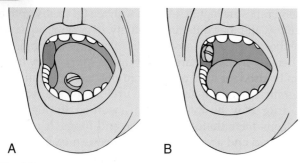

Fig. 7.5 Placing medication in the mouth. (A) Under the tongue (sublingual). (B) In the buccal pouch.

3. Remove the glove and dispose of it in accordance with institutional policy.
4. Perform hand hygiene.

PATIENT TEACHING

Explain the exact placement of the medication, the dosage, and the frequency of doses. The patient should be informed of adverse effects, where to carry the medication, how to store the medication, the medication's expiration date, and how to refill the prescription when needed.

DOCUMENTATION

Provide the right documentation of the medication administration and the patient's responses to drug therapy.
1. Chart the date, time, drug name, dose, site, and route of administration.
2. Perform and record regular patient assessments for the evaluation of therapeutic effectiveness (e.g., blood pressure, pulse, degree and duration of pain relief, number of doses taken).
3. Chart and report any signs and symptoms of adverse drug effects.
4. Perform and validate essential patient education about the drug therapy and other essential aspects of intervention for the disease process that is affecting the individual.

NOTE: When the patient is self-administering a medication, the nurse is still responsible for all aspects of the charting and monitoring parameters to document the drug therapy and the response achieved.

ADMINISTRATION OF EYEDROPS AND OINTMENT

DOSE FORM

Medications for use in the eye are labeled *ophthalmic*. If a drug is not labeled as such, it should not be administered to the eye. Ophthalmic solutions are sterile and easily administered, and they usually do not interfere with vision when they are instilled. Allow eye medication to warm to room temperature before administration.

Ophthalmic ointments do cause alterations in visual acuity. However, they have a longer duration of action than solutions. Always use a separate bottle or tube of eye medication for each patient.

Perform premedication assessment; see individual drug monographs for details.

EQUIPMENT

- Clean gloves
- Eyedrops, ointment prescribed (check strength carefully)
- Dropper (use only the dropper supplied by the manufacturer)
- Tissues and sterile eye dressing (pad), as appropriate
- Normal saline solution, if needed, for cleaning off exudates
- MAR and medication profile

SITE

Eye(s)

TECHNIQUES

1. Follow the procedure protocol described earlier.
2. Assemble the ophthalmic medication and equipment. Ensure that the medication is labeled for "Ophthalmic" or "Eye" use.
3. Position the patient so that the back of his or her head is firmly supported on a pillow and so his or her face is directed toward the ceiling. With a child, restraints may be necessary if the child is too young to cooperate voluntarily. Always ensure patient safety.
4. Apply clean gloves.
5. Inspect the affected eye to determine the current status. As appropriate, remove exudate from the eyelid and eyelashes with the use of sterile saline solution. A clean washcloth may be used, with a separate part of the cloth used for each eye. Start at the inner canthus and wipe outward.
6. Expose the lower conjunctival sac by applying gentle traction to the lower lid at the bony rim of the orbit.
7. Approach the eye from below with the medication dropper or tube of ointment. (Never touch the eyedropper or ointment tip to the eye or the face.)

Instilling Drops
- Have the patient look upward over your head (Fig. 7.6).
- Drop the specified number of drops into the conjunctival sac. Never drop the medication directly onto the eyeball.
- After instilling the drops, apply gentle pressure using a clean tissue to the inner canthus of the eyelid against the bone for approximately 1 to 2 minutes. This prevents the medication from entering the canal, where it would be absorbed in the vascular mucosa of the nose and produce systemic effects. It also ensures an adequate concentration of medication in the eye.
- When more than one type of eyedrop is ordered for the same eye, wait 1 to 5 minutes between the

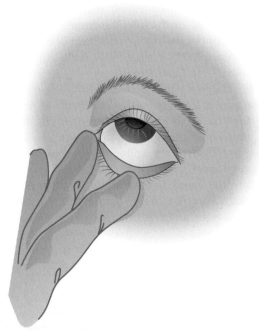

Fig. 7.6 To administer ophthalmic drops, gently pull down the skin below the eye to expose the conjunctival sac. (From Kee JL, Hayes ER, McCuistion LE. *Pharmacology: A Nursing Process Approach.* 7th ed. St. Louis: Saunders; 2012.)

instillation of the different medications. Use only the dropper provided by the manufacturer. Apply a sterile dressing as ordered.

Applying Ointment
- Gently squeeze the ointment in a strip fashion into the conjunctival sac (Fig. 7.7), from the inner canthus to the outer canthus. *Do not* allow the tip of the medication dispenser to touch the patient.
- Tell the patient to close the eyes gently and to move the eyes with the lids shut, as if looking around the room, to spread the medication.
8. At the conclusion of either procedure, remove gloves and dispose of them in accordance with institutional policy.
9. Perform hand hygiene.

PATIENT TEACHING
1. Teach the patient how to apply his or her own ophthalmic medication.
2. Tell the patient to wipe the eyes gently from the nose outward to prevent contamination between the eyes, as well as the possible spread of infection, and to use a separate tissue to wipe each eye.
3. Have the patient wash his or her hands often and avoid touching the eyes or the immediate surrounding areas, especially when an infection is present. Dispose of tissues in a manner that prevents the spread of infection.
4. Stress punctuality with regard to the administration of eye medications, especially when the medications are being used to treat infections or increased intraocular pressure.

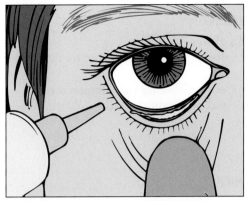

Fig. 7.7 Administering ophthalmic ointment. To instill the ointment, gently pull the lower lid down as the patient looks upward. Squeeze the ophthalmic ointment into the lower sac. Avoid touching the tube to the eyelid.

5. Tell the patient to discard eye medications that have changed color or become cloudy or that contain particles. (If the patient's visual acuity is reduced, someone else should check the medications for clarity.)
6. The patient must not use over-the-counter eyewashes without first consulting the healthcare provider who is managing the eye disorder.
7. Emphasize the need for the careful follow-up examination of any eye disorder until the healthcare provider releases the patient from further care.

DOCUMENTATION
Provide the right documentation of the medication administration and the patient's responses to drug therapy.
1. Chart the date, time, drug name, dosage, site, and route of administration.
2. Perform and record regular patient assessments for the evaluation of therapeutic effectiveness (e.g., redness, discomfort, visual acuity, changes in infection or inflammatory reaction, degree and duration of pain relief).
3. Chart and report any signs and symptoms of adverse drug effects.
4. Perform and validate essential patient education about the drug therapy and other essential aspects of intervention for the disease process that is affecting the individual.

ADMINISTRATION OF EARDROPS

DOSE FORM
Eardrops are a solution that contains a medication that is used for the treatment of localized infection or inflammation of the ear. Medications for use in the ear are labeled *otic*. If a drug is not labeled as such, it should not be administered to the ear. Eardrops should be warmed to room temperature before use, and a separate bottle of eardrops should be used for each patient.

Perform premedication assessment; see individual drug monographs for details.

EQUIPMENT

- Clean gloves
- Otic solution prescribed. Ensure that it is labeled for use
- Dropper provided by the manufacturer
- MAR and medication profile

SITE

Ear(s)

TECHNIQUE

1. Follow the procedure protocol described earlier.
2. Assemble the otic medication and dropper. Ensure that the medication is labeled for "Otic" or "Ear" use. Allow the medication to warm to room temperature.
2. Position the patient so that the affected ear is directed upward.
3. Review the policy of the practice setting and follow guidelines regarding whether gloves are to be worn during the instillation of ear medications. Apply clean gloves in accordance with institutional policy.
4. Assess the ear canal for wax accumulation. If wax is present, obtain an order to irrigate the canal before instilling the eardrops.
5. Shake the medication well and then draw it up into the dropper.
6. Administer the medication.
   - For children who are less than 3 years old, restrain the child, turn the child's head to the appropriate side, and then gently pull the lower earlobe *downward* and *back* (Fig. 7.8A) to straighten the external auditory canal. Instill the prescribed number of drops into the canal. Do not allow the dropper tip to touch any part of the ear. After administration, press gently on the tragus to help disperse the medicine.
   - For children who are more than 3 years old and for adults, enlist cooperation or restrain as necessary. Turn the head to the appropriate side, and then gently pull the upper earlobe *vertically* and *back* (Fig. 7.8B) to straighten the external auditory canal. Instill the prescribed number of drops into the canal. Do not allow the dropper tip to touch any part of the ear. After administration, press gently on the tragus to help disperse the medicine.
7. Instruct the patient to remain on his or her side for a few minutes after instillation; insert a cotton plug *loosely*, if ordered.
8. If eardrops are ordered for both ears, allow 5 to 10 minutes between administrations with the ear that received the medicine first remaining "up." Then repeat the procedure in the other ear.
9. Remove gloves and dispose of them in accordance with institutional policy.
10. Perform hand hygiene.

Clinical Goldmine

Remember, for children who are less than 3 years old, pull the lower earlobe downward and back. For adults and children who are 3 years old and older, pull the upper earlobe up and back (see Fig. 7.8).

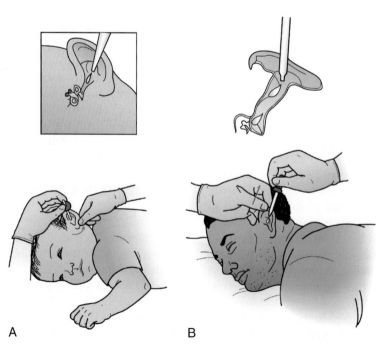

Fig. 7.8 Administering eardrops. (A) Pull the lower earlobe downward and back for children who are less than 3 years old. (B) Pull the upper earlobe upward and back for patients who are more than 3 years old.

PATIENT TEACHING

1. Explain the importance of administering the medication as prescribed.
2. Teach the patient self-administration, or teach the administration technique to another person, as appropriate.

DOCUMENTATION

Provide the right documentation of the medication administration and the patient's responses to drug therapy.

1. Chart the date, time, drug name, dosage, site, and route of administration.
2. Perform and record regular patient assessments for the evaluation of therapeutic effectiveness (e.g., redness, pressure, degree and duration of pain relief, color and amount of drainage).
3. Chart and report any signs and symptoms of adverse drug effects.
4. Perform and validate essential patient education about the drug therapy and other essential aspects of intervention for the disease process that is affecting the individual.

ADMINISTRATION OF NOSE DROPS

Nasal solutions are used to treat temporary disorders that affect the nasal mucous membranes. Always use the dropper provided by the manufacturer, and give each patient a separate bottle of nose drops.

Perform premedication assessment; see individual drug monographs for details.

EQUIPMENT

- Clean gloves
- Nose drops prescribed
- Dropper supplied by the manufacturer
- Tissue to blow the nose
- Penlight
- MAR and medication profile

SITE

Nostril(s)

TECHNIQUES

1. Follow the procedure protocol described earlier.
2. Review institutional policy and follow the appropriate guidelines regarding whether gloves are to be used during the instillation of nose drops to prevent possible contact with body fluid secretions. Apply clean gloves in accordance with institutional policy.
3. Explain the steps in the procedure to help the individual learn future self-administration.
4. Administer the medication (Fig. 7.9).

For Adults and Older Children

- Instruct the patient to blow the nose gently unless this is contraindicated (e.g., nosebleeds, risk of increased intracranial pressure). Use a penlight to assess the nares.
- Have the patient *lie down and hang the head backward* over the edge of the bed or over a pillow placed under the shoulders.
- Draw the medication into the dropper. Hold the dropper just above the nostril, and instill the medication.
- After a brief time, repeat the administration process in the second nostril, if needed.
- Have the patient remain in this position for 2 to 3 minutes to allow the drops to remain in contact with the nasal mucosa.

For Infants and Young Children

- Position the infant or small child with the head over the edge of a bed or pillow, or use the "football" hold to immobilize the infant.
- Administer nose drops in the same manner as is used for an adult.
- For a child who is cooperative, offer praise. Provide appropriate comforting and personal contact for all children and infants.

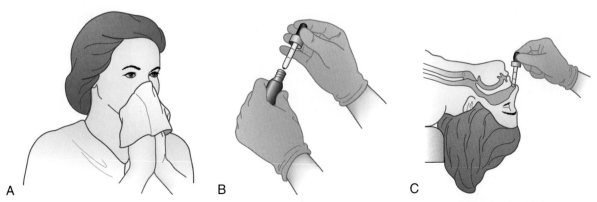

Fig. 7.9 Administering nose drops. (A) Have the patient gently blow the nose. (B) Open the medication bottle and draw the medication up to the calibration mark on the dropper. (C) Instill the medication. Have the patient remain in this position for 2 to 3 minutes. Repeat in the other nostril, if necessary.

- Have paper tissues available for use if it is absolutely necessary for the patient to blow his or her nose.
5. Remove gloves and dispose of them in accordance with institutional policy.
6. Perform hand hygiene.

PATIENT TEACHING

Teach the patient about the self-administration of nose drops, if necessary. Tell the patient that the overuse of nose drops can cause a rebound effect, which causes symptoms to become worse. If symptoms have not resolved after a week of nasal drop therapy, then the healthcare provider should be consulted again.

DOCUMENTATION

Provide the right documentation of the medication administration and the patient's responses to drug therapy.
1. Chart the date, time, drug name, dosage, site, and route of administration.
2. Perform and record regular patient assessments for the evaluation of the therapeutic effectiveness (e.g., nasal congestion, degree and duration of relief achieved, improvement in overall status), and reassess the condition of the nares periodically.
3. Chart and report any signs and symptoms of adverse drug effects.
4. Perform and validate essential patient education about the drug therapy and other essential aspects of intervention for the disease process that is affecting the individual.

ADMINISTRATION OF NASAL SPRAY

The mucous membranes of the nose absorb aqueous solutions very well. When applied as a spray, the small droplets of a solution that contains medication coat the membranes and are rapidly absorbed. The advantage of spray over drops is that there is less waste of medication because some of the drops often run down the back of the patient's throat before absorption can take place. Each patient should have a personal container of spray.

Perform premedication assessment; see individual drug monographs for details.

EQUIPMENT

- Clean gloves
- Nasal spray prescribed
- Paper tissues to blow the nose
- Penlight
- MAR and medication profile

SITE

Nostril(s)

TECHNIQUE

1. Follow the procedure protocol described earlier.
2. Review institutional policy and follow the appropriate guidelines regarding whether gloves are to be used during the instillation of nasal sprays. Apply clean gloves in accordance with institutional policy.
3. Instruct the patient to gently blow the nose (Fig. 7.10A), unless this is contraindicated (e.g., nosebleeds, risk of increased intracranial pressure).
4. Have the patient assume the *upright sitting position*. Use a penlight to inspect the nares.
5. Block one nostril.
6. Shake the spray bottle while holding it upright.
7. Immediately after shaking the bottle, insert the tip into the nostril (Fig. 7.10B). Ask the patient to inhale through the open nostril, and squeeze a puff of spray into the nostril at the same time.
8. Repeat the administration process in the second nostril, if needed (Fig. 7.10C).
9. Have paper tissues available for use if it is absolutely necessary for the patient to blow his or her nose after use of the nasal spray.
10. Remove gloves and dispose of them in accordance with institutional policy.
11. Perform hand hygiene.

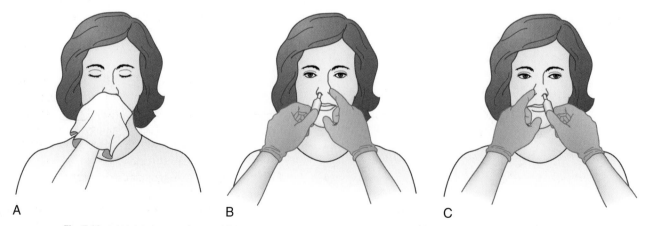

A   B   C

Fig. 7.10 Administering nasal spray. (A) Have the patient gently blow the nose. (B) Block one nostril; shake the medication bottle. Insert the tip of the bottle into the patient's nostril and squeeze a puff of spray while the patient inhales through the open nostril. (C) Repeat procedure on other nostril.

PATIENT TEACHING

Teach the patient the self-administration of nasal spray, if necessary. Tell the patient that the overuse of nasal spray can cause a rebound effect, which causes the symptoms to become worse. If symptoms have not resolved after a week of nasal spray therapy, then the healthcare provider should be consulted again.

DOCUMENTATION

Provide the right documentation of the medication administration and the patient's responses to drug therapy.

1. Chart the date, time, drug name, dosage, site, and route of administration.
2. Perform and record regular patient assessments for the evaluation of therapeutic effectiveness (e.g., nasal congestion, degree and duration of relief achieved, improvement in overall status).
3. Chart and report any signs and symptoms of adverse drug effects.
4. Perform and validate essential patient education about the drug therapy and other essential aspects of intervention for the disease process that is affecting the individual.

ADMINISTRATION OF MEDICATIONS BY INHALATION

The respiratory mucosa may be medicated via the inhalation of sprays or aerosols. **Aerosols** use a flow of air or oxygen under pressure to disperse the drug throughout the respiratory tract. Oily preparations should not be applied to the respiratory mucosa, because the oil droplets may be carried to the lungs and cause lipid pneumonia. Although saliva as a body fluid has not been implicated in the transmission of the human immunodeficiency virus, institutional protocols should reflect current standards of universal precautions for all patients and healthcare personnel. Follow these procedures faithfully to prevent the transmission of this disease.

Perform premedication assessment; see specific drug monographs for details. Assess the patient's ability to manipulate the nebulizer.

EQUIPMENT

- Clean gloves
- Liquid aerosol or spray forms of medications
- MAR and medication profile

SITE

Respiratory tract

TECHNIQUE

1. Follow the procedure protocol described earlier.
2. Review institutional policy and follow the appropriate guidelines regarding whether gloves are to be used during the administration of medication by inhalation. Apply clean gloves in accordance with institutional policy.
3. Have the patient assume a sitting position. This allows for maximum lung expansion.
4. Prepare the medication according to the prescribed directions, and fill the nebulizer with diluent. (This may be done before sitting the patient up if time is a factor for the patient's well-being.)
5. Activate the nebulizer with compressed oxygen or air until a fine mist is flowing; this will usually take up to 8 to 10 liters of oxygen or air.
6. Place nebulizer mask over patient's nose and mouth and ask patient to breathe normally.
7. Allow enough time for all the medication in the nebulizer to be administered; this should take approximately 10 minutes.
8. Assess the patient while still sitting to determine effectiveness.
9. Clean the equipment in accordance with the manufacturer's directions.
10. Remove gloves and dispose of them in accordance with institutional policy.
11. Perform hand hygiene.

PATIENT TEACHING

1. As appropriate to the circumstances, teach the patient, a family member, or a significant other how to operate the nebulizer that is to be used at home.
2. Explain the operation and cleansing of the equipment.
3. Before the patient is discharged, have the patient, a family member, or a significant other demonstrate using the equipment correctly and verbalize the medications that have been prescribed for at-home use.
4. Stress the need to perform the procedure exactly as prescribed and to report any difficulties that are experienced after discharge for the healthcare provider's evaluation.

DOCUMENTATION

Provide the right documentation of the medication administration and the patient's responses to drug therapy.

1. Chart the date, time, drug name, dosage, and route of administration.
2. Perform and record regular patient assessments for the evaluation of therapeutic effectiveness (e.g., blood pressure, pulse, improvement or quality of breathing, cough and productivity, lung sounds, degree and duration of pain relief, ability to operate the nebulizer, activity and exercise restrictions).
3. Chart and report any signs and symptoms of adverse drug effects.
4. Perform and validate essential patient education about the drug therapy and other essential aspects of intervention for the disease process that is affecting the individual.

ADMINISTRATION OF MEDICATIONS BY ORAL INHALATION

DOSE FORMS

Bronchodilators and corticosteroids may be administered by inhalation through the mouth with the use of an aerosolized, pressurized metered-dose inhaler (MDI) or a dry powder inhaler (DPI) (Fig. 7.11). The advantages of the inhalers are that the medications can be applied directly to the site of action (the bronchial smooth muscle), smaller doses are used, and the drug is rapidly absorbed. The valve of the pressurized container (i.e., the MDI) or the dry powder pack of the DPI also helps to ensure that the same dose of medication is administered with each inhalation.

Approximately 25% of patients do not use MDIs properly and therefore do not receive the maximal benefit of the medication. Devices known as *extenders* or *spacers* (Fig. 7.12) have been designed for patients who cannot coordinate the release of the medication with inhalation. The extender devices can be adapted to most pressurized canisters of MDIs. These devices trap the aerosolized medication in a chamber through which the patient inhales within a few seconds after releasing the medication into the chamber.

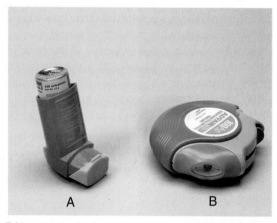

Fig. 7.11 (A) Metered-dose inhaler (MDI). (B) Dry powder inhaler (DPI).

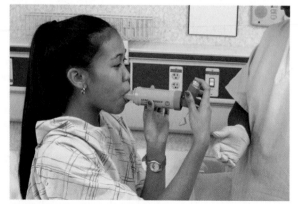

Fig. 7.12 Metered-dose inhaler with an extender or spacer. (From Lilley LL, Collins SR, Snyder JS. *Pharmacology and the Nursing Process.* 7th ed. St. Louis: Mosby; 2014.)

Perform premedication assessment; see individual drug monographs for details.

EQUIPMENT

- Clean gloves
- Prescribed medication packaged in an MDI or DPI
- MAR and medication profile

SITE

Respiratory tract

TECHNIQUES

Aerosolized Metered-Dose Inhaler

1. Follow the procedure protocol described earlier.
2. Review institutional policy and follow the appropriate guidelines regarding whether gloves are to be used during the administration of medication by oral inhalation. Apply clean gloves in accordance with institution policy.
3. The following principles apply to all MDIs. Read and adapt these techniques to the directions provided by the manufacturer for a specific inhaler and extender, if needed.
   - If the medication is a suspension, shake the canister. This disperses and mixes the active bronchodilator and propellant.
   - Have the patient open his or her mouth and then place the canister outlet 2 to 4 inches in front of the mouth. This space allows the propellant to evaporate and prevents large particles from settling in the mouth. When using an extender, have the patient place one end of the extender in the mouth and close the lips around it. Attach the other end of the extender to the inhaler device.
   - Activate the MDI, and instruct the patient to inhale deeply over 10 seconds to ensure that airways are open and that the drug is dispersed as deeply as possible.
   - Have the patient hold his or her breath and then exhale slowly to permit the drug to settle into pulmonary tissue.
   - If prescribed, repeat in 2 to 3 minutes. Using small doses with two or three inhalations helps the drug disperse into the smaller peripheral airways for a longer therapeutic effect.
   - If the inhaled medication is a corticosteroid, have the patient rinse the mouth with water when administration is complete.
4. Cleanse the apparatus according to the manufacturer's recommendations.
5. Remove gloves and dispose of them in accordance with institutional policy.
6. Perform hand hygiene.

Dry Powder Inhaler

1. Follow the procedure protocol described earlier.
2. Review institutional policy and follow the appropriate guidelines regarding whether gloves are to be used

during the administration of medication by oral inhalation. Apply clean gloves in accordance with institutional policy.

3. The following principles apply to all DPIs. Read and adapt these techniques to the directions provided by the manufacturer for a specific inhaler and extender, if needed.
   - Remove the cover, and check that the device and the mouthpiece are clean.
   - Make the medication available according to the manufacturer's instructions for each specific product. Keep the inhaler horizontal.
   - Have the patient breathe out, away from the device.
   - Place the mouthpiece gently into the patient's mouth, and have the patient close the lips around it.
   - Have the patient breathe in quickly, forcefully, and deeply until a full breath has been taken.
   - Remove the inhaler from the patient's mouth.
   - Have the patient hold the breath for about 10 seconds before breathing out.
   - Always check the number in the dose counter window to see how many doses remain.
   - If the patient drops the inhaler or breathes into it after the dose has been loaded, the dose may be lost. To ensure proper dosage, load another dose into the inhaler before using it.

4. Clean the device according to the manufacturer's instructions.
5. Remove gloves and dispose of them in accordance with institutional policy.
6. Perform hand hygiene.

 Health Promotion

Refilling the Prescription

The patient should not wait until the canister is empty before having the prescription refilled. The last few doses in a canister are often subtherapeutic because of an imbalance in the remaining amounts of medication and propellant. Consult the manufacturer's information on how to determine whether the canister is almost empty. The commonly used float test is inaccurate for many aerosolized MDIs.

PATIENT TEACHING

Explain the procedure, and allow the patient to demonstrate the technique. Teaching aids for MDIs and DPIs without active ingredients are available from the pharmacy department to encourage patients to practice the technique before medication administration. In addition to technique, the patient should be informed about adverse effects, how to carry the medication, how to store it, and how to have it refilled when needed.

Have the patient perform the self-administration of the prescribed amount of ordered medication. Have the patient demonstrate the ability to read the canister counter to determine the amount of medication remaining in the container.

DOCUMENTATION

Provide the right documentation of the medication administration and the patient's responses to drug therapy.

1. Chart the date, time, drug name, dose, site, and route of administration.
2. Perform and record regular patient assessments for the evaluation of therapeutic effectiveness (e.g., blood pressure, pulse, improvement of quality of breathing, cough and productivity, degree and duration of pain relief, ability to operate the MDI or DPI, activity and exercise restrictions).
3. Chart and report any signs and symptoms of adverse drug effects.
4. Perform and validate essential patient education about the drug therapy and other essential aspects of intervention for the disease process that is affecting the patient.

Life Span Considerations

Medicines Administered by Inhalation

When muscle coordination is not fully developed (e.g., in a younger child or when dexterity has diminished in an older adult patient), it may be beneficial to use an extender or spacer device (see Fig. 7.12) for medicines that are administered by aerosol inhalation. When administering medicines by aerosol therapy to an older adult, make sure that the patient has the strength and dexterity to self-operate the equipment before discharge.

ADMINISTRATION OF VAGINAL MEDICATIONS

Women with gynecologic disorders may require the administration of a medication intravaginally. Vaginal medications may be creams, jellies, tablets, foams, suppositories, or irrigations (i.e., douches; see Administration of a Vaginal Douche later). The creams, jellies, tablets, and foams are inserted with the use of special applicators that are provided by the manufacturer; suppositories are usually inserted with a gloved index finger.

Perform premedication assessment; see individual drug monographs for details.

EQUIPMENT

- Prescribed medication
- Vaginal applicator
- Perineal pad
- Water-soluble lubricant (for suppository)
- Clean gloves
- Paper towels
- MAR and medication profile

SITE

Vagina

TECHNIQUE

1. Follow the procedure protocol described earlier.
2. Have the patient void to ensure that the bladder is empty.
3. Apply clean gloves.
4. Fill the applicator with the prescribed tablet, jelly, cream, or foam.
5. Place the patient in the lithotomy position, and elevate her hips with a pillow. Drape the patient to prevent unnecessary exposure.
6. Administer the medication.
   - *For tablets, creams, foams, and jellies,* use the gloved nondominant hand to spread the labia and expose the vagina. Assess the status of the presenting symptoms (e.g., color and volume of discharge, odor, level of discomfort). Lubricate the applicator. Gently insert the vaginal applicator as far as possible into the vagina, and push the plunger to deposit the medication (Fig. 7.13). Remove the applicator, and wrap it in a paper towel for cleaning later.
   - *For suppositories,* unwrap a vaginal suppository that has been warmed to room temperature, and lubricate it with a water-soluble lubricant. Lubricate the gloved index finger of the dominant hand. With the gloved nondominant hand, spread the labia to expose the vagina. Insert the suppository (rounded end first) as far into the vagina as possible with the dominant index finger.
7. Remove the glove by turning it inside out; place it on a paper towel for later disposal.

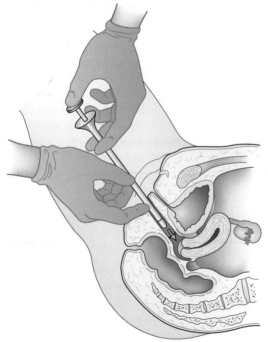

Fig. 7.13 Applying vaginal medication. Gently insert the vaginal applicator as far as possible into the vagina, and then push the plunger to deposit the medication.

8. Apply a perineal pad to prevent drainage onto the patient's clothing or bed.
9. Instruct the patient to remain in a supine position with the hips elevated for 5 to 10 minutes to allow for the melting and spreading of the medication.
10. Dispose of all waste in accordance with institutional policy.
11. Perform hand hygiene.

PATIENT TEACHING

1. Teach the patient how to administer the medication correctly.
2. The applicator should be washed in warm soapy water *after each use.*
3. Review personal hygiene measures such as wiping from the front to the back after voiding or defecating.
4. Tell the patient not to douche and to abstain from sexual intercourse after inserting the medication.
5. With most types of infections, both male and female partners require treatment. To prevent reinfection, patients should abstain from sexual intercourse until all partners are cured.

DOCUMENTATION

Provide the right documentation of the medication administration and the patient's responses to drug therapy.

1. Chart the date, time, drug name, dosage, and route of administration.
2. Perform and record regular patient assessments for the evaluation of the therapeutic effectiveness (e.g., type of discharge present, irritation of labia, discomfort, degree and duration of pain relief).
3. Chart and report any signs and symptoms of adverse drug effects.
4. Perform and validate essential patient education about the drug therapy and other essential aspects of intervention for the disease process that is affecting the individual.

ADMINISTRATION OF A VAGINAL DOUCHE

Douches (i.e., irrigants) are used to wash the vagina. This procedure is not necessary for normal female hygiene, but it may be required if a vaginal infection and discharge are present. It should also be noted that douching is not an effective method of birth control.

Perform premedication assessment; see individual drug monographs for details.

EQUIPMENT

- IV pole
- Clean gloves
- Water-soluble lubricant
- Douche bag with tubing and nozzle
- Douche solution
- MAR and medication profile

SITE

Vagina

TECHNIQUE

1. Follow the procedure protocol described earlier.
2. Ask the patient to void before the procedure.
3. If the nurse is teaching this procedure to a patient for home use, the patient would customarily recline in a bathtub. Depending on the patient's condition in the hospital, this too could occur. However, it may be necessary to place the patient on a bedpan and drape for privacy.
4. Fill the douche bag with douche solution and hang the douche bag on an IV pole, at a level about 12 inches above the vagina. Apply clean gloves. Apply water-soluble lubricant to a plastic vaginal tip.
5. Cleanse the vulva by allowing a small amount of solution to flow over the vulva and between the labia.
6. Gently insert the nozzle into the vagina, directing the tip backward and downward 2 to 3 inches.
7. Hold the labia together to facilitate filling the vagina with solution. Rotate the nozzle periodically to help irrigate all parts of the vagina.
8. Intermittently release the labia, allowing the solution to flow out.
9. When all of the solution has been used, remove the nozzle. Have the patient sit up and lean forward to empty the vagina thoroughly.
10. Pat the external area dry.
11. Clean all equipment with warm soapy water *after every use;* rinse the equipment with clear water, and allow it to dry.
12. Thoroughly clean and disinfect the bathtub, if used.
13. Remove gloves and dispose of them in accordance with institutional policy.
14. Perform hand hygiene.

PATIENT TEACHING

1. Teach the patient how to administer the douche correctly.
2. Explain that the bag and tubing should be washed in warm soapy water after each use so that they do not become a source of reinfection.
3. Review personal hygiene measures, such as wiping from the front to the back after voiding or defecating.
4. Explain that douching is not recommended during pregnancy.
5. With most types of infections, both male and female partners require treatment. To prevent reinfection, patients should abstain from sexual intercourse until all partners are cured.

DOCUMENTATION

Provide the right documentation of the medication administration and the patient's responses to drug therapy.

1. Chart the date, time, drug name, dosage, and route of administration.
2. Perform and record regular patient assessments for the evaluation of therapeutic effectiveness (e.g., type of discharge present, irritation of labia, discomfort, degree and duration of pain relief).
3. Chart and report any signs and symptoms of adverse drug effects.
4. Perform and validate essential patient education about the drug therapy and other essential aspects of intervention for the disease process that is affecting the individual.

Get Ready for the NCLEX® Examination!

Key Points

- Topical forms of medication include creams, lotions, ointments, and powders and may require the use of sponges, cotton-tipped applicators, or a tongue blade to apply.
- Patch testing is performed to determine the presence of allergy. Allergens are applied to the skin using a patch test kit, and results are read 24 to 72 hours later.
- Nitroglycerin ointment is applied using specific dose-measuring ointment paper, covered with plastic, and taped in place. Patient education includes proper application technique and timing of the nitroglycerin ointment.
- Patient education involving the transdermal patch medications includes discussing rotating the site of application and emphasizing the timing of the medication.
- Medications administered via the mucous membranes include sublingual and buccal tablets, eye and ear and nose drops, inhaled medications, and vaginal medications.
- Eardrops administered to a patient younger than 3 years old require the lower earlobe to be pulled down and back, compared with patients 3 years and older, where the upper earlobe is pulled upward and back.
- Patient education necessary for inhaled medications includes demonstrating the proper use of the equipment.
- Vaginal medications come in the form of creams, foams, and jellies that are applied using an applicator.

Additional Learning Resources

SG Go to your Study Guide for additional Review Questions for the NCLEX® Examination, Critical Thinking Clinical Situations, and other learning activities to help you master this chapter content.

Go to your Evolve website (https://evolve.elsevier.com/Clayton) for additional online resources.

Review Questions for the NCLEX® Examination

1. The nurse was teaching a patient how to apply the prescribed powder under a skinfold for a yeast infection. The nurse knows that further teaching is needed after the patient made which statement?
   1. "I know that I need to wash the area first and dry it thoroughly before I apply this powder."
   2. "I will need to watch for any changes in my rash and notify my physician if it gets worse."
   3. "I should shake the container first before I apply this powder."
   4. "I can sprinkle this powder all over to prevent the infection from spreading."

2. When performing a patch test for allergens, the nurse knows what is important? (*Select all that apply.*)
   1. To know what allergen is causing the symptoms
   2. To recognize when a wheal has formed
   3. To cleanse the area for testing with alcohol before applying the patches
   4. To have emergency equipment available in case of an anaphylactic response
   5. To ask the patient if he or she has taken any antihistamines or antiinflammatory agents

3. When nitroglycerin ointment is prescribed, how long is the typical recommended drug-free period?
   1. 3 to 4 hours off every 24 hours
   2. 5 to 10 hours off every 24 hours
   3. 10 to 12 hours off every 24 hours
   4. 12 to 14 hours off every 24 hours

4. Fentanyl patches do not usually achieve a sufficient blood level for pain control until how many hours after their initial application?
   1. 6 hours
   2. 12 hours
   3. 18 hours
   4. 24 hours

5. A patient is to receive a medication via the buccal route. Which action does the nurse plan to implement?
   1. Place the medication inside the pouch between the patient's lower molar and the cheek.
   2. Crush the medication before administration.
   3. Offer the patient a glass of water or juice after administration.
   4. Use sterile technique to administer the medication.

6. A patient is ordered to have eyedrops administered daily to both eyes. Into which part of the eye are eyedrops instilled?
   1. The sclera
   2. The outer canthus
   3. The lower conjunctival sac
   4. The opening of the lacrimal duct

7. A nurse is preparing to administer eardrops to a 5-year-old child. What is the proper technique to use for this patient?
   1. Pull the earlobe downward and back.
   2. Pull the earlobe forward and up.
   3. Pull the earlobe upward and back.
   4. Pull the earlobe downward and straight.

8. The nurse was teaching a patient how to use an inhaler prescribed for asthma. The nurse knows that further teaching is needed after the patient made which statement?
   1. "I will hold my breath for 10 seconds before breathing out."
   2. "I will take a slow deep breath and let it out quickly."
   3. "I will check the number on the dose counter window to see how many more puffs I have left."
   4. "I will notify my physician if I notice that I am coughing a lot more than usual."

9. When administering vaginal medications, the nurse knows the patient needs to be in which position?
   1. Sims position
   2. Trendelenburg position
   3. Lithotomy position
   4. Prone position

10. The nurse assesses the patient for the treatment effectiveness of the percutaneous medication nitroglycerin, and documents which assessment findings? (*Select all that apply.*)
    1. Blood pressure
    2. Pulse
    3. Pain relief
    4. Location of patch
    5. Urine output

Enteral Administration

Objectives

1. Describe general principles of administering solid forms of oral medications.
2. Compare the different techniques that are used with a unit-dose distribution system and a computer-controlled dispensing system.
3. Identify general principles used for liquid-form oral medication administration.
4. Cite the equipment needed, techniques used, and precautions necessary when administering medications via a nasogastric tube.
5. Cite the equipment needed and the technique required when administering rectal suppositories and disposable enemas.

Key Terms

capsules (KĂP-sŭlz) (p. 101)
lozenges (LŎ-zĕn-jĕz) (p. 102)
tablets (TĂB-lĕts) (p. 102)
caplet (KĂP-lĭt) (p. 102)
orally disintegrating tablet (ŌR-ăl-ē dĭs-ĬN-tĕ-grāt-ĭng) (p. 102)
elixirs (ĕ-LĬK-sŭrz) (p. 103)
emulsions (ĕ-MŬL-shĕnz) (p. 103)
suspensions (sŭ-SPĔN-shĕnz) (p. 103)

syrups (SĬR-ĕps) (p. 103)
unit-dose packaging (YŪ-nĭt DŌS PĂK-ĕj-ĭng) (p. 103)
bar code (BĂR KŌD) (p. 103)
soufflé cup (sū-FLĀ KŬP) (p. 103)
medicine cup (MĔD-ĭ-sĭn KŬP) (p. 104)
medicine dropper (MĔD-ĭ-sĭn DRŎ-pŭr) (p. 104)
oral syringe (ŌR-ăl sĭ-RĬNJ) (p. 104)
nasogastric tube (nā-sō-GĂS-trĭk) (p. 108)
suppository (sŭ-PŎZ-ĭ-tōr-ē) (p. 112)

The routes of drug administration can be classified into three categories: enteral, parenteral, and percutaneous. With the *enteral route*, drugs are administered directly into the gastrointestinal tract by the oral, rectal, percutaneous endoscopic gastrostomy (PEG), or nasogastric (NG) methods. The oral route is safe, convenient, and relatively economical, and dose forms are readily available for most medications. In case of a medication error or an intentional drug overdose, much of the drug can be retrieved for a reasonable time after administration. The major disadvantage of the oral route is that it has the slowest and least dependable rate of absorption of the commonly used routes of administration because of frequent changes in the gastrointestinal environment that are produced by food, emotion, and physical activity. Another limitation of this route is that a few drugs (e.g., insulin, gentamicin) are destroyed by digestive fluids and must be given parenterally for therapeutic activity. The enteral route should not be used if the drug may harm or discolor the teeth or if the patient is vomiting, has gastric or intestinal suction, is likely to aspirate, or is unconscious and unable to swallow.

For patients who cannot swallow or who have had oral surgery, the NG or PEG method may be used. The primary purpose of the NG method is to bypass the mouth and the pharynx. Advantages and disadvantages are similar to those of the oral route. The irritation caused by the tube in the nasal passage and throat must be weighed against the relative immobility associated with continuous intravenous (IV) infusions, the expense, and the pain and irritation of multiple injections. For patients who require long-term NG methods, a permanent gastrostomy tube is placed for ongoing drug and feeding administration.

The administration of drugs via the rectal route has the advantages of bypassing the digestive enzymes and avoiding the irritation of the mouth, the esophagus, and the stomach. It may also be an acceptable alternative when nausea or vomiting is present. Absorption via this route varies depending on the drug product, the ability of the patient to retain the suppository or enema, and the presence of fecal material.

ADMINISTRATION OF ORAL MEDICATIONS

DOSE FORMS

Capsules

Capsules are small, cylindrical, gelatin containers that hold dry powder or liquid medicinal agents (Fig. 8.1). They are available in a variety of sizes, and they are a

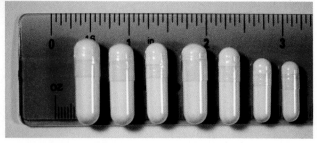

Fig. 8.1 Various sizes and numbers of gelatin capsules (actual size). (Courtesy Oscar H. Allison, Jr.)

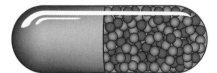

Fig. 8.2 Timed-release capsule.

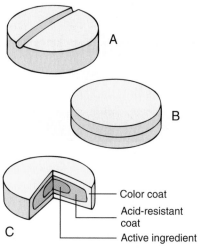

Fig. 8.3 (A) Scored tablet. (B) Layered tablet. (C) Enteric-coated tablet.

convenient way of administering drugs that have an unpleasant odor or taste. They do not require coatings or additives to improve the taste. The color and shape of the capsules, as well as the manufacturer's symbol on the capsule surface, are means of identifying the product.

Timed-release capsules and tablets. Timed-release or sustained-release capsules and tablets provide a gradual but continuous release of a drug because the granules in the capsule or the ingredients of a tablet dissolve at different rates (Fig. 8.2). The advantage of this delivery system is that it reduces the number of doses administered per day, usually to every 12 or 24 hours.

 Medication Safety Alert

Timed-release capsules and tablets should *not* be crushed or chewed or have their contents emptied into food or liquids because this may alter the absorption rate and could result in a drug overdose or subtherapeutic activity.

Lozenges

Lozenges are flat disks that contain a medicinal agent in a suitably flavored base. The base may be a hard sugar candy or a combination of sugar with sufficient gelatinous substances to give it form. Lozenges are held in the mouth to dissolve slowly, thereby releasing the therapeutic ingredients.

Pills

Pills are an obsolete dose form that is no longer manufactured because of the development of capsules and compressed tablets. However, the term is still used to refer to tablets and capsules.

Tablets

Tablets are dried powdered drugs that have been compressed into small disks. In addition to the drug,

tablets contain one or more of the following ingredients: binders, which are adhesive substances that allow the tablet to hold together; disintegrators, which are substances that encourage dissolution in body fluids; lubricants, which are required for efficient manufacturing; and fillers, which are inert ingredients that make the size of the tablet convenient. Tablets are sometimes scored or grooved (Fig. 8.3A); the indentation may then be used to divide the dose. When possible, it is best to request that the exact dose be prescribed rather than to attempt to divide even a scored tablet. A **caplet** is a tablet shaped in the form of a capsule. Many products that were previously sold in capsule form have been reformulated to caplets (solid dosage forms in the shape of a capsule) to prevent the ability to open a capsule and contaminate the contents of the capsule. (Author's note: Search online for the Chicago Tylenol murders.)

Tablets can be formed in layers (Fig. 8.3B). This method allows otherwise incompatible medications to be administered at the same time.

An enteric-coated tablet has a special coating that resists dissolution in the acidic pH of the stomach but that is readily dissolved in the alkaline pH of the intestines (Fig. 8.3C). Enteric-coated tablets are often used for administering medications that are destroyed in an acid pH environment such as the stomach.

A tablet that rapidly dissolves (usually within seconds) when placed on the tongue is known as an *orally disintegrating tablet.* These are differentiated from lozenges and from sublingual and buccal tablets, which take more than a minute to dissolve. Orally disintegrating tablets may be used for their rapid onset of action (e.g., for the treatment of migraine headache); for patients who have difficulty swallowing (e.g., patients with parkinsonism or Alzheimer's disease, or after a stroke); and for those for whom administration must be ensured (e.g., patients with schizophrenia, who often attempt to avoid prescribed medication).

A new dosage form first available in 2014 is the sublingual film. The film is placed under the tongue

For the Figure 8.3 labels:

Color coat
Acid-resistant coat
Active ingredient

for very rapid disintegration. This dosage form is used to administer Suboxone (buprenorphine plus naloxone), which is used to manage opiate addiction. The rapid disintegration of the film prevents retrieval of the product for later sale on the street.

 Medication Safety Alert

Enteric-coated tablets must *not* be crushed or chewed because their active ingredients will be released prematurely and destroyed in the stomach.

Elixirs

Elixirs are clear liquids that are composed of drugs that have been dissolved in alcohol and water. Elixirs are used primarily when the drug will not dissolve in water alone. After the drug is dissolved in the elixir, water and flavoring agents are often added to improve taste. The alcohol content of elixirs is highly variable, depending on the solubility of the drug. Many cough medicines and mouthwashes are elixirs containing alcohol.

Emulsions

Emulsions are dispersions of small droplets of water in oil or small droplets of oil in water. The dispersion is maintained by an emulsifying agent such as sodium lauryl sulfate, gelatin, or acacia. Emulsions are used to mask bitter tastes, to make the product feel better (palatable) in the mouth and throat (thus improving adherence), or to make certain drugs more soluble.

Suspensions

Suspensions are liquid dose forms that contain solid, insoluble drug particles dispersed in a liquid base. All suspensions should be shaken well before administration to ensure the thorough mixing of the particles. Many oral liquid antacids (Maalox, Riopan Plus) and liquid antibiotics (Cefaclor, Augmentin, erythromycin) are suspensions.

Syrups

Syrups contain medicinal agents that have been dissolved in a concentrated solution of sugar (usually sucrose) and water. Syrups are particularly effective for masking the bitter taste of a drug. Many preparations for pediatric patients are syrups because children tend to like the sweeter flavored base.

EQUIPMENT

Unit Dose or Single Dose

Unit-dose packaging, or single-dose packaging, provides a single dose of medication in one package that is ready for dispensing (Fig. 8.4). The package is labeled with both the generic and brand names, the manufacturer, the lot number, and the date of expiration. Depending on the distribution system, the patient's name may be added to the package by the pharmacy. Most unit-dose

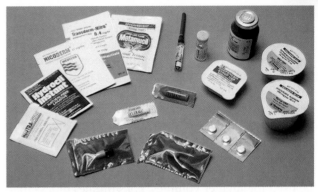

Fig. 8.4 Unit-dose packages. (Courtesy Chuck Dresner.)

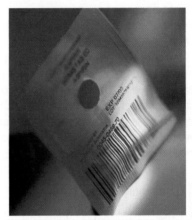

Fig. 8.5 Most unit-dose package labels include a bar code for the electronic charting of medication administration and inventory control. (Copyright 2003, McKesson Corporation, San Francisco, CA and/or one of its subsidiaries. All rights reserved.)

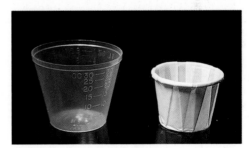

Fig. 8.6 Medicine cup *(left)* and soufflé cup *(right)*. (Courtesy Chuck Dresner.)

package labels include a **bar code** for administration, the electronic charting of medication administration, and inventory control (Fig. 8.5).

Soufflé Cup

A **soufflé cup** is a small paper cup that is used to transport solid medication forms such as capsules and tablets to the patient to prevent contamination by handling (Fig. 8.6). A tablet that must be crushed can be placed between two soufflé cups and then crushed with a pestle. This powdered form of the tablet can then be administered in a solution, if soluble, or it may be mixed with a small amount of food (e.g., applesauce).

Medicine Cup

A medicine cup is a plastic container with scales (metric, household) for measuring liquid medications (Fig. 8.7). Examine the medicine cup carefully before pouring any medication to ensure that the proper scale is being used for measurement (Table 8.1). The medicine cup should be placed on a hard surface when measuring liquid medication and then read at eye level. The medicine cup is inaccurate for measuring doses of less than 1 teaspoon, although it is reasonably accurate for larger volumes. A syringe comparable to the volume to be measured should be used for smaller volumes. For volumes of less than 1 mL, a tuberculin syringe should be used.

Medicine Dropper

The medicine dropper may be used to administer eye-drops, eardrops, and, occasionally, pediatric medications (Fig. 8.8). There is great variation with regard to the size of the drop formed, so it is important to use only the dropper supplied by the manufacturer for a specific liquid medication. Before drawing medication into a dropper, it is necessary to become familiar with the calibrations on the barrel. After the medication is drawn into the barrel, the dropper should not be tipped upside down because the medication will run into the bulb, thereby causing some loss of the medication. Medications should not be drawn into the dropper and then transferred to another container for administration because part of the medication will adhere to the second container, thus diminishing the dose delivered.

Teaspoon

Doses of most liquid medications are prescribed in terms using the teaspoon as the unit of measure (Fig. 8.9). However, there is great variation between the volumes measured by various spoons in the home. In the hospital, 1 teaspoon is converted to 5 mL (see Table 8.1), and this is read on the metric scale of the medicine cup. For home use, an oral syringe is recommended. If this is not available, a teaspoon that is used specifically for baking may be used as an accurate measuring device.

Oral Syringe

A plastic oral syringe may be used to measure liquid medications accurately (Fig. 8.10). Various sizes are available to measure volumes from 0.1 to 15 mL. Note that a needle will not fit on the tip.

Nipple

An infant feeding nipple with additional holes may be used for administering oral medications to infants (Fig. 8.11). (See also General Principles of Liquid-Form

Table 8.1	Commonly Used Measurement Equivalents	
HOUSEHOLD MEASUREMENT[a]	**METRIC MEASUREMENT**
2 Tbsp	30 mL
1 Tbsp	15 mL
2 tsp	10 mL
1 tsp	5 mL

[a]3 tsp = 1 Tbsp; 2 Tbsp = 30 mL = 1 oz.
mL, Milliliter; *oz*, ounce; *Tbsp*, Tablespoon; *tsp*, teaspoon.

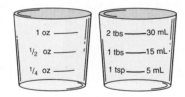

Fig. 8.7 Measuring scales on a medicine cup.

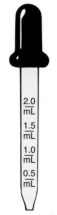

Fig. 8.8 Medicine dropper.

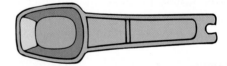

Fig. 8.9 Measuring teaspoon.

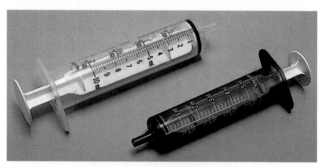

Fig. 8.10 Plastic oral syringes. (Courtesy Chuck Dresner.)

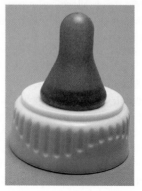

Fig. 8.11 Nipple. (Courtesy Chuck Dresner.)

Oral Medication Administration—For an Adult or Child later in this chapter.)

ADMINISTRATION OF SOLID-FORM ORAL MEDICATIONS

PROCEDURE PROTOCOL

The term *procedure protocol* will be used as part of the medication administration technique for the routes of administration described in this chapter. This term includes the following nursing interventions:

1. Assemble the appropriate equipment and then perform hand hygiene.
2. Use the *seven rights* of medication preparation and administration throughout the procedure: right patient, right drug, right indication, right route, right dose, right time, and right documentation.
3. Provide privacy for the patient and give a thorough explanation of the procedure and what to expect.
4. Perform a premedication assessment before administering any enteral medication. See individual drug monographs for more information.

UNIT-DOSE SYSTEM

Perform premedication assessment; see individual drug monographs for details.

EQUIPMENT

- Medication cart
- Medication profile

TECHNIQUE

1. Follow the procedure protocol described earlier.
2. Read the patient medication profile for the prescribed drugs and times of administration.
3. Obtain the prescribed medication from the drawer in the medication cart that is assigned to the patient.
4. Compare the label on the unit-dose package with the patient medication profile. Check the expiration date on all medication labels.
5. Check the number of doses remaining in the drawer. (If the number of doses remaining is not consistent, investigate.)
6. *Recheck* the seven rights of medication administration against the patient medication profile and the unit-dose package as it is removed from the drawer.
7. Proceed to the patient's bedside.
   - Check the patient's identification bracelet and verify it against the medication profile. Have the patient state his or her name and birth date or two other identifiers.
   - Carefully explain to the patient the drugs being given; state their names and provide education about the drugs being administered.

- Check pertinent patient monitoring parameters (e.g., apical pulse, respiratory rate).
8. Hand the medication to the patient and allow him or her to read the package label.
9. Offer the patient a sip of water to facilitate the swallowing of the medication. Retrieve the unit-dose package, open it, and place the contents in the patient's hand or a medication cup for placement into the mouth.
10. Perform hand hygiene.

COMPUTER-CONTROLLED DISPENSING SYSTEM

Perform premedication assessment; see individual drug monographs for details.

EQUIPMENT

- Computer-controlled dispensing system
- Medication profile

TECHNIQUE

1. Follow the procedure protocol described earlier.
2. Read the medication profile for the prescribed drugs and times of administration.
3. Access the computer-controlled dispensing system using the security access code and password.
4. Select the patient's name from the list of patients on the unit.
5. Review the patient's on-screen profile and select the medications to be administered at this time.
6. Check all aspects of the on-screen order against the medication profile.
7. Check the label on the unit-dose package against the patient medication profile. Check the expiration dates on all medication labels.
8. *Recheck* the seven rights of medication administration against the patient medication profile and the unit-dose package as it is removed from the drawer.
9. Proceed to the patient's bedside.
   - Check the patient's identification bracelet and verify it against the medication profile. Have the patient state his or her name and birth date or two other identifiers.
   - With a computerized scanner system, scan the patient identification, the bar code on the unit-dose medication package, and the nurse's badge, or use the protocol for the institution.
   - Carefully explain to the patient the drugs being given; state their names and provide education about the drugs being administered.
   - Check pertinent patient monitoring parameters (e.g., apical pulse, respiratory rate).
10. Hand the medication to the patient and allow him or her to read the package label.
11. Offer the patient a sip of water to facilitate the swallowing of the medication. Retrieve the unit-dose package, open it, and place the contents in the

patient's hand or a medication cup for placement into the mouth.

12. Perform hand hygiene.

GENERAL PRINCIPLES OF SOLID-FORM MEDICATION ADMINISTRATION

1. Allow the patient to drink a small amount of water to moisten the mouth so that swallowing the medication is easier.
2. Have the patient place the medication well toward the back of his or her tongue. Offer appropriate assistance.
3. Give the patient liquid to swallow the medication. Encourage the patient to keep his or her head forward while swallowing.
4. Drinking a full glass of fluid should be encouraged to ensure that the medication reaches the stomach and that it is diluted to decrease the potential for irritation.
5. Always remain with the patient while the medication is taken. *Do not* leave the medication at the bedside unless an order exists to do so (e.g., medication such as nitroglycerin may be ordered for the bedside).
6. Discard the medication container (e.g., a soufflé cup, a unit-dose package).
7. If the patient has difficulty swallowing and if liquid medications are not an option, use a tablet-crushing device (Fig. 8.12). Ensure that the medication is not a capsule and that it is not a timed-release or enteric-coated product. Follow the guidelines for using the crushing device. Mix the crushed medication in a small amount of soft food such as applesauce, ice cream, custard, or jelly; this will help to counteract the bitter taste and consistency of the mixture.

DOCUMENTATION

Provide the right documentation of medication administration and of the patient's responses to drug therapy. If using an computer-controlled dispensing system, the date, time, drug name, dose, and route of administration are automatically charted in the electronic medication administration record when the nurse signs in, scans the patient's identification bracelet, and the bar-coded unit-dose medication package.

1. Chart the date, time, drug name, dosage, and route of administration.
2. Perform and record regular patient assessments for the evaluation of the therapeutic effectiveness (e.g., blood pressure, pulse, intake and output, improvement or quality of cough and productivity, degree and duration of pain relief).
3. Chart and report any signs or symptoms of adverse drug effects.
4. Perform and validate essential patient education about the drug therapy and other essential aspects of intervention for the disease process that is affecting the individual.

ADMINISTRATION OF LIQUID-FORM ORAL MEDICATIONS

UNIT-DOSE SYSTEM

Perform premedication assessment; see individual drug monographs for details.

EQUIPMENT

- Medication cart
- Medication profile

TECHNIQUE

1. Follow the procedure protocol described earlier.
2. Read the patient medication profile for the prescribed drugs and times of administration.
3. Obtain the prescribed medication from the drawer in the medication cart that is assigned to the patient.
4. Check the label on the unit-dose package against the patient medication profile. Check the expiration dates on all medication labels.
5. Check the number of doses remaining in the drawer. (If the number of doses remaining is not consistent, investigate.)
6. *Recheck* the seven rights of medication administration against the patient medication profile and the unit-dose package as it is removed from the drawer.
7. Proceed to the patient's bedside.
   - Check the patient's identification bracelet and verify it against the medication profile. Have the patient state his or her name and birth date or two other identifiers.
   - Carefully explain to the patient the drugs being given; state their names and provide education about the drugs being administered.
   - Check pertinent patient monitoring parameters (e.g., apical pulse, respiratory rate).
8. Hand the medication to the patient and allow him or her to read the package label.

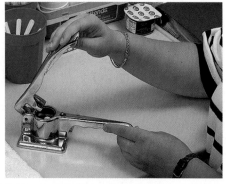

Fig. 8.12 Tablet crusher. (From Potter PA, Perry AG. *Fundamentals of Nursing.* 7th ed. St. Louis: Mosby; 2008.)

9. Retrieve the unit-dose package, open it, and place the container in the patient's hand for the placement of the contents into the patient's mouth.
10. Perform hand hygiene.

LIQUID-FORM ORAL MEDICATIONS IN MULTIDOSE CONTAINERS

Some liquid dosage forms (e.g., pediatric dosages) are not available in unit-dose packaging because the volume is too small. A small multidose container may be included in the unit-dose drawer with instructions on measuring the dose in a medicine cup or an oral syringe.

1. Follow the procedure protocol described earlier.
2. Read the patient medication profile for the prescribed drugs and times of administration.
3. Obtain the prescribed medication from the drawer in the medication cart that is assigned to the patient.
4. Check the label on the multidose container against the patient medication profile. Check the expiration dates on all medication labels.
5. Check the number of doses remaining in the container. (If the number of doses remaining is not consistent, investigate.) Remove the lid from the container.

Measuring With a Medicine Cup

- Hold the bottle of liquid so that the label is in the palm of the hand; this prevents the contents from smearing the label during pouring.
- Examine the medicine cup and locate the exact place where the measured volume should be measured.
- Place the medicine cup on a hard surface; pour the prescribed volume at eye level.
- Read the volume accurately at the level of the meniscus (Fig. 8.13).

Measuring With an Oral Syringe

- See Chapter 9 for more information about reading the calibrations of a syringe.
- Select a syringe of a size that is comparable to the volume to be measured.
  - *Method 1:* With a large-bore needle attached to the syringe, draw up the prescribed volume of medication (Fig. 8.14). The needle is not necessary if the bottle opening is large enough to receive the syringe.
  - *Method 2:* Pour the amount of medication needed into a medicine cup; then use a syringe to draw up the prescribed volume (Fig. 8.15).
6. Replace the lid on the container.
7. *Recheck* the seven rights of medication administration against the patient medication profile and the multidose container as it is removed from the drawer.
8. Return the medication container to the unit-dose cart.
9. Proceed to the patient's bedside when all medications are assembled for administration.
   - Check the patient's identification bracelet and verify it against the medication profile. Have the patient state his or her name and birth date or two other identifiers.

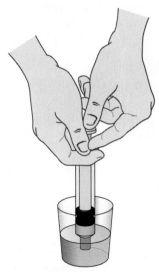

Fig. 8.14 Filling a syringe with medication directly from a bottle.

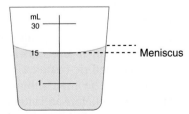

Fig. 8.13 Reading a meniscus. The meniscus is caused by the surface tension of the solution against the walls of the container. The surface tension causes the formation of a concave or hollowed curvature on the surface of the solution. Read the level at the lowest point of the concave curve.

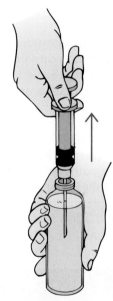

Fig. 8.15 Filling a syringe with medication directly from a medicine cup.

- Carefully explain to the patient the drugs being given; state their names and provide education about the drugs being administered.
- Check pertinent patient monitoring parameters (e.g., apical pulse, respiratory rate).

10. Hand the medication cup to the patient for the placement of the contents into his or her mouth, or administer the medication via the oral syringe.
11. Perform hand hygiene.

GENERAL PRINCIPLES OF LIQUID-FORM ORAL MEDICATION ADMINISTRATION

FOR AN ADULT OR CHILD

1. Never dilute a liquid medication unless specifically ordered to do so.
2. Always remain with the patient while the medication is taken. *Do not* leave the medication at the bedside unless an order exists to do so.

FOR AN INFANT

1. Check the infant's identification bracelet and verify it against the medication card or profile.
2. Be certain that the infant is alert.
3. Position the infant so that his or her head is slightly elevated (Fig. 8.16).
4. Administration:
   - *Oral syringe or dropper:* Place the syringe or dropper between the patient's cheek and gums, halfway back into the mouth. This placement will reduce the chance that the infant will spit out the medication with tongue movements. Slowly inject the medication and allow the infant to swallow it.

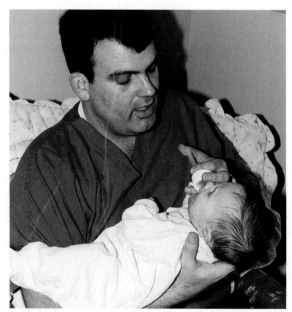

Fig. 8.16 Position the infant in a "football hold" with the head slightly elevated. Place the nipple in the infant's mouth. When the baby starts to suck, place the medication in the back of the nipple, and allow the baby to suck.

(Rapid administration may cause choking and aspiration.)
   - *Nipple:* When the infant is awake (and preferably hungry), place the nipple in the infant's mouth. When the baby starts to suck, place the medication in the back of the nipple with a syringe or dropper, and allow the baby to suck it in (see Fig. 8.16). (NOTE: The size of the nipple hole may need to be enlarged for suspensions and syrups.) Follow the medication with milk or formula, if necessary.
5. Perform hand hygiene.

DOCUMENTATION

Provide the right documentation of the medication administration and the patient's responses to drug therapy.

1. Chart the date, time, drug name, dosage, and route of administration.
2. Perform and record regular patient assessments for the evaluation of therapeutic effectiveness (e.g., blood pressure, pulse, output, improvement or quality of cough and productivity, degree and duration of pain relief).
3. Chart and report any signs and symptoms of adverse drug effects.
4. Perform and validate essential patient education about the drug therapy and other essential aspects of intervention for the disease process that is affecting the individual. If the medication is for a child, provide and validate essential patient education to the caregiver and child, keeping in mind the child's developmental level. This should address the drug therapy and other essential aspects of intervention for the disease process that is affecting the individual.

ADMINISTRATION OF MEDICATIONS BY NASOGASTRIC, NASODUODENAL, NASOJEJUNAL TUBE

Medications are administered via a **nasogastric (NG) tube,** nasoduodenal (ND) tube, or nasojejunal (NJ) tube (Fig. 8.17) to patients who have impaired swallowing, to those who are comatose, or to those who have a disorder of the esophagus. Whenever possible, the liquid form of a drug should be used for NG administration. If it is necessary to use a tablet or capsule, then the tablet should be crushed or the capsule pulled apart and the powder sprinkled in approximately 10 to 15 mL of water. (*Do not* crush enteric-coated tablets or open timed-release capsules.) The tube should be flushed with at least 30 mL of water before and after the medicine is administered. This serves to clear the tube for drug delivery, it facilitates drug transport to the intestine, and it indicates whether the tube has been cleared. When more than one medication is to be administered at about the same time, flush 5 to 10 mL of water between each

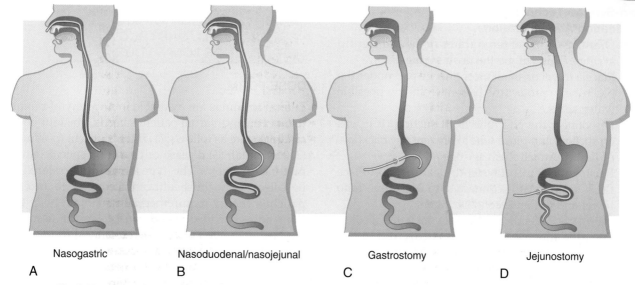

A Nasogastric   B Nasoduodenal/nasojejunal   C Gastrostomy   D Jejunostomy

Fig. 8.17 Types of gastrointestinal tubes. (A) Nasogastric tube is passed from the nose into the stomach. (B) Weighted nasoduodenal/nasojejunal tube is passed through the nose into duodenum/jejunum. (C) Gastrostomy tube is introduced through a temporary or permanent opening on the abdominal wall (stoma) into the stomach. (D) Jejunostomy tube is passed through a stoma directly into the jejunum.

medication. (Remember to include the water that is used to flush the tubing as part of the total water requirements for the patient for a 24-hour period.)

Perform premedication assessment; see individual drug monographs for details.

EQUIPMENT
- Glass of water
- Two 60-mL catheter tip syringes
- Measuring container or graduated cylinder
- Pill crusher (as needed when medications are not liquid)
- Towel or small incontinence pad
- pH tape and color verification
- Gloves

TECHNIQUE
Refer to the sections about the administration of solid-form or liquid-form oral medications for information about the preparation of doses.
1. Follow the procedure protocol described earlier.
2. Proceed to the patient's bedside when all medications are assembled for administration.
   - Check the patient's identification bracelet and verify it against the medication profile. Have the patient state his or her name and birth date or two other identifiers.
   - Carefully explain to the patient the procedure for the administration of medications into the NG tube. State the drug names and provide education about the drugs being administered.
3. Apply clean gloves.
4. Position the patient upright and check the location of the NG tube before administering any liquid.

(NOTE: Radiographic confirmation of NG tube placement is performed when the tube is initially inserted. Thereafter, pH and color testing may be used to confirm placement.)

pH and Color Testing of Gastric Contents to Check for Tube Placement
- Aspirate part of the stomach contents using the 60-mL catheter tip syringe. If unable to aspirate the stomach contents, reposition the patient on his or her left side and try aspirating again.
- Check the color of the aspirated fluid. Color verification guidelines are as follows:
  - Gastric fluid = green with sediment or off-white
  - Intestinal fluid = yellow (bile-colored)
  - Pleural fluid = clear to straw-colored
  - Tracheobronchial fluid = off-white or tan
- Check the pH of the gastric contents. The stomach pH is less than 3, the intestinal fluid pH is 6 to 7, and the respiratory fluid pH is greater than 7. Histamine-2 (H_2) antagonists (e.g., ranitidine, cimetidine, famotidine, nizatidine) affect the pH of the aspirated fluid in the following ways:
  - People not receiving H_2 blockers:
    - Gastric pH = 1 to 4
    - Intestinal pH ≥6
  - People receiving H_2 blockers:
    - Gastric pH = 1 to 6
    - Intestinal pH ≥6
    - Tracheobronchial or pleural aspirate pH ≥7
- Return the stomach contents after the confirmation of correct tube placement.
5. After the placement of the NG tube in the stomach is confirmed, administer the medication.

Two-Syringe Technique for Medication Administration

- Draw up 60 mL of tepid water in the catheter tip syringe. This will be the flush syringe.
- Place a towel or small incontinence pad under the NG tube to protect the patient from any possible water spills.
- Disconnect the NG tube from suction (if it was on suction) and pinch tube to prevent any backflow of liquid. Attach flush syringe.
- Flush with 30 mL of water to clear the tube. Place flush syringe, still connected to NG tube, onto towel and obtain second syringe.
- With second 60-mL syringe, draw up liquid medication to be administered; or (if needed) crush tablets, suspend in water (approximately 5 to 10 mL), and then draw up into syringe.
  - When administering multiple medications, give them one at a time. Do not mix the medications together in one syringe because this may clog the NG tube.
  - It is best to have multiple medication syringes laid out in orderly fashion for ease of administration.
- When second syringe is prepared, pinch the NG tube, disconnect the flush syringe, attach syringe with medication, and administer medication, keeping catheter tip vertical.
- Pinch NG tube to prevent backflow, switch to flush syringe, and flush tube with 10 mL of water following medication administration.
- Continue administering medications and flushing between them until all medications are administered.
- Flush the NG tube with 30 mL of water when finished and clamp tube. Tube should remain clamped for 30 to 60 minutes to allow for absorption.
- Provide oral hygiene for the patient, if needed.
6. Remove gloves and perform hand hygiene.

DOCUMENTATION

Provide the right documentation of medication administration and the patient's responses to drug therapy.
1. Chart the verification of the NG tube placement.
2. Chart the date, time, drug name, dosage, and route of administration. Include all fluids given (including the fluid used to flush the tube) on the intake record.
3. Perform and record regular assessments for therapeutic effectiveness (e.g., blood pressure, pulse, output, improvement or quality of cough and productivity, degree and duration of pain relief).
4. Chart and report any signs and symptoms of adverse drug effects.
5. Perform and validate essential patient education about the drug therapy and other critical aspects of intervention for the disease process affecting the individual.

ADMINISTRATION OF ENTERAL FEEDINGS VIA GASTROSTOMY OR JEJUNOSTOMY TUBE

DOSE FORM

Enteral formulas are available in a variety of mixtures to meet the individual patient's needs. The four general categories are as follows: (1) intact nutrient (polymeric); (2) elemental; (3) disease or condition specific; and (4) modular nutrient. The type of formula ordered will be selected by the healthcare provider to meet the patient's energy requirements to maintain body functions and growth demands and to repair tissue that has been damaged or depleted by illness or injury (see Chapter 46).

EQUIPMENT

- Prescribed enteral formula
- Disposable or ready-to-hang bag for continuous administration
- Infusion pump specific for enteral formulas
- Blood glucose testing materials (if blood glucose levels ordered)
- 60-mL catheter tip syringe
- 50 mL of water
- Measuring container or graduated cylinder
- pH indicator tape
- Clamp (C clamp or ostomy plug)
- Towel or small incontinence pad

Optional Supplies to Cleanse Stoma Area
- Clean basin
- 4 × 4-inch gauze sponges
- Sterile saline or water
- Tape
- Gloves

TECHNIQUE

Position the patient in a semi-Fowler's position with a 30-degree head-of-bed elevation.
1. Follow the procedure protocol described earlier.
2. Proceed to the patient's bedside.
   - Check the patient's identification bracelet and verify it against the medication profile. Have the patient state his or her name and birth date or two other identifiers.
   - Carefully explain to the patient the procedure used for administering enteral feedings and provide education about the formula being instilled.
3. Check patient positioning and drape the patient to avoid unnecessary exposure. Place a towel or small incontinence pad under the feeding tube area to protect the area in case of accidental spills.
4. Apply clean gloves.

5. If the stoma site needs cleansing, complete this at least once daily or as needed, proceeding as follows:
   - If the area around the stoma is crusted, soak 4 × 4-inch gauze sponges in a solution of normal saline or water.
   - Place saturated sponges around the stoma area, and then allow the solution to soften the crusted exudate.
   - Remove the sponges and wipe from the tube or stoma area outward.
   - Rinse the area with saline- or water-soaked gauze sponges; pat dry.
   - Cleanse as per institutional policy.
6. Verify tube placement and initiate the feeding:
   - *Gastrostomy tube* (Fig. 8.17C): Attach a 60-mL catheter tip syringe to the clamped tube; release the clamp. Slowly withdraw the plunger to aspirate the residual material. Observe the color and check the pH of the aspirated contents. (Use the principles described previously in the section on pH and Color Testing of Gastric Contents to Check for Tube Placement under Administration of Medications by Nasogastric Tube to aspirate gastric contents.) Notify the healthcare provider if the residual is greater than 100 mL (or amount specified) since the last bolus feeding 4 hours earlier. Reintroduce the gastric contents that were aspirated.
   - *Jejunostomy tube* (Fig. 8.17D): Aspirate the intestinal secretions using the same method as described for a gastrostomy tube. Observe the color and check the pH.
7. Flush the tube with 30 mL of water.
8. Clamp the tube (gastrostomy or jejunostomy).
9. Proceed with one of the following feeding techniques.

Intermittent Tube Feeding

- Using a disposable or ready-to-hang bag, fill the bag with the prescribed amount of formula and allow to infuse by gravity by hanging the bag on an IV pole. In general, this will infuse over 30 minutes. Check frequently to ensure that the formula is running.
- Flush the tubing with 50 to 60 mL of water after the bag is empty and the formula is gone. This removes the formula from the tubing, maintains the patency of the tube, and prevents the formula that remains in the tube from supporting bacterial growth.
- Clamp or plug the ostomy tube. Tell the patient to remain in a semi-Fowler's position or turn onto his or her right side for 30 to 60 minutes to help with the normal digestion of formula and to prevent gastric reflux (with possible aspiration) or leakage.
- Wash and dry all reusable equipment and store it in a clean area in the patient's environment until the next feeding. Change the equipment

(e.g., syringes) in accordance with institutional policy (often every 24 hours).

Continuous Tube Feeding

- Fill a disposable feeding container with enough of the prescribed formula for an 8-hour period. Store the remaining formula in the refrigerator. Label the container with the date and time that the feeding was initiated. The formula must be at room temperature at the time of initiation.
- Hang the container on an IV pole, clear air from the tubing, and thread the tubing through the pump in the manner prescribed by the pump's manufacturer.
- Connect the tube from the enteral feeding source to the end of the feeding tube. Release the clamp from the tube.
- Set the flow rate of the enteral formula at the prescribed rate to deliver the formula in the correct volume over the specified time span. When initiating tube feedings, the rate is initially slow and gradually increased at specified intervals.
- Wash and dry all reusable equipment and store it in a clean area in the patient's environment until the next feeding. Change the equipment every 24 hours.
10. Blood glucose determination may be performed and the level recorded every 6 hours during the initiation of tube feedings. Assessments are continued until glucose levels are maintained within a specified range for a 24-hour period after the rate of enteral feeding has reached the prescribed maximum flow.
11. When patients have an NG tube, inspect the nares at regular intervals to detect any pressure irritation created by the feeding tube. Inspect the tissue surrounding a PEG tube for signs of breakdown or infection.
12. Before the next scheduled feeding, a gastric residual volume should be checked with the use of a catheter tip syringe for aspiration to ensure that the formula is leaving the stomach and passing into the intestine for absorption. For residual volumes of less than 100 mL the residual can be readministered and the feeding can be resumed. If the residual volume is greater than 100 mL, the healthcare provider should be notified. If the residual is "coffee-ground" in color, the healthcare provider should also be notified because this may be an indication of bleeding developing.
13. Perform hand hygiene.

DOCUMENTATION

Provide the right documentation of the formula administered, the cleansing of the stoma, and the patient's therapeutic response to the enteral feedings.

1. Chart the date and time; the amount, color, and pH of the residual that is aspirated; the amount, type, and strength of the formula that is instilled; and the amount of water that is used to rinse the tubing.

⚠ Medication Safety Alert

Enteral formulas should be properly labeled with the time, date, type of formula, and strength. Check the date and time of preparation on a formula that is mixed in the hospital pharmacy, and discard any unused portion after 24 hours. Commercially prepared vacuum-sealed formulas are generally stored at room temperature until used. Check the expiration date and return the product if it is outdated. If the product has been opened, discard it in accordance with the manufacturer's recommendations or institutional policy.

For patients who are receiving enteral nutrition via intermittent tube feedings (using institutional guidelines), remember the following:

- Check the residual volume before each feeding.
- Check to ensure the presence of bowel sounds. The absence of bowel sounds indicates the need to contact the healthcare provider for orders before proceeding.
- Check the position of the tube to ensure that it is still in the stomach.
- During the initiation of enteral feedings by intermittent or continuous methods, blood glucose testing may be ordered.

ADMINISTRATION OF RECTAL SUPPOSITORIES

DOSE FORM

A **suppository** (Fig. 8.18) is a solid form of medication that is designed for introduction into a body orifice. At body temperature, the substance dissolves and is absorbed by the mucous membranes. Suppositories should be stored in a cool place to prevent softening. If a suppository becomes soft and the package has not yet been opened, hold the foil-wrapped suppository under cold running water or place it in ice water for a short time until it hardens. Rectal suppositories should generally not be used for patients who have had recent prostate or rectal surgery or for those who have experienced recent rectal trauma.

Perform premedication assessment; see individual drug monographs for details.

EQUIPMENT

- Gloves
- Water-soluble lubricant
- Prescribed suppository

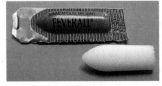

Fig. 8.18 Rectal suppositories.

TECHNIQUE

1. Follow the procedure protocol described earlier.
2. Proceed to the patient's bedside.
   - Check the patient's identification bracelet and verify it against the medication profile. Have the patient state his or her name and birth date or two other identifiers.
   - Explain carefully to the patient the procedure used for administering suppositories. Tell the patient the drug's name and provide education about the drug being administered.
   - Check pertinent patient monitoring parameters (e.g., time of last defecation, severity of nausea or vomiting, respiratory rate) as appropriate to the medication to be administered.
3. Whenever possible, have the patient defecate before the suppository is administered.
4. Provide for patient privacy; position and drape the patient to avoid unnecessary exposure (Fig. 8.19A). Generally, the patient is placed on his or her left side (i.e., Sims' position).
5. Apply clean gloves.
6. Ask the patient to bend the uppermost leg toward the waist.
7. Unwrap the suppository, and apply a small amount of water-soluble lubricant to its tip (Fig. 8.19B and C). If lubricant is not available, use plain water to moisten the medication. *Do not* use petroleum jelly or mineral oil because it may reduce the absorption of the medicine.
8. Place the tip of the suppository at the rectal entrance. Ask the patient to take a deep breath and to then exhale through the mouth (many patients will experience an involuntary rectal gripping when the suppository is pressed against the rectum). Gently insert the suppository about an inch beyond the orifice and past the internal sphincter (Fig. 8.19D). When inserting the suppository, use the index finger for an adult or the fourth finger for an infant.
9. Ask the patient to remain lying on his or her side for 15 to 20 minutes to allow for the melting and absorption of the medication.
   - For children, it is necessary to compress the buttocks gently but firmly and to hold them in place for 15 to 20 minutes to prevent expulsion.
10. Discard used materials and remove gloves.
11. Perform hand hygiene.

DOCUMENTATION

Provide the right documentation of medication administration and the patient's responses to drug therapy.

1. Chart the date, time, drug name, dosage, and route of administration.
2. Perform and record regular patient assessments for the evaluation of therapeutic effectiveness. For example, when a medication is given as a laxative, chart the color, amount, and consistency of stool. If

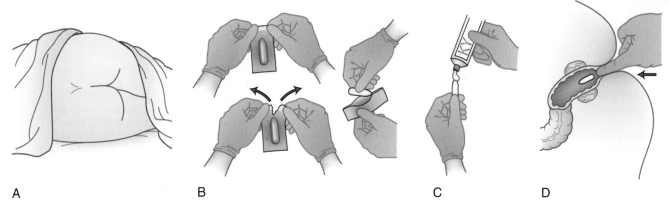

Fig. 8.19 Administering a rectal suppository. (A) Position the patient on his or her left side and then drape the patient. (B) Unwrap the suppository and remove it from its package. (C) Apply water-soluble lubricant to the suppository. (D) Gently insert the suppository about 1 inch past the internal sphincter. (Courtesy Chuck Dresner.)

a drug is given for pain relief, chart the degree and duration of pain relief. If the suppository is given as an antiemetic, chart the degree and duration of relief of nausea and vomiting.

3. Chart and report any signs and symptoms of adverse drug effects.
4. Perform and validate essential patient education about the drug therapy and other essential aspects of intervention for the disease process that is affecting the individual.

ADMINISTRATION OF A DISPOSABLE ENEMA

DOSE FORM

The dose form is a prepackaged, disposable enema solution of the type prescribed by the healthcare provider.

Perform premedication assessment; see individual drug monographs for details.

EQUIPMENT

- Toilet tissue
- Bedpan, if patient is not ambulatory
- Water-soluble lubricant
- Gloves
- Prescribed disposable enema kit

TECHNIQUE

1. Follow the procedure protocol described earlier.
2. Proceed to the patient's bedside.
   - Check the patient's identification bracelet and verify it against the medication profile. Have the patient state his or her name and birth date or two other identifiers.
   - Explain carefully to the patient the procedure used for administering an enema and provide education about the solution being administered. Depending on the purpose of the enema, ask the patient to defecate if there is an urge prior to the procedure.
   - Check pertinent patient monitoring parameters (e.g., the time of last defecation).
3. Position the patient on his or her left side, and drape the patient to avoid unnecessary exposure (Fig. 8.20A).
4. Apply clean gloves. Remove protective covering from the end of the enema and lubricate the end (Fig. 8.20B).
5. Insert the lubricated end into the patient's rectum and then dispense the solution by compressing the plastic container (Fig. 8.20C).
6. Replace the used container in its original package for disposal (Fig. 8.20D).
7. Encourage the patient to hold the solution for about 30 minutes before defecating.
8. Assist the patient to a sitting position on the bedpan or to the bathroom, as orders permit.
9. Tell the patient *not* to flush the toilet. The results of the enema need to be documented. Instruct the patient regarding the location of the call light in case assistance is needed.
10. Remove and discard gloves.
11. Perform hand hygiene.

DOCUMENTATION

Provide the right documentation of medication administration and the patient's responses to drug therapy.

1. Chart the date, time, drug name, dosage, and route of administration.
2. Perform and record regular patient assessments for the evaluation of the therapeutic effectiveness (e.g., color, amount, and consistency of stool).
3. Chart and report any signs and symptoms of adverse drug effects.
4. Perform and validate essential patient education about the drug therapy and other essential aspects of intervention for the disease process that is affecting the individual.

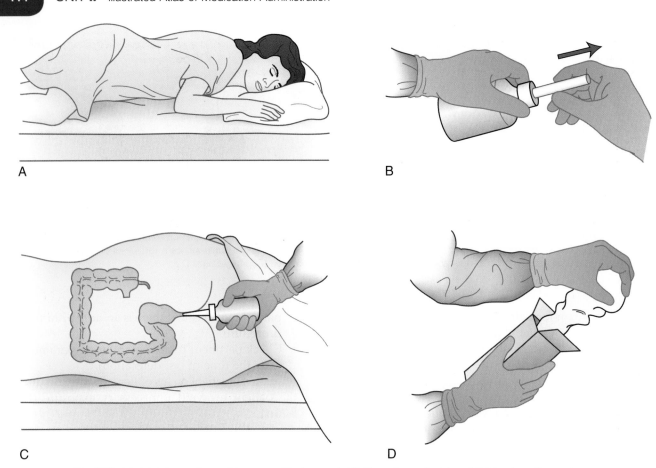

A

B

C

D

Fig. 8.20 Administering a disposable enema (Fleet enema). (A) Place the patient in a left lateral position, unless a knee-chest position has been specified. (B) Remove the protective covering from the end of the enema and lubricate the end. (C) Insert the lubricated end into the patient's rectum and dispense the solution by compressing the plastic container. (D) Replace the used container in its original wrapping for disposal.

Get Ready for the NCLEX® Examination!

Key Points

- Solid dose forms of medications include capsules, timed-release capsules, lozenges, tablets, caplets, and orally disintegrating tablets and films.
- Liquid dose forms for medications include elixirs, emulsions, suspensions, and syrups.
- The unit-dose system uses individual packaged medications that are distributed to each patient using a medication cart. The computer-controlled dispensing system uses unit-dose medications distributed in a locked, password-protected medication system using a computer and bar code scanner system.
- Liquid forms of medications are administered by unit-dose container or oral syringe, or by gastric tube.
- Nasogastric tube medication administration requires checking placement of the tube before administration and correct technique to ensure all medication is given accurately.
- Rectal suppositories and enemas are administered with the patient positioned on his or her left side and inserted with a water-based lubricant.

Additional Learning Resources

SG Go to your Study Guide for additional Review Questions for the NCLEX® Examination, Critical Thinking Clinical Situations, and other learning activities to help you master this chapter content.

Go to your Evolve website (https://evolve.elsevier.com/Clayton) for additional online resources.

Review Questions for the NCLEX® Examination

1. The prescriber has changed the route of the patient's medication from an intravenous route to an oral route. What effect (in general) does the change in route have on the drug dosage and the absorption time?
   1. Decreased dosage and increased absorption time
   2. Increased dosage and increased absorption time
   3. Increased dosage and decreased absorption time
   4. Decreased dosage and decreased absorption time

32415

2. With regard to the administration of oral medications, put the following actions that the nurse takes in chronologic order.
   1. Give the patient water to drink.
   2. Identify the patient.
   3. Check all aspects of the medication order.
   4. Sit the patient upright.
   5. Document the administration.

3. Which of the following nursing principles apply to administering guaifenesin syrup to a 5-year-old? *(Select all that apply.)*
   1. The correct amount of liquid should be measured in a medicine cup by reading the meniscus at eye level.
   2. Hold the bottle containing the liquid so the label is covered with the palm of the hand.
   3. Use a syringe that compares closely to the volume to be measured.
   4. The expiration date does not need to be checked on liquids.
   5. A syringe can be used when giving an infant medications.

4. The nurse is to administer several medications to the patient via an NG tube. What is the nurse's first action?
   1. Add the medication to the tube feeding being given.
   2. Crush all tablets and capsules before administration.
   3. Administer all of the medications mixed together.
   4. Check for the placement of the tube.

5. When administering an intermittent enteral feeding to an adult patient, the nurse finds that the residual aspirate obtained is "coffee-ground" in color. What does the nurse do?
   1. Administers the next scheduled feeding
   2. Stops feeding the patient for 30 minutes
   3. Reinstills the aspirate and starts a new feeding
   4. Notifies the healthcare provider

6. When administering a rectal suppository, the patient needs to be in which position?
   1. Semi-Fowler's
   2. Lithotomy
   3. Left side-lying
   4. Right side-lying

7. Why is it important not to crush medications that are considered long acting?
   1. Medications that are crushed are harder to swallow, making it harder to activate the effect.
   2. Medications that are crushed release the drug immediately, inactivating the long-acting effect and potentially causing an overdose.
   3. Medications that are crushed will not be absorbed properly, inactivating the long-acting effect.
   4. Medications that are crushed will become powder and lose all the effectiveness of the drug.

8. The nurse was aspirating the patient's NG tube to check the contents. What can the nurse expect for results if the contents are gastric fluid?
   1. pH of 8, clear colored
   2. pH of 3, green with sediment
   3. pH of 7, yellow colored
   4. pH of 4, off-white colored

Parenteral Administration: Safe Preparation of Parenteral Medications

Objectives

1. Identify the parts of a syringe and needle, as well as examples of the safety-type syringes and needles.
2. Describe how to select the correct needle gauge and length and how the needle gauge is determined.
3. Compare and contrast the volumes of medications that can be measured in a tuberculin syringe and those of larger-volume syringes.
4. Compare and contrast the advantages and disadvantages of using prefilled syringes.
5. Differentiate among ampules, vials, and Mix-O-Vials.
6. Describe the technique used to prepare two different drugs in one syringe (e.g., insulin).

Key Terms

barrel (BĂ-rŭl) (p. 117)
plunger (PLŬN-jŭr) (p. 117)
tip (p. 117)
milliliter scale (MĬL-ĭ-lē-tŭr) (p. 117)
tuberculin syringe (tū-BĔR-kū-lĭn sĭ-RĬNJ) (p. 117)
insulin syringe (ĬN-sŭ-lĭn) (p. 118)
prefilled cartridges and syringes (prē-FĬLD) (p. 119)

insulin pen (p. 119)
needle gauge (NĒ-dŭl GĀJ) (p. 119)
safety devices (SĀF-tē dĕ-VĪ-sĕz) (p. 123)
ampules (ĀM-pyūlz) (p. 123)
vials (VĪ-ălz) (p. 125)
Mix-O-Vials (MĬKS Ō VĪ-ălz) (p. 125)

The routes of drug administration can be classified into three categories: enteral, parenteral, and percutaneous. The term *parenteral* means administration by any route other than the enteral—or gastrointestinal—tract. As ordinarily used, the term *parenteral route* refers to intradermal (ID), subcutaneous (subcut), intramuscular (IM), or intravenous (IV) injections.

When drugs are given parenterally rather than orally, the following factors are involved: (1) the onset of drug action is generally more rapid but of shorter duration; (2) the dosage is often smaller because drug potency tends not to be altered immediately by the stomach or liver; and (3) the cost of drug therapy is often higher. Drugs are administered by injection when all of the drug must be absorbed as rapidly and completely as possible, when the drug must be absorbed at a steady and controlled rate, or when a patient is unable to take a medication orally because of nausea and vomiting.

SAFE PREPARATION, ADMINISTRATION, AND DISPOSAL OF PARENTERAL MEDICATIONS AND SUPPLIES

Drug preparation and administration errors have been identified as contributing factors to the high incidence of adverse drug events as discussed in Chapter 6. The actual rate of errors that occur during the preparation

and administration of medications is not known, but the potential is high. Thus the nurse must be diligent to prevent errors from occurring.

The role of the nurse in providing accurate drug administration requires attention to detail in all facets of pharmacotherapy. It is essential that nurses who are preparing and administering medications focus on the following: (1) the basic knowledge needed regarding the individual drugs being ordered, prepared, and administered; (2) the symptoms for which the medication is prescribed and the collection of baseline data to be used for the evaluation of the therapeutic outcomes desired for the prescribed medicine; and (3) the nursing assessments necessary to detect, prevent, or ameliorate adverse events. Finally, the nurse must exercise clinical judgment regarding the scheduling of new drug orders, missed doses, modified drug orders, the substitution of therapeutically equivalent medicines by the pharmacy, or changes in the patient's condition that require consultation with a physician, healthcare provider, or pharmacist.

Injection of drugs requires skill and special care because of the trauma at the site of needle puncture, the possibility of infection, the chance of allergic reaction, and the fact that, after it is injected, the drug is irretrievable. Therefore medications must be prepared and administered carefully and accurately. Aseptic technique is used during injection to avoid infection. Correct rate of drug administration and correct site of injection are followed to avoid injuries such as abscess formation, necrosis, skin sloughing, nerve injuries, and prolonged pain. Thus the parenteral administration of medications requires specialized knowledge and manual skills to ensure safety and therapeutic effectiveness for patients.

Healthcare professionals place the safety of their patients first, but the Occupational Safety and Health Administration (OSHA) has reported that more than 5 million workers in the healthcare industry and related occupations are at risk for occupational exposure to blood-borne pathogens that can cause devastating diseases, including human immunodeficiency virus, hepatitis B virus, and hepatitis C virus. Studies have indicated that as many as one-third of all sharps injuries (i.e., from needles, lancets, and scalpels) are related to the disposal process and that nurses sustain the majority of these injuries. Consequently, nurses have three primary safety concerns: for the patient, for themselves, and for other healthcare workers. Paramount to the safe administration of medicines is the need for nurses to follow established policies and procedures while checking and transcribing orders; preparing, administering, recording, and monitoring therapeutic responses to drug therapy; and properly disposing of parenteral supplies and equipment.

EQUIPMENT USED FOR PARENTERAL ADMINISTRATION

SYRINGES

Syringes are generally made of hard plastic; glass syringes are rarely used in clinical practice. A syringe has three parts (Fig. 9.1). The **barrel** is the outer portion on which the calibrations for the measurement of the drug volume are located (Fig. 9.2). The **plunger** is the inner cylindrical portion that fits snugly into the barrel. This portion is used to draw up and eject the solution from the syringe. The **tip** is the portion that holds the needle. Syringes are considered to be sterile when the package is still intact from the manufacturer. The nurse will remove the outer sheath that covers the syringe and then hold the barrel; the outside of the barrel is then considered unsterile or contaminated, whereas the inside of the barrel remains sterile. Nurses must keep the tip of the syringe sterile when connecting needles.

All syringes, regardless of their manufacturer, are available with a Luer-Slip or Luer-Lok tip. The Luer system consists of two parts: the male tapered end (Fig. 9.3A) and the reverse-tapered female connector with an outer flange (Fig. 9.3B).

The two types of syringe tips are the Luer-Slip, which has a male tapered end (Fig. 9.4A), and the Luer-Lok (Fig. 9.4B), which has a threaded locking collar outside of the male Luer-Slip that will lock the flange of the female connector securely. When the female connector is placed on a male Luer-Slip with a locking collar and given a half twist, it is securely locked in place (see Fig. 9.3C or Fig. 9.4B). However, if a female adapter is placed on a male Luer-Slip without a collar (see Fig. 9.4A), the connection is only relatively secure.

Syringe Calibration

A syringe is calibrated in milliliters (mL) (see Fig. 9.2). The most commonly used syringes are 1, 3, and 5 mL, but syringes of 10, 20, and 50 mL are also available. (NOTE: Technically, the milliliter is a measure of volume.)

Reading the calibration of the syringe

Milliliter (mL) scale. The **milliliter scale** represents the units whereby medications are routinely ordered. For volumes of 1 mL or less, use a 1-mL or tuberculin syringe for the more precise measurement of the drug (Fig. 9.5). Milliliters are read on the scale marked "mL" (see Figs. 9.2 and 9.5). The shorter lines represent 0.1 mL, and the longer lines each represent 0.5 mL.

Tuberculin syringe. The **tuberculin syringe**, or 1-mL syringe, was originally designed to administer tuberculin inoculations (see Fig. 9.5). Today it is used to measure small volumes of medication accurately. This type of syringe holds a total of 1 mL; each of the longest lines represents 0.1 ($\frac{1}{10}$) mL, the intermediate lines represent

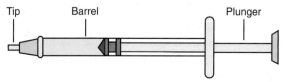

Fig. 9.1 Parts of a syringe.

Tip   Barrel   Plunger

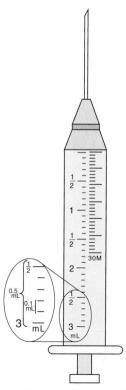

Fig. 9.2 Reading the calibrations of a 3-mL syringe.

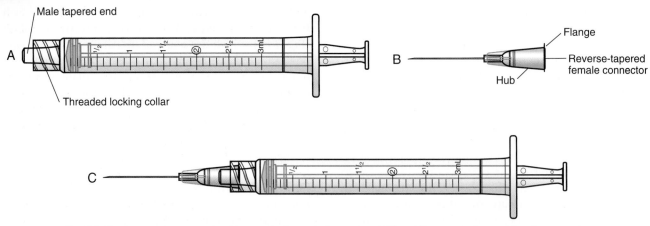

Fig. 9.3 The Luer system consists of two parts: the male tapered end (A) and the reverse-tapered female connector with an outer flange (B). (C) When the two components are joined together, the hub of the female connector slips over the male tapered end and is twisted so that the flange on the hub locks into the threads of the locking collar.

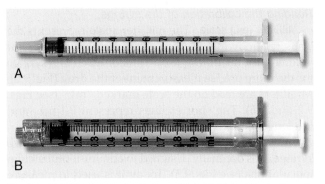

Fig. 9.4 (A) Male slip adapter tip (Luer-Slip). (B) Male slip adapter with outer locking collar (Luer-Lok). (Courtesy and © Becton, Dickinson and Company, Franklin Lakes, NJ.)

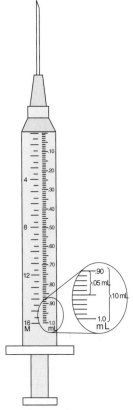

Fig. 9.5 Tuberculin syringe calibration.

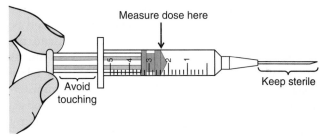

Fig. 9.6 Reading the measured amount of medication in a plastic syringe.

0.05 ($\frac{5}{100}$) mL, and the shortest lines represent 0.01 ($\frac{1}{100}$) mL.

Volumes in disposable plastic syringes are read at the point where the rubber flange of the syringe plunger is parallel to the calibration scale of the barrel (Fig. 9.6). In addition, note the area of the needle to keep sterile and the area on the syringe plunger to avoid touching.

Insulin syringe. The insulin syringe has a scale that has been specifically calibrated for the measurement of insulin. Insulin is now manufactured with a U-100 concentration in the United States. The U-100 syringe (Fig. 9.7A) holds 100 units of insulin per milliliter. Variations may be noticed in the way that units are marked on the scale, but in general the shorter lines represent 2 units of insulin, whereas the longer lines measure 10 units of insulin. Low-dose insulin syringes (Fig. 9.7B) may be used for patients who are receiving 50 units or less of U-100 insulin. The shorter lines on the scale of the low-dose insulin syringe measure 1 unit, whereas the longer lines each represent 5 units. When traveling abroad, patients should be aware that U-40 concentration insulin (i.e., 40 units of insulin/mL) is commonly available. A specific insulin syringe that has been calibrated for U-40 insulin should be used with the U-40 insulin.

Insulin delivery aids (e.g., nonvisual insulin measurement devices, syringe magnifiers, needle guides, vial stabilizers) are available for people with visual impairments. Information about these products is available

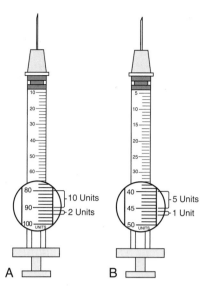

Fig. 9.7 Calibration of insulin syringes. (A) U-100 insulin syringe. (B) Low-dose insulin syringe. Low-dose syringes are available in 25-, 30-, and 50-unit sizes to measure U-100 insulin more accurately.

in the American Diabetes Association's annual diabetes resource guide, which is published each January.

 Life Span Considerations

Tuberculin Syringe

The tuberculin syringe (see Fig. 9.5), which makes use of the metric system of measurement, will provide the most accurate measurement for doses of parenteral medications of 1 mL or less. The practice of adding 0.2 mL of air bubbles to thoroughly empty all of the medication contained in the needle of a syringe can significantly increase a drug dose, especially when small volumes of medicine are being administered to neonates or infants. Check institutional policy regarding medication administration for the procedure to be used.

Prefilled Cartridges and Syringes

Several manufacturers supply a premeasured amount of medication either in presealed cartridge-needle units or in prefilled complete syringes. Both are used once and then discarded. Advantages of the **prefilled cartridges and syringes** include the time saved in preparing a standard amount of medication for one injection and the diminished chance of contamination between patients and hospital personnel. Disadvantages include additional expense and the limitation of the volume if a second medication is to be added to the cartridge or syringe.

The prefilled cartridge-needle units are marketed under the brand name Carpuject. The cartridge contains the amount of drug for one standard dose of medication. The drug name, concentration, and volume are clearly printed on the cartridge. The Carpuject prefilled cartridges require a holder that corresponds with the type of cartridge used (Fig. 9.8). Examples of drugs dispensed in prefilled cartridges are morphine, ketorolac, hydromorphone, ondansetron, and heparin. Other medicines (e.g., specific vaccines, enoxaparin, dalteparin, diclofenac,

amiodarone) are shipped from the manufacturer in a syringe for ease of use. Many hospital pharmacies prefill syringes for specific doses of medication for patients with specific conditions. The syringe is labeled with the drug name and dosage, the patient's name and room number, and the dates of preparation and expiration.

Insulin is also available in a prefilled syringe known as an **insulin pen** (Fig. 9.9). When capped, these pens look very much like ink pens, which allows the patient to carry insulin in a discreet manner. When needed, the cap is removed, a needle is attached, air bubbles are removed, the dose is dialed in, the needle is inserted into the subcut tissue, and a trigger is pushed to inject the measured dose. When finished, the needle is removed and the cap replaced, and the device again takes on the appearance of a pen. These pens are available in a variety of colors and styles, including a prefilled, disposable model; a smaller, low-dose model; and a refillable model into which a new cartridge can be inserted when needed. The patient should be instructed regarding the correct method of holding the pen and reading the dosing dial as indicated by the manufacturer; this will help to prevent dosing errors.

Another type of prefilled syringe is the EpiPen (Fig. 9.10). This syringe is a disposable automatic injection device that has been prefilled with epinephrine for use in an emergency, such as that caused by an allergic reaction to insect stings or bites, foods, or drugs. When held perpendicularly against the thigh and activated, a needle penetrates the skin into the muscle, and a single dose of epinephrine is injected into the muscle. This product is available in adult and pediatric dosages for use at home or when traveling for those who have strong reactions when they are exposed to allergens. It is important to educate those who are carrying these prefilled syringes to monitor the expiration date of this medication on a regular basis. After the epinephrine has been administered, the person should go to a hospital emergency department because additional treatment may be necessary. Other recently released products of injectable epinephrine for allergies are Auvi-Q and Impax.

THE NEEDLE

Parts of the Needle

The needle parts are the hub, the shaft, and the beveled tip (Fig. 9.11). The angle of the bevel can vary; the longer the bevel, the easier the needle penetration.

Needles are sterile when they arrive from the manufacturer. Nurses must pay careful attention to keep the parts of the needle sterile and to avoid contamination. If contamination is suspected during the process of withdrawing medications, discard the needle in a sharps container and start again with a new one.

Needle Gauge

The **needle gauge** is the diameter of the hole through the needle. The larger the gauge number, the smaller

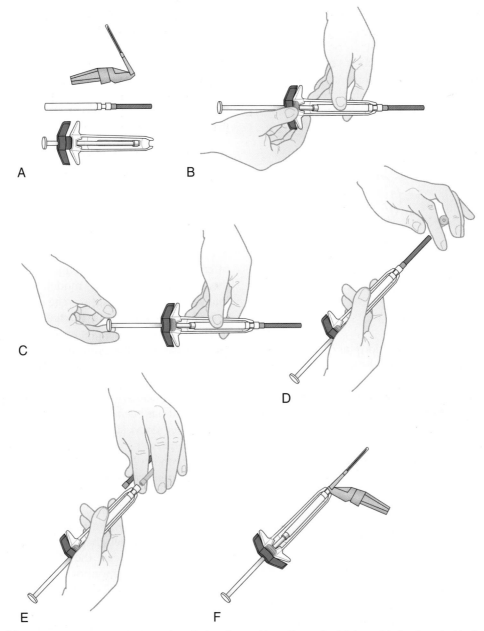

A B C D E F

Fig. 9.8 (A) Carpuject cartridge holder and prefilled sterile cartridge with needle. (B) Assemble the Carpuject by inserting the prefilled cartridge inside the Carpuject holder; lay the white flange of the syringe over one end and lock the blue end down to keep the syringe in place. (C) Twist the white end to screw into the prefilled cartridge. (D and E) Remove the green cover from the tip of the cartridge (D); keeping this end sterile, attach the needle to the cartridge (E). (F) Needle is now attached to the prefilled cartridge in a Carpuject cartridge holder.

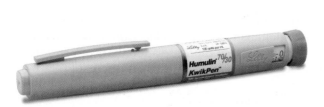

Fig. 9.9 An insulin pen. (Copyright Eli Lilly and Company, Indianapolis, IN. All rights reserved. Used with permission.)

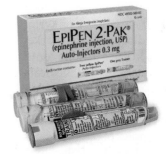
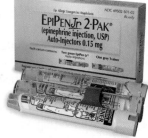

Fig. 9.10 Prefilled syringe and needle containing epinephrine for use during emergencies. (Courtesy Mylan Inc., Canonsburg, PA.)

the hole. The gauge number is marked on the hub of the needle and on the outside of the disposable package. The proper needle gauge is usually selected on the basis of the viscosity (thickness) of the solution to be injected. A thicker solution requires a larger diameter, so a smaller gauge number is chosen (Fig. 9.12). Finer needles (e.g., 27, 29, 31, and 32 gauge) are available for specialty use.

SELECTION OF THE SYRINGE AND NEEDLE

The size of the syringe used is determined by the volume of medication to be administered, the degree of accuracy needed for the measurement of the dose, and the type of medication to be administered.

Needle selection should be based on the correct gauge for the viscosity of the solution and the correct needle length for the delivery of the medication to the correct site (e.g., intradermal, subcut, IM, or IV). Table 9.1 may be used as a guide to select the proper volume of syringe and the length and gauge of needle for adult patients.

In small children and older infants, the usual maximum volume for an IM injection at one site is 1 mL. In small infants, the muscle mass may only be able to tolerate a volume of 0.5 mL using a ½-inch–long needle. For older children, the volume should be individualized; generally, the larger the muscle mass, the greater the similarity to the adult volume for one injection site. Pediatric IM injections routinely use a 25- to 27-gauge needle that is 1 to 1½ inches long, depending on the assessment of the depth of the muscle

mass of the child. Also available for pediatric use are 31-gauge, ½-inch needles.

Selection of Needle Length

Assess the depth of the patient's tissue for administration (e.g., muscle tissue for IM administration, subcutaneous tissue for subcut injection), and choose a needle length that corresponds to the findings.

Example of How to Select Needle Length

Compare the muscle depth of a 250-pound, obese, sedentary woman with the muscle depth of a 105-pound, debilitated adult patient. The obese individual may require a 2½- to 3-inch needle, and the frail person may need a 1- to 1½-inch needle. A child may require a 1-inch needle (Fig. 9.13).

PACKAGING OF SYRINGES AND NEEDLES

The sterility of the syringe and needle to be used should always be inspected and verified when preparing and administering a parenteral medication. Wrappers should be checked for holes, signs of moisture penetration of the wrapper, and the expiration date. With prepackaged disposable items, the continuity of the wrapper, loose lids or needle guards, and any penetration of the paper or plastic container by the needle should also be checked.

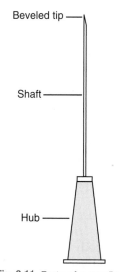

Fig. 9.11 Parts of a needle.

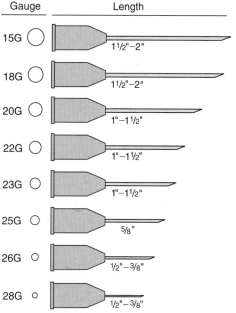

Fig. 9.12 Needle length and gauge.

Table **9.1**   Selection of Syringe and Needle

ROUTE	VOLUME (mL)	GAUGE	LENGTH[a]
Intradermal	0.01-0.1	26-29	⅜ to ½ inch
Subcutaneous	0.5-2	25-27	Individualized on the basis of the depth of the appropriate tissue at the site
Intramuscular	0.5-2[b]	20-23	Individualized on the basis of the depth of the appropriate tissue at the site

[a]When judging the needle length, allow an extra ¼ to ½ inch to remain above the skin surface when the injection is administered. In the rare event of a needle breaking, this allows a length of needle to protrude above the skin to grasp for removal.
[b]Divided doses are generally recommended for volumes that exceed 2 to 3 mL, particularly for medications that are irritating to the tissues.

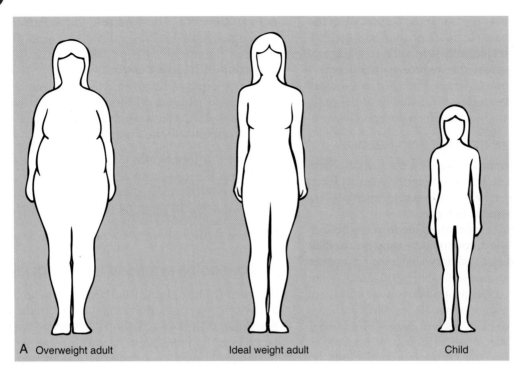

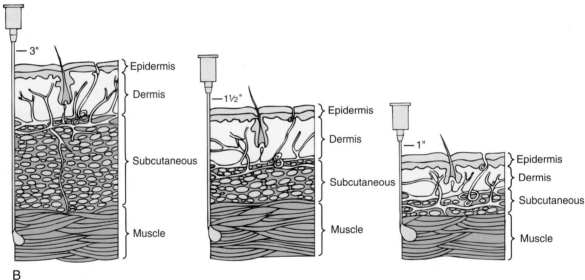

Fig. 9.13 Use body size (A) to estimate needle length for an intramuscular injection (B).

Should contamination be suspected, do not use the syringe; return it to the pharmacy for replacement.

SAFETY SYSTEMS FOR PARENTERAL PREPARATION, ADMINISTRATION, AND DISPOSAL

The US Congress passed the Needlestick Safety and Prevention Act in 2000 in response to sharps injuries from medical devices, most commonly needlesticks. This act requires OSHA to update its standards on blood-borne pathogens for the closer monitoring and reporting of needlestick injuries and to mandate the development of new safety equipment for the healthcare industry. One of the major developments has been the broader use of needleless systems. In accordance with OSHA regulations, needleless systems are required for the following: (1) for the collection of body fluids or the withdrawal of body fluids after initial venous or arterial access is established; (2) for the administration of medication or fluids; or (3) for any other procedure involving the potential for occupational exposure to blood-borne pathogens as a result of percutaneous injuries from contaminated sharps. Needleless systems provide an alternative to needles for routine procedures, thereby reducing the risk of injury involving contaminated sharps. Another delivery system under development is a jet injection system that delivers subcut injections of liquid medication (e.g., insulin, vaccine) through the skin without requiring the use of a needle.

BLUNT ACCESS DEVICES

The blunt access device (e.g., the spike) is a safety innovation that was created to reduce the frequency of needle injuries (Fig. 9.14). Note in that needleless access devices do not have a stainless steel needle that is suitable for injection (Fig. 9.14A). The spike is used when drawing liquid from a rubber-diaphragm–covered vial (Fig. 9.14B). Another type of blunt access device that is more commonly known as a *filter needle* looks similar to other spikes, but it contains an internal filter. This device is used to withdraw liquid from a glass ampule. The filter screens out glass particles that may have fallen into the ampule when the top was broken off (see Fig. 9.23). In addition to preventing needlestick injuries, these blunt access devices have the advantage of drawing larger fluid volumes from the container more rapidly. After the spike is used to draw up a medication, it is removed and the appropriately sized needle is attached to the syringe if the medication is intended for injection directly into the patient.

SAFETY DEVICES

Safety devices have been developed for syringes and needles. Some products have a sleeve that is stored

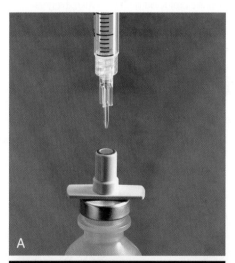

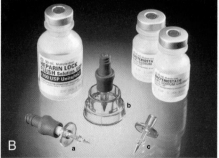

Fig. 9.14 Needle-free access devices. (A) INTERLINK Vial Access Cannula entering a universal vial adapter. (B) CLAVE Access System. *a*, A needle-free multidose vial adapter. *b*, The device snaps onto the top of a standard 20-mm medication vial. *c*, A single-dose vial adapter. (*A*, Courtesy Baxter Healthcare Corporation, Mountain Home, AR. All rights reserved. *B*, Courtesy ICU Medical Inc., San Clemente, CA.)

around the syringe barrel while the syringe is being filled through the needle (Fig. 9.15). After administration, the sleeve is pulled forward fully to lock the shield permanently in place to cover the needle. Another type of safety shielding device attaches to the needle hub (Fig. 9.16). After the medicine is injected, the healthcare provider pushes the hinged shield forward, thereby covering the needle. Other safety shield devices are also available for short needles (Fig. 9.17) and for closure with "hands-free" devices (Fig. 9.18). The BD Integra Syringe System is a spring-loaded syringe that retracts the needle into the syringe after injection. This system also uses a technology called Tru-Lok technology, which involves an apparatus that is similar to Luer-Lok technology. It allows for the changing of the needle between aspiration and administration, it locks the syringe and needle together securely, and it has a very low waste space in the hub (Fig. 9.18). Like all safety-designed syringes and needles, it is necessary to read the accompanying literature for adjustments that need to be made when operating these devices.

APPROPRIATE DISPOSAL

The appropriate disposal of used syringes and needles—including those with needle protection devices—is crucial to the prevention of needle injury and the transfer of blood-borne pathogens. To help minimize accidental needlesticks, a needle disposal container is commonly used for all sharps (Fig. 9.19). When the container is full, the lid stays in place and the entire container is disposed of in a specific manner to comply with OSHA standards. It is important to teach self-injecting patients how to protect themselves and others from accidental needlestick injury. Patients are encouraged to purchase a Sharps Disposal by Mail System at their pharmacy for the disposal of syringes, needles, and lancets. It is critical that patients use these systems to prevent the accidental exposure of sanitation workers to needles. The mail system includes a sharps container, an outer shipping box, and a prepaid postage label so that, when the container is filled, it can be mailed to an appropriate disposal center. If a patient is uncertain about the safest procedure for the disposal of used syringes and needles, he or she should contact the local sanitation service or department.

PARENTERAL DOSE FORMS

All parenteral drug dose forms are packaged so that the drug is sterile and ready for reconstitution (if needed) and administration.

AMPULES

Ampules are glass containers that usually contain a single dose of a medication. The container may be scored (Fig. 9.20A) or have a darkened ring around the neck (Fig. 9.20B) to indicate where the ampule should be broken open for withdrawing the medication.

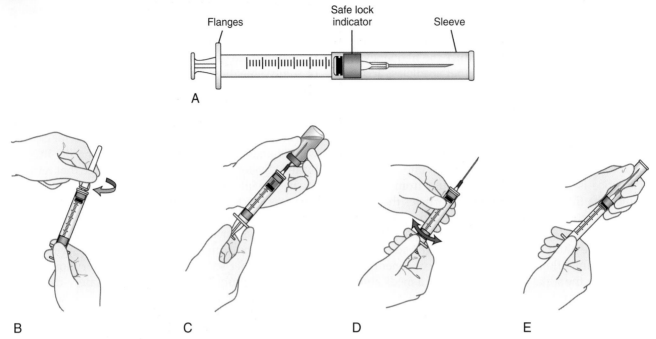

Fig. 9.15 An example of a safety syringe that includes a full protective sheath. (A) Syringe showing a sheath that covers the needle with a safe lock indicator. (B) Assemble the device by holding the needle and the syringe by the flanges (wings) and twisting the needle until it is firmly seated. (C) During aspiration, press the index finger against the flanges to prevent sleeve movement. (NOTE: If it is necessary to transport a filled syringe to the point of administration, use a safe, passive, one-handed recapping technique, per Occupational Safety and Health Administration standards, to cover the needle before transporting it to the point of use.) (D) After injection, grasp the sleeve firmly, and twist the flanges to loosen the sleeve. (E) Fully retract the needle into the sleeve until it locks in the protected position. When the green band fully covers the red band and an audible click is heard, the sleeve is locked into position. Place in sharps container.

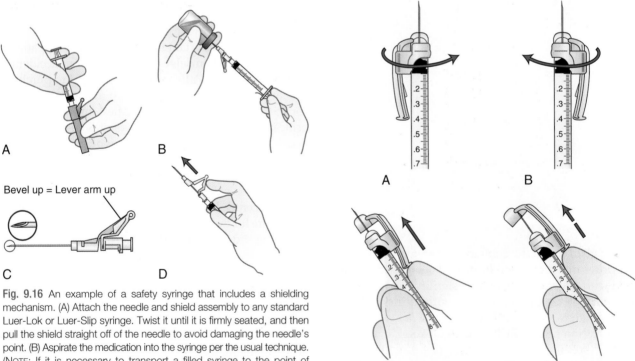

Fig. 9.16 An example of a safety syringe that includes a shielding mechanism. (A) Attach the needle and shield assembly to any standard Luer-Lok or Luer-Slip syringe. Twist it until it is firmly seated, and then pull the shield straight off of the needle to avoid damaging the needle's point. (B) Aspirate the medication into the syringe per the usual technique. (NOTE: If it is necessary to transport a filled syringe to the point of administration, use a safe, passive, one-handed recapping technique, per Occupational Safety and Health Administration standards, to cover the needle before transporting it to the point of use.) (C) Administer the injection in accordance with established technique. Note that the needle bevel is oriented to the lever arm. (D) After injection, immediately apply a single finger stroke to the activation-assist lever arm to activate the shielding mechanism. Place in sharps container. (NOTE: Activate the device away from yourself and others, listen for the click, and visually confirm that the needle tip is fully covered.)

Fig. 9.17 Another example of a safety syringe that includes a shielding mechanism. (A) Aspirate the medication into the syringe per the usual technique. The safety arm can be rotated for scale readability. (B) Administer the injection. To facilitate a low angle of injection, the safety arm can be rotated so that it is oriented to the needle bevel. (C) After injection, apply a single finger stroke to activate the safety arm by moving it completely forward. (D) The safety arm is locked and fully extended when you hear the click and the needle tip is covered.

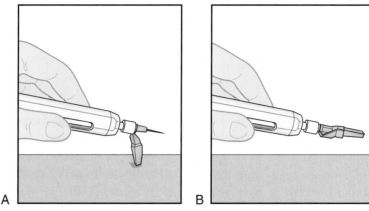

Fig. 9.18 Hands-free safety device.

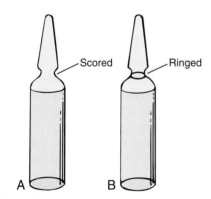

Fig. 9.19 Needle disposal container, also known as a sharps container.

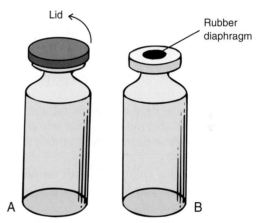

Fig. 9.21 (A) Vial protected by metal lid. (B) Rubber diaphragm exposed when lid is removed.

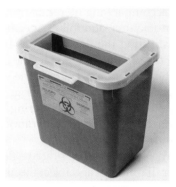

Fig. 9.20 (A) Scored ampule. (B) Ringed ampule.

VIALS

Vials are glass or plastic containers that contain one or more doses of a sterile medication. The unused vial is sealed with a metal lid to ensure sterility (Fig. 9. 21A). The mouth of the vial is covered with a thick rubber diaphragm through which a needle is passed to remove the medication (Fig. 9. 21B). The medication in the vial may be in solution, or it may be a sterile powder to be reconstituted just before administration. The drug also can be withdrawn from the vial using a spike attached to the syringe (see Fig. 9.14).

MIX-O-VIALS

Mix-O-Vials are glass containers with two compartments (Fig. 9.22). The lower chamber contains the drug (solute),

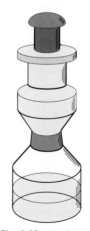

Fig. 9.22 Mix-O-Vial.

and the upper chamber contains a sterile diluent (solvent); between the two areas is a rubber stopper. A single dose of medication is normally contained in the Mix-O-Vial. At the time of use, pressure is applied to the top rubber diaphragm plunger. This forces the solvent and the rubber stopper to fall into the bottom chamber, where the diluent mixes with the powder, thereby dissolving the drug.

PREPARATION OF PARENTERAL MEDICATION

EQUIPMENT
- Drug in a sterile, sealed container
- Syringe of the correct volume
- Needles of the correct gauge and length
- Needleless access device
- Antiseptic alcohol wipe
- Medication profile

PROCEDURE PROTOCOL
The standard procedures for preparing all parenteral medications are as follows:

1. Perform hand hygiene *before* preparing any medication or handling sterile supplies. During the actual preparation of a parenteral medication, the primary rule to remember is "sterile to sterile" and "unsterile to unsterile" when handling the syringe and the needle.
2. Use the *seven rights* of medication preparation and administration throughout the procedure: right patient, right drug, right indication, right route, right dose, right time, and right documentation.
3. Check the drug dose form ordered against the source available.
4. Check compatibility charts or contact the pharmacist before mixing two medications or before adding medication to an IV solution.
5. Check medication calculations. When in doubt about a dose, check it with another qualified nurse. (Most hospital policies require fractional doses of medications and doses of heparin and insulin to be checked by two qualified personnel before administration.)
6. Know the institutional policy regarding limitations on the types of medications to be administered by nursing personnel.
7. Check the expiration date on the medication container.
8. After completing the standard procedures for preparing all parenteral medications, concentrate on the procedure at hand to ensure accuracy during preparation.
9. Prepare the drug in a clean, well-lit area and use aseptic technique throughout the entire procedure.

TECHNIQUES

Preparing a Medication From an Ampule
1. Move all the solution to the bottom of the ampule, and flick the side of the glass container with the fingers to displace the medication from the top portion of the ampule (Fig. 9.23A).
2. Cover the ampule neck area with an antiseptic alcohol wipe in its sleeve while breaking the top off (Fig. 9.23B-D). Discard the wipe and the ampule top in a sharps container.
3. With the use of a filter needle, withdraw all the medication from the ampule (Fig. 9.23E and F).
4. Remove the filter needle from the ampule and point it vertically. Pull back on the plunger (this allows air to enter the syringe), and then replace the filter needle with a new sterile needle of the appropriate gauge and length for administration.
5. Push the plunger slowly until the medication appears at the tip of the needle or measure the amount of air to be included to allow for the total clearance of the medication from the needle when injected. (Never add air to a syringe that is to be used to administer an IV medication.)

Drugs in a vial may be in solution ready for administration, or they may be in powdered form for reconstitution before administration.

Preparing a Medication From a Vial
Reconstitution of a sterile powder

1. Read the accompanying literature from the medication's manufacturer, and follow specific instructions for reconstituting the drug that has been ordered. Add only the diluent specified by the manufacturer.
2. Cleanse the rubber diaphragm of the vial of diluent with an antiseptic alcohol wipe (Fig. 9.24A).
3. Pull back on the plunger of the syringe to fill it with an amount of air equal to the volume of solution to be withdrawn (Fig. 9.24B).
4. Insert the needle or needleless access device through the rubber diaphragm and inject the air (Fig. 9.24C).
5. Withdraw the measured volume of diluent required to reconstitute the powdered drug (Fig. 9.24D and E). Remove the needle from the diaphragm of the diluent container.
6. Recheck the type and volume of diluent to be injected against the type and amount required.
7. Tap the vial containing the powdered drug to break up the caked powder (Fig. 9.24F). Wipe the rubber diaphragm of the vial of powdered drug with a new alcohol wipe (Fig. 9.24G).
8. Insert the needle or needleless access device in the diaphragm and inject the diluent into the powder (Fig. 9.24H).
9. Remove the syringe and needle from the rubber diaphragm.
10. *Mix the powdered drug and diluent thoroughly* to ensure that the powder is entirely dissolved *before* withdrawing the dose (Fig. 9.24I).
11. Label the reconstituted medication, and include the date and time of reconstitution, the volume and type of diluent added, the name of the reconstituted drug, the concentration of the reconstituted drug, the expiration date and time, and the name of the person who reconstituted the drug. Store the medication in accordance with the manufacturer's instructions.

Removal of a volume of liquid from a vial
(see Fig. 9.24A-E)

1. Calculate the volume of medication required for the prescribed dose of medication to be administered.
2. Cleanse the rubber diaphragm of the vial of drug with an antiseptic alcohol wipe.

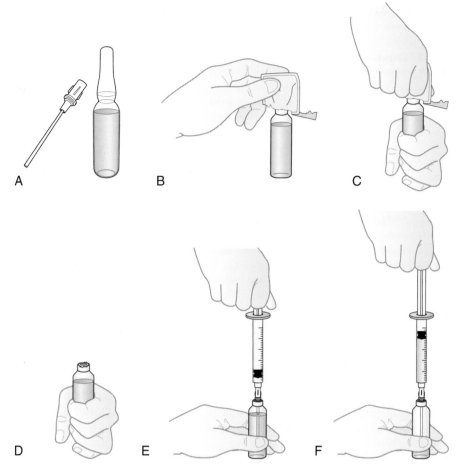

Fig. 9.23 Withdrawing from an ampule with a filter needle. (A) Obtain a filter needle and displace the medication from the top portion of the ampule. (B) Cover the ampule neck area with an antiseptic alcohol wipe remaining in its cover. (C and D) Snap off the top of the ampule sharply in one swift motion. (E) Using a filter needle, withdraw the medication from the ampule. (F) Note that the needle must be lowered to withdraw all of the solution from the ampule.

3. Pull back on the plunger of the syringe to fill it with an amount of air equal to the volume of solution to be withdrawn.
4. Insert the needle or needleless access device through the rubber diaphragm and inject the air.
5. Withdraw the volume of drug required to administer the prescribed dose.
6. Recheck all aspects of the drug order.
7. Remove the needle or the needleless access device from the syringe. Attach a new sterile needle of the appropriate gauge and length to administer the medication to the patient.

Preparing a Drug From a Mix-O-Vial
1. Check the drug order against the medication available for administration.
2. Tap the container in your hand a few times to break up the caked powder.
3. Remove the plastic lid protector (Fig. 9.25A) to access the diaphragm plunger (Fig. 9.25B).
4. Push down firmly on the diaphragm plunger. The downward pressure will dislodge the divider between the two chambers (Fig. 9.25C).

5. Mix thoroughly to ensure that the powder is *completely dissolved* before drawing up the medication for administration.
6. Cleanse the rubber diaphragm and remove the drug in the same manner as described for the removal of a volume of liquid from a vial (see Fig. 9.24A-E).

Preparing Two Medications in One Syringe
Occasionally, two medications may be drawn into the same syringe for a single injection. This is usually done when preparing a preoperative medication or when two types of insulin are ordered to be administered at the same time. Mixing insulin is a routine procedure, so it will be used to illustrate this technique. Before administering insulin, the nurse always evaluates the patient's blood glucose level.
1. Check the compatibility of the two types of insulin to be mixed before starting to prepare the medications.
2. Check the labels of the insulin vials against the insulin order. Check the insulin order and the calculations of the preparation with another qualified nurse in accordance with institutional policy.

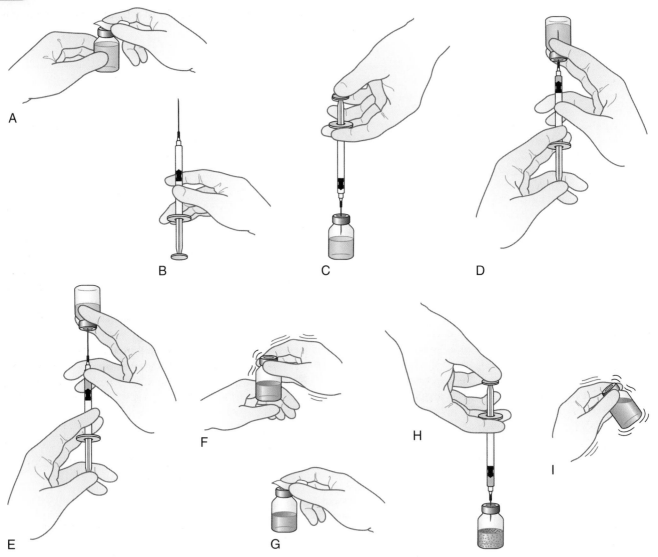

Fig. 9.24 Removal of a volume of liquid from a vial for reconstitution of a powder. (A) Cleanse the rubber diaphragm of the vial. (B) Pull back on the plunger of the syringe to fill with an amount of air that is equal to the volume of the solution to be withdrawn. (C) Insert the needle through the rubber diaphragm; inject the air with the vial sitting in a downward position. (D) Invert the syringe and vial and withdraw the volume of diluent required to reconstitute the drug. (E) Move the needle downward within the rubber diaphragm to facilitate the removal of all of the diluent. (F) Tap the container with the powdered drug to break up the caked powder. (G) Wipe the rubber diaphragm of the vial of the powdered drug with a new antiseptic alcohol wipe. (H) Insert the needle of the syringe with the diluent into the rubber diaphragm, and inject the diluent into the powdered drug. (I) Mix thoroughly to ensure that the powdered drug is dissolved before withdrawing the prescribed dose.

3. Check the following:
   - *Type:* regular, neutral protamine Hagedorn (NPH), other
   - *Concentration:* U-100 (U-100 = 100 units/mL)
   - *Expiration date:* Do NOT use the insulin if the expiration date has passed.
   - *Appearance:* Clear? Cloudy? Precipitate present? Insulin suspensions should be cloudy. All other insulin solutions should be clear. See Table 35.5.
   - *Temperature:* The insulin should be at room temperature.
4. To resuspend insulin suspensions, (NPH, Humulin, Novolin, Humalog, Novolog insulin), roll the vial or pen between the palms of the hands or gently invert the vial several times to mix the contents thoroughly. See Table 35.6 on compatibility of combining insulins
5. The American Diabetes Association's 2017 guidelines recommend drawing up the rapid-acting insulin into the syringe then adding the intermediate-acting insulin.
   - When teaching a patient to mix insulin for self-administration, using a consistent method of preparing the mixture should be stressed so that this becomes a habit for the patient. This can help to prevent the patient from inadvertently reversing the dose of rapid- and longer-acting insulin in the mixture.
6. Cleanse the tops of *both* vials with separate antiseptic alcohol wipes (Fig. 9.26A).

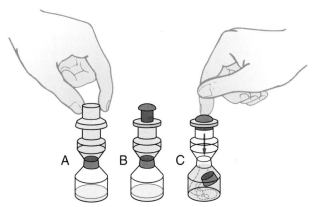

Fig. 9.25 Using a Mix-O-Vial. (A) Remove the plastic lid protector to expose the diaphragm plunger. (B) The powdered drug is in the lower half; the diluent is in the upper half. (C) Push firmly on the diaphragm plunger; downward pressure dislodges the divider between the two chambers.

7. Pull back the plunger on the syringe to an amount that is equal to the volume of the longer-acting insulin that has been ordered (Fig. 9.26B).
8. Insert the needle through the rubber seal of the longer-acting insulin bottle, and inject the air (Fig. 9.26C). Do not bubble air through the insulin solution, because it might break up insulin particles. Remove the syringe and needle. Do not withdraw insulin at this time.
9. Pull back the plunger on the syringe to an amount that is equal to the volume of the shorter-acting insulin that has been ordered (Fig. 9.26D).
10. Insert the needle through the rubber seal of the second bottle and inject the air (Fig. 9.26E).
11. Invert the bottle, and withdraw the volume of rapid-acting insulin (Fig. 9.26F). (NOTE: Leaving the needle in the bottle, check for bubbles in the insulin in the syringe. Flick the side of the syringe with the fingers to displace the bubbles, and then recheck the amount of insulin in the syringe.) Remove the syringe and needle. Check the medication order against the label of the container and the amount in the syringe.
12. Wipe the lid of the longer-acting insulin container again (Fig. 9.26G). Recheck the drug order against this container.
13. Insert the needle of the syringe containing the rapid-acting insulin, and withdraw the specified amount of longer-acting insulin (Fig. 9.26H). Be careful *not* to inject any of the first type of insulin already in the syringe into the longer-acting insulin vial.
14. Remove the syringe and needle. Recheck the drug order against the labels on the insulin containers and the amount in the syringe (Fig. 9.26I).
15. Draw back a small amount of air into the syringe, and then mix the two medications. Remove air carefully so that part of the medication is not displaced.

16. Administer the insulin to the patient by the subcut route.

GUIDELINES FOR PREPARING MEDICATIONS FOR USE IN THE STERILE FIELD DURING A SURGICAL PROCEDURE
Drugs Used in the Operating Room
- All medications used during an operative procedure must remain sterile.
- All medication containers (e.g., ampules, vials, piggyback containers, blood bags) used during the surgical procedure should remain in the operating room until the entire procedure is completed. If a question arises, the container is then available.
- *Do not save* any unused portion of medication for use during another surgical procedure. Discard this unused medication at the end of the surgical procedure, or send the patient's medication to the patient care unit with the patient, if appropriate (e.g., antibiotic ointment for a patient who is having ophthalmic surgery).
- Adhere to hospital policies that address the handling and storage of medications in the operating room.
- *Always* tell the surgeon the name and dosage or concentration of the medication or solution that is being handed to him or her.
- *Always* repeat the entire medication order back to the surgeon when the request is made to verify all aspects of the order. If in doubt, repeat this information again until accuracy is certain.

Drugs Used in the Sterile Surgical Field
- Prepare the drug prescribed in accordance with the directions.
- Always check the accuracy of the drug order against the medication being prepared at least three times during the preparation phase: (1) when it is first removed from the drug storage area; (2) immediately before removing the solution for use in the sterile field; and (3) immediately after completing the transfer of the medication or solution to the sterile field. *Always* tell the surgeon the name and dose or concentration of the medication or solution when passing it to him or her for use.
- The circulating (nonsterile) nurse retrieves the medication from storage, reconstitutes it as needed, and turns the medication container so that the scrubbed (sterile) person can read the label. It is best to read the label aloud to ensure that both individuals are verifying the contents against the verbal order from the surgeon.
- The medication is transferred to the sterile field by one of two methods.

Method 1
1. The circulating (nonsterile) nurse cleanses the top of the vial or breaks off the top of the ampule, as described previously.

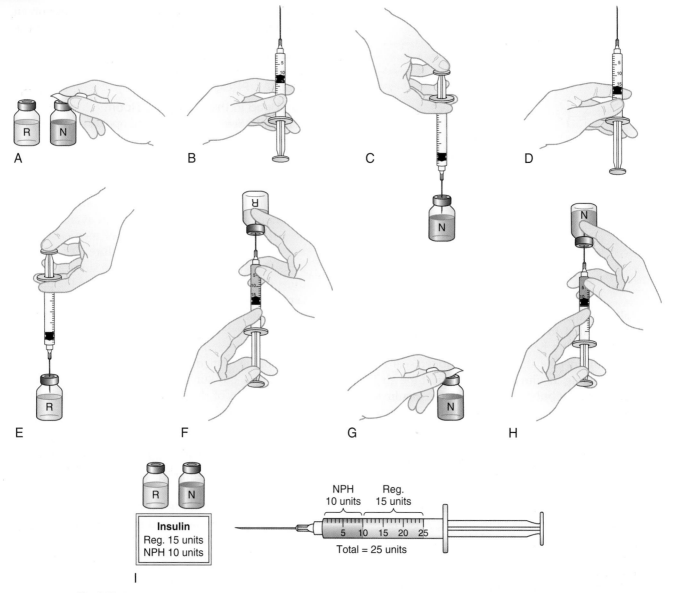

Fig. 9.26 Preparing two drugs in one syringe. (A) Check the insulin order and then cleanse the tops of both vials with an antiseptic alcohol wipe. (B) Pull back on the plunger to an amount that is equal to the volume of the longer-acting insulin. (C) Insert the needle through the rubber diaphragm of the longer-acting insulin and inject the air. Remove the syringe and needle; do not remove the insulin. (D) Pull back the plunger on the syringe to a point that is equal to the volume of the shorter-acting insulin ordered. (E) Insert the needle through the rubber diaphragm and inject the air. (F) Invert the bottle and withdraw the volume of the rapid-acting insulin ordered. Remove the syringe and needle. Check the amount withdrawn against the amount ordered. (G) Rewipe the top of the longer-acting insulin vial. (H) Insert the needle; withdraw the specified amount of longer-acting insulin. (I) Remove the syringe and needle. Recheck the drug order against the labels on the insulin containers and the amount in the syringe. *R,* Regular insulin; *N,* neutral protamine Hagedorn (NPH) insulin.

2. The scrubbed (sterile) person chooses a syringe of the correct volume for the medication to be withdrawn and attaches a large-bore needle to facilitate the removal of the solution from the container.
3. The circulating (nonsterile) nurse holds the ampule or vial in such a way that the scrubbed (sterile) person can easily insert the sterile needle tip into the medication container (Fig. 9.27A).
4. The scrubbed person pulls back the plunger on the syringe until all of the medication prescribed has been withdrawn from the container and from the needle used to withdraw the medication.

5. The needle is disconnected from the syringe and left in the vial or ampule (see Fig. 9.27B).
6. The medication container is again shown to the scrubbed person and read aloud to verify all components of the drug prepared against the medication or solution requested.

Method 2
1. The circulating (nonsterile) nurse removes the entire lid of the vial with a bottle opener, cleanses the rim of the vial, and pours the medication directly into a sterile medicine cup held by the scrubbed nurse.

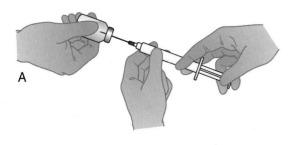

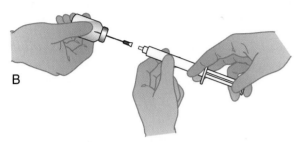

Fig. 9.27 Preparing a medication in the operating room. (A) The circulating (nonsterile) nurse holds the vial to facilitate the scrubbed (sterile) person inserting the sterile needle tip into the medication container. (B) The needle is disconnected from the syringe and left in the vial.

2. The scrubbed person continues drug preparation on the sterile field in accordance with the intended use (e.g., irrigation, injection).

Regardless of the method used to transfer the medication to the sterile field, both the sterile scrubbed person and the nonsterile circulating nurse should know the location and the exact disposition of each medication on the sterile field.

Get Ready for the NCLEX® Examination!

Key Points

- A syringe has three parts: the barrel, the plunger, and the tip that holds the needle. Types of safety syringes and needles include the Luer-Lok and needleless systems of blunt needles and shields over the needles.
- To correctly determine the gauge and length of the needle to use, the site of injection and the size of the patient are factored in, as well as the volume of medication to be administered.
- The tuberculin syringe is used to measure volumes of less than 1 mL; the standard syringe sizes are 1, 3, and 5 mL.
- Prefilled cartridge-needle units and syringes contain a standard dose of a medication and are a time saver for the nurse, but more expensive than a multidose vial of medication. Cartridges require a special cartridge holder to administer the medication.
- *Ampules* are glass containers of medications that need to be opened by snapping (breaking) the neck of the ampule before use.
- *Vials* have a rubber diaphragm that a needle passes through to access the medication.
- *Mix-O-Vials* are glass containers with two compartments. The lower compartment contains the medicine in powder form, and the upper compartment contains the diluent needed to dissolve the medicine. The two chambers are separated by a rubber plug. To mix the medicine, a rubber stopper on the top chamber is pushed, forcing the rubber stopper between the chambers to drop into the lower chamber, along with the diluent. Shaking the container dissolves the medicine, allowing it to be drawn up into a syringe for administration.

- Insulin can be mixed in one syringe by drawing up the short-acting insulin first, then adding the longer-acting insulin to the same syringe using a specific method.

Additional Learning Resources

SG Go to your Study Guide for additional Review Questions for the NCLEX® Examination, Critical Thinking Clinical Situations, and other learning activities to help you master this chapter content.

Go to your Evolve website (https://evolve.elsevier.com/Clayton) for additional online resources.

Review Questions for the NCLEX® Examination

1. Which parts of the syringe and needle are considered sterile? *(Select all that apply.)*
   1. The tip of the needle
   2. The outer barrel of the syringe
   3. The plunger tip of the syringe
   4. The Luer-Lok end
   5. The inner barrel of the syringe
2. The nurse was preparing to give an injection into her patient's abdomen for his early morning insulin dose. Which needle length and gauge are appropriate to use?
   1. 18 gauge, 1½ inch
   2. 20 gauge, 1 inch
   3. 22 gauge, ⅝ inch
   4. 25 gauge, ⅝ inch

31245

3. The nurse is preparing an IM injection of 0.5 mL of influenza vaccine for an average adult patient and will be using which needle length and syringe size when administering the dose?
   1. ⅝ inch, 3 mL
   2. 1 inch, 3 mL
   3. 1½ inch, 5 mL
   4. ⅝ inch, 5 mL

4. What are the advantages of the prefilled cartridge-needle units and syringes? *(Select all that apply.)*
   1. They require special cartridge holders.
   2. They diminish the chance of contamination of the medication.
   3. They are cheaper than the multidose vials.
   4. They save the nurse the time it takes to prepare the injection.
   5. They contain a standard amount of medication.

5. When removing a parenteral medication from an ampule, what must the nurse do?
   1. Inject air equal to the amount of medication to be removed.
   2. Use a needleless spike for removing the medication.
   3. Use a filter needle or filter straw to ensure that no glass particles are drawn into the syringe.
   4. Depress the top rubber diaphragm to displace the stopper.

6. The nurse is teaching the patient how to prepare 10 units of regular insulin and 5 units of NPH insulin for injection. List in the correct order the proper sequence for preparation that the nurse will describe to the patient.
   1. Inject appropriate volumes of air into the NPH vial and the regular insulin vial.
   2. Withdraw 10 units of regular insulin into the syringe.
   3. Wipe the tops of the insulin vials with alcohol.
   4. Withdraw 5 units of NPH insulin into the syringe to mix with the regular insulin.
   5. Inject the insulin in the proper subcut site.

7. Which of these routes are classified as "parenteral administration"?
   1. subcutaneous, intramuscular, intradermal, intravenous
   2. subcutaneous, intermuscular, interdermal, intervenous
   3. oral, rectal, sublingual, buccal
   4. oral, nasogastric, transdermal, nasal

8. List in order the steps necessary to mix two medications in one syringe.
   1. Withdraw the medication from the second vial.
   2. Wipe off the tops of both vials.
   3. Check the compatibility of the two drugs.
   4. Inject air into each vial equal to the amount to be withdrawn.
   5. Withdraw the medication from the first vial.

Objectives

1. Describe the technique that is used to administer a medication via the intradermal route.
2. List the equipment needed and describe the technique that is used to administer a medication via the subcutaneous route.
3. Describe the technique used to administer medications intramuscularly.
4. Describe the landmarks that are used to identify the vastus lateralis muscle, the rectus femoris muscle, the ventrogluteal area, and the deltoid muscle sites before medication is administered.
5. Identify suitable sites for the intramuscular administration of medication in an infant, a child, an adult, and an older adult.

Key Terms

intradermal (ĭn-tră-DŬR-măl) (p. 133)
erythema (ĕr-ĭ-THĒ-mă) (p. 135)
induration (ĭn-dĕ-RĀ-shĕn) (p. 135)
anergic (ăn-ĔR-jĭk) (p. 135)
subcutaneous (sŭb-kū-TĀ-nē-ŭs) (p. 135)
intramuscular (ĭn-tră-MŬS-kyū-lăr) (p. 137)

vastus lateralis (VĂS-tŭs lăt-ĕr-Ă-lĭs) (p. 138)
rectus femoris (RĔK-tŭs FĔ-mŭr-ĭs) (p. 138)
ventrogluteal area (vĕn-trō-GLOO-tē-ăl) (p. 139)
deltoid muscle (DĔL-tōyd MŬS-ŭl) (p. 139)
Z-track method (ZĒ TRĂK MĚTH-ĭd) (p. 141)

ADMINISTRATION OF MEDICATION BY THE INTRADERMAL ROUTE

Intradermal injections are made into the dermal layer of skin just below the epidermis (Fig. 10.1). Small volumes, usually 0.1 mL, are injected. The absorption from intradermal sites is slow, thereby making it the route of choice for allergy sensitivity tests, desensitization injections, local anesthetics, and vaccinations.

Perform premedication assessments; see individual drug monographs for details.

EQUIPMENT

- Medication to be injected or solutions of suspected allergens
- Tuberculin syringe with 26-gauge, ¼-inch, or 28-gauge, ½-inch needle, or a special needle and syringe for allergens
- Metric ruler, if performing skin-testing procedure
- Gloves
- Record for charting data about the substances applied and the patient's responses
- Antiseptic alcohol wipe
- Prescriber's order or medication profile

SITES

Intradermal injections may be made on any skin surface, but the site should be hairless and receive little friction from clothing. The upper chest, the scapular areas of the back, and the inner aspect of the forearms are the most commonly used areas (Fig. 10.2A and B).

TECHNIQUE

This example of an intradermal injection technique involves allergy sensitivity testing. Two methods can be used to administer allergy testing. One method requires the intradermal injection of the allergens; the other is completed by using the skin prick method.

Caution: Do not start any type of allergy testing unless emergency equipment (including epinephrine) is available in the immediate area in case of an anaphylactic response. Nurses should be familiar with the procedure to follow if an emergency does arise.

1. Follow the procedure protocol in Chapter 9 (see Preparation of Parenteral Medication).
2. Verify the identity of the patient using two identifiers.
3. Check with the patient before starting the testing to ensure that he or she has not taken any antihistamines or antiinflammatory agents (e.g., aspirin, ibuprofen, corticosteroids) and that he or she has not received immunosuppressant therapy for 24 to 48 hours before the tests. If the patient has taken antihistamines, certain sleep medications (e.g., doxylamine, diphenhydramine), or antiinflammatory agents, check with the healthcare provider before proceeding with the testing.

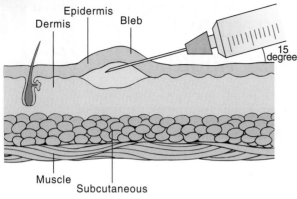

Fig. 10.1 Intradermal injection technique.

4. Provide for patient privacy.
5. Perform hand hygiene and apply clean gloves.
6. Cleanse the area selected for testing thoroughly with an antiseptic alcohol wipe. Use circular motions, starting at the planned site of injection and continuing outward in circular motions to the periphery. Allow the area to air-dry.

Intradermal Injection Method

• Prepare the designated solutions for injection using aseptic technique. Usual volumes to be injected range between 0.01 and 0.05 mL. A positive-control solution that contains histamine and a negative-control solution that contains saline or the diluent of the allergen are also administered.

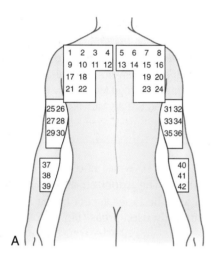

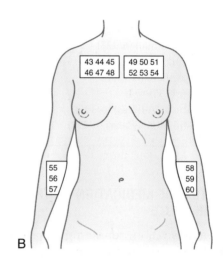

Reading Chart for Intradermal Testing

Patient Name:_____

Identification Number:_____

Physician Name:_____

DATE:	TIME:	AGENT	CONCENTRATION	DOSAGE	SITE NUMBER[a]	Reading Time in Hours or Minutes, 30 min or 24, 48, or 72 hr		

[a]Refer to diagram of sites (Fig.10.2A–B).
• Follow directions for the "reading" of the skin testing performed.
• Inspect sites in a good light.
• Record reaction in upper half of box using the following guidelines, e.g., [2+]
  + (1+)   No wheal, 3 mm flare
  ++ (2+)   2 to 3 mm wheal with flare
  +++ (3+) 3 to 5 mm wheal with flare
  ++++ (4+) >5 mm wheal
• Record measurement of induration (process of hardening) in mm in lower half of box, e.g., [5 mm]

C

Fig. 10.2 Intradermal sites. (A) Posterior view. (B) Anterior view. (C) Reading chart for intradermal testing.

- Insert the needle at a 15-degree angle with the needle bevel upward. (NOTE: There is a controversy regarding whether the needle bevel should be upward or downward. Check the procedure manual for facility policy.) The solution being injected is deposited in the space immediately below the skin; remove the needle quickly. A small bleb will appear on the surface of the skin as the solution enters the intradermal area (see Fig. 10.1). Be careful not to inject into the subcutaneous space and do not wipe the site with alcohol after injection.
- *Do not* recap any needles that have been used. Activate the safety device if on the syringe. Dispose of used needles and syringes into a puncture-resistant needle disposal container in accordance with institutional policy.

Skin Prick Test Method
- Make a grid of at least four squares, more if needed, on the test site at 2-cm intervals with a pen.
- Place a drop of each allergen in one of the grid squares of the testing site. A positive-control solution that includes histamine and a negative-control solution that includes saline or the diluent of the allergen are also administered.
- Using a lancet with a 1-mm point, prick the skin through the allergen drop. Wipe the lancet with dry gauze between each prick to prevent the carryover of the allergen from the previous site.
- Gently blot the excess allergen off of the site.
- The skin prick test can be read 10 to 20 minutes after administration, depending on protocol.

7. Remove gloves and dispose of them in accordance with institutional policy. Perform hand hygiene.
8. Chart the times, agents, concentrations, and amounts administered (see Fig. 10.2C). Make a diagram in the patient's chart, and number each location. Record what agent at what concentration was injected at each site. (Subsequent readings of each area are then performed and charted on this record.)
9. Follow the directions regarding the time of the reading of the skin testing being performed. The inspection of the injection sites should be performed in good light. Generally, a positive reaction (i.e., the development of a wheal) to a diluted strength of a suspected allergen is considered clinically significant. Measure the diameter of the wheal and any **erythema** (i.e., redness at the site of injection) in millimeters, and palpate and measure the size of any **induration** (i.e., the hardening of an area of the body in response to inflammation). No reaction to the allergens, especially to the positive control, is known as an *anergic reaction.* Anergy is associated with immunodeficiency disorders.
10. Record the information from the skin test reading in the patient's chart. The following is a list of commonly used readings of reactions and their appropriate symbols:

+	(1+)	No wheal, 3-mm flare
++	(2+)	2- to 3-mm wheal with flare
+++	(3+)	3- to 5-mm wheal with flare
++++	(4+)	>5-mm wheal

Generally, a positive reaction to delayed hypersensitivity skin testing (to evaluate in vivo cell-mediated immunity) requires an induration of at least 5 mm in diameter.

PATIENT TEACHING
1. For intradermal injections, tell the patient the time, date, and place to return to have the test sites read.
2. Tell the patient not to wash or scrub the area until the injections have been read.
3. If the patient develops an area of severe burning or itching, he or she should try not to scratch it. Tell the patient to report immediately the development of any breathing difficulty, severe hives, or rashes and to go to the nearest emergency department if he or she is unable to reach the healthcare provider who prescribed the skin tests.

DOCUMENTATION
Provide the right documentation of the allergen testing sites and the patient's responses to the allergens that were injected.
1. Chart the date, time, allergens (including agent, concentration, and amount), and site of administration (see Fig. 10.2).
2. Perform a reading of each site after the application of the test as directed by the healthcare provider or the policy of the healthcare agency.
3. Chart and report any signs and symptoms of adverse allergen effects.
4. Perform and validate essential patient education about the testing and other essential aspects of intervention for the allergy that is affecting the individual.

ADMINISTRATION OF MEDICATION BY THE SUBCUTANEOUS ROUTE

Subcutaneous (subcut) injections are made into the loose connective tissue between the dermis and the muscular layer (Fig. 10.3). Absorption is slower and drug action is generally longer with subcut injections as compared with intramuscular (IM) or intravenous (IV) injections. If the patient's circulation is adequate, then the drug is completely absorbed from the tissue.

Many drugs cannot be administered by this route because ordinarily no more than 2 mL can be deposited at a subcut site. The drugs must be quite soluble and potent enough to be effective in a small volume without causing significant tissue irritation. Drugs commonly injected into the subcut tissue are heparin, enoxaparin, and insulin.

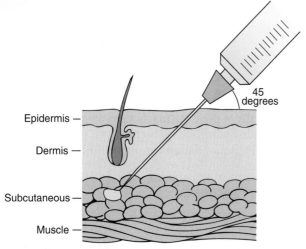

Fig. 10.3 Subcutaneous injection. Inject at a 45- to 90-degree angle depending on the depth of subcutaneous tissue, the length of the needle, and the volume to be injected.

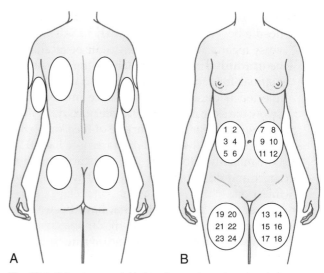

Fig. 10.4 Subcutaneous injection sites and rotation plan. (A) Posterior view. (B) Anterior view illustrating commonly used subcutaneous sites for self-administration. The anterior view also provides an example of a numbered rotation schedule for insulin injection, using one site systematically before proceeding to the next site of administration.

Perform premedication assessments; see individual drug monographs for details.

EQUIPMENT

- Medication to be injected
- Syringe of correct volume
- Needle of correct length and gauge
- Gloves
- Antiseptic alcohol wipe
- Prescriber's order
- Medication profile

Syringe Size

Choose a syringe that corresponds with the volume of drug to be injected at one site. The usual amount injected subcutaneously at one site is 0.5 to 2 mL. Correlate the syringe size with the size of the patient and the tissue mass.

Needle Length

Assess each patient so that the needle length selected will deposit the medication into the subcut tissue rather than the muscle tissue. Needle lengths of ⅜, ½, and ⅝ inch are routinely used. It is prudent to leave an extra ¼ inch of needle extending above the skin surface in case the needle breaks.

Needle Gauge

Commonly used gauges for subcut injections are 25 to 29 gauge.

SITES

Common sites used for the subcut administration of medications include the upper arms, the anterior thighs, and the abdomen (Fig. 10.4). Less common areas are the buttocks and the upper back or scapular region.

A plan for rotating injection sites should be developed for all patients who require repeated injections (see Fig. 10.4). The anterior view (see Fig. 10.4B) illustrates areas

that are easily accessible for self-administration. The posterior view (see Fig. 10.4A) illustrates less commonly used areas that may be used by a caregiver who is injecting the medication into the patient.

When administering insulin subcutaneously, it is important to rotate the injection sites to prevent lipohypertrophy or lipoatrophy, which slows the absorption rate of the insulin. The American Diabetes Association Clinical Practice Recommendations state that insulin injection sites should be rotated systematically within one area before progressing to a new site for injection (see Fig. 10.4B); it is thought that this will decrease variations in insulin absorption. Absorption is known to be fastest when the insulin is administered in the abdomen; this is followed by the arms, thighs, and buttocks. Because exercise is also known to affect the rate of insulin absorption, site selection should take this factor into consideration.

TECHNIQUE

1. Follow the procedure protocol in Chapter 9 (see Preparation of Parenteral Medication).
2. Verify the identity of the patient using two identifiers. Ensure that the patient does not have an allergy to the medication.
3. Check the accuracy of the drug order against the medication being prepared at least three times during the preparation phase: (1) when first removing the drug from the storage area, (2) immediately after preparation, and (3) immediately before administration.
4. Consult the master rotation schedule for the patient so that the drug is administered at the correct site.
5. Explain carefully to the patient what to expect.
6. Provide for the patient's privacy and position the patient appropriately.

7. Perform hand hygiene and apply clean gloves.
8. Expose the selected site and locate the landmarks.
9. Cleanse the skin surface with an antiseptic alcohol wipe starting at the injection site and working outward in a circular motion toward the periphery. Allow the area to air-dry.
10. Check the site of injection and the length of the needle. Assess whether the injection is most appropriately administered at a 45- to 90-degree angle for subcutaneous delivery.
11. Insert the needle quickly at a 45- to 90-degree angle; slowly inject the medication. The American Diabetes Association Clinical Practice Recommendations state that "thin individuals or children may need to pinch the skin and inject at a 45-degree angle to avoid IM injection, especially in the thigh area."
12. Withdraw the needle. Gentle pressure may be applied to the site with an antiseptic alcohol wipe, but *do not* rub.
13. *Do not* recap any needles that have been used. Activate the safety device. Dispose of used needles and syringes into a puncture-resistant needle disposal container in accordance with institutional policy.
14. Remove gloves and dispose of them according to facility policy. Perform hand hygiene.

PATIENT TEACHING

Perform appropriate patient teaching as described in the related drug monographs.

DOCUMENTATION

Provide the right documentation of the medication administration and the patient's response to drug therapy.
1. Chart the date, time, drug name, dose, site, and route of administration.
2. Perform and record regular patient assessments for the evaluation of the therapeutic effectiveness (e.g., blood pressure, pulse, output, improvement or quality of cough and productivity, degree and duration of pain relief).
3. Chart and report any signs and symptoms of adverse drug effects.
4. Perform and validate essential patient education about the drug therapy and other essential aspects of intervention for the disease process that is affecting the individual.

ADMINISTRATION OF MEDICATION BY THE INTRAMUSCULAR ROUTE

Intramuscular injections are made by penetrating a needle through the epidermis, dermis, and subcut tissue into the muscle layer. The injection deposits the medication deep within the muscle mass (Fig. 10.5). Absorption is more rapid than that associated with subcut injections because muscle tissue has a greater blood supply. Site

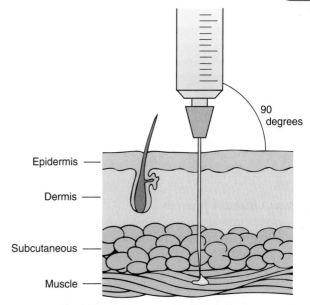

Fig. 10.5 Intramuscular injection technique.

selection is especially important with IM injections because the incorrect placement of the needle may cause damage to nerves or blood vessels. Complications from improper technique of IM injections include hematoma (when a vein is punctured) and pain (when a nerve is touched). A large, healthy muscle that is free from infections and wounds should be used.

Perform premedication assessments; see individual drug monographs for details.

EQUIPMENT

- Medication to be injected
- Syringe of correct volume
- Needle of correct length and gauge
- Gloves
- Antiseptic alcohol wipe
- Prescriber's order
- Medication profile

Syringe Size

Choose a syringe that corresponds with the volume of drug to be injected at one site. The usual amount injected intramuscularly at one site is 0.5 to 3 mL. In infants and children the amount should range between 0.5 and 1 mL, and it should not exceed 1 mL. Correlate the syringe size with the size of the patient and the tissue mass. In adults, divided doses are generally recommended for amounts in excess of 3 mL; 1 mL is the maximum amount to be injected in the deltoid area. Other factors that influence syringe size and needle gauge include the type of medication, the site of administration, the thickness of the subcut fatty tissue, and the age of the individual.

Needle Length

Assess each patient so that the needle length selected will deposit the medication into the muscular tissue (see Fig. 10.5). There is a significant difference among the needle lengths that are appropriate for an obese patient, an infant, or an emaciated or debilitated patient. Needles that are commonly used are 1 to 1½ inches long, although longer lengths may be required for obese patients.

Needle Gauge
Commonly used gauges for IM injections are 20 to 23 gauge.

SITES

Vastus Lateralis Muscle
The **vastus lateralis** muscle is located on the anterior lateral thigh, away from nerves and blood vessels (Fig. 10.6). The midportion is one handbreadth below the greater trochanter and one handbreadth above the knee (see Fig. 10.6B). This is generally the preferred site for IM injections in infants because it has the largest muscle mass for that age group. This muscle is also a good choice for an injection site in healthy, ambulatory adults. It accommodates a large volume of medication, and it allows for good drug absorption. In the older, debilitated, or nonambulatory adult, the muscle should be carefully assessed before injection because significantly less muscle mass may be present. If muscle mass is insufficient, an alternative site should be selected.

Rectus Femoris Muscle
The **rectus femoris** muscle (Fig. 10.7) lies just medial to the vastus lateralis muscle, but it does not cross the midline of the anterior thigh. The injection site is located

in the same manner as is used for the vastus lateralis muscle. This muscle may be used in both children and adults when other sites are unavailable. A primary advantage to its use is that it may be used more easily by patients for self-administration. A disadvantage is that the medial border is close to the sciatic nerve and major blood vessels (see Fig. 10.7). If the muscle is not well developed, injections into this site may also cause considerable discomfort and potential injury.

> ### Life Span Considerations
> **Injection Sites**
> - The *vastus lateralis* site is preferred in infants. In the older, debilitated, or nonambulatory adult, carefully assess the sufficiency of the muscle mass before using this site for injection.
> - The *ventrogluteal* site is also appropriate for infants and adults, and it may be used as often as needed because of the convenience of the thigh muscle.
> - The *deltoid* site is preferred when administering 1 mL or less because of the convenience of the arm muscle.

Gluteal Area
The gluteal area is a commonly used site of injection because it is free of major nerves and blood vessels. The dorsogluteal area must not be used in children who are less than 3 years old because the muscle has not yet been well developed from walking. The ventrogluteal area is an appropriate site for injections in children who are less than 3 years old; however, this site is not used as often as the vastus lateralis muscle because of the

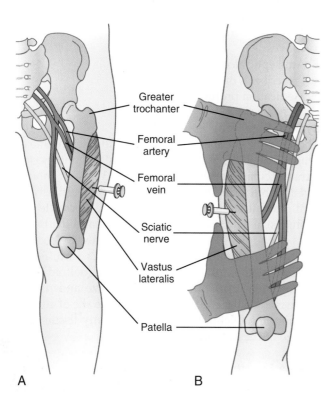

Fig. 10.6 Vastus lateralis muscle. (A) Child or infant. (B) Adult.

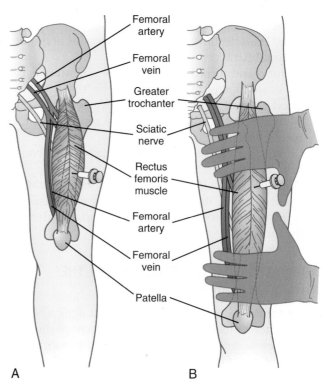

Fig. 10.7 Rectus femoris muscle. (A) Child or infant. (B) Adult.

convenience of the that muscle. The area may be divided into two distinct injection sites: (1) the ventrogluteal area and (2) the dorsogluteal area.

Ventrogluteal area. The **ventrogluteal area** is easily accessible when the patient is in a prone, supine, or side-lying position. It is located by placing the palm of the hand on the lateral portion of the greater trochanter with the thumb pointing toward the groin, the index finger on the anterior superior iliac spine, and the middle finger extended to the iliac crest. The injection is made into the center of the "V" that is formed between the index and middle fingers, with the needle directed slightly upward toward the crest of the ilium (Fig. 10.8). Pain on injection can be minimized if the muscle is relaxed. The patient can help with this relaxation by pointing the toes inward while lying in a prone position (Fig. 10.9) or by flexing the upper leg if lying on his or her side (Fig. 10.10).

Dorsogluteal area. The use of this site is discouraged and not practiced to any great extent because of the possible damage to the sciatic nerve.

Deltoid Muscle

The **deltoid muscle** is often used because of the ease of access to this area when the patient is in the standing, sitting, or prone position. However, it should be used in infants only when the volume to be injected is small, the drug is nonirritating, and the dose will be quickly absorbed. In adults, the volume should be limited to 1 mL or less and the substance must not cause irritation. Caution must also be exercised to avoid the clavicle, the humerus, the acromion, the brachial vein and artery, and the radial nerve. The injection site (Fig. 10.11) of the deltoid muscle is located by palpating the acromion process or top of the shoulder and measuring down two to three fingerbreadths. It is advisable to palpate the muscle of the deltoid, which is roughly triangular in shape, to determine the thickest part of the muscle, which will then be the area for the injection.

SITE ROTATION

A master plan for site rotation should be developed and used for all patients who require repeated injections (Fig. 10.12).

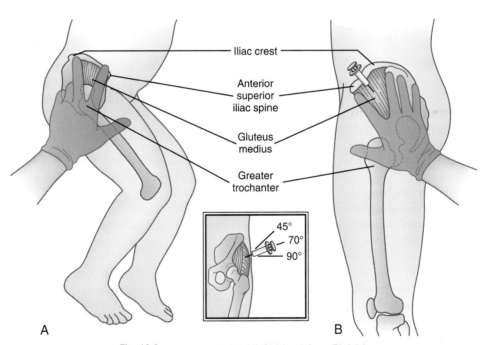

Fig. 10.8 Ventrogluteal site. (A) Child or infant. (B) Adult.

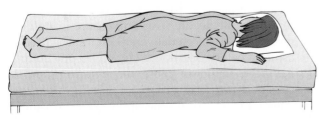

Fig. 10.9 Patient lying in the prone position. The toes are pointed inward to promote muscle relaxation.

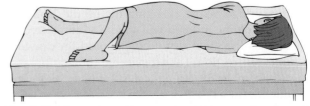

Fig. 10.10 Patient lying on the side. Flexing the upper leg promotes muscle relaxation.

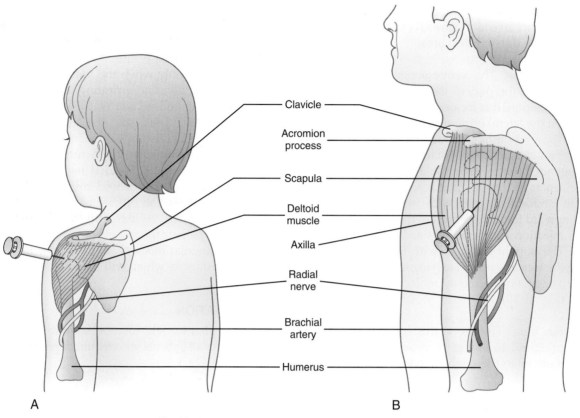

Fig. 10.11 Deltoid muscle site. (A) Child or infant. (B) Adult.

TECHNIQUE

Standard Method

1. Follow the procedure protocol in Chapter 9 (see Preparation of Parenteral Medication).
2. Verify the identity of the patient using two identifiers. Ensure that the patient does not have an allergy to the medication.
3. Check the accuracy of the drug order against the medication being prepared at least three times during the preparation phase: (1) when first removing the drug from the storage area, (2) immediately after preparation, and (3) immediately before administration.
4. Calculate and draw up the medication. Check the institutional policy regarding whether 0.1 or 0.2 mL of air should be added to the syringe *after* accurately measuring the prescribed volume of drug for administration. (NOTE: The rationale for adding the air is that it will result in the needle being completely cleared of all medication at the time of injection. Conversely, if the volume is completely drawn into the syringe before changing the needle, then the drug volume ordered will still be administered as long as the same size needle is used for drawing up and injection. Thus the needle should not need to be completely cleared of medication by air during administration. This issue can be critical when small volumes of potent drugs are repeatedly administered to infants.)
5. Consult the master rotation schedule for the patient so that the drug is administered at the correct site (see Fig. 10.12).
6. Explain carefully to the patient what will be done.
7. Provide for the patient's privacy; position the patient appropriately (see Figs. 10.9 and 10.10 for relaxation techniques).
8. Perform hand hygiene and apply clean gloves.
9. Expose the selected site and locate the landmarks.
10. Cleanse the skin surface with an antiseptic alcohol wipe starting at the injection site and working outward in a circular motion toward the periphery. Allow the area to air-dry.
11. Using the nondominant hand, spread the skin and hold down to push subcut tissue away and allow greater needle penetration.
12. Insert the needle at a 90-degree angle using a quick, dart-throwing action.
13. Inject the medication using gentle, steady pressure on the plunger and wait for a count of 3 before removing the needle. This will ensure that all the medication has been delivered. (NOTE: The need to aspirate before injection is no longer practiced; it has been found to cause more damage and is considered unnecessary.)
14. After removing the needle, apply gentle pressure to the site. Massage can increase the pain if the muscle mass is stressed by the amount of medication given.

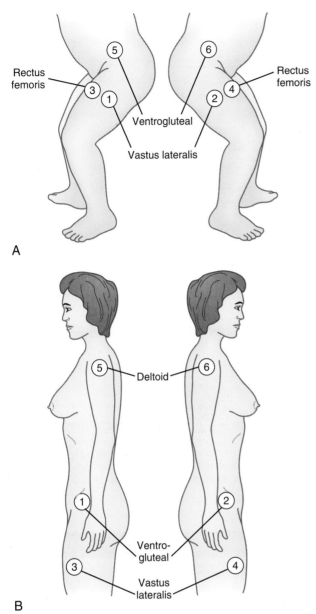

A

B

Fig. 10.12 Intramuscular master rotation plan. (A) Infant or child. Note that the deltoid site may also be used in an infant or child; however, the volume of medication must be small and the drug nonirritating. (B) Adult. In an adult, avoid using the rectus femoris site because of the pain produced.

15. *Do not* recap any needles that have been used. Activate the safety device. Dispose of used needles and syringes into a puncture-resistant needle disposal container in accordance with institutional policy.
16. Apply a small bandage to the site.
17. Provide emotional support to the patient. Children should be comforted during and after the injection. Sometimes letting a child hold your hand or say "ouch" helps. Praise the patient for his or her assistance and cooperation.
18. Remove gloves and perform hand hygiene.

Z-Track Method

The use of a **Z-track method** (Fig. 10.13) may be appropriate for medications that are particularly irritating or that stain the tissue. Check facility policy regarding which personnel may administer medications using this method.

1. Provide for the patient's privacy; position the patient appropriately.
2. Perform hand hygiene and apply clean gloves.
3. Expose the ventrogluteal site or vastus lateralis site (Fig. 10.13A). Never inject into the patient's arm.
4. Calculate and draw up the medication; add 0.5 mL of air to ensure that the drug will clear the needle.
5. Cleanse the skin surface with an antiseptic alcohol wipe starting at the injection site and working outward in a circular motion toward the periphery. Allow the area to air-dry.
6. Stretch the patient's skin approximately 1 inch to one side (Fig. 10.13B).
7. Insert the needle. It is important to choose a needle of sufficient length to ensure deep muscle penetration.
8. Gently inject the medication and then wait approximately 10 seconds (Fig. 10.13C).
9. Remove the needle and allow the skin to return to its normal position (Fig. 10.13D).
10. *Do not* massage the injection site.
11. If further injections are to be made, alternate among sites per the master rotation schedule.
12. *Do not* recap any needles that have been used. Dispose of used needles and syringes into a puncture-resistant needle disposal container in accordance with institutional policy.
13. Remove gloves and dispose of them according to facility policy. Perform hand hygiene.
14. Teach the patient that walking will help with the medication's absorption. Vigorous exercise or pressure on the injection site (e.g., tight-fitting clothing) should be temporarily avoided.

PATIENT TEACHING

Perform appropriate patient teaching as described in related drug monographs.

DOCUMENTATION

Provide the right documentation of the medication administration and the patient's response to drug therapy.

1. Chart the date, time, drug name, dose, site, and route of administration.
2. Perform and record regular patient assessments for the evaluation of the therapeutic effectiveness (e.g., blood pressure, pulse, output, improvement or quality of cough and productivity).
3. Chart and report any signs and symptoms of adverse drug effects.
4. Perform and validate essential patient education about the drug therapy and other essential aspects of intervention for the disease process that is affecting the individual.

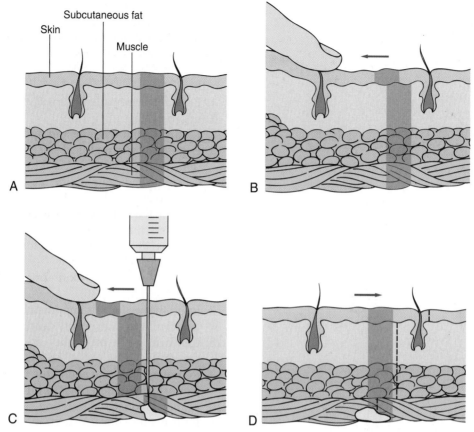

Fig. 10.13 Z-track method of intramuscular injection. (A) Alignment of layers before starting Z-tracking. (B) Stretch the skin slightly to one side by approximately 1 inch. (C) Inject the medication and then wait approximately 10 seconds. (D) Remove the needle and allow the skin to return to its normal position. Do not massage the injection site.

Get Ready for the NCLEX® Examination!

Key Points

- Intradermal injections are made into the dermal layer just below the epidermis and are usually 0.1 mL in volume.
- Subcutaneous injections are made into the subcutaneous tissue or fatty layer between the dermis and the muscle.
- Intramuscular injections are made into the muscle below the subcutaneous tissue. Care must be taken to ensure that the muscle is injected.
- The sites for administration of IM injections include the vastus lateralis muscle, the rectus femoris muscle, the ventrogluteal area, and the deltoid muscle.
- The most suitable sites for an IM injection for children are the vastus lateralis muscle, the rectus femoris muscle, or the ventrogluteal area. In adults, the sites are the same as for a child, but also include the deltoid muscle.

Additional Learning Resources

SG Go to your Study Guide for additional Review Questions for the NCLEX® Examination, Critical Thinking Clinical Situations, and other learning activities to help you master this chapter content.

Go to your Evolve website (https://evolve.elsevier.com/Clayton) for additional online resources.

Review Questions for the NCLEX® Examination

1. The instructor asks the student nurse to gather the equipment needed to perform an intradermal injection. Which items are appropriate? *(Select all that apply.)*
   1. 3-mL syringe
   2. Tuberculin syringe
   3. ¼-inch needle
   4. 21-gauge needle
   5. 26-gauge needle

53214

2. A student nurse has been practicing subcutaneous injections in the laboratory and is about to administer her first injection. List in correct order the proper sequence to follow when administering a subcut injection.
   1. Remove the needle.
   2. Inject the insulin.
   3. Dart the needle in at a 90-degree angle.
   4. Document the administration.
   5. Cleanse the site with alcohol.

3. Why will a nurse who administers an IM medication of iron use the Z-track method of administration?
   1. It will provide faster absorption of the medication.
   2. It will reduce discomfort from the needle.
   3. It can provide more even absorption of the drug.
   4. It will prevent the drug from staining or irritating sensitive tissue.

4. The nurse was finding the landmark of the acromion process and measuring down two to three fingerbreadths to administer an IM injection into which site?
   1. Vastus lateralis muscle
   2. Rectus femoris muscle
   3. Ventrogluteal area
   4. Deltoid muscle

5. A student nurse reads an order to give a 69-year-old patient an IM injection. Which muscles would be the preferred injection sites for an adult? *(Select all that apply.)*

   1345

   1. Deltoid
   2. Dorsogluteal
   3. Ventrogluteal
   4. Vastus lateralis
   5. Rectus femoris

6. The nurse needs to administer an IM injection and chose the rectus femoris muscle. What landmarks will the nurse use for the injection?
   1. Two fingerbreadths below the acromion process
   2. One handbreadth below the greater trochanter and one handbreadth above the knee
   3. Between the V of the index finger and middle finger when on the trochanter
   4. Between the anterior superior iliac spine and the iliac crest

7. The nurse is preparing to administer an IM injection to an elderly patient; what considerations need to be practiced?
   1. The muscle needs to be palpated to determine if the muscle mass is sufficient.
   2. The length of the needle needs to be at least $1\frac{1}{2}$ inches, since the patient is older.
   3. The amount of the injection must be limited to 1 mL or less.
   4. The injection needs to be in the deltoid muscle only.

Objectives

1. Define intravenous (IV) therapy and describe the three intravascular compartments and the three fluid compartments of the body.
2. Discuss the different IV access devices used for IV therapy.
3. Differentiate between isotonic, hypotonic, and hypertonic IV solutions and explain their clinical uses.
4. Identify the general principles for administering medications via the IV route.
5. Compare and contrast the differences between a peripheral IV line and a central IV line.
6. Describe the correct techniques for administering medications by means of a saline lock, an IV bag, an infusion pump, and a secondary piggyback set.
7. Describe the recommended guidelines and procedures for IV catheter care.
8. Identify baseline assessments for IV therapy and proper maintenance of patency of IV lines and implanted access devices.
9. Explain the signs, symptoms, and treatment of the complications associated with IV therapy (e.g., phlebitis, thrombophlebitis, localized infection, septicemia, infiltration, extravasation, air in tubing, pulmonary edema, catheter embolism, and "speed shock").

Key Terms

intravenous (ĭn-tră-VĒ-nŭs) (p. 145)
intracellular (ĭn-tră-SĔL-yĕ-lĕr) (p. 145)
intravascular (ĭn-tră-VĂS-cū-lĕr) (p. 145)
interstitial (ĭn-tĕr-STĬ-shĕl) (p. 145)
extracellular (ĕk-strĕ-SĔL-yĕ-lĕr) (p. 145)
IV administration set (p. 145)
macrodrip (p. 145)
microdrip (p. 145)
programmable infusion pumps (prō-GRĂM-ă-bŭl ĭn-FŪ-zhăn PŬMPZ) (p. 147)
syringe pumps (sĭ-RĬNJ) (p. 148)
peripheral devices (pĕ-RĬF-ĕr-ăl dĕ-VĪ-sĕz) (p. 148)
midline catheters (MĬD-līn KĂTH-ĕ-tŭrz) (p. 148)
central devices (SĔN-trŭl dĕ-VĪ-sĕz) (p. 148)
implantable venous infusion ports (ĭm-PLĂNT-ă-bŭl VĒ-nŭs ĭn-FŪ-zhăn PŌRTS) (p. 148)
winged, butterfly, or scalp needles (WĬNGD, BŬT-ŭr-flī, SKĂLP NĒ-dŭlz) (p. 148)
over-the-needle catheters (p. 148)
saline lock or medlock (SĀ-lēn-lŏk, MĔD-lŏk) (p. 149)
in-the-needle catheters (p. 149)
peripherally inserted central venous catheters (PICCs) (pĕ-RĬF-ŭr-ăl-ē ĭn-SŬR-tĕd SĔN-trŭl VĒ-nŭs KĂTH-ĕ-tŭrz) (p. 149)

tunneled central venous catheters (TŬN-ŭld) (p. 149)
implantable infusion ports (ĭm-PLĂNT-ă-bŭl ĭn-FŪ-zhăn PŌRTZ) (p. 150)
intravenous (IV) solutions (ĭn-tră-VĒ-nŭs sŏl-Ū-shŭnz) (p. 151)
electrolytes (ĕ-LĔK-trō-līts) (p. 151)
isotonic (ī-sō-TŎN-ĭk) (p. 151)
hypotonic (hī-pō-TŎN-ĭk) (p. 151)
hypertonic (hī-pĕr-TŎN-ĭk) (p. 151)
tandem setup, piggyback, or IV rider (TĂN-dĕm, PĬ-gē-băk, RĪ-dŭr) (p. 152)
SASH guideline (SĂSH GĪD-līn) (p. 155)
phlebitis (flĕ-BĪ-tĭs) (p. 172)
thrombophlebitis (thrŏm-bō-flĕ-BĪ-tĭs) (p. 172)
Infiltration Scale (ĭn-fĭl-TRĀ-shŭn SKĀL) (p. 172)
septicemia (sĕp-tĭ-SĒ-mē-yŭ) (p. 173)
infiltration (ĭn-fĭl-TRĀ-shŭn) (p. 173)
extravasation (ĕks-tră-vă-SĀ-shŭn) (p. 173)
air embolism (ĀR ĔM-bō-līz-ŭm) (p. 173)
pulmonary edema (PŬL-mō-nār-ē ĕ-DĒ-mŭ) (p. 174)
pulmonary embolism (PŬL-mō-nār-ē ĔM-bō-līz-ŭm) (p. 174)
"speed shock" (SPĒD SHŎK) (p. 174)

The term **intravenous** (IV) administration refers to the introduction of fluids directly into the venous bloodstream. The advantage of this technique is that large volumes of fluids can be rapidly administered into the vein for volume expansion in cases of shock, or more rapid onset of medications administered intravenously in cases of emergency. Intravenous administration is the most rapid of all parenteral routes because it bypasses all barriers to drug absorption. Drugs may be given by direct injection with a needle in the vein, but they are more commonly administered intermittently or by continuous infusion through an established peripheral or central IV line.

An advantage of IV administration compared with other forms of parenteral administration is that it is generally more comfortable for the patient, especially when several doses of medications must be administered daily. However, disadvantages to the IV route include nurses needing the skill to establish and maintain an IV site. In addition, the patient tends to be less mobile with IV administration, and there is a greater possibility for infection and for severe adverse reactions to the drug.

From a physiologic standpoint, the water in the body is distributed among three compartments: (1) the **intracellular** compartment—within the cells (Fig. 11.1A); (2) the **intravascular** compartment—within the vascular system (e.g., the arteries, veins, and capillaries) (Fig. 11.1B); and (3) the **interstitial** compartment—within the spaces between the cells that are outside of the vascular compartment (Fig. 11.1C). The **extracellular** compartment (the spaces outside the cells) is composed of the intravascular and interstitial compartments, and it contains about one-third of the total body water, whereas the intracellular compartment (within the cells) contains about two-thirds of the total body water.

All IV therapy requires a written order from a healthcare provider that is dated and that specifies the type of solution or medication to be administered, the dosage, and the rate and frequency of administration.

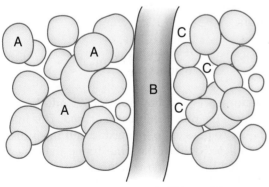

Fig. 11.1 Fluid compartments of the body. (A) Intracellular spaces (e.g., the spaces within the cells). (B) Vascular spaces (e.g., within arteries, veins, and capillaries). (C) Interstitial spaces (e.g., the spaces between the cells). The body maintains a water and electrolyte balance among these compartments for homeostasis.

Some hospitals use infusion therapy teams for administration via the IV system, but many now assign the responsibility for infusion therapy to nurses with earned credentials. The nurse who is performing venipuncture (initiation of an IV line) and infusion therapy must be well versed in the guidelines established by the Infusion Nurses Society.

The Infusion Nurses Society, a professional nursing organization, publishes the Infusion Nursing Standards of Practice related to quality assurance, technology and application, fluids and electrolytes, pharmacology, infection control, pediatrics, oncology, and parenteral nutrition. Most state laws recognize the role of the licensed practical nurse/licensed vocational nurse (LPN/LVN) in IV therapy, but delegate the scope of practice to be defined in the policies and procedures of individual clinical practice settings. The nurse should check with his or her particular state board of nursing to determine the current guidelines and education requirements. In general, LPN/LVN responsibilities do not include the administration of IV medication, blood products, or antineoplastic agents.

Before any nurse administers IV therapy, he or she should ask the following questions:

- "Does the law in this state delegate this function to the nurse?"
- "Does the written policy of the institution or agency through which I am employed, with the approval of the medical staff, permit a nurse with my level of education and experience to administer IV therapy?"
- "Does the institution or agency policy limit the types of fluids and medications that I may administer?"

EQUIPMENT USED FOR INTRAVENOUS THERAPY

INTRAVENOUS ADMINISTRATION SETS

An **IV administration set** is an apparatus that connects a large volume of parenteral solution with the IV access device in the patient's vein. All sets (Fig. 11.2) have an insertion spike, a drip chamber, plastic tubing with a rate-control clamp, a rubber injection portal (also referred to as a Y port), a needle adapter, and a protective cap over the needle adapter. Depending on the manufacturer, the sets are available in a variety of styles (e.g., different volumes and sizes of drip chamber, "piggyback" portals, filters, and styles of control clamps [Fig. 11.3]).

The type of system used by a particular institution is usually determined by the manufacturer of the IV solutions used by the institution. Each manufacturer makes adapters to fit a specific type of plastic or glass large-volume solution container. A crucial point to remember about administration sets is that the drops delivered by drip chambers vary among manufacturers. **Macrodrip** chambers (see Fig. 11.2A and B) provide 10, 15, or 20 drops/mL of solution, whereas **microdrip** chambers (see Fig. 11.2C) deliver 60 drops/mL of solution.

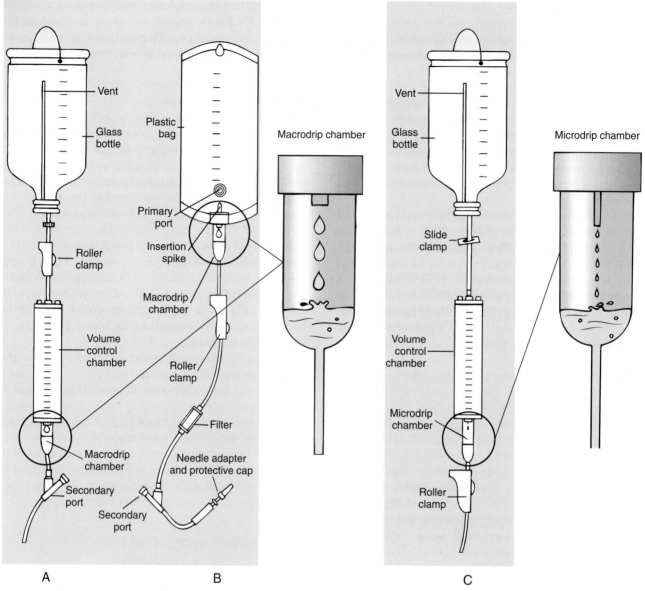

Fig. 11.2 (A and B), Different types of intravenous (IV) administration sets that make use of a macrodrip chamber. (C) An IV administration set that includes a microdrip chamber.

Microdrip administration sets are used when a small volume of fluid is being administered, particularly when accuracy of volume administration is indicated (e.g., with neonatal and pediatric populations; for those patients with fluid volume concerns). Volume-control chambers (see Fig. 11.2A and C) are also used as a safety factor to limit the volume administered. In many clinical settings, microdrip sets are used for all volumes of IV fluid ordered that are administered at less than 100 mL/hr. It is essential to read the label on the box before opening it to ensure that the correct IV administration set has been selected.

The nurse must be able to calculate the flow rate for any IV solution. The flow rates that are used for infusion pumps are generally in milliliters per hour (mL/hr). A typical flow rate problem would be as follows: At what rate will the nurse set the infusion pump if the order

reads, "Infuse 1000 mL of D5W over 8 hours"? Calculate the rate of infusion using a simple formula: mL divided by hours.

$$\frac{1000\ \text{mL}}{8\ \text{hours}} = 125\ \text{mL/hr}$$

The nurse sets the pump rate for 125 mL/hr, making sure to note the time the infusion started. This information is key to pass on to the next shift if the infusion is not completed within the time frame that the nurse who started the infusion will be present. The primary parts of the IV administration set need to be labeled; the IV fluid needs a label that indicates when it needs to be changed (usually in 24 to 48 hours), and the IV tubing needs a label indicating when it needs to be changed (usually in 72 to 96 hours).

Equipment Used in Conjunction With Intravenous Therapy

A large variety of connector and access devices are available for various components of infusion therapy. The nurse must become familiar with the IV access

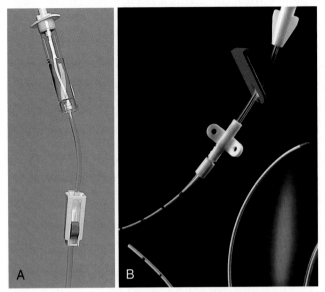

Fig. 11.3 Control clamps for intravenous administration sets. (A) Roller clamp. (B) Slide clamp. (A, From Perry AG, Potter PA, Ostendorf WR. *Clinical Nursing Skills and Techniques.* 8th ed. St. Louis: Mosby; 2014. B, From Otto SE. *Pocket Guide to Intravenous Therapy.* 4th ed. St. Louis: Mosby; 2001.)

systems and the terms used for these systems at the clinical practice setting. Knowing which parts of the system are clean and which parts are to remain sterile is crucial for the provision of safe IV therapy.

TYPES OF INFUSION-CONTROL PUMPS

Precise infusion rates are important for certain therapeutic effects (e.g., with a continuous heparin infusion for anticoagulation) or when monitoring the administration of medications to prevent toxicity (e.g., nephrotoxicity, ototoxicity). Programmable infusion pumps are used to ensure the safe administration of IV fluids and medications (Fig. 11.4).

Pumps

The **programmable infusion pumps** apply external pressure to the administration set tubing to squeeze the solution through the tubing at a specific rate (e.g., a certain number of mL/min or mL/hr). These pumps are programmed for a specific volume over time. These pumps have an alarm system that sounds if there is resistance in the IV line caused by a developing occlusion as a result of thrombus formation or a kink in the administration set line caused by patient movement. Disadvantages of pumps are the cost of the equipment and the training of personnel, the cost of maintenance, the need for more equipment at the bedside, and the potential for serious IV infiltration.

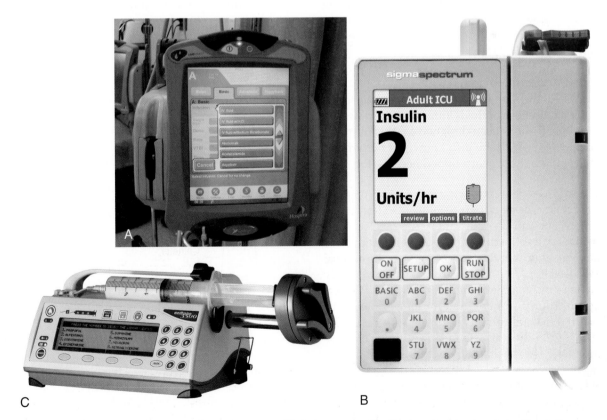

Fig. 11.4 (A) Infusion controller. (B) Infusion pump. (C) Syringe pump. (A, Courtesy Hospira, Inc., Lake Forest, IL. B, Courtesy Baxter Healthcare Corporation, Mountain Home, AR. All rights reserved. C, Courtesy Smiths Medical, Minneapolis, MN.)

Syringe Pumps

Syringe pumps hold a prefilled syringe and apply positive pressure to the plunger to deliver a specific volume of medicine over a set time. Syringe pumps are more commonly used when small volumes need to be administered (Fig. 11.4C). Examples of small syringe pumps are those that continually infuse insulin into the subcutaneous tissue of patients with diabetes mellitus and patient-controlled analgesia pumps, which allow patients who are receiving pain medications to administer continual infusions and intermittent boluses of the medicine for comfort.

Syringe pumps are easy to use, and their use is taught to patients needing home infusion therapy, when patients self-administer medications through an implanted infusion port. It is important that the nurse become familiar with the specific devices that are used in the clinical setting for safe and efficient patient care.

INTRAVENOUS ACCESS DEVICES

Intravenous access devices are often subdivided into four groups on the basis of the location of the terminal tip of the access device: (1) **peripheral devices** are for short-term use in peripheral veins in the hand or forearm; (2) **midline catheters** are for use over 2 to 4 weeks and are inserted into intermediate-sized veins and advanced into larger vessels; (3) **central devices** are inserted into intermediate-sized vessels and advanced into central veins where the tip of the catheter typically will be in the superior vena cava to allow for maximal mixing with large volumes of blood; and (4) **implantable venous infusion ports**, which are surgically placed into central veins for long-term therapy.

Peripheral Access Devices

All needles—if they are long enough—may be used to administer medications or fluids intravenously. However, special equipment has been designed for this purpose. **Winged needles**, which are also known as *butterfly* or *scalp needles*, are short, sharp-tipped needles (Fig. 11.5)

that were originally designed for venipuncture of small veins in infants and for geriatric use. These needles are available in sizes that range from 17 to 29 gauge, and have been designed to minimize tissue injury during insertion. The winged area is pinched together to form a handle while the needle is being inserted. The wings are then laid flat against the skin to form a base that can be anchored with tape. Two types of these needles are now available: one with a short length of plastic tubing and a permanently attached resealable injection port and one with a variable length of plastic tubing with a female Luer adapter for the attachment of a syringe or an administration set (see Fig. 11.5). The patency of the needle is maintained with the use of a heparin or saline flush routine in accordance with facility policy.

Over-the-needle catheters, which are also known as *short peripheral venous catheters*, are recommended for routine peripheral infusion therapy. The needles are stainless steel and coated with a Teflon-like plastic catheter (Fig. 11.6A). After the needle penetrates the vein in the hand or forearm, the catheter is advanced into the vein and the metal needle is removed, thereby leaving the plastic catheter in place. An IV administration set is then attached to the catheter for continuous infusion. This unit is used when IV therapy is expected to continue for a few days. The rationale for the use of the plastic catheter is that it does not have a sharp tip that could cause venous irritation and extravasation.

When a patient no longer requires IV fluid therapy but venous access is still needed for medication

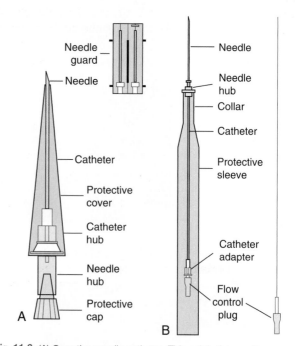

Fig. 11.6 (A) Over-the-needle catheter. This unit is the most commonly used type of catheter when intravenous therapy is expected to continue for several days. (B) In-the-needle catheters make use of a large-bore needle for venipuncture. A 4- to 6-inch sterile, small-gauge, plastic catheter is then advanced through the needle and into the vein. The needle is withdrawn, and the skin forms a seal around the plastic catheter. The intracatheter is infrequently used today.

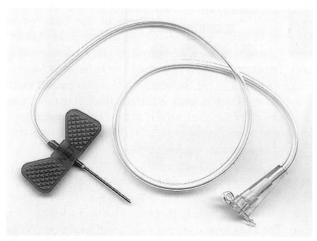

Fig. 11.5 Winged needle with a female Luer adapter. (Courtesy Narang Medical Limited, New Delhi, India.)

administration, an extension tube with an injection port is attached to the catheter and the IV fluid is discontinued. This type of IV access device is called a *saline lock* or a *medlock* (i.e., *medication lock*). Normal saline flushing rather than heparin is sufficient to prevent clotting and maintain the peripheral catheter integrity. Generally, peripheral catheters should be changed every 72 to 96 hours to prevent infection and phlebitis. Blood samples should not be drawn from peripheral catheters. If sites for venous access are limited and no evidence of infection is present, peripheral venous catheters can remain in place, although the patient and the insertion site should be monitored closely for signs and symptoms of phlebitis, infiltration, and infection. The Centers for Disease Control and Prevention (CDC) recommends that peripheral catheters not be changed for pediatric patients unless this is clinically indicated.

In-the-needle catheters make use of large-bore needles for venipuncture (Fig. 11.6B). A 4- to 6-inch sterile, smaller-gauge, plastic catheter is then advanced through the needle into the vein. The needle is withdrawn, and the skin forms a seal around the plastic catheter. The IV administration set is attached directly to the plastic catheter. In-the-needle catheters are seldom used today for peripheral IVs because of the risk of shearing the through-the-needle catheter.

Midline access catheters are selected for use if it is anticipated that IV access will be needed for 7 days or more. These catheters are often left in place for 2 to 4 weeks. Midline catheters are flexible and 3 to 8 inches long, and are inserted at the antecubital fossa into the cephalic or basilic vein and advanced to the distal subclavian vein. They do not enter the superior vena cava. Midline catheters appear to be associated with lower rates of phlebitis than short peripheral catheters; they have a lower rate of infection, and they cost less than central venous catheters. The CDC recommends the replacement of the catheter and the rotation of the injection site no more frequently than every 72 to 96 hours, but the CDC does not provide recommendations regarding the maximum length of time that the catheter may remain in place. Many institutions require that the healthcare provider write an order that indicates that the IV infusion may be left in place for more than 72 hours. Midline catheters are used for continuous access, repeated access, or IV solutions with high flow rates. This type of catheter needs to be flushed with saline and heparin solution after each use, or at least once daily if it is not in use. Blood should not be drawn through this catheter.

Central Access Devices

Central IV access devices, which are also known as *indwelling catheters*, are used in the following situations: when the purpose of therapy dictates their use (e.g., large volumes of medication, for irritating medicine such as chemotherapy, or when hypertonic solutions such as total parenteral nutrition [TPN] are to be infused); when peripheral sites have been exhausted as a result of repeated use or the condition of the veins for access is poor; when long-term or home therapy is required; or when emergency conditions mandate adequate vascular access.

The central venous sites that are most commonly used for central venous catheters are the subclavian and jugular veins. When the upper body veins are not acceptable, the femoral veins may be accessed for short-term or emergency use. A physician can also elect to perform a venisection or a cutdown to insert this type of catheter into the basilic or cephalic veins in the antecubital fossa. Three types of devices, based on the placement of the catheter's proximal tip, are routinely used for central catheters: peripheral devices, tunneled devices, and implantable devices.

Peripherally inserted central venous catheters (PICCs) are inserted into the superior vena cava or just outside the right atrium by way of the cephalic or basilar veins of the antecubital space, thereby providing an alternative to subclavian or jugular venous catheterization. PICCs are available in sizes that range from 14 to 28 gauge, with various lengths, thereby making them available for pediatric use. The catheter itself can have an open tip or a valved (Groshong) tip, and it comes with a single or double lumen. The PICC line has the advantage of ease of insertion because the procedure can be performed at the bedside by a qualified nurse. PICCs are associated with fewer mechanical complications (e.g., thrombosis, hemothorax), they cost less than other central venous catheters, they are easier to maintain than short peripheral catheters (because there is less frequent infiltration and phlebitis), and they require less frequent site rotation. PICC lines routinely remain in place for 1 to 3 months, but they can last for 1 year or more if they are cared for properly. When the device is not in use, the IV infusion is disconnected and the catheter is flushed and capped. The line should be flushed with a saline-heparin solution after every use or daily, if not used, in accordance with institutional policy.

Tunneled central venous catheters are surgically placed during an outpatient procedure with the patient under local anesthesia. The terminal tip of the catheter is inserted through an incision and into the subclavian vein, where it is then advanced to the superior vena cava. The proximal end of the catheter is tunneled about 6 inches away under the skin on the chest to exit near a nipple. A Dacron cuff is often placed around the catheter under the skin, which anchors the catheter and forms a seal around the catheter as the skin heals, thereby helping to keep the tunnel sterile.

Three types of catheters that are frequently used are the Hickman, Broviac, and Groshong catheters (Fig. 11.7). The Broviac catheter is a single-lumen catheter with a larger external diameter and a standard end hole. The Hickman catheter is larger in diameter than the Broviac catheter, but it contains two or three lumens; it also has a standard end hole. When they are not in

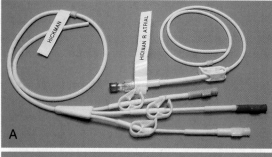

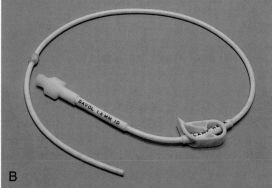

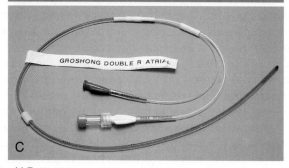

Fig. 11.7 (A) Hickman catheter. (B) Broviac catheter. (C) Groshong catheter. (Courtesy Chuck Dresner.)

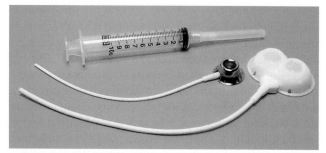

Fig. 11.8 Silicone venous catheter with infusion ports. (From Potter PA, Perry AG. *Basic Nursing: Theory and Practice.* 5th ed. St. Louis: Mosby; 2001.)

double-lumen catheter is attached to a single- or double-lumen access port (Fig. 11.8) and then implanted and sutured into a subcutaneous pocket in the chest area or the upper arm. The double ports are designed to allow for the administration of two IV solutions, two IV medications, or one of each simultaneously. One port can also be reserved for drawing blood samples. The ports contain a self-sealing silicone rubber septum that has been specifically designed for repeated injections over an extended period of time. A special noncoring, 90-degree-angle Huber needle is used to penetrate the skin and the septum of the implanted device to minimize damage to the self-sealing septum. To prolong the life of the septum, only the smallest-gauge noncoring needles should be used. The chest port is estimated to withstand up to 2000 punctures, whereas the arm port has an estimated life of 1000 punctures.

An implanted central venous access catheter may remain in place for more than 1 year, and it requires only a saline-heparin solution flush after every access or once monthly. Because the entire port and catheter are under the skin, no daily maintenance is needed, although the site should be monitored visually on a regular basis to check for swelling, redness, or drainage. This type of central venous catheter gives the patient the greatest flexibility in terms of daily activities and exercise, including swimming; however, contact sports should be avoided.

All central venous access devices require postinsertion radiography to verify the location of the device and to check for the presence of a pneumothorax for catheters that are tunneled on the chest. The CDC recommends that central venous catheters not be routinely replaced to prevent catheter-related infection.

INTRAVENOUS DOSE FORMS

Review Chapter 9 for information about the use of ampules, vials, and Mix-O-Vials. All parenteral drug dose forms are packaged so that the drug is sterile and ready for reconstitution (if needed) and administration.

TYPES OF INTRAVENOUS SOLUTIONS

Under normal and healthy conditions, the body loses water and electrolytes daily through urine, perspiration,

use, both of these catheters are clamped to prevent contamination, clotting, and air embolism. These catheters must also be flushed with a saline-heparin solution after every medication administration, or at least once daily if they are not in use. The Groshong catheter contains one to three lumens, and each one has a rounded valved tip. The Groshong valve opens inward for blood sampling and outward for infusion, but it remains closed when it is not in use. Because the valve remains closed when it is not in use, it seals the fluid inside the catheter and prevents it from coming into contact with the patient's blood. Thus weekly flushing with saline solution is all that is required to keep the catheter patent. The valve also eliminates the need for routine clamping of the catheter, although it should remain capped when it is not being used.

Implantable infusion ports (e.g., Infus-A-Port, Port-A-Cath) are used when long-term therapy is required and intermittent accessing of the central vein is required for the administration of IV fluids, medications, TPN, chemotherapy, and blood products. The implantable devices are similar to tunneled devices with regard to placement; however, the proximal end of the single- or and feces. Fluids are replenished as a result of the absorption of water in the gastrointestinal tract from the liquids and foods that are consumed. However, as a result of many different disease states (e.g., vomiting, diarrhea, gastrointestinal suctioning, hemorrhage, drainage from a wound, decreased intake, nausea, anorexia, fever, excess loss from disease [e.g., uncontrolled diabetes mellitus, diabetes insipidus]), patients are unable to ingest sufficient quantities of fluid and electrolytes to offset these losses. When this happens, the IV infusion of solutions may be necessary for replacement. See a medical-surgical nursing textbook for more information about patient assessments for deficient fluid volume.

Intravenous (IV) solutions (Box 11.1) consist of water (e.g., a solvent) that contains one or more types of

---

Box 11.1	**Types of Intravenous Solutions and Their Ingredients**[a]

ELECTROLYTE SOLUTIONS
- 5% dextrose in water (D5W)
- 10% dextrose in water (D10W)
- 0.45% sodium chloride (0.45 NS)
- 0.9% sodium chloride (normal saline; NS)
- Lactated Ringer's solution (LR)
- 5% dextrose in 0.2% sodium chloride (D5/0.2 NS)
- 5% dextrose in 0.45% sodium chloride (D5/0.45 NS)
- 5% dextrose in 0.9% sodium chloride (D5/0.9 NS)
- 5% dextrose in lactated Ringer's solution (D5/LR)
- 5% dextrose in 0.2% sodium chloride with 20 mEq of potassium chloride (D5/0.2 NS + 20 KCl)

NUTRIENT SOLUTION
Carbohydrate
- Dextrose 5% to 25% (D5-25)
Amino Acids (Trade Names)
- Aminosyn
- Travasol
- ProcalAmine
- NephrAmine
- TrophAmine
- HepatAmine
Lipids (Trade Name)
- Intralipid
- Liposyn II
Blood-Volume Expanders
- Hetastarch
- Dextran
- Albumin
- Plasma
- Tetrastarch
Alkalinizing Solutions
- Sodium bicarbonate
- Tromethamine (tris[hydroxymethyl]aminomethane [THAM])
- Citrate citric acid solutions
- Sodium lactate
Acidifying Solution
- Ammonium chloride

[a]This is a representative listing; it is not intended to be complete.

---

dissolved particles (e.g., solutes). The solutes that are most commonly dissolved in IV solutions are sodium chloride, dextrose, and potassium chloride. The solutes that dissolve in water and dissociate into ion particles (e.g., Na^+, K^+, Cl^-) are called **electrolytes** because these ions give water the ability to conduct electricity. Total parenteral solutions contain all the electrolytes necessary in addition to enough carbohydrates (usually dextrose), amino acids, and fatty acids to sustain life.

The spontaneous movement of water across the intravascular compartment capillary membranes to the interstitial spaces and across the cell membranes and back to the intravascular capillary space is called *osmosis.* The water moves from an area of high concentration of water (e.g., of low electrolyte concentration) to an area of low water concentration (e.g., of high electrolyte concentration). The electrolyte and protein concentrations of each fluid compartment are what draw water into the compartment until there is equilibrium between compartments. The force caused by the electrolytes and proteins is called *osmotic pressure.* The concentration of the dissolved particles in each compartment is known as the *osmolality.* Normal blood serum osmolality is 295 to 310 milliosmoles per liter (mOsm/L). Because IV solutions also contain dissolved particles, they also have an osmolality. If the IV solution and the blood have approximately the same osmolality, then the solution is said to be isotonic. Solutions that have fewer dissolved particles than the blood are considered to be hypotonic, and those with a higher concentration of dissolved particles are thought of as hypertonic. A 0.9% solution of sodium chloride, which is also known as *normal saline* (NS) or *physiologic saline,* is an isotonic solution with an osmolality of 308 mOsm/L. Table 11.1 lists commonly used IV solutions, their electrolyte concentrations, and their osmolalities. Those solutions with osmolalities below 270 mOsm/L are hypotonic, those with values from 270 to 310 mOsm/L are isotonic, and those with values of more than 310 mOsm/L are hypertonic.

Isotonic solutions (e.g., 0.9% sodium chloride, lactated Ringer's) are ideal replacement fluids for the patient with an intravascular fluid deficit (e.g., acute blood loss as a result of hemorrhage, gastrointestinal bleeding, or trauma). This type of fluid is used for hypovolemic, hypotensive patients to increase vascular volume to support blood pressure; however, these patients must be monitored for fluid overload (potential pulmonary edema), especially if the patient has congestive heart failure. Another isotonic solution, dextrose 5% with 0.2% sodium chloride (D5/0.2 NS), is a standard solution for maintaining hydration and electrolytes (e.g., potassium chloride), administering continuous infusion IV medications, and to keep open (TKO) IV therapy for the intermittent administration of medications. D5/0.2 NS solutions are infused as isotonic solutions, but they rapidly become hypotonic solutions as the dextrose is metabolized. Therefore D5/0.2 NS solutions—even though they are initially isotonic—should not be used

Table 11.1 Intravenous Solutions, Electrolyte Concentrations, and Osmolality

SOLUTION	Na⁺ (mEq/L)	Cl⁻ (mEq/L)	GLUCOSE (g/L)	OSMOLALITY (mOsm/L)
0.45 Normal saline	77	77	0	154
0.9 Normal saline	154	154	0	308
5% Dextrose in 0.2% sodium chloride	34	34	50	320
5% Dextrose in 0.45% sodium chloride	77	77	50	405
5% Dextrose in 0.9% sodium chloride	154	154	50	560
Lactated Ringer's solution[a]	130	109	0	273

[a]Also contains the following: K^+ (4 mEq/L), lactate (28 mEq/L), Ca^{2+} (3 mEq/L).

to maintain vascular volume in a patient who is hypovolemic and hypotensive.

Hypotonic solutions (e.g., 0.2% or 0.45% sodium chloride) have lower osmolality than serum. This type of solution contains fewer electrolytes and more free water, so the water is rapidly pulled from the vascular compartment into the interstitial and intracellular fluid compartments. Although these solutions are useful in conditions of cellular dehydration, administering them too rapidly may cause a sudden shift of fluids being drawn from the intravascular space into the other compartments.

Hypertonic solutions have an osmolality that is higher than that of the serum. Although hypotonic and isotonic solutions are used in particular situations because of their tonicity, hypertonic solutions are rarely used in this way because they have the potential to pull fluid from the intracellular and interstitial compartments into the intravascular compartment, thereby causing cellular dehydration and vascular volume overload. In cases of extravascular volume overload, these solutions are used to diurese patients because these solutions will draw fluid into the vascular compartment, which then can be excreted by the kidneys, usually with the help of diuretics such as furosemide. Hypertonic solutions also have the disadvantage of causing phlebitis and venous spasm, with infiltration and extravasation occurring in the peripheral veins. In general, solutions with osmolalities of more than approximately 600 to 700 mOsm/L should not be administered in peripheral veins. Hypertonic solutions (e.g., parenteral nutrition solutions) must be administered through central infusion lines, where the solution can be rapidly diluted by large volumes of rapidly flowing blood (e.g., in the superior vena cava near the entrance to the right atrium).

LARGE-VOLUME SOLUTION CONTAINERS

Intravenous solutions are available in both plastic and glass containers in a variety of types and concentrations (see Table 11.1 and Box 11.1) and in volumes that range from 100 to 2000 mL. Both the glass and plastic containers are vacuum sealed. The glass bottles are sealed with a hard rubber stopper and then a metal disk, and this is followed by a metal cap. Right before use, the metal cap and disk are removed, thereby exposing the hard rubber stopper. The insertion spike of the IV administration set is pushed into a specifically marked area on the rubber stopper. Some brands also have another opening in the rubber stopper that serves as an air vent (see Fig. 11.2A and C). As the solution runs out of the container, it is replaced with air. Other brands make use of a flexible plastic container (see Fig. 11.2B). As the solution runs out of the bag, the flexible container collapses.

Plastic bags are somewhat different in that the entire bag and solution are sealed inside another plastic bag that is removed just before administration. When the insertion spike is forced into the specially marked portal, an internal seal is broken, which allows the solution to flow into the tubing.

SMALL-VOLUME SOLUTION CONTAINERS

Some medicines (e.g., antibiotics) are administered by intermittent infusion through an apparatus known as a *tandem setup*, *piggyback*, or *IV rider* (Fig. 11.9). These medicines are given by a setup that is hung in tandem and connected with the primary setup. The secondary setup may consist of a drug infusion from a small volume of fluid in a small bag or bottle (≤250 mL; see Fig. 11.9) or from a volume control set (Buretrol, Volutrol; see Fig. 11.2A and C). A volume control set is composed of a calibrated chamber that is hung under the primary IV solution container and that can provide the necessary 50 to 250 mL of diluent per dose of drug. Most intermittent diluted drug infusions are infused over 20 to 60 minutes.

ADMINISTRATION OF MEDICATIONS BY THE INTRAVENOUS ROUTE

DOSE FORMS

Medications for IV administration are available in ampules, vials, prefilled syringes, and large-volume IV solution bags. Be certain that the label specifically states that the medication is for IV use. Intravenous fluid and electrolyte solutions come in a variety of volumes and concentrations in glass and plastic containers (see Box 11.1).

EQUIPMENT

- Medication profile
- Prescriber's order
- Gloves

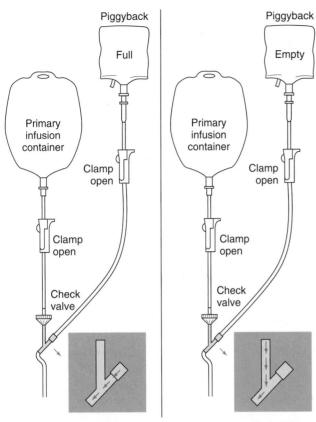

Fig. 11.9 Piggyback intermittent administration setup. Note that the smaller bag is hung higher than the primary bag.

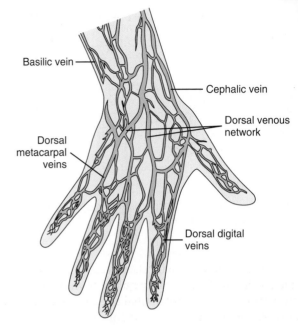

Fig. 11.10 Intravenous sites on the hand. (Redrawn from Williams PL, Warwick R, Dyson M, Bannister LH, eds. *Gray's Anatomy*. 37th ed. New York: Churchill Livingstone; 1989.)

- Tourniquet
- Administration set with syringe, appropriate needle or needleless connector (if giving by bolus), drip chamber, and filter
- Medication
- Physiologic solution ordered
- Sterile dressing materials
- Antiseptic solution
- Saline lock adapter
- Arm board (if indicated)
- Tape
- Standard IV pole
- Saline solution, piggyback, and additional solutions as appropriate

Additional supplies may be required to access, flush, or change IV administration sets, inline filters, or dressings, depending on the type of peripheral, central, or implantable device being used.

SITES

Peripheral Intravenous Access

When selecting an IV site, consider the following: the length of time that the IV infusion will be required; the condition and location of the veins; the purpose of the infusion (e.g., rehydration; delivery of nutritional needs [e.g., TPN], chemotherapy, and antibiotics); and the patient's status, cooperation level, and preference for and amount of self-care needed for the injection site (if appropriate).

Peripheral IV devices include the wing-tipped needle (see Fig. 11.5), the over-the-needle catheter (see Fig. 11.6A), and the in-the-needle catheter (see Fig. 11.6B). The over-the-needle catheters are the most commonly used venous access systems for entering the peripheral veins.

If a prolonged course of treatment is anticipated, start the first IV infusion in the hand (Fig. 11.10). The metacarpal veins, the dorsal vein network, the cephalic vein, and the basilic vein are commonly used. To avoid irritation and leakage from a previous puncture site, the subsequent venipuncture sites should be made above the earlier site. Fig. 11.11 shows the veins of the forearm area that could be used for additional venipuncture sites.

Central Intravenous Access

Central IV access devices are used for the following situations: when the purpose of therapy dictates (e.g., large-volume, high-concentration, or hypertonic solutions are to be infused); when peripheral sites have been exhausted as a result of repeated use or when the condition of the veins for access is poor; when long-term or home therapy is required; or when an emergency condition mandates adequate vascular access.

The central veins that are most commonly used for central venous catheters are the subclavian and jugular veins. When upper body veins are not acceptable, the femoral veins may be accessed for short-term or emergency use.

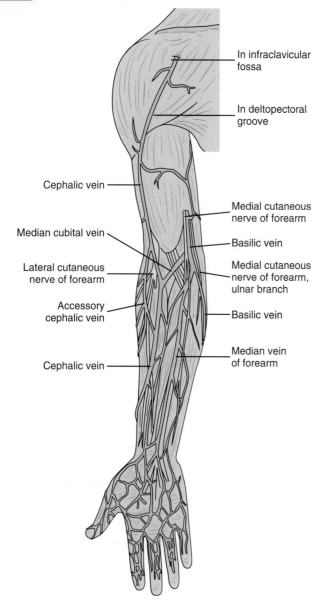

In infraclavicular fossa

In deltopectoral groove

Cephalic vein

Medial cutaneous nerve of forearm

Median cubital vein

Basilic vein

Lateral cutaneous nerve of forearm

Medial cutaneous nerve of forearm, ulnar branch

Accessory cephalic vein

Basilic vein

Median vein of forearm

Cephalic vein

Fig. 11.11 Veins in the forearm that are used as intravenous sites. (Redrawn from Williams PL, Warwick R, Dyson M, Bannister LH, eds. *Gray's Anatomy.* 37th ed. New York: Churchill Livingstone; 1989.)

GENERAL PRINCIPLES OF INTRAVENOUS MEDICATION ADMINISTRATION

- The nurse shall have passed a skill competency that demonstrates his or her knowledge of the IV administration procedure.
- If it is institutional policy to use a local anesthetic to anesthetize the IV site before insertion, the nurse must determine the patient's allergies to anesthetic agents.
- Use appropriate barrier precautions (e.g., universal blood and body fluid precautions) to prevent the transmission of any infectious diseases, including human immunodeficiency virus, as recommended by the CDC.
- Gloves should be worn throughout the venipuncture procedure. Care should be taken to wash the skin surface if the area is contaminated with blood.

- When the procedure is complete, remove the gloves and dispose of them in accordance with the policies of the practice setting. Perform hand hygiene as soon as the gloves are removed. Care should be taken to avoid contaminating the IV tubing and the rate regulator.
- Any used needles, syringes, venipuncture catheters, or vascular access devices should be placed in a puncture-resistant needle disposal container in the immediate vicinity for disposal in accordance with the policies of the practice setting. Needle safety devices should be activated before placing in the disposal container.
- Never recap, bend, or break used needles because of the danger of inadvertently puncturing the skin.
- Whenever possible, use needle protector systems such as blunt needles, injection ports, needle sheaths, or needleless systems to prevent inadvertent needle-sticks, as well as the risk of introducing pathogens into oneself.
- Be certain that medications to be administered intravenously are thoroughly dissolved in the correct volume and type of solution. Always follow the manufacturer's recommendations.
- Most clinical practice settings now use transparent dressings over the IV insertion site that are changed in accordance with hospital policies, generally every 72 to 96 hours. Some clinical practice settings still use gauze dressings. When gauze is used, the four edges of the dressing should be sealed with tape. Always check the specific policies of the employing institution, as well as the healthcare provider's orders, with regard to the frequency of dressing changes.
- Do not use topical antibiotic ointments or creams on insertion sites because of the potential to promote fungal infections and antimicrobial resistance.
- At the time of the dressing change for any type of IV site, the area should be thoroughly inspected for any drainage, redness, tenderness, irritation, or swelling. The presence of any of these symptoms should be reported to the healthcare provider immediately. (In addition, take the patient's vital signs and report these at the same time.)
- Use inline filters as recommended by the manufacturer of the drug to be infused.
- *Do not* administer any drug or IV solution that is hazy or cloudy or that has foreign particles or precipitate in it.
- *Do not* mix any other drugs with blood or blood products (e.g., albumin).
- *Do not* administer a drug in an IV solution if the compatibility is not known.
- Use aseptic technique, including the use of a cap, mask, sterile gown, sterile gloves, and a large sterile sheet, for the insertion of central venous catheters (including PICCs) and for guidewire exchanges.
- A drug must be entirely infused through the IV line before adding a second medication to the IV line.

- Drugs that are given by IV push or bolus generally are given in accordance with the **SASH guideline**—*S*aline flush first; *A*dminister the prescribed drug; *S*aline flush after the drug; *H*eparin flush the line (depending on the type of line [e.g., Hickman catheter]; check institutional policy).
- The SAS technique is similar to the SASH guideline but without the heparin: *S*aline flush first; *A*dminister the prescribed drug; *S*aline flush after the drug.
- After a medication has been mixed, know the length of time that it remains stable; all unused IV solutions should be returned to the pharmacy if they are not used within 24 hours.
- Check the institutional policy for the definition of TKO. It is usually interpreted as an infusion rate of 10 to 20 mL/hr, and less than 500 mL/24 hr should be infused.
- Shade IV solutions that contain drugs that should be protected from light. All IV solution bags or bottles should be changed every 24 to 48 hours (check institutional policy) to minimize the development of new infections. Label all IV solutions with the date and time initiated and the nurse's initials. *Do not* use marking pens directly on plastic IV containers, because the ink may penetrate the plastic and enter the IV solution.
- Intravenous administration sets that are used to deliver blood or blood products should be changed after the unit is administered. Sets that have been used to infuse lipids or TPN should be changed every 24 hours. Administration sets that are used only for physiologic IV fluids (e.g., D5/0.2 NS) may be changed every 72 to 96 hours (check institutional policy). The sets or tubing must be labeled with the

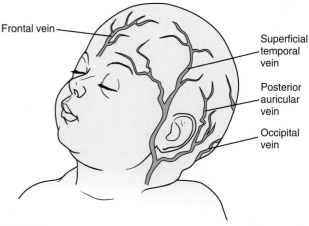

Fig. 11.12 Veins in infants and children that are used as intravenous sites. (Redrawn from Hankins J, Lonsway RA, Hedrick C, Perdue M, eds. *Infusion Therapy in Clinical Practice.* 2nd ed. Philadelphia: Saunders; 2001.)

date and time initiated, the date upon which to change the set, and the nurse's initials.
- Whenever a patient is receiving IV fluids, monitor his or her intake and output accurately. Report declining hourly outputs, as well as those of less than 30 mL/hr.
- Never speed up an IV flow rate to catch up when the volume to be infused has fallen behind. In certain cases this could be dangerous. The healthcare provider should be consulted, particularly for pediatric patients and for those who have cardiac, renal, or circulatory impairment.

PREPARING AN INTRAVENOUS SOLUTION FOR INFUSION

DOSE FORM

Check the healthcare provider's order for the specific IV solution ordered and for any medication to be added to the container. If the order has not already been prepared by the pharmacy, check the accuracy of the drug order against the medication or solution being prepared at least three times during the preparation phase: (1) when first removing the drug or solution from the storage area; (2) immediately after preparation; and (3) immediately before administration. Check the expiration date on any additives and on the primary solution. If an IV medication is to be added, ensure that the drug is approved for administration by nurses.

Perform pre–IV access assessments (see under Venipuncture pg. 157).

EQUIPMENT

- Prescriber's order
- Administration set with appropriate needle or needleless connector, appropriate drip chamber (microdrip or macrodrip; see Fig. 11.2), IV catheter, and inline filter (if used); the primary line administration set is usually labeled "universal" or "continuous flow"

Clinical Pitfalls

- NOTE: Never start an IV infusion in an artery!
- Whenever possible, initiate the IV infusion in accordance with the patient's preference or in his or her nondominant arm.
- Do not initiate an IV infusion in an arm with compromised lymphatic or venous flow (e.g., after mastectomy or axillary node dissection) or in an extremity with a dialysis or apheresis catheter or shunt inserted.
- Avoid the use of blood vessels over bony prominences or joints unless absolutely necessary.
- In the older adult, using the veins in the hand area may be a poor choice because of the fragility of the skin and veins in this area.
- Veins that are commonly used in infants and children for IV administration are on the back of the hand, the dorsum of the foot, or the temporal region of the scalp (Fig. 11.12). The scalp veins are to be used as a last resort for infants.
- When possible, avoid using the veins of the lower extremities because of the danger of the development of thrombi and emboli.

- Medications for IV delivery and labels
- Physiologic solution ordered
- IV pole or pump

TECHNIQUE

1. Assemble equipment and perform hand hygiene.
2. Check the patient's vein for the size and type of needle required to access the vein selected for venipuncture or for the type of needle required to access an implanted access device for the delivery of the IV solution or medication.
3. Check the healthcare provider's order against the physiologic solution chosen for administration.
4. Inspect the IV container for cloudiness, discoloration, and the presence of any precipitate. Verify the expiration date on the IV fluid container.
5. Remove the plastic cover from the IV container, and inspect the plastic IV bag to be certain that it is intact; squeeze it gently to detect any punctures. Inspect a glass container of IV solution for any cracks.
6. Choose the administration set that is appropriate for the type of solution ordered, for the rate of delivery requested (e.g., microdrip or macrodrip), and for the type of IV container being used. Plastic bag IV containers *do not* require an air vent in the administration set. Glass containers for IV delivery must be vented or have an administration set with an air filter vent in it. Remove the administration set from its container, and inspect it for any faults or contamination.
7. Move the roller or slide clamp to the upper portion of the IV line 6 to 8 inches from the drip chamber; close the clamp.
8. Connect the IV administration set or tubing to the IV solution.
   - *Plastic IV bags:* Remove the tab from the spike receiver port, remove the tab from the administration set spike, and insert the spike firmly into the bag port. Maintain the sterility of the port and spike throughout the process.
   - *Glass IV bottle:* Peel back the metal tab and lift the protective metal disk from the container; remove the latex-type covering (if present) from the top of the rubber stopper. As the latex diaphragm is removed, a sudden noise should be heard as the vacuum within the glass container is released. If the noise is not heard, the contents of the IV container may not be sterile and should be discarded. Remove the tab from the administration set spike; insert the spike firmly into the port in the rubber stopper. Maintain the sterility of the port and spike throughout the process.
   - NOTE: When additive medications are ordered, they should be added to the large-volume container before tubing is attached to help ensure a uniform mixing of the medication and the physiologic solution. If medication is added to an existing IV solution, clamp the line before adding the medication to the container, and make sure that adequate mixing takes place before the infusion is started again. (See Adding a Medication to an Intravenous Bag, Bottle, or Volume Control Device, pg. 164.)
9. Hang the solution on an IV pole, squeeze the drip chamber, and fill it halfway. Prime the IV line by removing the protective tab or cap from the distal end of the IV line, invert the Y port, open the roller or slide clamp, and allow the solution to run until all of the air is removed from the line. If using a pump, prime the tubing in accordance with institutional policy. Cover the end of the IV tubing with a sterile cap. Inspect the entire length of tubing to be certain that all air is removed from the line. (NOTE: It may be necessary to add inline filters to the setup if this is recommended for the administration of the ordered medication. Purge air from the line before attaching the filter, then run solution through the filter to remove air from the filter.)
10. Label the container with the patient's name along with the date and time of preparation. If medication has been added, all details of the medication must be marked on the container's label: the drug name and dose, the rate of administration requested in the healthcare provider's order.
11. Label the IV tubing with the date and time that it is opened and the date and time that it is to be changed. The CDC recommends that IV tubing be changed every 72 hours. Administration sets that are used to deliver blood or blood products may be changed after each unit is infused, as defined by institutional policy, or within 24 hours of initiating the infusion. Lipid solutions have special tubing that should be changed every 24 hours if they are administered by continuous infusion or after every unit if they are administered intermittently. Follow institutional policies.
12. The IV solution can now be taken to the bedside for attachment after a venipuncture is performed or for addition to an existing IV system. For safety, all aspects of the IV order should be checked again immediately before attaching the IV solution for infusion.

INTRAVENOUS FLUID MONITORING

The infusion of IV fluids requires careful monitoring for patients of all ages. The microdrip chamber, which delivers 60 drops (gtt)/mL, is used whenever a small volume of IV solution is ordered to be infused over a specific time. Many clinical practice settings interpret a small volume as less than 100 mL/hr. In pediatric units, volume control chamber devices (e.g., a Buretrol, a SoluSet) and syringe pump controllers are commonly used to regulate the volume of fluid that is infused.

BASIC GUIDELINES FOR THE INTRAVENOUS ADMINISTRATION OF MEDICATIONS

EQUIPMENT

- Medication profile
- Prescriber's order
- Tourniquet
- Clean gloves
- Drug in a sterile, sealed container
- Syringe of the correct volume
- Needles of the correct gauge and length
- Antiseptic alcohol wipes
- Tape
- Change label
- Special equipment based on the route of administration (e.g., a radiopaque over-the-needle catheter for insertion; infusion pump)
- Transparent dressing supplies

PREMEDICATION ASSESSMENT

1. Know basic patient data, the patient's diagnosis, the symptoms of the disorder or disease process for which the medication is ordered, and the desired action of the drug for the particular individual.
2. Obtain baseline vital signs.
3. Check for any tape, latex, and drug allergies or prior drug reactions.
4. Check the accuracy of the drug order against the medication or solution being prepared at least three times during the preparation phase: (1) when first removing the drug or solution from the storage area; (2) immediately after preparation; and (3) immediately before administration.
5. Check for leaks, clarity, and expiration date on the IV solution and on the drug to be added to the solution.
6. Review the individual drug monograph to identify laboratory studies recommended before or intermittently during therapy, the calculation of the dose, the adverse effects, the monitoring parameters recommended for the specific drug prescribed, and other considerations. (With certain light-sensitive medications [e.g., amphotericin B, nitroprusside], it is necessary to shield the IV bag with a dark plastic bag to prevent the degradation of the drug.)
7. Know the type of IV access that the patient has in place, the date and time of insertion, the type of IV fluid or medication running, and the rate of flow prescribed.

PROCEDURE PROTOCOL

The standard procedures for preparing all parenteral medications are as follows:
1. Perform hand hygiene before preparing any medication or handling sterile supplies. During the actual preparation of a parenteral medication, the primary rule is "sterile to sterile" and "unsterile to unsterile" when handling the syringe and needle.
2. Use the *seven rights* of medication preparation and administration throughout the procedure: right patient, right drug, right indication, right route, right dose, right time, and right documentation.
3. Check the drug dose form ordered against the source used for the preparation.
4. Check compatibility charts or contact the pharmacist before mixing two medications or adding medications to an IV solution.
5. Check medication calculations. When in doubt about a dose, check it with another qualified nurse. (Most institutional policies require fractional doses of medications and doses of heparin and insulin to be checked by two qualified individuals before administration.)
6. Know the institutional policy regarding limitations on the types of medications to be administered by nursing personnel. Before administering an IV drug, the nurse should check the list of drugs approved for administration by nurses in the clinical care setting.
7. Prepare the drug in a clean, well-lighted area with the use of aseptic technique throughout the entire procedure.
8. Concentrate on the procedure; ensure accuracy during preparation.
9. Check the expiration date of the medication.
10. Research the medication ordered as an IV additive; this procedure also applies for direct push or bolus administration.
    - Name of drug.
    - Usual dose (take into consideration the patient's age, weight, and hydration state).
    - Compatibility of the drug with existing IV drugs that are currently infusing.
    - For IV push or bolus, does the drug need to be diluted, or can it be given undiluted? If it should be diluted, what types and amounts of diluent can be used? If it is being added to an existing IV infusion, is the drug compatible with the primary solution?
    - Recommended rate of infusion.

VENIPUNCTURE

Perform the following pre–IV access assessments:
- Assess the patient's demeanor. Does the patient appear cooperative, or will assistance be needed? (Always have sufficient assistance when working with pediatric patients.)
- Check for and avoid previously used IV sites, areas of impaired circulation, and any fistulas that may be present in the extremities.
- Examine the extremities for potential sites and estimate the size of the veins that are available for use.

EQUIPMENT

- Medication profile
- Prescriber's order
- IV start set
- Antiseptic alcohol wipes
- One pair of gloves
- Site label
- Tape
- Transparent dressing materials
- Two gauze sponges, 2 × 2 inches
- One roll of transparent tape
- Latex tourniquet
- One change label
- Arm board (when indicated)
- As appropriate, medications and physiologic solutions ordered for IV delivery and IV equipment needed (see Preparing an Intravenous Solution for Infusion pg. 155)
- For a saline lock or a medlock, obtain the correct extension tubing and injection cap, as appropriate (see Administration of Medication by a Saline Lock or Medlock later); use saline and heparin flush solutions in accordance with institutional policy (use 10-mL syringes that contain an appropriate volume of solution for flushing)
- IV pump, if required

Selection of the Catheter or Butterfly Needle

When selecting a catheter or butterfly needle for use, choose the smallest size that is feasible for administering the specific type of fluid that has been ordered. Catheters are available in sizes ranging from 27 gauge, ⅝ inch to 14 gauge, ½ inch, and butterfly needles are available in sizes 17 to 29 gauge. A more viscous fluid such as blood requires a larger-diameter catheter. As with other needles, the lower the number of the gauge, the larger the diameter of the opening of the catheter. During the assessment process, the nurse notes the size of the vein to be accessed.

TECHNIQUE FOR ESTABLISHING AN IV LINE

1. Perform the premedication assessment and follow the procedure protocol described.
2. Assemble the necessary equipment and perform hand hygiene.
3. Check all aspects of the healthcare provider's orders.
4. Recheck the size and type of catheter or butterfly needle needed to access the vein selected and any extension tubing or injection caps that are needed to prepare the site for future intermittent or continuous use for the prescribed IV therapy.
5. If ordered, the IV solution and medication should be prepared and taken to the bedside for attachment after a venipuncture has been performed. For safety, all aspects of the IV therapy orders should be checked again immediately before initiating the venipuncture and before attaching the IV solution for infusion. (NOTE: Always identify the patient by checking his or her ID bracelet before initiating any procedure. Have the patient state his or her name and birth date or other identifiers. Explain the procedure, and provide education about the drug being administered.)
6. Position the patient appropriately. Immobilize an infant or child for patient safety, if necessary. (Be sure that the patient is wearing the type of hospital gown that has openings on the shoulder seams.)
7. Cut tape for stabilizing the IV catheter or butterfly needle before starting the procedure. Turn the ends of the tape back on themselves to form a tab that will not adhere to a glove when the tape is to be applied or removed. (NOTE: The nurse must consider his or her gloves to be contaminated when they come into contact with blood. If the gloves come into contact with the tape and dressing materials that have been used at the venipuncture site, the outside of the dressings and tape are then potentially contaminated. Therefore during the procedure, the nurse must focus on allowing contamination only of the dominant gloved hand; the nondominant hand must be maintained as uncontaminated to handle the taping and stabilization of the peripheral access device. After the needle or catheter is stabilized, the gloves can be removed; perform hand hygiene and apply the gauze or the occlusive type of dressing materials in accordance with practice setting policies.)
8. When extension tubing is used with the catheter or the butterfly needle, fill the extension tubing with saline and purge it of all air.
9. Apply the tourniquet using a slipknot 2 to 6 inches above the site chosen (this is the shaded area in Fig. 11.13A). Inspect the area to identify a vein of sufficient size to accommodate the catheter and provide adequate anchorage.
10. Put on nonsterile gloves. As the vein dilates, palpate the vein to feel its depth and direction (Fig. 11.13B and C). To dilate the vein, it may be necessary to place the extremity in a dependent position. Massage the vein against the direction of blood flow, have the patient open and close the hand repeatedly, or remove the tourniquet and apply a heating pad or warm wet towels to the extremity for 15 to 20 minutes, and then restart the process.
11. Cleanse the skin surface with the antiseptic alcohol wipe, starting at the site of entry and working outward in a circular motion toward the periphery (Fig. 11.13D). Do not retouch the area where the puncture site will be made. (Alternatives are to put a sterile glove on one hand so that the site can be touched again or to prepare the fingertip with antiseptic.)
12. Allow the area to air-dry.

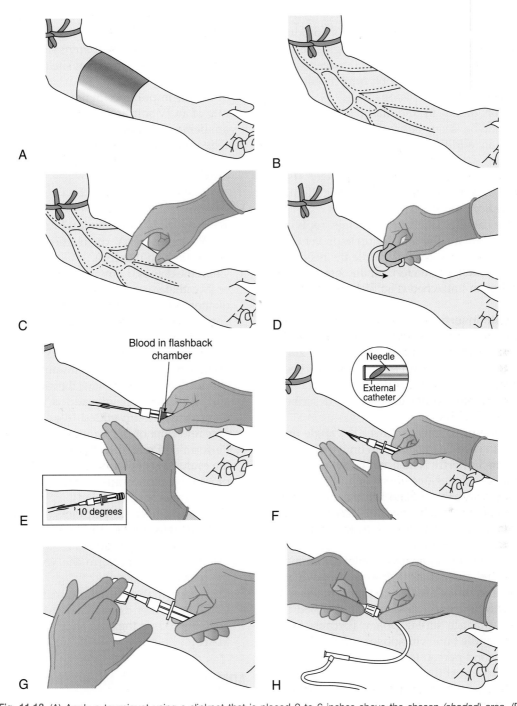

Fig. 11.13 (A) Apply a tourniquet using a slipknot that is placed 2 to 6 inches above the chosen *(shaded)* area. (B) Allow the veins to dilate. (C) Palpate the vein to feel its depth and direction. (D) Cleanse the skin surface with an antiseptic alcohol wipe, starting at the anticipated site of entry and working outward in a circular motion to the periphery. (E) For an over-the-needle catheter, hold the flashback chamber with the thumb and forefinger and insert the catheter with the needle at a 10- to 30-degree angle (or at the angle as specified in manufacturer's directions), with the bevel up. (F) Withdraw the needle from the catheter. (G) Apply gentle pressure over the catheter tip to prevent the excessive backflow of blood while the needle is removed and the intravenous line is attached. (H) Secure the connection of the intravenous tubing to the hub of the catheter.

13. Hold the catheter or butterfly needle to be inserted in the dominant hand, and remove the protective cover while maintaining the sterility of the needle. Approach the vein directly from above or from slightly to one side of the vein. Provide tension on the skin surface to stretch the skin and stabilize the vein.

Peripheral Over-the-Needle Catheter Insertion (See Fig. 11.6A)

- Inspect the IV catheter and loosen the catheter needle by rotating the catheter.
- Hold the flashback chamber with the thumb and forefinger and insert the catheter with the needle

at a 10- to 30-degree angle with the bevel up (Fig. 11.13E). Check the manufacturer's product instructions for the recommended angle of entry and assess the depth of the vein; the deeper the vein, the greater the angle of entry needed to puncture the skin and venous wall.

- Watch for blood in the flashback chamber; after blood is seen, advance the needle and catheter an additional $\frac{1}{16}$ to $\frac{1}{4}$ inch into the vein.
- Withdraw the needle from the catheter (Fig. 11.13F), lower the angle of the catheter slightly, and advance the catheter into the vein.
- Hold the catheter hub in place while applying gentle pressure on the catheter tip to prevent the excessive backflow of blood while the needle is removed from the catheter and the catheter and IV solution are attached (Fig. 11.13G).

Butterfly Needle Insertion

- Prepare the site as described previously.
- Hold the butterfly needle by the tabs and align the needle, bevel up, with the vein that has been selected.
- Puncture the skin and vein surface as described previously.
- After the vein is entered, lower the angle and advance the needle into the vein until the tabbed area of the butterfly is adjacent to the puncture site.

14. Release the tourniquet and secure the connection of the IV tubing to the over-the-needle plastic needle hub (Fig. 11.13H) or to the butterfly apparatus.
15. Cleanse the area to eliminate any blood that may have contacted the skin or IV tubing. Remove the gloves and anchor the needle and tubing to the arm or hand with tape and dressing, as prescribed by the clinical practice setting policy. (Because it is difficult to handle tape with gloves on, it is helpful to have a second person to anchor the needle and tubing and to adjust the flow rate.)
16. If no continuously flowing IV solution is attached, flush the catheter in accordance with clinical practice setting policy.
17. The individual who is performing the venipuncture can dispose of all soiled dressings and contaminated supplies in accordance with the clinical practice setting's policy.
18. Adjust the rate of flow solution or set the rate on the pump.
19. Regardless of the apparatus used, mark the label with the date and time of insertion.
20. In a way that is appropriate to the age, site, and physical orientation of the individual, attach a padded arm board to support and stabilize the infusion site.

PATIENT TEACHING

1. Teach the patient about any symptoms that should be reported at the insertion site (e.g., pain, swelling, discomfort).
2. Stress the importance of not trying to self-adjust the rate of an IV solution or of any IV medications that are being administered.
3. Explain the purpose of the dressing that has been applied to the IV site and the need to leave the dressing intact.

DOCUMENTATION

Provide the right documentation of the venipuncture (e.g., IV started or IV medication administered and response to drug therapy).

1. Chart the date and time; the size and type of butterfly or IV catheter used; the site accessed; and the number of attempts made to perform the venipuncture. Make entries on the appropriate IV site flow sheets that are used at the clinical practice setting.
2. On the patient's medication administration record (MAR), chart the type and amount of IV fluid started or added to an existing line; the rate of administration; and, if medication was added, the date, the drug name, the amount added (e.g., the dose), and the date and time of preparation and initiation.
3. Perform and record regular patient assessments for the evaluation of therapeutic effectiveness (e.g., blood pressure, pulse, output, lung field sounds, degree and duration of pain relief).
4. Chart any signs and symptoms of the adverse effects of the drugs given or problems encountered during the venipuncture procedure. If more than one attempt was required to perform the venipuncture, record the relevant details.
5. Record any patient teaching that was done.
6. If the IV access device was flushed, it should be documented on the flow sheet and on the patient's MAR.

ADMINISTRATION OF MEDICATION BY A SALINE LOCK OR A MEDLOCK

A saline lock or medlock may be used for administration of medications or withdrawing blood samples (Fig. 11.14). Perform premedication assessments and follow procedure protocol as described earlier in this chapter. In addition, refer to the individual drug monographs.

EQUIPMENT

- Medication profile
- Prescriber's order
- Medication for IV delivery and label
- Extension tubing and injection cap, as appropriate
- Syringes and needleless connectors
- Saline and heparin flush solutions

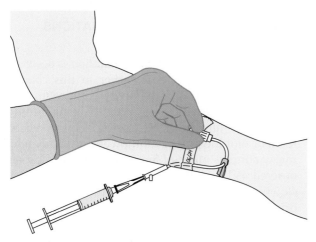

Fig. 11.14 Heparin lock/saline lock/medlock with an extension tubing taped in place and ready for access.

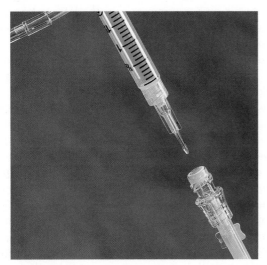

Fig. 11.15 Syringe with a blunt-access cannula, attached by a Luer-Lok, approaching a portal on an intravenous administration set. (Courtesy Baxter Healthcare Corporation, Mountain Home, AR. All rights reserved.)

- Gloves
- Antiseptic alcohol wipes
- Sharps safety container for used needle and receptacle for old dressing material that is removed

TECHNIQUE FOR IV BOLUS MEDICATIONS WITH CAPPED IV LINE

1. Select a syringe that is several milliliters larger than required for the volume of the drug. This allows room for the aspiration of blood to ensure the proper placement of the needle or catheter in the vein and to allow blood to mix with the drug solution. Place a needleless access device on the syringe (Fig. 11.15) or use a syringe that is used with a needleless system (Fig. 11.16).
2. Research and prepare the medication as described previously. Prepare the saline in syringes with needleless access devices to flush the line before and after medication administration in accordance with institutional policy. It is recommended that

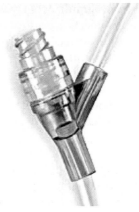

Fig. 11.16 The Baxter CLEARLINK Access System features an integrated clamp to help protect patients from the effects of accidental disconnection and ensure minimal fluid displacement with proper technique. Clear housing allows easy identification of residuals, which may indicate need for replacement. A double seal provides effective barrier to microbial ingress. A flat septum with tight fit to housing helps reduce the risk of microbial contamination and eases cleansing. (Courtesy Baxter Healthcare Corporation, Mountain Home, AR. All rights reserved.)

10-mL syringes that contain a few milliliters of flush solution be used for flushing to reduce the pressure exerted in the vein or catheter.
3. Identify the patient by checking his or her ID bracelet. Recheck the medication order, explain the procedure, and provide education about the drug being administered. Have the patient state his or her name and birth date or two other identifiers.
4. Apply clean gloves.
5. Swab the self-sealing portal of the injection site with an antiseptic alcohol wipe for 15 seconds, and attach the syringe via the injection cap.
6. Access the injection portal or cap with a syringe that contains flush solution and gently pull back on the plunger for blood return. If return is not obtained or if resistance is felt, stop and evaluate the cause. Do not force the insertion of the solution or a clot could be dislodged.
7. When blood return is established, inject the saline for the flush followed by the medication at the rate specified by the manufacturer. *Always carefully check the drug order and a reliable reference for the proper dilution and recommended rate of administration of the drug. Watch the clock and time the injection rate as accurately as possible!*
8. Observe the IV site at the catheter tip for swelling and monitor the patient for complaints of discomfort.
9. After administration, withdraw the needleless device from the injection port and dispose of it in a sharps safety container.
10. Access the injection cap and insert another syringe that contains (usually) 1 to 2 mL of normal saline to flush the remaining drug from the catheter.
11. *Optional:* In accordance with institutional policy, flush the lock with 1 mL of heparin (10 to 100 units/mL). Maintain constant pressure on the plunger of

the syringe while simultaneously withdrawing the needle from the injection port to prevent the back-flow of blood. Always verify the heparin dose with another qualified nurse.

12. Cleanse the site of any blood or fluids. Remove gloves and dispose of them properly. Perform hand hygiene. Dispose of equipment in accordance with Occupational Safety and Health Administration standards.

The saline lock or medlock should be flushed when it is initially placed, after administration of medications, after withdrawing blood samples, or daily if medications are not administered more frequently. Check the institutional policy to determine how long a lock may remain in place before it is changed. Monitor the venipuncture site for any adverse effects or complications.

PATIENT TEACHING

Explain to the patient the purpose of the medication administered and any adverse effects for that medication that should be reported.

DOCUMENTATION

1. In the patient's MAR, document the date, time, drug, and dosage; the flushing procedure; and any assessment data that are pertinent (e.g., how well the procedure was tolerated, observations of the venipuncture site).
2. Perform and record regular patient assessments for the evaluation of therapeutic effectiveness.
3. Chart any signs and symptoms of the adverse effects of the drugs given or problems encountered during the procedure.
4. Record any patient teaching that was done.

 Life Span Considerations

Benzyl Alcohol Preservative

Do not use bacteriostatic water or saline that contains the preservative benzyl alcohol to reconstitute or dilute medications or to flush the IV catheters of newborns because this preservative is toxic to these patients.

ADMINISTRATION OF MEDICATIONS INTO AN ESTABLISHED INTRAVENOUS LINE

Perform premedication assessments and follow procedure protocol as described earlier. In addition, refer to the individual drug monographs.

EQUIPMENT

- Medication profile
- Prescriber's order
- Medication for IV delivery and label
- Gloves
- Antiseptic alcohol wipes
- Syringe and needleless connector
- Saline solution as appropriate

TECHNIQUE FOR IV BOLUS MEDICATIONS WITH IV SOLUTION RUNNING

1. Research and then prepare the medication as described in the procedure protocol earlier in this chapter. Ensure that the drug to be prepared is compatible with the IV solution that is currently being infused. Always carefully check the drug order and a reliable reference for the proper dilution and recommended rate of administration of the drug. Many medications ordered as IV push or bolus must be administered slowly over several minutes. An excessive rate of administration can result in shock and cardiac arrest.
2. Identify the patient by checking his or her ID bracelet. Explain the procedure and provide education about the drug being administered. Have the patient state his or her name and birth date or two other identifiers.
3. Recheck the medication order.
4. Put on gloves when there is a potential for exposure to blood or body fluids. It is helpful to keep one gloved hand uncontaminated.
5. Swab the self-sealing portal of the injection site with an antiseptic alcohol wipe for 15 seconds and attach a syringe via the injection cap.
6. Using a needleless device on the syringe, puncture the Y port site (see Fig. 11.15). Alternatively, for an injection cap (see Fig. 11.16), attach the syringe with medication directly.
7. Inject the prescribed medication into the IV line at the rate recommended by the manufacturer.
   If the medication and the IV solution are not compatible:
   - Swab the injection port nearest the catheter with an alcohol wipe for 15 seconds.
   - Insert a needleless device into the port; stop the primary infusion and inject 2 mL of 0.9% NS (e.g., saline flush), in accordance with institutional policy, via IV push.
   - Swab the port with an alcohol wipe; insert the needleless device that contains medication and administer the drug at the prescribed rate.
   - Remove the medication syringe, swab the port again, and inject 2 mL of 0.9% NS (e.g., saline flush), in accordance with institutional policy, via IV push. If injecting into a central line, follow institutional policy regarding the need to irrigate with a saline and heparin solution.
8. When all of the medication has been administered, open the established IV line and readjust the flow rate to correspond with the healthcare provider's order. Remove gloves and perform hand hygiene.

PATIENT TEACHING

Explain to the patient the purpose of the medication administered and discuss any potential adverse effects of the medication.

DOCUMENTATION

1. In the patient's MAR, document the date, time, drug, and dosage and any assessment data that are pertinent (e.g., how well the procedure was tolerated, observations of the venipuncture site).
2. Perform and record regular patient assessments for the evaluation of therapeutic effectiveness.
3. Chart any signs and symptoms of the adverse effects of the drugs given or problems encountered during the procedure.
4. Record any patient teaching that was done.

 Clinical Pitfall

Flushing the IV line by accelerating the IV infusion rate is not recommended because the medication that is still in the line will be administered too rapidly. This is contrary to the manufacturer's safety recommendation. Sudden boluses of certain medications may also cause severe hypotension or other signs of toxicity.

ADMINISTRATION OF MEDICATION THROUGH AN IMPLANTED VENOUS ACCESS DEVICE

Perform premedication assessments and follow procedure protocol as described on pg. 157 in this chapter. In addition, refer to the individual drug monographs.

EQUIPMENT

- Medication profile
- Prescriber's order
- Medication for IV delivery and label
- IV piggyback bag
- Dressing kits (at some clinical practice settings)
- Two pairs of sterile gloves
- Two 10-mL syringes with 0.9% NS, 2 to 10 mL; consult the institutional policy manual for the volume used in the facility
- One 10-mL syringe with heparin (10 to 100 units/mL), usually 2.5 to 5 mL; consult the institutional policy manual for the volume used in the facility
- Sterile 10-mL syringe
- Needleless access device
- 18- to 22-gauge (⅝-inch) needle
- Antiseptic solution or swab sticks per institutional policy
- Alcohol swabs
- Huber needle
- Extension tubing
- Sharps safety container for used needle and receptacle for old dressing material that is removed

TECHNIQUE FOR IV MEDICATIONS VIA IMPLANTED VENOUS ACCESS DEVICE

1. Research and prepare the medication as described in the procedure protocol earlier in this chapter.
2. Prepare a syringe with the medication or add the medication to an IV piggyback bag.
3. Insert the administration set into the IV container, prime the IV line to remove all air, and then cover the end of the IV line with a sterile cap. Leave the prescribed medication in a sterile syringe.
4. Take all supplies and the IV medication to the patient's bedside.
5. Identify the patient by checking his or her ID bracelet. Explain the procedure and provide education about the drug being administered. Have the patient state his or her name and birth date or two other identifiers.
6. Recheck all aspects of the medication order.
7. Perform hand hygiene.
8. If the implanted port is not already accessed, palpate the site to identify landmarks.
9. Open the dressing kit, set up and prepare the flushing supplies, and prime the infusion set while maintaining the sterility of the Huber needle.
10. Apply sterile gloves.
11. Use the nondominant gloved hand to cleanse the skin over the implanted port with alcohol; cleanse from the intended site of insertion outward in widening circles. Repeat the cleansing process two more times. Allow the alcohol to dry and then repeat the cleansing process with the use of antiseptic swab sticks.
12. Using the sterile gloved hand, grasp the Huber needle by the winged flanges, attach it to the syringe that contains saline, and insert the needle perpendicular to the patient's skin until the needle tip comes into contact with the bottom of the port. Support the Huber needle with folded 2 × 2-inch sponges.
13. Withdraw the plunger of the saline syringe slightly until blood returns. Inject normal saline (to flush the port of heparin, left from a previous flush) and then attach the syringe that contains medication or the IV piggyback container with medicine. If administering from the syringe, use the IV bolus technique. If administering as an infusion with the IV piggyback container (see Adding a Medication With a Piggyback Set later in this chapter), attach the primed administration set to the Huber needle and adjust the rate of infusion. Provide support for the IV line. Apply transparent or gauze dressing and tape it in place. When the medication administration is completed, flush the line with saline and heparin in accordance with institutional policy. Maintain steady pressure on the plunger of the syringe as the needle is withdrawn from the access device to prevent the backflow of blood.
14. Label the site with the date of access, the size and length of the Huber needle, the nurse's initials, and the date.
15. If the Huber needle is removed from a healed site at this time, cleanse the injection site with an alcohol wipe and apply an adhesive bandage.

16. Dispose of used needles into a sharps safety container. Dispose of used extension tubing and other supplies in accordance with institutional policy.

17. Remove and dispose of gloves properly. Perform hand hygiene.

PATIENT TEACHING

1. Explain to the patient the purpose of the medication being administered and discuss the potential adverse effects of that medication.

2. Stress the importance of preventing infection in the port; the patient should avoid touching the site. If medication is being given intermittently with the use of a pump, have the patient put the call light on when the machine alarm sounds.

DOCUMENTATION

1. In the patient's MAR, document the date, time, drug, and dosage and any assessment data that are pertinent (e.g., how well the procedure was tolerated, observations of the injection site).

2. Perform and record regular patient assessments for the evaluation of therapeutic effectiveness.

3. Chart any signs and symptoms of the adverse effects of the drugs given or problems encountered during the procedure.

4. Record any patient teaching that was done.

ADDING A MEDICATION TO AN INTRAVENOUS BAG, BOTTLE, OR VOLUME-CONTROL DEVICE

Perform premedication assessments and follow procedure protocol as described earlier. In addition, refer to the individual drug monographs.

EQUIPMENT

- Medication profile
- Prescriber's order
- Medication for IV delivery and label
- Gloves
- Antiseptic alcohol wipes
- Needleless connector

TECHNIQUE FOR ADDING MEDICATIONS TO IV SOLUTIONS

1. Research and prepare the medication as described in the procedure protocol earlier in this chapter.

2. Identify the patient by checking his or her ID bracelet. Explain the procedure and provide education about the drug being administered. Have the patient state his or her name and birth date or two other identifiers.

3. Recheck all aspects of the medication order.

4. Perform hand hygiene and apply gloves.

5. Identify the injection port on the specific type of IV container or volume control set that is being used; cleanse the portal with an antiseptic swab.

6. Clamp the IV tubing.

7. Insert the sterile access device into the port and slowly add the prescribed medication to the IV solution. Always check to be certain that the medication is being added to a compatible solution of sufficient volume to ensure the proper dilution of the medication as specified by the manufacturer. Agitate the bag, bottle, or volume control device to disperse the medication in the fluid thoroughly.

8. For a volume control apparatus, fill the volume chamber with the specified amount of IV solution (see Fig. 11.2A and C) and then clamp the tubing between the IV bottle or bag and the volume control chamber. Add the medication, as described previously, via the cleansed injection port. Be sure that the medication is dispersed in the solution and adjust the rate of the flow solution.

9. Affix a label to the container. Indicate the medication's name and dose, the date and time, the prepared rate of infusion, and the length of infusion time, and include the nurse's signature.

 Clinical Pitfall

When IV medications are administered by a volume control apparatus, the calculation of the rate of infusion for administering the drug over the proper time must include an allowance for the volume of the fluid in the IV tubing and for the volume of medication.

PATIENT TEACHING

Explain to the patient the purpose of the medication administered and advise him or her of any adverse effects of the medication.

DOCUMENTATION

1. In the patient's MAR, document the date, time, drug, and dosage; the rate of administration if a volume-control apparatus is used; and any assessment data that are pertinent (e.g., how well the procedure was tolerated).

2. Perform and record regular patient assessments for the evaluation of therapeutic effectiveness.

3. Chart any signs and symptoms of the adverse effects of the drugs given or problems encountered during the procedure.

4. Record any patient teaching that was done.

ADDING A MEDICATION WITH A PIGGYBACK SET

Perform premedication assessments and follow procedure protocol. In addition, refer to the individual drug monographs.

EQUIPMENT

- Medication profile
- Prescriber's order
- Medication for IV delivery and label

- IV piggyback bag
- Administration set with needleless connector
- Antiseptic alcohol wipes

TECHNIQUE FOR IV PIGGYBACK MEDICATIONS

1. Research and then prepare the medication as described in the procedure protocol earlier in this chapter and then add it to an IV piggyback bag.
   - Reconstitute a powder using a preassembled IV medication system such as the ADD-Vantage System (Fig. 11.17). This is a needleless system with two distinctly separate components: (1) an ADD-Vantage diluent container (e.g., a plastic piggyback bag) that contains 0.9% NS, D5W, or 0.45% sodium chloride; and (2) an ADD-Vantage drug vial that contains medication (e.g., ampicillin powder).
     - Hold the ADD-Vantage vial and plastic container in a vertical position by the bottom of the attached drug vial (the vial is actually upside down).
     - Reach through the flexible container of diluent, grasp the inner stopper in the vial by the plastic ring that surrounds it, and pull straight down on the ring; the stopper disconnects and falls into the diluent solution. The drug powder also falls out and, with a few squeezes of the diluent bag, mixes with the diluent to reconstitute the drug.
     - The ADD-Vantage container is now ready for the attachment of the secondary IV tubing when it is taken to the bedside.
   - Immediately before use, check all aspects of the drug order against the drug container.

2. Identify the patient by checking his or her ID bracelet. Explain the procedure and provide education about the drug being administered. Have the patient state his or her name and birth date or two other identifiers.
3. Determine the compatibility of the primary IV solution and its additives with that of the piggyback medication or solution.
4. Recheck all aspects of the medication order.
5. Perform hand hygiene.
6. Insert the administration set into the piggyback container and attach a needleless device.
7. Connect to the primary IV tubing by arranging the piggyback container so that it is elevated higher than the primary container (see Fig. 11.9). Cleanse the portal on the primary line with an antiseptic swab for 15 seconds and insert the needleless device connector (Fig. 11.18) by attaching the piggyback tubing to the port of the tubing of the primary solution. Secure this in place.
8. Lower the piggyback container below the level of the primary solution, open the secondary tubing clamp, and slowly purge the secondary tubing of air with the use of the backflow method; this will allow the primary solution to fill the secondary tubing. Place the piggyback solution higher than the primary IV solution before administration.
9. Check the specific orders for the infusion rate and the sequence of the solution or medication administration.
10. Affix a label to the container. Indicate the medication name and dose, the date and time that it was prepared, the rate of infusion, and the length of infusion time, and include the nurse's signature.

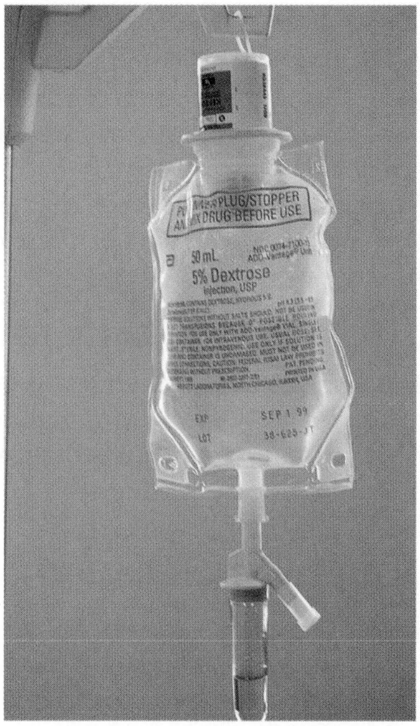

Fig. 11.17 The ADD-Vantage drug delivery system. (Courtesy Bruce Clayton.)

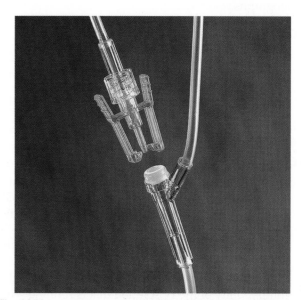

Fig. 11.18 A male Luer-Lok with an INTERLINK lever lock cannula attached. This illustrates how a (needle-free) blunt plastic cannula-tipped adapter can be used to attach a piggyback container to the portal of a primary intravenous administration set. (Courtesy Baxter Healthcare Corporation, Mountain Home, AR. All rights reserved.)

11. When the piggyback empties, the check valve in the primary line releases and the primary infusion resumes. If a pump is used, the primary infusion will resume when the piggyback or secondary infusion is complete.

 Clinical Pitfall

One of the most common mistakes when using preassembled IV medication containers (for safety and ease of reconstitution) is forgetting to activate the system and mix the drug powder with the diluent before hanging it for administration.

PATIENT TEACHING

Explain to the patient the purpose of the medication that is being administered and discuss with him or her any potential adverse effects of the medication.

DOCUMENTATION

1. In the patient's MAR, document the date, time, drug, and dosage and any assessment data that are pertinent (e.g., how well the procedure was tolerated).
2. Perform and record regular patient assessments for the evaluation of therapeutic effectiveness.
3. Chart any signs and symptoms of the adverse effects of the drugs given or problems encountered during the procedure.
4. Record any patient teaching that was done.

CHANGING TO THE NEXT CONTAINER OF INTRAVENOUS SOLUTION

Perform premedication assessments and follow procedure protocol. In addition, refer to the individual drug monographs.

EQUIPMENT

- Medication profile
- Prescriber's order
- IV solution ordered
- Administration set with appropriate needle or needleless connector, drip chamber, and filter
- Change label

TECHNIQUE FOR CHANGING IV SOLUTIONS

1. Monitor the rate of infusion and the IV insertion site at least once hourly. When the container nears completion, notify the nurse who is responsible for adding the next container.
2. Slow the rate to keep the vein open if the level of solution in the container is low.
3. Check the IV site, the dates on the IV lines, and the compatibility of the IV solution that is running with the new container of IV solution to be added. (Medications may have been added to the IV solution per the healthcare provider's orders.)
4. Perform hand hygiene.

5. Prepare the IV solution as described previously. Hang the new IV bag on the IV pole.
   - *If the same tubing is used,* clamp the tubing on the primary IV line. Using aseptic technique, quickly exchange the new container for the empty one.
   - *If new tubing is used,* attach the administration set to the solution container, fill the chamber on the IV line half full, prime the line to purge the air, and attach it to the venous access device. Date and initial the new tubing with the label that is used in the clinical practice setting. If a pump is used, prime the IV tubing, connect the tubing to the venous access device, and start the pump.
6. Unclamp the tubing and adjust the flow rate as previously described; inspect the venipuncture site.
7. Recheck all aspects of the IV order.

PATIENT TEACHING

Explain to the patient the purpose of the IV solution.

DOCUMENTATION

1. In the patient's MAR, document the date and time, the IV solution used, and the rate of administration.
2. Record the amount of fluid infused on the intake and output sheet, as well as on any flow sheets maintained at the clinical practice setting.
3. Record pertinent assessment data collected.

CARE OF PERIPHERAL SITES, CENTRAL VENOUS CATHETERS, AND IMPLANTED PORTS

- Gauze and transparent semipermeable membranes are the two types of dressing materials that are most frequently used for IV dressings. When using gauze dressings, always seal all of the edges with tape.
- Always label the dressing with the date, the time of the dressing change, the gauge and length of the catheter, and the name of the nurse who inserted the catheter or changed the dressing.
- Always stabilize the catheter when changing a dressing to prevent the movement of the catheter and irritation of the vein.

FLUSHING OF PERIPHERAL CATHETERS

See the section on General Principles of Intravenous Medication Administration for information about the SAS and SASH procedures, and consult the procedures used at the clinical practice setting.

PERIPHERAL SITE DRESSING CHANGES

The CDC recommends that venipuncture site dressings be changed when they become damp, loose, or soiled or whenever the venipuncture site is changed. Most clinical practice settings use this procedure for midline catheters as well.

EQUIPMENT

- Nonsterile gloves
- Dressing change kit
- Sterile gloves

TECHNIQUE FOR PERIPHERAL IV SITE DRESSING CHANGES

1. Gather the necessary supplies and check the healthcare provider's order and the clinical practice setting guidelines.
2. Identify the patient by checking his or her ID bracelet. Explain what is to be done. Have the patient state his or her name and birth date or two other identifiers.
3. Perform hand hygiene.
4. Put on unsterile gloves to remove and discard the existing dressing. Stabilize the catheter to minimize movement and irritation.
5. Remove gloves and perform hand hygiene again.
6. Open dressing change kit using sterile technique.
7. Apply sterile gloves.
8. Assess the IV insertion site and the surrounding tissues for redness, swelling, drainage, and warmth.
9. Maintaining sterile technique, cleanse the site with 70% alcohol swabs or chlorhexidine swabs (whatever is available in the kit). When using alcohol swabs, start at the insertion site and continue outward in concentric circles until an area approximately 6 inches in diameter is covered; when using chlorhexidine swabs, use a back-and-forth motion for 15 seconds over an area of about $2\frac{1}{2} \times 2\frac{1}{2}$ inches to cleanse the area. Allow the area to air-dry for 30 seconds.
10. Cover the site with transparent dressing or sterile gauze dressing in accordance with clinical practice setting guidelines. Affix a label to the site as appropriate, with the date and time, the catheter gauge and length, and the initials of the person performing the procedure.

PATIENT TEACHING

The patient and significant others should be taught the signs and symptoms of infection of an IV site (e.g., elevated temperature, redness, swelling, pain, drainage). If the patient is immunocompromised or receiving corticosteroids, analgesics, or antipyretics (e.g., acetaminophen), then his or her temperature may not be elevated or may only be minimally elevated.

DOCUMENTATION

1. Document the dressing change in the patient record and on any IV flow sheets maintained by the clinical practice setting. State the date, the time, and the name of the nurse who performed the procedure. The nurse should also record his or her observations of the peripheral site whenever the procedure is performed and at least once per shift daily.

2. If the IV access device was flushed, it should be documented on the flow sheet and on the patient's MAR.

FLUSHING OF CENTRAL VENOUS CATHETERS

EQUIPMENT

- Two 10-mL syringes with 0.9% NS, usually 5 to 10 mL; consult the institutional policy manual for the volume used in the facility
- One 10-mL syringe with heparin (10 units/mL), usually 2.5 to 5 mL; consult the institutional policy manual for the volume used in the facility
- Alcohol wipes

TECHNIQUE FOR FLUSHING A CAPPED CENTRAL VENOUS CATHETER

1. Gather the necessary equipment and check the healthcare provider's order.
2. Identify the patient by checking his or her ID bracelet. Explain what is to be done. Have the patient state his or her name and birth date or two other identifiers.
3. Perform hand hygiene and prepare the equipment. Check the condition of the insertion site, the dates on the insertion site, and all IV tubing in use.
4. Cleanse the injection cap with an alcohol wipe for 15 seconds and allow it to air-dry.
5. Eliminate all air from the syringes immediately before performing the SAS (for Groshong catheter) or SASH (for non-Groshong catheter) procedure (see under Monitoring Intravenous Therapy).
6. Insert the syringe into the center of the injection cap, release the clamp, aspirate a small amount of blood, and then inject the flush solution using a push-pause technique.
7. Repeat steps 4 through 6 until the SAS or SASH procedure of flushing is completed. Always close the clamp as the last 0.5 mL of solution is inserted into non-Groshong catheters to prevent backflow.
8. Check the injection cap to be sure that it is securely in place and then resume IV therapy as prescribed. Check the rate of any infusing IV solutions before leaving the area.

PATIENT TEACHING

During the flushing procedure, explain to the patient what is being done and why and offer him or her reassurance.

DOCUMENTATION

1. Document the condition of the insertion site and the dressing in the patient record. Record any IV tubing changes, if they are done at this time, on the IV flow sheets maintained by the institution.
2. Document the flushes used on the patient's MAR.
3. Document any problems with catheter function in the record and the measures taken to rectify the

problem. Always record any notification of the healthcare provider, additional orders obtained, and the patient's condition.

DRESSING CHANGES FOR CENTRAL LINES

Check individual institutional guidelines regarding the frequency of dressing changes. In general, gauze dressings on central venous access sites are changed every 48 hours and semipermeable transparent dressings are changed every 3 to 7 days. However, it should be emphasized that whenever the site dressing is loose or sterility is compromised, the dressing should be changed.

EQUIPMENT

- Dressing change kit
- Face masks
- Nonsterile gloves
- Sterile gloves
- Dressing materials: transparent or gauze, in accordance with institutional guidelines

TECHNIQUE FOR CENTRAL VENOUS CATHETER SITE DRESSING CHANGES

1. Gather the necessary supplies and check the healthcare provider's order and the institutional guidelines.
2. Identify the patient by checking his or her ID bracelet. Explain what is to be done. Have the patient state his or her name and birth date or two other identifiers.
3. Perform hand hygiene and put on the mask; offer a mask to the patient. (NOTE: Some institutions require that the patient also wear a mask during the central line dressing change.)
4. Put on the unsterile gloves to remove and discard the existing dressing; stabilize the catheter to minimize movement.
5. Assess the IV insertion site and the surrounding tissue for redness, swelling, drainage, and warmth.
6. Remove the unsterile gloves and perform hand hygiene again.
7. Open dressing change kit using sterile technique then put on the sterile gloves.
8. Maintaining sterile technique, cleanse the site with 70% alcohol swabs or chlorhexidine swabs (whatever is available in the kit). When using alcohol swabs, start at the proposed insertion site and continue outward in concentric circles until an area approximately 6 inches in diameter is covered; when using chlorhexidine swabs, use a back-and-forth motion for 15 seconds over an area of about $2\frac{1}{2} \times 2\frac{1}{2}$ inches to cleanse the area. Allow the area to air-dry for 30 seconds.
9. Cover the site with transparent dressing or sterile gauze dressing in accordance with institutional guidelines. Affix a label to the site as appropriate, with the date, the time, and the initials of the person performing the procedure.

PATIENT TEACHING

The patient and significant others should be taught the signs and symptoms of infection of the IV site (e.g., elevated temperature, redness, swelling, pain, drainage). If the patient is immunocompromised or receiving corticosteroids, analgesics, or antipyretics (e.g., acetaminophen), then his or her temperature may not be elevated or may only be minimally elevated.

DOCUMENTATION

1. Document the dressing change in the appropriate patient records. State the date, the time, and the name of the nurse who performed the procedure. The nurse should also record his or her observations of the peripheral site whenever the procedure is performed and at least once per shift daily.
2. If the IV access device was flushed, it should be documented on the flow sheet and on the patient's MAR.

CARE OF VENOUS PORTS

Generally, Huber infusion sets are changed every 7 days or when contaminated or not functioning. Check the IV flow sheet and the labeling on the dressing for the date of insertion of the Huber needle.

EQUIPMENT

- Appropriate dressing kit
- Noncoring Huber needle infusion set of the correct size and length. (NOTE: For flushing an arm port, a $\frac{1}{2}$- or $\frac{3}{4}$-inch Huber needle of 20 gauge or smaller is preferred.)
- SAS or SASH flushing equipment, depending on whether the catheter has a Groshong valve and on institutional policy; use a 10-mL or larger syringe for routine flushing and medication administration
- 2×2-inch gauze pads to support the Huber needle
- Tape
- Sharps safety container for used needle and receptacle for old dressing material that is removed
- Face masks for nurse and patient
- Sterile gloves

TECHNIQUE FOR IMPLANTED ASSESS DEVICE DRESSING CHANGE

1. Gather the necessary equipment and check the healthcare provider's order.
2. Identify the patient by checking his or her ID bracelet. Carefully explain what you plan to do. Have the patient state his or her name and birth date or two other identifiers.
3. The nurse and the patient should put on masks. (Explain to the patient that this is to keep microorganisms in the respiratory tract from depositing on the site.)

4. Maintain aseptic technique throughout the procedure.

5. Perform hand hygiene, put on sterile gloves, and palpate the port. Hold the port firmly in place with the thumb and middle finger to stabilize it as the dressing is removed. Remove the Huber infusion set and needle. Keep the needle in a straight line while pulling it upward; do not twist or bend it from side to side to prevent an inadvertent needle-stick or the causing of discomfort or a scratch to the patient as the needle is withdrawn.

6. Remove the sterile gloves and perform hand hygiene again.

7. Open the sterile dressing kit and prepare the flushing supplies.

8. Put on a new pair of sterile gloves.

9. Use the gloved dominant hand to handle the sterile supplies. Use the nondominant gloved hand for nonsterile supplies.

10. Attach an access or injection cap to the extension tubing and prime the infusion set with 0.9% NS (leave the saline syringe attached) while maintaining the sterility of the Huber infusion set.

11. Maintaining sterile technique, cleanse the site with 70% alcohol swabs or chlorhexidine swabs (whatever is available in the dressing kit). When using alcohol swabs, start at the insertion site and continue outward in concentric circles until an area approximately 6 inches in diameter is covered; when using chlorhexidine swabs, use a back-and-forth motion for 15 seconds over an area of about $2\frac{1}{2} \times 2\frac{1}{2}$ inches to cleanse the area. Allow the area to air-dry for 30 seconds.

12. Grasp the Huber needle firmly. Support the edges of the port as the Huber needle is inserted in a straight line through the skin into the septum until the needle reaches the bottom of the port reservoir. Support the Huber needle with folded 2 × 2-inch gauze sponges.

13. Aspirate to view a small amount of blood return.

14. Flush the port with 10 mL 0.9% NS in a 10-mL syringe; use the push-pause technique to create turbulence in the reservoir and then thoroughly flush the port. If the port is not going to be used immediately, flush it with 5 mL of heparin (100 units/mL) in a 10-mL syringe, or follow institutional policy. Anchor the Huber needle with sterile tape and 2 × 2-inch folded gauze pads to support the needle and to keep it from shifting.

15. Apply the transparent dressing.

16. Remove the gloves, anchor the edges of the dressings with tape, and then tape the infusion set to anchor it in place.

17. Fill out the label with the date, the time of access, the size and length of the Huber needle, and the initials of the nurse who performed the procedure.

18. Discard the used Huber needle in a sharps safety container and the dressing materials in the proper biohazard receptacle as established by institutional policy.

19. Perform hand hygiene.

PATIENT TEACHING

1. Explain throughout the procedure what is being done and why.

2. The patient and significant others should be taught the signs and symptoms of infection of an IV site (e.g., elevated temperature, redness, swelling, pain, drainage at the port site) and the actual catheter care procedures.

3. At the time of discharge, flush the port with saline and heparin. Have specific orders regarding the when, where, and who of the future care of the port. Stress the importance of keeping appointments to maintain port function.

DOCUMENTATION

1. Document the insertion and dressing change in the patient record and on any IV flow sheets maintained by the institution.

 Clinical Pitfalls

- The flushing of central lines is an important aspect of maintaining the patency of the central venous access device. Two types of solutions are used to maintain the patency of vascular access devices: heparin is used to prevent clot formation, and 0.9% NS is used to clean the interior diameter of the device of blood or particles of medication. It is recommended that a 10-mL syringe be used for flushing lines and medication administration to prevent excessive pressure within the catheter that could result in rupture. Always follow institutional guidelines for recommended procedures to maintain line patency.

- Preventing infection is a major concern with all IV devices. Appropriate procedures for cleansing the area and the access device with the recommended antiseptics are mandatory.

- If unable to aspirate blood when performing a flush procedure, the catheter may be occluded. Never force the solution into the IV line.
  - Start interventions by doing the simple things, like checking that the clamp is open and that the catheter and IV tubing are not kinked. Reposition the patient's upper body, and have the patient perform a Valsalva maneuver.
  - It may be necessary to remove the injection cap, attach a 20-mL syringe, and aspirate the blood clot. (Check institutional policy regarding the removal and replacement of the injection cap.) Immediately after the aspiration of the blood clot, replace the injection cap with a new sterile cap and institute 0.9% NS and heparin (100 units/mL) flushing of the catheter in accordance with institutional guidelines.

- Report any malfunctioning of the catheter to the healthcare provider. Radiographic evaluation and the instillation of a thrombolytic agent (e.g., urokinase) may be necessary.

2. Include the date, the time of access, the size and length of the Huber needle, and the initials of the nurse who performed the procedure. The nurse should also record any observations about the port site whenever the procedure is performed and at least once per shift daily.
3. Document the flushes used on the patient's MAR.
4. Document the dressing changes and the condition of the port site in the patient's MAR.

DISCONTINUING AN INTRAVENOUS INFUSION

EQUIPMENT

- Tourniquet (if used in the healthcare agency)
- Sterile sponges
- Gloves
- Dressing materials
- Tape
- Sharps safety container for needles and butterfly or other types of IV catheters
- Extension tubing with cap and a saline flush in a 10-mL syringe if the infusion device is being converted to a saline lock or a medlock

TECHNIQUE FOR REMOVING AN IV

If the IV site is being discontinued completely, the following should be done:

1. Review institutional policy regarding the placement of a tourniquet. (Some healthcare agencies state that a tourniquet should be applied before the removal of the needle or IV catheter in case the tip breaks during removal. Other agencies state that the tourniquet should be loosely attached to the limb but not tightened unless necessary.)
2. Check the healthcare provider's orders. Verify that all IV solutions and medications have been completed.
3. Check the patient's identity using his or her ID bracelet. Carefully explain what is being done and why. Have the patient state his or her name and birth date or two other identifiers.
4. Perform hand hygiene.
5. Adequately expose the IV site.
6. Clamp the IV tubing and turn off the electronic controller or pump.
7. Prepare a gauze sponge and tape for use on the venipuncture site.
8. Loosen the tape at the site while simultaneously stabilizing the needle to prevent venous damage. If the IV site is contaminated by blood or drainage, put on gloves before handling the tape.
9. Apply clean gloves.
10. With the use of a gauze pad, gently apply pressure with the nondominant hand to the venipuncture site. Withdraw the needle or catheter, pulling it out parallel to the skin surface. Inspect the tip of the needle or catheter to be sure that it is intact. Release the tourniquet, if one is in place. Place the needle or catheter in the sharps safety container.

11. Cleanse the area if it has been contaminated with any blood or fluid.
12. Continue to hold the IV site firmly until all bleeding ceases. If the venipuncture site was in the antecubital fossa, have the patient flex the elbow to hold the gauze in place.
13. Check for bleeding after 1 to 2 minutes. Remove the gauze, and discard it with other contaminated dressings. Cleanse the area as appropriate.
14. Remove and discard the gloves in accordance with institutional policy, and perform hand hygiene.
15. Apply a small dressing or adhesive bandage as stated by institutional policy.
16. Provide patient comfort.

If the IV site is to be converted to a saline lock when the large-volume solution is discontinued, the following should be done:

1. Perform steps 1 through 5 as described for discontinuing the IV site.
2. Prepare a saline flush, attach the syringe to the extension tubing, purge air from the tubing, and then clamp the extension tubing. Leave the syringe attached.
3. Clamp the tubing on the IV line, and then shut off the infusion equipment, if present.
4. Put on gloves and cleanse the connector site with antiseptic alcohol wipe. Let air-dry.
5. Stabilize the catheter hub while disconnecting the IV primary tubing and then quickly connect the extension tubing.
6. Unclamp the extension tubing and flush the catheter with saline in accordance with institutional policy; clamp the tubing as the last 0.5 mL is injected.
7. Tape the site securely and label and date the extension tubing.

DOCUMENTATION

Provide the right documentation of the termination of IV therapy.

1. Chart the date and time of the termination of the IV site or of the conversion to a saline lock.
2. Perform and record regular patient assessments (e.g., site data, size of site, color of skin at venipuncture site).
3. Chart and report any signs of adverse effects (e.g., redness, warmth, swelling, pain at venipuncture site).
4. Record the total amount infused on the intake and output record and on any flow sheets used in the clinical practice setting.
5. Record the saline flush on the patient's MAR.

MONITORING INTRAVENOUS THERAPY

Before initiating therapy, perform baseline patient assessments to evaluate the patient's current status. Report at appropriate intervals throughout the course of treatment.

Immediately after receiving a report regarding assigned patients, check the MAR or Kardex for IV medications and IV infusion orders for those patients. Make rounds to perform a baseline assessment. Data that should be gathered and analyzed with reference to IV therapy include the following:

- Check that the ordered IV solution (with or without medications) is being administered to the correct patient at the correct rate of infusion.
- Check the total amount infused against the amount that should have been infused. Is the volume of infused IV solution or IV medication "on target," "ahead," or "behind"?
- Calculate the drip rate to administer the medicine over the appropriate time interval. With a programmable infusion pump, ensure that the pump is set to deliver the prescribed volume (mL) per hour.
- Check for inline filters. If one is recommended for the medicine being infused, is it being used?
- Check the date and time that the infusing IV solution or IV medication was hung. Identify when the infusing IV solution, administration set and tubing, IV site, IV catheters, and dressings are to be changed in accordance with the policies of the clinical practice setting. The CDC recommends that venipuncture site dressings be changed when they become damp, loose, or soiled or whenever the venipuncture site is changed.
- Check the date and time that procedures are ordered to maintain the patency of the established IV lines. (Follow institutional policies.) The following are general guidelines:
  - Peripheral intermittent IV lines are usually flushed every 8 to 12 hours with the use of 1 to 2 mL of saline solution. Use positive pressure to prevent the backflow of blood and possible occlusion.
  - Central venous IV lines are usually flushed with a minimum of 10 mL of normal saline solution whenever they are irrigated. Use a push-pause method to irrigate (rather than continuous pressure). To prevent excessive pressure within the line, always use at least a syringe with a 10-mL capacity to irrigate and maintain the patency of a central line. Follow institutional policy for the use of saline and heparin solutions.
  - Groshong catheters have a two-way valve that prevents backflow; therefore these catheters do not require heparin. Groshong catheters are flushed with 5 mL of NS weekly or at an interval determined by institutional policy for lumens that are not in use. After medication administration or TPN infusion, flush with 10 mL of NS. After blood sample draws or blood product infusion, flush with 20 mL of sterile NS.
  - The amount of solution used to flush a Hickman, Broviac, or Groshong catheter varies and must be sufficient to equal two times the volume required to fill the catheter lumen plus the volume of any extension tubing that is being used.
  - Implantable vascular access ports (e.g., Port-A-Cath, Infus-A-Port) require that the port be filled with sterile heparinized solution, usually 100 units/mL, after each use. If the port is not accessed regularly, flushes may only be performed once each month or at an interval cited by institutional policy.
- Prevent damage to central venous catheters by clamping only the catheter with a padded hemostat or a smooth-edged clamp.
- Change the injection caps for lumen hubs on central venous catheters every 72 hours or as stated in the institutional policy.
- Check the IV tubing for any obstructions or air in the line. The patient and the venipuncture site should be checked at least every hour for flow rate, infiltration (e.g., tenderness, redness, puffiness), and adverse effects. Report and take immediate action if the infusion is infiltrated, if it is improperly infusing, or if signs of infection exist. If the flow rate is falling behind schedule, do the following:
  1. Check for mechanical obstruction of the tubing (e.g., closed clamp, kinking) or filter, and either irrigate or change the tubing.
  2. Check the drip chamber. If it is less than half full, squeeze it to fill it more completely. Do not overfill.
  3. Check to make sure that the IV container is not empty. Also, check to make sure that the container is more than 3 feet above the venipuncture site. The height may be inadvertently incorrect if the patient is repositioned or if the bed height is readjusted.
  4. Check for tubing that has fallen below the venipuncture site. If a significant length has fallen, elevate and carefully coil the tubing near the site of the venipuncture.
- Wear gloves to inspect the IV site. Check the transparent dressing for the date that the infusion device was started. Palpate gently around the catheter or needle for edema, coolness, or pain, which indicate infiltration. Check for any signs of redness or heat, which indicate that an inflammatory process is occurring.
- Check to determine whether the bevel of the needle is pushing against the wall of the vein. Do this by *cautiously* raising or lowering the angle of the needle slightly to see if flow is restored. If so, reposition the needle slightly with the use of a gauze pad in the most appropriate location.
- Check the temperature of the solution that is being infused. Cold solutions can cause spasms in the vein.
- Check to ensure that a restraint or blood pressure cuff applied to the arm has not interfered with the flow.

- If it appears that the IV access device is clotted, *do not* attempt to clear the needle by flushing it with fluid. This will dislodge the clot, which may cause a thromboembolism. The aspiration of the needle or catheter with a syringe to dislodge the clot is no longer recommended; rather, the site should be discontinued and the IV infusion restarted.
- Remain alert at all times for complications associated with IV therapy of any type (e.g., phlebitis, infection, air in the tubing, circulatory overload, pulmonary edema, pulmonary embolism, drug reactions from the IV medications).
- Document all findings and procedures performed in association with IV therapy.
- During shift report, identify the exact volume of IV solution or medication that has been infused on the current shift and the volume remaining to be infused during the next shift. In addition, report any IV sites that are functioning poorly or IV lines that require frequent site changes.

COMPLICATIONS ASSOCIATED WITH INTRAVENOUS THERAPY

Complications that can occur with IV therapy include phlebitis, thrombophlebitis, localized infection, septicemia, infiltration, extravasation, air in the tubing, air embolism, circulatory overload, pulmonary edema, catheter embolism, and "speed shock."

Phlebitis, Thrombophlebitis, and Localized Infection

Phlebitis is the inflammation of a vein; thrombophlebitis is the inflammation of a vein with the formation of a thrombus in the area of inflammation. The three primary causes of phlebitis are as follows:

1. Irritation of the vein by the catheter (e.g., catheter that is too large for the vein, improper insertion, improper anchoring with excessive movement of the catheter).
2. Chemical irritation from medicines (e.g., solution infused too rapidly or at a volume that was too large for the vein, solution is irritating to the vein).
3. Infection caused by improper aseptic technique during accessing or dressing changes, or from long-term catheter placement.

If signs of redness (erythema), warmth, tenderness, swelling, and burning pain along the course of the vein are present, phlebitis or thrombophlebitis and infection may be developing (Table 11.2). Confirm the presence of these signs with the supervising nurse. The treatment of phlebitis depends on the cause of venous irritation. If the IV line is peripheral and there is evidence of infiltration using the Infiltration Scale (Table 11.3), then the IV catheter is discontinued and a new IV line using all new equipment is inserted at a different location. For people with any type of midline catheter (e.g., PICC), the healthcare provider should be notified. Not all midline catheters are removed when infection occurs;

Table 11.2	Assessing the Severity of Phlebitis
SCORE	**DESCRIPTORS**
0	No clinical symptoms
1	Erythema at access site, with or without pain
2	Pain at the access site with erythema and/or edema
3	Pain at the access site with erythema, streak formation, and/or palpable venous cord ±1 inch long
4	Pain at the access site with erythema, streak formation, palpable venous cord >1 inch long, and/or purulent drainage

From Infusion Nurses Society. Infusion nursing standards of practice. *J Infus Nurs.* 2016, S45.

Table 11.3	Infiltration Scale
GRADE	**CLINICAL CRITERIA**
0	No symptoms
1	Skin blanched Edema <1 inch in any direction Cool to touch With or without pain
2	Skin blanched Edema 1-6 inches in any direction Cool to touch With or without pain
3	Skin blanched, translucent Gross edema >6 inches in any direction Cool to touch Mild to moderate pain Possible numbness
4	Skin blanched, translucent Skin tight, leaking Skin discolored, bruised, swollen Gross edema >6 inches in any direction Deep pitting tissue edema Circulatory impairment Moderate to severe pain Infiltration of any amount of blood product, irritant, or vesicant

From Infusion Nurses Society. Infusion nursing standards of practice. *J Infus Nurs.* 2016, S46.

some may be treated with antibiotic therapy. Many institutions also require that the infection control nurse be notified. If purulent drainage is present, a sample of the drainage is obtained for culture and sensitivity. If a fever and chills (e.g., signs of septicemia) accompany these symptoms, cultures of the patient's blood and the catheter tip may also be indicated. Check institutional policies regarding whether a healthcare provider's order is necessary to do this or whether standing orders exist as part of infection control procedures. Generally, follow-up treatment includes elevation and the application of warm, moist compresses to the site. Document the findings, the treatment that is administered, and the results of ongoing assessments.

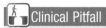
Septicemia

When pathogens that are associated with a local infection invade the bloodstream, are carried to other parts of the body, and trigger an inflammatory response (e.g., fever, chills), the infection is no longer local; it is now systemic, and this condition is called septicemia. People who already have an infection or who are immunocompromised are at higher risk for the development of septicemia. The importance of maintaining aseptic technique throughout all aspects of catheter insertion and maintenance care cannot be overemphasized. The potential for contamination exists during every aspect of IV therapy, starting at the time of the manufacture and packaging of IV fluids and equipment and continuing throughout the actual preparation and administration of the IV therapy. The risk of septicemia also increases with the frequency with which the catheter and site are manipulated and with how long an IV catheter remains in place. Perform catheter site inspections in accordance with institutional policy. Suspect localized infection at the catheter site if redness, edema, or purulent drainage is present at the entry site or if the patient has an elevated temperature or an elevated white blood cell count. Keep in mind that immunocompromised patients or those who are receiving an antipyretic (e.g., acetaminophen, ibuprofen) may not develop a fever.

Suspect septicemia if the patient develops the following: a sudden onset of flushing, fever, chills, general malaise, headache, nausea, vomiting, hypotension, shock, or a weak, rapid pulse. Obtain the patient's vital signs and notify the healthcare provider immediately of all findings. Obtain the healthcare provider's orders, which will usually include blood cultures, the discontinuation of the IV catheter, and antibiotic therapy after cultures are obtained. Return the unused portion of the IV solution to the pharmacy or laboratory for testing as specified by institutional policy.

Document the findings, the treatment administered, and the ongoing assessments.

Infiltration and Extravasation

Infiltration is the leakage of an IV solution into the tissue that surrounds the vein; extravasation is the leakage of an irritant chemical (e.g., the medicine being infused) into the tissue that surrounds the vein. Infiltration or extravasation may be accompanied by redness and warmth, coolness and blanching of the skin, swelling, and a dull ache to a severe pain at the venipuncture site (see Table 11.3). Infiltration or extravasation occurs most commonly when a needle tip punctures the vein and the IV solution leaks into the tissue that surrounds the vein. Serious tissue damage may occur, particularly if the medicine in the solution is irritating to the tissue

(e.g., a calcium salt) or causes vasoconstriction (e.g., levarterenol) to the vasculature in the area.

The nurse should always educate the patient regarding the signs and symptoms of these conditions so that the patient can report early discomfort and thus early interventions can be initiated in the event that infiltration or extravasation does occur.

Inspect the IV site at regular intervals for infiltration. Whenever a change in the limb's color, size, or skin integrity is observed, make a comparison with the opposite limb. General guidelines are as follows:

- For infiltration, stop the infusion and elevate the affected limb. Assess for circulatory compromise: check capillary refill and pulses proximal and distal to the area of infiltration. If the infiltration is caused by an IV solution, remove the catheter as directed by policy and as described earlier. Whether cold or heat is applied to the site depends on the specific type of IV solution and the type of medication that has infiltrated. Consult institutional guidelines and describe the patient's condition using the infiltration scale (see Table 11.3).
- For extravasation, the protocol will call for the IV infusion to be stopped, but the catheter is left in place. With authorization from the healthcare provider, attempts may be made to aspirate the medication, with orders that an antidote may be injected or infused to minimize tissue damage. Elevate the extremity. Apply ice (per institutional policy) rather than heat for 24 hours, except for treatment of vincristine or vinblastine extravasation, which requires heat rather than cold. Document the condition on the patient's chart as 4+ infiltration, and describe the visual appearance and measurements of the size of the site where extravasation has occurred. Photographs of the site may be part of the protocol. After the protocol for extravasation is complete, restart the IV solution at a new site proximal to the area of extravasation.
- Document the findings, the treatment administered, and the ongoing assessments.

Air in the Tubing or Air Embolus

If an air bubble is found in the IV tubing, clamp the tubing immediately. Swab the injection site in the rubber hub near the needle or the piggyback portal—whichever is closer to the air bubble—with an alcohol wipe. Using sterile technique, insert a needleless access device on a syringe into the portal below the air bubble, and withdraw the air pocket.

Air embolism occurs as a result of an air bubble entering the cardiovascular system. Symptoms of an air embolism may include patient complaints of palpitations, chest pain, shortness of breath, cyanosis, hypotension, and a weak, thready pulse. If air has actually entered the patient via the IV tubing, turn the patient onto his or her left side with the head in a dependent position. Administer oxygen and notify the healthcare provider immediately. Monitor vital signs. Be prepared for possible orders to draw arterial blood gases and for ventilatory support, if necessary. Air emboli can be prevented by clamping catheters when they are not in use, instructing the patient to perform the Valsalva maneuver during tubing and injection cap changes, using proper inline filters, not allowing IV containers to run dry, and removing all air from tubing or syringes before connecting them to an IV access device. Always purge the flush or medication syringe of air before attachment and injection.

Document the findings, the treatment administered, and the ongoing assessments.

Circulatory Overload and Pulmonary Edema

Circulatory overload that leads to pulmonary edema is caused by infusing fluid too rapidly or by giving too much fluid, particularly to older adults, infants, or patients with cardiovascular disease. Signs of circulatory overload are engorged neck veins, dyspnea, reduced urine output, edema, bounding pulse, and shallow, rapid respirations. The signs of pulmonary edema are dyspnea, cough, anxiety, coarse crackles, possible cardiac dysrhythmias, thready pulse, elevation or drop in blood pressure (depending on severity), and frothy sputum. When these symptoms develop, slow the IV infusion immediately to a TKO rate. Place the patient in a high Fowler's position, start oxygen, obtain vital signs, and summon the healthcare provider immediately. During severe respiratory distress, the patient may require intubation and a mechanical ventilator to improve oxygen delivery. Anticipate the healthcare provider's orders for medications such as diuretics, vasodilators, and morphine sulfate.

Document the findings, the treatment administered, and the ongoing assessments.

Pulmonary Embolism

A pulmonary embolism may occur as a result of foreign materials being injected into the vein or from a blood clot that breaks loose and travels to the lungs, where it lodges in the arterioles. Symptoms include the sudden onset of apprehension and dyspnea, pleuritic pain, sweating, tachycardia, cough, unexplained hemoptysis, low-grade fever, and cyanosis. When this condition is suspected, immediately place the patient in a semi-Fowler's position, administer oxygen, obtain vital signs, and notify the healthcare provider. Anticipate orders for the drawing of blood for arterial blood gases, performing a lung scan to verify the presence of the pulmonary embolism, and determining the baseline prothrombin time before initiating anticoagulant therapy.

Foreign-particle emboli can be prevented by using an inline filter, using proper diluents for reconstitution, ensuring the complete dissolution of any medications that are added to a solution, and ensuring that there are no visible signs of foreign matter in IV solutions.

Thromboemboli can be avoided by not using the veins in the lower extremities in adults and by using a 10-mL syringe when flushing all central lines. A 10-mL syringe decreases the pressure that is exerted within the vascular system. (The smaller the syringe, the greater the pressure exerted.) When flushing a catheter, never force the flush solution because this may dislodge a clot.

Document the findings, the treatment administered, and the ongoing assessments.

"Speed Shock"

"Speed shock" occurs as a systemic reaction to a foreign substance that is given too rapidly into the bloodstream. This can occur when an IV drug is administered too rapidly into the circulation, most commonly by IV push. The rapid delivery of the IV drug creates a concentrated plasma level in the patient that may result in shock, syncope, and cardiac arrest. Different resources (e.g., *AHFS Drug Information, Physicians' Desk Reference*) and package inserts that accompany medications state the recommended rate of injection or flow rate to prevent complications that may result from a rapid infusion rate. The nurse needs to time the administration of an IV push medication by observing the infusion time on a clock or watch directly. The nurse also needs to frequently check the flow rate of IV infusions, use infusion control devices, and resist speeding up medications or IV rates when therapy is behind schedule. Assess the patient before initiating an IV drug to obtain baseline data (e.g., vital signs), and continue monitoring during IV therapy for dizziness; flushing; tightness in the chest; rapid, irregular pulse; hypotension; and anaphylactic shock. When speed shock is suspected, immediately stop the infusion, maintain IV patency at a TKO rate, obtain the patient's vital signs, and notify the healthcare provider. Anticipate the treatment of shock by checking institutional policy.

PATIENT TEACHING

Always teach the patient and his or her significant others about the signs and symptoms of complications that should be reported immediately to the healthcare provider. Depending on the type of IV delivery system that is used to administer the medication, instruct those being treated on an outpatient basis or in a home health setting when to return for the catheter to be changed and when to return for the next visit to the healthcare provider or clinic.

DOCUMENTATION

Provide the right documentation of the medication administration, the patient's responses to drug therapy, and any complications of or untoward reactions to the prescribed therapy.
1. Chart the date and time, the drug name and dosage, and the route of administration.
2. Perform and record regular patient assessments for the evaluation of therapeutic effectiveness (e.g., blood

pressure, pulse, intake and output, lung field sounds, respiratory rate, pain at infusion site).

3. Perform regular assessments of the patient and the IV access sites for complications associated with IV therapy or the administration of IV drug therapy.

4. Chart and report any signs and symptoms of adverse drug effects related to therapy. Notify the healthcare provider of any complications.

5. Chart any dressing changes performed and record any signs and symptoms of complications at the insertion site (e.g., redness, tenderness, swelling, drainage).

6. Chart any difficulty with irrigation of any venous access device and notify the healthcare provider as appropriate.

7. Chart the dates and times that procedures are performed to maintain the patency of the IV site, needle, peripheral or midline catheter, central venous catheter, or port (e.g., heparinized flush; saline flush for a Groshong catheter).

8. Perform and validate essential patient education regarding the drug therapy and other essential aspects of intervention for the disease process that is affecting the individual.

9. Perform and validate essential patient education regarding the drug therapy, site or central venous catheter care, dressing care, and the flushing of the IV system that is being used to administer medication.

Get Ready for the NCLEX® Examination!

Key Points

- Intravenous therapy involves the administration of fluids and medications directly into the bloodstream. The three intravascular compartments are veins, arteries, and capillaries. The three fluid compartments are intracellular spaces, intravascular spaces (e.g., arteries, veins, and capillaries), and interstitial spaces.
- Intravenous access devices include peripheral IV lines, central catheters, and implantable infusion ports.
- Intravenous solutions that are hypotonic are used for dehydration, isotonic solutions are used to maintain hydration, and hypertonic solutions may be used to draw fluid into the intravascular compartment to support blood pressure and promote diuresis.
- Principles of IV administration include:
  - Review the chart to determine the medical and nursing diagnosis, the patient's history and allergies, and the significant presenting symptoms.
  - Review the assessment of the patient's baseline data, current vital signs, laboratory and diagnostic data, and type and use of any IV access. After the IV site is established, the IV solution or blood product is hung, or an IV medication is administered, an ongoing assessment is required to monitor the patient's condition, the IV site, and response to the IV therapy that is being delivered.
- Patient education needs to be implemented. All aspects of the patient's care needs must be explained to the patient and his or her family. In addition, community resources must be arranged to assist with home infusion therapy.
- Complications of IV therapy include phlebitis, thrombophlebitis, localized infection, septicemia, infiltration, extravasation, air in the tubing, air embolism, circulatory overload, pulmonary edema, catheter embolism, and "speed shock."

Additional Learning Resources

SG Go to your Study Guide for additional Review Questions for the NCLEX® Examination, Critical Thinking Clinical Situations, and other learning activities to help you master this chapter content.

Go to your Evolve website (https://evolve.elsevier.com/Clayton) for additional online resources.

Review Questions for the NCLEX® Examination

1. When determining the patency of an IV access device, the nurse recognizes that the fluid runs into an area known as what?
   1. The interstitial compartment
   2. The intracellular compartment
   3. The extracellular compartment
   4. The intravascular compartment

2. A nurse is starting a peripheral IV line for the first time in an extremity of an elderly patient and knows which is the best site for an IV line?
   1. Near the antecubital space
   2. In the biggest vein that is visible
   3. In the dominant hand
   4. In the metacarpal vein, if it is large enough

3. The nurse notified the healthcare provider that a patient had signs of peripheral dehydration. Which type of IV solution would be anticipated to be ordered for this condition?
   1. Isotonic
   2. Hypertonic
   3. Hypotonic
   4. Piggyback

4. After changing a primary IV bag, the nurse finds that it will not run. What does the nurse check for first?
   1. Type of IV solution hung
   2. Clamps not being released
   3. Height of container
   4. Piggyback or rider set needed

5. A patient's skin at the site of a running peripheral IV line appears swollen and feels cool, and the patient reports discomfort. What does the nurse do next?
   1. Flushes the site with saline
   2. Instructs the patient to perform the Valsalva maneuver
   3. Applies warm compresses to the area
   4. Discontinues the IV infusion

6. The technique used to flush central lines is known as what?
   1. The ASA technique
   2. The SAS technique
   3. The SASH technique
   4. The SHAS technique

7. To minimize the risk of air embolism with IV therapy, the nurse should routinely do which of the following? *(Select all that apply.)*
   1. Cap off the IV catheter when not in use.
   2. Instruct the patient to perform the Valsalva maneuver during tubing and injection cap changes.
   3. Always use proper inline filters.
   4. Allow IV containers to run dry to ensure all fluid/medication is given.
   5. Remove all air from tubing or syringes before connecting to an IV access device.

8. When inserting a Huber needle into a port, what is the next step the nurse takes?
   1. Cover the site with a clean pad.
   2. Use clean technique throughout the procedure.
   3. Wear latex examination gloves.
   4. Put on a mask and use sterile technique with gloves and supplies.

9. The nurse knows to watch for which of the following signs and symptoms of phlebitis in an IV site? *(Select all that apply.)*
   1. Redness over insertion site
   2. Sudden onset of flushed skin
   3. A weak, rapid pulse
   4. Fluid leaking around the IV site
   5. Swollen, puffy area around the IV site

10. The nurse has completed the administration of an IV injection of furosemide (Lasix) and will document this on the MAR by including what? *(Select all that apply.)*
    1. The time of administration
    2. The date of administration
    3. The drug administered
    4. The dosage administered
    5. The IV site used

Drugs Affecting the Autonomic Nervous System

12

https://evolve.elsevier.com/Clayton

Objectives

1. Describe how the central nervous system differs from the peripheral nervous system.
2. Name the most common neurotransmitters known to affect central nervous system function and identify the two major neurotransmitters of the autonomic nervous system.
3. Explain how drugs inhibit the actions of cholinergic and adrenergic fibers.
4. Identify two broad classes of drugs used to stimulate the adrenergic nervous system.
5. Review the actions of adrenergic agents and the conditions that require the use of these drugs.
6. Describe the benefits of using beta-adrenergic blocking agents for hypertension, angina pectoris, cardiac dysrhythmias, and hyperthyroidism.
7. Identify diseases in which beta-adrenergic blocking agents should not be used, and discuss why they should not be used.
8. Describe clinical uses and the predictable adverse effects of cholinergic agents and anticholinergic agents.

Key Terms

central nervous system (SĔN-trŭl NŬR-vŭs SĬS-tĕm) (p. 177)
peripheral nervous system (pĕ-RĬF-ĕr-ăl) (p. 177)
afferent nerves (ĂF-ĕ-rĕnt NŬRVZ) (p. 177)
efferent nerves (ĔF-ĕ-rĕnt) (p. 177)
autonomic nervous system (ŏ-tō-NŎM-ĭk) (p. 177)
neurons (NYŪR-ŏn) (p. 178)
synapse (SĬN-ăps) (p. 178)
neurotransmitters (nyŭr-ō-TRĂNZ-mĭ-tŭrz) (p. 178)
receptors (rē-SĔP-tŭrz) (p. 178)
norepinephrine (nōr-ĕp-ĭ-NĔF-rĭn) (p. 178)
acetylcholine (ăs-ē-tĭl-KŌ-lēn) (p. 178)
cholinergic fibers (kō-lĭn-ŬR-jĭk FĪ-bŭrz) (p. 178)

adrenergic fibers (ăd-rĭn-ŬR-jĭk) (p. 178)
cholinergic agents (kō-lĭn-ŬR-jĭk Ā-jĕnts) (p. 178)
adrenergic agents (ăd-rĭn-ŬR-jĭk) (p. 178)
anticholinergic agents (ăn-tē-kō-lĭn-ŬR-jĭk) (p. 178)
adrenergic blocking agents (ăd-rĭn-ŬR-jĭk BLŎ-kĭng Ā-jĕnts) (p. 178)
catecholamines (kăt-ĕ-KŌL-ă-mēnz) (p. 178)
alpha receptors (ĂL-fă rē-SĔP-tŭrz) (p. 178)
beta receptors (BĀ-tă rē-SĔP-tŭrz) (p. 178)
dopaminergic receptors (dō-pă-mĭn-ŬR-jĭk rē-SĔP-tŭrz) (p. 178)

THE CENTRAL AND AUTONOMIC NERVOUS SYSTEMS

The control of the human body as a living organism comes primarily from two major systems: the nervous system and the endocrine system. In general, the endocrine system controls the body's metabolism. The nervous system regulates the body's ongoing activities (e.g., heart and respiratory muscle contractions), its rapid response to sudden changes in the environment (e.g., skeletal muscles contracting to help an individual to avoid danger), and the rates of secretion of some glands.

The nervous system is composed of the **central nervous system** (CNS), which is made up of the brain and the spinal cord, and the **peripheral nervous system**, which includes the peripheral nerves subdivided into the afferent and efferent nerves. The **afferent (peripheral) nerves** conduct signals from sensory receptors (e.g., vision, pressure, pain, cold, warmth, touch, smell) throughout the body to the CNS. The CNS processes these signals and controls the body's response by sending signals back through the **efferent nerves** of the peripheral nervous system. The peripheral nervous system is further subdivided into the somatic nervous system, which controls voluntary movement (e.g., skeletal muscle contractions), and the **autonomic nervous system**, which, as suggested by the name, works automatically and is not under voluntary control.

Each nerve of the central and peripheral nervous systems is actually composed of a series of segments called *neurons*. The junction between one neuron and the next is called a *synapse*. The transmission of nerve signals or impulses occurs because of the activity of chemical substances called *neurotransmitters* (e.g., transmitters of nerve impulses). A neurotransmitter is released into the synapse at the end of one neuron, thereby activating **receptors** on the next neuron in the chain or, at the end of the nerve chain, stimulating receptors on the end organ (e.g., the heart, smooth muscle, or gland). Neurotransmitters can be excitatory, which means that they stimulate the next neuron, or inhibitory, which means that they inhibit electrical impulses through the neuron. Because a single neuron releases only one type of neurotransmitter, the CNS is composed of different types of neurons that secrete separate neurotransmitters. Research indicates that there are more than 30 different types of neurotransmitters; the more common ones throughout the CNS are acetylcholine, norepinephrine, epinephrine, dopamine, glycine, gamma-aminobutyric acid, and glutamic acid. Substance P and the enkephalins and endorphins regulate the sensation of pain, and serotonin and dopamine regulate mood. Other neurotransmitters include prostaglandins, histamine, cyclic adenosine monophosphate, amino acids, and peptides. Neurotransmitter regulation by pharmacologic agents (e.g., medicines) is a major mechanism that allows for the control of disease processes caused by an excess or deficiency of these neurotransmitters. The use of inhibitory and excitatory neurotransmitters to control illnesses is explained in the rest of the chapters in this unit.

THE AUTONOMIC NERVOUS SYSTEM

With the exception of skeletal muscle, the autonomic nervous system controls most tissue function. This nervous system helps to control blood pressure, gastrointestinal (GI) secretion and motility, urinary bladder function, sweating, and body temperature. In general, it maintains a constant internal environment (homeostasis) and responds to emergency situations.

There are two main branches of the autonomic nervous system: the sympathetic branch and the parasympathetic branch. The sympathetic and parasympathetic branches typically function in opposition with each other. However, this can be considered complementary in nature rather than antagonistic. The sympathetic branch speeds up normal processes, and the parasympathetic branch slows down these processes. The sympathetic division typically functions in actions that require quick responses during the "fight-or-flight" response. The parasympathetic division functions as part of actions that do not require immediate reaction during the "rest-and-digest" response.

The two major neurotransmitters of the autonomic nervous system are **norepinephrine** and **acetylcholine**. The nerve endings that liberate acetylcholine are called *cholinergic fibers*; those that secrete norepinephrine are called *adrenergic fibers*. Most organs are innervated by both adrenergic and cholinergic fibers, but these fibers produce opposite responses. For example, in the heart, the stimulation of adrenergic fibers increases the heart rate, and the stimulation of cholinergic fibers slows the heart rate; in the eyes, the stimulation of adrenergic fibers causes pupillary dilation, and the stimulation of cholinergic fibers causes pupillary constriction (Table 12.1).

Medications that cause effects in the body similar to those produced by acetylcholine are called *cholinergic agents* or *parasympathomimetic agents,* because they mimic the action produced by the stimulation of the parasympathetic division of the autonomic nervous system. Medications that cause effects similar to those produced by the adrenergic neurotransmitter are called *adrenergic agents* or *sympathomimetic agents.* Agents that block or inhibit cholinergic activity are called *anticholinergic agents*, and those that inhibit the adrenergic system are referred to as *adrenergic blocking agents*. Fig. 12.1 presents a diagram of the autonomic nervous system and its representative stimulants and inhibitors.

DRUG CLASS: ADRENERGIC AGENTS

Actions

The adrenergic nervous system may be stimulated by two broad classes of drugs: **catecholamines** and noncatecholamines. The body's naturally occurring neurotransmitter catecholamines are norepinephrine, epinephrine, and dopamine. Norepinephrine is secreted primarily from nerve terminals, epinephrine comes primarily from the adrenal medulla, and dopamine is found at selected sites in the brain, the kidneys, and the GI tract. All three agents are also synthetically manufactured and may be administered to produce the same effects as those that are naturally secreted. Noncatecholamines have actions that are somewhat similar to those of the catecholamines; however, they are more selective for certain types of receptors, they are not quite as fast acting, and they have a longer duration of action.

As illustrated in Fig. 12.1, the adrenergic side of the autonomic nervous system can be subdivided into the **alpha receptors, beta receptors,** and **dopaminergic receptors**. In general, the stimulation of the alpha-1 receptors causes the vasoconstriction of blood vessels. The alpha-2 receptors appear to serve as mediators of negative feedback, thereby preventing the further release of norepinephrine. Stimulation of beta-1 receptors causes an increase in the heart rate, and stimulation of beta-2 receptors causes the relaxation of smooth muscle in the bronchi (bronchodilation), the uterus (relaxation), and the peripheral arterial blood vessels (vasodilation). Stimulation of the dopaminergic receptors in the brain improves the symptoms associated with Parkinson's disease. Dopamine also increases urine output as a result of the stimulation of specific receptors in the kidneys that results in better renal perfusion.

Table 12.1 Actions of Autonomic Nerve Impulses on Specific Tissues

TISSUE	RECEPTOR TYPE	ADRENERGIC RECEPTORS (SYMPATHETIC)	CHOLINERGIC RECEPTORS (PARASYMPATHETIC)
Blood Vessels			
Arterioles			
Coronary	α; β_2	Constriction; dilation	Dilation
Skin	α	Constriction	Dilation
Renal	α_1; β_1 and β_2	Constriction; dilation	—
Skeletal muscle	α; β_2	Constriction; dilation	Dilation
Veins (systemic)	α_1; β_2	Constriction; dilation	—
Eye			
Radial muscle, iris	α_1	Contraction (mydriasis)	—
Sphincter muscle, iris	—	—	Contraction (miosis)
Ciliary muscle	β	Relaxation for far vision	Contraction for near vision
Gastrointestinal Tract			
Smooth muscle	α; β_1 and β_2	Relaxation	Contraction
Sphincters	α	Contraction	Relaxation
Heart	β_1	Increased heart rate, force of contraction	Decreased heart rate
Kidney	Dopamine	Dilates renal vasculature, thereby increasing renal perfusion	—
Lung			
Bronchial muscle	β_2	Smooth muscle relaxation (opens airways)	Smooth muscle contraction (closes airways)
Bronchial glands	α_1; β_2	Decreased secretions; increased secretions	Stimulation
Metabolism	β_2	Glycogenolysis (increases blood glucose)	—
Urinary Bladder			
Fundus (detrusor)	β_3	Relaxation	Contraction
Trigone and sphincter	α	Contraction	Relaxation
Uterus	α; β_2	Pregnancy: contraction (α); relaxation (β_2)	Variable

α, Alpha receptor; α_1, alpha-1 receptor; β, beta receptor; β_1, beta-1 receptor; β_2, beta-2 receptor; β_3, beta-3 receptor.

Uses

As noted in Table 12.2, many drugs act on more than one type of adrenergic receptor. Fortunately, each agent can be used for a specific purpose without many adverse effects. If recommended doses are exceeded, however, certain receptors may be stimulated excessively, which can cause serious adverse effects. An example of this is terbutaline, which is primarily a beta stimulant. With normal doses, terbutaline is an effective bronchodilator. However, in addition to bronchodilation, higher doses of terbutaline cause CNS stimulation, which results in insomnia and wakefulness. See Table 12.2 for a list of the clinical uses of the adrenergic agents.

❖ Nursing Implications for Adrenergic Agents

See Chapters 29 and 30 for more information about the nursing implications for respiratory tract disease, bronchodilators, and decongestants.

◆ Premedication assessment

1. Obtain baseline vital signs: heart rate and blood pressure.

2. See Chapters 29 and 30 for the premedication assessments for respiratory tract disease, bronchodilators, and decongestants.

◆ Availability

See Table 12.2.

◆ Common adverse effects.

Adverse effects associated with adrenergic agents are usually dose related and resolve when the dosage is reduced or the medication discontinued. Patients who are potentially more sensitive to adrenergic agents are those with impaired hepatic function, thyroid disease, hypertension, and heart disease. Patients with diabetes mellitus may also have an increased frequency of episodes of hyperglycemia.

Cardiovascular

Palpitations, tachycardia, skin flushing, dizziness, tremors. These adverse effects are usually mild, and they tend to resolve with continued therapy. Encourage the patient not to discontinue therapy without first consulting the healthcare provider.

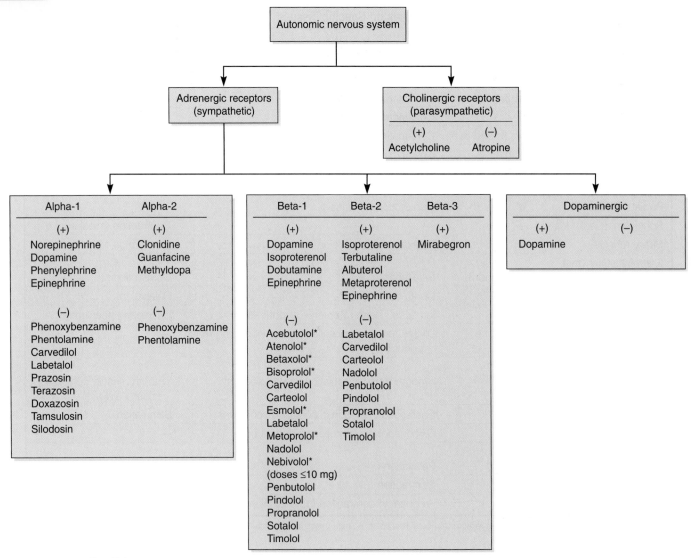

Fig. 12.1 Receptors of the autonomic nervous system. (+) Stimulates receptors; (−) inhibits receptors; asterisks (*) indicate selective beta-1 antagonists.

Orthostatic hypotension. Although this condition is infrequent and generally mild, adrenergic agents may cause some degree of orthostatic hypotension, which is manifested by dizziness and weakness, particularly when therapy is initiated. Monitor the blood pressure daily with the patient in both the supine and standing positions. Anticipate the development of postural hypotension, and take measures to prevent an occurrence. Teach the patient to rise slowly from a supine or sitting position; encourage the patient to sit or lie down if he or she feels faint.

◆ **Serious adverse effects**

Cardiovascular

Dysrhythmias, chest pain, severe hypotension, hypertension, anginal pain. Discontinue therapy immediately and notify the healthcare provider. Ask the patient if there has been a recent change in his or her regimen of prescription, nonprescription, or herbal medicines.

Gastrointestinal

Nausea, vomiting. Notify the healthcare provider. Ask the patient if there has been a recent change in his or her regimen of prescription, nonprescription, or herbal medicines.

◆ **Drug interactions**

Agents that may increase therapeutic and toxic effects. Monoamine oxidase inhibitors (e.g., phenelzine, tranylcypromine), tricyclic antidepressants (e.g., amitriptyline, imipramine), atropine, and halothane anesthesia may increase both therapeutic and toxic effects. Many over-the-counter medications (e.g., cold remedies, appetite suppressants/diet pills [e.g., pseudoephedrine, ephedrine, ma huang]) contain adrenergic medicines that can have an additive effect when they are taken with a prescribed adrenergic agent. Monitor patients for tachycardia, serious dysrhythmias, hypotension, hypertension, and chest pain.

Table 12.2   Adrenergic Agents

GENERIC NAME	BRAND NAME	AVAILABILITY	ADRENERGIC RECEPTOR	ACTION	CLINICAL USES
albuterol[a]	Proventil HFA, Ventolin HFA, ProAir HFA, ProAir RespiClick	Aerosol: 90 mcg/puff Tablets: 2, 4 mg Syrup: 2 mg/5 mL Tablets, extended release: 4, 8 mg Nebulizer solution: 0.083%/3-mL ampule, 0.5%/0.5-mL ampule and 20-mL bottle; 0.63-mg/3-mL ampule, 1.25-mg/3-mL ampule	β_2	Bronchodilator	Asthma, emphysema
arformoterol[a]	Brovana	Nebulizer: 15 mcg/2 mL in 2-mL vials	β_2	Bronchodilator	Emphysema, chronic bronchitis
dobutamine ⊕	—	IV: 1 mg/mL (250 mL); 2 mg/mL (250 mL); 4 mg/mL (250 mL); 12.5 mg/mL in 250-mg/20-mL vial; 500-mg/40-mL vial	β_1	Cardiac stimulant	Inotropic agent
dopamine ⊕	—	IV: 40, 80, 160 mg/mL in 5-, 10-mL ampules; 200, 400, and 800 mg in D5W (various volumes available)	α, β_1, dopaminergic	Vasopressor	Shock, hypotension; inotropic agent
ephedrine[a] ⊕	Akovaz	IV: 50 mg/mL	α, β	Vasoconstrictor	Anesthesia-induced hypotension
epinephrine[a] ⊕	Adrenalin	IV: 1:1000 in 1-mL ampules; 1:10,000 in 10-mL prefilled syringes	α, β	Allergic reactions, vasoconstrictor, cardiac stimulant	Anaphylaxis, cardiac arrest; topical vasoconstrictor, bronchodilator, cardiac stimulant
formoterol[a]	Perforomist Oxeze 🍁	Nebulizer: 20 mcg/2 mL in 2-mL container	β_2	Bronchodilator	Asthma, emphysema, chronic bronchitis
indacaterol[a]	Arcapta Neohaler Onbrez Breezhaler 🍁	Capsule for inhalation: 75 mcg	β_2	Bronchodilator	Emphysema, chronic bronchitis
isoproterenol ⊕	Isuprel	Subcut, IM, IV: 0.2 mg/mL solution; 1-, 5-mL vials	β	Bronchodilator, cardiac stimulant	Shock, digitalis toxicity, bronchospasm
metaproterenol	—	Tablets: 10, 20 mg Syrup: 10 mg/5 mL	β_2	Bronchodilator	Bronchospasm
norepinephrine (levarterenol) ⊕	Levophed	IV: 1 mg/mL in 4-mL ampules	α_1	Vasoconstrictor	Shock, hypotension
phenylephrine[b]		Subcut, IM, IV: 10 mg/mL in 1-mL ampules and 5-mL vial ⊕ Ophthalmic drops: 2.5%, 10% Nasal solutions: 0.25%, 0.5%, 1% Tablets: 10 mg Syrup: 2.5 mg/5 mL	α_1	Vasoconstrictor	Shock, hypotension, nasal decongestant; ophthalmic vasoconstrictor, mydriatic
salmeterol	Serevent Diskus	Aerosol powder: 50 mcg/dose	β_2	Bronchodilator	Asthma, emphysema, chronic bronchitis
terbutaline[a]		Tablets: 2.5, 5 mg Subcut: 1 mg/mL in 1-mL ampules	β_2	Bronchodilator, uterine relaxant	Emphysema, asthma

[a]See also bronchodilators (Chapter 30).
[b]See also decongestants (Chapter 29).
α, Alpha; β, beta; IM, intramuscular; IV, intravenous; Subcut, subcutaneous.
🍁 Available in Canada.   ⊕ High-alert medication.

Agents that inhibit therapeutic activity. The concurrent use of beta-adrenergic blocking agents (e.g., propranolol, nadolol, timolol, pindolol, atenolol, metoprolol), alpha-adrenergic blocking agents (e.g., phenoxybenzamine, phentolamine), and reserpine with adrenergic agents is not recommended.

DRUG CLASS: ALPHA- AND BETA-ADRENERGIC BLOCKING AGENTS

Actions
The alpha- and beta-adrenergic blocking agents act by plugging the alpha or beta receptors, which prevents other agents—usually the naturally occurring catecholamines—from stimulating the specific receptors.

The beta blockers can be subdivided into nonselective and selective beta antagonists. The nonselective blocking agents have an equal affinity for beta-1 and beta-2 receptors, and they inhibit both. These agents are propranolol, nadolol, pindolol, penbutolol, carteolol, sotalol, and timolol. The selective beta-1 blocking agents exhibit action against the heart's beta-1 receptors (cardioselective) and do not readily affect the beta-2 receptors of the bronchi. The selective beta-1 antagonists are esmolol, metoprolol, acebutolol, betaxolol, bisoprolol, and atenolol. This selective action is beneficial for patients in whom nonselective beta blockers may induce bronchospasm (e.g., those with asthma). However, it is important to note that the selectivity of these agents is only relative. In larger doses, these agents will also inhibit the beta-2 receptors. There are no selective beta-2 blockers available. Labetalol and carvedilol exhibit selective alpha-1 and nonselective beta-adrenergic blocking activity. The alpha and beta blockers are listed in Fig. 12.1.

Uses
Because one of the primary actions of the alpha-receptor stimulants is vasoconstriction, it would be expected that alpha-blocking agents are indicated for patients with diseases that are associated with vasoconstriction. Alpha blockers (e.g., prazosin, terazosin, doxazosin) are sometimes used to treat hypertension (see Chapter 22). Alfuzosin, doxazosin, and tamsulosin are used to relax the smooth muscle of the bladder and prostate; they are used to treat urinary obstruction caused by benign prostatic hyperplasia (see Chapter 40).

Beta-adrenergic blocking agents (e.g., beta blockers) are used extensively to treat post–myocardial infarction. They may also be used for hypertension, angina pectoris, cardiac dysrhythmias, symptoms of hyperthyroidism, and stage fright. Nonselective beta blockers must be used with extreme caution in patients with respiratory conditions such as bronchitis, emphysema, asthma, or allergic rhinitis. A beta blockade produces severe bronchoconstriction and may aggravate wheezing, especially during pollen season.

Beta blockers should be used with caution in patients with diabetes and in those who are susceptible to

hypoglycemia. Beta blockers further induce the hypoglycemic effects of insulin and reduce the release of insulin in response to hyperglycemia. All beta blockers mask most of the signs and symptoms of acute hypoglycemia.

Beta-adrenergic blocking agents should be used only in patients with controlled heart failure. Further hypotension, bradycardia, or heart failure may develop.

❖ Nursing Implications for Beta-Adrenergic Blocking Agents
See also the nursing implications for patients with antidysrhythmic therapy (Chapter 23) and for those with hypertension (Chapter 22).

◆ *Premedication assessment*
1. Obtain baseline vital signs: heart rate and blood pressure.
2. See also the premedication assessments for patients with antidysrhythmic therapy (Chapter 23) and for those with hypertension (Chapter 22).

◆ *Availability, dosage, and administration*
See Table 12.3.

Individualization of dosage. Although the onset of activity is fairly rapid, it may take several days to weeks for a patient to show optimal improvement and to become stabilized on an adequate maintenance dosage. Patients must be periodically reevaluated to determine the lowest effective dosage that is necessary to control the disorder.

Sudden discontinuation. Patients must be counseled against poor adherence or the sudden discontinuation of therapy without a healthcare provider's advice. Sudden discontinuation has resulted in an exacerbation of anginal symptoms, and this has been followed in some cases by myocardial infarction. When discontinuing chronically administered beta blockers, the dosage should be gradually reduced over 1 to 2 weeks, with careful patient monitoring. If anginal symptoms develop or become more frequent, beta blocker therapy should be restarted temporarily.

◆ *Common adverse effects.* Most of the adverse effects associated with beta-adrenergic blocking agents are dose related. Response by individual patients is highly variable. Many of the adverse effects that do occur may be transient. Strongly encourage patients to see their healthcare providers before discontinuing therapy. Minor dosage adjustment may be all that is required to eliminate most adverse effects.

Endocrine
Patients with diabetes. Monitor for symptoms of hypoglycemia, including headache, weakness, decreased coordination, general apprehension, diaphoresis, hunger, or blurred or double vision. Many of these symptoms may be masked by beta-adrenergic blocking agents. Notify the healthcare provider if any of the symptoms described appear intermittently.

Table 12.3   Beta-Adrenergic Blocking Agents

GENERIC NAME	BRAND NAME	AVAILABILITY	CLINICAL USES	DOSAGE RANGE
acebutolol	Sectral ✤	Capsules: 200, 400 mg	Hypertension, ventricular dysrhythmias	PO: initial, 400 mg daily; maintenance, 600-1200 mg daily
atenolol	Tenormin Apo-Atenol ✤	Tablets: 25, 50, 100 mg	Hypertension, angina pectoris, after myocardial infarction	PO: initial, 50 mg daily; maintenance, ≤200 mg daily
betaxolol		Tablets: 10, 20 mg	Hypertension	PO: initial, 10 mg daily; maintenance, 20 mg daily
bisoprolol	PMS-Bisoprolol ✤	Tablets: 5, 10 mg	Hypertension	PO: initial, 5 mg daily; maintenance, 10-20 mg daily
carvedilol	Coreg, Coreg CR Apo-Carvedilol ✤	Tablets: 3.125, 6.25, 12.5, 25 mg Capsules, extended release: 10, 20, 40, 80 mg	Hypertension, heart failure, myocardial infarction	PO: initial, 6.25 mg twice daily; maintenance, ≤50 mg daily PO: initial, 10 mg daily; maintenance, ≤80 mg daily Extended release: 10 mg daily
esmolol ⬤	Brevibloc	Injection: 10 mg/mL in 10-mL ampules; 10 mg/mL in 250-mL bag; 20 mg/mL in 100-mL bag	Supraventricular tachycardia, hypertension	IV: initial, 500 mcg/kg/min for 1 min followed by 50 mcg/kg/min for 4 min and then adjusted to patient's needs
labetalol ⬤	Trandate ✤	Tablets: 100, 200, 300 mg Injection: 5 mg/mL in 4-, 20-, 40-mL vials	Hypertension	PO: initial, 100 mg twice daily; maintenance, ≤2400 mg daily
metoprolol ⬤	Lopressor, Toprol-XL Betaloc ✤	Tablets: 25, 37.5, 50, 100 mg Injection: 1 mg/mL in 5-mL ampules	Hypertension, myocardial infarction, angina pectoris, heart failure	PO: 50 mg twice daily; maintenance dosing of ≤450 mg daily, divided
nadolol	Corgard	Tablets: 20, 40, 80 mg	Angina pectoris, hypertension	PO: initial, 40 mg daily; maintenance, 40-80 mg daily; maximum, 320 mg daily for hypertension; maximum, 240 mg for angina.
nebivolol	Bystolic	Tablets: 2.5, 5, 10, 20 mg	Hypertension	PO: initial, 5 mg daily; maintenance, ≤40 mg daily
penbutolol		Tablets: 20 mg	Hypertension	PO: initial, 20 mg daily; maintenance, 20-40 mg daily Maximum: 80 mg daily
pindolol	Apo-pindol ✤ Pindolol ✤ Visken ✤	Tablets: 5, 10, 15 mg	Hypertension	PO: initial, 5 mg twice daily; maintenance, 10-30 mg daily; maximum, 60 mg daily
propranolol ⬤	propranolol, Inderal LA Teva-propranolol ✤	Tablets: 10, 20, 40, 60, 80 mg Solution: 20, 40 mg/5 mL Capsules, sustained release: 60, 80, 120, 160 mg IV: 1 mg/mL in 1-mL ampules	Dysrhythmias, hypertension, angina pectoris, myocardial infarction, migraine, tremor, hypertrophic subaortic stenosis	PO, immediate release: initial, 40 mg twice daily; maintenance, 120-640 mg daily in two to four divided doses PO, sustained release: 80-160 mg daily; maximum 640 mg daily IV: 1-3 mg with close electrocardiographic monitoring
sotalol	Betapace, Sorine Riva-Sotalol ✤	Tablets: 80, 120, 160, 240 mg IV: 150 mg/10 mL Oral solution: 5 mg/mL	Dysrhythmias	PO: initial, 80 mg twice daily; maintenance, ≤320 mg daily
timolol	Timolol ✤	Tablets: 5, 10, 20 mg	Hypertension, myocardial infarction, migraine	PO: initial, 10 mg twice daily; maintenance, ≤30 mg twice daily

IV, Intravenous; *PO,* by mouth.
✤ Available in Canada.   ⬤ High-alert medication.

◆ **Serious adverse effects**
Cardiovascular
Bradycardia, peripheral vasoconstriction (e.g., purple, mottled skin). Discontinue further doses until the patient is evaluated by a healthcare provider.

Heart failure. Monitor patients for an increase in edema, dyspnea, crackles, bradycardia, and orthopnea. Notify the healthcare provider if these symptoms develop.
Respiratory
Bronchospasm, wheezing. Withhold additional doses until the patient has been evaluated by a healthcare provider.

◆ **Drug interactions**
Antihypertensive agents. All beta-blocking agents have hypotensive properties that are additive with antihypertensive agents (e.g., angiotensin-converting enzyme inhibitors, calcium channel blockers, diuretics, angiotensin receptor blockers, methyldopa, hydralazine, clonidine, reserpine). If it is decided to discontinue therapy in patients who are receiving beta blockers and clonidine concurrently, the beta blocker should be withdrawn gradually and discontinued for several days before gradually withdrawing the clonidine.

Beta-adrenergic agents. Depending on the dosage, the beta stimulants (e.g., isoproterenol, metaproterenol, terbutaline, albuterol) may inhibit the action of beta-blocking agents and vice versa.

Lidocaine, phenytoin, disopyramide, digoxin. When these drugs are occasionally used concurrently with beta-blocking agents, the patient must be monitored carefully for additional arrhythmias, bradycardia, and signs of heart failure.

Enzyme-inducing agents. Enzyme-inducing agents (e.g., cimetidine, phenobarbital, pentobarbital, rifampin, phenytoin) enhance the metabolism of propranolol, metoprolol, pindolol, and timolol. This reaction probably does not occur with nadolol or atenolol because they are not metabolized but rather are excreted unchanged. The dosage of the beta blocker may have to be increased to provide therapeutic activity. If the enzyme-inducing agent is discontinued, the dosage of the beta blocker will also require reduction.

Nonsteroidal antiinflammatory agents. Indomethacin, salicylates, and possibly other prostaglandin inhibitors reduce the antihypertensive activity of propranolol and pindolol. This results in a loss of hypertensive control. The dose of the beta blocker may have to be increased to compensate for the antihypertensive inhibitory effect of indomethacin and perhaps other prostaglandin inhibitors.

DRUG CLASS: CHOLINERGIC AGENTS

Actions
Cholinergic agents, which are also known as *parasympathomimetic agents,* produce effects that are similar to those of acetylcholine. Some cholinergic agents act by directly stimulating the parasympathetic nervous system, whereas others inhibit acetylcholinesterase, which is the enzyme that metabolizes acetylcholine after it has been released by the nerve ending. These latter agents are known as *indirect-acting cholinergic agents.* Some of the cholinergic actions are slow heartbeat; increased GI motility and secretions; increased contractions of the urinary bladder, with relaxation of the muscle sphincter; increased secretions and contractility of the bronchial smooth muscle; sweating; miosis (constriction) of the pupil, which reduces intraocular pressure; increased force of the contraction of skeletal muscle; and, sometimes, decreased blood pressure.

Uses
See Table 12.4.

❖ **Nursing Implications for Cholinergic Agents**
See also the nursing implications for patients with disorders of the eyes (Chapter 42), glaucoma (Chapter 42), urinary system disease (Chapter 41), and respiratory tract disease (Chapters 29 and 30).

◆ **Premedication assessment**
1. Obtain baseline vital signs: heart rate and blood pressure.
2. See also the premedication assessments for patients with disorders of the eyes (Chapter 42), glaucoma (Chapter 42), urinary system disease (Chapter 41), and respiratory tract disease (Chapters 29 and 30).

◆ **Availability, dosage, and administration**
See Table 12.4.

◆ **Common adverse effects.** Because cholinergic fibers innervate the entire body, effects in most body systems can be expected. Fortunately, because all receptors do not respond to the same dosage, adverse effects are not always seen. The higher the dosage, however, the greater the likelihood of adverse effects.
Gastrointestinal
Nausea, vomiting, diarrhea, abdominal cramping. These symptoms are extensions of the pharmacologic effects of the medication, and they are dose related. Reducing the dosage may be effective for controlling these adverse effects without eliminating the desired pharmacologic effect.
Cardiovascular
Dizziness, hypotension. Monitor the patient's blood pressure and pulse. To minimize hypotensive episodes, instruct the patient to rise slowly from a supine or sitting position, and have him or her perform exercises to prevent blood from pooling while he or she is standing or sitting in one position for a prolonged period. Teach the patient to sit or lie down if he or she feels faint.

◆ **Serious adverse effects**
Respiratory
Bronchospasm, wheezing. Withhold the next dose until the patient is evaluated by a healthcare provider.

Table 12.4 Cholinergic Agents

GENERIC NAME	BRAND NAME	AVAILABILITY	CLINICAL USES
bethanechol	Urecholine Duvoid ❦	Tablets: 5, 10, 25, 50 mg	Urinary retention
edrophonium	Enlon	Injection: 10 mg/mL in 15-mL vial	Diagnosis of myasthenia gravis; reverse nondepolarizing muscle relaxants (e.g., tubocurarine)
neostigmine		Injection: 0.5, 1 mg/mL	Reverse nondepolarizing muscle relaxants (e.g., tubocurarine)
physostigmine	—	Injection: 1 mg/mL in 2-mL ampules	Reverse toxicity of overdoses of anticholinergic agents (e.g., pesticides, insecticides)
pilocarpine	Salagen Tablets Isopto Carpine	Tablets: 5, 7.5 mg Ophthalmic solution: 1, 2, 4%	Treat symptoms of dry mouth due to salivary gland hypofunction following radiation therapy Glaucoma
pyridostigmine	Mestinon Mestinon-SR ❦ Regonol	Tablets: 60 mg Syrup: 60 mg/5 mL Tablets, sustained release: 180 mg Injection: 5 mg/mL	Treatment of myasthenia gravis Reversal of nondepolarizing muscle relaxants

❦ Available in Canada.

Table 12.5 Anticholinergic Agents

GENERIC NAME	BRAND NAME	AVAILABILITY	CLINICAL USES
atropine	Atropine Sulfate	Injection: 0.05, 0.1, 0.4, 0.8, 1 mg/mL	Presurgery: to reduce salivation and bronchial secretions; to minimize bradycardia during intubation; adjuvant use with anticholinesterases (e.g., neostigmine) to decrease their adverse effects during reversal of neuromuscular blockade
dicyclomine	Bentyl Bentylol ❦	Tablets: 20 mg Capsules: 10 mg Injection: 10 mg/mL Solution: 10 mg/5 mL	Irritable bowel syndrome
glycopyrrolate	Robinul	Tablets: 1, 2 mg Injection: 0.2 mg/mL	Presurgery: to reduce salivation and bronchial secretions and to minimize bradycardia during intubation

❦ Available in Canada.

Cardiovascular
Bradycardia. Withhold the next dose until the patient is evaluated by a healthcare provider.

◆ *Drug interactions*

Atropine, antihistamines. Atropine, other anticholinergic agents, and most antihistamines antagonize the effects of cholinergic agents.

DRUG CLASS: ANTICHOLINERGIC AGENTS

Actions
Anticholinergic agents, which are also known as *cholinergic blocking agents* or *parasympatholytic agents,* block the action of acetylcholine in the parasympathetic nervous system. These drugs act by occupying receptor sites at parasympathetic nerve endings, which prevent the action of acetylcholine. The parasympathetic response is reduced, depending on the amount of anticholinergic drug that is blocking the receptors. The inhibition of cholinergic activity (e.g., anticholinergic effects) includes the following: mydriasis (dilation) of the pupil with increased intraocular pressure in patients with glaucoma; dry, tenacious secretions of the mouth, nose, throat, and bronchi; decreased secretions and motility of the GI tract; increased heart rate; and decreased sweating.

Uses
See Table 12.5.

❖ **Nursing Implications for Anticholinergic Agents**
See also the nursing implications for patients with Parkinson's disease (Chapter 14) and disorders of the eyes (Chapter 42), and for antihistamines (Chapter 29).

◆ *Premedication assessment*
1. All patients should be screened for closed-angle glaucoma because anticholinergic agents may precipitate an acute attack. Patients with open-angle glaucoma can safely use anticholinergic agents in conjunction with miotic therapy.
2. Check the patient's history for an enlarged prostate. If this condition is present, anticholinergic agents may cause the patient to have a temporary inability to void.

3. Obtain baseline vital signs: heart rate and blood pressure.

4. See also the premedication assessments for patients with Parkinson's disease (Chapter 14), disorders of the eyes (Chapter 42), and antihistamines (Chapter 29).

◆ *Availability dosage and administration*
See Table 12.5.

◆ *Common adverse effects.* Because cholinergic fibers innervate the entire body, effects from blocking this system occur throughout most systems. Fortunately, because all receptors do not respond to the same dose, all adverse effects are not seen to the same degree with all cholinergic blocking agents. The higher the dosage, however, the greater the likelihood of more adverse effects. The following symptoms are the anticholinergic effects that are produced by these agents. Patients who are taking these medications should be monitored for the development of these adverse effects.

Sensory
Blurred vision. Warn the patient that blurred vision may occur and make appropriate suggestions for the patient's personal safety.

Gastrointestinal
Constipation; dryness of the mucosa of the mouth, nose, and throat. Mucosal dryness may be alleviated by sucking hard candy or ice chips or by chewing gum. Give the patient stool softeners as prescribed. Encourage adequate fluid intake and the eating of foods that provide sufficient bulk.

Genitourinary
Urinary retention. If the patient develops urinary hesitancy, assess him or her for bladder distention. Contact the healthcare provider for further evaluation.

◆ *Serious adverse effects*
Sensory
Glaucoma. All patients should be screened for closed-angle glaucoma before the initiation of therapy. Patients with open-angle glaucoma can safely use anticholinergic agents. Monitor the patient's intraocular pressures regularly.

Psychological
Confusion, depression, nightmares, hallucinations. Perform a baseline assessment of the patient's degree of alertness and orientation to name, place, and time before initiating therapy. Make regularly scheduled subsequent evaluations of the patient's mental status and compare findings. Report the development of alterations and provide for patient safety during these episodes. A reduction in the daily medication dosage may control these adverse effects.

Cardiovascular
Orthostatic hypotension. Although orthostatic hypotension occurs infrequently and is generally mild, all anticholinergic agents may cause some degree of this condition, which is manifested by dizziness and weakness, particularly when therapy is initiated. Monitor the patient's blood pressure daily in both the supine and standing positions. Anticipate the development of postural hypotension and take measures to prevent it. Teach the patient to rise slowly from a supine or sitting position, and encourage the patient to sit or lie down if he or she feels faint.

Palpitations, dysrhythmias. Contact the healthcare provider for further evaluation.

◆ *Drug interactions*
Amantadine, tricyclic antidepressants, phenothiazines. These agents may potentiate anticholinergic adverse effects. Confusion and hallucinations are characteristic of excessive anticholinergic activity.

Get Ready for the NCLEX® Examination!

Key Points

- The nervous system is one of two primary regulators of body homeostasis and defense. The CNS is composed of the brain and the spinal cord.
- The peripheral nervous system is subdivided into the afferent and efferent nerve pathways. The afferent (peripheral) nerves conduct signals from sensory receptors (e.g., vision, pressure, pain, cold, warmth, touch, smell) throughout the body to the CNS. The CNS processes these signals and controls the body's response by sending signals back through the efferent nerves of the peripheral nervous system. The efferent nervous system is subdivided into the motor nervous system, which controls skeletal muscle, and the autonomic nervous system, which regulates smooth muscle and heart muscle and controls secretions from certain glands.
- Nerve impulses are passed between neurons and from neurons to end organs by neurotransmitters. The main neurotransmitters of the autonomic nervous system are acetylcholine and norepinephrine. Nerve endings that liberate acetylcholine are called *cholinergic fibers;* those that secrete norepinephrine are called *adrenergic fibers.*
- The CNS is composed of systems of different types of neurons that secrete separate neurotransmitters, such as acetylcholine, norepinephrine, epinephrine, dopamine, serotonin, and gamma-aminobutyric acid.
- The control of neurotransmitters is a primary way to alleviate the symptoms that are associated with many diseases. As shown in Table 12.1, the administration of one type of autonomic nervous system drug can

affect several organ systems, and adverse effects can be numerous. Therefore the use of these drugs requires the monitoring of more than just the symptoms for which the medicine was prescribed.

Additional Learning Resources

SG Go to your Study Guide for additional Review Questions for the NCLEX® Examination, Critical Thinking Clinical Situations, and other learning activities to help you master this chapter content.

Go to your Evolve website (https://evolve.elsevier.com/Clayton) for additional online resources.

Review Questions for the NCLEX® Examination

1. The peripheral nervous system includes which of the following components? *(Select all that apply.)*
   1. Afferent nerves
   2. Brain
   3. Efferent nerves
   4. Spinal cord
   5. Skeletal muscles

2. What are the two major neurotransmitters of the autonomic nervous system?
   1. Norepinephrine and epinephrine
   2. Dopamine and serotonin
   3. Acetylcholine and norepinephrine
   4. Endorphins and enkephalins

3. Cholinergic agents are drugs that have which of these effects? *(Select all that apply.)*
   1. Slowing the heart rate
   2. Increasing the heart rate
   3. Dilating the pupils
   4. Constricting the pupils
   5. Increasing gastric motility

4. What are the two broad classes of drugs used to stimulate the adrenergic nervous system?
   1. Dopamine and norepinephrine
   2. Epinephrine and serotonin
   3. Catecholamines and noncatecholamines
   4. Dopaminergic receptors and beta blockers

5. Adrenergic agents that stimulate the beta receptors of the autonomic nervous system have which of the following effects? *(Select all that apply.)*
   1. Constriction of the coronary arterioles
   2. Relaxation of the urinary bladder
   3. Increased renal perfusion
   4. Increased heart rate
   5. Increased blood glucose

6. A patient who has recently been prescribed a beta-adrenergic blocking agent presents to the emergency department with a serious adverse effect. Which adverse effect is the patient likely exhibiting?
   1. Hypertension
   2. Angina pectoris
   3. Bronchoconstriction
   4. Cardiac dysrhythmias

7. Which data in the patient's history and physical examination cause the nurse to question a preoperative medication order for atropine sulfate and morphine?
   1. Excessive oral secretions
   2. Bradycardia
   3. Increased gastric motility
   4. Prostatic enlargement

8. The cholinergic agent pilocarpine is used for which common condition?
   1. Glaucoma
   2. Hypertension
   3. Peptic ulcer disease
   4. Constipation

9. The nurse teaching a patient about the drug pyridostigmine (Mestinon) for myasthenia gravis knows the patient needs further teaching after which statement by the patient?
   1. "I understand I need this to drug because it will help improve my symptoms."
   2. "If I develop the side effect of dizziness, I will be sure not to get up too fast."
   3. "I can reduce the dose of the medication when I feel any side effects."
   4. "I can expect to take this drug long term for my condition."

13

Drugs Used for Sleep

Objectives

1. Differentiate among the terms *sedative* and *hypnotic*; *initial*, *intermittent*, and *terminal insomnia*; *transient*, *short-term*, and *chronic insomnia*; and *rebound sleep*.
2. Identify alterations found in the sleep pattern when hypnotics are discontinued.
3. Cite nursing interventions that can be implemented as an alternative to administering a sedative-hypnotic medication.

4. Compare the effects of benzodiazepines and nonbenzodiazepines on the central nervous system.
5. Identify the antidote drug used for the management of benzodiazepine overdose.
6. Identify laboratory tests that should be monitored when benzodiazepines are administered for an extended period.

Key Terms

rapid eye movement (REM) sleep (p. 188)
insomnia (ĭn-SŎM-nē-ă) (p. 189)
hypnotic (hĭp-NŎT-ĭk) (p. 189)

sedative (SĔD-ă-tĭv) (p. 189)
rebound sleep (RĒ-bŏwnd SLĒP) (p. 189)

SLEEP AND SLEEP PATTERN DISTURBANCE

Sleep is a state of unconsciousness from which a patient can be aroused by an appropriate stimulus. It is a naturally occurring phenomenon that occupies about one-third of an adult's life.

Adequate sleep that progresses through the normal stages is important to maintain body function, including psychiatric equilibrium and the strengthening of the immune system to ward off disease. A normal sleep duration of 7 to 8 hours per night is thought to be optimal for good health. Studies also show that a reduced amount of sleep is associated with overweight and obesity, as well as the development of metabolic syndrome (see Chapter 20). Obesity itself is also detrimental to healthy sleep patterns, and it can contribute to the development of sleep apnea. Other studies show a strong connection between a shortened duration of sleep and cardiovascular disease. Individuals who sleep less than 5 hours per night have a threefold increased risk of heart attacks. The National Health Interview Survey also demonstrates a close relationship between symptoms of insomnia and common adverse physical and mental health conditions, including obesity, diabetes mellitus, hypertension, heart failure, anxiety, and depression. The *Healthy People 2020* program has as one of its objectives the promotion of sleep health, which includes promoting optimal sleep durations and reducing the prevalence and effect of sleep disorders.

Natural sleep rhythmically progresses through phases that provide both physical and mental rest. On the basis of brain-wave activity, muscle activity, and eye movement, normal sleep can be divided into two phases: non–rapid eye movement (NREM) sleep and rapid eye movement (REM) sleep. The NREM phase can be further divided into four stages, each of which is characterized by a specific set of brain-wave activities. Stage 1 is a transition phase between wakefulness and sleep that lasts only a few minutes. Some people experience it as wakefulness, whereas others feel it as drowsiness. Approximately 2% to 5% of sleep is stage 1 sleep. Stage 2 sleep comprises about 50% of normal sleep time. People often experience a drifting or floating sensation, and if they are awakened during this stage, they will often deny being asleep, responding, "I was just resting my eyes." Stages 1 and 2 are light sleep periods from which a person is easily aroused. Stage 3 is a transition from the lighter to deeper sleep state of stage 4. Stage 4 sleep is dreamless, very restful, and associated with a 10% to 30% decrease in blood pressure, respiratory rate, and basal metabolic rate. Stage 4 sleep is also referred to as *delta sleep* on the basis of the pattern of brain waves that are observed during this stage. Stage 4 sleep comprises 10% to 15% of sleep time in young, healthy adults. Stage 4 sleep diminishes in length as people age, and many people who are more than 75 years old do not demonstrate any stage 4 sleep patterns. Older adults also take longer to cycle through the relaxation stages of NREM sleep, with an increased frequency and duration of awakenings.

During a normal night of sleep, a person will rhythmically cycle from wakefulness through stages 1, 2, 3, and 4; he or she will then go back to stage 3, then to stage 2, and then to REM sleep over the course of about 90 minutes. The early episodes of REM sleep last only a few minutes. However, as sleep progresses, the amount of REM sleep increases, with REM periods becoming longer and more intense around 5 AM. This type of sleep represents 20% to 25% of sleep time, and it is characterized by REM, dreaming, increased heart rate, irregular breathing, the secretion of stomach acids, and some muscular activity. REM sleep appears to be an important time for the subconscious mind to release anxiety and tension and reestablish a psychiatric equilibrium.

Insomnia is defined as the inability to sleep. It is the most common sleep disorder known; 95% of all adults experience insomnia at least once during their lives, and up to 35% of adults will have insomnia during a given year. In general, insomnia is not a disease but rather a symptom of physical or mental stress. It is usually mild and lasts only a few nights. Common causes are changes in lifestyle or environment (e.g., hospitalization), pain, illness, the excess consumption of products that contain caffeine (e.g., coffee, energy drinks) or alcohol, eating large or rich meals shortly before bedtime, and stress. *Initial insomnia* is the inability to fall asleep when desired, *intermittent insomnia* is the inability to stay asleep, and *terminal insomnia* is characterized by early awakening with the inability to fall asleep again. Insomnia is also classified in accordance with its duration. A sleep disturbance that lasts only a few nights is considered to be *transient insomnia*. A sleep disturbance that lasts less than 3 weeks is referred to as *short-term insomnia*, and it is usually associated with travel across time zones, illness, or anxiety (e.g., job-related changes, financial stress, examinations, emotional relationships). *Chronic insomnia* requires at least 1 month of sleep disturbance before the individual is diagnosed with a sleep disorder. About 10% of adults and up to 20% of older people report having chronic insomnia. Women report experiencing insomnia twice as frequently as men. A higher incidence of insomnia is reported by older adults, the unemployed, those of lower socioeconomic status, and the recently separated or widowed. As many as 40% of patients with chronic insomnia also have psychiatric disorders (e.g., anxiety, depression, substance abuse). People with chronic insomnia often develop fatigue or drowsiness that interferes with daytime functioning and employment responsibilities.

SEDATIVE-HYPNOTIC THERAPY

Drugs that are used in conjunction with altered patterns of sleep are known as *sedative-hypnotic agents*. A **hypnotic** is a drug that produces sleep; a **sedative** quiets the patient and gives him or her a feeling of relaxation and rest, but this is not necessarily accompanied by sleep. A good hypnotic should provide the following actions within a short period of time: the onset of restful, natural sleep; a duration of action that allows a patient to awaken at the usual time; a natural awakening with no "hangover" effects; and no danger of habit formation. Unfortunately, the ideal hypnotic is not available. The most commonly used sedative-hypnotic agents increase total sleeping time, especially the time spent in stage 2 sleep (i.e., light sleep); however, they also decrease the number of REM periods and the total time spent in REM sleep. Rapid eye movement sleep is needed to help maintain a mental balance during daytime activities. When REM sleep is decreased, there is a strong physiologic tendency to make it up. Compensatory REM sleep, or **rebound sleep**, seems to occur even when hypnotic agents are used for only 3 or 4 days. After the chronic administration of sedative-hypnotic agents, REM rebound may be severe and accompanied by restlessness and vivid nightmares. Depending on the frequency of hypnotic administration, normal sleep patterns may not be restored for weeks. The effects of REM rebound may enhance an individual's chronic use of and dependence on these agents to avoid the unpleasant consequences of rebound sleep. Because of this, a vicious cycle occurs as the normal physiologic need for sleep is not met and the body attempts to compensate.

Because sedative-hypnotic agents have many adverse effects, especially with long-term use, medications that are recognized for other primary uses are being used by healthcare providers for the treatment of insomnia. Antidepressants such as amitriptyline, trazodone, and mirtazapine are prescribed in lower dosages for their sedative effects to assist patients with getting to sleep (see Chapter 16). Anticonvulsants that are used in this way include gabapentin and topiramate (see Chapter 18). Antipsychotic agents such as quetiapine and olanzapine are prescribed for patients with psychoses who also have insomnia (see Chapter 17). However, it is important to note that no extensive studies have been completed regarding the use of these antidepressants, antipsychotics, and anticonvulsants for insomnia, so their long-term effects are unknown and their use for treating chronic insomnia cannot be recommended.

ACTIONS

Sedatives, which are used to produce relaxation and rest, and hypnotics, which are used to produce sleep, are not always different drugs. Their effects may depend on the dosage and the condition of the patient. A small dose of a drug may act as a sedative, whereas a larger dose of the same drug may act as a hypnotic and produce sleep.

Sedative-hypnotic medications may be classified into two groups: benzodiazepines and nonbenzodiazepine sedative-hypnotic medications.

USES

The primary uses of sedative-hypnotic medications are as follows: (1) to improve sleep patterns for the temporary treatment of insomnia; and (2) to decrease the level of anxiety and increase relaxation or sleep before diagnostic or operative procedures.

❖ NURSING IMPLICATIONS FOR SEDATIVE-HYPNOTIC THERAPY

◆ Assessment

Central nervous system function. Because sedative-hypnotic drugs depress overall central nervous system (CNS) function, identify the patient's level of alertness and orientation as well as his or her ability to perform various motor functions.

Vital signs. Obtain the patient's current blood pressure, pulse, and respiration rates before initiating drug therapy.

Sleep pattern. Assess the patient's usual pattern of sleep, and obtain information about the pattern of sleep disruption (e.g., difficulty falling asleep, inability to remain asleep the entire night, awakening during the early morning hours and unable to return to a restful sleep).

Ask about the amount of sleep (i.e., number of hours) that the patient considers normal and how his or her insomnia is managed at home. Does the patient have a regular time to go to bed and wake up? If the patient is taking medications, determine the drug, dosage, and frequency of administration and whether this may be contributing to sleeplessness. (Medicines that may induce or aggravate insomnia include theophylline, caffeine, pseudoephedrine, nicotine, levodopa, corticosteroids, and selective serotonin reuptake inhibitor antidepressants.)

Patients with persistent insomnia should be carefully monitored for the number of naps taken during the day. Investigate the type of activities that the patient performs immediately before going to bed.

Anxiety level. Assess the patient's exhibited degree of anxiety. Is it really a sedative-hypnotic medication that the patient needs, or does the patient just need someone to listen to him or her? Ask about the stressors that the patient has been experiencing in his or her personal and work environments.

Environmental control. Obtain data related to possible disturbances present in the individual's sleeping environment that may interfere with sleep (e.g., room temperature, lights, noise, traffic, restlessness, a snoring partner).

Nutritional needs. Obtain a dietary history to identify sources of caffeinated products that may act as stimulants.

Alcohol intake. Although alcohol causes sedation, it disrupts sleep patterns and may cause early-morning awakening.

Exercise. Obtain data related to the patient's usual degree of physical activity and at what times during the day he or she is most active.

Respiratory status. People with respiratory disorders and those who snore heavily may have low respiratory reserves and should not receive hypnotic agents because of their potential to cause respiratory depression.

◆ Implementation

Vital signs. Obtain the patient's vital signs periodically as the situation indicates.

Preoperative medication. Give the patient preoperative medications at the specified time.

Monitoring effects. When a medication is administered, carefully assess the patient at regular intervals for the drug's therapeutic and adverse effects.

As-needed medications. If giving the patient as-needed (PRN) medications, ask the patient about the effectiveness of previously administered therapy. It is sometimes necessary to repeat a medication if an order permits doing so. This is done at the nurse's discretion on the basis of the evaluation of a particular patient's needs.

◆ Patient Education: Promote Good Sleep Hygiene

Bedtime. Encourage the patient to choose a standard time to go to bed to help the body establish a rhythm and routine.

Nutrition. Teach the patient appropriate nutrition information concerning the Food and Drug Administration's (FDA's) recommendations of MyPlate, adequate fluid intake, and vitamin use. Communicate the information at the educational level of the patient.

Avoiding heavy meals during the evening. Alcohol and caffeine consumption should be reduced or discontinued, especially within several hours of bedtime. Educate the patient about decaffeinated or herbal products that can be substituted for caffeinated foods. Help the patient to avoid products that contain caffeine, such as coffee, tea, energy drinks, soft drinks, and chocolate. Limit the total daily intake of these items, and provide the patient with warm milk and crackers as a bedtime snack. Protein foods and dairy products contain an amino acid that synthesizes serotonin, which is a neurotransmitter that has been found to increase sleep time and decrease the time required to fall asleep.

For insomnia, suggest that the patient drink warm milk about 30 minutes before going to bed.

Personal comfort. Position the patient for maximum comfort, provide a back rub, encourage the patient to empty the bladder, and be certain that the bedding is clean and dry. Take time to meet the patient's individual needs and to calm his or her fears. Foster a trusting relationship.

Environmental control. Tell the patient to sleep in an environment that promotes sleep, such as a quiet, darkened room free from distractions, and to avoid using the bedroom for watching television, responding to e-mails, preparing work for the following day, eating, and paying bills. Provide adequate ventilation, subdued lighting, and a comfortable room temperature and control traffic in and out of the patient's room.

For safety, instruct the patient to leave a night-light on and not smoke in bed after taking medication.

Activity and exercise. Suggest the inclusion of exercise in the patient's daily activities so that the patient obtains sufficient exercise and is tired enough to sleep. For some individuals, plan a quiet "unwinding" time before retiring for the night. For children, assist with sleep by providing a warm bath and structure before bedtime. Try a bedtime story that is pleasant and soothing (rather than one that may cause anxiety or fear).

Stress management
- Explore personal and work stressors that could have a bearing on the patient's insomnia. Some stressors may exist in the work environment; therefore the involvement of the occupational health nurse, along with a thorough exploration of work factors, may be appropriate. Stress produced within the dynamics of the family may require professional counseling.
- Teach the patient relaxation techniques and personal comfort measures (e.g., a warm bath) to relieve stress. Playing soft music may also promote relaxation.
- Make referrals for the mastery of biofeedback, meditation, or other techniques to reduce stress levels.
- Encourage the patient to openly express feelings about his or her stress and insomnia. The adjustment to this situation involves working through great personal fears, frustrations, hostilities, and resentments.
- Explore the coping mechanisms that the person uses in response to stress, and identify methods of channeling these toward positive realistic goals and alternatives to the use of medication.

Fostering health maintenance. Throughout the course of treatment, discuss medication information and how it will benefit the patient. Stress the importance of nonpharmacologic interventions and the long-term effects that compliance with the treatment regimen can provide.

Provide the patient or the patient's significant others with important information that is contained in the specific drug monographs for the medicines prescribed.

Additional health teaching and nursing interventions for the common adverse effects and serious adverse effects that require contact with the healthcare provider are described in the following drug monographs (benzodiazepines, nonbenzodiazepine sedative-hypnotic medications).

Patient self-assessment. Enlist the patient's help with developing and maintaining a written record of monitoring parameters (e.g., extent and frequency of insomnia); see the Patient Self-Assessment Form for Sleeping Medication on the Evolve website. Complete the Premedication Data column for use as a baseline to track the patient's response to drug therapy. Ensure that the patient understands how to use the form, and instruct the patient to bring the completed form to follow-up visits. During these follow-up visits, focus on issues that will foster the patient's adherence with the therapeutic interventions that have been prescribed.

DRUG THERAPY FOR SLEEP DISTURBANCE

DRUG CLASS: BENZODIAZEPINES

Benzodiazepines have been extremely successful products from both the therapeutic and safety standpoints. A major advantage of the benzodiazepine sedative-hypnotic agents is the wide safety margin between therapeutic and lethal doses. Intentional and unintentional overdoses well above the normal therapeutic doses are well tolerated and not fatal.

More than 2000 benzodiazepine derivatives have been identified, and more than 100 have been tested for sedative-hypnotic or other therapeutic activity. Although there are many similarities among the benzodiazepines, they are difficult to characterize as a class. Some benzodiazepines are effective anticonvulsants, others serve as antianxiety and muscle-relaxant agents, and others are used as sedative-hypnotic drugs.

Actions

Benzodiazepines exert their effects through stimulation of the gamma-aminobutyric acid (GABA)–benzodiazepine receptor complex. GABA is an inhibitory neurotransmitter that exerts its effects at specific receptor subtypes designated GABA-A and GABA-B. GABA-A is the primary receptor subtype in the CNS. Specific benzodiazepine (BZD) receptor subtypes are thought to be coupled to GABA-A receptors. The BZD_1 receptors are located in the cerebellum and cerebral cortex, the BZD_2 receptors in the cerebral cortex and spinal cord, and the BZD_3 receptors in the peripheral tissues. Activation of the BZD_1 receptors is thought to mediate sleep, and the BZD_2 receptor affects muscle relaxation, anticonvulsant activity (see Chapter 18), motor coordination, and memory.

Uses

Estazolam, flurazepam, quazepam, temazepam, and triazolam are the benzodiazepines that have been marketed for hypnosis. Triazolam, which is a shorter-acting hypnotic, as well as estazolam and temazepam, which are intermediate-acting hypnotic agents, do not contain active metabolites and therefore do not accumulate as readily after several nights of dosing. Flurazepam and quazepam have long half-lives and active metabolites, thus making patients much more susceptible to hangovers the day after use. Benzodiazepines that are used as sedative-hypnotic agents increase stage 2 sleep and decrease stages 3 and 4 sleep and, to a lesser extent, REM sleep.

When benzodiazepine therapy is started, patients experience deep and refreshing sleep. However, benzodiazepine-induced sleep varies from normal sleep in that there is less REM sleep. With the chronic administration of benzodiazepines, the amount of REM sleep gradually increases as tolerance develops to the REM-suppressant effects of the drugs. When benzodiazepines are discontinued, a rebound increase in REM sleep may occur despite the patient's tolerance. During the rebound period, the number of dreams stays about the same, but many of the dreams are reported to be bizarre. After long-term use of most benzodiazepines, there is also a rebound in insomnia. Consequently, it is important to use these agents only for short courses (i.e., usually no more than 4 weeks) of therapy.

The short-acting benzodiazepines (e.g., midazolam, lorazepam) are used parenterally as preoperative sedatives and intravenously for conscious sedation before short diagnostic procedures or for the induction of general anesthesia. Midazolam has a more rapid onset of action, produces a greater degree of amnesia, and has a much shorter duration compared with diazepam. Lorazepam is used as an antianxiety agent in general, but it is particularly useful before diagnostic procedures when a longer duration of action is required; a parenteral dosage form is available. It also has no active metabolites that may prolong sedation.

Flumazenil is an antidote that is administered intravenously for the complete or partial reversal of the effects of benzodiazepines that are used as general anesthetics or during diagnostic or therapeutic procedures. Flumazenil is also used for the management of an intentional or accidental overdose of benzodiazepines.

Therapeutic Outcomes

The primary therapeutic outcomes sought from benzodiazepine therapy are as follows:

1. To produce mild sedation
2. For short-term use, to produce sleep
3. Preoperative sedation with amnesia

❖ Nursing Implications for Benzodiazepines
◆ Premedication assessment
1. Record the patient's baseline vital signs (e.g., blood pressure, pulse, respirations); measure the patient's blood pressure in both sitting and lying positions.
2. Check for a history of blood dyscrasias or hepatic disease, and determine whether the patient is in the first trimester of pregnancy.
3. Assess the patient's level of pain.

◆ Availability, dosage, and administration. See Table 13.1.
The habitual use of benzodiazepines may result in physical and psychological dependence. The rapid discontinuance of benzodiazepines after long-term use may result in symptoms that are similar to those of alcohol withdrawal, such as weakness, anxiety, delirium, and grand mal seizures. These symptoms may not appear for several days after discontinuation. Discontinuation of benzodiazepines consists of gradual withdrawal over 2 to 4 weeks.

Pregnancy and lactation. It is generally recommended that benzodiazepines not be administered during at least the first trimester of pregnancy. There may be an increased incidence of birth defects if these drugs are taken because these agents readily cross the placenta and enter the fetal circulation.

Mothers who are breastfeeding should not receive benzodiazepines regularly. These agents readily cross into breast milk and exert a pharmacologic effect on the infant.

◆ Common adverse effects
Neurologic
Drowsiness, hangover, sedation, lethargy, decreased level of alertness. Patients may complain of "morning hangover" and blurred vision. If the hangover effect continues and becomes troublesome, there should be a reduction in the drug dosage, a change in the medication, or both. People who work around machinery, drive a car, pour and give medications, or perform other duties for which they must remain mentally alert should not take these medications while working.

Cardiovascular
Transient hypotension when arising. Explain to the patient the need to first rise to a sitting position, to then stay sitting for several moments until any dizziness or lightheadedness passes, and to then stand up slowly. Assistance with ambulation may be required.

◆ Serious adverse effects
Psychological
Confusion, agitation, hallucinations, amnesia. All benzodiazepines have the potential to cause these symptoms, particularly in older patients who have been taking higher doses or taking the drugs for prolonged periods. Discuss the case with the healthcare provider and make plans to cooperatively approach the gradual reduction of the medication to prevent withdrawal symptoms and rebound insomnia.

Excessive use or abuse. The habitual use of benzodiazepines may result in physical dependence. Discuss the case with the healthcare provider and make plans to cooperatively approach the gradual withdrawal of the medications that are being abused. Assist the patient

Table 13.1 Benzodiazepines Used for Sedation and Hypnosis

GENERIC NAME	BRAND NAME	AVAILABILITY	ADULT ORAL DOSAGE RANGE	COMMENTS
estazolam	—	Tablets: 1, 2 mg	Hypnosis: 1-2 mg at bedtime	Intermediate acting; Schedule IV; used to treat insomnia; tapering therapy recommended to reduce rebound insomnia; minimal morning hangover
flurazepam	Flurazepam, Apo-Flurazepam ♣	Capsules: 15, 30 mg	Hypnosis: 15-30 mg at bedtime	Long acting; Schedule IV; used for short-term treatment of insomnia for up to 4 wk; morning hangover may be significant; rebound insomnia and rapid eye movement sleep occur less frequently
lorazepam ❶ ⇄ Do not confuse lorazepam with loperamide.	Ativan ⇄ Do not confuse Ativan with Ambien, or Atarax ♣ Apo-Lorazepam ♣	Tablets: 0.5, 1, 2 mg Oral solution: 2 mg/mL Injection: 2, 4 mg/mL in 1-, 10-mL vials; 2 mg/mL in prefilled syringes	Hypnosis: 2-4 mg at bedtime	Used primarily to treat insomnia but may also be used for preoperative anxiety, status epilepticus; IM and IV administration also available
midazolam	—	Syrup: 2 mg/mL Suspension: 1 mg/ml Injection: 1, 5 mg/mL in 1-, 2-, 5-, 10-mL vials; 2 mg/2 mL, 4 mg/2 mL in prefilled syringes IV: 1, 2 mg/mL in 100 mL container	Preoperatively: 0.07-0.08 mg/kg IM 1 hr before surgery Induction of anesthesia: 0.2-0.3 mg/kg IV Conscious sedation: 0.5-2 mg IV slowly over 2 min; repeat every 2-3 min as needed	Short acting; Schedule IV; causes amnesia in most patients; lower dosages for patients more than 55 yr old Onset: IM, 15 min; IV, 3-5 min Duration: IM, 30-60 min; IV, 2-6 hr
quazepam	Doral	Tablets: 15 mg	Hypnosis: 7.5-15 mg at bedtime	Long acting; Schedule IV; used to treat insomnia; tapering therapy recommended to reduce rebound insomnia; morning hangover may be significant
temazepam	Restoril ⇄ Do not confuse Restoril with Remeron, Risperdal, or Vistaril. Novo-Temazepam ♣	Capsules: 7.5, 15, 22.5, 30 mg	Hypnosis: 15-30 mg at bedtime	Intermediate acting; Schedule IV; used to treat insomnia; minimal if any morning hangover; rebound insomnia may occur
triazolam	Halcion ⇄ Do not confuse Halcion with Haldol. Apo-Triazo ♣	Tablets: 0.125, 0.25 mg	Hypnosis: 0.125-0.5 mg at bedtime	Short acting; Schedule IV; used to treat insomnia but tends to lose effectiveness within 2 wk; tapering therapy recommended to reduce rebound insomnia; rapid onset of action; no morning hangover

IM, Intramuscular(ly); *IV,* intravenous(ly).

♣ Available in Canada.   ⇄ Do not confuse.   ❶ High-alert medication.

with recognizing the abuse problem. Identify the patient's underlying needs and plan for the more appropriate management of those needs. Provide for the emotional support of the individual and display an accepting attitude. Be kind but firm.

Blood dyscrasias. Blood dyscrasias are rare but have been reported. Routine laboratory studies (e.g., red blood cell count, white blood cell [WBC] count, differential and platelet counts) should be scheduled. Stress that the patient should return for these tests. Monitor the patient for the development of a sore throat, fever, purpura, jaundice, or excessive and progressive weakness.

Hepatotoxicity. The symptoms of hepatotoxicity are anorexia, nausea, vomiting, jaundice, hepatomegaly, splenomegaly, and abnormal liver function tests (e.g., elevated levels of bilirubin, aspartate aminotransferase [AST], alanine aminotransferase [ALT], gamma-glutamyltransferase [GGT], and alkaline phosphatase; increased prothrombin time).

◆ *Drug interactions*

Antihistamines, alcohol, analgesics, anesthetics, tranquilizers, narcotics, cimetidine, disulfiram, isoniazid, rifampin, erythromycin, and other sedative-hypnotics. All of these agents increase the toxic effects of these drugs.

Smoking. Smoking enhances the metabolism of benzodiazepines. Larger doses may be necessary to maintain sedative effects in patients who smoke.

DRUG CLASS: NONBENZODIAZEPINE SEDATIVE-HYPNOTIC AGENTS

Actions

The nonbenzodiazepine sedative-hypnotic drugs are listed in Table 13.2. They represent a variety of chemical classes, all of which cause CNS depression. These include the histamine-1 blockers diphenhydramine and doxylamine (i.e., antihistamines); doxepin, which is a tricyclic antidepressant; benzodiazepine receptor agonists (zaleplon, zolpidem, eszopiclone); melatonin, which is a hormone secreted from the pineal gland (see Chapter 47); melatonin-receptor stimulants (ramelteon, tasimelteon); and valerian, which is an herbal medicine (see Chapter 47). The newest agent used for insomnia is the novel orexin receptor antagonist, suvorexant. All of these drugs have somewhat variable effects on REM sleep, tolerance development, rebound REM sleep, and insomnia.

Uses

Antihistamines—particularly diphenhydramine and doxylamine—have sedative properties that may be used for the short-term treatment of mild insomnia. These drugs are common ingredients in over-the-counter sleep aids. Because tolerance develops after only a few nights of use, increasing the dose actually causes a more restless and irregular sleep pattern. Doxylamine has a longer half-life of approximately 10 hours, which frequently causes a morning hangover.

Doxepin is a tricyclic antidepressant. At lower doses it works on histamine-1 receptors, which is thought to promote and maintain sleep. It can cause dry mouth and constipation.

Suvorexant is an orexin receptor antagonist. Orexins promote wakefulness; suvorexant blocks binding to orexins. It is a Schedule IV controlled substance. It has been shown to improve falling asleep and maintaining sleep.

Melatonin is available over the counter as a sleep aid. It appears to be particularly useful for patients who have been traveling through time zones and who are experiencing jet lag. Because this medicine is classified as a dietary supplement and thus is not regulated by the FDA, there may be inconsistencies with regard to its potency (see Chapter 47).

Ramelteon and tasimelteon are melatonin receptor stimulants and are the first members of this class to be approved by the FDA. Ramelteon is used to treat patients with insomnia who have difficulty falling asleep. Tasimelteon is used to help blind persons, who are not sensitive to night and day, maintain a circadian rhythm and normal sleep patterns.

Valerian, which is an herbal medicine, has been used for hundreds of years as a mild sedative. Its mechanism of action is unknown, but it may inhibit the enzyme that metabolizes GABA, thereby prolonging the inhibitory neurotransmitter's duration of action. Like melatonin, valerian is classified as a dietary supplement, and thus it is not regulated by the FDA. There may be differences in the strength and potency of this substance among distributors.

As a result of their effect on sleep patterns and REM sleep, the use of benzodiazepines is diminishing in favor of the newer benzodiazepine receptor agonists such as zaleplon, zolpidem, and eszopiclone, which bind to different GABA receptors in the CNS. In contrast to benzodiazepines, zaleplon, zolpidem, and eszopiclone have less effect on sleep stages 3 and 4 and REM sleep. These agents are used as hypnotics to produce sleep. The recommended period of use for these benzodiazepine receptor agonists is 7 to 10 days, with reevaluation of the patient if use exceeds 2 to 3 weeks. Daytime drowsiness is generally not a problem with these agents because of their short half-lives, although it is more likely with eszopiclone. The return of insomnia has been reported after the discontinuation of these drugs. Zaleplon has a short onset of action and duration of 2 to 4 hours. It is used clinically for people who have difficulty getting to sleep and for those who awaken in the middle of the night. Zolpidem has a similar onset of action but duration of 3 to 5 hours. It is more effective for helping patients get to sleep and for prolonging sleep duration without causing a morning hangover.

Eszopiclone is the newest of these agents. Its onset of action is somewhat slower than that of the other two agents, but its duration of action is 5 to 8 hours, thus

| | Table 13.2 | **Nonbenzodiazepine Sedative-Hypnotic Agents** |

GENERIC NAME	BRAND NAME	AVAILABILITY	ADULT ORAL DOSAGE RANGE	COMMENTS
dexmedetomidine ❶	Precedex	Infusion: 100, 200 mcg/mL in 2-mL vials; 200 mcg/50 mL vials; 400 mcg/100 mL vials	Intravenous sedation: 1 mcg/kg over 10 min followed by the infusion of 0.2-0.7 mcg/kg/hr with the use of a controlled-infusion device	For the sedation of initially intubated and mechanically ventilated patients in the intensive care setting; infusion should not continue for more than 24 hr
diphenhydramine ⇄ *Do not confuse diphenhydramine with dicyclomine or dipyridamole.*	Banophen, Diphenhist Simply Sleep 🍁	Tablets: 25, 50 mg Capsules: 25, 50 mg Liquid: 12.5 mg/5 mL; 6.25 mg/mL in 30 mL bottle Syrup: 12.5 mg/5 mL in 237 mL bottle	Sedation: 25-50 mg at bedtime	Over-the-counter availability; used for mild insomnia for up to 1 wk; tolerance develops, and increased dosage causes more adverse effects with no additional efficacy
doxepin	Silenor	Tablets: 3, 6 mg	Hypnosis: 3-6 mg once daily within 30 min of bedtime	Avoid doses > 6 mg/day. It is also used in depression but in higher doses.
doxylamine	Sleep Aid	Tablets: 25 mg	Sedation: 25 mg at bedtime	Over-the-counter availability; morning hangover may be significant; see diphenhydramine on p. 194
eszopiclone	Lunesta	Tablets: 1, 2, 3 mg	Hypnosis: 2-3 mg	Onset within 45 min; duration 5-8 hr Older adult patients should start with 1 mg; see "Drug Interactions" on p. 194
melatonin	—	—	—	See Chapter 47
ramelteon ⇄ *Do not confuse ramelteon with Remeron, Remegel, Reminyl, or Renagel.*	Rozerem ⇄ *Do not confuse Rozerem with Remeron, Remegel, Reminyl, or Renagel.*	Tablets: 8 mg	Hypnosis: 8 mg within 30 min of bedtime	Do not take with or immediately after a high-fat meal
suvorexant	Belsomra	Tablets: 5, 10, 15, 20 mg	Hypnosis: 10 mg once daily within 30 min of bedtime; may increase to a maximum of 20 mg once daily	Schedule IV drug; may be beneficial in patients having problems falling asleep and staying asleep
valerian ⇄ *Do not confuse valerian with Valium*	—	—	—	See Chapter 47

Continued

Table 13.2   Nonbenzodiazepine Sedative-Hypnotic Agents—cont'd

GENERIC NAME	BRAND NAME	AVAILABILITY	ADULT ORAL DOSAGE RANGE	COMMENTS
tasimelteon	Hetlioz	Capsule: 20 mg	Hypnosis: 20 mg once daily at the same time each night before bedtime	Used to treat non–24-hour sleep-wake disorder in blind persons; may take weeks to months to be effective due to variation in circadian rhythms
zaleplon ⇄ Do not confuse zaleplon with zolpidem.	Sonata ⇄ Do not confuse Sonata with Soma.	Capsules: 5, 10 mg	Hypnosis: 10 mg at bedtime; Maintenance: 5-20 mg	Schedule IV; short acting; onset within 30 min, duration 2-4 hr; older adults or low-weight patients should start with 5 mg
zolpidem ⇄ Do not confuse zolpidem with zaleplon.	Ambien ⇄ Do not confuse Ambien with Ativan or Atarax. ♣	Tablets: 5, 10 mg	Hypnosis: Women: 5 mg at bedtime Men: 5-10 mg at bedtime	Schedule IV; short acting; onset within 30 min, duration 3-5 hr; older adult patients should start with 5-mg immediate-release tablets or 6.25-mg controlled-release tablets; place a sublingual tablet under tongue, where it will disintegrate in seconds; do not chew, break, or split the tablet; sublingual tablets and oral spray should not be administered with or immediately after a meal
	Ambien CR	Tablets, controlled-release: 6.25, 12.5 mg	Hypnosis: Women: 6.25 mg at bedtime Men: 6.25-12.5 mg at bedtime	
	Edluar	Tablets, sublingual: 1.75, 3.5, 5, 10 mg	Hypnosis: Women: 5 mg Men: 5-10 mg	
	Zolpimist	Oral spray: 5 mg/actuation		
	Intermezzo	Tablets, sublingual 1.75, 3.5 mg		

♣ Available in Canada.   ⇄ Do not confuse.   ❶ High-alert medication.

making it more effective for patients who wake up during the night or early morning. It has been reported to cause morning hangover, especially among older patients and with higher doses.

Therapeutic Outcomes
The primary therapeutic outcomes sought from miscellaneous sedative-hypnotic agents are as follows:
1. To produce mild sedation
2. For short-term use to produce sleep

❖ **Nursing Implications of Nonbenzodiazepine Sedative-Hypnotic Agents**
◆ *Premedication assessment*
1. Record the patient's baseline vital signs (i.e., blood pressure, pulse, and respirations); measure the patient's blood pressure with him or her in both sitting and lying positions.
2. Check for the patient's history of hepatic disease.
3. Ask female patients if they are pregnant or breastfeeding if age appropriate.

◆ *Availability, dosage, and administration.* See Table 13.2. The habitual use of sedative-hypnotic agents may result in physical dependence. Rapid discontinuance after long-term use may result in symptoms that are similar to those of alcohol withdrawal, such as weakness, anxiety, delirium, and generalized seizures. Discontinuation consists of gradual withdrawal over 2 to 4 weeks.

Zaleplon, zolpidem, and eszopiclone have a very rapid onset of action. These agents should be taken only immediately before going to bed or after the patient has gone to bed and then has difficulty falling asleep.

◆ *Common adverse effects*
Neurologic
Hangover, sedation, lethargy, decreased level of alertness. General adverse effects include drowsiness, lethargy, headache, muscle or joint pain, and mental depression. Some people experience transient restlessness and anxiety before falling asleep. Morning hangover commonly occurs after the administration of hypnotic doses of doxylamine, as well as the long-acting benzodiazepines quazepam and

flurazepam, and it is also being reported with eszopiclone. Patients may display dulled affect, subtle distortion of mood, and impaired coordination.

Patients may complain of morning hangover, blurred vision, and transient hypotension upon arising. If the hangover effect becomes troublesome, the dosage should be reduced, the medication should be changed, or both. People who work around machinery, drive a car, pour and give medications, or perform other duties for which they must remain mentally alert should not take these medications while working.

Cardiovascular

Transient hypotension when arising. Explain to the patient the need to first rise to a sitting position, to then stay sitting for several moments until any dizziness or lightheadedness passes, and to then stand up slowly. Assistance with ambulation may be required.

Psychological

Restlessness, anxiety. These adverse effects are usually mild and do not warrant discontinuing the medication. Encourage the patient to try to relax and to let the sedative effect take over. Older patients and those in severe pain may respond paradoxically with excitement,

euphoria, restlessness, and confusion. Safety measures such as the maintenance of bed rest, side rails, and observation should be used during this period. Pain medications may also be administered, if indicated.

◆ *Drug interactions*

Antihistamines, alcohol, analgesics, anesthetics, tranquilizers, narcotics, cimetidine, disulfiram, isoniazid, rifampin, erythromycin, ketoconazole, and other sedative-hypnotics. All these agents increase the toxic effects of all sedative-hypnotic agents.

Fluvoxamine. Fluvoxamine specifically inhibits the metabolism of ramelteon, thus causing excessive sedation. Patients who are receiving fluvoxamine should not take ramelteon.

Rifampin. Rifampin significantly enhances the metabolism of eszopiclone and ramelteon, thereby reducing the therapeutic effect. Consider the use of zolpidem instead.

Food. The presence of food—particularly food with a high fat content—slows the absorption of zolpidem, zaleplon, eszopiclone, and ramelteon, slowing the onset of action. For a faster onset of action, do not administer these drugs with or immediately after a meal.

Get Ready for the NCLEX® Examination!

Key Points

- There are many types of sleep disorders, but the most common is insomnia.
- Most cases of insomnia are short lived and can be effectively treated by nonpharmacologic methods, such as a back rub, eating a lighter meal in the evening, eliminating naps, and reducing the use of alcohol and stimulants such as caffeine and nicotine.
- People who have insomnia that lasts for more than 1 month and who also experience daytime impairment of their social and employment responsibilities should be referred to a healthcare provider for a complete history and physical assessment. There may be other underlying conditions that must be treated before the patient resorts to the use of sedative-hypnotic agents.
- A variety of sedative-hypnotic drugs are available for pharmacologic treatment; however, the drugs of choice are the nonbenzodiazepines (e.g., zaleplon, zolpidem, eszopiclone) because of their wide margin of safety.

Additional Learning Resources

SG Go to your Study Guide for additional Review Questions for the NCLEX® Examination, Critical Thinking Clinical Situations, and other learning activities to help you master this chapter content.

Go to your Evolve website (https://evolve.elsevier.com/Clayton) for additional online resources.

Review Questions for the NCLEX® Examination

1. A patient was discussing a recent development of nightmares and restlessness since the discontinuation of triazolam (Halcion) with the nurse, who recognized the symptoms of which sleep disorder?
   1. Rebound insomnia
   2. Terminal insomnia
   3. Paradoxical excitement
   4. Initial insomnia
2. The nurse is reviewing an order for a sleep aid for a patient who was complaining of insomnia. The nurse understands that a sedative is different from a hypnotic in which manner?
   1. The sedative causes feelings of relaxation and rest, and the hypnotic agent causes feelings of restlessness and anxiety.
   2. The sedative causes feelings of relaxation and rest, and the hypnotic agent produces sleep.
   3. The hypnotic agent produces sleep, and the sedative causes no hangover effect.
   4. The hypnotic agent causes feelings of relaxation and rest, and the sedative produces sleep.

3. A patient who has been receiving benzodiazepines for several years was told by the nurse that this may cause which condition as a complication?
   1. Nephrotoxicity
   2. A rush of morning energy with repeated usage
   3. Withdrawal symptoms if the drug is discontinued rapidly
   4. Seizures during the time that the drug is being administered

4. The nurse is making rounds at 0200 on the unit during the night shift and notes that one of the older patients is awake. The nurse reviews the patient's bedtime medication and sees that 5 mg of zolpidem (Ambien) was administered at 2100. What interventions are appropriate for the nurse to do next? *(Select all that apply.)*
   1. Repeat the dose if ordered.
   2. Provide patient comfort measures (i.e., back rub, quiet room, etc.).
   3. Determine what the patient normally does at home when unable to sleep.
   4. Keep the patient awake to prevent rebound sleep.
   5. Assess for paradoxical symptoms and provide safety measures.

5. The nurse was discussing the difference between temazepam (Restoril) and zolpidem (Ambien) with a patient requesting drug therapy for sleep disturbance. Which of the following statements are appropriate? *(Select all that apply.)*
   1. "When you take Restoril, it can cause rebound insomnia if you abruptly stop taking it without tapering the drug."
   2. "There is no difference between these drugs; you can take them without any worries."
   3. "Ambien is also available in a sublingual tablet form, which disintegrates in seconds."
   4. "The side effect of morning drowsiness is only caused by Restoril, not Ambien."
   5. "Ambien is used for short-term treatment of insomnia."

6. The nurse taking care of a patient who was admitted for an overdose of lorazepam (Ativan) knows which antidote will be used?
   1. Fluvoxamine
   2. Temazepam (Restoril)
   3. Flumazenil
   4. Selegiline (Eldepryl)

7. The nurse is monitoring laboratory results for a patient who has been taking quazepam (Doral) for several years. Which of the following tests need to be followed to monitor for hepatotoxicity? *(Select all that apply.)*
   1. AST
   2. Platelet count
   3. Alkaline phosphatase
   4. WBC
   5. ALT

8. A patient came in to the clinic complaining of not being able to get a good night's sleep for the past month, as he finds that he frequently awakens throughout the night. The nurse recognizes this condition as which sleep disorder?
   1. Initial insomnia
   2. Intermittent insomnia
   3. Terminal insomnia
   4. Transient insomnia

Drugs Used to Treat Neurodegenerative Disorders

14

Objectives

1. Identify the signs and symptoms of Parkinson's disease.
2. Identify the neurotransmitter that is found in excess and the neurotransmitter that is deficient in people with parkinsonism.
3. Describe the reasonable expectations of the medications that are prescribed for the treatment of Parkinson's disease.
4. Cite the action of carbidopa, levodopa, and apomorphine on the neurotransmitters involved in Parkinson's disease.
5. Explain the action of entacapone and of the monoamine oxidase inhibitors (selegiline, safinamide, and rasagiline) as it relates to the treatment of Parkinson's disease.
6. Cite the specific symptoms that should show improvement when anticholinergic agents are administered to the patient with Parkinson's disease.
7. Explain the action of the agents used in the treatment of Alzheimer's disease.

Key Terms

Parkinson's disease (PĂR-kĭn-sĕnz dĭ-ZĒZ) (p. 199)
dopamine (DŌ-pă-mēn) (p. 199)
neurotransmitter (nyū-rō-TRĂNZ-mĭ-tĕr) (p. 199)
acetylcholine (ăs-ē-tĭl-KŌ-lēn) (p. 199)
anticholinergic agents (ĂN-tē-kō-lĭn-ŬR-jĭk) (p. 201)
tremors (TRĔ-mŭrz) (p. 202)

dyskinesia (dĭs-kĭ-NĒ-zhă) (p. 202)
propulsive, uncontrolled movement (prō-PŬL-sĭv ŭn-kŏn-TRŌLD MŬV-mĕnt) (p. 203)
akinesia (ă-kĭ-NĒ-zhă) (p. 203)
livedo reticularis (lĭ-VĒ-dō rĭ-tĭk-yĕ-LĀR-ĭs) (p. 209)
Alzheimer's disease (ĂLZ-hī-mŭrz) (p. 217)

PARKINSON'S DISEASE

Parkinson's disease is a chronic, progressive disorder of the central nervous system. It is the second most common neurodegenerative disease after Alzheimer's disease. An estimated 1% of the US population that is more than 50 years old, 2% of the population that is more than 60 years old, and 4% to 5% of the population 85 years old or older have this disorder. Thirty percent of patients report an onset of symptoms before the age of 50 years; 40% report that the onset occurred between the ages of 50 and 60 years; and the remainder report that their symptoms began after the age of 60 years. The incidence is slightly higher in men than women, and all races and ethnic groups are affected. Characteristic motor symptoms include muscle tremors, slowness of movement (i.e., bradykinesia) when performing activities of daily living (ADLs), muscle weakness with rigidity, and alterations in posture and equilibrium.

The symptoms associated with parkinsonism are caused by a deterioration of the dopaminergic neurons in the substantia nigra pars compacta, which results in a depletion of dopamine along the nigrostriatal pathway that extends into neurons in the autonomic ganglia, the basal ganglia, and the spinal cord and causes progressive neurologic deficits. These areas of the brain are responsible for maintaining posture and muscle tone, as well as for regulating voluntary smooth muscle activity and other nonmotor activities. Normally, a balance exists between **dopamine**, which is an inhibitory **neurotransmitter**, and **acetylcholine**, which is an excitatory neurotransmitter. With a deficiency of dopamine, a relative increase in acetylcholine activity occurs and causes the symptoms of parkinsonism. About 80% of the dopamine in the neurons of the substantia nigra pars compacta of the brain must be depleted for symptoms to develop.

Whereas the motor symptoms associated with parkinsonism have been considered to be the hallmarks of the disease, subtle nonmotor symptoms are now being recognized as occurring as much as 10 years before the onset of motor symptoms. Nonmotor symptoms usually start with constipation, progressing over the next few years with orthostatic hypotension, nocturnal sleep disturbances with daytime somnolence, depression, and progressing dementia. It is not known yet whether early treatment with medicines that control the symptoms of Parkinson's disease will slow the progression of the disease.

There are two types of parkinsonism. Primary or idiopathic parkinsonism is caused by a reduction in dopamine-producing cells in the substantia nigra pars compacta. The causes are not yet known, but there appear to be both genetic and environmental factors associated with its development. Approximately 10% to 15% of cases appear to be inherited. Secondary parkinsonism is caused by head trauma, intracranial infections, tumors, and recurrent exposure to drugs and pesticides. Medicines that deplete dopamine and thus cause secondary parkinsonism include dopamine antagonists such as haloperidol, phenothiazines, reserpine, methyldopa, and metoclopramide. In most cases of drug-induced parkinsonism, recovery is complete if the drug is discontinued.

Life Span Considerations
Parkinson's Disease

Parkinson's disease, which is most often seen in geriatric patients, causes a relative excess of acetylcholine as a result of a deficiency of dopamine. Drug therapy with dopaminergic agents increases dopamine availability, whereas anticholinergic medicines may be taken to counterbalance the excess availability of acetylcholine. Approximately 40% of patients with parkinsonism have some degree of clinical depression as a result of the reduced availability of the active metabolites of dopamine in the brain.

All drugs that are prescribed for the treatment of Parkinson's disease produce a pharmacologic effect on the central nervous system. An assessment of the patient's mental status and physical functioning before the initiation of therapy is essential to serve as a baseline so that comparisons can be made with subsequent evaluations.

Parkinson's disease is both progressive and incurable. The goals of treatment are to moderate the symptoms and to slow the progression of the disease. It is important to encourage the patient to take the medications as scheduled and to stay as active and involved in ADLs as possible.

Orthostatic hypotension is common with most of the medicines that are used to treat Parkinson's disease. To provide for patient safety, teach the patient to rise slowly from a supine or sitting position, and encourage the patient to sit or lie down if he or she is feeling faint.

Constipation is a frequent problem among patients with Parkinson's disease. Instruct the patient to drink six to eight 8-ounce glasses of liquid daily and to increase bulk in the diet to prevent constipation. Bulk-forming laxatives may also need to be added to the daily regimen.

The motor symptoms of parkinsonism start insidiously and are almost imperceptible at first, with weakness and tremors gradually progressing to involve movement disorders throughout the body (Fig. 14.1). The symptoms usually begin on one side of the body (i.e., asymmetric onset and progression) as a tremor of a finger or hand, and they then progress to become bilateral. The upper part of the body is usually affected

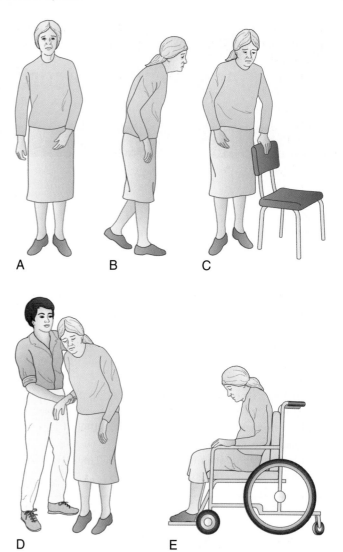

Fig. 14.1 **Stages of Parkinsonism.** (A) Flexion of the affected arm. The patient leans toward the unaffected side. (B) Slow, shuffling gait. (C) The patient has increased difficulty walking and looks for sources of support to prevent falls. (D) Further progression of weakness. The patient requires assistance from another person for ambulation. (E) Profound disability. The patient may be confined to a wheelchair as a result of increasing weakness.

first. Eventually the individual has postural and gait alterations that result in the need for assistance with total care needs. Varying degrees of depression are the most common (i.e., 40% to 50%) nonmotor symptom associated with Parkinson's disease. Most patients with depression also develop feelings of anxiety, and this sometimes includes panic attacks. Chronic fatigue, which is another common symptom, may also contribute to depression. Dementia that resembles Alzheimer's disease occurs in a significant number of patients, but there is continuing debate as to whether it is part of the Parkinson's disease process or if it is caused by concurrent drug therapy, Alzheimer's disease, or other factors. Dementia is characterized by the slowing of the thought processes, lapses in memory, and a loss of impulse control. The diagnosis of Parkinson's disease is based on a careful history taking, a physical examination, and a positive response to dopaminergic treatment. There are no laboratory tests or imaging studies that can confirm the diagnosis.

Nurses can have a major influence in the positive use of coping mechanisms as the patient and family express varying emotional responses. The primary goal of nursing interventions should be to keep the patient socially interactive and participating in ADLs. This can be accomplished through physical therapy, adherence to the drug regimen, and management of the course of treatment.

DRUG THERAPY FOR PARKINSON'S DISEASE

ACTIONS

The goal of the treatment of parkinsonism is minimizing the symptoms because there is no cure for the disease. Pharmacologic goals are to relieve symptoms and to restore dopaminergic activity and neurotransmitter function to as close to normal as possible. Treatment is usually started when symptoms progress to the point that they interfere with the patient's ability to perform at work or to function in social situations or they impair quality of life. The goal is to improve motor and nonmotor symptoms to optimize quality of life. Drug therapy includes the use of the following: monoamine oxidase type B (MAO-B) inhibitors (rasagiline, safinamide, selegiline), possibly to slow the deterioration of dopaminergic nerve cells; dopamine agonists (carbidopa-levodopa, ropinirole, pramipexole, rotigotine, apomorphine), amantadine (dopamine reuptake inhibitor that increases dopamine release and may have anticholinergic properties), or a catechol-*O*-methyltransferase (COMT) inhibitor (entacapone, which reduces metabolism of dopamine) in various combinations to enhance dopaminergic activity; and anticholinergic agents to inhibit the relative excess of cholinergic activity (e.g., tremor).

Therapy must be individualized, and realistic goals must be set for each patient. It is not possible to eliminate all symptoms of the disease because the medications' adverse effects would not be tolerated. The trend is to use the lowest possible dose of medication so that, as the disease progresses, dosages can be increased and other medicines added to obtain a combined effect. Unfortunately, as the disease progresses, drug therapy becomes more complex in terms of the number of medicines, dosage adjustments, the frequency of dosage administration, and the frequency of adverse effects. Therapies often have to be discontinued because of the impact of adverse effects on the quality of life.

USES

The MAO-B inhibitors may be used to slow the course of Parkinson's disease by possibly slowing the progression of the deterioration of dopaminergic nerve cells. A dopamine receptor agonist—often carbidopa-levodopa—is initiated when the patient develops functional impairment. Carbidopa-levodopa continues to be the most effective drug for the relief of symptoms; however, after 3 to 5 years, the drug's effect gradually wears off and the patient suffers from "on-off" fluctuations in levodopa activity. A COMT inhibitor (entacapone) or MAO-B inhibitor (safinamide) may be added to carbidopa-levodopa therapy to prolong the activity of the dopamine by slowing its rate of metabolism. Apomorphine may also be administered to treat off periods. Although seldom used in older adults, **anticholinergic agents** provide symptomatic relief from excessive acetylcholine. These agents are often used in combination to promote optimal levels of motor function (e.g., to improve gait, posture, or speech) and to decrease disease symptoms (e.g., tremors, rigidity, drooling). Fig. 14.2 presents an algorithm for the treatment for Parkinson's disease.

❖ NURSING IMPLICATIONS FOR PARKINSON'S DISEASE THERAPY

◆ Assessment

Unified Parkinson's disease rating scale. The Unified Parkinson's Disease Rating Scale (UPDRS) is often used to identify the baseline of Parkinson's disease symptoms at the time of diagnosis and to monitor changes in symptoms that may require medicine dosage adjustment. The UPDRS evaluates the following: (1) mentation, behavior, and mood; (2) self-evaluation of ADLs; (3) motor examination; (4) complications of therapy; (5) modified Hoehn and Yahr staging; and (6) the Schwab and England ADL Scale.

History of parkinsonism. Obtain a history of the patient's exposure to known conditions associated with the development of parkinsonian symptoms, such as head trauma, encephalitis, tumors, and drug exposure (e.g., phenothiazines, reserpine, methyldopa, metoclopramide, pesticides). In addition, ask if the person has a history of being exposed to toxic levels of metals or carbon monoxide.

Obtain data to classify the extent of parkinsonism that the patient is exhibiting. A rating scale such as the UPDRS may be used to assess the severity of Parkinson's disease on the basis of the degree of disability exhibited by the patient:

- Stage 1: Involvement of one limb; slight tremor or minor change in speech, facial expression, posture, or movement; mild disease
- Stage 2: Involvement of two limbs; early postural changes; some social withdrawal; possible depression
- Stage 3: Significant gait disturbances; moderate generalized disability
- Stage 4: Akinesia (i.e., an abnormal state of motor and psychic hypoactivity or muscle paralysis), rigidity, and severe disability; still able to walk or stand unassisted

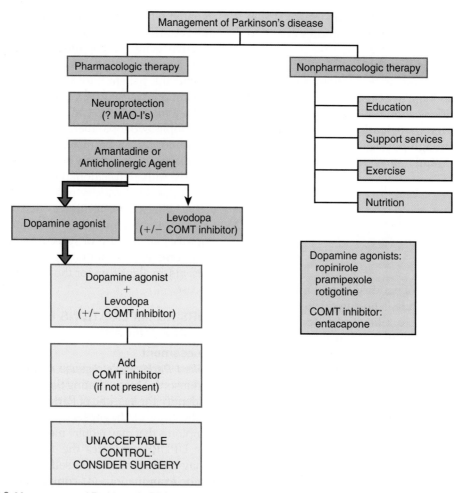

Fig. 14.2 Management of Parkinson's Disease. Consider neuroprotective therapy as soon as the diagnosis is made. When functional impairment starts, initiate a dopamine agonist; supplement this with levodopa when dopamine agonist monotherapy no longer provides satisfactory clinical control. Consider introducing supplemental levodopa in combination with a catechol-*O*-methyl transferase (COMT) inhibitor to extend levodopa's duration of action. Consider surgical intervention when parkinsonism cannot be satisfactorily controlled with medical therapies. (Modified from Olanow CW, Watts RL, Koller WC. An algorithm (decision tree) for the management of Parkinson's disease (2001): treatment guidelines. *Neurology.* 2001;56(11 suppl 5):S84; Chen JJ, Swope DM. Parkinson's disease. In DiPiro JT, Talbert RL, Yee GC, Matzke GR, Wells BG, Posey LM, eds. *Pharmacotherapy: A Pathophysiologic Approach.* 9th ed. New York: McGraw-Hill; 2014.)

- Stage 5: Unable to stand or walk or to perform all ADLs; wheelchair bound or bedridden unless aided

Motor function. Patients with Parkinson's disease progress through the following symptoms.

Tremor. Tremors (uncontrolled shaking) are initially so minor that they are observed only by the patient. They occur primarily when the individual is at rest, but they are more noticeable during emotional turmoil or periods of increased concentration. The tremors are often observed in the hands and may involve the jaw, lips, and tongue. A pill-rolling motion in the fingers and thumbs is characteristic. Tremors are usually reduced with voluntary movement.

Assess the degree of tremor involvement and specific limitations in activities that are being affected by the tremors. Obtain a history of the progression of the symptoms from the patient.

Dyskinesia. Dyskinesia is the impairment of the individual's ability to perform voluntary movements. This symptom commonly starts in one arm or hand. It is usually most noticeable because the patient ceases to swing the arm on the affected side while walking. Involuntary movements of muscles can cause jerking, spastic symptoms that characterize *chorea,* which is often an adverse response to treatment.

As dyskinesia progresses, movement—especially in the small muscle groups—becomes slow and jerky. This motion is often referred to as *cogwheel rigidity.* Muscle soreness, fatigue, and pain are associated with the prolonged muscle contractions. The patient develops a shuffling gait and may have difficulty with halting steps while walking (i.e., festination). When starting movement, there may be brief moments of immobility called *freezing.* Movements that were formerly automatic, such as getting out of a chair or walking, require a concentrated effort.

In addition to the shuffling gait, the head and spine flex forward, and the shoulders become rounded and stooped. As mobility deteriorates, the steps quicken and become shorter. **Propulsive, uncontrolled movement** forward or backward is evident, and patient safety becomes a primary consideration. Obtain antislip pads for chairs and other positioning devices. Perform a safety check of the patient's environment to prevent accidents and falls.

Bradykinesia. Bradykinesia is the extremely slow body movement that may eventually progress to akinesia (i.e., a lack of movement).

Facial appearance. The patient typically appears to be expressionless, as if wearing a mask. The eyes are wide open and fixed in position.

Nutrition. Complete an assessment of the person's dietary habits, any recent weight loss, and any difficulties with eating.

Salivation. As a result of excessive cholinergic activity, patients will salivate profusely. As the disease progresses, patients may be unable to swallow all secretions, and they will frequently drool. If the pharyngeal muscles are involved, the patient will have difficulty chewing and swallowing.

Psychological. The chronic nature of the disease and its associated physical impairment produce mood swings and serious depression. Patients commonly display a delayed reaction time.

Stress. Obtain a detailed history of the manner in which the patient has controlled his or her physical and mental stress.

Safety and self-care. Assess the level of assistance that is needed by the patient for mobility and for the performance of ADLs and self-care.

Family resources. Determine what family resources are available, as well as the closeness of the family, during both daily and stress-producing events.

◆ **Implementation**
- Implement planned interventions that are consistent with assessment data; identify the individual needs of the patient.
- Monitor and record the patient's vital signs, especially blood pressure, during the course of therapy. Report significant changes in blood pressure; these are most likely to occur during periods of dosage adjustment. Emphasize measures to prevent orthostatic hypotension.
- Monitor the patient's bowel function and implement measures to prevent constipation (e.g., adequate fluid intake, bulk in diet, exercise, use of stool softeners).

- Support the patient's efforts to remain mobile. Provide a safe environment by removing clutter and throw rugs; use correct equipment and supportive devices.
- Minimize deformities by encouraging the patient to maintain an erect posture. Maintain joint mobility with the use of both active and passive range-of-motion exercises.
- Nutritional needs must be carefully assessed, because dietary modifications will be required as the disease progresses. Be vigilant for difficulty with swallowing and realize that the patient may be prone to the aspiration of food or water. Weigh the patient weekly; evaluate and report fluctuations in body weight to the dietitian or healthcare provider.
- Provide a restful environment and attempt to keep stressors at a minimum.
- Monitor the patient's mood and affect and be alert for signs of depression. Mood alterations and depression are secondary to disease progression (e.g., lack of ability to participate in sex, immobility, incontinence) and may be expected, but they should not be ignored.
- Provide for patient safety during ambulation and delivery of care.
- Stress that the effectiveness of medication therapy may take several weeks.

◆ **Patient Education**
Nutrition. Teach the patient to drink at least six to eight glasses of water or fluid per day to maintain adequate hydration. Because constipation is often a problem, instruct the patient to include bulk in the diet and to use stool softeners as needed. As the disease progresses, the type and consistency of the foods eaten will need to be adjusted to meet the individual's needs. Because of fatigue and difficulty with eating, give assistance that is appropriate to the patient's degree of impairment. Do not rush the individual when he or she is eating, and cut foods into bite-sized pieces. Teach swallowing techniques to prevent aspiration. Plan six smaller meals daily rather than three larger meals.

Instruct the patient to weigh himself or herself weekly. Ask the patient to state the guidelines for weight loss or gain that should be reported to the healthcare provider.

Stress that vitamins should not be taken unless they have been prescribed by the healthcare provider. Pyridoxine (vitamin B$_6$) will reduce the therapeutic effect of levodopa.

Stress management. Explain to the patient and caregivers about the importance of maintaining an environment that is as free from stress as possible. Explain that symptoms such as tremors are enhanced by anxiety.

Self-reliance. Encourage patients to perform as many ADLs as they can. Parkinson's disease is a progressive disorder; explain to caregivers that it is important not to take over and that they should encourage patients' self-maintenance, continued social involvement, and participation in activities such as hobbies. Use adaptive devices to help the patient with dressing, and purchase clothing with easy closures or fasteners such as Velcro. As mobility diminishes, use a bath chair and handheld shower nozzle to help the patient maintain his or her cleanliness.

Exercise. Instruct the patient and caregiver about the importance of maintaining correct body alignment, walking as erect as possible, and practicing the gait training taught by the physical therapy department. Gait training is essential if the patient is to delay the onset of shuffling and gait propulsion. Patients should wear sturdy, supportive shoes and use a cane, walker, or other assistive device to maintain mobility. Exercises to maintain the strength of facial muscles and of the tongue help the patient to maintain speech clarity and the ability to swallow. Active and passive range-of-motion exercises of all joints help to minimize deformities. Explain that maintaining the exercise program can increase the patient's long-term well-being.

Mood alterations. Explain to the patient and the caregiver that depression and mood alterations are secondary to disease progression (e.g., inability to participate in sex, immobility, incontinence) and are to be expected. Changes in mental outlook should be discussed with the healthcare provider.

Fostering health maintenance. Provide the patient and his or her significant others with important information contained in the specific drug monographs for the medicines that are prescribed, including the name of the medication; its dosage, route, and administration time; potential adverse effects; and drug-specific patient education.

Provide information to the patient, family, and caregivers about resources, including the American Parkinson Disease Association and the services and information available from this source. There are support groups for patients and families that can serve as caring environments for people with similar experiences and concerns. Respite care may also be available, which provides temporary services to the dependent older adult either at home or in an institutional setting to give the family relief from the demands of daily patient care.

Patient self-assessment. Enlist the patient's help with developing and maintaining a written record of monitoring parameters (e.g., degree of tremor relief, stability, changes in mobility and rigidity, sedation, constipation, drowsiness, mental alertness, deviations from the norm); see the Patient Self-Assessment Form for Antiparkinson Agents on the Evolve website. Complete the Premedication Data column for use as a baseline to track the patient's response to drug therapy. Ensure that the patient understands how to use the form, and instruct the patient to bring the completed form to follow-up visits. During follow-up visits, focus on issues that will foster adherence with the therapeutic interventions that have been prescribed.

DRUG CLASS: MONOAMINE OXIDASE TYPE B INHIBITORS

rasagiline (ra SA ji leen)
  Azilect (az a LECt)
safinamide (sa FIN a mide)
  Xadago (Ex a da go)
selegiline (se LE ji leen)
  Eldepryl (El da pril)

Actions

Selegiline, safinamide, and rasagiline are potent MAO-B inhibitors that reduce the metabolism of dopamine in the brain, thus allowing for greater dopaminergic activity. Although there are reports that these agents may be neuroprotective, there is currently no conclusive proof of this from clinical trials.

Uses

A combination of carbidopa and levodopa is the current drug of choice for the treatment of Parkinson's disease. Unfortunately, these agents lose effectiveness (i.e., the "on-off" phenomenon) and develop more adverse effects (i.e., dyskinesias) over time. It is often necessary to add other dopamine receptor agonists (e.g., pramipexole, ropinirole) or a COMT inhibitor (e.g., entacapone) to improve the patient's response and tolerance. The MAO-B inhibitors have adjunctive activity similar to carbidopa-levodopa for the treatment of Parkinson's disease. The combination of an MAO-B inhibitor and carbidopa-levodopa improves memory and motor speed, and it may also increase life expectancy.

The MAO-B inhibitors may be used early during the treatment of Parkinson's disease to slow the progression of symptoms and to delay the initiation of levodopa therapy. Selegiline was also recently approved for the treatment of depression.

Selegiline, rasagiline, and safinamide have different metabolic pathways and therefore somewhat different adverse effect profiles. Selegiline tablets and capsules, when swallowed, are metabolized to amphetamines that cause cardiovascular and psychiatric adverse effects. The orally disintegrating tablet dosage form allows the drug to be absorbed from the buccal area in the mouth, thereby avoiding much of the formation of these active metabolites. There is a notable difference in strength between the tablets and the orally disintegrating tablets. A 10-mg tablet of selegiline is approximately equal in potency to a 1.25-mg orally disintegrating tablet of selegiline. Rasagiline and safinamide are not metabolized to amphetamines, so cardiovascular and psychiatric adverse effects are minimal.

Therapeutic Outcomes

The primary therapeutic outcomes sought from MAO-B inhibitors for the treatment of parkinsonism are as follows:

1. Slowing the development of symptoms and the progression of the disease
2. Establishing a balance of dopamine and acetylcholine in the basal ganglia of the brain by enhancing the delivery of dopamine to brain cells

❖ Nursing Implications for Monoamine Oxidase Type B Inhibitor Therapy

◆ *Premedication assessment*

1. Perform a baseline assessment of parkinsonism with the use of the UPDRS.
2. Obtain a history of gastrointestinal (GI) symptoms.
3. Perform a baseline assessment of the patient's degree of alertness and orientation to name, place, and time before the initiation of therapy.
4. Check for any antihypertensive therapy that is currently prescribed. Monitor the patient's blood pressure daily in both the supine and standing positions. If antihypertensive medications are being taken, report this to the healthcare provider for possible dosage adjustment.
5. Check other medications prescribed; see Drug Interactions for MAO-B inhibitors later in this section.

◆ *Availability, dosage, and administration.* The dosage must be adjusted according to the patient's response and tolerance.

Adult: *PO* (see Table 14.1). Selegiline orally disintegrating tablets should be taken in the morning before breakfast, without liquid. Patients should not attempt to push selegiline orally disintegrating tablets through the foil backing. Patients should peel back the backing off one or two blisters (as prescribed) with dry hands and gently remove the tablets. Patients should immediately place the orally disintegrating selegiline tablets on top of the tongue, where they will disintegrate in seconds. Patients should avoid ingesting food or liquids for 5 minutes before and 5 minutes after taking orally disintegrating selegiline tablets.

After 2 to 3 days of treatment, the dosage of carbidopa-levodopa should start being titrated downward. Carbidopa-levodopa dosages may be able to be reduced by 10% to 30%.

◆ *Common adverse effects.* Selegiline and rasagiline cause relatively few adverse effects. They may increase the adverse dopaminergic effects of levodopa (e.g., chorea, confusion, hallucinations). Dosage reduction of levodopa is usually the optimal treatment.

Gastrointestinal

Constipation, stomach upset. Both of these effects may be minimized by a temporary reduction in dosage, administration with food, and the use of stool softeners for constipation.

◆ *Serious adverse effects*

Neurologic

Chorea, confusion, hallucinations. Selegiline and rasagiline may increase these adverse dopaminergic effects of levodopa, but these can be controlled by reducing the dosage of levodopa. Make regularly scheduled subsequent evaluations of the patient's mental status and

Table 14.1 Monoamine Oxidase Inhibitors Type B

GENERIC NAME	BRAND NAME	AVAILABILITY	INITIAL DOSAGE (PO)	MAXIMUM DAILY DOSAGE
rasagiline ⇄ Do not confuse rasagiline with repaglinide, raloxifene, Risperdal, or risperidone.	Azilect	Tablets: 0.5, 1 mg	Monotherapy: 1 mg once daily Adjunctive therapy: 0.5 mg once daily	1 mg 1 mg
selegiline ⇄ Do not confuse selegiline with Serentil, sertraline, or Salagen.	Eldepryl ⇄ Do not confuse Eldepryl with enalapril. Zelapar	Tablets and capsules: 5 mg Tablets, orally disintegrating: 1.25 mg	5 mg daily 1.25 mg once daily for at least 6 weeks with concomitant levodopa/carbidopa dissolved on the tongue; withhold food and liquid for at least 5 min	5 mg twice daily 2.5 mg before breakfast, at least 5 min before any liquid or breakfast
safinamide	Xadago	Tablets: 50, 100 mg	50 mg once daily	After 2 wk may increase to 100 mg once daily

⇄ Do not confuse.

compare findings. Report alterations in mood. Provide patient safety, be emotionally supportive, and assure the patient that these adverse effects usually dissipate as tolerance develops over the next few weeks.

Cardiovascular

Orthostatic hypotension. Monitor the patient's blood pressure daily in both the supine and standing positions. Anticipate the development of postural hypotension and take measures to prevent such an occurrence. Teach the patient to rise slowly from a supine or sitting position and encourage the patient to sit or lie down if feeling faint.

◆ Drug interactions

Levodopa. MAO-B inhibitors and levodopa have additive neurologic effects. These interactions may be beneficial because they often allow for a reduction in the dosage of levodopa.

Meperidine, tramadol, methadone. Fatal drug interactions have been reported between monoamine oxidase inhibitors (MAOIs) and these agents. Although these interactions have not been reported with selegiline, safinamide, or rasagiline, it is recommended that selegiline, safinamide, and rasagiline not be administered with any of these agents.

Dextromethorphan. Episodes of psychosis and bizarre behavior have been reported with selegiline and dextromethorphan. Do not administer these drugs concurrently.

Food. Patients should avoid foods and beverages with high tyramine content (e.g., Chianti wine, fava beans, cheeses), particularly if they are receiving selegiline in excess of 9 mg/day. Rare cases of hypertensive reactions have been reported.

Antihypertensive agents. A dosage adjustment of the antihypertensive agent is often necessary in response to excessive orthostatic hypotension.

Ciprofloxacin. This antibiotic inhibits the metabolism of rasagiline, thus significantly raising rasagiline serum levels and potentially causing significant hypertension. Use the combination very cautiously. Reduce the dose of rasagiline by half to avoid complications.

Antidepressants (tricyclic antidepressants, selective serotonin reuptake inhibitors, serotonin-norepinephrine reuptake inhibitors, St. John's Wort). Use these drugs with extreme caution in conjunction with MAO-B inhibitor therapy. Although rare, there is a potential for serotonin syndrome, which is manifested by behavioral and mental status changes, diaphoresis, muscular rigidity, hypertension, syncope, and death. Many patients are receiving antidepressants for the treatment of depression that frequently accompanies parkinsonism. Closely monitor patients for these symptoms.

Sympathomimetic amines (ephedrine, pseudoephedrine, phenylephrine). Cases of hypertensive crisis have rarely been reported among patients who are concurrently taking sympathomimetic amines and MAO-B inhibitors. Concurrent therapy is not recommended.

DRUG CLASS: DOPAMINE AGONISTS

carbidopa (kăr-bĭ-DŌ-pă)
levodopa (lē-vō-DŌ-pă)
  Sinemet (SĬN-ĕ-mĕt)
  ⇄ *Do not confuse Sinemet with Senokot.*
  Rytary (rye-TAR-ee)

Actions

Dopamine, when administered orally, does not enter the brain. However, levodopa *does* cross into the brain, where it is metabolized to dopamine and replaces the dopamine deficiency in the basal ganglia. Dopamine stimulates D_1, D_2, and D_3 dopamine receptors.

Sinemet and Rytary are combination products of carbidopa and levodopa that are used for treating the symptoms of Parkinson's disease. Carbidopa is an enzyme inhibitor that reduces the metabolism of levodopa, thus allowing for a greater portion of the administered levodopa to reach the desired receptor sites in the basal ganglia. Carbidopa has no effect when it is used alone; it must be used in combination with levodopa.

Uses

About 75% of patients with parkinsonism respond favorably to levodopa therapy. However, after a few years the response diminishes and becomes more uneven, and it is accompanied by many more adverse effects. This loss of therapeutic effect reflects the progression of the underlying disease process.

Carbidopa is used to reduce the dose of levodopa required by approximately 75%. When administered with levodopa, carbidopa increases plasma levels and the plasma half-life of levodopa.

Therapeutic Outcome

The primary therapeutic outcome sought from carbidopa-levodopa for the treatment of parkinsonism is the establishment of a balance of dopamine and acetylcholine in the basal ganglia of the brain by enhancing the delivery of dopamine to brain cells.

❖ Nursing Implications for Carbidopa-Levodopa Therapy

◆ Premedication assessment

1. Perform a baseline assessment of parkinsonism with the use of the UPDRS.
2. Obtain a history of GI and cardiovascular symptoms, including baseline vital signs (e.g., blood pressure, pulse).
3. Ask specifically about any symptoms of hallucinations, nightmares, dementia, or anxiety. Inquire about any urine testing that is being done.
4. All patients should be screened for the presence of closed-angle glaucoma before initiating therapy.

Patients with open-angle glaucoma can safely use levodopa. Do not administer the medicine to people with a history of glaucoma unless it has been specifically approved by the patient's healthcare provider.

5. Review the medicines that have been prescribed that may require dose adjustments. Plan to perform focused assessments to detect responses to therapy that would need to be reported to the healthcare provider.

◆ *Availability.* **PO:** Sinemet is a combination product that contains both carbidopa and levodopa. The combination product is available in ratios of 10/100, 25/100, and 25/250 mg of carbidopa and levodopa, respectively. There is also a sustained-release tablet (Sinemet CR) that contains either 25/100 mg or 50/200 mg of carbidopa and levodopa, respectively.

Rytary is an oral extended-release combination product that contains both carbidopa and levodopa. It is available in capsules in ratios of 23.75/95, 36.25/145, 48.75/195, and 61.25/245 mg of carbidopa and levodopa, respectively.

◆ *Dosage and administration.* **Adult:** *PO:* For patients who are not receiving levodopa initially, give Sinemet 10/100 or 25/100 mg three times daily, increasing by 1 tablet every other day, until a dosage of 6 tablets daily is attained. As therapy progresses and patients show indications of needing more levodopa, substitute Sinemet 25/250 mg, 1 tablet three or four times daily. Increase by 1 tablet every other day to a maximum of 8 tablets daily. See the manufacturer's guidelines for converting a patient from the immediate-release to the sustained-release formulation of Sinemet.

Administer this medication with food or milk to reduce gastric irritation. Therapy for at least 6 months may be necessary to determine this medication's full therapeutic benefits.

Extended-Release Formulations: Sinemet Extended-Release Tablets: For patients not currently receiving levodopa initially, start with Sinemet CR 50 mg/200 mg twice daily at intervals of 6 hours or more. Following an interval of at least 3 days between dosage adjustments, increase or decrease dosage based on response. Most patients are adequately treated with a dose that provides 400 to 1600 mg of levodopa per day in divided doses at intervals of 4 to 8 hours while awake. If an interval of less than 4 hours is used and/or if the divided doses are not equal, give the smaller doses at the end of the day.

Rytary Extended-Release Capsules: For patients not currently receiving levodopa initially, start with Rytary 23.75/95 mg three times daily for 3 days; on day 4, increase to 36.25/145 mg three times daily. The dose may be increased up to 97.5/390 mg three times daily, and the frequency of dosing may be increased to a maximum of five times daily if needed and tolerated (maximum: 612.5/2450 mg per day).

See the manufacturer's guidelines for converting a patient from immediate-release formulations to extended-release capsules.

◆ *Common adverse effects.* Levodopa causes many adverse effects, but most are dose related and reversible. Adverse effects vary greatly depending on the stage of the disease.

Gastrointestinal
Nausea, vomiting, anorexia. These effects can be reduced by slowly increasing the dose, dividing the total daily dosage into four to six doses, and administering the medication with food or antacids.

Cardiovascular
Orthostatic hypotension. Although the effects are generally mild, levodopa may cause some degree of orthostatic hypotension; this is manifested by dizziness and weakness, particularly when therapy is initiated. Tolerance usually develops after a few weeks of therapy. Monitor the patient's blood pressure daily in both the supine and standing positions. Anticipate the development of postural hypotension and take measures to prevent such an occurrence. Teach patients to rise slowly from a supine or sitting position, and encourage them to sit or lie down if feeling faint.

◆ *Serious adverse effects*
Neurologic
Chewing motions, bobbing, facial grimacing, rocking movements. These involuntary movements occur in about half of the patients who take levodopa for more than 6 months. A reduction in dosage may be beneficial.

Psychological
Nightmares, depression, confusion, hallucinations. Perform a baseline assessment of the patient's degree of alertness and orientation to name, place, and time before initiating therapy. Make regularly scheduled subsequent evaluations of mental status, and compare findings. Report alterations in mood. Provide for patient safety during these episodes. Reducing the daily dosage may control these adverse effects.

Cardiovascular
Tachycardia, palpitations. Take the patient's pulse at regularly scheduled intervals. Report any changes for further evaluation.

◆ *Drug interactions.* Sinemet and Rytary may be used to treat parkinsonism in conjunction with dopamine agonists, COMT inhibitors, or anticholinergic agents. The dosages of all medications may need to be reduced as a result of combined therapy.

Monoamine oxidase inhibitors (phenelzine, tranylcypromine, isocarboxazid, selegiline). These MAOIs unpredictably exaggerate the effects of levodopa. They should be discontinued at least 14 days before the administration of levodopa.

Isoniazid. Use this drug with caution in conjunction with levodopa. Discontinue isoniazid if patients who are taking levodopa develop hypertension, flushing, palpitations, and tremor.

Pyridoxine. Pyridoxine (vitamin B_6) in oral doses of 5 to 10 mg may reduce the therapeutic and toxic effects of levodopa. Normal diets contain less than 1 mg of pyridoxine, so dietary restrictions are not necessary. However, the ingredients of multiple vitamins should be considered.

Diazepam, chlordiazepoxide, clonidine, phenytoin. These agents appear to cause a deterioration of the therapeutic effects of levodopa. Use them with caution for patients with parkinsonism, and discontinue them if the patient's clinical status deteriorates.

Phenothiazines, haloperidol, risperidone, metoclopramide. An adverse effect associated with these agents is a Parkinson's-like syndrome. Because this condition will nullify the therapeutic effects of levodopa, do not use the drugs concurrently.

Epinephrine, amphetamines. Levodopa may increase the therapeutic and toxic effects of these agents. Monitor the patient for tachycardia, dysrhythmias, and hypertension. Reduce the dosage of these agents if necessary.

Antihypertensive agents. A dosage adjustment of the antihypertensive agent is frequently necessary in response to excessive orthostatic hypotension.

Anticholinergic agonists (benztropine, diphenhydramine, trihexyphenidyl). Although these agents are used to treat parkinsonism, they increase gastric deactivation and decrease the intestinal absorption of levodopa. The administration of doses of anticholinergic agents and levodopa should be separated by 2 hours or more.

Toilet bowl cleaners. The metabolites of levodopa react with toilet bowl cleaners to turn the urine red to black. This may also occur if the urine is exposed to air for long periods. Inform the patient that there is no cause for alarm.

---

amantadine hydrochoride (a-MAN-ta-dēn)
Gocovri (go-cover-ee)
Osmolex ER (oz-MO'-lex ER)

Amantadine is a compound developed originally to treat viral infections. It was administered to a patient with influenza A who also had parkinsonism. During the course of therapy for influenza, the patient showed definite improvement in the parkinsonian symptoms.

Actions

The exact mechanism of action is unknown but appears to be unrelated to the drug's antiviral activity. Amantadine seems to slow the destruction of dopamine, thus making the small amount present more effective. It may also aid in the release of dopamine from its storage sites. Unfortunately, about half of the patients who benefit from amantadine therapy begin to notice a reduction in benefit after 2 or 3 months. A dosage increase or temporary discontinuation followed by a reinitiation of therapy several weeks later may restore the therapeutic benefits. When being discontinued, amantadine should be gradually withdrawn.

Uses

Amantadine is used for the relief of symptoms associated with Parkinson's disease and for the treatment of susceptible strains of viral influenza A.

Recently two extended-release products became available. Gocovir (amantadine) ER is indicated for the treatment of dyskinesia in patients with Parkinson's disease receiving levodopa-based therapy, with or without concomitant dopaminergic medications. Osmolex (amantadine) ER indicated for the treatment of Parkinson's disease and for the treatment of drug-induced extrapyramidal reactions in adult patients

Therapeutic Outcome

The primary therapeutic outcome sought from amantadine in treating parkinsonism is to establish a balance of dopamine and acetylcholine in the basal ganglia of the brain by enhancing delivery of dopamine to brain cells.

❖ **Nursing Implications for Amantadine Therapy**
◆ *Premedication assessment*
1. Perform a baseline assessment of parkinsonism using the UPDRS.
2. Amantadine should be used with caution in patients with a history of seizure activity, liver disease, uncontrolled psychosis, or congestive heart failure. Amantadine may cause an exacerbation of these disorders.
3. Take baseline blood pressures in supine and standing positions.

◆ *Availability. PO:* 100-mg tablets; 100-mg capsules; 50 mg/5 mL syrup; 68.5, 137 mg Extended-release (24 hr) capsules (Gocovri); 129, 193, 258 mg Extended-release (24 hr) tablets (Osmolex ER).

◆ *Dosage and administration.* **Adult:** *PO:* Initially 100 mg two times daily; maximum daily dose is 400 mg. Because of the possibility of insomnia, plan the last dose to be administered in the afternoon, not at bedtime.

Gocovri (amantadine) ER: Initially 137 mg; after 1 week, increase to the recommended daily dosage of 274 mg

Osmolex (amantadine) ER: Initially 129 mg orally once daily in the morning; may be increased in weekly intervals to a maximum daily dose of 322 mg once daily in the morning

◆ *Common adverse effects.* Most of the adverse effects of amantadine therapy are dose related and reversible.

Neurologic

Confusion, disorientation, hallucinations, mental depression. Perform a baseline assessment of the patient's degree of alertness and orientation to name, place, and time before initiating therapy. Make regularly scheduled subsequent evaluations of mental status and compare findings. Report alterations.

Dizziness, lightheadedness. Provide patient safety during periods of dizziness or lightheadedness.

Gastrointestinal

Anorexia, nausea, abdominal discomfort. These side effects are usually mild and tend to resolve with continued therapy. Encourage the patient not to discontinue therapy without first consulting the healthcare provider.

Cardiovascular

Livedo reticularis (skin mottling). A dermatologic condition known as livedo reticularis is occasionally observed in conjunction with amantadine therapy. It is characterized by diffuse rose-colored mottling of the skin, often accompanied by ankle edema, predominantly in the extremities. It is more noticeable when the patient is standing or exposed to cold. It is reversible within 2 to 6 weeks after discontinuation of amantadine. However, discontinuing therapy is generally not necessary.

These side effects are usually mild and tend to resolve with continued therapy. Symptoms are enhanced by exposure to the cold or by prolonged standing. Encourage the patient not to discontinue therapy without first consulting the healthcare provider.

◆ *Serious adverse effects*

Gastrointestinal

Hepatotoxicity. The symptoms of hepatotoxicity are anorexia, nausea, vomiting, jaundice, hepatomegaly, splenomegaly, and abnormal liver function tests (elevated bilirubin, aspartate aminotransferase, alanine aminotransferase, gamma-glutamyltransferase, alkaline phosphatase, prothrombin time).

Neurologic

Seizure disorders, psychosis. Provide patient safety during episodes of dizziness; report symptoms for further evaluation.

Cardiovascular

Dyspnea/edema. If amantadine is used with patients who have a history of heart failure, assess lung sounds, additional edema, and weight gain on a regular basis.

◆ *Drug interactions*

Anticholinergic agents (trihexyphenidyl, benztropine, procyclidine, diphenhydramine) Amantadine may exacerbate the side effects of anticholinergic agents that may also be used to control the symptoms of parkinsonism. Confusion and hallucinations may gradually develop.

---

apomorphine (ă-pō-MŌR-fēn)
⇄ Do not confuse apomorphine with morphine.
Apokyn (ă-PŌ-kĭn)

The dosage of amantadine or the anticholinergic agent should be reduced.

Actions

Apomorphine is a nonergot dopamine agonist. It is thought to stimulate dopamine receptors in the brain, thereby temporarily restoring motor function. It is chemically related to morphine, but it does not have any opioid activity.

Uses

As Parkinson's disease progresses, patients often experience episodes of lower responsiveness to levodopa, which causes periods of hypomobility (e.g., inability to rise from a chair, speak, or walk). Apomorphine is used to treat the hypomobility associated with the "wearing off" of dopamine agonists, either near the end of a dosage cycle or at unpredictable times (i.e., the "on-off" phenomenon).

Therapeutic Outcomes

The primary therapeutic outcomes sought from apomorphine for the treatment of parkinsonism are improving motor and ADL scores and decreasing off time.

❖ **Nursing Implications for Apomorphine Therapy**
◆ *Premedication assessment*

1. Perform a baseline assessment of parkinsonism with the use of the UPDRS.
2. Obtain a history of cardiovascular symptoms, including the baseline vital signs (e.g., blood pressure, heart rate).
3. Perform a baseline assessment of the patient's degree of mobility, alertness, and orientation to name, place, and time before initiating therapy. Ask specifically whether he or she may be taking any other sedating medicines. Make regularly scheduled subsequent evaluations of blood pressure, pulse, mental status, and mobility and compare findings.

◆ *Availability.* *Subcutaneous:* 10 mg/mL in 3-mL cartridges.

◆ *Dosage and administration.* Apomorphine is administered most commonly with the use of a manual, reusable, multidose injector pen that holds a 3-mL cartridge of medicine. To avoid potential confusion with the use of the pen and inadvertent overdose, it is recommended that the dose of the drug be identified in milliliters rather than in milligrams. The pen is adjustable in 0.02-mL increments. A training pamphlet that addresses the use of the injector pen is available for patient use.

> ⚠ **Medication Safety Alert**
>
> *Do not administer apomorphine intravenously.* This drug may crystallize in the vein and form a thrombus or embolism.

Adult

Use of an antiemetic. One of the pharmacologic actions of apomorphine is emesis. The antiemetic trimethobenzamide (Tigan) should be administered orally at a dosage of 300 mg three times daily for at least 3 days before the initial dose of apomorphine. Discontinue trimethobenzamide as soon as it is needed for emesis, but no longer than 2 months. About 50% of patients are able to discontinue the antiemetic while continuing therapy with apomorphine. Do not use prochlorperazine or ondansetron (Zofran) as antiemetics (see Drug Interactions for apomorphine later in this section).

Subcutaneous: Initially, a test dose of 0.2 mL (2 mg) should be administered in the stomach area, upper leg, or upper arm. Both supine and standing blood pressures should be determined before administering the dose and again at 20, 40, and 60 minutes after administration. If significant orthostatic hypotension develops, therapy should be discontinued and the patient should receive no further doses of apomorphine.

If the patient tolerates the 0.2-mL dose and responds, then the starting dose should be 0.2 mL used on an as-needed (PRN) basis to treat off times. If needed, the dose can be increased in 0.1-mL (1-mg) increments every few days on an outpatient basis. The maximum recommended dose is 0.6 mL (6 mg).

If a patient discontinues therapy for longer than 1 week and then wishes to go back to the use of apomorphine, therapy should be reinitiated at the starting dose of 0.2 mL, with gradual increases in dosage to optimal therapy.

◆ *Common adverse effects.* Most adverse effects observed with apomorphine are direct extensions of its pharmacologic properties.

Gastrointestinal

Nausea, vomiting. These effects can be reduced by premedicating the patient with trimethobenzamide and then slowly increasing the dosage.

Cardiovascular

Orthostatic hypotension. Apomorphine commonly causes orthostatic hypotension, which is manifested by dizziness and weakness, particularly when therapy is initiated. Patients with Parkinson's disease are at risk for falling because of the underlying postural instability associated with the disease; apomorphine may increase the risk of falling by lowering blood pressure and altering mobility. Anticipate the development of postural hypotension and provide assistance when necessary. Monitor the patient's blood pressure before and during apomorphine therapy in both the supine and standing positions. Teach patients to rise slowly from a supine or sitting position; encourage them to sit or lie down if feeling faint.

◆ *Serious adverse effects*

Neurologic

Chewing motions, bobbing, facial grimacing, rocking movements. These involuntary movements (dyskinesias) occur in some patients, especially if they are also taking levodopa. A reduction in the dosage of the levodopa or apomorphine may be beneficial.

Sudden sleep events. Sleep episodes have been reported with the dopamine agonists (e.g., apomorphine, pergolide, pramipexole, ropinirole). These episodes are described as "sleep attacks" or "sleep episodes," and they include daytime sleep. Some sleep events have been reported as sudden and irresistible; other sleep events have been preceded by sufficient warning to prevent accidents. Patients who are taking dopamine agonists should be informed about the possibility of daytime sleepiness and outright sleep attacks with these medicines and allowed to make their own decisions about driving on the basis of their past experiences with the medicines. The assessment of patients who are at risk for sleep attacks is possible with the Epworth Sleepiness Scale.

Psychological

Nightmares, depression, confusion, hallucinations. Perform a baseline assessment of the patient's degree of alertness and orientation to name, place, and time before initiating therapy. Make regularly scheduled subsequent evaluations of mental status, and compare findings. Report alterations in mood. Provide for patient safety during these episodes. Reducing the daily medication dosage may control these adverse effects.

Cardiovascular

Tachycardia, palpitations. Take the patient's pulse at regularly scheduled intervals. Report any changes for further evaluation.

Genitourinary

Penile erection, priapism. Apomorphine may cause penile erection and, rarely, priapism (i.e., prolonged, painful erection). Apomorphine has been overused because of its ability to induce erection and increase libido. Indications of abuse include frequent erections, atypical sexual behavior, heightened libido, dyskinesias, agitation, confusion, and depression.

◆ *Drug interactions*

Serotonin antagonists (ondansetron, dolasetron, granisetron, palonosetron, alosetron). The use of serotonin antagonists with apomorphine is contraindicated. Profound hypotension and loss of consciousness have been reported.

Phenothiazines, including prochlorperazine, butyrophenones (e.g., haloperidol), thioxanthenes, metoclopramide. These medicines are dopamine antagonists. They will block the dopaminergic effect of apomorphine, thereby aggravating parkinsonian symptoms.

Ethanol, antihypertensive agents, vasodilators (e.g., nitrates). The use of these agents concurrently with apomorphine significantly increases the frequency of orthostatic hypotension. Alcohol should be avoided when taking apomorphine. Dosage adjustment of the antihypertensive agent is often necessary because of excessive orthostatic hypotension.

pramipexole (pră-mĭ-PĔKS-ŏl)
Mirapex (MĬR-ă-pĕks)
Mirapex ER
⇌ *Do not confuse Mirapex with MiraLAX.*

Actions

Pramipexole is a nonergot dopamine agonist that stimulates D_2 and D_3 dopamine receptors.

Uses

Pramipexole may be used alone to manage the early signs and symptoms of parkinsonism by improving ADLs and motor manifestations such as tremor, rigidity, bradykinesia, and postural stability. It may also be used in combination with levodopa for advanced parkinsonism to manage similar signs and symptoms of the disease.

Therapeutic Outcomes

The primary therapeutic outcomes sought from pramipexole for the treatment of parkinsonism are as follows:

1. Improved motor and ADL scores
2. Decreased off time
3. Reduced dosage of levodopa

❖ **Nursing Implications for Pramipexole Therapy**
◆ *Premedication assessment*

1. Perform a baseline assessment of parkinsonism with the use of the UPDRS.
2. Obtain a history of GI and cardiovascular symptoms, including baseline vital signs (e.g., blood pressure, pulse).
3. Ask specifically about any symptoms of hallucinations, nightmares, dementia, or anxiety.

◆ *Availability.* **PO:** tablets: 0.125, 0.25, 0.5, 0.75, 1, and 1.5 mg; tablets, extended release (24 hour): 0.375, 0.75, 1.5, 2.25, 3, 3.75, and 4.5 mg.

◆ *Dosage and administration.* ***Adult: PO:***
NOTE: Dosage adjustment is required for patients with a serum creatinine clearance of 30 mL/min or lower. See manufacturer's recommendations.

Immediate-release tablets: Initially, give 0.125 mg three times daily for 1 week. If tolerated, increase the dosage to 0.25 mg three times daily the second week. If tolerated, increase by increments of 0.25 mg three times daily through the seventh week. The usual maintenance dosage is 0.5 to 1.5 mg three times daily, with or without levodopa therapy. When pramipexole is used with levodopa, consider reducing the levodopa dose.

Extended-release tablets: Initially, 0.375 mg orally once a day. Increase gradually no more than every 5 to 7 days. The first dose increase should be to 0.75 mg once daily, followed by incremental increases of 0.75 mg;

assess therapeutic response and tolerability at a minimum of 5 days after each dose increase.

Administer medication with food or milk to reduce gastric irritation.

If pramipexole is to be discontinued, the dosage should be gradually reduced over 1 week.

◆ *Common adverse effects.* Pramipexole causes many adverse effects, but most are dose related and are reversible. Adverse effects vary greatly depending on the stage of the disease and the concurrent use of other medicines.

Gastrointestinal

Nausea, vomiting, anorexia. These effects can be reduced by slowly increasing the dosage, dividing the total daily dose into three doses, and administering the medication with food.

Cardiovascular

Orthostatic hypotension. Although it is generally mild, pramipexole may cause some degree of orthostatic hypotension; this is manifested by dizziness and weakness, particularly when therapy is being initiated. Tolerance usually develops after a few weeks of therapy. Monitor the patient's blood pressure daily in both the supine and standing positions. Anticipate the development of postural hypotension and take measures to prevent such an occurrence. Teach patients to rise slowly from a supine or sitting position, and encourage them to sit or lie down if feeling faint.

◆ *Serious adverse effects*

Neurologic

Chewing motions, bobbing, facial grimacing, rocking movements. These involuntary movements occur in some patients, especially if they are also taking levodopa. A reduction in dosage of the levodopa may be beneficial.

Sudden sleep events. Sleep episodes have been reported with the dopamine agonists (e.g., pramipexole, ropinirole). These episodes are described as "sleep attacks" or "sleep episodes," and they include daytime sleep. Some sleep events have been reported as sudden and irresistible; other sleep events have been preceded by sufficient warning to prevent accidents. Patients who are taking dopamine agonists should be informed about the possibility of daytime sleepiness and outright sleep attacks with these medicines and be allowed to make their own decisions about driving on the basis of their past experiences with the medicines. The assessment of patients who are at risk for sleep attacks is possible with the Epworth Sleepiness Scale.

Psychological

Nightmares, depression, confusion, hallucinations. Perform a baseline assessment of the patient's degree of alertness and orientation to name, place, and time before initiating therapy. Make regularly scheduled subsequent evaluations of mental status, and compare findings. Report alterations in mood. Provide for patient safety during these episodes. Reducing the daily dosage may control these adverse effects.

Impulse control/compulsive behaviors. While taking pramipexole and other dopamine agonists, patients can experience an intense urge to gamble, increased sexual urge, an intense urge to spend money uncontrollably, binge eating, and/or other intense urges with the inability to control these urges. Patients may not recognize these behaviors as abnormal. It is important to notify healthcare providers about the development of impulsive behaviors.

Cardiovascular

Tachycardia, palpitations. Take the pulse at regularly scheduled intervals. Report any changes for further evaluation.

◆ *Drug interactions*

Cimetidine, ranitidine, diltiazem, verapamil, quinidine, triamterene. These agents inhibit the urinary excretion of pramipexole. A dose reduction of pramipexole is often required to prevent toxic effects.

Dopamine antagonists. Dopamine antagonists include phenothiazines, butyrophenones, thioxanthenes, and metoclopramide. As dopamine antagonists, these agents will diminish the effectiveness of pramipexole, which is a dopaminergic agonist.

Antihypertensive agents. A dosage adjustment of the antihypertensive agent is often necessary in response to excessive orthostatic hypotension.

---

ropinirole (rō-PĬN-ĭ-rŏl)
⇌ **Do not confuse ropinirole with raloxifene or risperidone.**
Requip (RĒ-kwĭp)
Requip XL
⇌ **Do not confuse Requip with Risperdal.**

Actions

Ropinirole is a nonergot dopamine agonist that stimulates D_2 and D_3 dopamine receptors.

Uses

Ropinirole may be used alone to manage the early signs and symptoms of parkinsonism by improving ADLs and motor manifestations such as tremor, rigidity, bradykinesia, and postural stability. It may also be used in combination with levodopa for advanced parkinsonism to manage similar signs and symptoms of the disease and to reduce the degree of "on-off" fluctuations that are often associated with the long-term use of levodopa.

Therapeutic Outcomes

The primary therapeutic outcomes sought from ropinirole for the treatment of parkinsonism are as follows:
1. Improved motor and ADL scores
2. Decreased off time
3. Reduced dosage of levodopa

❖ **Nursing Implications for Ropinirole Therapy**
◆ *Premedication assessment*
1. Perform a baseline assessment of parkinsonism with the use of the UPDRS.
2. Obtain a history of GI and cardiovascular symptoms, including baseline vital signs (e.g., blood pressure, pulse).
3. Ask specifically about any symptoms of hallucinations, nightmares, dementia, or anxiety.

◆ *Availability.* **PO:** tablets: 0.25, 0.5, 1, 2, 3, 4, and 5 mg; tablets, extended release (24 hour): 2, 4, 6, 8, and 12 mg.

◆ *Dosage and administration.* **Adult:** *PO:* Initially, give 0.25 mg three times daily for 1 week. If tolerated, increase to 0.5 mg three times daily the second week. If tolerated, increase to 0.75 mg three times daily for the third week and then to 1 mg three times daily through the fourth week. If necessary, the daily dosage may be increased by 1.5 mg/day on a weekly basis up to a daily dosage of 9 mg/day. Dosages may be further adjusted at weekly intervals up to a total dosage of 24 mg/day.

Administer medication with food or milk to reduce gastric irritation.

Extended-release tablet PO: Initially 2 mg once daily for 1 to 2 weeks, followed by increases of 2 mg/day at weekly or longer intervals based on therapeutic response and tolerability; there was no additional benefit shown for doses greater than 8 mg/day in advanced Parkinson's disease or 12 mg/day in early Parkinson's disease; maximum: 24 mg/day.

When ropinirole is used with levodopa, consider reducing the levodopa dosage. If ropinirole is to be discontinued, the dosage should be gradually reduced over the course of 1 week.

◆ *Common adverse effects.* Ropinirole causes many adverse effects, but most are dose related and are reversible. Adverse effects vary greatly depending on the stage of the disease and the concurrent use of other medicines.

Gastrointestinal

Nausea, vomiting, anorexia. These effects can be reduced by slowly increasing the dosage, dividing the total daily dosage into three doses, and administering the medication with food.

Cardiovascular

Orthostatic hypotension. Ropinirole may cause some degree of orthostatic hypotension, although it is generally mild; this is manifested by dizziness and weakness, particularly when therapy is being initiated. Tolerance usually develops after a few weeks of therapy.

Monitor the patient's blood pressure daily in both the supine and standing positions. Anticipate the development of postural hypotension and take measures to prevent such an occurrence. Teach patients to rise slowly from a supine or sitting position, and encourage them to sit or lie down if feeling faint.

◆ **Serious adverse effects**
Neurologic
Chewing motions, bobbing, facial grimacing, rocking movements. These involuntary movements occur in some patients, especially if they are also taking levodopa. Reducing the dosage of levodopa may be beneficial.

Sudden sleep events. Sleep episodes have been reported with the dopamine agonists (e.g., pramipexole, ropinirole). These episodes are described as "sleep attacks" or "sleep episodes," and they include daytime sleep. Some sleep events have been reported as sudden and irresistible, whereas other sleep events have been preceded by sufficient warning to prevent accidents. Patients who are taking dopamine agonists should be informed about the possibility of daytime sleepiness and outright sleep attacks with these medicines and be allowed to make their own decisions about driving on the basis of their past experiences with the medicines. The assessment of patients who are at risk for sleep attacks is possible with the Epworth Sleepiness Scale.

Psychological
Nightmares, depression, confusion, hallucinations. Perform a baseline assessment of the patient's degree of alertness and orientation to name, place, and time before initiating therapy. Make regularly scheduled subsequent evaluations of mental status and compare findings. Report alterations in mood. Provide patient safety during these episodes. Reducing the daily dosage may control these adverse effects.

Impulse control/compulsive behaviors. Patients can experience an intense urge to gamble, increased sexual urge, an intense urge to spend money uncontrollably, binge eating, and/or other intense urges with the inability to control these urges while taking ropinirole and other dopamine agonists. Patients may not recognize these behaviors as abnormal. It is important to notify healthcare providers about the development of impulsive behaviors.

Cardiovascular
Tachycardia, palpitations. Take the pulse at regularly scheduled intervals. Report any changes for further evaluation.

◆ **Drug interactions**
Ciprofloxacin. This antibiotic inhibits the metabolism of ropinirole. A dosage reduction of ropinirole is often required to prevent toxic effects.

Estrogens (primarily ethinyl estradiol). Estrogen inhibits ropinirole excretion. If estrogen therapy is started or stopped during treatment with ropinirole, it may be necessary to adjust the dosage of ropinirole.

Dopamine antagonists. Dopamine antagonists include phenothiazines, butyrophenones, thioxanthenes, and metoclopramide. As dopamine antagonists, these agents will diminish the effectiveness of ropinirole, which is a dopaminergic agonist.

Antihypertensive agents. A dosage adjustment of the antihypertensive agent is often necessary in response to excessive orthostatic hypotension.

---

rotigotine (rō-TĬG-ō-tēen)
Neupro (new-PRO)
⇌ *Do not confuse Neupro with Neupogen.*

Actions
Rotigotine is a nonergot dopamine agonist with specificity for D_3, D_2, and D_1 dopamine receptors.

Uses
Rotigotine is used to manage early-stage and late-stage Parkinson's disease.

Therapeutic Outcomes
The primary therapeutic outcomes sought from rotigotine for the treatment of parkinsonism are improved motor and ADL scores.

❖ **Nursing Implications for Rotigotine Therapy**
◆ *Premedication assessment*
1. Perform a baseline assessment of parkinsonism with the use of the UPDRS.
2. Obtain a history of GI and cardiovascular symptoms, including baseline vital signs (e.g., blood pressure, pulse).
3. Ask specifically about any symptoms of hallucinations, nightmares, dementia, or anxiety.

◆ *Availability.* **Transdermal:** 1, 2, 3, 4, 6, and 8 mg/24 hr patch.

◆ *Dosage and administration.* **Adult, early-stage:** *Transdermal: Initial:* Apply 2 mg/24 hr patch once daily; may increase by 2 mg/24 hr weekly based on clinical response and tolerability.
Lowest effective dose: 4 mg/24 hr (manufacturer recommends a maximum dose of 6 mg/24 hr).
Adult, late-stage: *Transdermal: Initial:* Apply 4 mg/24 hr patch once daily; may increase by 2 mg/24 hr weekly based on clinical response and tolerability.
Recommended dose: 8 mg/24 hr; in clinical trials maximum doses up to 16 mg/24 hr were used.
When rotigotine is used with levodopa, consider reducing the levodopa dosage. If rotigotine is to be

---

⚠ Medication Safety Alert

The backing layer of rotigotine contains aluminum. To avoid skin burns, the patch should be removed prior to magnetic resonance imaging or cardioversion.

Heat application has been shown to increase absorption severalfold with other transdermal products. Patients should be advised to avoid exposing the rotigotine application site to external sources of direct heat, such as heating pads or electric blankets, heat lamps, saunas, hot tubs, heated water beds, and prolonged direct sunlight.

discontinued, the dosage should be decreased by less than 2 mg/24 hr preferably every other day until withdrawal is complete.

◆ *Common adverse effects.* Rotigotine causes many adverse effects, but most are dose related and are reversible. Adverse effects vary greatly depending on the stage of the disease and the concurrent use of other medicines.

Gastrointestinal

Nausea, vomiting, anorexia. These effects can be reduced by slowly increasing the dosage.

Cardiovascular

Orthostatic hypotension. Although it is generally mild, rotigotine may cause some degree of orthostatic hypotension; this is manifested by dizziness and weakness, particularly when therapy is being initiated. Tolerance usually develops after a few weeks of therapy.

Monitor the patient's blood pressure daily in both the supine and standing positions. Anticipate the development of postural hypotension and take measures to prevent such an occurrence. Teach patients to rise slowly from a supine or sitting position, and encourage them to sit or lie down if feeling faint.

Skin

Application site reactions may be seen with rotigotine transdermal patches. The signs and symptoms of these reactions generally are erythema, edema, or pruritus limited to the patch area. Daily rotation of rotigotine application sites has been shown to reduce the incidence. If the patient reports a persistent application site reaction (of more than a few days), reports an increase in severity, or reports a skin reaction spreading outside the application site, contact the healthcare provider.

◆ *Serious adverse effects*

Neurologic

Chewing motions, bobbing, facial grimacing, rocking movements. These involuntary movements occur in some patients, especially if they are also taking levodopa. Reducing the dosage of levodopa may be beneficial.

Sudden sleep events. Sleep episodes have been reported with the dopamine agonists. These episodes are described as "sleep attacks" or "sleep episodes," and they include daytime sleep. Some sleep events have been reported as sudden and irresistible, whereas other sleep events have been preceded by sufficient warning to prevent accidents. Patients who are taking dopamine agonists should be informed about the possibility of daytime sleepiness and outright sleep attacks with these medicines and be allowed to make their own decisions about driving on the basis of their past experiences with the medicines. The assessment of patients who are at risk for sleep attacks is possible with the Epworth Sleepiness Scale.

Psychological

Nightmares, depression, confusion, hallucinations. Perform a baseline assessment of the patient's degree of alertness

and orientation to name, place, and time before initiating therapy. Make regularly scheduled subsequent evaluations of mental status and compare findings. Report alterations in mood. Provide patient safety during these episodes. Reducing the daily dosage may control these adverse effects.

Impulse control/compulsive behaviors. Patients can experience an intense urge to gamble, increased sexual urge, an intense urge to spend money uncontrollably, binge eating, and/or other intense urges with the inability to control these urges while taking rotigotine and other dopamine agonists. Patients may not recognize these behaviors as abnormal. It is important to notify healthcare providers about the development of impulsive behaviors.

Cardiovascular

Tachycardia, palpitations. Take the pulse at regularly scheduled intervals. Report any changes for further evaluation.

◆ *Drug interactions*

Dopamine antagonists. Dopamine antagonists include phenothiazines, butyrophenones, thioxanthenes, and metoclopramide. As dopamine antagonists, these agents will diminish the effectiveness of rotigotine, which is a dopaminergic agonist.

Antihypertensive agents. A dosage adjustment of the antihypertensive agent is often necessary in response to excessive orthostatic hypotension.

DRUG CLASS: CATECHOL-*O*-METHYLTRANSFERASE INHIBITORS

---

entacapone (ĕn-TĂK-ă-pōn)
  Comtan (CŎM-tăn)
entacapone/levodopa/carbidopa
  Stalevo (stă-LĒ-vō)

Actions

Entacapone is a potent COMT inhibitor that reduces the destruction of dopamine in the peripheral tissues, thereby allowing significantly more dopamine to reach the brain to eliminate the symptoms of parkinsonism.

Uses

Carbidopa-levodopa is the current drug combination of choice for the longer-term treatment of Parkinson's disease. Unfortunately, these agents lose effectiveness (i.e., the "on-off" phenomenon) and result in the development of more adverse effects (i.e., dyskinesias) over time. Adding entacapone inhibits the metabolism of dopamine, which results in more constant dopaminergic stimulation in the brain. This stimulation reduces motor fluctuations, increases on time, reduces off time, and often results in a reduction in the dosage of levodopa. Entacapone should always be administered with carbidopa-levodopa. Entacapone has no antiparkinsonian effect when it is used alone. Stalevo is a combination product that contains levodopa, carbidopa, and entacapone.

Therapeutic Outcomes

The primary therapeutic outcomes sought from entacapone for the treatment of parkinsonism are as follows:

1. Reduced motor fluctuations
2. Increased on time and reduced off time
3. Reduced total daily dosage of carbidopa-levodopa

❖ Nursing Implications for Entacapone Therapy

◆ Premedication assessment

1. Perform a baseline assessment of parkinsonism with the use of the UPDRS.
2. Obtain a history of bowel patterns and any ongoing GI symptoms.
3. Perform a baseline assessment of the patient's degree of alertness and orientation to name, place, and time before initiating therapy.
4. Check for any antihypertensive therapy that is currently prescribed. Monitor the patient's blood pressure daily in both the supine and standing positions. If antihypertensive medications are being taken, report this to the healthcare provider for possible dosage adjustment.
5. Check the patient's hepatic function before the initiation of therapy and periodically throughout the course of administration.

◆ Availability. PO: Entacapone (Comtan): 200-mg tablets (do not administer entacapone without levodopa/carbidopa; it has no pharmacologic effect of its own).

Stalevo 50: 12.5 mg carbidopa, 50 mg levodopa, and 200 mg entacapone;
Stalevo 75: 18.75 mg carbidopa, 75 mg levodopa, and 200 mg entacapone;
Stalevo 100: 25 mg carbidopa, 100 mg levodopa, and 200 mg entacapone;
Stalevo 125: 31.25 mg carbidopa, 125 mg levodopa, and 200 mg entacapone;
Stalevo 150: 37.5 mg carbidopa, 150 mg levodopa, and 200 mg entacapone;
Stalevo 200: 50 mg carbidopa, 200 mg levodopa, and 200 mg entacapone.

◆ Dosage and administration. Dosage must be adjusted in accordance with the patient's response and tolerance.

Adult: *PO:* Initially, start therapy by adding entacapone to already existing levodopa/carbidopa therapy: give one 200-mg tablet of Comtan with each carbidopa-levodopa dose to a maximum of eight times daily (1600 mg of entacapone). The dosage of carbidopa-levodopa will need to be reduced, particularly if the levodopa dose is higher than 600 mg/day and if the

patient has moderate or severe dyskinesias before the entacapone is started.

Once the patient has been stabilized on a new combination of entacapone, levodopa, and carbidopa, the patient may be switched to a Stalevo product that most closely matches the dosage of levodopa/carbidopa and entacapone being taken.

◆ Common adverse effects. Entacapone may increase the adverse dopaminergic effects of levodopa (e.g., chorea, confusion, hallucinations), but these can be controlled by reducing the dosage of levodopa.

Gastrointestinal

Diarrhea. Diarrhea of usually mild to moderate severity may develop 1 to 12 weeks after the initiation of therapy, especially when higher doses are used. These effects may be minimized by a temporary reduction in dosage.

Neurologic

Sedative effects. Patients may complain of drowsiness and lethargy, especially during the initiation of therapy. People should not drive or operate complex machinery or perform duties for which they must remain mentally alert until they have gained enough experience with entacapone to know whether it affects their mental or motor performance.

Genitourinary

Urine discoloration. Patients should be advised that entacapone may change the color of their urine to a brownish orange but that this is harmless and there is no cause for alarm.

◆ Serious adverse effects

Neurologic

Neurologic effects. Entacapone may increase the adverse dopaminergic effects of levodopa, such as chorea, confusion, and hallucinations. Make regularly scheduled subsequent evaluations of mental status and compare findings. Report alterations in mood. A reduction of the carbidopa-levodopa dosage may be required to alleviate these effects. Provide for patient safety, be emotionally supportive, and assure the patient that these effects usually dissipate as tolerance to the drug develops over the subsequent few weeks.

Cardiovascular

Orthostatic hypotension. Monitor the patient's blood pressure daily in both the supine and standing positions. Anticipate the development of postural hypotension and take measures to prevent such an occurrence. Teach the patient to rise slowly from a supine or sitting position, and encourage the patient to sit or lie down if feeling faint.

◆ Drug interactions

Levodopa. Entacapone and levodopa have additive neurologic effects. This interaction may be beneficial because it often allows for a reduction in the dosage of the levodopa.

Antihypertensive agents. A dosage adjustment of the antihypertensive agent is often necessary in response to excessive orthostatic hypotension.

Apomorphine, isoproterenol, epinephrine, norepinephrine (levarterenol), dopamine, dobutamine, methyldopa. These agents are metabolized by COMTs. The concurrent administration of entacapone with these agents may prolong their duration of activity. Monitor the patient's blood pressure and heart rate.

DRUG CLASS: ANTICHOLINERGIC AGENTS

Actions
Parkinsonism is induced by the imbalance of neurotransmitters in the basal ganglia of the brain. The primary imbalance appears to be a deficiency of dopamine, which results in a relative excess of the cholinergic neurotransmitter acetylcholine. Anticholinergic agents are thus used to reduce the hyperstimulation that is caused by excessive acetylcholine.

Uses
The anticholinergic agents reduce the severity of the tremor and drooling that are associated with parkinsonism. Anticholinergic agents are more useful for patients with minimal symptoms and no cognitive impairment. Combination therapy with levodopa and anticholinergic agents is also successful for controlling symptoms of the disease more completely in about half of patients who are already stabilized on levodopa therapy. Anticholinergic agents have little effect on rigidity, bradykinesia, or postural abnormalities. If anticholinergic therapy is to be discontinued, it should be done so gradually to avoid withdrawal effects and the acute exacerbation of parkinsonian symptoms, even for patients in whom there appears to have been no clinical response.

Therapeutic Outcome
The primary therapeutic outcome sought from anticholinergic agents for the treatment of parkinsonism is a reduction in the severity of the tremor and drooling that are caused by a relative excess of acetylcholine in the basal ganglia.

❖ **Nursing Implications for Anticholinergic Agent Therapy**

◆ *Premedication assessment*
1. Perform a baseline assessment of parkinsonism with the use of the UPDRS.
2. Obtain baseline data related to patterns of urinary and bowel elimination.
3. Perform a baseline assessment of the patient's degree of alertness and orientation to name, place, and time before initiating therapy.
4. Take the patient's blood pressure in both the supine and standing positions. Record the pulse rate, rhythm, and regularity.
5. All patients should be screened for the presence of closed-angle glaucoma before the initiation of therapy. Anticholinergic agents may precipitate an acute attack of closed-angle glaucoma. Patients with open-angle glaucoma can safely use anticholinergic agents. Monitor intraocular pressure regularly.

◆ *Availability, dosage, and administration.* **Adult:** *PO* (see Table 14.2). Administer medication with food or milk to reduce gastric irritation.

◆ *Common adverse effects*
Gastrointestinal
Constipation; dryness of the mucosa of the mouth, throat, and nose. These symptoms are the result of the anticholinergic effects that are produced by these agents. Patients who are taking these medications should be monitored

---

Table 14.2 Anticholinergic Agents

GENERIC NAME	BRAND NAME	AVAILABILITY	INITIAL DOSAGE RANGE (PO)	MAXIMUM DAILY DOSAGE RANGE
benztropine mesylate ⇄ *Do not confuse benztropine with benzonatate.*	Cogentin -PMS-Benztropine 🍁	Tablets: 0.5, 1, 2 mg Injection ❶: 1 mg/mL in 2-mL ampules	0.5-1 mg at bedtime	6 mg
diphenhydramine hydrochloride ⇄ *Do not confuse diphenhydramine with dicyclomine or dipyridamole.*	Benadryl Allergy Aler-Dryl ❶ ⇄ *Do not confuse Benadryl Allergy with benazepril or Bentyl.*	Tablets: 25, 50 mg Capsules: 25, 50 mg Strips, orally disintegrating: 12.5 mg Tablets, orally disintegrating: 25 mg Elixir: 12.5 mg/5 mL Syrup: 12.5 mg/5 mL Injection ❶: 50 mg/mL in 1-, 10-mL vials; 1-mL cartridges	25-50 mg three or four times daily	PO: 300 mg IM/IV: 400 mg
trihexyphenidyl hydrochloride		Tablets: 2, 5 mg Elixir: 2 mg/5 mL	1-2 mg daily	12-15 mg

🍁 Available in Canada.   ⇄ Do not confuse.   ❶ High-alert medication.

for the development of these adverse effects. Milder adverse effects (e.g., dry mouth) may subside with continued treatment.

Dryness of the mucosa may be relieved by sucking hard candy or ice chips or by chewing gum. Give stool softeners as prescribed. Encourage adequate fluid intake, foods that provide sufficient bulk, and exercise as tolerated.

Genitourinary

Urinary retention. If patients develop urinary hesitancy, assess them for bladder distention. Report to the healthcare provider any symptoms of urinary retention for further evaluation. This symptom is a result of the anticholinergic effects produced by these agents. Patients who are taking these medications should be monitored for the development of this adverse effect.

Sensory

Blurred vision. This symptom may subside with continued treatment. Provide for patient safety.

◆ *Serious adverse effects*

Psychological

Nightmares, depression, confusion, hallucinations. Make regularly scheduled subsequent evaluations of mental status and compare findings. Report the development of alterations in mood. Provide patient safety during these episodes. Reducing the daily dosage may control these adverse effects.

Cardiovascular

Orthostatic hypotension. Although this condition is infrequent and generally mild, all anticholinergic agents may cause some degree of orthostatic hypotension, which is manifested by dizziness and weakness, particularly when therapy is being initiated.

Monitor the patient's blood pressure daily in both the supine and standing positions. Anticipate the development of postural hypotension and take measures to prevent such an occurrence. Teach the patient to rise slowly from a supine or sitting position and encourage the patient to sit or lie down if feeling faint.

Palpitations, dysrhythmias. Report any changes for further evaluation.

◆ *Drug interactions*

Amantadine, tricyclic antidepressants, phenothiazines. These agents may enhance the anticholinergic adverse effects. Confusion and hallucinations are characteristic of excessive anticholinergic activity. A dosage reduction may be required.

Levodopa. Large doses of anticholinergic agents may slow gastric emptying and inhibit the absorption of levodopa. An increase in the dosage of levodopa may be required.

ALZHEIMER'S DISEASE

Alzheimer's disease is a progressive neurodegenerative disease that affects older adults. The probability of being diagnosed with Alzheimer's disease nearly doubles every 5 years after age 65. According to the Alzheimer's Association, more than 5 million Americans are living with Alzheimer's disease. It is the most common type of dementia. Other types of dementia are dementia with Lewy bodies, vascular (multi-infarct) dementia, Parkinson's disease dementia, and frontotemporal disorders. Patients with Alzheimer's disease will develop cognitive dysfunction (memory loss), psychiatric and behavioral problems, and difficulty performing ADLs. The neuropathology appears to be an accumulation of amyloid plaques and neurofibrillary tangles that cause neuronal injury. Included in this neuronal injury are cholinergic neurons that are critical in memory, cognition, and other cortical functions. Disturbances in glutamate neurotransmission have been linked with the pathophysiologic processes underlying Alzheimer's disease. Elevated concentrations of glutamate have been associated with increased sensitivity and/or activity of the glutamatergic system, resulting in neuronal dysfunction and cell death in Alzheimer's disease. Although there is no cure for this disease, medications can decrease some of the symptoms by increasing acetylcholine and inhibiting glutamate.

DRUG THERAPY FOR ALZHEIMER'S DISEASE

Drug therapy is focused on improving cognitive function. Two classes of drugs are currently used to treat Alzheimer's disease: acetylcholinesterase inhibitors (donepezil, galantamine, rivastigmine) and an *N*-methyl-D-aspartate (NDMA) inhibitor (memantine). To date, no drugs are available to slow the degenerative process.

❖ NURSING IMPLICATIONS FOR ALZHEIMER'S DISEASE THERAPY

Patients start to have difficulty with memory, problem solving, attention, counting, and language. As the disease progresses, behavioral symptoms of Alzheimer's disease such as wandering, agitation, anxiety, sleeplessness, and aggression are manifested. Families and caregivers need to learn effective management of these behaviors to make patients more comfortable. The focus of patient care is to maintain mental function, manage behavioral symptoms, and slow or delay the symptoms of disease. Be alert for these symptoms of Alzheimer's disease:

- Impaired memory and judgment; often these patients can no longer drive
- Confusion or disorientation; redirecting and calming the patient is an effective intervention
- Inability to recognize family or friends; reminding and calming the patient is used
- Aggressive behavior
- Depression; often accompanies anxiety
- Psychoses, including paranoia and delusions
- Anxiety

Because this disease is progressive and the patient will continue to have worsening memory and cognitive function changes, this takes its toll on the caregiver of the patient. Developing good coping skills and a strong support system, as well as utilizing respite care, can help caregivers handle the stress of caring for a loved one with Alzheimer's disease. Eventually, patients are cared for in a memory care unit, usually a separate section of a nursing home designed to care for Alzheimer's disease patients exclusively.

◆ **Assessment**
- Obtain baseline assessments of presenting symptoms.
- Record baseline pulse, respirations, and blood pressure.
- Assess for and record any GI symptoms present before initiation of therapy.
- Assess the patient's ability to receive and understand instructions.

Safety and self-care. Caregivers are taught to repeat, reassure, and redirect the Alzheimer's disease patient as the cognitive decline progresses. Safety issues should always be a concern. Allowing the patient to be as independent as long as possible is also considered.

Stress. The Alzheimer's disease patient can become agitated, anxious, and aggressive as the disease progresses. Recognize the need for calming reassurance and repeating instructions. The memory loss leads to confusion and frustration. Continue to reassure and redirect behavior that can be stressful.

Family resources. Help families connect with programs designed to teach them about the various stages of Alzheimer's disease and about ways to deal with difficult behaviors and other caregiving challenges.

◆ **Implementation**
- Implement planned interventions that are consistent with assessment data, and identify the individual needs of the patient.
- Monitor and record the patient's vital signs, especially blood pressure, during the course of therapy. Report significant changes in blood pressure; these are most likely to occur during periods of dosage adjustment. Emphasize measures to prevent orthostatic hypotension.

◆ **Patient Education**
Education is focused on the caregiver with regard to how to manage the declining cognitive abilities of the patient. Caregivers should remember the three Rs—repeat, reassure, and redirect; these are key concepts to keep in mind when dealing with Alzheimer's disease patients. Allow the patient to continue to perform ADLs as long as possible, and supervise all household ADLs such as cooking and cleaning.

Fostering health maintenance
- Throughout the course of treatment, discuss medication information and how it will benefit the patient.

- Provide the patient and significant others with the important information contained in the specific drug monographs for the drugs prescribed. Additional health teaching and nursing interventions for common and serious adverse effects will be found in each drug monograph.
- Seek cooperation and understanding of the following points so that medication compliance is increased: name of medication; dosage, routes, and times of administration; and common and serious adverse effects.

Patient self-assessment. Enlist the patient's aid in developing and maintaining a written record of monitoring parameters (e.g., blood pressures, weight, exercise; see the Patient Self-Assessment Form for anticholinesterase inhibitors on the Evolve website). Complete the Premedication Data column for use as a baseline to track response to drug therapy. Ensure that the patient understands how to use the form, and instruct the patient to bring the completed form to follow-up visits. During follow-up visits, focus on issues that will foster adherence with the therapeutic interventions prescribed.

DRUG CLASS: ACETYLCHOLINESTERASE INHIBITORS

donepezil (dŏn-ĔP-ĭ-zĭl)
  Aricept (ĀR-ĭ-sĕpt)
rivastigmine (riva-STIG-men)
  Exelon
galantamine (ga-lanta-mēn)
  Razadyne; Razadyne ER

Actions
Donepezil, galantamine, and rivastigmine are acetylcholinesterase inhibitors that allow acetylcholine to accumulate at cholinergic synapses, causing a prolonged and exaggerated cholinergic effect.

Uses
Although the causes are unknown, Alzheimer's disease is characterized by a loss of cholinergic neurons in the central nervous system, resulting in memory loss and cognitive deficits (dementia). Donepezil and rivastigmine (only the patch) are used in patients with mild to severe dementia to enhance cholinergic function. Galantamine is used in patients with mild to moderate dementia to enhance cholinergic function. Their function diminishes with ongoing loss of cholinergic neurons. Donepezil, galantamine, and rivastigmine do not prevent or slow the neurodegeneration caused by Alzheimer's disease.

Therapeutic Outcome
The primary therapeutic outcome expected from donepezil, galantamine, and rivastigmine therapy is improved cognitive skills (e.g., word recall, object naming, language, word finding, task performance).

❖ **Nursing Implications for Donepezil, Galantamine, and Rivastigmine Therapy**

◆ *Premedication assessment*

1. Obtain baseline assessments of presenting symptoms.
2. Record baseline pulse, respirations, and blood pressure.
3. Assess for and record any GI symptoms present before initiation of therapy.

◆ *Availability*

Donepezil. *PO:* 5-, 10-, and 23-mg tablets; 5- and 10-mg orally disintegrating tablets.

Galantamine. *PO:* 4-, 8-, 12-mg tablets; 4-mg/ml oral solution; 8-, 16-, 24-mg extended release 24 hr capsules.

Rivastigmine. *Transdermal:* 4.6, 9.5, and 13.3 mg/24 hr patch.

◆ *Dosage and administration*

Donepezil. *PO:* Initial dosage is 5 mg daily at bedtime. After 4 to 6 weeks of therapy, dosage may be increased to 10 mg daily to assess therapeutic benefit. After 3 months, dose may be increased to 23 mg in moderate to severe Alzheimer's disease. Donepezil may be taken with or without food. The orally disintegrating tablets may be helpful for patients who have difficulty swallowing. Allow tablets to dissolve on the tongue and follow with a glass of water.

Galantamine. *Adult: PO:* Immediate release initial dosage 4 mg twice a day. After a minimum of 4 weeks, dosage may be increased to 8 mg twice a day. Then after 4 weeks, dose should be increased to 12 mg twice a day.

Adult: PO: Extended release initial dosage 8 mg once daily. After a minimum of 4 weeks, dosage may be increased to 16 mg once a day. Then after 4 weeks dose should be increased to 24 mg once a day.

Rivastigmine. *Transdermal: Initial:* Apply 4.6 mg/24 hr patch once daily; if well tolerated, dose may be titrated (no sooner than every 4 weeks) to 9.5 mg/24 hr (continue as long as therapeutically beneficial), and then to 13.3 mg/24 hr patch (maximum dose).

Recommended effective dose: Apply 9.5 mg/24 hr or 13.3 mg/24 hr patch once daily; remove old patch and replace with a new patch every 24 hours.

◆ *Common adverse effects*

Gastrointestinal

Nausea, vomiting, dyspepsia, diarrhea. These are natural extensions of the pharmacologic effects of cholinergic agents. The dosage may need to be reduced if the patient has difficulty with these adverse effects. Symptoms are less common with lower doses and tend to subside after 2 to 3 weeks of therapy. Gradually increasing the dose may help avoid these complications.

◆ *Serious adverse effects*

Cardiovascular

Bradycardia. Cholinergic agents cause a slowing of the heart. These agents may enhance the bradycardiac effects of beta blockers. Notify the healthcare provider if the heart rate is regularly less than 60 beats/min.

◆ *Drug interactions*

Anticholinergic agents. As a cholinergic agent, donepezil has the potential to reduce the activity of anticholinergic agents (e.g., benztropine, diphenhydramine, orphenadrine, procyclidine, trihexyphenidyl).

Succinylcholine-type muscle relaxants, cholinergic agents. As a cholinesterase inhibitor, donepezil is likely to exaggerate the actions of the depolarizing muscle relaxant (succinylcholine) during anesthesia and enhance the pharmacologic activity of cholinergic agents such as bethanechol.

DRUG CLASS: NMDA RECEPTOR INHIBITOR

memantine (MĚM-ăn-tēn)
Namenda (năm-ĚN-dă)

Actions

Memantine is an inhibitor of the NMDA receptor, a type of glutamate receptor.

Uses

Although the causes are unknown, one of the neurochemical characteristics of Alzheimer's disease is persistent activation of NMDA receptors in the central nervous system. Memantine blocks these receptors and is used alone or in combination with an acetylcholinesterase inhibitor for the treatment of dementia associated with moderate to severe Alzheimer's disease. Patients taking memantine show improvement in cognitive function and behavioral symptoms and a slower decline in ADLs, but memantine does not prevent or slow the neurodegeneration of Alzheimer's disease.

Therapeutic Outcome

The primary therapeutic outcome expected from memantine therapy is improved cognitive skills (e.g., word recall, object naming, language, word finding, task performance).

❖ **Nursing Implications for Memantine Therapy**

◆ *Premedication assessment*

1. Obtain baseline assessments of presenting symptoms.
2. Record baseline pulse, respirations, and blood pressure.

◆ *Availability.* *PO:* 5- and 10-mg tablets; 7-, 14-, 21-, and 28-mg capsules, extended release (24 hour); 2 mg/mL in 360-mL oral solution.

◆ *Dosage and administration.* **Adult:** *PO:* 5 mg once daily. The dose should be increased in 5-mg increments to 10, 15, and 20 mg daily. The minimal interval between dose increases is 1 week. Memantine can be taken with or without food.

Conversion: Patients taking 10-mg immediate-release tablets twice daily may switch to a 28-mg extended-release capsule once daily the day following the last dose of a 10-mg immediate-release tablet.

Reduction in dose for renal impairment: A target dose of 14 mg/day is recommended in patients with severe renal impairment (creatinine clearance of 5 to 29 mL/min, based on the Cockcroft-Gault equation).

◆ **Common and serious adverse effects**
Neurologic

Headache, dizziness, akathisia, insomnia, restlessness, increased motor activity, excitement, agitation. Many of these symptoms decline with continued therapy and can be reduced with a longer dosage titration. Dosage may need to be reduced if the patient has difficulty with these adverse effects.

◆ **Drug Interactions**

Acetazolamide, sodium bicarbonate. Medicines that alkalinize the pH of the urine will reduce excretion of memantine. Severe medical conditions such as renal tubular acidosis and severe urinary tract infections also may cause alkalization of the urine, with potential toxicity of memantine.

Get Ready for the NCLEX® Examination!

Key Points

- Parkinson's disease is a progressive neurologic disorder that is caused by the deterioration of dopamine-producing cells in the portion of the brain that is responsible for the maintenance of posture and muscle tone and the regulation of voluntary smooth muscle.
- Normally, a balance exists between dopamine, which is an inhibitory neurotransmitter, and acetylcholine, which is an excitatory neurotransmitter. The symptoms associated with Parkinson's disease develop because of a relative excess of acetylcholine in the brain.
- The goal of treatment is to restore dopamine neurotransmitter function to as close to normal as possible and to relieve the symptoms that are caused by excessive acetylcholine.
- Therapy must be individualized, but selegiline therapy is often started first to slow the development of symptoms. As selegiline becomes less effective, levodopa is started, with or without selegiline.
- Dopamine agonists (e.g., ropinirole, pramipexole) may be added to directly stimulate dopamine receptors.
- Entacapone may be added to levodopa therapy to reduce the metabolism of levodopa, thus prolonging its action.
- Anticholinergic agents may be added at any time to reduce the effects of the "excessive" acetylcholine.
- The nonpharmacologic treatment (e.g., diet, exercise, physical therapy) of Parkinson's disease is equally important as medication for maintaining the long-term well-being of the patient.
- Although there is no cure for Alzheimer's disease, acetylcholinesterase inhibitors (donepezil, rivastigmine) and memantine are used to help improve cognitive skills.

Additional Learning Resources

SG Go to your Study Guide for additional Review Questions for the NCLEX® Examination, Critical Thinking Clinical Situations, and other learning activities to help you master this chapter content.

Go to your Evolve website (https://evolve.elsevier.com/Clayton) for additional online resources.

Review Questions for the NCLEX® Examination

1. The nurse suspects that a patient is manifesting early Parkinson's disease because of the development of which of these symptoms?
   1. Weakness and tremors involving one limb
   2. Drooling and having difficulty chewing and swallowing
   3. Gait alterations causing moderate generalized disability
   4. Expressionless facial features
2. Which neurotransmitters are responsible for Parkinson's disease symptoms?
   1. Excess serotonin and deficient amounts of dopamine
   2. Excess acetylcholine and deficient amounts of dopamine
   3. Excess dopamine and deficient amounts of acetylcholine
   4. Excess epinephrine and deficient amounts of acetylcholine
3. What is the primary purpose of selegiline (Eldepryl) therapy during the early treatment of Parkinson's disease?
   1. Reducing excessive acetylcholine
   2. Increasing dopamine in the basal ganglia
   3. Slowing symptom progression and delaying the initiation of levodopa therapy
   4. Reducing the metabolism of levodopa, thereby making more available

4. Possible adverse effects of carbidopa-levodopa therapy for a patient with Parkinson's disease include which of the following? *(Select all that apply.)*
   1. Urinary retention
   2. Sudden sleep events
   3. Orthostatic hypotension
   4. Involuntary movements such as chewing and bobbing
   5. Depression

5. How is carbidopa used for the treatment of Parkinson's disease?
   1. As a successful monotherapy
   2. In conjunction with levodopa to reduce the dose of levodopa
   3. In conjunction with levodopa to increase plasma levels of levodopa
   4. As a parenteral supplement

6. The drug apomorphine (Apokyn) is chemically related to morphine but does not work the same. It stimulates what in the brain instead?
   1. Dopamine receptors
   2. Acetylcholine receptors
   3. GABA receptors
   4. Serotonin receptors

7. Drugs classified as anticholinergic agents are used to treat symptoms of Parkinson's disease because they have which effect?
   1. They decrease the amount of dopamine available.
   2. They decrease the amount of acetylcholine available.
   3. They increase the amount of acetylcholine available.
   4. They increase the amount of dopamine available.

8. The nurse is educating the family of an elderly patient on the mechanism of action for donepezil (Aricept). Which statement by the family indicated further teaching is needed?
   1. "As I understand it, this drug will improve the cognitive skills of my dad."
   2. "So you are saying that this drug is used in patients with mild to moderate dementia caused by Alzheimer's disease."
   3. "Are you saying that the enzyme that normally breaks down acetylcholine is inhibited by this medication?"
   4. "As I understand it, this medication will slow the progress of the neurodegeneration caused by Alzheimer's disease."

15 Drugs Used for Anxiety Disorders

Objectives

1. Compare and contrast the differences between generalized anxiety disorder, panic disorder, phobias, and obsessive-compulsive disorder.
2. Describe the essential components included in a baseline assessment of a patient's mental status.
3. Cite the drug therapy used to treat anxiety disorders.
4. Identify adverse effects that may result from drug therapy used to treat anxiety.
5. Discuss psychological and physiologic drug dependence.

Key Terms

anxiety (ăng-ZĪ-ĭ-tē) (p. 222)
generalized anxiety disorder (JĔN-ŭr-ăl-īzd ăng-ZĪ-ĭ-tē dĭs-ŌR-dŭr) (p. 222)
panic disorder (PĂN-ĭk) (p. 222)
phobias (FŌ-bē-ăz) (p. 223)

obsessive-compulsive and related disorders (ŏb-SĔS-ĭv kŏm-PŬL-sĭv) (p. 223)
compulsion (kŏm-PŬL-shŭn) (p. 223)
anxiolytics (ăng-zē-ō-LĬ-tĭks) (p. 223)
tranquilizers (TRĂN-kwĕ-lī-zŭrz) (p. 223)

ANXIETY DISORDERS

Anxiety is a normal human emotion that is similar to fear. It is an unpleasant feeling of apprehension or nervousness caused by the *perception* of potential or actual danger that threatens a person's security, whereas fear is an emotional response to a real or perceived threat. *Mild anxiety* is a state of heightened awareness of one's surroundings and is seen in response to day-to-day circumstances. This type of anxiety can be beneficial as a motivator for the individual to take action in a reasonable and adaptive manner. It is sometimes said that people find the inner strength to meet their challenges or "rise to the occasion."

Patients are considered to have *anxiety disorders* when their responses to stressful situations are abnormal or irrational and impair normal daily functioning. The National Institute of Mental Health identifies anxiety disorders as the most commonly encountered mental health disorders in clinical practice; 16% of the general population will experience anxiety disorders during their lifetime. Anxiety disorders usually begin before the age of 30 years and are more common among women than men. Anxiety is a primary symptom of many psychiatric disorders, including schizophrenia, mania, depression, dementia, and substance abuse. Therefore the evaluation of the anxious patient requires a thorough history and physical and psychiatric examinations to determine whether the anxiety is a primary condition or secondary to another illness. Patients who develop anxiety disorders often have more than one. Patients may also have major depression or develop substance abuse problems. The most common disorders are generalized anxiety disorder, panic disorder, social phobia, simple phobia, and obsessive-compulsive disorder.

Generalized anxiety disorder is described as excessive and unrealistic worry about two or more life circumstances (e.g., finances, illness, misfortune) for 6 months or more. Symptoms are both psychological (e.g., tension, fear, difficulty concentrating, apprehension) and physical (e.g., tachycardia, palpitations, tremor, sweating, gastrointestinal upset). The disease has a gradual onset, usually among individuals in the 20- to 30-year-old age group, and it has twice the frequency among women as among men. This illness usually follows a chronic fluctuating course of exacerbations and remissions that are triggered by stressful events in the person's life. Persistent irrational anxiety or episodic anxiety generally requires medical and psychiatric treatment. Patients with generalized anxiety disorder often develop other psychiatric disorders (e.g., panic disorder, obsessive-compulsive disorder, social anxiety disorder, major depression) at some time during their lives.

Panic disorder is recognized as a separate entity and not as a more severe form of chronic generalized anxiety disorder. A panic attack is an abrupt surge of intense fear or intense discomfort that reaches a peak within minutes. During the attack, at least four of the following symptoms arise: palpitations, tachycardia, or pounding heart; sweating; shaking or trembling; sensations of shortness of breath or smothering; feelings of choking; chest pain or discomfort; nausea or abdominal distress; feeling dizzy, unsteady, lightheaded, or faint; chills or heat sensation; numbness or tingling sensations; feelings of unreality or depersonalization; fear of losing control; and fear of dying. The average age of onset is during the early 20s; the disorder is often relapsing, and it may require lifetime treatment. Panic disorder is estimated to affect 1% to 2% of Americans at some time during their lives. Women are affected two to three times more frequently than men. Genetic factors appear to play a significant role in the disease; 15% to 20% of patients will have a close relative with a similar illness. Panic disorder begins as a series of acute or unprovoked anxiety (panic) attacks that involve an intense, terrifying fear. The attacks do not occur as a result of exposure to anxiety-causing situations, as phobias do. Initially the panic attacks are spontaneous, but later during the course of the illness they may be associated with certain actions (e.g., driving a car, being in a crowded place). Patients with panic disorder often develop other psychiatric disorders (e.g., generalized anxiety disorder, personality disorders, substance abuse, obsessive-compulsive disorder, social anxiety disorder, major depression) at some time during their lives.

Phobias are irrational fears of specific objects, activities, or situations. Unlike other anxiety disorders, the object or activity that creates the feeling of fear is recognized by the patient, who also realizes that the fear is unreasonable. The fear persists, however, and the patient seeks to avoid the situation. *Social phobia* is described as a fear of certain social situations in which the person is exposed to scrutiny by others and fears doing something embarrassing. A social phobia involving public speaking is fairly common, and the activity is usually avoided. If public speaking is unavoidable, it is done with intense anxiety. Social phobias are rarely incapacitating, but they do cause some interference with social or occupational functioning. A *simple phobia* is an irrational fear of a specific object or situation, such as heights (acrophobia), closed spaces (claustrophobia), air travel, or driving. Phobias that involve animals such as spiders, snakes, and mice are particularly common. If the person with the phobia is exposed to the object, there is an immediate feeling of panic, sweating, and tachycardia. People are aware of their phobias, and they simply avoid the feared objects.

Obsessive-compulsive disorder is not classified under anxiety disorders in the new *Diagnostic and Statistical Manual of Mental Disorders*, 5th edition (DSM-5). The DSM-5 added a new category of disorders called **Obsessive-Compulsive and Related Disorders** (OCRDs). The OCRDs category includes the familiar obsessive-compulsive disorder (OCD). Although anxiety remains a key feature in OCRDs, there are enough unique differences between anxiety disorders and OCRDs to justify a separate category. The primary features of obsessive-compulsive disorder are recurrent obsessions or compulsions that cause significant distress and interfere with normal occupational responsibilities, social activities, and relationships. The average age of onset of the symptoms of obsessive-compulsive disorder is during late adolescence to the early 20s. The condition occurs with twice the frequency in men as in women, and there also appears to be a genetic component to the disease. It is estimated that 2% to 8% of the general population suffers from obsessive-compulsive disorder, making it one of the most common personality disorders. An *obsession* is an unwanted thought, idea, image, or urge that the patient recognizes as time consuming and senseless but that repeatedly intrudes into that patient's consciousness, despite his or her attempts to ignore, prevent, or counteract it. Examples of obsessions are recurrent thoughts of dirt or germ contamination, a fear of losing things, a need to know or remember something, a need to count or check something, blasphemous thoughts, or concerns about something happening to the self or others. An obsession produces a tremendous sense of anxiety in the affected person. A **compulsion** is a repetitive, intentional, purposeful behavior that must be performed to decrease the anxiety associated with an obsession. The act is done to prevent a vague dreaded event, but the person does not derive pleasure from the act. Common compulsions deal with cleanliness, grooming, and counting. When patients are prevented from performing a compulsion, there is a sense of mounting anxiety. In some individuals the compulsion can become the patient's lifetime activity. Obsessive-compulsive disorder is a complex condition that requires a highly individualized and integrated approach to treatment that includes pharmacologic, behavioral, and psychosocial components.

DRUG THERAPY FOR ANXIETY DISORDERS

A great many medications have been used over the decades to treat anxiety. They range from the purely sedative effects of ethanol, bromides, chloral hydrate, and barbiturates to drugs with more specific antianxiety and less sedative activity, such as benzodiazepines, buspirone, hydroxyzine, and propranolol (a beta-adrenergic antagonist). More recently, tricyclic antidepressants (e.g., imipramine), selective serotonin reuptake inhibitors (SSRIs), serotonin-norepinephrine reuptake inhibitors (duloxetine, extended-release venlafaxine), and serotonin antagonists (e.g., ondansetron) have been studied for the treatment of anxiety disorders. The treatment of anxiety disorders usually requires a combination of pharmacologic and nonpharmacologic therapies. When it is decided to treat the anxiety in addition to the other medical or psychiatric diagnoses, antianxiety medications—also known as *anxiolytics* or *tranquilizers*—are prescribed. See the individual drug monographs later in this chapter for the mechanisms of action of these agents.

USES

Generalized anxiety disorder is treated with psychotherapy and the short-term use of antianxiety agents. The US Food and Drug Administration (FDA) has approved four classes of compounds or medications for treatment: (1) specific benzodiazepines (alprazolam, chlordiazepoxide, clobazam, clonazepam, clorazepate, diazepam, lorazepam, oxazepam); (2) SSRIs (paroxetine and escitalopram); (3) duloxetine and extended-release venlafaxine; and (4) buspirone. To some extent, the beta-adrenergic blocking agents (see Chapter 12) are also used. The antihistamine hydroxyzine is infrequently prescribed. *Panic disorders* may be treated with a variety of agents in addition to behavioral therapy. Alprazolam and clonazepam (benzodiazepines), as well as sertraline, paroxetine, and fluoxetine (SSRIs), are approved by the FDA for the treatment of panic disorder. Other agents that show benefit are the tricyclic antidepressants desipramine and clomipramine, as well as mirtazapine (see Chapter 16). *Phobias* are treated with the use of avoidance, behavior therapy, and benzodiazepines or beta-adrenergic blockers such as propranolol or atenolol. *Obsessive-compulsive related disorders* are treated with behavioral and psychosocial therapy in addition to paroxetine, sertraline, fluoxetine, or fluvoxamine.

❖ NURSING IMPLICATIONS FOR ANTIANXIETY THERAPY

◆ Assessment

History of behavior. Obtain a history of the precipitating factors that may have triggered or contributed to the individual's current anxiety. Has the individual been using alcohol or drugs? Has the patient had a recent adverse event, such as a job or relationship loss, the death of a loved one, or a divorce? Has the individual witnessed or survived a traumatic event? Does the individual have any medical problems (e.g., hyperthyroidism) that could be related to these symptoms? Are there symptoms present that could be attributed to a panic attack, such as a feeling of choking, palpitations, sweating, chest pain or discomfort, nausea, abdominal distress, or fear of losing control, going crazy, or dying? Does the patient have symptoms of obsessions or compulsions? Does the individual have a history of agoraphobia (i.e., situations in which he or she feels trapped or unable to escape)? Did the attack occur in response to a social or performance situation? Is the patient also depressed? What specific fears does the individual have?

Take a detailed history of all medications that the individual is taking. Is there any use of central nervous system (CNS) stimulants (e.g., cocaine, amphetamines) or CNS depressants (e.g., sedatives, opioids, alcohol)? Adverse effects of medications being taken may be aggravating the patient's anxiety level.

Ask for details regarding how long the individual has been exhibiting anxiety. Has the patient been treated for anxiety previously? When did the symptoms start? Did they begin during intoxication or withdrawal from a substance?

Basic mental status. Note the patient's general appearance and appropriateness of attire. Is the individual clean and neat? Is the posture stooped, erect, or slumped? Is the patient oriented to date, time, place, and person? Determine whether the patient is at risk for harming herself or himself or others. Is he or she able to participate in self-directed activities of daily living, including eating and providing the self-care that is required to sustain life? These areas are regularly assessed to determine whether acute hospitalization is indicated. Otherwise, the outpatient setting is the most common setting for the treatment of anxiety disorders.

What coping mechanisms has the individual been using to deal with the situation? Are these mechanisms adaptive or maladaptive? Identify the individual's ability to understand new information, follow directions, and provide self-care.

Identify events that trigger anxiety in the individual. Discuss the patient's behavior and thoughts, and foster an understanding of this with his or her family members. Involve the family and significant others in the discussion of the anxiety-producing events or circumstances, and explain how these individuals can help the patient to reduce anxiety or cope more adaptively with stressors. Identify support groups.

Mood and affect. Is the individual tearful, excessively excited, angry, hostile, or apathetic? Is the facial expression tense, fearful, sad, angry, or blank? Ask the patient to describe his or her feelings. Is there worry about real-life problems? Are the patient's responses displayed as an intense fear, detachment, or absence of emotions? If the patient is a child, are there episodes of tantrums or clinging?

Patients who are experiencing altered thinking, behavior, or feelings require the careful evaluation of their verbal and nonverbal actions. Often, the thoughts, feelings, and behaviors that are displayed are inconsistent with the so-called normal responses of individuals in similar circumstances. Identify management techniques for handling anxiety-producing situations effectively.

Assess whether the mood being described is consistent with or appropriate for the circumstances being described. For example, is the patient speaking of death while smiling?

Clarity of thought. Evaluate the coherency, relevancy, and organization of the patient's thoughts. Ask specific questions about the individual's ability to make judgments and decisions. Is there any memory impairment? Identify areas in which the patient is capable of having input into setting goals and making decisions. (This will help the patient to overcome a sense of powerlessness over certain life situations.) When the patient is unable to make decisions, set goals to involve the patient to the degree of his or her capability because abilities change with treatment.

Psychomotor functions. Ask specific questions regarding the activity level that the patient has maintained. Is the patient able to work or go to school? Is the patient able to fulfill responsibilities at work, socially, or within the family? How have the patient's normal responses to daily activities been altered? Is the individual irritable, angry, easily startled, or hypervigilant? Observe the patient for gestures, gait, hand tremors, voice quivering, and actions such as pacing or the inability to sit still.

Obsessions or compulsions. Does the individual experience persistent thoughts, images, or ideas that are inappropriate and cause increased anxiety? Are there repetitive physical or mental behaviors, such as handwashing, needing to arrange things in perfect symmetrical order, praying, or silently repeating words? If obsessions or compulsions are present, how often do these occur? Do the obsessions or compulsions impair the patient's social or occupational functioning?

Sleep pattern. What is the patient's normal sleep pattern, and how has it varied since the onset of the symptoms? Ask specifically whether insomnia is present. Ask the individual to describe the amount and quality of the sleep. What is the degree of fatigue that is present? Is the individual having recurrent stressful dreams (e.g., after a traumatic event)? Is there difficulty falling or staying asleep?

Dietary history. Ask questions about the individual's appetite and note weight gains or losses not associated with intentional dieting.

◆ Implementation
- Deal with problems as they occur; practice reality orientation.
- Identify signs of escalating anxiety; decrease the escalation of anxiety.
- Provide a safe, structured environment for the release of energy; set limits on aggressive or destructive behaviors.
- Establish a trusting relationship with the patient by providing support and reassurance.
- Reduce stimulation by having interactions with the patient in a quiet, calm environment. Provide a nonstimulating environment for patients who are having sleeping difficulties (e.g., dim lighting, quiet area) that will encourage drowsiness and sleep.
- Provide an opportunity for the individual to express his or her feelings. Use active listening and therapeutic communication techniques. Be especially aware of cues that would indicate that the patient may be

considering self-harm. (If suicidal ideation is suspected, ask the patient directly if suicide is being considered. If necessary, intervene to provide for safety.)

Allow the patient to make decisions of which he or she is capable, make decisions when the patient is not capable, and provide a reward for progress when decisions are initiated appropriately. Involve the patient in self-care activities. During periods of severe anxiety or during escalating anxiety, the individual may be unable to have insight or to make decisions appropriately.

Encourage the individual to develop coping skills with the use of various techniques, such as rehearsing or role-playing responses to threatening stressors. Have the individual practice problem solving, and discuss the possible consequences of the solutions that are offered by the patient.

Assist individuals with nonpharmacologic measures, such as music therapy, relaxation techniques, or massage therapy.

◆ Patient Education
For those patients who are attending an outpatient clinic or hospitalized, orient the individual to the unit and the rules of the unit. Explain the process of privileges and how they are obtained or lost. (The extent of the orientation and explanations given will depend on the individual's orientation to date, time, place, and abilities.)

Explain activity groups and resources that are available within the community. A variety of group process activities (e.g., social skills groups, self-esteem groups, work-related groups, physical exercise groups) exist in particular therapeutic settings. Meditation, biofeedback, and relaxation therapy may also be beneficial.

Involve the patient and his or her family in goal setting, and integrate them into the available group processes to develop positive experiences for the individual to enhance his or her coping skills.

Patient education should be individualized and based on assessment data to provide the individual with a structured environment in which to grow and enhance self-esteem. Initially, the individual may not be capable of understanding lengthy explanations; therefore the approaches used should be based on the patient's capabilities.

Explore the coping mechanisms that the patient uses in response to stressors, and identify methods of channeling these toward positive realistic goals as an alternative to the use of medication.

Fostering health maintenance. Throughout the course of treatment, discuss medication information and how the medication will benefit the patient. Stress the importance of the nonpharmacologic interventions and the long-term effects that compliance with the treatment regimen can provide. Additional health teaching and nursing interventions for adverse effects are described in the drug monographs later in this chapter. Seek cooperation and understanding regarding the following points so that medication compliance is increased: the name of the medication; its dosage, route, and times of administration; and its adverse effects. Instruct the patient not to suddenly discontinue prescribed medications after having been on long-term therapy. Withdrawal should be undertaken with instructions from a healthcare provider, and it usually requires 4 weeks of gradual reduction in dosage and widening the intervals of administration.

Patient self-assessment. Enlist the patient's help with developing and maintaining a written record of monitoring parameters (see the Patient Self-Assessment Form for Antianxiety Medication on the Evolve website). Complete the Premedication Data column for use as a baseline to track patient response to drug therapy. Ensure that the patient understands how to use the form, and instruct the patient to bring the completed form to follow-up visits. During follow-up visits, focus on issues that will foster adherence with the therapeutic interventions that have been prescribed.

DRUG CLASS: BENZODIAZEPINES

Benzodiazepines are most commonly used because they are more consistently effective, are less likely to interact with other drugs, are less likely to cause overdose, and have less potential for abuse than other antianxiety agents. They account for perhaps 75% of the 100 million prescriptions that are written annually for anxiety. Six benzodiazepine derivatives are used as antianxiety agents (Table 15.1).

Actions

It is thought that the benzodiazepines have mechanisms of action similar to CNS depressants, but individual drugs in the benzodiazepine family act more selectively at specific sites, which allows for a variety of uses (e.g., sedative-hypnotic, muscle relaxant, antianxiety agent,

Table 15.1 Benzodiazepines Used to Treat Anxiety

GENERIC NAME	BRAND NAME	AVAILABILITY	INITIAL DOSAGE RANGE (PO)	MAXIMUM DAILY DOSAGE RANGE
alprazolam	Xanax Apo-Alpraz ♦ ⇄ Do not confuse Xanax with Zantac or Zyrtec.	Tablets: 0.25, 0.5, 1, 2 mg Tablets, orally disintegrating: 0.25, 0.5, 1, 2 mg Solution: 1 mg/mL	0.25-0.5 mg three times daily	4 mg for anxiety management 10 mg for panic disorder
	Xanax XR	Tablets, extended release, 24 hr: 0.5, 1, 2, 3 mg	0.5-1 mg daily	10 mg maximum for extended-release tablets; usual range is 3-6 mg daily
chlordiazepoxide ❶ ⇄ Do not confuse chlordiazepoxide with chlorpromazine.		Capsules: 5, 10, 25 mg	5-10 mg three or four times daily	300 mg
clorazepate	Tranxene T Clorazepate ♦	Tablets: 3.75, 7.5, 15 mg	10 mg once to three times daily	60 mg
diazepam ❶ ⇄ Do not confuse diazepam with Ditropan.	Valium Apo-Diazepam ♦ ⇄ Do not confuse Valium with valerian.	Tablets: 2, 5, 10 mg Liquid: 5 mg/5 mL Concentrate: 5 mg/mL Injection: 5 mg/mL in 2-mL prefilled syringe Rectal gel: 2.5, 10, 20 mg/rectal delivery system	2-10 mg two to four times daily	—
lorazepam ❶ ⇄ Do not confuse lorazepam with loperamide.	Ativan Ativan ♦ ❶ Do not confuse Ativan with Ambien or Atarax.	Tablets: 0.5, 1, 2 mg Liquid: 2 mg/mL Injection: 2, 4 mg/mL in 1-, 10-mL vials	2-3 mg divided two or three times daily	10 mg
oxazepam		Capsules: 10, 15, 30 mg	10-15 mg three or four times daily	120 mg

♦ Available in Canada.   ⇄ Do not confuse.   ❶ High-alert medication.

anticonvulsant). The benzodiazepines reduce anxiety by stimulating BNZ$_2$ benzodiazepine receptors to stimulate the inhibitory neurotransmitter gamma-aminobutyric acid (GABA), which improves symptoms of sleep disturbance, tremor, and muscle tension. (See Chapter 13 for more discussion of the actions of benzodiazepines.)

In patients with reduced hepatic function or in older adults, lorazepam and oxazepam may be most appropriate because they have a relatively short duration of action and no active metabolites. Oxazepam has been the most thoroughly investigated. The other benzodiazepines all have active metabolites that significantly prolong the duration of action and that may accumulate to the point of excessive adverse effects with chronic administration.

Uses

Patients with anxiety reactions to recent events and those with treatable medical illnesses that induce anxiety respond most readily to benzodiazepine therapy. In general, benzodiazepines are equally effective for the treatment of anxiety. Patients generally respond to therapy within 1 week. Because all benzodiazepines have similar mechanisms of action, the selection of the appropriate derivative depends on how the benzodiazepine is metabolized (see Actions previously). Oxazepam, lorazepam, chlordiazepoxide, diazepam, and clorazepate are approved for the treatment of anxiety associated with alcohol withdrawal. Oxazepam and lorazepam are the drugs of choice because they have no active metabolites. However, their use is somewhat limited for patients who cannot tolerate oral administration as a result of nausea and vomiting. Diazepam or lorazepam may be administered intramuscularly in this case (see Chapter 48).

Use of benzodiazepines whether for anxiety (Table 15.1) or for sedation (Table 13.2) during pregnancy should be avoided. Benzodiazepines are pregnancy category D and X. Animal studies indicate the possibility of increased risk of congenital malformations if prescribed in the first trimester of pregnancy. Benzodiazepines are also not recommended for breastfeeding mothers. The benzodiazepines transfer to breast milk and can accumulate in breast-fed infants, acting as a sedative.

Therapeutic Outcome

The primary therapeutic outcome expected from the benzodiazepine antianxiety agents is a decrease in the level of anxiety to a manageable level (i.e., coping is improved; physical signs of anxiety such as a look of anxiety, tremor, and pacing are reduced).

❖ Nursing Implications for Benzodiazepines
◆ Premedication assessment
1. Record baseline data regarding the level of anxiety that is present.
2. Record the patient's baseline vital signs, particularly blood pressure in both the sitting and supine positions.
3. Check for a history of blood dyscrasias or hepatic disease.
4. Determine whether the individual is pregnant or breastfeeding.

◆ *Availability, dosage, and administration.* See Table 15.1. Habitual benzodiazepine use may result in physical and psychological dependence. Rapidly discontinuing benzodiazepines after long-term use may result in symptoms that are similar to those of alcohol withdrawal. Mild withdrawal symptoms have been reported in almost half of patients who received therapeutic doses for as little as 4 to 6 weeks. Common symptoms of withdrawal include restlessness, worsening of anxiety and insomnia, tremor, muscle tension, increased heart rate, and auditory hypersensitivity. More serious withdrawal symptoms include delirium and tonic-clonic seizures. Symptoms may not appear for several days after discontinuation. Prevention consists of the gradual withdrawal of benzodiazepines over the course of 4 weeks.

Pregnancy and lactation. It is recommended that benzodiazepines not be administered during at least the first trimester of pregnancy. There may be an increased incidence of birth defects because these agents readily cross the placenta and enter the fetal circulation. If benzodiazepines are taken regularly during pregnancy, the infant should be monitored closely after delivery for signs of withdrawal, including sedation and hypotonia.

Mothers who are breastfeeding should not receive benzodiazepines regularly. The benzodiazepines readily cross into the breast milk and exert a pharmacologic effect on the infant.

◆ *Common adverse effects*
Neurologic
Drowsiness, hangover, sedation, lethargy. Patients may complain of morning hangover, blurred vision, and transient hypotension on arising. Explain to the patient the need for rising first to a sitting position for several moments until any dizziness or lightheadedness passes and then standing slowly. Assist the individual with ambulation, if necessary. If hangover becomes troublesome, the dosage should be reduced, the medication changed, or both.

People who work around machinery, drive, administer medication, or perform other duties for which they must remain mentally alert should not take these medications while working.

◆ *Serious adverse effects*
Psychological
Excessive use or abuse. Habitual benzodiazepine use may result in physical dependence. Discuss the case with the healthcare provider and make plans to cooperatively approach the gradual withdrawal of the medications that are being abused. Assist the patient with recognizing the abuse problem. Identify underlying

needs and plan for the more appropriate management of those needs. Provide emotional support of the individual, display an accepting attitude, and be kind but firm.

Hematologic

Blood dyscrasias. Routine laboratory studies (e.g., red blood cell and white blood cell counts, differential counts) should be scheduled. Stress the patient's need to return for these tests. Monitor the patient for sore throat, fever, purpura, jaundice, or excessive and progressive weakness.

Gastrointestinal

Hepatotoxicity. The symptoms of hepatotoxicity are anorexia, nausea, vomiting, jaundice, hepatomegaly, splenomegaly, and abnormal liver function tests (e.g., elevated bilirubin, aspartate aminotransferase, alanine aminotransferase, and gamma-glutamyltransferase, alkaline phosphatase levels; increased prothrombin time).

◆ *Drug interactions*

Antihistamines, alcohol, analgesics, anesthetics, probenecid, tranquilizers, opioids, cimetidine, other sedative-hypnotics. All these agents increase the toxic effects of benzodiazepines and may cause excessive sedation and impaired psychomotor function.

Oral contraceptives, cimetidine, fluoxetine, metoprolol, propranolol, isoniazid, ketoconazole, valproic acid. These agents inhibit the metabolism of alprazolam, chlordiazepoxide, clonazepam, and diazepam. Pharmacologic effects of the benzodiazepines may be increased and excessive sedation and impaired psychomotor function may result.

Smoking, rifampin. Smoking and rifampin enhance the metabolism of benzodiazepines. Larger doses may be necessary to maintain anxiolytic effects in patients who smoke.

DRUG CLASS: AZASPIRONES

buspirone (byū-SPĪ-rŏn)
⇄ *Do not confuse buspirone with bupropion.*

Actions

Buspirone is an antianxiety agent that comes from the chemical class known as the *azaspirones,* which are chemically unrelated to benzodiazepines or other anxiolytic agents. The mechanism of action of buspirone is not fully understood. It is a partial serotonin and dopamine agonist, and it interacts in several ways with nerve systems in the midbrain; therefore it is sometimes called a *midbrain modulator.* It does not affect GABA receptors. Its advantages over other antianxiety agents are that it has lower sedative properties and it does not alter psychomotor functioning. It requires 7 to 10 days of treatment before initial signs of improvement are

evident, and it takes 3 to 4 weeks of therapy for optimal effects to occur.

Uses

Buspirone is approved for use in the treatment of anxiety disorders and for the short-term relief of the symptoms of anxiety. Buspirone has no antipsychotic activity, and it should not be used in place of appropriate psychiatric treatment. Because there is minimal potential for abuse with buspirone, it is not a controlled substance.

Therapeutic Outcome

The primary therapeutic outcome expected from buspirone is a decrease in the level of anxiety to a manageable level (i.e., coping is improved; physical signs of anxiety such as a look of anxiety, tremor, and pacing are reduced).

❖ **Nursing Implications for Buspirone Therapy**
◆ *Premedication assessment.* Record baseline data regarding the level of anxiety present.

◆ *Availability. PO:* tablets: 5, 7.5, 10, 15, and 30 mg. Schedule assessments periodically throughout therapy for the development of slurred speech or dizziness, which are signs of excessive dosing.

◆ *Dosage and administration.* **Adult:** *PO:* Initially, 5 mg three times daily. Doses may be increased by 5 mg every 2 to 3 days. Maintenance therapy often requires 30 mg daily in divided doses. Do not exceed 60 mg daily.

◆ *Common adverse effects*

Neurologic

Sedation, lethargy. The most common adverse effects of buspirone therapy are CNS disturbances (3.4%), which include dizziness, insomnia, nervousness, drowsiness, and lightheadedness. People who work around machinery or who perform other duties for which they must remain mentally alert should not take this medication while working. Slurred speech and dizziness are signs of excessive dosing. Report to the healthcare provider for further evaluation. Provide patient safety during these episodes.

◆ *Drug interactions*

Itraconazole, erythromycin, nefazodone, clarithromycin, diltiazem, verapamil, fluvoxamine, grapefruit juice. These substances potentiate the toxicity of buspirone by inhibiting its metabolism. If any of these are used together, the dose of buspirone should be reduced by half for a few weeks and then adjusted as needed.

Rifampin, phenytoin, phenobarbital, carbamazepine. These drugs enhance the metabolism of buspirone. An increase in the dose of buspirone may be needed.

Alcohol. Buspirone and alcohol generally do not have additive CNS depressant effects, but individual patients may be susceptible to impairment. Tell patients to use alcohol with extreme caution.

DRUG CLASS: SELECTIVE SEROTONIN REUPTAKE INHIBITORS

fluvoxamine (flū-VŎKS-ă-mēn)
⇄ *Do not confuse fluvoxamine with fluoxetine.*
Luvox (LŪ-vŏks)
⇄ *Do not confuse Luvox with Lasix, Levoxyl, or Lovenox.*

Actions
Fluvoxamine inhibits the reuptake of serotonin at nerve endings, thus prolonging serotonin activity.

Uses
Fluvoxamine is used for the treatment of OCRDs when obsessions or compulsions cause marked distress, are time consuming, or interfere substantially with social or occupational responsibilities. Fluvoxamine reduces the symptoms of these disorders but does not prevent obsessions and compulsions. However, patients indicate that the obsessions are less intrusive and that they have more control over them.

Therapeutic Outcome
The primary therapeutic outcome expected from fluvoxamine is a decrease in the level of anxiety to a manageable level (i.e., coping with obsession is improved; frequency of compulsive activity is reduced).

❖ **Nursing Implications for Fluvoxamine Therapy**
See Serotonin-Norepinephrine Reuptake Inhibitors section in Chapter 16.

DRUG CLASS: MISCELLANEOUS ANTIANXIETY AGENTS

hydroxyzine (hī-DRŎKS-ĭ-zēn)
⇄ *Do not confuse hydroxyzine with hydroxyurea.*
Vistaril (VĬS-tă-rĭl)
⇄ *Do not confuse Vistaril with Restoril or Zestril.*

Actions
When defined strictly by chemical structure, hydroxyzine is considered an antihistamine. It acts within the CNS to produce sedation and antiemetic, anticholinergic, antihistaminic, antianxiety, and antispasmodic activity, thus making it a somewhat multipurpose agent.

Uses
Hydroxyzine is used as a mild tranquilizer for psychiatric conditions that are characterized by anxiety, tension, and agitation. It is also occasionally used as a preoperative or postoperative sedative to control vomiting, diminish

anxiety, and reduce the amount of opioids that are needed for analgesia. Hydroxyzine may also be used as an antipruritic agent to relieve the itching that is associated with allergic reactions.

Therapeutic Outcomes
The primary therapeutic outcomes expected from hydroxyzine are as follows:
1. A decrease in the level of anxiety to a manageable level (i.e., coping is improved; physical signs of anxiety such as a look of anxiety, tremor, and pacing are reduced)
2. Sedation, relaxation, and reduction in analgesics before and after surgery
3. Absence of vomiting when used as an antiemetic
4. Itching controlled during allergic reactions

❖ **Nursing Implications for Hydroxyzine Therapy**
◆ *Premedication assessment*
1. Perform a baseline assessment of anxiety symptoms.
2. Determine the patient's level of anxiety present before and after surgical intervention; record and intervene appropriately.
3. For nausea and vomiting, administer when nausea first starts and determine the effectiveness of control before giving subsequent doses.
4. For allergic reactions, perform a baseline assessment of physical symptoms before administering the dose; repeat this assessment before the administration of subsequent doses to determine the medication's effectiveness.
5. Monitor the patient for the level of sedation present, slurred speech, or dizziness; report to the healthcare provider if these symptoms are excessive before administering repeat doses.

◆ *Availability.* **PO:** 10-, 25-, and 50-mg tablets; 25-, 50-, and 100-mg capsules; 10 mg/5 mL syrup.
IM: 25 and 50 mg/mL.

◆ *Dosage and administration.* **Adult:**
- Antianxiety: *PO:* 25 to 100 mg three or four times daily; *IM:* 50 to 100 mg every 4 to 6 hours
- Preoperatively and postoperatively: *IM:* 25 to 100 mg
- Antiemetic: *IM:* 25 to 100 mg

◆ *Common adverse effects.* These symptoms are the anticholinergic effects that are produced by hydroxyzine. Patients who are taking these medications should be monitored for the development of these adverse effects.
Sensory
Blurred vision. Caution the patient that blurred vision may occur and make appropriate suggestions for personal safety.
Gastrointestinal
Constipation; dryness of the mucosa of the mouth, throat, and nose. Mucosal dryness may be relieved by sucking

hard candy or ice chips or by chewing gum. The use of stool softeners (e.g., docusate) may be required for constipation.

Neurologic

Sedation, slurred speech, dizziness. People who work around machinery, drive, administer medication, or perform other duties for which they must remain mentally alert should not take these medications while working. Slurred speech and dizziness are signs of excessive dosing. Report to the healthcare provider for further evaluation. Provide patient safety during these episodes.

◆ *Drug interactions*

Antihistamines, alcohol, analgesics, anesthetics, tranquilizers, opioids, other sedative-hypnotics. These all are agents that can increase toxic effects. Monitor the patient for excessive sedation, and reduce the dosage of hydroxyzine if necessary.

Get Ready for the NCLEX® Examination!

Key Points

- Anxiety is an unpleasant feeling of apprehension or nervousness that is caused by the perception of danger threatening the patient's security. In most cases, it is a normal human emotion.
- When a patient's response to anxiety is irrational and impairs his or her daily functioning, then he or she is said to have an anxiety disorder. Some 16% of the general population will experience an anxiety disorder during their lifetime.
- The most common types of anxiety disorders are generalized anxiety disorder, panic disorder, social phobia, simple phobia, and obsessive-compulsive disorder.
- Anxiety is a component of many medical illnesses that involve the cardiovascular, pulmonary, digestive, and endocrine systems. It is also a primary symptom of many psychiatric disorders. Therefore the evaluation of the anxious patient requires a thorough history and physical and psychiatric examination to determine whether the anxiety is the primary condition or secondary to another illness. Persistent irrational anxiety or episodic anxiety usually requires medical and psychiatric treatment.
- The treatment of anxiety disorders usually requires a combination of pharmacologic and nonpharmacologic therapies.
- It is the responsibility of the nurse to educate patients about their therapy, to monitor for therapeutic benefits and common and serious adverse effects, and to intervene whenever possible to optimize therapeutic outcomes.

Additional Learning Resources

SG Go to your Study Guide for additional Review Questions for the NCLEX® Examination, Critical Thinking Clinical Situations, and other learning activities to help you master this chapter content.

Go to your Evolve website (https://evolve.elsevier.com/Clayton) for additional online resources.

Review Questions for the NCLEX® Examination

1. A nurse is determining the type of anxiety that a patient is experiencing. The patient states that he always counts the number of steps that it takes to walk to his car. What is this an example of?
   1. Generalized anxiety disorder
   2. Obsessive-compulsive disorder
   3. Phobia related to walking
   4. A panic attack

2. A nurse performing a baseline mental status assessment on a patient includes which of the following details? *(Select all that apply.)*
   1. General appearance and appropriateness of attire
   2. Clarity of thought
   3. Mood and affect
   4. Obsessions or compulsions
   5. Job history

3. The nurse caring for a patient with an anxiety disorder knows which drug is used most often for treatment of anxiety disorders?
   1. fluvoxamine (Luvox)
   2. hydroxyzine (Vistaril)
   3. sertraline (Zoloft)
   4. lorazepam (Ativan)

4. The nurse will monitor which of these laboratory values for a patient receiving a benzodiazepine?
   1. Complete blood cell count with differential and liver function
   2. Complete blood cell count and renal function
   3. White blood cell count and biochemical profile
   4. Blood glucose and electrolytes

5. The patient is exhibiting the symptoms of restlessness, worsening of anxiety, and insomnia, along with tremors. The patient has recently stopped taking Ativan; the nurse suspects the patient is experiencing what?
   1. Generalized anxiety disorder
   2. Benzodiazepine dependence
   3. Obsessive-compulsive disorder
   4. Panic attack

6. After discussing with the patient and the family the drug management of alprazolam (Xanax) for anxiety, the nurse knows further teaching is needed after the patient makes which statement?
   1. "I know that I need to avoid drinking any alcohol while taking this Xanax."
   2. "I understand that this drug may make me drowsy during the day and I should not work around machinery while taking it."
   3. "I understand that I can stop the drug at any time that I feel I do not need it anymore."
   4. "I know that Xanax will start to work within a week."

16 Drugs Used for Depressive and Bipolar Disorders

Objectives

1. Describe the essential components of the baseline assessment of a patient with depression or bipolar disorder.
2. Identify the premedication assessments that are necessary before the administration of monoamine oxidase inhibitors (MAOIs), selective serotonin reuptake inhibitors (SSRIs), serotonin-norepinephrine reuptake inhibitors (SNRIs), tricyclic antidepressants (TCAs), and antimanic agents.
3. Compare the mechanism of action of SSRIs with that of other antidepressant agents.
4. Cite the common adverse effects that may develop for patients who are taking MAOIs.
5. Cite the common adverse effects that may develop for patients who are taking SNRIs.
6. Cite the common adverse effects that may develop for patients who are taking TCAs.
7. Cite the common adverse effects that may develop for patients who are taking lithium.

Key Terms

mood (MŪD) (p. 232)
mood disorder (MŪD dĭs-ŌR-dŭr) (p. 232)
neurotransmitters (nū-rō-TRĂNZ-mĭ-tŭrz) (p. 233)
dysthymia (dĭs-THĬ-mē-ă) (p. 233)
depression (dē-PRĔSH-ŭn) (p. 233)
cognitive symptoms (KŎG-nĭ-tĭv) (p. 233)
psychomotor symptoms (sī-kō-MŌ-tŭr) (p. 233)
bipolar disorder (bī-PŌ-lăr) (p. 233)

mania (MĀ-nē-ă) (p. 233)
euphoria (yū-FŎR-ē-ă) (p. 234)
labile mood (LĀ-bīl) (p. 234)
grandiose delusions (GRĂN-dē-ōs dĕ-LŪ-zhŭnz) (p. 234)
cyclothymia (sī-klō-THĬ-mē-ă) (p. 234)
suicidal ideation (sū-ĭ-SĪ-dĕl ī-dē-Ā-shĕn) (p. 234)
antidepressants (ăn-tī-dē-PRĔS-ăntz) (p. 235)

DEPRESSIVE AND BIPOLAR DISORDERS

The new *Diagnostic and Statistical Manual of Mental Disorders,* 5th edition (DSM-5), recognizes major psychiatric disorders on a continuum, with depressive disorders and psychotic spectrum at the ends of the continuum and with bipolar disorders serving as a bridge between the two diagnostic classes in terms of symptomatology, family history, and genetics. The common feature among depressive and bipolar disorders is the presence of sad, empty, or irritable mood, accompanied by changes that significantly affect the individual's capacity to function. Duration, timing, and assumed etiology are what differ between the disorders (DSM-5).

Mood is a sustained emotional feeling perceived along a normal continuum of sad to happy that affects our perception of our surroundings. A mood disorder (or affective disorder) is present when certain symptoms impair a person's ability to function for a time. Mood disorders are characterized by abnormal feelings of depression or euphoria. They involve the prolonged and inappropriate expression of emotion that goes beyond brief emotional upset from negative life experiences. In severe cases, other psychotic features may also be present. About 15% to 20% of the US population will have a diagnosable mood disorder during their lifetime.

In *Mental Health: A Report of the Surgeon General* (US Department of Health and Human Services, 1999) it was recognized that the effect of mental illness on health and productivity has been profoundly underestimated. Major depression currently ranks as the second leading cause of disease burden (i.e., years lived with the disability) in the United States; the leading cause is ischemic heart disease. Unfortunately, the majority of people with depression receive no treatment. Undertreatment of mood disorders stems from many factors, including social stigma, financial barriers, underrecognition by healthcare providers, and underappreciation by the general public of the potential benefits of treatment. The symptoms of depression, such as feelings of worthlessness, excessive guilt, and lack of motivation, deter people from seeking treatment. Members of racial and ethnic minority groups often encounter additional barriers.

The underlying causes of mood disorders are still unknown. They are too complex to be completely explained by a single social, developmental, or biologic theory. A variety of factors appear to work together to cause depressive disorders. It is known that patients with depression have changes in the brain **neurotransmitters** norepinephrine, serotonin, dopamine, acetylcholine, and gamma-aminobutyric acid, but other unexpected negative life events (e.g., the sudden death of a loved one, unemployment, medical illness, other stressful events) also play a role. Endocrine abnormalities, such as excessive secretion of cortisol and abnormal thyroid-stimulating hormone, have been found in 45% to 60% of patients with depression. Genetic factors also predispose patients to developing depression. Depressive disorders and suicide tend to cluster in families, and relatives of patients with depression are two to three times more likely to develop depression. Medicines being taken for other diseases may also contribute to depression, including antihypertensives (e.g., reserpine, methyldopa, clonidine, beta-adrenergic blocking agents), antiparkinsonian medicines (e.g., levodopa), and hormones (e.g., estrogens, progestins, corticosteroids).

DEPRESSIVE DISORDER

Major depressive disorder (MDD) and dysthymia are known as *unipolar disorders,* manifested by varying degrees of depression. Patients with MDD experience one or more specific episodes of depression, whereas patients with **dysthymia** suffer from more chronic, ongoing symptoms of depression that last for at least 2 years.

The onset of a depressive disorder tends to occur during the late 20s, although it can occur at any age. The lifetime frequency of depressive symptoms appears to be as high as 26% for women and 12% for men. Risk factors for depression include a personal or family history of depression, prior suicide attempts, female gender, lack of social support, stressful life events, substance abuse, and medical illness. The American Psychiatric Association classifies episodes of depression as mild, moderate, and severe. Mild depression causes only minor functional impairment. Moderate depression involves an intermediate degree of impairment and affects both symptomatology and functionality. Patients with severe depression have several symptoms that exceed the minimum diagnostic criteria and daily functioning is significantly impaired; hospitalization may be required.

It is beyond the scope of this text to discuss mood disorders in detail, but this discussion describes general types of symptoms associated with mood disorders. Patients experiencing **depression** display varying degrees of emotional, physical, cognitive, and psychomotor

symptoms. Emotionally, the depression is characterized by a persistent, reduced ability to experience pleasure in life's usual activities, such as hobbies, family, and work. Patients frequently appear sad, and a personality change is common. They may describe their mood as sad, hopeless, or blue. Patients often feel that they have let others down, although these feelings of guilt are unrealistic. Anxiety symptoms (see Chapter 15) are present in almost 90% of depressed patients. Physical symptoms often motivate the person to seek medical attention. Common physical symptoms seen in patients with depression include chronic fatigue, sleep disturbances such as frequent early morning awakening (terminal insomnia), appetite disturbances (weight loss or gain), and other symptoms such as stomach complaints or heart palpitations. **Cognitive symptoms**, such as the inability to concentrate, slowed thinking, confusion, and poor memory of recent events, are particularly common in older patients with depression. **Psychomotor symptoms** of depression include slowed or retarded movements, thought processes, and speech or, conversely, agitation manifesting as purposeless, restless motion (e.g., pacing, hand wringing, outbursts of shouting). Comorbid conditions such as substance-related disorders, panic disorder, obsessive-compulsive related disorders, and anorexia nervosa are commonly present in patients with MDD.

Life Span Considerations
Depression

The patient and caregivers must understand the importance of continuing to take the prescribed antidepressant medication despite a minimal initial response. The lag time of 1 to 4 weeks between the initiation of therapy and the therapeutic response must be emphasized. In most cases, the symptoms of depression may improve within a few days (e.g., improved appetite, sleep, psychomotor activity). However, the depression still exists, and monitoring should be continued for negative thoughts, feelings, and behaviors. Suicide precautions should be maintained until assessment indicates that suicidal ideation is no longer present.

Suicide statistics are varied and not well documented. Adolescents and older adults with depression are more likely to have suicidal ideation, and older adults commit suicide more frequently than depressed people of other age groups. It appears that older adults are quite serious when attempting suicide because one in two attempts is successful.

Suicide is the third leading cause of death in adolescents; the incidence may be even higher because of underreporting. Suicide is a call for help; however, it is permanent when successfully completed. All comments about suicide or suicide gestures should be taken seriously.

Bipolar disorder (formerly known as *manic depression*) is characterized by distinct episodes of **mania** (elation, euphoria) and depression separated by intervals without mood disturbances. The patient displays extreme changes in mood, cognition, behavior, perception, and sensory experiences. At any one time, a patient with bipolar disorder may be manic or depressed, exhibit symptoms of both mania and depression (mixed), or be between episodes.

Symptoms of acute mania usually begin abruptly and escalate over several days. These symptoms include a heightened mood (**euphoria**), quicker thoughts (flight of ideas), more and faster speech (pressured speech), increased energy, increased physical and mental activities (psychomotor excitement), decreased need for sleep, irritability, heightened perceptual acuity, paranoia, increased sexual activity, and impulsivity. There is often a **labile mood**, with rapid shifts toward anger and irritability. The attention span is short, resulting in an inability to concentrate. Anything in the environment may change the topic of discussion, leading to flight of ideas. Social inhibitions are lost, and the patient may become disruptive and loud, departing suddenly from the social interaction and leaving everything in disarray. As the manic phase progresses, approximately two-thirds of patients with bipolar disorder develop psychotic symptoms (see Chapter 17), primarily paranoid or **grandiose delusions** (the delusion that one has great talents or special powers), if treatment interventions have not been initiated. Unfortunately, most manic patients do not recognize the symptoms of illness in themselves and may resist treatment. **Cyclothymia** is a milder form of bipolar illness characterized by episodes of depression and hypomania that are not severe enough to meet the full criteria for bipolar disorder, but the symptoms of which last at least 2 years.

Bipolar disorder occurs equally in men and women, with a prevalence rate of 0.4% to 1.6% in the adult population of the United States. The onset of bipolar disorder is usually during late adolescence or the early 20s. It is rare before adolescence, and it may occur as late as age 50. Approximately 60% to 80% of patients with bipolar disease will begin with a manic episode. Without treatment, episodes last from 6 months to a year for depression and for approximately 4 months for mania. Patients with bipolar disorder commonly have co-occurring conditions such as anxiety disorders (panic attacks, phobias, social anxiety), attention-deficit/hyperactivity disorder, and substance use disorder (e.g., alcohol).

People with depressive and bipolar disorders have a high incidence of attempting suicide. The frequency of successful suicide is 15%, which is 30 times higher than that of the general population. All patients with depressive symptoms should be assessed for suicidal thoughts or **suicidal ideation**. Factors that increase the risk of suicide include increasing age, being widowed, being unmarried, unemployment, living alone, substance abuse, previous psychiatric admission, and feelings of hopelessness. The presence of a detailed plan with the intention and ability to carry it out indicate strong intent and a high risk for suicide. Other hints of potential suicidal intent include changes in personality, a sudden decision to make a will or give away possessions, and the recent purchase of a gun or hoarding a large supply of medications, including antidepressants, tranquilizers, or other toxic substances.

The prognosis for depressive and bipolar disorders is highly variable. Of patients with major depression, 20% to 30% recover fully and do not experience another bout of depression. Another 50% have recurring episodes, often with a year or more separating the events. The remaining 20% have a chronic course with persistent symptoms and social impairment. Most treated episodes of depression last approximately 3 months; untreated ones last 6 to 12 months. Patients with bipolar illness are more likely to have multiple subsequent episodes of symptoms.

TREATMENT OF DEPRESSIVE AND BIPOLAR DISORDERS

Mood disorders are treated with nonpharmacologic and pharmacologic therapy. Cognitive behavior therapy, psychodynamic therapy, and interpersonal therapy with pharmacologic treatment have been more successful than any one treatment alone. Psychotherapy improves psychosocial function, interpersonal relationships, and day-to-day coping. Patients and family members should be taught to recognize the signs and symptoms of mania, as well as those of depression, and the importance of treatment compliance to minimize the recurrence of the illness should be stressed. Patients should be encouraged to target symptoms that help them recognize mood changes and to seek treatment as soon as possible.

Most patients pass through three phases—acute, continuation, and maintenance—before full function is restored. The acute phase is the period from diagnosis to initial treatment response. The initial response occurs when the symptoms become so significantly reduced that the person no longer fits the criteria for the illness. Medication response in the acute phase typically takes 10 to 12 weeks, during which time the patient is seen by the healthcare provider weekly or biweekly to monitor symptoms and adverse effects, to make dosage adjustments, and to provide support. Psychotherapies are initiated at the same time. Treatment of the acute phase is often prolonged because about half of patients become noncompliant with the medication and the psychotherapy or abandon the program. The goals of the continuation phase of therapy are to prevent relapse and to consolidate the initial response into a complete recovery (defined as being symptom free for 6 months). The continuation phase involves 4 to 9 months of combined pharmacotherapy and psychotherapy for patients with a first episode of MDD. Maintenance-phase therapy is recommended for individuals with a history of three or more depressive episodes, chronic depression, or bipolar disorder. The goal of maintenance-phase therapy is to prevent recurrences of the mood disorder;

patients may receive pharmacologic and nonpharmacologic therapy for this condition for a year or more.

Another form of nonpharmacologic treatment for depression and bipolar illness is electroconvulsive therapy (ECT). When performed under the guidelines provided by the American Psychiatric Association, ECT is safe and effective for all subtypes of major depression and bipolar disorders. It is more effective, more rapid in onset of effect, and safer for patients with cardiovascular disease than many drug therapies. A course of ECT usually consists of 6 to 12 treatments, but the number is individualized to the needs of the patient. Patients are now premedicated with anesthetics and neuromuscular blocking agents to prevent many of the adverse effects previously associated with ECT. Although it has been misused, ECT should be viewed as a treatment option that can be lifesaving for patients who otherwise would not recover from depressive illness. It is usually followed by drug therapy to minimize the rate of relapse.

DRUG THERAPY FOR DEPRESSIVE AND BIPOLAR DISORDERS

ACTIONS

Pharmacologic treatment of depression is recommended for patients with symptoms of moderate to severe depression, and it should be considered for patients who do not respond well to psychotherapy. Several classes of drugs, collectively known as *antidepressants*, are used for treatment. Patients diagnosed with bipolar disorder showing symptoms of mania may be treated pharmacologically with an antimanic agent, lithium (see Antimanic agent, p. 251), valproate, or an atypical antipsychotic agent (see USES later).

Antidepressants can be subdivided into three categories:

1. First-generation antidepressants: monoamine oxidase inhibitors (MAOIs) and tricyclic antidepressants (TCAs)
2. Second-generation antidepressants: selective serotonin reuptake inhibitors (SSRIs) and serotonin-norepinephrine reuptake inhibitors (SNRIs)
3. Miscellaneous agents: bupropion, mirtazapine, nefazodone, trazodone, vilazodone, and vortioxetine

The second-generation antidepressants have efficacy similar to and lower toxicity with overdose than the first-generation antidepressants, so they are recommended as first-line agents.

All antidepressants have varying degrees of effects on norepinephrine, dopamine, and serotonin by blocking reuptake and reducing destruction of these neurotransmitters, thereby prolonging their action. The development of a clinical antidepressant response requires at least 2 to 4 weeks of therapy at adequate dosages. In general, the antidepressant used for therapy should be

changed if there is no clear effect within 4 to 6 weeks. Although much is known about the pharmacologic actions of antidepressants, the exact mechanism of action of these agents for treating depressive and bipolar disorders is still unknown. However, it is now understood that these disorders are not simply a deficiency of neurotransmitters, but very complex diseases associated with genetics, life stressors, and altered physiologic pathways in the brain.

USES

Two factors are important when selecting an antidepressant drug: the patient's history of response to previously prescribed antidepressants and the potential for adverse effects associated with different classes of antidepressants. Contrary to marketing claims, there are no differences among antidepressant drugs (with the exception of the MAOIs) in relative overall therapeutic efficacy and onset caused by full therapeutic dosages. However, there are substantial differences in the adverse effects caused by different agents. It is not possible to predict which drug will be the most effective for an individual patient, but patients do show a better response to a specific drug, even within the same class of drugs. About 30% of patients do not show appreciable therapeutic benefit with the first agent used, but they may have a high degree of success with a change in medication. The history of previous treatment is helpful during the selection of new treatment if illness returns. Approximately 65% to 70% of patients respond to antidepressant therapy, and 30% to 40% achieve remission. Therapy is based on a patient's history of previous response or the successful response of a first-degree relative who responded to antidepressant therapy. Concurrent medical conditions such as obesity, seizure history, potential for dysrhythmias, presence of anxiety, and potential for drug interactions must also be considered in therapy selection. Certain types of mood disorders respond to medication more readily than others. Therapeutic success with TCAs and lithium can be improved by monitoring and maintaining therapeutic serum levels and adjusting dosages as needed. Serum levels of other classes of antidepressants generally do not correlate well with success in therapy, but they may be helpful to determine whether the patient is adhering to the dosage regimen or suffering from toxicities associated with higher serum levels. Recent changes in practice guidelines emphasize the need for continuing drug therapy for all patients; lifelong maintenance therapy will be required for some patients. The dosages of continuance and maintenance therapy must also be the same as the acute dose effective for eliminating depressive symptoms. When patients are given lower maintenance dosages, the risk of relapse is significantly greater than when doses are maintained at acute dose levels.

Antidepressants increase the risk of suicidal thinking and behavior (suicidality) in short-term studies of children and adolescents with MDD and other psychiatric disorders. Anyone considering the use of an antidepressant for a child or an adolescent must balance the risk with the clinical need. When therapy is started, patients must be closely observed for clinical worsening, suicidality, or unusual changes in behavior. Families and caregivers need to be advised about the need for close observation and communication with the prescriber. Pooled analyses of short-term (4 to 16 weeks) placebo-controlled trials of nine antidepressant drugs (SSRIs and others) in children and adolescents with MDD, obsessive-compulsive related disorders, or other psychiatric disorders—a total of 24 trials involving more than 4400 patients—have revealed a greater risk for adverse reactions representing suicidal thinking or behavior during the first few months of treatment in those receiving antidepressants. The average risk of such reactions in patients receiving antidepressants was 4%, which was twice the placebo risk of 2%. No suicides occurred during these trials.

Patients must be counseled about expected therapeutic benefits and adverse effects to be tolerated because of antidepressant therapy. The physiologic manifestations of depression (e.g., sleep disturbance, change in appetite, loss of energy, fatigue, palpitations) begin to be alleviated within the first week of therapy. The psychological symptoms (e.g., depressed mood, lack of interest, social withdrawal) will improve after 2 to 4 weeks of therapy at an effective dosage. Therefore it may take 4 to 6 weeks to adjust the dosage to optimize therapy and to minimize adverse effects. Unfortunately, some adverse effects develop early in therapy, and patients who are already pessimistic because of their illness have a tendency to become noncompliant.

The pharmacologic treatment of bipolar disorder must be individualized because the clinical presentation, severity, and frequency of episodes vary widely among patients. Acute mania is initially treated with lithium, valproate, or an atypical antipsychotic agent (e.g., olanzapine, risperidone) as monotherapy. Options with the best evidence to support use as maintenance treatments include antipsychotics, lithium, and valproate; possible alternatives include lamotrigine, carbamazepine, or oxcarbazepine.

❖ NURSING IMPLICATIONS FOR MOOD DISORDER THERAPY

◆ Assessment

History of mood disorder
- Obtain a history of the patient's mood disorder. Is it depressive only, or are there both manic and depressive phases interspersed with periods of normalcy? What precipitating factors contribute to the changes in mood? Is it associated with a particular season? How often do the depressive, normal, and manic moods persist? Are there better or worse times of day? Has the patient been treated previously for a mood disorder? What is the patient's current status? Has the individual been using alcohol or drugs? Has

there been a recent loss (e.g., job loss, end of a relationship, death of a loved one)?
- Obtain a detailed history of all medications that the individual is currently taking and those taken within the past 2 months to evaluate the patient's adherence to the treatment regimen. How compliant has the patient been with the treatment regimen?

Basic mental status
- Note the patient's general appearance and appropriateness of attire. Is the individual clean and neat? Is the posture erect, stooped, or slumped? Is the individual oriented to date, time, place, and person?
- What coping mechanisms have been used to deal with the mood disorder? How adaptive are these coping mechanisms? If these coping mechanisms are maladaptive, initiate changes by guiding the individual in the use of more adaptive coping strategies.
- Review standardized instruments or tools completed by the patient, such as the Beck Depression Inventory II (Beck, Steer, and Brown, 1996), a widely used assessment tool when screening for depression.

Interpersonal relationships
- Assess the patient's interpersonal relationships. Identify people in the patient's life who are supportive.
- Identify whether interpersonal relationships have declined between the patient and family members, at work, or in social settings.

Mood and affect
- Is the individual elated, overjoyed, angry, irritable, crying, tearful, or sad? Is the facial expression tense, worried, sad, angry, or blank? Ask the person to describe his or her feelings. Be alert for expressions of loneliness, apathy, worthlessness, or hopelessness. Moods may change suddenly.
- Be brief, direct, and to the point with patients experiencing the manic phase who have become argumentative and aggressive. Setting limits will be necessary. Plan to approach the individual in a quiet, safe environment with other staff available in case the patient is aggressive or threatens harm to self or others.
- Patients with altered thinking, behavior, or feelings must be carefully evaluated for verbal and nonverbal actions. Often the thoughts, feelings, and behaviors displayed by these patients are inconsistent with the so-called normal responses of persons in similar circumstances.
- Assess whether the mood being described is consistent with the circumstances being described. For example, is the person speaking of death while smiling?

Clarity of thought.
Evaluate the coherency, relevancy, and organization of the patient's thoughts; observe for flight of ideas, hallucinations, delusions, paranoia, or

grandiose ideation. Ask specific questions about the individual's ability to make judgments and decisions. Is there evidence of memory impairment? Identify areas in which the patient is capable of providing input to set goals and make decisions. (This will help the individual overcome a sense of powerlessness regarding life situations.) When the patient is unable to make decisions, plan to make them. Set goals to involve the patient because abilities change with treatment. Provide an opportunity to plan for self-care.

Suicidal ideation. If the individual is suspected of being suicidal, ask the patient whether he or she has ever had thoughts about suicide. If the response is "yes," get more details. Has a specific plan been formulated? How often do these thoughts occur? Does the patient make direct or indirect statements regarding death (e.g., "things would be better" if death occurred)?

Psychomotor function. Ask specific questions about the activity level the patient has maintained. Is the person able to work or go to school? Is the person able to fulfill responsibilities at work, socially, and within the family? How have the person's normal responses to daily activities been altered? Is the individual withdrawn and isolated or still involved in social interactions? Check gestures, gait, pacing, presence or absence of tremors, and ability to perform gross or fine motor movements. Is the patient hyperactive or impulsive? Note the speech pattern. Are there prolonged pauses before answers are given or altered levels of volume and inflection?

Sleep pattern. What is the patient's normal sleep pattern, and how does it vary with mood swings? Ask specifically whether insomnia is present and whether it is initial (falling asleep) or terminal (staying asleep) in nature. Ask the individual to describe the perception of the amount and quality of sleep nightly. Are naps taken regularly?

Dietary history. Ask questions about the patient's appetite, and note weight gains or losses not associated with intentional dieting. During the manic phase, the individual may become anorexic. Is the person able to sit down to eat a meal, or does he or she only eat small amounts while pacing?

Nonadherence. Nonadherence is usually expressed by the denial of the severity of the disease. In addition, listen for excuses that the patient may make for not taking prescribed medicine (e.g., cannot afford it, asymptomatic, "I don't like the way it changes me. I want to be myself!").

◆ **Implementation**
- Nursing interventions must be individualized and based on patient assessment data.

- Provide an environment of acceptance that focuses on the individual's strengths while minimizing weaknesses. Sometimes it is necessary to provide a new environment for the patient during a period of depression. The individual may not be able to work and may need a new peer group. The patient may also need to be away from the family while restructuring and regrouping personal resources, identifying strengths, and achieving a therapeutic drug level.
- Provide an opportunity for the patient to express feelings. Use active listening and therapeutic communication techniques. Allow the patient to express feelings in nonverbal ways, such as involvement in physical activities or occupational therapy. Recognize that patients are hyperactive and talkative during the manic phase; it may be necessary to interrupt talking and give concise, simple directions.
- Remain calm, direct, and firm when providing care. Because patients in the manic phase tend to be argumentative, avoid getting involved in an argument. State the unit rules in a matter-of-fact manner and enforce them.
- Allow the patient to make decisions, if capable; make those decisions that the patient is not capable of making. Provide a reward for progress when decisions are initiated appropriately. Involve the patient in self-care activities.
- If the patient is suicidal, ask for details about the plan being formulated. Follow up on details obtained with appropriate family members or significant others (e.g., have guns removed from the home if this is part of the suicide plan). Provide for patient safety and supervision, and record observations at specified intervals consistent with the severity of the suicide threat and the policies of the practice site. This is the highest priority for those with severe mood disorders.
- Manic patients may harm others; it may be necessary to limit their interactions with other patients. Patients in the manic phase may require a quiet room.
- Stay with patients who are highly agitated.
- Administer as-needed drugs as ordered for hyperactivity. Make necessary observations about patient responses to the medications administered.
- ECT may be ordered to treat severe depression. Check the healthcare provider's orders specific to the pretreatment and posttreatment care of the patient receiving ECT.
- Use physical restraints within the guidelines of the clinical setting as appropriate to the behaviors being exhibited. Use the least restrictive alternative possible for the circumstances. Have sufficient staff available to assist with violent behavior to demonstrate the ability to control the situation while providing for the safety and well-being of the patient and fellow staff members.

- Provide for nutritional needs by having high-protein, high-calorie foods appropriate for the individual to eat while pacing or highly active. Have nutritious snacks that the patient is known to like available on the unit, and offer them throughout the day. Give vitamins and liquid supplemental feedings as ordered.
- Manipulative behavior must be handled in a consistent manner by all staff members. Set limits and use consequences that are agreed to by all staff members. When the patient attempts to blame others, refocus on the patient's responsibilities. Give positive reinforcement for nonmanipulative behaviors when they occur.
- Sleep deprivation (i.e., missing one or more night's sleep) is a possibility with manic patients and can be life threatening. Provide a quiet, nonstimulating environment for the patient to sleep. For patients with depression, do not allow the individual to sleep continually. Design activities during the day that will stimulate the individual and promote sleep at night. Schedule specific rounds to evaluate the individual's sleep and safety.

◆ **Patient Education**
- Orient the individual to the unit. Explain the rules and the process of privileges and how they are obtained or lost. (The extent of the orientation and explanations given will depend on the patient's orientation to date, time, and place, as well as his or her abilities.)
- Describe the variety of group activities (e.g., social skills, self-esteem, physical exercise) available within particular therapeutic settings.
- Involve the patient and the family in goal setting, and integrate the patient into the appropriate group processes to develop positive experiences and enhance coping skills.
- Base patient education on the assessment data and individualize teaching to provide the patient with a structured environment in which to grow and enhance his or her self-esteem.
- Before discharge, make sure the patient and the family understand the desired treatment outcomes and the entire follow-up plan (e.g., frequency of therapy sessions, prescribed medications, physician visits, return-to-work goals).

Fostering health maintenance
- Throughout the course of treatment, discuss medication information and how it will benefit the patient. Drug therapy is not immediately effective in treating depression; therefore the patient and significant others must understand the importance of continuing to take the prescribed medications despite minimal initial response. The lag time of 2 to 4 weeks between the initiation of drug therapy and the therapeutic response must be stressed.

- Encourage the patient, family, and caregivers to be alert to the emergence of anxiety, agitation, panic attacks, insomnia, irritability, hostility, aggressiveness, impulsivity, akathisia (psychomotor restlessness), hypomania, mania, unusual changes in behavior, worsening of depression, and suicidality, especially at the start of antidepressant treatment and when the dosage is adjusted up or down. Advise the family and caregivers to observe for the emergence of such symptoms on a daily basis because changes may be abrupt. Such symptoms should be reported to the patient's prescriber, especially if they are severe, are abrupt in onset, or were not part of the patient's presenting symptoms. Symptoms such as these may be associated with an increased risk of suicidal thinking and behavior and may indicate the need for very close monitoring and possible changes in the medication regimen.
- Emphasize the need for the lithium blood level to be measured at specified intervals. Give the patient details regarding the date, time, and place for the test to be performed.
- Stress the importance of adequate hydration (i.e., six to eight 8-ounce glasses of water per day) and sodium intake when receiving lithium therapy.
- Instruct the patient to weigh himself or herself daily.
- Provide the patient or significant others with important information contained in the specific drug monographs for the medicines prescribed. The monographs also contain health teaching and nursing interventions for common and serious adverse effects.
- Seek cooperation and understanding of the following points so that medication adherence is increased: name of the medication; its dosage, route, and time of administration; and its common and serious adverse effects. Encourage the patient not to discontinue or adjust the drug dosage without consulting the healthcare provider.
- Children and adolescent patients must be closely observed for clinical worsening, suicidality, or unusual changes in behavior. Families and caregivers need to be advised of the need for close observation and communication with the prescriber.
- Provide patients and families with information about available community resources, including the National Alliance on Mental Illness.

Patient self-assessment. Enlist the patient's help with developing and maintaining a written record of monitoring parameters. See the Patient Self-Assessment Form for Antidepressants on the Evolve website, and complete the Premedication Data column for use as a baseline to track the patient's response to drug therapy. Ensure that the patient understands how to use the form, and instruct the patient to bring the completed form to follow-up visits. During follow-up visits, focus on issues that will foster adherence with the therapeutic interventions prescribed.

Clinical Pitfall

Antidepressants may increase the risk of suicidal thinking and behavior (suicidality) in patients of all ages who are experiencing MDD. Patients who are started on antidepressants should be monitored daily by family members and caregivers for the emergence of agitation, irritability, unusual changes in behavior, and suicidality. Such symptoms should be immediately reported to healthcare providers.

DRUG THERAPY FOR DEPRESSIVE DISORDERS

DRUG CLASS: MONOAMINE OXIDASE INHIBITORS

During the early 1950s, isoniazid and iproniazid were developed to treat tuberculosis. It was soon reported that patients treated with iproniazid exhibited mood elevation. After further investigation, it was discovered that iproniazid—in addition to having antitubercular properties—inhibited monoamine oxidase, whereas isoniazid did not. Other MAOIs were synthesized and used extensively to treat depression until the 1960s, when the TCAs became available.

Actions

Monoamine oxidase inhibitors block the metabolic destruction of epinephrine, norepinephrine, dopamine, and serotonin neurotransmitters by the enzyme monoamine oxidase in the presynaptic neurons of the brain. As a result, the concentration of these central nervous system (CNS) neurotransmitters becomes increased. Although MAO inhibition starts within a few days after initiating therapy, the antidepressant effects require 2 to 4 weeks to become evident. Approximately 60% of the clinical improvement of symptoms of depression occurs after 2 weeks, and maximum improvement is usually attained within 4 weeks.

Uses

The MAOIs used today are phenelzine, tranylcypromine, isocarboxazid, and selegiline (Table 16.1). They are equally effective and have similar adverse effects. They are most effective for atypical depression, panic disorder, obsessive-compulsive related disorders, and some phobic disorders. Selegiline is approved for treatment of MDD. They are also used when TCA therapy is unsatisfactory and when ECT is inappropriate or refused. Selegiline is available as a transdermal patch that should be changed once every 24 hours. Patients using the lowest strength available (6 mg) do not have dietary restrictions. However, dietary restrictions are required for those using the 9- and 12-mg patches.

Therapeutic Outcomes

The primary therapeutic outcomes expected from MAOIs are elevated mood and the reduction of symptoms of depression.

❖ Nursing Implications for Monoamine Oxidase Inhibitors

◆ Premedication assessment

1. Obtain the patient's blood pressure and pulse rate before and at regular intervals after initiating therapy.
2. If the patient has diabetes, monitor the blood glucose level to establish baseline values and assess this periodically during therapy. Because MAOIs cause hypoglycemia, a dosage adjustment in insulin or oral hyperglycemic therapy may be required. If the patient has a history of severe renal disease, liver disease, cerebrovascular disease, or congestive heart failure, do not give the medication and consult with the prescriber.
3. Complete a diet history to ensure that the patient has not ingested meals with a high tyramine content during the past few days.
4. Complete a medication history to ensure that the patient has not taken any of the following medicines during the past few days: SSRIs, SNRIs, TCAs, dextromethorphan, ephedrine, amphetamines, methylphenidate, levodopa, tramadol, St. John's wort, cyclobenzaprine, carbamazepine, or meperidine.

◆ Availability. See Table 16.1.

◆ Dosage and administration

1. Instruct the patient how to limit tyramine-containing foods, which could cause a life-threatening hypertensive crisis if they are ingested concurrently with MAOIs.
2. The dosage should be taken in divided doses, with the last dose administered no later than 6 PM to prevent drug-induced insomnia. Caution the patient not to discontinue the medicine abruptly. If a dose is missed, take it immediately when this is realized and then space the remainder of the daily dosage throughout the rest of the day.
3. Make certain that the patient is not receiving any of the medications listed in the premedication assessment shown previously.

◆ Common adverse effects
Cardiovascular
Orthostatic hypotension. The most common adverse effect of MAOIs is hypotension; it is more significant with phenelzine than with tranylcypromine. Orthostatic hypotension, manifested by dizziness and weakness, is generally mild and is more common when therapy is started. Daily divided doses help minimize the hypotension, and tolerance usually develops after a few weeks of therapy. Monitor the patient's blood pressure daily in both the supine and standing positions. Anticipate the development of postural hypotension and take measures to prevent its occurrence. Teach the patient to rise slowly from a supine or sitting position, and encourage sitting or lying down if feeling faint.

Table 16.1   Antidepressants

GENERIC NAME	BRAND NAME	AVAILABILITY	INITIAL DOSAGE RANGE (ORAL UNLESS OTHERWISE NOTED)	DAILY MAINTENANCE DOSAGE RANGE (MG)	MAXIMUM DAILY DOSAGE RANGE (MG)
Monoamine Oxidase Inhibitors					
isocarboxazid	Marplan	Tablets: 10 mg	10 mg twice daily	40	60
phenelzine	Nardil	Tablets: 15 mg	15 mg three times daily	15-60	90
selegiline ⇄ *Do not confuse selegiline with sertralineor Salagen.*	Emsam	Patch, transdermal: 6, 9, 12 mg/24 hr	6-mg patch daily	6	12
tranylcypromine	Parnate	Tablets: 10 mg	30 mg daily divided	30	60
Selective Serotonin Reuptake Inhibitors					
citalopram	Celexa ⇄ *Do not confuse Celexa with Zyprexa or Celebrex.*	Tablets: 10, 20, 40 mg Liquid: 10 mg/5 mL	20 mg daily	20-40	40
escitalopram	Lexapro ⇄ *Do not confuse Lexapro with loxapine.*	Tablets: 5, 10, 20 mg Liquid: 1 mg/mL	10 mg daily	10-20	20
fluoxetine ⇄ *Do not confuse fluoxetine with fluphenazine, fluvoxamine, famotidine, fluvastatin, or paroxetine.*	Prozac Riva-Fluoxetine ❦ ⇄ *Do not confuse Prozac with Prilosec or Proscar.*	Capsules: 10, 20, 40 mg Tablets: 10, 20, 60 mg Solution: 20 mg/5 mL Capsules, delayed release, weekly: 90 mg	20 mg in the morning	20-60	80
fluvoxamine ⇄ *Do not confuse fluvoxamine with fluoxetine.*	Luvox ⇄ *Do not confuse Luvox with Lasix, Levoxyl, or Lovenox.*	Tablets: 25, 50, 100 mg Capsules, 24 hr sustained release: 100, 150 mg	50 mg at bedtime	50-300	300
paroxetine ⇄ *Do not confuse paroxetine with fluoxetine, paclitaxel, or pyridoxine.*	Paxil ⇄ *Do not confuse Paxil with paclitaxel, Plavix, or Taxol.* Paxil CR	Tablets: 10, 20, 30, 40 mg Suspension: 10 mg/5 mL Tablets, sustained release: 12.5, 25, 37.5 mg	20 mg daily	20-50	50-75
sertraline ⇄ *Do not confuse sertraline with selegiline, Seroquel, or Singulair.*	Zoloft Apo-Sertraline ❦ ⇄ *Do not confuse Zoloft with Zocor or Zyloprim.*	Tablets: 25, 50, 100 mg Oral concentrate: 20 mg/mL	50 mg daily	50-200	200

Table 16.1   Antidepressants—cont'd

GENERIC NAME	BRAND NAME	AVAILABILITY	INITIAL DOSAGE RANGE (ORAL UNLESS OTHERWISE NOTED)	DAILY MAINTENANCE DOSAGE RANGE (MG)	MAXIMUM DAILY DOSAGE RANGE (MG)
Serotonin-Norepinephrine Reuptake Inhibitors					
desvenlafaxine	Pristiq, Khedezla	Tablets, 24 hr sustained release: 25, 50, 100 mg	50 mg daily at the same time	50-400	400
duloxetine	Cymbalta ⇄ Do not confuse Cymbalta with Zyprexa or Celebrex.	Capsules, sustained release: 20, 30, 40, 60 mg	40 mg daily	60	120
levomilnacipran	Fetzima	Capsules, extended release: 20, 40, 80, 120 mg	20 mg once daily for 2 days; then 40 mg once daily	40-120	120
venlafaxine	Effexor Riva-Venlafaxine XR ♣	Tablets: 25, 37.5, 50, 75, 100 mg Capsules, tablets, sustained release: 37.5, 75, 150, 225 mg	75 mg in two or three doses daily, taken with food	75-225	225 (outpatients) 375 (inpatients)
Tricyclic Antidepressants					
amitriptyline ⇄ Do not confuse amitriptyline with aminophylline.	—	Tablets: 10, 25, 50, 75, 100, 150 mg	25-75 mg daily, divided as needed	75-200	200 (outpatients) 300 (inpatients)
amoxapine	—	Tablets: 25, 50, 100, 150 mg	50 mg two or three times daily	200-300	400 (outpatients) 600 (inpatients)
clomipramine	Anafranil Apo-Clomipramine ♣	Capsules: 25, 50, 75 mg	25 mg once daily	100-150	250
desipramine	Norpramin	Tablets: 10, 25, 50, 75, 100, 150 mg	50-75 mg daily, divided in one to four doses	75-200	300
doxepin ⇄ Do not confuse doxepin with digoxin.	Apo-Doxepin ♣	Capsules: 10, 25, 50, 75, 100, 150 mg Oral concentrate: 10 mg/mL	25 mg three times daily	75-150	300 (inpatients)
imipramine hydrochloride	Tofranil Impril ♣	Tablets: 10, 25, 50 mg	30-75 mg daily in one to four divided doses	50-150	200 (outpatients) 300 (inpatients)
imipramine pamoate	—	Capsules: 75, 100, 125, 150 mg	75-150 mg daily at bedtime	75-150	200 (outpatients) 300 (inpatients)
nortriptyline	Pamelor PMS-Nortriptyline ♣	Capsules: 10, 25, 50, 75 mg Solution: 10 mg/5 mL Capsules: 10, 25 mg	25-50 mg in one to four divided doses	50-75	150
protriptyline	Vivactil	Tablets: 5, 10 mg	5-10 mg three times daily	20-40	60
trimipramine	Surmontil	Capsules: 25, 50, 100 mg	25 mg three times daily	50-150	200 (outpatients) 300 (inpatients)

♣ Available in Canada.   ⇄ Do not confuse.

Neurologic

Drowsiness, sedation. Phenelzine has mild to moderate sedating effects. These symptoms tend to disappear with continued therapy and with the possible readjustment of the dosage. Inform the patient of possible sedative effects. The patient should use caution while driving or performing other tasks that require alertness. Consult with the healthcare provider to consider moving the daily dose to bedtime if sedation continues to be a problem.

Restlessness, agitation, insomnia. These effects are more common with tranylcypromine and are transient as the dosage is being adjusted. Have the patient take the last dose before 6 PM to minimize insomnia.

Sensory

Blurred vision. Caution the patient that blurred vision may occur and make appropriate suggestions for the patient's personal safety.

Gastrointestinal

Constipation; dryness of mucosa of the mouth, throat, nose. Mucosal dryness may be relieved by sucking hard candy or ice chips or by chewing gum. Give the patient stool softeners as prescribed. Encourage adequate fluid intake and foods that will provide sufficient bulk.

Genitourinary

Urinary retention. If the patient develops urinary hesitancy, assess for bladder distention. Report this to the healthcare provider for further evaluation.

◆ *Serious adverse effects*

Cardiovascular

Hypertension. Hypertensive crisis is a major potential complication with MAOI therapy, particularly with tranylcypromine. Because MAOIs block amine metabolism in tissues outside of the brain, patients who consume foods or medications (see Drugs That Increase Toxic Effects under Drug Interactions later in this section) containing indirect-acting sympathomimetic amines are at considerable risk for a hypertensive crisis. Foods containing significant quantities of tyramine include well-ripened cheeses (e.g., Camembert, Edam, Roquefort, Parmesan, mozzarella, cheddar); yeast extract; red wines; pickled herring; sauerkraut; overripe bananas, figs, and avocados; chicken liver; and beer. Foods containing other vasopressors include fava beans, chocolate, coffee, tea, and colas. Common prodromal symptoms of hypertensive crisis include severe occipital headache, stiff neck, sweating, nausea, vomiting, and sharply elevated blood pressure.

◆ *Drug interactions*

Drugs that increase toxic effects. Dextromethorphan, carbamazepine, cyclobenzaprine, methylphenidate, tryptophan, amphetamines, ephedrine, methyldopa, levodopa, epinephrine, and norepinephrine potentiate the toxicity of MAOIs by raising neurotransmitter levels.

Tricyclic antidepressants. Monoamine oxidase inhibitors and TCAs, especially imipramine and desipramine,

should not be administered concurrently. It is recommended that at least 14 days lapse between the discontinuation of MAOIs and the initiation of another antidepressant.

Selective serotonin reuptake inhibitors, serotonin-norepinephrine reuptake inhibitors. Severe reactions—such as convulsions, hyperpyrexia, and death—have been reported with concurrent use of these drugs. It is recommended that at least 14 days lapse between discontinuing an MAOI and starting SSRI or SNRI therapy. A 5-week interval is recommended between discontinuing fluoxetine and starting MAOIs.

General anesthesia, diuretics, antihypertensive agents. Monoamine oxidase inhibitors may potentiate the hypotensive effects of general anesthesia, diuretics, and antihypertensive agents.

Insulin, oral hypoglycemic agents. Monoamine oxidase inhibitors have an additive hypoglycemic effect when combined with insulin and oral sulfonylureas. Monitor the patient's blood glucose level and lower the hypoglycemic dosage, if necessary.

Meperidine, tramadol. When MAOIs are used concurrently with meperidine or tramadol, patients may suffer from hyperpyrexia, restlessness, hypertension, hypotension, convulsions, and coma. The effects of this interaction may occur for several weeks after discontinuing an MAOI. Morphine might be an alternative at lower doses, but monitoring is needed.

DRUG CLASS: SELECTIVE SEROTONIN REUPTAKE INHIBITORS

Actions

Selective serotonin reuptake inhibitors (see Table 16.1) are a newer class of antidepressants chemically unrelated to other antidepressants. They inhibit the reuptake of serotonin from the synaptic cleft, thereby increasing the serotonin concentration that enhances neurotransmission.

Uses

Selective serotonin reuptake inhibitors have become the most widely used class of antidepressants and have been shown to be as effective in treating depression as TCAs. A particular advantage of the SSRIs is that they do not have the anticholinergic and cardiovascular adverse effects that often limit the use of TCAs. As with other antidepressants, it takes 2 to 4 weeks of therapy to obtain the full therapeutic benefit when treating depression. Fluoxetine is the only SSRI that has been approved for use in treating depression in children and adolescents. The US Food and Drug Administration has recommended that paroxetine not be given to patients younger than 18 years.

Selective serotonin reuptake inhibitors are also being studied for treatment of obsessive-compulsive related disorders, obesity, eating disorders (e.g., anorexia nervosa, bulimia nervosa), bipolar disorder, panic disorder, autism, and several other disorders.

Fluvoxamine, paroxetine, sertraline, and fluoxetine are approved for use in patients with obsessive-compulsive related disorders. Fluoxetine is marketed under the brand name Sarafem for treatment of premenstrual dysphoric disorder. Duloxetine is also approved for treatment of generalized anxiety disorder and diabetic peripheral neuropathic pain.

Therapeutic Outcomes

The primary therapeutic outcomes expected from the SSRIs are elevated mood and reduction of the symptoms of depression.

❖ Nursing Implications for Selective Serotonin Reuptake Inhibitor Therapy

◆ *Premedication assessment*
1. Obtain the patient's baseline blood pressures in the supine, sitting, and standing positions; record and report significant lowering to the healthcare provider before administering the drug.
2. Obtain the patient's baseline weight and schedule weekly weight measurements.
3. Note any gastrointestinal (GI) symptoms present before the start of therapy.
4. Monitor any CNS symptoms present, such as insomnia or nervousness.
5. Check the patient's hepatic studies before initiating the medication and periodically throughout the course of administration.

◆ *Availability, dosage, and administration.* See Table 16.1.
Observation. Symptoms of depression may improve (e.g., increased appetite, sleep, and psychomotor activity) within a few days. However, the depression still exists, and it usually takes several weeks of the patient receiving therapeutic dosing before improvement is noted. Suicide precautions should be maintained during this time.

◆ *Common adverse effects*
Neurologic
Restlessness, agitation, anxiety, insomnia. These effects usually occur early in therapy and may require short-term treatment with sedative-hypnotic agents. Avoiding bedtime doses may also help decrease the incidence of insomnia.

Sedative effect. Tell the patient about possible sedative effects. The patient should use caution while driving or performing other tasks that require alertness. Consult with the healthcare provider to consider moving the daily dose to bedtime if sedation continues to be a problem.
Gastrointestinal
Nausea, anorexia. Most of these effects may be minimized by temporarily reducing the dosage and taking the dose with food. Encourage the patient not to discontinue therapy without consulting the healthcare provider first.

Psychological
Suicidal ideation. Monitor the patient for changes in thoughts, feelings, and behaviors during the initial stages of therapy.

◆ *Drug interactions*
Tricyclic antidepressants. The interaction between SSRIs and TCAs is very complex. An increased toxicity results from TCAs. Observe the patient for signs of toxicity, such as dysrhythmias, seizure activity, and CNS stimulation.

Lithium. Lithium may enhance the serotonergic effect of SSRIs, thereby increasing the risk of serotonin toxicity (serotonin syndrome). Use the combination of SSRIs and lithium very cautiously, monitoring closely for signs of serotonin toxicity such as irritability, hallucinations, delirium, increased muscle tone, shivering, myoclonus, and reduced consciousness.

Monoamine oxidase inhibitors. Severe reactions—including excitement, diaphoresis, rigidity, convulsions, hyperpyrexia, and death—have been reported with the concurrent use of MAOIs and SSRIs. It is recommended that at least 14 days lapse between discontinuing an MAOI and starting SSRI therapy. A 5-week stop interval is recommended between discontinuing fluoxetine and starting MAOIs.

Haloperidol. Fluoxetine and fluvoxamine increase haloperidol levels and the frequency of extrapyramidal symptoms (EPSs). If used concurrently, the dosage of haloperidol may need to be decreased.

Phenytoin, phenobarbital. Complex interactions occur when phenobarbital and phenytoin enhance the metabolism of paroxetine, thereby requiring a dosage increase in paroxetine for therapeutic effect. In a similar fashion, paroxetine increases the metabolism of phenytoin, thus requiring an increase in the dosage of phenytoin to maintain the therapeutic effect. Conversely, fluoxetine may diminish the metabolism of phenytoin, thereby resulting in potential phenytoin toxicity.

Carbamazepine. Fluoxetine and fluvoxamine can increase carbamazepine concentrations, which can result in signs of toxicity such as vertigo, tremor, headache, drowsiness, nausea, and vomiting. The dosage of carbamazepine may need to be reduced. Carbamazepine may enhance the excretion of citalopram, thereby leading to a decreased therapeutic effect. The dosage of citalopram may need to be increased.

Alprazolam. Fluoxetine, fluvoxamine, and sertraline prolong the activity of alprazolam, which results in excessive sedation and impaired motor skills.

Propranolol, metoprolol. Fluvoxamine and citalopram significantly inhibit the metabolism of these beta-adrenergic blocking agents. Monitor the patient closely for bradycardia and hypotension. Reduce the dosage of the beta blocker as needed.

Cimetidine. Cimetidine inhibits the metabolism of paroxetine and sertraline. Patients should be closely monitored when cimetidine is added to paroxetine or sertraline therapy.

Warfarin. Fluoxetine, paroxetine, sertraline, citalopram, and fluvoxamine may enhance the anticoagulant effects of warfarin. Observe the patient for petechiae, ecchymoses, nosebleeds, bleeding gums, dark tarry stools, and bright red or coffee-ground emesis. Monitor the international normalized ratio (INR) of warfarin; reduce the dosage of warfarin if necessary.

Smoking. Cigarette smoking enhances the metabolism of fluvoxamine. Dosages of fluvoxamine may need to be increased to achieve full therapeutic response.

Amphetamines, tryptophan, dextromethorphan, ephedrine, pseudoephedrine, epinephrine. All of these agents increase serotonin levels, potentially causing serotonin syndrome when taken by a person receiving SSRIs. Symptoms of serotonin syndrome include irritability, hallucinations, delirium, increased muscle tone, shivering, myoclonus, and reduced consciousness. These medications should be used together only under the supervision of a healthcare provider.

DRUG CLASS: SEROTONIN-NOREPINEPHRINE REUPTAKE INHIBITORS

Actions
Serotonin-norepinephrine reuptake inhibitors (see Table 16.1) are a newer class of antidepressants that act by inhibiting the reuptake of serotonin and norepinephrine—and, to a lesser extent, dopamine—from the synaptic cleft, thereby prolonging the action of the neurotransmitters.

Uses
Serotonin-norepinephrine reuptake inhibitors have become a widely used class of antidepressants. As with other antidepressants, it takes 2 to 4 weeks of therapy to obtain the full therapeutic benefit in treating depression.

Venlafaxine is approved for treatment of depression, generalized anxiety disorder, social anxiety disorder, and panic disorder. Duloxetine is approved for treatment of MDD, generalized anxiety disorder, fibromyalgia, chronic musculoskeletal pain, and diabetic peripheral neuropathic pain. Desvenlafaxine and levomilnacipran are approved for treatment of MDD.

Therapeutic Outcomes
The primary therapeutic outcomes expected from the SNRIs are elevated mood and reduction of symptoms of depression.

❖ **Nursing Implications for Serotonin-Norepinephrine Reuptake Inhibitor Therapy**
◆ *Premedication assessment*
1. Obtain the patient's baseline weight and blood pressure.
2. Note any GI symptoms before starting therapy.
3. Monitor any CNS symptoms present, such as insomnia or nervousness.

4. Report any history of hypertension, substance abuse, or renal or hepatic disease to the healthcare provider.

◆ *Availability, dosage, and administration.* See Table 16.1.
   Discontinuation of therapy. If the patient has taken the medicine for more than 1 week before discontinuation, the dosage should be tapered over the next few days. If venlafaxine has been taken for more than 6 weeks, the dosage should gradually be tapered over the next 2 weeks.
   Observation. Symptoms of depression may improve (e.g., increased appetite, sleep, and psychomotor activity) within a few days. However, the depression still exists, and it usually takes several weeks of the patient receiving therapeutic dosing before improvement is noted. Suicide precautions should be maintained during this time.

◆ *Common adverse effects*
   Neurologic
   Dizziness, drowsiness. The patient should be warned to not work with machinery, operate a motor vehicle, administer medication, or perform other duties that require mental alertness until it is known whether this adverse effect impairs judgment.
   Restlessness, agitation, anxiety, insomnia. These effects usually occur early in therapy, and the patient may require short-term treatment with sedative-hypnotic agents. Avoiding bedtime doses may help decrease the incidence of insomnia.
   Gastrointestinal
   Nausea, anorexia. Most of these effects may be minimized by temporarily reducing the dosage and taking the doses with food.

◆ *Serious adverse effects*
   Psychological
   Suicidal ideation. Monitor the patient for changes in thoughts, feelings, and behaviors during the initial stages of therapy.

◆ *Drug interactions*
   Monoamine oxidase inhibitors. Severe reactions—including excitement, diaphoresis, rigidity, convulsions, hyperpyrexia, and death—have been reported with the concurrent use of MAOIs and SNRIs. It is recommended that at least 14 days lapse between discontinuing an MAOI and starting SNRI therapy (and vice versa).
   Cimetidine. Cimetidine inhibits the metabolism of venlafaxine and duloxetine. Patients should be closely monitored for excessive effects of these two drugs when cimetidine is added to the therapeutic regimen.
   Trazodone. Serotonin syndrome may develop when trazodone is used in conjunction with venlafaxine. Symptoms of serotonin syndrome include irritability, hallucinations, delirium, increased muscle tone, shivering, myoclonus, and reduced consciousness. Use trazodone

cautiously; initiate therapy at a lower dosage and closely monitor for the adverse effects listed.

Haloperidol. Venlafaxine increases haloperidol levels and increases the frequency of EPSs, such as akathisia, dystonia, pseudoparkinsonism, and dyskinesia (see Chapter 17 for more information). If these drugs are used concurrently, the dosage of haloperidol may need to be decreased.

DRUG CLASS: TRICYCLIC ANTIDEPRESSANTS

Actions

Until recently, TCAs (see Table 16.1) were the most widely used medications for the treatment of depression. Selective serotonin reuptake inhibitors now have that distinction, but their long-term effects are yet to be completely determined. Tricyclic antidepressants prolong the action of norepinephrine, dopamine, and serotonin to varying degrees by blocking the reuptake of these neurotransmitters in the synaptic cleft between neurons. The exact mechanism of action when these drugs are used as antidepressants is unknown.

Uses

Tricyclic antidepressants produce antidepressant and mild tranquilizing effects. After 2 to 4 weeks of therapy, these drugs elevate mood, improve appetite, and increase alertness in approximately 80% of patients with endogenous depression. Combination therapy with phenothiazine derivatives may be beneficial for treating depression associated with schizophrenia or moderate to severe anxiety and depression observed with psychosis.

All TCAs are equally effective for treating depression, assuming that appropriate dosages are used for an adequate period. Consequently the selection of an antidepressant is based primarily on the characteristics of each agent. Sedation is more notable with amitriptyline, doxepin, and trimipramine. Protriptyline has no sedative properties, and it may actually produce mild stimulation in some patients. All tricyclic compounds display anticholinergic activity, with amitriptyline displaying the most and desipramine the least. This factor should be considered in patients with cardiac disease, prostatic hyperplasia, or glaucoma. Other factors to consider are that men tend to respond better to imipramine than women and older adults tend to respond better to amitriptyline than younger patients.

Doxepin is also approved for treating anxiety, and imipramine is approved for treating enuresis in children who are 6 years old and older. Clomipramine is not used to treat depression, but it is approved for treating obsessive-compulsive related disorders.

Selected TCAs are also used to treat phantom limb pain, chronic pain, cancer pain, peripheral neuropathy with pain, postherpetic neuralgia, arthritic pain, eating disorders, premenstrual symptoms, and obstructive sleep apnea.

Therapeutic Outcomes

The primary therapeutic outcomes expected from TCAs are elevated mood and reduction of symptoms of depression.

❖ Nursing Implications for Tricyclic Antidepressants
◆ *Premedication assessment*

1. Note the consistency of the patient's bowel movements; constipation is common when taking TCAs.
2. Obtain the patient's baseline blood pressures in supine and standing positions; record and report significant hypotension to the healthcare provider before administering the drug.
3. Check the patient's history for symptoms of dysrhythmias, tachycardia, or congestive heart failure; if present, consult the healthcare provider before starting therapy (the patient may require electrocardiography before therapy is started).
4. If the patient has a history of seizures, check with the healthcare provider to see if the dosage of anticonvulsant therapy medications needs to be adjusted.

◆ *Availability, dosage, and administration.* **Adult:** *PO:* See Table 16.1. The medication should be initiated at a low dosage level and increased gradually, particularly for older or debilitated patients. Dosage increases should be made in the evening because increased sedation often occurs.

Observation. Symptoms of depression may improve (e.g., increased appetite, sleep, and psychomotor activity) within a few days. However, the depression still exists, and it usually takes several weeks of the patient receiving therapeutic dosing before improvement is noted. Suicide precautions should be maintained during this time.

◆ *Common adverse effects*
  Cardiovascular
  Orthostatic hypotension. All TCAs may cause some degree of orthostatic hypotension, manifested by dizziness and weakness, particularly when therapy is first begun. Monitor the patient's blood pressure daily in both the supine and standing positions. Anticipate the development of postural hypotension and take measures to prevent such an occurrence. Teach the patient to rise slowly from a supine or sitting position and encourage the patient to sit or lie down if feeling faint.
  Neurologic
  Sedative effects. Tell the patient about possible sedative effects. These effects usually occur early in therapy. Taking a single dose at bedtime may diminish or relieve the sedative effects.
  Sensory
  Blurred vision. Caution the patient that blurred vision may occur and make appropriate suggestions to ensure the patient's personal safety.
  Gastrointestinal
  Constipation; dryness of mucosa of the mouth, throat, nose. Mucosal dryness may be relieved by sucking hard

candy or ice chips or by chewing gum. The use of stool softeners such as docusate or the occasional use of a stimulant laxative such as bisacodyl may be required for constipation.

◆ **Serious adverse effects**

Neurologic

Tremor. Approximately 10% of patients develop this adverse effect. Tremor can be controlled with small doses of propranolol.

Numbness, tingling. Report these symptoms to the healthcare provider for further evaluation.

Parkinsonian symptoms. If these symptoms develop, the TCA dosage must be reduced or discontinued. Antiparkinsonian medications will not control symptoms induced by TCAs.

Seizure activity. High doses of antidepressants lower the seizure threshold. Adjustment of anticonvulsant therapy may be required, especially for seizure-prone patients.

Cardiovascular

Dysrhythmias, tachycardia, heart failure. Report these symptoms to the healthcare provider for further evaluation.

Psychological

Suicidal ideation. Monitor the patient for changes in thoughts, feelings, and behaviors during the initial stages of therapy.

◆ **Drug interactions**

Enhanced anticholinergic activity. Antihistamines, phenothiazines, trihexyphenidyl, and benztropine enhance the anticholinergic activity associated with TCA therapy. The adverse effects are usually not severe enough to warrant discontinuing therapy, but stool softeners may be required.

Enhanced sedative activity. Ethanol, barbiturates, narcotics, tranquilizers, antihistamines, anesthetics, and sedative-hypnotics enhance the sedative activity associated with TCA therapy. Concurrent therapy is not recommended.

Phenobarbital. Phenobarbital may stimulate the metabolism of TCAs. Dosage adjustments of the antidepressant may be necessary.

Bupropion. Bupropion may increase serum levels of TCAs. Dosages may need to be reduced.

Carbamazepine. Tricyclic antidepressants can increase carbamazepine concentrations, resulting in signs of toxicity such as vertigo, tremor, headache, drowsiness, nausea, and vomiting. The dosage of carbamazepine may need to be reduced. Carbamazepine may also reduce serum levels of TCAs. Dosages of the TCA may need to be increased.

Valproic acid, methylphenidate. These medications may increase the serum levels of the TCAs. This reaction has been advantageous in attempts to gain a faster onset of antidepressant activity, but an increased incidence of dysrhythmias also has been reported.

Clonidine. Tricyclic antidepressants inhibit the antihypertensive effects of clonidine and may enhance the hypertension seen with the abrupt discontinuation of clonidine. Concurrent therapy should be avoided.

Monoamine oxidase inhibitors. Severe reactions—including convulsions, hyperpyrexia, and death—have been reported with concurrent use. It is recommended that 2 weeks lapse between discontinuing an MAOI and starting TCAs.

Selective serotonin reuptake inhibitors. The interaction between SSRIs and TCAs is complex. The net result is that there is an increased toxicity from the TCAs. Observe patients for signs of toxicity, such as dysrhythmias, seizure activity, and CNS stimulation.

Amphetamines, tryptophan, dextromethorphan, ephedrine, pseudoephedrine, epinephrine. All of these agents increase serotonin levels, potentially causing serotonin syndrome when taken by a person receiving TCAs. Symptoms of serotonin syndrome include irritability, hallucinations, delirium, increased muscle tone, shivering, myoclonus, and reduced consciousness. These medications should be used together only under the supervision of a healthcare provider.

Cimetidine. Cimetidine inhibits the metabolism of TCAs. Patients should be closely monitored for additional anticholinergic symptoms. In general, cimetidine therapy should be avoided in patients taking TCAs. Ranitidine and famotidine may be used without drug interactions.

Smoking. Cigarette smoking enhances the metabolism of TCAs. Dosages of the TCA may need to be increased to achieve a full therapeutic response.

DRUG CLASS: MISCELLANEOUS AGENTS

---

bupropion hydrochloride (byū-PRŌ-pē-ŏn)
⇄ *Do not confuse bupropion with buspirone.*
Wellbutrin (wĕl-BYŪ-trĭn)
Zyban (ZĪ-băn)

Actions

Bupropion is a monocyclic antidepressant. Its mechanism of action is not fully known. Compared with TCAs, it is believed to be a weak inhibitor of the reuptake of the neurotransmitters norepinephrine and dopamine. It has no monoamine oxidase inhibition or serotonin reuptake inhibition effect.

Uses

Bupropion is approved for use in patients who are unresponsive to TCAs and who cannot tolerate the adverse effects of TCAs. Disadvantages include seizure activity and the requirement of multiple doses daily. It must not be used in patients with psychotic disorders because its dopamine agonist activity causes increased psychotic symptoms.

Bupropion is also approved (as Zyban) as an aid to support someone who is trying to quit smoking. Treatment should be initiated while the patient is still smoking because approximately 1 week of treatment is required to achieve steady-state blood levels of bupropion. Patients should set a target quit date during the first 2 weeks of treatment with bupropion, generally in the second week. Treatment should be continued for 7 to 12 weeks; longer treatment should be guided by the relative benefits and risks for individual patients.

Therapeutic Outcomes

The primary therapeutic outcomes expected from bupropion therapy when used for depression are elevated mood and reduction of symptoms of depression. When it is used for smoking cessation, the expected outcome is the termination of smoking.

❖ **Nursing Implications for Bupropion Therapy**
◆ *Premedication assessment*

1. Obtain the patient's baseline weight.
2. Use the Dyskinesia Identification System: Condensed User Scale (DISCUS) or the Abnormal Involuntary Movement Scale (AIMS) (see Evolve website) at specified intervals to detect or check up on EPSs; record and report in accordance with institutional policy.

◆ *Availability.* **PO:** 75- and 100-mg tablets; 100-, 150-, and 200-mg 12-hour extended-release tablets; 150, 174, 300, 348, 450 24-hour extended-release tablets.

◆ *Dosage and administration for depression.* **Adult: PO:** Initially, 100 mg twice daily. This may be increased to 100 mg three times daily (at least every 6 hours) after several days of therapy. No single dose of bupropion should exceed 150 mg; do not exceed 450 mg daily. Avoid taking a dose shortly before bedtime.

◆ *Dosage and administration for smoking cessation.* **Adult: PO:** Dosing should begin at 150 mg/day given every day for the first 3 days, followed by a dosage increase for most patients to the recommended usual dosage of 300 mg/day. There should be an interval of at least 8 hours between successive doses. Dosages above 300 mg/day should not be used. Bupropion should be swallowed whole, not crushed, divided, or chewed.

Treatment should continue for 7 to 12 weeks; longer treatment should be guided by the relative benefits and risks for individual patients. If a patient has not made significant progress toward abstinence by the seventh week of therapy with bupropion, it is unlikely that he or she will quit during that attempt and treatment should probably be discontinued. Conversely, a patient who successfully quits after 7 to 12 weeks of treatment should be considered for ongoing therapy with bupropion. Dosage tapering of bupropion is not required when discontinuing treatment. The patient should

continue to receive counseling and support throughout treatment with bupropion and for a period of time thereafter.

Individualization of therapy. The smoking cessation patient is more likely to quit smoking and remain abstinent if seen frequently and receiving support from the healthcare provider. Ensure that the patient reads the instructions provided and has any questions answered. The patient's healthcare provider should review the overall smoking cessation program, including treatment with bupropion. The patient should be advised about the importance of participating in the behavioral interventions, counseling, and support services to be used in conjunction with bupropion.

Observation. In the patient with depression, symptoms of depression may improve within a few days (e.g., improved appetite, sleep, and psychomotor activity). However, the depression still exists, and it usually takes several weeks of the patient receiving therapeutic dosing before improvement is noted. Suicide precautions should be maintained during this time.

◆ *Common adverse effects*
Gastrointestinal
Anorexia, constipation, diarrhea, nausea, vomiting. Most GI effects may be minimized by temporarily reducing the dosage, giving with food, and using stool softeners for constipation.
Neurologic
Restlessness, agitation, anxiety, insomnia. These effects usually occur early in therapy, and the patient may require short-term treatment with sedative-hypnotic agents. Avoiding bedtime doses may help decrease the incidence of insomnia.

◆ *Serious adverse effects*
Neurologic
Seizures. See Assessment: History of Seizure Activity in the Antiepileptic Therapy section of Chapter 18.
Psychological
Suicidal ideation. Monitor the patient for changes in thoughts, feelings, and behaviors during the initial stages of therapy.

◆ *Drug interactions*
Cimetidine. Cimetidine inhibits the metabolism of bupropion and increases bupropion blood levels. A decrease in the bupropion dosage may be necessary.
Carbamazepine, phenobarbital, phenytoin. Carbamazepine, phenobarbital, and phenytoin may decrease bupropion serum levels, leading to decreased pharmacologic effect. It may be necessary to adjust the dosage of bupropion.
Nicotine replacement. Although bupropion is used in combination with nicotine replacement products to help with smoking cessation, coadministration of nicotine replacement products with bupropion may cause hypertension. Monitor the patient's blood pressure when

products such as nicotine patches or nicotine gum are being used.

Ritonavir. Ritonavir may stimulate the metabolism of bupropion, causing a reduction in serum concentrations of bupropion. An increase in the bupropion dosage may be necessary.

Levodopa. Bupropion has some mild dopaminergic activity and may result in an increase in the adverse effects caused by levodopa. If bupropion is to be added to levodopa therapy, it should be initiated at a lower dosage with small increases in the dosage of bupropion.

---

mirtazapine (mĭr-TĂZ-ĕ-pĕn)
Remeron (RĔ-mĕr-ŏn)
⇌ *Do not confuse Remeron with Restoril.*

Actions

Mirtazapine is a tetracyclic antidepressant that is a serotonin antagonist. The mechanism of action is unknown, but the pharmacologic response is similar to that of tricyclic antidepressants.

Uses

Mirtazapine is used to treat depression.

Therapeutic Outcomes

The primary therapeutic outcomes expected from mirtazapine therapy are elevated mood and reduction of symptoms of depression.

❖ **Nursing Implications for Mirtazapine Therapy**

◆ *Premedication assessment*

1. Obtain the patient's baseline blood pressures in the supine, sitting, and standing positions; record and report significant hypotension to the healthcare provider before administering the drug.
2. Obtain the patient's baseline weight and schedule weekly weight measurements.
3. Check for a history of seizures. If present, notify the healthcare provider before starting therapy.
4. Check the patient's hepatic studies before initiating therapy and periodically throughout the course of administration.
5. Use the DISCUS or the AIMS (see Evolve website) at specified intervals to detect or check up on EPSs; record and report in accordance with institutional policy.
6. Obtain the patient's white blood cell count before and at regular intervals after initiating therapy because agranulocytosis has been reported.

◆ *Availability.* **PO:** 7.5-, 15-, 30-, and 45-mg tablets; 15-, 30-, and 45-mg orally disintegrating tablets (Remeron SolTab).

◆ *Dosage and administration.* **Adult:** *PO:* Initially, 15 mg daily. Every 1 to 2 weeks the dosage may be increased

up to a maximum of 45 mg daily. Increases in dosage should be made in the evening because increased sedation is often present.

Observation. See Tricyclic Antidepressants on p. 245. Symptoms of depression may improve (e.g., increased appetite, sleep, and psychomotor activity) within a few days. However, the depression still exists, and it usually takes several weeks of the patient receiving therapeutic dosing before improvement is noted. Suicide precautions should be maintained during this time.

🌿 Herbal Interactions

St. John's Wort

St. John's wort may increase the toxic effects of antidepressant medications. The use of St. John's wort with other antidepressants should be done only with close supervision by a healthcare provider.

---

trazodone hydrochloride (TRĂ-zō-dōn)
⇌ *Do not confuse trazodone with amiodarone or tramadol.*

Actions

Trazodone was the first of the triazolopyridine antidepressants to be released for clinical use. The triazolopyridines are chemically unrelated to the other classes of antidepressants. The exact mechanisms of action of trazodone are unknown, but it potentiates serotonin activity by inhibiting reuptake and destruction of serotonin. The actions are complex and in some ways resemble those of the TCAs, benzodiazepines, and phenothiazines; however, the overall activity of trazodone is different from that of each of these classes of drugs.

Uses

Trazodone has been shown to be as effective as TCAs in treating depression; depression associated with schizophrenia; and depression, tremor, and anxiety associated with alcohol dependence. Compared with other antidepressants, trazodone has a low incidence of anticholinergic adverse effects, which makes it particularly useful in patients whose antidepressant dosages are limited by anticholinergic adverse effects and in patients with severe closed-angle glaucoma, prostatic hyperplasia, organic mental disorders, or cardiac dysrhythmias. Trazodone is commonly used to treat insomnia in patients with substance abuse because it is sedating, improves sleep continuity, and has minimal potential for tolerance and addiction.

Therapeutic Outcomes

The primary therapeutic outcomes expected from trazodone therapy are elevated mood and reduction of symptoms of depression.

❖ Nursing Implications for Trazodone Therapy
◆ Premedication assessment
1. Obtain the patient's baseline blood pressures in the supine, sitting, and standing positions.
2. Record and report significant hypotension to the healthcare provider before administering the drug.

◆ Availability. *PO:* 50-, 100-, 150-, and 300-mg tablets.

◆ Dosage and administration. **Adult:** *PO:* Initially, 150 mg in three divided doses. Increase the dosage in increments of 50 mg daily every 3 to 4 days while monitoring the clinical response. Do not exceed 400 mg daily in outpatients or 600 mg daily in hospitalized patients.

Trazodone therapy should be initiated at a low dosage and increased gradually, particularly in older adults or debilitated patients. Dosage increases should be made in the evening because increased sedation often occurs. Administer the medication shortly after a meal or with a light snack to reduce adverse effects.

Observation. Symptoms of depression may improve (e.g., increased appetite, sleep, and psychomotor activity) within a few days. However, the depression still exists, and it usually takes several weeks of the patient receiving therapeutic dosing before improvement is noted. Suicide precautions should be maintained during this time.

◆ Common adverse effects
Cardiovascular

Orthostatic hypotension. Although episodes are infrequent and generally mild, trazodone may cause some degree of orthostatic hypotension, manifested by dizziness and weakness, particularly when therapy is initiated. Monitor the patient's blood pressure daily in both the supine and standing positions. Anticipate the development of postural hypotension and take measures to prevent an occurrence. Teach the patient to rise slowly from a supine or sitting position, and encourage the patient to sit or lie down if feeling faint.

Neurologic

Drowsiness. The patient should be warned to not work with machinery, operate a motor vehicle, administer medication, or perform other duties that require mental alertness until it is known whether this adverse effect impairs judgment.

◆ Serious adverse effects
Cardiovascular

Dysrhythmias, tachycardia. Report these symptoms to a healthcare provider for further evaluation.

Neurologic

Confusion. Before initiating therapy, perform a baseline assessment of the patient's degree of alertness and orientation to name, place, and time. Make regularly scheduled subsequent evaluations of the patient's mental status and compare findings. Report any significant alterations to the prescriber.

Dizziness, lightheadedness. Provide for patient safety during episodes of dizziness and report these symptoms to the prescriber for further evaluation.

◆ Drug interactions

Enhanced sedative activity. Ethanol, narcotics, tranquilizers, antihistamines, anesthetics, phenothiazines, and sedative-hypnotics enhance the sedative effects associated with trazodone therapy. Concurrent therapy is not recommended.

MAOIs, SSRIs, SNRIs. Serotonin syndrome may develop when trazodone is used in conjunction with any of these agents. Symptoms of serotonin syndrome include irritability, hallucinations, delirium, increased muscle tone, shivering, myoclonus, and reduced consciousness. Use trazodone cautiously; initiate therapy at a lower dosage and closely monitor for the adverse effects listed.

---

vilazodone (vĭl-ĂZ-zō-dōn)
⇌ ***Do not confuse vilazodone with trazodone or nefazodone.***
Viibryd (vī-brĭd)

Actions
Vilazodone is a newer medication that acts as an SSRI and a partial agonist of serotonin (5-hydroxytryptamine) 5-HT_{1A} receptors, thereby enhancing serotonin activity.

Uses
Vilazodone is approved to treat MDD in adults.

Therapeutic Outcomes
The primary therapeutic outcomes expected from vilazodone therapy are elevated mood and reduction of symptoms of depression.

❖ Nursing Implications for Vilazodone Therapy
◆ Premedication assessment
1. Note any GI symptoms present before the start of therapy.
2. Monitor any CNS symptoms present (e.g., insomnia, restlessness).

◆ Availability. *PO:* 10-, 20-, and 40-mg tablets.

◆ Dosage and administration. **Adult:** *PO:* Initially, 10 mg once daily with food, followed by 20 mg once daily with food for the next 7 days, and then increased to the recommended dosage of 40 mg once daily. Vilazodone should be taken with food for optimal absorption.

Observation. Symptoms of depression may improve (e.g., increased appetite, sleep, and psychomotor activity) within a few days. However, the depression still exists, and it usually takes several weeks of the patient receiving therapeutic dosing before improvement is noted. Suicide precautions should be maintained during this time.

◆ *Common adverse effects*

Gastrointestinal

Diarrhea, nausea, vomiting. These adverse effects should be mild, particularly if the dose is administered with food. They should also resolve with continued therapy. Patients with persistent vomiting should be evaluated for other causes, as well as for the development of electrolyte imbalance.

Neurologic

Dizziness, drowsiness. Provide for patient safety during episodes of dizziness and report these symptoms to the healthcare provider for further evaluation. The patient should not take these medications while working with machinery, operating a motor vehicle, administering medication, or performing other duties that require mental alertness.

◆ *Serious adverse effects*

Neurologic

Confusion. Before initiating therapy, perform a baseline assessment of the patient's degree of alertness and orientation to name, place, and time. Make regularly scheduled subsequent evaluations of the patient's mental status and compare findings. Report any significant alterations to the prescriber.

Dizziness, lightheadedness. Provide for patient safety during episodes of dizziness and report these symptoms to the healthcare provider for further evaluation.

Psychological

Suicidal ideation. Monitor the patient for changes in thoughts, feelings, and behaviors, especially during the initial stages of therapy.

◆ *Drug interactions*

Monoamine oxidase inhibitors. Severe reactions—including excitement, diaphoresis, rigidity, convulsions, hyperpyrexia, and death—may result from the concurrent use of MAOIs and vilazodone. It is recommended that at least 14 days lapse between discontinuing an MAOI and starting vilazodone. It is further recommended that there be a 14-day drug-free interval between discontinuing vilazodone and starting MAOI therapy.

Enhanced sedative activity. Ethanol, narcotics, tranquilizers, antihistamines, anesthetics, phenothiazines, and sedative-hypnotics enhance the sedative effects that are associated with vilazodone therapy. Concurrent therapy is not recommended.

Trazodone, MAOIs, SSRIs, SNRIs, tramadol, triptans. Serotonin syndrome may develop when vilazodone is used in conjunction with any of these agents. Symptoms of serotonin syndrome include irritability, hallucinations, delirium, increased muscle tone, shivering, myoclonus, and reduced consciousness. Use these drugs cautiously; initiate therapy at a lower dosage and closely monitor for the adverse effects listed.

Aspirin, nonsteroidal antiinflammatory drugs, warfarin. Serotonin release by platelets plays an important role in hemostasis. Selective serotonin reuptake inhibitors may enhance the anticoagulant effects of warfarin and enhance the potential for GI bleeding caused by nonsteroidal antiinflammatory drugs or aspirin. Observe the patient for petechiae, ecchymoses, nosebleeds, bleeding gums, dark tarry stools, and bright red or coffee-ground emesis. Monitor prothrombin time and the INR of warfarin, and reduce the dosage of warfarin if necessary.

Phenytoin, phenobarbital, carbamazepine. These agents may enhance the metabolism of vilazodone, reducing serum levels and leading to decreased pharmacologic effect.

Erythromycin, clarithromycin, fluoxetine, grapefruit juice. These drugs inhibit the metabolism of vilazodone, causing an increase in serum levels and the potential for toxicity. Dosages of the antidepressant may need to be reduced by up to 50% to avoid toxicities.

---

vortioxetine (vōr-tē-ŎX-ĕt-ēn)
⇄ *Do not confuse vortioxetine with atomoxetine.*
Trintellix (trĭn-TĔL-ĭx)

Actions

Vortioxetine is a new medication that acts as an SSRI, an agonist of the serotonin 5-HT$_{1A}$ receptors that enhances serotonin activity and antagonizes the serotonin 5-HT$_3$ receptors.

Uses

Vortioxetine is approved to treat MDD in adults.

Therapeutic Outcomes

The primary therapeutic outcomes expected from vortioxetine therapy are elevated mood and reduction of symptoms of depression.

❖ **Nursing Implications for Vortioxetine Therapy**

◆ *Premedication assessment*

1. Note any GI symptoms present before the start of therapy.
2. Monitor any CNS symptoms present (e.g., insomnia, restlessness).

◆ *Availability.* **PO:** 5-, 10-, and 20-mg tablets.

◆ *Dosage and administration.* **Adult: PO:** Initially, 10 mg once daily, followed by 20 mg once daily as tolerated. For those not tolerating 10 mg daily, therapy may be reduced to 5 mg daily. Maximum daily dose is 20 mg. If the drug is well tolerated, patients should remain on therapy for several months.

When discontinuation is planned, the dose should be tapered to monitor closely for development of withdrawal symptoms and to detect the development of depressive symptoms. The manufacturer recommends that doses of 15 mg daily or higher should be reduced to 10 mg daily for 1 week before full discontinuation to prevent withdrawal symptoms.

◆ *Common adverse effects*
Gastrointestinal
Diarrhea, nausea, vomiting, dry mouth. These adverse effects should be mild and should resolve with continued therapy. Patients with persistent vomiting should be evaluated for other causes, as well as for the development of electrolyte imbalance (syndrome of inappropriate secretion of antidiuretic hormone or serotonin syndrome).

Neurologic
Dizziness, abnormal dreams. Provide for patient safety during episodes of dizziness. Provide comfort and patient safety in those reporting abnormal dreams. Report these symptoms to the healthcare provider for further evaluation. The patient should not take these medications while working with machinery, operating a motor vehicle, administering medication, or performing other duties that require mental alertness.

◆ *Serious adverse effects*
Psychological
Suicidal actions, hypomania, mania, serotonin syndrome. Monitor the patient for changes in thoughts, feelings, and behaviors, especially during the initial stages of therapy. Symptoms of depression may improve (e.g., increased appetite, sleep, and psychomotor activity) within a few days. However, the depression still exists, and it usually takes several weeks of the patient receiving therapeutic dosing before improvement is noted. Suicide precautions should be maintained during this time.

Review patient history for a personal or family history of bipolar disorder because vortioxetine may induce latent bipolar disorder. Vortioxetine is not approved for treatment of bipolar depression.

◆ *Drug interactions*
Monoamine oxidase inhibitors. Severe reactions—including excitement, diaphoresis, rigidity, convulsions, hyperpyrexia, and death—may result from the concurrent use of MAOIs and vortioxetine. It is recommended that at least 14 days lapse between discontinuing an MAOI and starting vortioxetine. It is further recommended that there be a 14-day drug-free interval between discontinuing vortioxetine and starting MAOI therapy.

Trazodone, MAOIs, SSRIs, SNRIs, tramadol, triptans, buspirone, St. John's wort, linezolid, fentanyl. Serotonin syndrome may develop when vortioxetine is used in conjunction with any of these agents. Symptoms of serotonin syndrome include irritability, hallucinations, delirium, reduced consciousness, increased muscle tone, myoclonus, and shivering. Use these drugs cautiously; initiate therapy at a lower dosage and closely monitor for the adverse effects listed.

Aspirin, nonsteroidal antiinflammatory drugs, warfarin. Serotonin release by platelets plays an important role in hemostasis. Selective serotonin reuptake inhibitors may enhance the anticoagulant effects of warfarin and enhance the potential for GI bleeding caused by nonsteroidal antiinflammatory drugs or aspirin. Observe the patient for petechiae, ecchymoses, nosebleeds, bleeding gums, dark tarry stools, and bright red or coffee-ground emesis. Monitor prothrombin time and the INR of warfarin and reduce the dosage of warfarin if necessary.

Buspirone. Buspirone inhibits the metabolism of vortioxetine, causing an increase in serum levels and the potential for toxicity. Dosages of vortioxetine should be reduced by up to 50% to avoid toxicities.

DRUG CLASS: ANTIMANIC AGENTS

lithium carbonate (LĬTH-ē-um)

Actions
Lithium is a monovalent cation that competes with other monovalent and divalent cations (i.e., potassium, sodium, calcium, magnesium) at cellular binding sites that are sensitive to changes in cation concentration. Lithium replaces intracellular and intraneuronal sodium, stabilizing the neuronal membrane. It also reduces the release of norepinephrine and increases the uptake of tryptophan, the precursor to serotonin. It also interacts with second-messenger cellular processes to inhibit intracellular concentrations of cyclic adenosine monophosphate. Because of the complexity of the CNS, the exact mechanisms of action of lithium for treating mood disorders are unknown. It has no sedative, depressant, or euphoric properties, which differentiates it from all other psychotropic agents.

Uses
Lithium is used to treat acute mania and for prophylactic treatment of recurrent manic and depressive episodes in patients with bipolar disorder. In patients with bipolar disorder, it is more effective in preventing signs and symptoms of mania than those of depression. It is also effective in some patients for reducing the recurrence of the depressive episodes associated with unipolar disorder.

Therapeutic Outcome
The primary therapeutic outcome expected from lithium therapy is maintaining the individual at an optimal level of functioning, with minimal exacerbations of mood swings.

❖ **Nursing Implications for Lithium Therapy**
◆ *Premedication assessment*
1. Before initiating lithium therapy, the following laboratory tests should be completed for baseline information: electrolytes, fasting blood glucose, blood urea nitrogen (BUN), serum creatinine, creatinine clearance, urinalysis, and thyroid function.
2. Obtain baseline blood pressures with the patient in the supine, sitting, and standing positions; record

and report significant hypotension to the healthcare provider before administering the drug.

3. Weigh the patient daily, check the hydration status (e.g., moistness of mucous membranes, skin turgor, firmness of eyeball), and monitor urine specific gravity.

4. Lithium may enhance sodium depletion, which increases lithium toxicity. Assess for early signs of lithium toxicity before giving the medication, including nausea, vomiting, abdominal pain, diarrhea, lethargy, speech difficulty, mild dizziness, muscle twitching, and tremor.

◆ *Availability. PO: Lithium carbonate:* 150-, 300-, 600-mg capsules; 300-mg tablets; 300- and 450-mg slow-release tablets. *Lithium citrate:* 8 mEq/5 mL solution.

◆ *Dosage and administration.* **Adult:** *PO:* 300 to 600 mg three or four times daily. Administer with food or milk. An adequate diet is important to maintain normal serum sodium levels and to prevent toxicity. The onset of the acute antimanic effect of lithium usually occurs within 5 to 7 days; the full therapeutic effect often requires 10 to 21 days.

Serum lithium levels. Lithium levels are monitored once or twice weekly during the initiation of therapy and monthly while the patient is receiving a maintenance dosage. Blood should be drawn approximately 12 hours after the last dose was administered. The normal serum level is 0.4 to 1.2 mEq/L. Promptly report serum levels higher than these values to the healthcare provider.

Good nutrition. Lithium may enhance sodium depletion, which increases lithium toxicity. The patient should maintain a normal dietary intake of sodium and adequate maintenance fluids (i.e., 10 to 12 eight-ounce glasses of water daily)—especially when initiating therapy—to prevent toxicity.

◆ *Common adverse effects*
Gastrointestinal
Nausea, vomiting, anorexia, abdominal cramps. These adverse effects are usually mild and tend to resolve with continued therapy. Encourage the patient not to discontinue therapy without first consulting the healthcare provider. If gastric irritation occurs, administer the medication with food or milk. If symptoms persist or increase in severity, report them to the healthcare provider for evaluation. These also may be early signs of toxicity.

Excessive thirst. This adverse effect is usually mild and tends to resolve within a week with continued therapy. Encourage the patient not to discontinue therapy without first consulting the healthcare provider. If excessive thirst persists or becomes severe, the patient should consult the healthcare provider.

Neurologic
Fine hand tremor. If fine hand tremor persists or becomes severe, the patient should consult the healthcare provider.

Genitourinary
Excessive urination. This adverse effect is usually mild and tends to resolve within a week with continued therapy. Encourage the patient not to discontinue therapy without first consulting the healthcare provider. If excessive urination persists or becomes severe, the patient should consult the healthcare provider.

◆ *Serious adverse effects*
Gastrointestinal
Persistent vomiting, profuse diarrhea. These are symptoms of impending serious toxicity. Report them immediately and do not give the next dose of medication until administration has been reconfirmed by the healthcare provider.

Neurologic
Hyperreflexia, lethargy, weakness. These are signs of impending serious toxicity. Report them immediately and do not give the next dose of medication until administration has been reconfirmed by the healthcare provider.

Endocrine, metabolic
Progressive fatigue, weight gain. These may be early signs of hypothyroidism. Report these symptoms to the healthcare provider for further evaluation.

Hyperglycemia. Report this symptom to the healthcare provider for further evaluation.

Genitourinary
Nephrotoxicity. Monitor urinalysis and kidney function tests for abnormal results. Report an increasing BUN or creatinine level, increasing or decreasing urine output or decreasing specific gravity (despite adequate fluid intake), and casts or protein in the urine.

◆ *Rare adverse effects from lithium therapy*
Pruritus, ankle edema, metallic taste. Report these symptoms for further evaluation by the healthcare provider.

◆ *Drug interactions*
Reduced serum sodium levels. The therapeutic activity and toxicity of lithium are highly dependent on sodium concentrations. Decreased sodium levels significantly enhance the toxicity of lithium and high sodium levels result in low lithium levels. Patients who are to begin diuretic therapy, a low-sodium diet, or activities that produce excessive and prolonged sweating should be observed particularly closely.

Diuretics. Diuretics may reduce the elimination of lithium, resulting in lithium toxicity. Monitor the patient's lithium serum levels closely. Monitor patients receiving concurrent long-term therapy for signs of the development of lithium toxicity (e.g., nausea, vomiting, abdominal pain, diarrhea, lethargy, speech difficulty, mild dizziness, tremor). A lithium level may be necessary.

Methyldopa. Monitor patients receiving concurrent long-term therapy for signs of the development of lithium toxicity (e.g., nausea, vomiting, abdominal pain, diarrhea, lethargy, speech difficulty, mild dizziness, tremor). A lithium level may be necessary.

Indomethacin, piroxicam. Indomethacin and piroxicam reduce the renal excretion of lithium, allowing the lithium to accumulate to potentially toxic levels. Monitor for signs of lithium toxicity (e.g., nausea, vomiting, abdominal pain, diarrhea, lethargy, speech difficulty, mild dizziness, tremor). A lithium level may be necessary.

Get Ready for the NCLEX® Examination!

Key Points

- The new *Diagnostic and Statistical Manual of Mental Disorders,* 5th edition (DSM-5), recognizes major psychiatric disorders on a continuum, with depressive disorders and psychotic spectrum at the ends of the continuum and bipolar disorders serving as a bridge between the two diagnostic classes in terms of symptomatology, family history, and genetics. The common feature among depressive and bipolar disorders is the presence of sad, empty, or irritable mood, accompanied by changes that significantly affect the individual's capacity to function.
- Treatment of mood disorders requires both nonpharmacologic and pharmacologic therapy. Simultaneous psychotherapy and pharmacologic treatment are more successful than either treatment alone.
- Antidepressant medications act on a variety of receptors in the CNS, as well as peripheral tissues, and are associated with many adverse effects and drug interactions. It is the responsibility of the nurse to educate patients about therapy and to monitor for therapeutic benefit and common and serious adverse effects, as well as to intervene whenever possible to optimize therapeutic outcomes.

Additional Learning Resources

SG Go to your Study Guide for additional Review Questions for the NCLEX® Examination, Critical Thinking Clinical Situations, and other learning activities to help you master this chapter content.

Go to your Evolve website (https://evolve.elsevier.com/Clayton) for additional online resources.

Review Questions for the NCLEX® Examination

1. The nurse was assessing the patient who came in with depression. Which components are part of the baseline assessment? *(Select all that apply.)*
   1. Oral hygiene and number of dental cavities
   2. History of previous depression episodes and treatments
   3. Sleep pattern
   4. Suicidal ideation
   5. Tattoos present

2. Patients who are being treated for depression should continually be monitored for thoughts of suicide. Which behavior may indicate suicidal ideation?
   1. Excessive appetite
   2. Poor hygiene
   3. Comments from the patient such as, "Things will get better after I'm gone."
   4. Sleeping throughout the day

3. The nurse knows to assess for a severe reaction, such as excitement, diaphoresis, rigidity, and convulsions, that can occur between SSRIs and which drug(s)?
   1. MAOIs
   2. Lithium carbonate
   3. TCAs
   4. Antihistamines

4. The nurse is explaining to the patient taking an MAOI of the need to be aware of which condition developing?
   1. Hyperpyrexia
   2. Hyperglycemia
   3. Hypertension
   4. Hyperactivity

5. A patient came into the clinic complaining of drowsiness and nausea after being started on duloxetine (Cymbalta). The nurse knows that these symptoms from SNRIs may mean what?
   1. Serious adverse effects
   2. A drug interaction with haloperidol
   3. The dose needs to be adjusted
   4. Common adverse effects

6. Patients taking doxepin should be aware of which of the following adverse effects common to TCAs? *(Select all that apply.)*
   1. Orthostatic hypotension
   2. Parkinsonism symptoms
   3. Dry mouth and throat
   4. Hyperglycemia
   5. Blurred vision

7. The nurse who is discussing ways to prevent lithium toxicity with a patient currently on lithium will include which of the following statements? *(Select all that apply.)*
   1. "Be sure to report symptoms of persistent vomiting and/or profuse diarrhea."
   2. "You need to drink 10 glasses of water (8 ounces each) daily."
   3. "It is important to draw lithium blood levels weekly."
   4. "Because you are taking lithium, we can prevent lithium toxicity with diuretic therapy."
   5. "Be sure to report symptoms of lethargy and weakness."

8. The nurse knows that lithium can be used to treat which of these multiple different mental health issues? *(Select all that apply.)*
   1. Acute mania
   2. Bipolar disorder
   3. Unipolar disorder
   4. Phobias
   5. Obsessive-compulsive related disorders

Drugs Used for Psychoses

17

Objectives

1. Identify the signs and symptoms of psychotic behavior.
2. Describe the major indications for the use of antipsychotic agents.
3. Discuss the antipsychotic medications that are used for the treatment of psychoses.
4. Identify the common adverse effects that are observed with the use of antipsychotic medications.

Key Terms

psychosis (sī-KŌ-sĭs) (p. 255)
delusion (dĕ-LŪ-zhŭn) (p. 255)
hallucinations (hă-lū-sĭ-NĀ-shŭnz) (p. 255)
disorganized thinking (dĭs-ŌR-găn-īzd THĬN-kĭng) (p. 256)
loosening of associations (LŪ-sĕn-ĭng ŭv ăs-sō-sē-Ā-shŭnz) (p. 256)
disorganized behavior (dĭs-ŌR-gă-nīzd bē-HĀV-yŭr) (p. 256)
negative symptoms (NĚG-ĕ-tiv SĬMP-tĕmz) (p. 256)
target symptoms (TĂR-gĕt SĬMP-tĕmz) (p. 256)
typical (first-generation) antipsychotic agents (TĬP-ĭ-kŭl ăn-tī-sī-KŎT-ĭk) (p. 257)
atypical (second-generation) antipsychotic agents (ā-TĬP-ĭ-kŭl ăn-tī-sī-KŎT-ĭk) (p. 257)
equipotent doses (ĕk-wē-PŌ-tĕnt DŌS-ĕz) (p. 257)
extrapyramidal symptoms (EPSs) (ĕks-tră-pĭ-RĂM-ĭ-dăl) (p. 257)

dystonias (dĭs-TŌN-ē-ăz) (p. 261)
pseudoparkinsonian symptoms (SŪ-dō-păr-kĭn-SŌ-nē-ĭn) (p. 261)
akathisia (ă-kĕ-THĬ-zhă) (p. 261)
tardive dyskinesia (TĂR-dĭv dĭs-kĭ-NĒ-zē-ă) (p. 261)
Abnormal Involuntary Movement Scale (AIMS) (ăb-NŌR-mŭl ĭn-VŎL-ĕn-tār-ē MŌV-mĕnt SKĀL) (p. 262)
Dyskinesia Identification System: Condensed User Scale (DISCUS) (dĭs-kĭ-NĒ-zē-a ī-dĕn-tĭ-fĭ-KĀ-shŭn SĬS-tĕm: kŏn-DĔNST YŪ-zŭr SKĀL) (p. 262)
neuroleptic malignant syndrome (NMS) (nyū-rō-LĔP-tĭk mă-LĬG-nănt SĬN-drōm) (p. 262)
depot antipsychotic medicine (DĔ-pō ăn-tē-sī-KŎT-ĭk) (p. 262)

PSYCHOSIS

Psychosis does not have a single definition but is a clinical descriptor applied to someone who is out of touch with reality. Psychotic symptoms can be associated with many illnesses, including dementias and delirium, that may have metabolic, infectious, or endocrinologic causes. Psychotic symptoms are also common in patients with mood disorders such as major depression and bipolar disorder and schizophrenia spectrum. Psychosis can also be caused by many drugs (e.g., phencyclidine, opiates, amphetamines, cocaine, hallucinogens, anticholinergic agents, alcohol). Psychotic disorders are characterized by loss of reality, perceptual deficits such as hallucinations and delusions, and deterioration of social functioning. Schizophrenia is the most common of the several psychotic disorders defined by the American Psychiatric Association in the *Diagnostic and Statistical Manual of Mental Disorders,* 5th edition (DSM-5).

Psychotic disorders are extremely complex illnesses that are influenced by biologic, psychosocial, and environmental circumstances. Some of the disorders require several months of observation and testing before a final diagnosis can be determined. It is beyond the scope of this text to discuss psychotic disorders in detail, but general types of symptoms associated with psychotic disorders will be described.

A **delusion** is a false or irrational belief that is firmly held despite obvious evidence to the contrary. Delusions may be persecutory, grandiose, religious, sexual, or hypochondriacal. Delusions of reference—in which the patient attributes a special, irrational, and usually negative significance to other people, objects, or events, such as song lyrics or newspaper articles, in relation to self—are common. Delusions may be defined as "bizarre" if they are clearly irrational and do not derive from ordinary life experiences. A common bizarre delusion is the patient's belief that his or her thinking process, body parts, or actions or impulses are controlled or dictated by some external force.

Hallucinations are false sensory perceptions that are experienced without an external stimulus and seem real to the patient. Auditory hallucinations experienced as voices that are characteristically heard commenting negatively about the patient in the third person are prominent among patients with schizophrenia. Hallucinations of touch, sight, taste, smell, and bodily sensation also occur.

Disorganized thinking is commonly associated with psychoses. These thought disorders may consist of a **loosening of associations** or a flight of ideas so that the speaker jumps from one idea or topic to another unrelated one (derailment) in an illogical, inappropriate, or disorganized way. Answers to questions may be obliquely related or completely unrelated (tangentiality). At its most serious, this incoherence of thought extends into pronunciation itself and the speaker's words become garbled or unrecognizable. Speech may also be overly concrete (loss of ability to think in abstract terms) and inexpressive; it may be repetitive and may convey little or no real information.

Disorganized behavior is another common characteristic of psychosis. Problems may be noted with any form of goal-directed behavior, leading to difficulties with performing activities of daily living such as organizing meals or maintaining hygiene. The patient may appear markedly disheveled, may dress in an unusual manner (e.g., wearing several layers of clothing, scarves, and gloves on a hot day), or may display clearly inappropriate sexual behavior (e.g., public masturbation) or unpredictable, nontriggered agitation (e.g., shouting, swearing).

Negative symptoms, or changes in affect, may also be symptoms of psychosis. Emotional expressiveness is diminished; there is poor eye contact and reduced spontaneous movement. The patient appears to be withdrawn from others, and the face appears to be immobile and unresponsive. Speech is often minimal (alogia), with only brief, slow, monotone replies given in response to questions. There is a withdrawal from areas of functioning that affect interpersonal relationships, work, education, and self-care (asociality), and anhedonia, the decreased ability to experience pleasure from positive stimuli or reduced pleasure from previously positive stimuli.

TREATMENT OF PSYCHOSIS

The importance of the initial assessment for an accurate diagnosis cannot be underestimated for a patient with acute psychosis. A thorough physical and neurologic examination, a mental status examination, a complete family and social history, and a laboratory workup must be performed to exclude other causes of psychoses, including substance abuse. Both drug and nondrug therapies are critical to the treatment of most psychoses. Long-term outcome is improved for patients with an integrated drug and nondrug treatment regimen. Nonpharmacologic interventions beneficial to patients include (1) individual psychotherapy to improve insight into the illness and help the patient cope with stress; (2) group therapy to enhance socialization skills; (3) behavioral or cognitive therapy; and (4) vocational training. Referral to community resources such as the National Alliance on Mental Illness (NAMI) may provide additional support for the patient and family.

Before initiating therapy, the treatment goals and baseline level of functioning must be established and documented. **Target symptoms** must also be identified and documented. Target symptoms are critical monitoring parameters used to assess changes in an individual's clinical status and response to medications. Examples of target symptoms include frequency and type of agitation, degree of suspiciousness, delusions, hallucinations, loose associations, grooming habits and hygiene, sleep patterns, speech patterns, social skills, and judgment. The ultimate goal is to restore behavioral, cognitive, and psychosocial processes and skills to as close to baseline levels as possible so that the patient can be reintegrated into the community. Realistically, unless the psychosis is part of another medical diagnosis such as substance abuse, most patients will have recurring symptoms of the mental disorder for most of their lives. Therefore treatment is focused on decreasing the severity of the target symptoms that most interfere with functioning. A variety of scales have been developed to assist with the objective measurement of change in target symptoms in response to psychotherapy and pharmacotherapy. These include the Brief Psychiatric Rating Scale (BPRS), the Positive and Negative Syndrome Scale for Schizophrenia (PANSS), the Clinical Global Impression (CGI) scale, and the Rating of Aggression Against People and/or Property (RAAPP) scale.

DRUG THERAPY FOR PSYCHOSIS

Pharmacologic treatment of psychosis includes several classes of drugs. The most specific are the first- and second-generation antipsychotic agents, but benzodiazepines (see Chapter 15) are often used to control acute psychotic symptoms. Beta-adrenergic blocking agents (beta blockers; e.g., propranolol) (see Chapter 12), lithium (see Chapter 16), anticonvulsants (e.g., valproic acid) (see Chapter 18), carbamazepine (see Chapter 18), antiparkinsonian agents (see Chapter 14), and anticholinergic agents (see Chapters 12 and 14) occasionally play a role in controlling the adverse effects of medications used in antipsychotic therapy.

Antipsychotic (also known as *neuroleptic*) medications can be classified in several ways. Traditionally, they have been divided into phenothiazines and nonphenothiazines. Antipsychotic medications can also be classified as low-potency or high-potency drugs. The terms *low potency* and *high potency* refer only to the milligram doses used for these medicines and not to any difference in effectiveness (e.g., 100 mg of chlorpromazine, a low-potency drug, is equivalent in antipsychotic activity to 2 mg of haloperidol, a high-potency drug).

Chlorpromazine and thioridazine are low-potency drugs, whereas trifluoperazine, fluphenazine, thiothixene, haloperidol, and loxapine are high-potency drugs. Since 1990, antipsychotic medications have also been classified as **typical (first-generation) antipsychotic agents** or **atypical (second-generation) antipsychotic agents** on the basis of their mechanism of action (see Table 17.1 later in this chapter). The atypical antipsychotic agents are aripiprazole, asenapine, brexpiprazole, cariprazine, clozapine, iloperidone, lurasidone, olanzapine, paliperidone, pimavanserin, quetiapine, risperidone, and ziprasidone. All of the remaining antipsychotic agents listed in Table 17.1 are typical antipsychotic agents.

ACTIONS

The typical antipsychotic medications block the neurotransmitter dopamine in the central nervous system (CNS). The atypical antipsychotic agents block dopamine receptors, but they also block serotonin receptors to varying degrees. However, the exact mechanisms whereby these actions prevent psychotic symptoms are unknown. There is substantially more to the development of psychotic symptoms than elevated dopamine levels. There are at least five known types of dopamine receptors and several more types of serotonin receptors in various areas of the CNS. Antipsychotic medications also stimulate or block cholinergic, histaminic, nicotinic, alpha-adrenergic, and beta-adrenergic neurotransmitter receptors to varying degrees, accounting for many of the adverse effects of therapy.

Pimavanserin differs from other atypical antipsychotics in that it selectively blocks a serotonin (5-hydroxytryptamine) receptor (5-HT_{2A}) and lacks activity at dopamine receptors. It is effective in treating psychosis related to Parkinson's disease dementia. Using atypical antipsychotics for treatment of Parkinson's disease dementia-related psychosis can worsen Parkinson's disease motor symptoms. Due to pimavanserin's lack of activity at dopamine receptors, it does not aggravate Parkinson's disease motor symptoms.

Medication Safety Alert

Increased Mortality in Elderly Patients With Dementia-Related Psychosis

Antipsychotic drugs increase the all-cause risk of death in elderly patients with dementia-related psychosis.

USES

All antipsychotic medications are equal in efficacy when used in **equipotent doses**. There is some unpredictable variation among patients, however, and individual patients sometimes show a better response to particular drugs. In general, medication should be selected on the basis of the need to avoid certain adverse effects when dealing with concurrent medical or psychiatric disorders. Despite practice trends, no proof exists that agitation responds best to sedating drugs or that withdrawn patients respond best to nonsedating drugs. Medication history should be a major factor in drug selection. The final important factors in drug selection are the clinically important differences in the frequency of adverse effects. No single drug is least likely to cause all adverse effects; thus individual response should be the best determinant of which drug is to be used. The atypical antipsychotic agents tend to be more effective in relieving the negative and cognitive symptoms associated with schizophrenia and treating refractory schizophrenia, and they have a much lower incidence of **extrapyramidal symptoms (EPSs)** and hyperprolactinemia.

The initial goals of antipsychotic therapy are calming the agitated patient, who may be a physical threat to himself or herself or to others, and beginning the treatment of the psychosis and thought disorder. Combined therapy with benzodiazepines (often lorazepam) and antipsychotic medications allows lower dosages of the antipsychotic medication to be used, reducing the risk of serious adverse effects more commonly seen with higher-dose therapy. Some therapeutic effects, such as reduced psychomotor agitation and insomnia, are observed within 1 week of therapy, but reductions in hallucinations, delusions, and thought disorder often require 6 to 8 weeks of treatment to achieve the full therapeutic effect. Rapid increases in the dosing of antipsychotic medications will not reduce the antipsychotic response time. Patients, families, and the healthcare team must be informed about giving antipsychotic agents an adequate chance to work before unnecessarily escalating the dosage and increasing the risk of adverse effects.

Clinical Pitfall

During episodes of acute psychosis, the patient is out of touch with reality and often does not understand the need to take medicines that will help stabilize his or her condition. The nurse must ensure that the patient has actually swallowed the medication when it is administered and not just "mouthed" or "cheeked" it. Outpatients often require that medication administration be supervised to ensure adherence to the medication regimen. In some cases, it is necessary to inject long-acting medicines to overcome a patient's nonadherence problem. After an acute psychotic episode has resolved and the patient is free from overt psychotic symptoms, a decision must be made as to whether maintenance therapy is necessary. This will depend on the diagnosed psychotic disorder and the patient's tolerance of the adverse effects of the medication. However, most psychotic disorders are treated with lower maintenance dosages to minimize the risk of recurrence of the disorder's psychotic episodes (Box 17.1).

ADVERSE EFFECTS OF ANTIPSYCHOTIC DRUG THERAPY

EXTRAPYRAMIDAL SYMPTOMS

Many of the serious adverse effects of antipsychotic medications can be attributed to the pharmacologic

Table 17.1   Antipsychotic Agents

GENERIC NAME	BRAND NAME	AVAILABILITY	ADULT DOSAGE RANGE (MG)	MAJOR ADVERSE EFFECTS			
				SEDATION	EXTRAPYRAMIDAL SYMPTOMS	HYPOTENSION	ANTICHOLINERGIC EFFECTS
Typical (First-Generation) Antipsychotic Agents							
Phenothiazines							
chlorpromazine ⇅ *Do not confuse chlorpromazine with chlordiazepoxide, chlorhexidine, chlorpropamide, or chlorthalidone.*	Teva-Chlorpromazine ✦	Tablets: 10, 25, 50, 100, 200 mg; Injection: 25 mg/mL	25-2000	+++	++	+++	++
fluphenazine	– Modecate Concentrate ✦	Tablets: 1, 2.5, 5, 10 mg; Elixir: 2.5 mg/5 mL; Concentrate: 5 mg/mL; Injection: 2.5 mg/mL; 25 mg/mL	0.5-40	+	++++	+	+
perphenazine	—	Tablets: 2, 4, 8, 16 mg	12-64	+	+++	+	++
prochlorperazine	– PMS-Prochlorperazine ✦	Tablets: 5, 10 mg; Injection: 5 mg/mL; Suppository: 25 mg	15-150	+	+++	+	+
thioridazine	—	Tablets: 10, 25, 50, 100 mg	150-800	+++	+	+++	+++
trifluoperazine	—	Tablets: 1, 2, 5, 10 mg	2-40	+	+++	+	+
Thioxanthenes							
thiothixene	—	Capsules: 1, 2, 5, 10 mg	6-60	+	+++	+	+
Nonphenothiazines							
haloperidol	Haldol Apo-Haloperidol ✦	Tablets: 0.5, 1, 2, 5, 10, 20 mg; Concentrate: 2 mg/mL; Injection: 5 mg/mL; Injection, sustained release: 50, 100 mg	1-100	+	+++	+	+
loxapine ⇅ *Do not confuse loxapine with Lexapro.*	Xylac ✦	Capsules: 5, 10, 25, 50 mg	20-250	++	+++	++	+

Table 17.1   Antipsychotic Agents—cont'd

GENERIC NAME	BRAND NAME	AVAILABILITY	ADULT DOSAGE RANGE (MG)	MAJOR ADVERSE EFFECTS			
				SEDATION	EXTRAPYRAMIDAL SYMPTOMS	HYPOTENSION	ANTICHOLINERGIC EFFECTS
Atypical (Second-Generation) Antipsychotic Agents							
aripiprazole	Abilify, Abilify Discmelt, Abilify Maintena, Abilify Maintena, Aristada	Tablets: 2, 5, 10, 15, 20, 30 mg; Tablets, orally disintegrating: 10, 15 mg; Solution: 1 mg/mL; Injection Intramuscular suspension: 300, 400 mg; Prefilled syringes: 300, 400 mg; 441 mg/1.6 mL; 662 mg/2.4 mL; 882 mg/3.2 mL; 1064 mg/3.9 mL	10-30	+	+	+	0
asenapine	Saphris	Tablets, sublingual: 2.5, 5, 10 mg	5-20	++	++	++	+
brexpiprazole	Rexulti	Tablets: 0.25, 0.5, 1, 2, 3, 4 mg	2-4	+	+	0/+	0/+
cariprazine	Vraylar	Capsules: 1.5, 3, 4.5, 6 mg	1.5-6	+	++	0/+	0/+
clozapine	Clozaril, Gen-Clozapine ❋ *Do not confuse Clozaril with Colazal.*	Tablets: 25, 50, 100, 200 mg; Tablets, orally disintegrating: 12.5, 25, 100, 150, 200 mg; Oral Suspension: 50 mg/mL in 100 mL bottle	300-900	+++	+	+++	++
iloperidone	Fanapt	Tablets: 1, 2, 4, 6, 8, 10, 12 mg	2-24	++	+	++	++
lurasidone	Latuda	Tablets: 20, 40, 60, 80, 120 mg	20-160	++	++	++	++
olanzapine ⇅ *Do not confuse olanzapine with oxcarbazepine.*	Zyprexa ⇅ *Do not confuse Zyprexa with Celexa, Zaroxolyn, or Zyrtec.*	Tablets: 2.5, 5, 7.5, 10, 15, 20 mg; Tablets, orally disintegrating: 5, 10, 15, 20 mg; Injection: 10 mg; Injection, sustained release: 210, 300, 405 mg	PO: 5-20 IM: 30	++	+	++	+++
paliperidone	Invega, Invega Trinza, Invega Sustenna	Tablets, extended release: 1.5, 3, 6, 9 mg; IM injection suspension, extended release: 39, 78, 117, 156, 243, 273, 410, 546, 819 mg	3-12	+	+++	++	0

Continued

Table 17.1 Antipsychotic Agents—cont'd

GENERIC NAME	BRAND NAME	AVAILABILITY	ADULT DOSAGE RANGE (MG)	MAJOR ADVERSE EFFECTS			
				SEDATION	EXTRAPYRAMIDAL SYMPTOMS	HYPOTENSION	ANTICHOLINERGIC EFFECTS
pimavanserin	Nuplazid	Tablets: 10, 17 mg Capsules: 34 mg	34	+	0/+	++	+
quetiapine	Seroquel, Seroquel XR ⇅ Do not confuse Seroquel with or Sertraline.	Tablets: 25, 50, 100, 200, 300, 400 mg Tablets, 24-hr extended release: 50, 150, 200, 300, 400 mg	50-800	++	0	++	0
risperidone	Risperdal ⇅ Do not confuse Risperdal with estradiol, reserpine, Restoril, risedronate, or ropinirole. Risperdal Consta	Tablets: 0.25, 0.5, 1, 2, 3, 4 mg Tablets, orally disintegrating: 0.25, 0.5, 1, 2, 3, 4 mg PO solution: 1 mg/mL IM injection suspension: 12.5, 25, 37.5, 50 mg	2-16	+	++	++	+
ziprasidone ⇅ Do not confuse ziprasidone with zidovudine.	Geodon	Capsules: 20, 40, 60, 80 mg Injection: 20 mg	40-160	+	++	+	++

+, Low; ++, moderate; +++, high.
🍁 Available in Canada.   ⇅ Do not confuse.

| Box 17.1 | **Antipsychotic Medicines: Response Times and Adverse Effects** |

Patients who begin antipsychotic drug therapy can expect some therapeutic effects, such as reduced psychomotor agitation and insomnia, within 1 week of starting treatment. However, reduction in hallucinations, delusions, and thought disorders often requires 6 to 8 weeks for a full therapeutic response to be achieved. Rapid increases in dosages of antipsychotic medications will not reduce the antipsychotic response time but will increase the frequency of adverse effects.

Antipsychotic medicines may produce extrapyramidal effects. Tardive dyskinesia may be reversible during its early stages, but it becomes irreversible with continued use of the antipsychotic medication. Regular assessment for tardive dyskinesia should be performed for all patients receiving antipsychotic drugs. Older adult patients should be observed for hypotension and tardive dyskinesia.

effect of blocking dopaminergic, cholinergic, histaminic, serotonergic, and adrenergic neurotransmitter receptors. Although these agents block D_2 dopamine receptors in the mesolimbic area of the brain to stop psychotic symptoms, blockade of D_2 receptors in other areas of the brain explains the occurrence of EPSs.

EPSs are the most troublesome adverse effects and the most common cause of nonadherence associated with antipsychotic therapy. There are four categories of EPSs: dystonic reactions, pseudoparkinsonism, akathisia, and tardive dyskinesia.

Acute dystonia has the earliest onset of all the EPSs. **Dystonias** are spasmodic movements (prolonged tonic contractions) of muscle groups such as tongue protrusion, rolling back of the eyes (oculogyric crisis), jaw spasm (trismus), and neck torsion (torticollis). These symptoms are often frightening and painful for the patient. Approximately 90% of all dystonic reactions occur during the first 72 hours of therapy. Dystonic reactions are most frequent in male patients, younger patients, and patients receiving high-potency medications such as haloperidol. Dystonic reactions are generally brief and are the EPSs most responsive to treatment. Acute dystonic reactions may be controlled by intramuscular injections of diphenhydramine, benztropine, diazepam, or lorazepam. Rating scales for assessing patients with different forms of dystonias include the Toronto Western Spasmodic Torticollis Rating Scale (TWSTRS), the Global Dystonia Scale (GDS), the Unified Dystonia Rating Scale (UDRS), and the Fahn-Marsden Scale.

Pseudoparkinsonian symptoms of tremor, muscular rigidity, mask-like expression, shuffling gait, and loss or weakness of motor function typically begin after 2 to 3 weeks of antipsychotic drug therapy but may occur up to 3 months after starting therapy. They are more commonly seen in older adults. These symptoms result from a relative deficiency of dopamine, with cholinergic

excess, caused by antipsychotic medications and are well controlled by anticholinergic antiparkinsonian drugs (e.g., benztropine, diphenhydramine, trihexyphenidyl).

Akathisia is a syndrome consisting of subjective feelings of anxiety and restlessness and objective signs of pacing, rocking, and inability to sit or stand in one place for extended periods. Akathisia can increase aggression and is a frequent cause of noncompliance. It occurs more commonly when high-potency antipsychotic medications are used. The mechanism of action is unknown. Reducing the dosage of the antipsychotic medication or switching to a lower-potency drug should be considered. Treatment with anticholinergic agents, benzodiazepines (e.g., diazepam, lorazepam), beta blockers (e.g., propranolol), and clonidine has shown varying degrees of success.

Tardive dyskinesia is a syndrome of persistent and involuntary hyperkinetic abnormal movements. It develops in about 20% to 25% of patients receiving typical antipsychotic medications on a long-term basis (e.g., months to years). There appears to be a lower incidence in patients receiving atypical antipsychotic agents, but these agents are newer, and it sometimes takes years for tardive dyskinesia to develop. This drug-induced, late-appearing neurologic disorder is noted for such symptoms as buccolingual masticatory syndrome or orofacial movements. The buccolingual masticatory movements begin with mild forward, backward, or lateral tongue movement. As the disorder progresses, more obvious movements appear, including tongue thrusting, rolling, or "fly-catching" movements, as well as chewing or lateral jaw movements that produce smacking noises. Symptoms may interfere with the patient's ability to chew, speak, or swallow. Facial movements include frequent blinking, brow arching, grimacing, and upward deviation of the eyes. The severity of symptoms of tardive dyskinesia can fluctuate daily and symptoms often will remit during sleep. The clinical manifestations of tardive dyskinesia are similar to those of dystonias, but there are some significant differences. Tardive dyskinesia typically appears after antipsychotic dosage reduction or discontinuation, it improves when the antipsychotic dosage is increased, it worsens with the administration of anticholinergic agents, and it may persist for months or years after antipsychotic medicines are discontinued. The exact cause of tardive dyskinesia is unknown. Early signs may be reversible but, over time, they may become irreversible, even with discontinuation of the antipsychotic medicine.

The best treatment approach to tardive dyskinesia is prevention. Patients who receive maintenance antipsychotic drug therapy should be assessed for early signs of tardive dyskinesia at least semiannually and preferably quarterly. Findings should be documented in patient records to ensure continuity of care and medicolegal protection. Because of the variability in severity and presentation, rating scales have been developed to standardize assessments and diagnoses. The **Abnormal Involuntary Movement Scale (AIMS)** rates dyskinetic movements, but it is not exclusively diagnostic for tardive dyskinesia (see Evolve website). The **Dyskinesia Identification System: Condensed User Scale (DISCUS)** rates the presence and severity of abnormal movements and considers other variables when formulating a conclusion. The DISCUS evaluation specifically describes the type of tardive dyskinesia and allows diagnoses to change over time (see Evolve website).

Treatment of tardive dyskinesia is not particularly successful. The most beneficial treatments are anticholinergic withdrawal, adrenergic blocking agents (e.g., beta blockers, clonidine), and benzodiazepines. Antipsychotic dosages may be increased, but they may only mask symptoms, and they eventually will worsen tardive dyskinesia. Patients receiving typical antipsychotic therapy who have severe symptoms of tardive dyskinesia can be switched to an atypical antipsychotic agent. A new class of medicine targeted specifically to treat tardive dyskinesia are the vesicular monoamine transporter 2 (VMAT2) inhibitors. The two members of this class are valbenazine (Ingrezza) and deutetrabenazine (Austedo). More information on the use of these drugs will be forthcoming when more experience is gained on its use in the clinical setting.

Neuroleptic malignant syndrome (NMS) is a potentially fatal adverse effect of antipsychotic therapy in which the patient displays EPSs as part of the symptoms of the disorder. It occurs in 0.5% to 1.4% of patients receiving antipsychotic therapy and is reported most often with high-potency antipsychotic agents given intramuscularly. It typically occurs after 3 to 9 days of treatment with antipsychotic medications, and it is not related to dosage or previous drug exposure. Once NMS begins, symptoms rapidly progress over 24 to 72 hours. Symptoms usually last for 5 to 10 days after discontinuation of oral medications and 13 to 30 days with **depot antipsychotic medicine** (*depot:* injectable, slow-release dose form). Most cases of NMS occur in patients younger than 40 years old, and it occurs twice as often in men. The syndrome is characterized by the following: fever, severe EPSs (e.g., lead-pipe rigidity, trismus, choreiform movements, opisthotonos), autonomic instability (e.g., tachycardia, labile hypertension, diaphoresis, incontinence), and alterations in consciousness (e.g., stupor, mutism, coma). Mortality rates have been as high as 30%, but prompt recognition of the symptoms has reduced the mortality rate to 4% in recent years. It is hypothesized that the cause of the symptoms is excessive dopamine depletion. Treatment includes bromocriptine or amantadine as dopamine agonists and dantrolene as a muscle relaxant. Fever is treated with cooling blankets, adequate hydration, and antipyretics. After the patient's condition has stabilized, a thorough evaluation of the medications being prescribed must be made. Resumption of the antipsychotic medication may result in a recurrence of NMS; therefore the lowest dose possible of an antipsychotic agent is prescribed, and close observation of the patient's response is required.

SEIZURES

Antipsychotic agents may lower the seizure threshold in patients with seizure disorders and even in those with no previous history of seizures. The low-potency typical agents and clozapine, an atypical agent, have a higher incidence of inducing seizures.

WEIGHT GAIN

Antipsychotic drug therapy often causes substantial weight gain. There is a higher prevalence of obesity associated with schizophrenia, and the weight gain often contributes to nonadherence to therapy. Obesity leads to an increased risk of type 2 diabetes mellitus, dyslipidemia, hypertension, coronary heart disease, and stroke (see Chapter 20). The frequency and amount of weight gain are generally greater with atypical agents than with typical medications, although individual atypical agents vary in the extent to which they cause weight gain. Of the atypical agents, clozapine and olanzapine cause the most weight gain, moderate weight gain is reported with risperidone and quetiapine, and aripiprazole and ziprasidone cause the least weight gain.

HYPERGLYCEMIA

A relatively new adverse effect being reported—particularly with atypical antipsychotic agents—is hyperglycemia and the development of diabetes mellitus. The mechanism whereby this occurs is unknown, and research in this area is more difficult because patients with schizophrenia also have a two- to threefold higher incidence of diabetes mellitus than the general population. Hyperglycemia occurs more frequently with clozapine, olanzapine, and quetiapine, but development of hyperglycemia with the other atypical agents cannot yet be ruled out because these agents are new.

DYSLIPIDEMIA

Clozapine, olanzapine, and quetiapine appear to increase serum triglyceride levels. They do not increase cholesterol levels, although they may appear to do so because serum triglycerides are a component of total serum cholesterol values. The increase in serum triglyceride levels may occur without a change in weight, although increased body weight will contribute to the hypertriglyceridemia.

DYSRHYTHMIAS

Thioridazine, ziprasidone, haloperidol, quetiapine, olanzapine, asenapine, iloperidone, lurasidone, and risperidone have rarely been associated with torsades de pointes—a ventricular dysrhythmia associated with prolongation of the Q–Tc interval on the electrocardiogram, syncope, and sudden death. Bradycardia, electrolyte imbalance (hypokalemia, hypomagnesemia), presence of congenital prolongation of the Q–Tc interval, and concomitant use of other medications that may significantly prolong the Q–Tc interval (e.g., quinidine, sotalol, moxifloxacin, dofetilide) can increase the risk of torsades de pointes and sudden death in patients receiving antipsychotic agents.

OTHER ADVERSE EFFECTS

Other adverse effects of antipsychotic therapy can also be predicted on the basis of the receptor-blocking activity of the agents:

- Blocking the cholinergic (acetylcholine) receptors explains the anticholinergic effects (e.g., dry mouth, constipation, sinus tachycardia, blurred vision, inhibition or impairment of ejaculation, urinary retention) associated with antipsychotic agents.
- Blocking histamine-1 receptors causes sedation, drowsiness, and appetite stimulation and contributes to the hypotensive effects and potentiation of CNS depressant drugs. Antipsychotic agents also block alpha-1 and alpha-2 adrenergic receptors, causing postural hypotension, sexual dysfunction, reflex tachycardia, and potentiation of antihypertensive agents. The most potent alpha-1 blockers are chlorpromazine and thioridazine, whereas haloperidol has almost no effect on alpha-1 receptors.

Antipsychotic agents may produce many adverse effects other than those already listed, including hepatotoxicity, blood dyscrasias, allergic reactions, endocrine disorders, skin pigmentation, and reversible effects in the eyes. Patients receiving clozapine are particularly susceptible to developing agranulocytosis. Regularly scheduled white blood cell (WBC) counts are mandatory.

Clinical Pitfall

Antipsychotic medicines may have adverse effects such as seizure activity, pseudoparkinsonian symptoms, tardive dyskinesia, and hepatotoxicity that require management by the prescribing healthcare provider. The patient and those providing supervision need to understand the importance of reporting any of these symptoms promptly for appropriate interventions.

❖ NURSING IMPLICATIONS FOR ANTIPSYCHOTIC THERAPY

◆ Assessment

History of behavior

- Gather information from the patient and other individuals relating to the onset, duration, and progression of the patient's symptoms. Has the patient previously been treated for this or other mental disorders? Does the patient have any coexisting health conditions?
- Take a detailed history of all medications that the patient is taking or has taken during the past 3 months.
- Inquire about the use of substances.

Basic mental status

- Note the patient's general appearance and appropriateness of attire. Is the patient clean and neat? Is the posture erect, stooped, or slumped? Is the patient oriented to date, time, place, and person?
- What coping mechanisms has the patient been using to deal with the situation? How adaptive are the coping mechanisms? Initiate changes in maladaptive coping mechanisms by guiding the patient toward the use of more adaptive coping strategies.
- Has the patient been able to carry out self-care activities and social and work obligations?
- Are symptoms of depression present? Symptoms may not be evident during the acute phase of schizophrenia.

Interpersonal relationships. Assess the quality of the relationships in which the patient is involved. Identify people in the patient's life who are supportive. Ask the family and significant others to describe the relationship they have with the patient. Has there been deterioration in their closeness and their ability to interrelate effectively?

Mood and affect. Patients experiencing altered thinking, behavior, or feelings require careful evaluation of their verbal and nonverbal actions. Often the thoughts, feelings, and behaviors displayed are inconsistent with the so-called normal responses of individuals in similar circumstances.

- Is the facial expression worried, sad, angry, or blank?
- Is the patient displaying behaviors that are inappropriate or blunted? Does the patient have a flat affect?
- Is the patient apathetic to normal situations?
- Is there consistency when the patient is expressing feelings verbally and nonverbally?
- Does the patient overreact to situations at times?

Clarity of thoughts and perception

- Does the patient suffer from delusions, disorganized speech pattern, flight of ideas, autism, grandiose ideas, or mutism? Ask about the presence of hallucinations (auditory, visual, tactile).
- Does the patient talk about unrelated topics (loose association) as though they are connected and related?
- Is the patient self-absorbed and not in contact with reality?
- Does the patient display an interruption of thoughts?
- Does the patient display paranoid behavior?

Suicidal ideation. Ask the patient whether he or she has ever had thoughts about suicide. If the response is "yes," get more details. Has a specific plan been formulated? How often do these thoughts occur? Does the patient make direct or indirect statements regarding death (e.g., "things would be better" if death occurred)?

Psychomotor function. What is the patient's activity level? Is the individual unable to sit still and instead paces continually? Is the patient catatonic (i.e., immobile as a result of psychological dysfunction)?

Sleep pattern. What is the patient's normal sleep pattern, and how has it varied since the onset of the psychotic symptoms? Ask specifically whether insomnia is present. Ask the patient to describe his or her perception of the amount and quality of sleep nightly. What is the level of fatigue? Are naps taken regularly?

Dietary history. Ask questions about the patient's appetite and note weight gains or losses not associated with intentional dieting.

◆ Implementation

- Nursing interventions must be individualized and based on patient assessment data.
- Provide the individual with a structured environment that is safe and that decreases external stimuli.
- Provide an environment of acceptance that focuses on the individual's strengths while minimizing weaknesses.
- Provide an opportunity for the patient to express feelings. Use active listening and therapeutic communication techniques. Allow the patient to express feelings in nonverbal ways, such as involvement in physical activities or occupational therapy.
- Allow the patient to make decisions, if capable; make those decisions that the patient is not capable of making. Provide a reward for progress when decisions are initiated appropriately.
- Involve the patient in self-care activities. Assist with personal grooming as needed. Ensure that the patient is dressed appropriately.
- Set limits for the patient to handle inappropriate behaviors and enforce them in a kind, firm manner.
- Once the content is known, do not reinforce the patient's hallucinations or delusions.
- When the patient has altered perceptions, provide diversionary activities and minimize interactions, such as viewing television programs that may reinforce the distorted perceptions.
- Be open and direct when handling a patient who is highly suspicious. Speak distinctly to be heard; do not whisper or laugh in circumstances that the patient could misconstrue.
- If the patient is suicidal, ask for details about the plan being formulated. Follow up on details obtained with appropriate family members or significant others. Provide for patient safety and supervision as appropriate.
- Use physical restraints within the guidelines of the clinical setting as appropriate to the behaviors being exhibited. Use the least restrictive alternative possible for the circumstances.

- Provide for nutritional needs by having high-protein, high-calorie foods appropriate for the individual to eat while pacing or highly active. Give vitamins and liquid supplemental feedings as ordered.
- Provide an opportunity for the individual to be involved in selecting foods appropriate to needs (to lose or gain weight). If the person is paranoid and suspects being poisoned, allow the individual to self-serve food, open canned food, and perform other activities, as appropriate within the setting.
- Manipulative behavior must be handled in a consistent manner by all staff members. Set limits and use consequences that are agreed to in advance by all staff members. When the patient attempts to blame others, refocus on the patient's responsibilities. Give positive reinforcement for nonmanipulative behaviors when they occur.

◆ Patient Education

- Orient the individual to the unit. Explain the rules and the process of privileges and how they are obtained or lost. (The extent of the orientation and explanations given will depend on the patient's orientation to date, time, and place, as well as his or her abilities.)
- Base patient education on assessment data and individualize instruction to provide the patient with a structured environment.
- Explain the activity groups available and how and when the individual will participate in them.
- Involve the patient and family in establishing outcomes and integrate the patient into the appropriate group processes to develop positive experiences to enhance coping skills.
- Before discharge, make sure the patient and the family understand the desired treatment outcomes and the entire follow-up plan (e.g., frequency of therapy sessions, prescribed medications, physician visits, return-to-work goals).

Fostering health maintenance

- Throughout the course of treatment, discuss medication information and how it will benefit the patient's symptoms and circumstances. Drug therapy is a major portion of antipsychotic therapy. Although symptoms may improve, they may not be totally eliminated. The onset of a drug's effectiveness varies widely, depending on the drug and the route of administration.
- Nonadherence is a major problem in this group of patients; therefore tracking the medications being taken requires careful scrutiny. On an outpatient basis, many of these patients need their medications administered by another responsible individual. Nonadherence is thought to be a major cause of repeat hospitalization in these patients. Long-acting injections may be used for some patients in an attempt to overcome this problem. On an inpatient basis, the nurse must always check to be sure that the patient

is actually swallowing the medication because there is a high incidence of "cheeking" (i.e., hiding drugs between the teeth and gums).

- Use baseline clinical evaluation rating scales (e.g., BPRS, CGI, PANSS) and adverse effect scales (e.g., GDS, TWSTRS for dystonias, DISCUS or AIMS for EPSs) at specified intervals; record and report findings in accordance with agency policy.
- Seek cooperation and understanding of the following points so that medication adherence is increased: name of the medication; its dosage, route, and time of administration; and its common and serious adverse effects. Encourage the patient not to discontinue or adjust the drug dosage without consulting the healthcare provider. Provide the patient and family with information about available community resources, including the NAMI.

Patient self-assessment. Enlist the patient's help with developing and maintaining a written record of monitoring parameters. See the Template for Developing a Written Record for Patients to Monitor Their Own Therapy on the Evolve website, and complete the Premedication Data column for an assessment of the patient's physical and mental capabilities as a baseline to track the patient's response to drug therapy. Ensure that the patient understands how to use the form, and instruct the patient to bring the completed form to follow-up visits. Because there are a number of debilitating adverse effects and others that are life threatening if they are not acted on correctly, it is important to maintain open communication with healthcare providers, nurses, therapists, and pharmacists throughout the course of therapy.

DRUG CLASS: ANTIPSYCHOTIC AGENTS

Actions

Although the antipsychotic medications are from distinctly different chemical classes, all are similar in that they act by blocking the action of dopamine in the brain. The exception is pimavanserin, which selectively blocks the 5-HT$_{2A}$ serotonin receptor and lacks activity at dopamine receptors. The atypical antipsychotic agents block serotonin receptors in addition to dopamine receptors. Because all the antipsychotic agents work at different sites in the brain, adverse effects are observed in different body systems. Atypical antipsychotic agents tend to be more effective and have fewer adverse effects than typical agents.

Uses

Antipsychotic agents are used to treat psychoses associated with mental illnesses such as schizophrenia, mania, psychotic depression, and psychotic organic brain syndrome. Medications used to treat these disorders are grouped into two broad categories (Table 17.1): first-generation antipsychotic drugs, also known as

typical antipsychotic drugs, including the phenothiazines and nonphenothiazines (e.g., thioxanthenes, haloperidol, loxapine); and second-generation antipsychotic drugs, also known as *atypical antipsychotic drugs* (e.g., aripiprazole, olanzapine, quetiapine, risperidone). The atypical antipsychotics (except pimavanserin) are usually used first line to provide significant relief of active psychotic symptoms such as hallucinations, delusions, and thought disorganization for approximately 70% of patients with schizophrenia. In addition, several of the atypical antipsychotics are used for treatment of bipolar disorder (e.g., lurasidone) and as adjunctive treatment to major depressive disorders (e.g., aripiprazole). Clozapine is reserved for more resistant cases that do not respond adequately to the other atypical agents. All these antipsychotic medications also significantly reduce the risk of recurrence. Pimavanserin is used for the treatment of hallucinations and delusions associated with Parkinson's disease dementia-related psychosis.

As clinical experience is being gained with the relatively new second-generation antipsychotic drugs, dramatic weight gain, diabetes mellitus, electrocardiographic changes (e.g., Q–T interval prolongation), and dyslipidemia have been reported. The risk of these potentially serious adverse effects is not the same with all drugs, but the US Food and Drug Administration has issued precautionary statements to encourage close monitoring of body weight, blood glucose, and serum lipid levels in all patients receiving these antipsychotic agents.

Therapeutic Outcome

The primary therapeutic outcome expected from antipsychotic therapy is maintaining the individual at an optimal level of functioning, with minimal exacerbations of psychotic symptoms and minimal adverse effects from medicines.

❖ Nursing Implications for Antipsychotic Agent Therapy

◆ Premedication assessment

1. Obtain baseline blood pressures with the patient supine, sitting, and standing; record and report significant lowering to the healthcare provider before administering the medicine. Monitor on a yearly basis thereafter.
2. Check the patient's electrolyte levels, body weight, waist circumference, height, blood glucose level, lipid profile, hepatic function, cardiac function, and thyroid function before initiating therapy and periodically throughout the course of treatment. Weight should be monitored every 4 weeks until 12 weeks after initiating therapy and then every 3 months. Monitor waist circumference and fasting plasma glucose level annually and fasting lipid levels every 5 years.
3. Use baseline clinical evaluation rating scales (e.g., BPRS, CGI, PANSS) and adverse effect scales (e.g., GDS, TWSTRS for dystonias, DISCUS or AIMS for

EPSs) at specified intervals; record and report findings in accordance with agency policy.

4. Use of clozapine requires a baseline WBC count and weekly WBC counts for the first 6 months of treatment because of the high incidence of agranulocytosis. Thereafter, if WBC counts are acceptable (i.e., ≥3500/mm³) and if the absolute neutrophil count is more than 2000/mm³, WBC counts can be monitored every other week. WBC counts must be monitored weekly for at least 4 weeks after the discontinuation of clozapine.

◆ *Availability, dosage, and administration.* See Table 17.1. The dosage must be individualized according to the patient's degree of mental and emotional disturbance. It will often take several weeks for a patient to show optimal improvement and become stabilized on an adequate maintenance dosage. As a result of the cumulative effects of antipsychotic agents, the patient must be reevaluated periodically to determine the lowest effective dosage necessary to control psychiatric symptoms.

◆ *Common adverse effects*
Neurologic
Chronic fatigue, drowsiness. Chronic fatigue and drowsiness are common problems associated with medications used to treat psychoses. Sedative effects associated with antipsychotic therapy can be minimized by giving the dose of medication at bedtime. The patient should not take these medications while working with machinery, operating a motor vehicle, administering medication, or performing other duties that require mental alertness.
Cardiovascular
Orthostatic hypotension. All antipsychotic agents may cause some degree of orthostatic hypotension manifested by dizziness and weakness, particularly when therapy is initiated. Monitor the patient's blood pressure daily in the supine, sitting, and standing positions. Anticipate the development of postural hypotension and take measures to prevent an occurrence. Teach the patient to rise slowly from a supine or sitting position and encourage the patient to sit or lie down if feeling faint.
Sensory
Blurred vision. Caution the patient that blurred vision may occur and make appropriate suggestions to ensure the patient's personal safety.
Genitourinary
Urinary retention. Urinary retention may occur after the administration of antipsychotic agents.
Gastrointestinal
Constipation; dryness of mucosa of the mouth, throat, nose. Mucosal dryness may be relieved by sucking hard candy or ice chips or by chewing gum. A high-fiber diet, stool softeners (e.g., docusate), or the occasional use of a stimulant laxative (e.g., bisacodyl) may be required to treat constipation.

◆ *Serious adverse effects*
Neurologic
Seizure activity. Provide for patient safety during episodes of seizures; report this symptom to the healthcare provider for further evaluation. An adjustment of anticonvulsant therapy may be required, especially for seizure-prone patients.

Pseudoparkinsonian symptoms. Report the development of drooling, cogwheel rigidity, shuffling gait, mask-like expression, or tremors. Anticholinergic agents may be used to help control these symptoms.

Tardive dyskinesia. Tardive dyskinesia occurs much more commonly with the first-generation antipsychotic drugs. Report the development of fine tremors of the tongue, "fly-catching" tongue movements, and lip smacking. This is particularly important for patients who have been receiving antipsychotic drugs and anticholinergic medications for several years.
Gastrointestinal
Hepatotoxicity. The symptoms of hepatotoxicity are anorexia, nausea, vomiting, jaundice, hepatomegaly, splenomegaly, and abnormal liver function test results (e.g., elevated bilirubin, aspartate aminotransferase, alanine aminotransferase, gamma-glutamyltransferase, and alkaline phosphatase levels; increased prothrombin time).
Hematologic
Blood dyscrasias. Routine laboratory studies (e.g., red blood cell, WBC, and differential counts) should be scheduled. This is particularly important for patients receiving clozapine. Monitor for sore throat, fever, purpura, jaundice, or excessive and progressive weakness.
Hypersensitivity
Hives, pruritus, rash. Report these symptoms to the healthcare provider for further evaluation.
Other
Photosensitivity. The patient should be cautioned to avoid prolonged exposure to sunlight and ultraviolet light. Suggest that the patient wear long-sleeved clothing, a hat, and sunglasses when exposed to sunlight. Advise against using artificial tanning lamps.

◆ *Drug interactions*
Drugs that increase adverse effects. Antihistamines, alcohol, analgesics, anesthetics, tranquilizers, opiates, St. John's wort, and sedative-hypnotics increase the toxic effects of antipsychotic drugs. Monitor the patient for excessive sedation and reduce the dosage of the previously mentioned drugs if necessary.

 Herbal Interactions

St. John's Wort

St. John's wort increases the toxic effects of antipsychotic medications.

Drugs that decrease therapeutic effects

Dopamine agonists. Dopamine agonists (i.e., levodopa, bromocriptine, amantadine, ropinirole, pramipexole) block the dopamine antagonist effects of the antipsychotic agents. Avoid concurrent use.

Carbamazepine. Carbamazepine stimulates the metabolism of haloperidol, clozapine, aripiprazole, iloperidone, olanzapine, risperidone, and ziprasidone. Adjustment of the dosage of the antipsychotic medicine may be required.

Erythromycin, clarithromycin, fluoxetine, fluvoxamine, grapefruit juice, ketoconazole. All of these agents inhibit the metabolism of aripiprazole, asenapine, clozapine, iloperidone, quetiapine, and ziprasidone, causing an increase in serum levels and potential toxicity from the antipsychotic drug. Dosages of the antipsychotic drug may need to be reduced by up to 50% to avoid toxicities.

Cimetidine. Cimetidine inhibits the metabolism of quetiapine, clozapine, and risperidone. The dosage of these medicines may need to be reduced to prevent adverse effects.

Phenytoin. Phenytoin increases the metabolism of quetiapine, thioridazine, and haloperidol. Increases in dosage of the antipsychotic medication may be necessary.

Beta blockers. Beta blockers (e.g., propranolol, timolol, nadolol, pindolol) significantly enhance the hypotensive effects of antipsychotic agents. Concurrent therapy is not recommended unless it is used to treat the adverse effects of antipsychotic agents.

Insulin, oral hypoglycemic agents. Patients with prediabetes or diabetes must be monitored for the development of hyperglycemia, particularly during the early weeks of therapy. Assess patients regularly for glycosuria and report it to the healthcare provider if it occurs with any frequency. Patients receiving oral hypoglycemic agents or insulin may require a dosage adjustment.

Venlafaxine. Venlafaxine significantly inhibits the metabolism of haloperidol. Doses of haloperidol may have to be given less often to prevent potential toxicity.

Get Ready for the NCLEX® Examination!

Key Points

- Psychoses are symptoms of psychotic disorders—that is, illnesses in which the patient has lost touch with reality. The underlying illness must be treated, not just the psychosis.
- A combination of nonpharmacologic and pharmacologic therapies provides the most successful therapeutic outcomes.
- The emphasis on community treatment has ensured that almost all healthcare settings treat patients with psychotic symptoms. Community hospitals and health maintenance organizations now provide care to many psychiatric patients, and nurses increasingly serve residential care facilities. Many patients require years of antipsychotic drug treatment to prevent exacerbations of their illness.
- Although antipsychotic medications cause many adverse effects, most can be minimized by patient education, manipulation of dosage and administration, and sometimes adjunctive drug treatments. These patients require careful monitoring of target symptoms to maximize response and minimize adverse effects.

Additional Learning Resources

SG Go to your Study Guide for additional Review Questions for the NCLEX® Examination, Critical Thinking Clinical Situations, and other learning activities to help you master this chapter content.

Go to your Evolve website (https://evolve.elsevier.com/Clayton) for additional online resources.

Review Questions for the NCLEX® Examination

1. A nurse is assessing a patient who has been admitted to the psychiatric unit and who has been hearing voices that told her to lock all her doors and not answer any phone calls. The nurse should administer which scale specific for schizophrenia?
   1. AIMS
   2. TWSTRS
   3. PANSS
   4. DISCUS

2. Which premedication assessments does the nurse complete for patients who have been prescribed antipsychotic agents? *(Select all that apply.)*
   1. Baseline rating scales (e.g., BPRS, CGI)
   2. Height and waist circumference
   3. Positional blood pressure reading
   4. Allergy to sulfonamides
   5. Activity tolerance

3. A patient who has been taking an antipsychotic agent develops tongue protrusion, jaw spasms, and neck torsions. What are these extrapyramidal symptoms referred to as?
   1. Akathisia
   2. Dystonias
   3. Neuroleptic malignant syndrome
   4. Pseudoparkinsonian symptoms

4. What are the major adverse effects of antipsychotic medications? *(Select all that apply.)*
   1. Extrapyramidal symptoms
   2. Seizures
   3. Weight loss
   4. Chronic fatigue
   5. Dyslipidemia

5. A psychotic patient began taking antipsychotic medications 1 week ago. What will the nurse expect the patient to experience? *(Select all that apply.)*
   1. Reduced auditory hallucinations
   2. Reduced delusions
   3. Rapid weight gain
   4. Reduced agitation
   5. Reduced insomnia

6. The nurse reviewing a patient's medication list recognized which one as the antipsychotic?
   1. Trimipramine (Surmontil)
   2. Tranylcypromine (Parnate)
   3. Thiothixene
   4. Trazodone

neurotransmitters. Benzodiazepines, phenobarbital, tiagabine, gabapentin, and pregabalin enhance the inhibitory effect of gamma-aminobutyric acid (GABA), an inhibitory neurotransmitter that counterbalances the effect of excitatory neurotransmitters. Gamma-aminobutyric acid opens chloride channels, resulting in a hyperpolarized cell membrane that prevents excitation of the cell, stopping further propagation of the seizure. Seizure control medications are sometimes subdivided into broad-spectrum and narrow-spectrum agents in relation to their efficacy against different types of seizures. The broad-spectrum agents are levetiracetam, topiramate, valproic acid, zonisamide, and lamotrigine. These drugs are often used for the initial treatment of a patient with a newly diagnosed seizure disorder. The narrow-spectrum agents are phenytoin, carbamazepine, oxcarbazepine, tiagabine, gabapentin, and pregabalin (French and Pedley, 2008).

In general, antiepileptic therapy should start with the use of a single drug selected from a group of agents based on the type of seizure. In choosing an initial therapy, clinicians must weigh relative efficacy, pharmacokinetics, and potential for adverse effects of each drug, but other patient-specific factors need to be considered, including age, sex, childbearing potential, comorbidities, and concomitant medications. Comparative efficacy and tolerability data are limited, however, and trials that have been performed have not shown significant differences among various drugs in terms of efficacy. With more than 20 antiepileptic drugs and implantable antiseizure devices available to treat epilepsy in adults, opportunities to tailor drug therapy have never been greater, but the multitude of treatment options for seizures is a challenge.

In general, if treatment is not successful with the first agent chosen, that agent is discontinued and another agent is started. If treatment fails with the second agent, the healthcare provider may decide to discontinue the second agent and start a third agent, or combination therapy may be started by adding an alternative medication to one of the initial agents. Occasionally some patients will require multiple-drug therapy with a combination of agents and will still not be completely free of seizures. Those patients with newly diagnosed epilepsy who respond to treatment are referred to as "treatment responsive," and those who do not respond to initial agents are referred to as "treatment resistant." About half of patients with newly diagnosed epilepsy become free of seizures while using the first prescribed antiepileptic drug. Almost two-thirds of patients become free of seizures after receiving the second or third agent.

Nonpharmacologic treatment of refractory seizures includes surgical intervention, the use of an implantable vagus nerve stimulator for children who are 12 years old and older, and a ketogenic diet. The ketogenic diet is used for children, and it includes the restriction of carbohydrate and protein intake; fat is the primary fuel that produces acidosis and ketosis. Although the diet has been shown to reduce refractory seizures in children who have not achieved effective control with drug therapy, the adverse effects of this diet include high blood lipid levels with long-term effects that are not known.

According to a report by the US Food and Drug Administration (2008), patients who were receiving antiepileptic drugs had approximately twice the risk of suicidal behavior or ideation (0.43%) compared with patients receiving placebo (0.22%). The increased risk of suicidal behavior and suicidal ideation was observed as early as 1 week after starting the antiepileptic drug, and it continued through 24 weeks of use of the medication. Healthcare professionals should closely monitor all patients currently receiving antiepileptic drugs for notable changes in behavior that could indicate the emergence or worsening of suicidal thoughts or behavior or depression. The drugs included in the analysis were carbamazepine, felbamate, gabapentin, lamotrigine, levetiracetam, oxcarbazepine, pregabalin, tiagabine, topiramate, valproate, and zonisamide (from the FDA's "Statistical Review and Evaluation: Antiepileptic Drugs and Suicidality." Published online May 23, 2008).

Life Span Considerations
Antiepileptic Therapy

In children, antiepileptic therapy may cause a change in personality and possible indifference to both school and family activities. Behavioral differences must be discussed with the healthcare provider, family or caregivers, and teachers. The school nurse must be informed about the medications that have been prescribed.

Liquid dosage forms of antiepileptic medicines must be measured accurately to help maintain seizure control. It is extremely important to shake the liquid first to disperse the medication uniformly in the suspension. The dosage should then be measured with an oral syringe to ensure accuracy before administration.

Medications should be taken at the same time daily to maintain a consistent blood level. Dosages should not be self-adjusted, and drugs should not be discontinued suddenly.

Monitoring the patient's response to antiepileptic therapy is essential. Dosages may need to be adjusted weekly, especially during the initiation of therapy.

USES

Antiepileptic medicines are used to reduce the frequency of seizures.

❖ NURSING IMPLICATIONS FOR ANTIEPILEPTIC THERAPY

Nurses may play an important role in the correct diagnosis of seizure disorders. Accurate seizure diagnosis is crucial to the selection of the most appropriate medications for each patient. Because healthcare providers are not always able to observe patient seizures directly, nurses should learn to observe and record these events objectively.

◆ Assessment

History of seizure activity

- What activities was the patient engaged in immediately before the last seizure?
- Has the patient been ill recently?
- Is there a history of fever, unusual rash, or tick infestation?
- Has the patient noticed any particular activity that usually precedes the attacks?
- When was the last seizure before the current one?
- Did the patient have any changes in behavior before the onset of the seizure (e.g., increasing anxiety or depression)?
- Is the patient aware of a preseizure "aura" (i.e., a particular feeling or odor that occurs before a seizure onset)?
- Was there an "epileptic cry"?

Seizure description

- Record the exact time of seizure onset and the duration of each phase, a description of the specific body parts involved, and any progression of seizure action in the affected body parts.
- Did the patient lose consciousness?
- Were stiffening and/or jerking movements present?
- Describe the autonomic responses usually seen during the clonic phase: altered, jerky respirations; frothy salivation; dilated pupils; any eye movements; cyanosis; diaphoresis; incontinence.

Postictal behavior

- Record the level of consciousness (i.e., orientation to time, place, and person).
- Assess the degree of alertness, fatigue, or headache present.
- Evaluate the degree of weakness, any alterations in speech, and memory loss.
- Patients often have muscle soreness and an extreme need for sleep. Record the duration of sleep.
- Evaluate any bodily harm that occurred during the seizure (e.g., bruises, cuts, lacerations).

◆ Implementation

Management of seizure activity. Assist the patient during a seizure by doing the following:

- Do not leave the patient.
- Have drugs available to treat status epilepticus or know the procedure for obtaining them as quickly as possible.
- Protect the patient from further injury. Place padding around or under the patient's head; do not try to restrain the patient and loosen any tight clothing. If the patient is in a standing position initially, lower to a horizontal position.
- When the patient starts to relax after a seizure, turn slightly onto the side to allow secretions to drain out of the mouth.
- Remain calm and quiet, and give reassurance to the patient when the seizure is over.

- Have oxygen available as well as emergency equipment for suctioning and/or ventilating the patient.
- Suction the patient as needed and initiate ventilatory assistance if breathing does not return spontaneously.
- Provide a place for the patient to rest immediately after a seizure. Summon appropriate assistance after the seizure.
- Initiate nursing interventions appropriate to the underlying cause of the seizures (e.g., high fever, metabolic disorder, head trauma, drug or alcohol withdrawal).
- If the patient has another seizure or if a seizure lasts for more than 4 minutes, immediately summon assistance; the patient may be going into status epilepticus.
- Observe all aspects of the seizure for detailed recording: aura (if present), time started and ended, body parts affected, order of progression of seizure action, autonomic signs (e.g., altered breathing, diaphoresis, incontinence, salivation, flushing, pupil dilation), postictal period observations (e.g., vital signs; level of consciousness; speech pattern/ disorder; muscle soreness, weakness, or paralysis), and how long each phase lasted.

Psychological implications

Lifestyle. Encourage the patient to maintain a normal lifestyle. Provide for appropriate limitations (e.g., limits on operating power equipment or motor vehicles; swimming) to ensure patient safety. Make the patient aware of the Rehabilitation Act of 1973, which was initiated to ensure that individuals with disabilities do not experience discrimination in employment. Contact the Epilepsy Foundation of America and state vocational rehabilitation agencies for information about vocational rehabilitation and employment.

Expressing feelings. Allow the patient to ventilate his or her feelings. Seizures may occur in public, and they may be accompanied by incontinence. Patients are usually embarrassed about having a seizure in front of others. Provide for the expression of feelings about any discrimination that the patient feels at the workplace. Encourage the open discussion of self-concept issues related to the disease and its effect on daily activities, work, and the responses of others toward the patient.

School-age children. Acceptance by peers can present a problem to a patient in this age group. The school nurse can help teachers and other children to understand the patient's seizures.

Denial. Be alert for signs of denial of the disease, which are indicated by increased seizure activity in a previously well-controlled patient. Question the patient's adherence to the drug regimen.

Adherence. Determine the patient's current medication schedule, including the name of the medication, the dosage, and the time of the last dose. Have any doses been skipped? If so, how many? If adherence appears to be a problem, try to determine the reasons why so that appropriate interventions can be implemented.

Status epilepticus

1. Provide for patient protection and summon assistance to transport the patient to an emergency facility.
2. Administer oxygen. Have suction and resuscitation equipment available and attach cardiac and oxygen saturation monitors.
3. Establish an intravenous (IV) line and have drugs available for treatment (e.g., lorazepam, diazepam, phenytoin, phenobarbital). When administering IV drugs, monitor the patient for bradycardia, hypotension, and respiratory depression.
4. Monitor the patient's vital signs and neurologic status.
5. Insert a nasogastric tube if the patient is vomiting.

◆ Patient Education

Exercise and activity. Discuss what activities or actions trigger seizures and how to avoid them. Encourage the patient to maintain a regular lifestyle with moderate activity. Avoid excessive exercise that could lead to excessive fatigue.

Nutrition. Avoid excessive use of stimulants (e.g., caffeine-containing products). Seizures are also known to follow the significant intake of alcoholic beverages; therefore such ingestion should be avoided or limited. Ask the healthcare provider whether vitamin supplements are needed, because some anticonvulsants interfere with vitamin and mineral absorption.

Safety. Teach the patient to avoid operating power equipment or machinery. Driving may be minimized or prohibited. Check state laws regarding how or if an individual with a history of seizure activity may qualify for a driver's license. Be especially alert to signs of confusion and impaired coordination in older patients. Provide for the patient's safety.

Stress. The reduction of tension and stress within the individual's environment may reduce seizure activity in some patients.

Oral hygiene. Encourage daily oral hygiene practices and scheduling of regular dental examinations. **Gingival hyperplasia**, which is gum overgrowth associated with hydantoins (e.g., phenytoin, ethotoin), can be reduced with good oral hygiene, frequent gum massage, regular brushing, and proper dental care.

Medication considerations in pregnancy

- If pregnancy is suspected, consult an obstetrician as soon as possible.
- Inform the healthcare provider of seizure medications.
- Do not discontinue medications unless told to do so by the healthcare provider.
- The patient should carry an identification card or bracelet.

Fostering health maintenance. Throughout the course of treatment, discuss medication information and how it will benefit the patient. Recognize that nonadherence may be a means of denial. Explore underlying problems regarding the patient's acceptance of the disease and the need for strict adherence for maximum seizure control. Provide the patient and significant others with important information contained in the specific drug monographs for the medications prescribed. Additional health teaching and nursing interventions regarding the adverse effects are described in the drug monographs that follow. Seek cooperation and understanding of the following points so that medication adherence is increased: the name of the medication, its dosage, its route and times of administration, and its common and serious adverse effects.

Patient self-assessment. Enlist the patient's help with developing and maintaining a written record or seizure diary of monitoring parameters (e.g., degree of lethargy; sedation; oral hygiene for gum disorders; degree of seizure relief; any nausea, vomiting, or anorexia present). See the Patient Self-Assessment Form for Anticonvulsants on the Evolve website. Complete the Premedication Data column for use as a baseline to track the patient's response to drug therapy. Ensure that the patient and significant others understand how to use the form. Have others record the date, time, duration, and frequency of any seizure episodes. In addition, record the patient's behavior immediately before and after seizures. Emphasize taking medications at the same time daily to help maintain a consistent therapeutic drug level. The patient should consult with a pharmacist before taking over-the-counter medications to prevent drug interactions. Have the patient bring the completed form to follow-up visits.

DRUG THERAPY FOR SEIZURE DISORDERS

DRUG CLASS: BENZODIAZEPINES

Actions

The mechanisms of action for benzodiazepines are not fully understood, but it is thought that benzodiazepines stimulate BDZ_2 receptors to inhibit neurotransmission by enhancing the effects of GABA in the postsynaptic clefts between nerve cells. Increased levels of GABA open the chloride channel, resulting in a hyperpolarized cell membrane that prevents further excitation of the cell, thus preventing propagation of the seizure activity. (See Chapter 13 for more details on benzodiazepine activity.)

Uses

The four benzodiazepines approved for use as antiepileptic therapy are diazepam, lorazepam, clonazepam, and clorazepate. Clonazepam is useful for the oral treatment of absence, akinetic, and myoclonic seizures in children. Diazepam and lorazepam must be administered intravenously to control seizures; they are the drugs of choice for treating status epilepticus. Clorazepate is used with other antiepileptic agents to control partial seizures. Diazepam administered as a rectal gel may be used to prevent breakthrough seizures.

Therapeutic Outcomes

The primary therapeutic outcomes expected from the benzodiazepines are as follows:
1. Reduced frequency of seizures and reduced injury from seizure activity
2. Minimal adverse effects from therapy

❖ Nursing Implications for Benzodiazepines
◆ *Premedication assessment*
1. Review routine blood studies to detect blood dyscrasias and hepatotoxicity.
2. Perform a baseline assessment of the patient's speech patterns, degree of alertness, and orientation to name, place, and time before initiating therapy. Monitor the patient's behavioral responses to therapy.
3. Review the patient's medical record to document the frequency of seizure activity.

◆ *Availability, dosage, and administration.* See Table 18.1.

> ### Medication Safety Alert
>
> Rapidly discontinuing benzodiazepines after long-term use may result in symptoms similar to those of alcohol withdrawal. These may vary from weakness and anxiety to delirium and generalized tonic-clonic seizures. The symptoms may not appear for several days after discontinuation. Treatment consists of the gradual withdrawal of benzodiazepines over the course of 2 to 4 weeks.

Intravenous administration. Do not mix parenteral diazepam or lorazepam in the same syringe with other medications; do not add these to other IV solutions because of precipitate formation. Administer diazepam slowly at a rate of no more than 5 mg/min or lorazepam at a rate of no more than 2 mg/min. If at all possible, give these drugs with the patient under electrocardiographic (ECG) monitoring and observe closely for bradycardia. When bradycardia occurs, stop boluses until the heart rate returns to normal.

◆ *Common adverse effects*
Neurologic
Sedation, drowsiness, dizziness, fatigue, lethargy. The more common adverse effects of benzodiazepines are extensions of their pharmacologic properties. These symptoms tend to disappear with continued therapy and possible dosage readjustment. Encourage the patient not to discontinue therapy without first consulting the healthcare provider. The patient should be warned not to

work with machinery, operate a motor vehicle, administer medication, or perform other duties that require mental alertness. Provide for patient safety during episodes of dizziness and ataxia; report these changes to the healthcare provider for further evaluation.

>
> ### Clinical Pitfall
>
> Do not mix parenteral diazepam, lorazepam, or phenytoin with other medications in the same syringe, and do not add either medication to other IV solutions because of precipitate formation. Always check for IV incompatibility before administering either medication through an established IV line, and use the SAS (**S**aline flush first, **A**dminister the prescribed drug, **S**aline flush after the drug) technique. Administer diazepam slowly at a rate of 5 mg/min and lorazepam at a rate of 2 mg/min. Administer phenytoin slowly at a rate of 25 to 50 mg/min, preferably through a large vein or as an IV piggyback. Phenytoin can be quite irritating to small veins. During the administration of either medication, it is recommended that an ECG monitor be used to closely observe for bradycardia. If bradycardia occurs, stop the bolus infusion until the heart rate returns to normal. Observe the patient during administration for respiratory depression and hypotension.

Sensory
Blurred vision. Caution the patient that blurred vision may occur and make appropriate suggestions for the patient's personal safety.

◆ *Serious adverse effects*
Psychological
Behavioral disturbances. Behavioral disturbances such as aggressiveness and agitation have been reported, especially in patients who are mentally handicapped or who have psychiatric disturbances. Provide supportive physical care and safety during these responses. Assess the level of the patient's excitement, and deal calmly with the individual. During periods of excitement, protect the patient from harm and provide for the physical channeling of energy (e.g., walk with him or her). Seek a change in the medication order.

Hematologic
Blood dyscrasias. Routine laboratory studies (i.e., red blood cell [RBC], white blood cell [WBC], differential, and platelet counts) may be scheduled. Monitor the patient for sore throat, fever, purpura, jaundice, or excessive and progressive weakness. Blood dyscrasias are a rare but serious adverse effect.

Gastrointestinal
Hepatotoxicity. The symptoms of hepatotoxicity include anorexia, nausea, vomiting, jaundice, hepatomegaly, splenomegaly, and abnormal liver function test results (e.g., elevated bilirubin, aspartate aminotransferase [AST], alanine aminotransferase [ALT], gamma-glutamyltransferase [GGT], and alkaline phosphatase levels; increased prothrombin time [PT]).

Table 18.1   Antiepileptic Medicines

GENERIC NAME	BRAND NAME	AVAILABILITY	ADULT DOSAGE RANGE	USE FOR SEIZURES
Benzodiazepines				
clobazam	Onfi	Tablets: 10, 20 mg Oral suspension: 2.5 mg/mL (120 mL)	Up to 40 mg/day	Adjunct treatment of partial seizures in adolescents older than 16, and adults
clonazepam	Klonopin Rivotril ✤ ⇄ Do not confuse Klonopin with clonidine.	Tablets: 0.5, 1, 2 mg Tablets, orally disintegrating: 0.125, 0.25, 0.5, 1, 2 mg	Up to 20 mg/day	Absence and myoclonic seizures
clorazepate	Tranxene-T Apo-Clorazepate ✤	Tablets: 3.75, 7.5, 15 mg	Up to 90 mg/day	Focal seizures
diazepam ❶ ⇄ Do not confuse diazepam with Ditropan.	Valium Apo-Diazepam ✤ ⇄ Do not confuse Valium with valerian.	Tablets: 2, 5, 10 mg Intramuscular, intravenous: 5 mg/mL Concentrate: 5 mg/mL Gel, rectal: 2.5, 10, 20 mg	Initially 5-10 mg/day; up to 30 mg/day	All forms of epilepsy; used in conjunction with other agents
lorazepam ❶ ⇄ Do not confuse lorazepam with loperamide.	Ativan Novo-Lorazepam ✤ ⇄ Do not confuse Ativan with Ambien.	Tablets: 0.5, 1, 2 mg Oral solution: 2 mg/mL Intramuscular, intravenous: 2, 4 mg/mL	Intravenous: 4-8 mg, repeated at 10- to 15-min intervals, if seizing	Status epilepticus
Hydantoins				
ethotoin	Peganone	Tablets: 250 mg	2-3 g/day	Generalized tonic-clonic seizures; psychomotor seizures
fosphenytoin	Cerebyx ⇄ Do not confuse Cerebyx with Avelox, Celebrex, or Celexa.	Intravenous: 100 mg phenytoin in 2-mL vials; 500 mg phenytoin in 10-mL vials (75 mg/mL of fosphenytoin is equivalent to 50 mg/mL of phenytoin)	Same dosage as for phenytoin	Status epilepticus see also phenytoin
phenytoin ❶ ⇄ Do not confuse phenytoin with phenylephrine.	Dilantin ⇄ Do not confuse Dilantin with Diflucan. Novo-Phenytoin ✤	Tablets, chewable: 50 mg Capsules: 30, 100, 200, 300 mg Suspension: 125 mg/5 mL Injection: 50 mg/mL in 2- and 5-mL ampules	300-600 mg/day	Generalized tonic-clonic seizures; psychomotor seizures
Succinimides				
ethosuximide	Zarontin	Capsules: 250 mg Syrup: 250 mg/5 mL	1000-1250 mg/day	Absence seizures
methsuximide	Celontin	Capsules: 300 mg	900-1200 mg/day	Absence seizures

✤ Available in Canada.   ⇄ Do not confuse.   ❶ High-alert medication.

◆ *Drug interactions*

Drugs that increase toxic effects. Antihistamines, alcohol, analgesics, anesthetics, tranquilizers, narcotics, cimetidine, sedative-hypnotics, and other concurrent antiepileptic drugs increase the toxic effects of benzodiazepines. Monitor the patient for excessive sedation and eliminate other medicines not needed for antiepileptic therapy, if possible.

Smoking. Cigarette smoking enhances the metabolism of benzodiazepines. Increased dosages may be necessary to maintain effects in patients who smoke.

DRUG CLASS: HYDANTOINS

Actions

The primary site of action of the hydantoins is the motor cortex, where they inhibit the spread of seizure activity. The hydantoins stabilize the threshold of neuronal cell membranes against hyperexcitability caused by excessive stimulation by promoting sodium excretion from neurons. Phenytoin also reduces the maximal activity of brainstem centers responsible for the tonic phase of tonic-clonic seizures.

Uses

The hydantoins (e.g., phenytoin, ethotoin, fosphenytoin) are anticonvulsants used to control focal seizures and generalized tonic-clonic seizures. Phenytoin is the most commonly used antiepileptic of the hydantoins. Fosphenytoin is a prodrug that is converted to phenytoin after administration. Fosphenytoin is particularly useful when loading doses of phenytoin must be administered. Phenytoin causes less sedation than phenobarbital. In toxic concentrations, phenytoin can induce seizures.

Therapeutic Outcomes

The primary therapeutic outcomes expected from the hydantoins are as follows:

1. Reduced frequency of seizures and reduced injury from seizure activity
2. Minimal adverse effects from therapy

❖ Nursing Implications for Phenytoin

◆ *Premedication assessment*

1. Review routine blood studies to detect blood dyscrasias and hepatotoxicity.
2. Determine baseline blood sugar levels in patients with diabetes. Monitor these patients periodically at specified intervals because hyperglycemia may be caused by hydantoin therapy.
3. Perform a baseline assessment of the patient's speech patterns, degree of alertness, and orientation to name, place, and time before initiating therapy. Monitor the patient's behavioral responses to therapy.
4. Review the patient's medical record to document the frequency of seizure activity.

◆ *Availability, dosage, and administration.* See Table 18.1. Administer medication with food or milk to reduce gastric irritation. If an oral suspension is used, shake it well first. Encourage the use of an oral syringe for accurate measurement.

Intramuscular (IM): If at all possible, avoid IM administration. Absorption is slow and painful.

IV: Do not mix parenteral phenytoin in the same syringe with other medications; because of precipitate formation, do not add to other IV solutions.

Administer phenytoin slowly at a rate of 25 to 50 mg/min. Fosphenytoin may be administered at a rate of 150 mg/min. If at all possible, give these drugs under ECG monitoring and observe the patient closely for bradycardia. If bradycardia occurs, stop boluses until the heart rate returns to normal. Therapeutic blood levels for phenytoin are between 10 and 20 mg/L.

◆ *Common adverse effects*

Gastrointestinal

Nausea, vomiting, indigestion. These effects are common during the initiation of therapy. Gradual increases in dosage and administration with food or milk will reduce gastric irritation.

Neurologic

Sedation, drowsiness, dizziness, fatigue, lethargy. These symptoms tend to disappear with continued therapy and possible dosage adjustment. Encourage the patient not to discontinue therapy without first consulting the healthcare provider. The patient should be warned not to work with machinery, operate a motor vehicle, administer medication, or perform other duties that require mental alertness. Provide for patient safety during episodes of dizziness; report these changes to the healthcare provider for further evaluation.

Confusion. Perform a baseline assessment of the patient's degree of alertness and orientation to name, place, and time before initiating therapy. Make regularly scheduled subsequent evaluations of the patient's mental status and compare findings. Report significant alterations in mental status to the healthcare provider.

Sensory

Blurred vision. Caution the patient that blurred vision may occur and make appropriate suggestions for the patient's personal safety.

Nystagmus. Nystagmus is a back-and-forth movement of the eyeballs on the horizontal plain, particularly when looking laterally (out of the corners of the eyes). Patients may develop nystagmus as higher dosage levels are required to control seizures or as the drug accumulates in the body. Nystagmus may be used as an indicator of possible overdose. Monitor the patient closely for other signs of toxicity such as sedation, lethargy, nausea and vomiting, and ataxia. If nystagmus and other signs of toxicity become more prominent, bring this to the attention of the healthcare provider. Serum levels may be ordered and the dosage reduced.

Dental hygiene

Gingival hyperplasia. The frequency of gum overgrowth may be reduced by using good oral hygiene, including gum massage, frequent brushing, and proper dental care.

◆ *Serious adverse effects*

Metabolic

Hyperglycemia. Hydantoins may elevate blood glucose levels, especially if higher dosages are used; patients with diabetes mellitus are more susceptible to hyperglycemia. Particularly during the early weeks of therapy, diabetic or prediabetic patients must be monitored for the development of hyperglycemia. Assess the patient regularly for glycosuria and report it to the healthcare provider if it occurs with any frequency. Patients who are receiving oral hypoglycemic agents or insulin may require a dosage adjustment.

Hematologic

Blood dyscrasias. Routine laboratory studies (i.e., RBC, WBC, and differential counts) should be scheduled. Monitor the patient for sore throat, fever, purpura, jaundice, or excessive and progressive weakness.

Gastrointestinal

Hepatotoxicity. The symptoms of hepatotoxicity include anorexia, nausea, vomiting, jaundice, hepatomegaly, splenomegaly, and abnormal liver function tests (e.g., elevated bilirubin, AST, ALT, GGT, and alkaline phosphatase levels; increased PT).

Integumentary

Dermatologic reactions. Report a rash or pruritus immediately and withhold additional doses pending approval by the healthcare provider.

◆ *Drug interactions*

Drugs that enhance therapeutic and toxic effects. Warfarin, carbamazepine, oxcarbazepine (>1200 mg/day), topiramate, metronidazole, azole antifungal agents (e.g., itraconazole, voriconazole, fluconazole), omeprazole, phenothiazines, disulfiram, amiodarone, isoniazid, chloramphenicol, cimetidine, and sulfonamides enhance the therapeutic and toxic effects of phenytoin. Monitor patients with concurrent therapy for signs of phenytoin toxicity, such as nystagmus, sedation, or lethargy. Serum levels may be ordered; a reduced dosage of phenytoin may be required.

Drugs that decrease therapeutic effects. Loxapine, phenobarbital, nitrofurantoin, theophylline, ethanol (chronic ingestion), rifampin, sucralfate, folic acid, and antacids decrease the therapeutic effects of phenytoin. Monitor patients with concurrent therapy for increased seizure activity. Monitoring changes in the patient's serum levels should help predict possible increased seizure activity.

Disopyramide, quinidine, mexiletine. Phenytoin decreases the serum levels of these agents. Monitor patients for the redevelopment of dysrhythmias.

Prednisolone, dexamethasone. Phenytoin decreases the serum levels of these agents. Monitor patients for reduced antiinflammatory activity.

Estrogen-containing contraceptives. Phenytoin enhances the metabolism of estrogens. Spotting or bleeding may be an indication of reduced estrogen levels and reduced contraceptive activity with estrogen-containing contraceptives. Using alternative forms of birth control is recommended.

Theophylline. Phenytoin decreases the serum levels of theophylline derivatives. Monitor patients for a higher frequency of respiratory difficulty. The theophylline dosage may need to be increased by 50% to 100% to maintain the same therapeutic response.

Valproic acid. This agent may increase or decrease the activity of phenytoin. Monitor the patient for an increased frequency of seizure activity. Monitoring changes in serum levels should help predict possible increased seizure activity. Monitor patients with concurrent therapy for signs of phenytoin toxicity, including nystagmus, sedation, and lethargy. Serum levels may be ordered, and a reduced dosage of phenytoin may be required.

Ketoconazole. The concurrent administration with ketoconazole may alter the metabolism of one or both drugs. Monitoring the levels of both drugs is recommended.

> **❗ Medication Safety Alert**
>
> Phenytoin is associated with many drug interactions. Those listed earlier are the most common drug interactions recognized, but it is only a representative list. Consult a resource such as *Drug Interaction Facts* for a more complete description.

DRUG CLASS: SUCCINIMIDES

Actions

The succinimides elevate the seizure threshold by depression of nerve transmission in the cortex by reducing the current in the T-type calcium channels found in primary afferent neurons.

Uses

Succinimides (e.g., ethosuximide, methsuximide) are used to control absence seizures.

Therapeutic Outcomes

The primary therapeutic outcomes expected from the succinimides are as follows:

1. Reduced frequency of seizures and reduced injury from seizure activity
2. Minimal adverse effects from therapy

❖ **Nursing Implications for Succinimides**

◆ *Premedication assessment*

1. Perform a baseline assessment of the patient's speech patterns, degree of alertness, and orientation to name, place, and time before initiating therapy.
2. Monitor the patient's behavioral responses to therapy.
3. Review the patient's medical record to document the frequency of seizure activity.

◆ *Availability, dosage, and administration.* See Table 18.1.

◆ *Common adverse effects*

Gastrointestinal

Nausea, vomiting, indigestion. These effects are common during the initiation of therapy. Gradual increases in dosage and administration with food or milk will reduce gastric irritation.

Neurologic

Sedation, drowsiness, dizziness, fatigue, lethargy. These symptoms tend to disappear with continued therapy and possible dosage adjustment. Encourage the patient not to discontinue therapy without first consulting the healthcare provider. The patient should be warned not to work with machinery, operate a motor vehicle, administer medication, or perform other duties that require mental alertness. Provide for patient safety during episodes of dizziness; report these changes to the healthcare provider for further evaluation.

◆ *Drug interactions*

Drugs that enhance toxic effects. Antihistamines, alcohol, analgesics, anesthetics, tranquilizers, other antiepileptic drugs, and sedative-hypnotics enhance the toxic effects of succinimides.

DRUG CLASS: MISCELLANEOUS ANTIEPILEPTIC MEDICINES

carbamazepine (kăr-bă-MĀZ-ă-pēn)
Tegretol (TĔG-rĕ-tŏl)
⇌ *Do not confuse Tegretol with Toradol or Trileptal.*

Actions
Carbamazepine blocks the reuptake of norepinephrine and decreases the release of norepinephrine and the rate of dopamine and GABA turnover. Despite knowledge of these pharmacologic effects, the mechanisms of action as an antiepileptic, selective analgesic, and antimanic agent are not fully known. Carbamazepine is structurally related to the tricyclic antidepressants.

Uses
Carbamazepine is an antiepileptic often used in combination with other antiepileptic agents to control generalized tonic-clonic and focal seizures. It is not effective for controlling myoclonic or absence seizures. Carbamazepine has also been used successfully to treat the pain associated with trigeminal neuralgia (tic douloureux). It may also be used to treat manic-depressive disorders when lithium therapy has not been optimal.

In March 2008, the US Food and Drug Administration issued an alert to healthcare professionals about dangerous and possibly fatal skin reactions that may occur with carbamazepine in certain patient populations. These skin reactions are significantly more common among patients with a particular human leukocyte antigen: the HLA-B*1502 allele. This allele occurs almost exclusively in persons of Asian ancestry, including South Asian Indians. Patients with this ancestry should be screened with available genetic tests for the allele before starting treatment with carbamazepine. If test results are positive, the drug should not be started unless the expected benefit clearly outweighs the risk of serious skin reactions. Patients who test positive for the allele may also be at increased risk from other antiepileptic drugs that have caused serious skin reactions. More than 90% of all serious skin reactions occur within the first few months of treatment. This means that patients who have been on the drug for longer periods without developing skin reactions have a low risk of reaction in the future, even if they have tested positive for the allele.

Therapeutic Outcomes
The primary therapeutic outcomes expected from carbamazepine are as follows:
1. Reduced frequency of seizures and reduced injury from seizure activity
2. Minimal adverse effects from therapy

❖ **Nursing Implications for Carbamazepine**
◆ *Premedication assessment*
1. As a result of serious adverse reactions, the manufacturer recommends that the following baseline studies be repeated at regular intervals: complete blood count, liver function tests, urinalysis, blood urea nitrogen (BUN), serum creatinine, and ophthalmologic examination.
2. Review the patient's history to exclude Asian ancestry, including South Asian Indian ancestry. If the patient does have this ancestry, bring it to the prescriber's attention so that genetic testing may be completed.
3. Perform a baseline assessment of the patient's speech patterns, degree of alertness, and orientation to name, place, and time before initiating therapy. Monitor the patient's behavioral responses to therapy.
4. Review the patient's medical record to document the frequency of seizure activity.

◆ *Availability.* **PO:** 200-mg tablets; 100-mg chewable tablets; 100-, 200-, and 400-mg tablets, extended release (12 hr); 100-, 200-, and 300-mg capsules, extended release (12 hr); 100 mg/5 mL oral suspension.

◆ *Dosage and administration.* **Adult:** *PO:* Initial dosage is 200 mg twice daily on the first day. Dosage may be increased by 200 mg/day at weekly intervals. Maximum dosage 1000 mg/day in adolescents 12 to 15 years or 1200 mg/day in those younger than 15 years. In rare instances, doses of 1600 mg/day or higher in adults may be necessary. Therapeutic plasma levels for carbamazepine range from 4 to 12 mg/L.

◆ *Common adverse effects.* These effects can be reduced by slowly increasing the dosage. They are usually mild and tend to resolve with continued therapy. Encourage the patient not to discontinue therapy without first consulting the healthcare provider.
Gastrointestinal. Gastrointestinal effects include nausea and vomiting.
Neurologic
Drowsiness, dizziness. Provide for patient safety during episodes of drowsiness or dizziness. Patients must be warned not to work around machinery, operate motor vehicles, or perform other duties that require constant mental alertness until it is known how they are affected by this medication.

◆ *Serious adverse effects*
Cardiovascular
Orthostatic hypotension, hypertension. Monitor the patient's blood pressure daily in the supine and standing positions. Anticipate the development of postural hypotension and take measures to prevent an occurrence. Teach the patient to rise slowly from a supine or sitting position, and encourage the patient to sit or lie down if feeling faint.

Dyspnea, edema. If carbamazepine is used by a patient with a history of heart failure, monitor daily weights, lung sounds, and accumulation of edema.

Neurologic
Slurred speech, sedation, confusion. Perform a baseline assessment of the patient's speech patterns, degree of alertness, and orientation to name, place, and time before initiating therapy. Make regularly scheduled subsequent evaluations of the patient's mental status and compare findings. Report any significant alterations to the healthcare provider.

Genitourinary
Nephrotoxicity. Monitor the patient's urinalysis and kidney function tests for abnormal results. Report increasing BUN and creatinine levels, decreasing urine output or specific gravity despite the amount of fluid intake, casts or protein in the urine, frank blood or smoky-colored urine, or RBCs in excess of 0 to 3 on the urinalysis report.

Gastrointestinal
Hepatotoxicity. The symptoms of hepatotoxicity include anorexia, nausea, vomiting, jaundice, hepatomegaly, splenomegaly, and abnormal liver function tests (i.e., elevated bilirubin, AST, ALT, GGT, and alkaline phosphatase levels; increased PT).

Hematologic
Blood dyscrasias. Routine laboratory studies (i.e., RBC, WBC, and differential counts) should be scheduled. Monitor the patient for sore throat, fever, purpura, jaundice, or excessive and progressive weakness.

Integumentary
Dermatologic reactions. Report a rash or pruritus immediately and withhold additional doses pending approval by the healthcare provider.

◆ *Drug interactions*

Drugs that enhance therapeutic and toxic effects. Isoniazid, cimetidine, fluoxetine, fluvoxamine, ketoconazole, and macrolide antibiotics (e.g., erythromycin, clarithromycin) inhibit the metabolism of carbamazepine. Monitor the patient for signs of toxicity, such as disorientation, ataxia, lethargy, headache, drowsiness, nausea, and vomiting. Dosage reductions in carbamazepine may be necessary.

Verapamil, diltiazem, danazol, lamotrigine. These drugs increase serum levels of carbamazepine. Monitor the patient for signs of toxicity (e.g., disorientation, ataxia, lethargy, headache, drowsiness, nausea, vomiting). A 40% to 50% decrease in the carbamazepine dosage may be necessary.

Warfarin. Carbamazepine may diminish the anticoagulant effects of warfarin. Monitor the PT and increase the dosage of warfarin, if necessary.

Phenobarbital, phenytoin, valproic acid. Carbamazepine enhances the metabolism of these agents. Monitor the patient for an increased frequency of seizure activity. Monitoring changes in serum levels should help predict possible increased seizure activity.

Doxycycline. Carbamazepine enhances the metabolism of this antibiotic. Monitor the patient for signs of continued infection.

Estrogen-containing contraceptives. Carbamazepine enhances the metabolism of estrogens. Spotting or bleeding may be an indication of reduced estrogen levels and reduced contraceptive activity. The use of other forms of birth control is recommended.

---

gabapentin (găb-ă-PĔN-tĭn)
Neurontin (nyŭr-ŎN-tĭn)
⇄ *Do not confuse Neurontin with Neoral.*

Actions
The mechanism of action of gabapentin is unknown. It does not appear to enhance GABA.

Uses
Gabapentin is an antiepileptic usually used in combination with other antiepileptic drugs to control focal seizures. Gabapentin is also approved for use in patients with diabetic neuropathy, fibromyalgia, and postherpetic neuralgia.

Therapeutic Outcomes
The primary therapeutic outcomes expected from gabapentin are as follows:
1. Reduced frequency of seizures and reduced injury from seizure activity
2. Symptomatic relief from diabetic neuropathy, fibromyalgia, and postherpetic neuralgia
3. Minimal adverse effects from therapy

❖ **Nursing Implications for Gabapentin**
◆ *Premedication assessment*
1. Perform a baseline assessment of the patient's speech patterns, degree of alertness, and orientation to name, place, and time before initiating therapy. Monitor the patient's behavioral responses to therapy.
2. Review the patient's medical record to document the frequency of seizure activity.
3. When gabapentin is used as an analgesic, perform a pain assessment before administering it and at appropriate intervals during therapy. Report poor pain control, and obtain a modification in the patient's orders.

◆ *Availability.* *PO:* 100-, 300-, and 400-mg capsules; 300-, 600-, and 800-mg tablets; 25 mg/mL, 250 mg/5 mL, and 300 mg/6 mL oral solution.

◆ *Dosage and administration.* **Adult:** *PO:* 900 to 1800 mg daily. Initially administer 300 mg at bedtime on day 1, 300 mg two times on day 2, and then 300 mg three times on day 3. May increase using 300-, 400-, 600-, or 800-mg dosage forms given three times per day. Effective dose is 900 to 1800 mg/day, but up to 2400 mg/

day has been used long term. Dosages of 3600 mg/day have been given to limited patients for a relatively short duration. The maximum time between doses for the three-times-daily schedule should not exceed 12 hours. Therapeutic blood levels for gabapentin are 12 to 20 mg/L. If the patient also uses antacids, administer gabapentin at least 2 hours after the last dose of antacid, because antacids reduce the absorption of gabapentin.

◆ *Common adverse effects*
Neurologic
Sedation, drowsiness, dizziness. These symptoms tend to disappear with continued therapy and possible dosage adjustment. Encourage the patient not to discontinue therapy without first consulting the healthcare provider. Provide for patient safety during episodes of drowsiness or dizziness. Patients must be warned not to work around machinery, operate motor vehicles, or perform other duties that require constant mental alertness until it is known how they are affected by this medication.
Sensory
Blurred vision. Caution the patient that blurred vision may occur and make appropriate suggestions for the patient's personal safety.

◆ *Serious adverse effects*
Neurologic
Slurred speech, lethargy, confusion. Perform a baseline assessment of the patient's speech patterns, degree of alertness, and orientation to name, place, and time before initiating therapy. Make regularly scheduled subsequent evaluations of the patient's mental status and compare findings. Report any significant alterations.

◆ *Drug interactions*
Enhanced sedation. Central nervous system depressants—including sleep aids, analgesics, tranquilizers, and alcohol—enhance the sedative effects of gabapentin. Patients must be warned not to work around machinery, operate motor vehicles, or perform other duties that require constant mental alertness until it is known how they are affected by this medication. Provide for patient safety during episodes of drowsiness or dizziness.

Urine protein. False-positive readings for protein in the urine have been reported by patients who are taking gabapentin who use the Multistix 10-SG Reagent dipstick test (Siemens Healthcare, Erlangen, Germany). The manufacturer recommends that the more specific sulfosalicylic acid precipitation procedure be used to determine the presence of urine protein.

---

lamotrigine (lă-MŎ-trĭ-gēn)
 ⇌ *Do not confuse lamotrigine with lamivudine.*
Lamictal (lă-MĬK-tăl)
 ⇌ *Do not confuse Lamictal with labetalol, Lamisil, or Lomotil.*

Actions
Lamotrigine is a newer antiepileptic of the phenyltriazine class that is unrelated to other antiepileptic medications currently available. It is thought to act by blocking voltage-sensitive sodium and calcium channels in the neuronal membranes. This stabilizes the neuronal membranes and inhibits the release of excitatory neurotransmitters (e.g., glutamate), which may induce seizure activity.

Uses
Lamotrigine is used in combination with other antiepileptic therapy to treat focal seizures and the generalized seizures of Lennox-Gastaut syndrome in pediatric and adult patients. Lamotrigine is also approved for use in combination with other standard therapies to treat bipolar disorder to delay the time to the onset of mood episodes (i.e., depression, mania, mixed episodes).

Therapeutic Outcomes
The primary therapeutic outcomes expected from lamotrigine are as follows:
1. Reduced frequency of seizures and reduced injury from seizure activity
2. Treatment of bipolar disorder
3. Minimal adverse effects from therapy

❖ **Nursing Implications for Lamotrigine**
◆ *Premedication assessment*
1. Perform a baseline assessment of the patient's speech patterns, degree of alertness, and orientation to name, place, and time before initiating therapy. Monitor the patient's behavioral responses to therapy.
2. Review the patient's medication history to determine whether the patient is already taking valproic acid for seizure control.
3. Review the patient's medical record to document the frequency of seizure activity.

◆ *Availability.* **PO:** tablets: 25, 100, 150, 200, and 250 mg; chewable tablets: 5 and 25 mg; orally disintegrating tablets: 25, 50, 100, and 200 mg; tablets, 24-hr extended release: 25, 50, 100, 200, 250, and 300 mg.

◆ *Dosage and administration*
Seizure disorder. Adult: *PO:* If the patient is already taking valproic acid for seizure control, initiate lamotrigine therapy at 25 mg every other day for 2 weeks, followed by 25 mg daily for 3 to 4 weeks; then the dose may be increased by 25 to 50 mg PO daily every 1 to 2 weeks until the maintenance dosage is achieved. The usual maintenance dose is 100 to 400 mg/day PO, given in one to two divided doses. The usual maintenance dose for patients who add lamotrigine to valproic acid alone ranges from 100 to 200 mg/day.

If the patient is not already taking metabolism-inducing medications (e.g., valproic acid, carbamazepine, phenytoin, phenobarbital, rifampin) for seizure control, initiate lamotrigine therapy at 25 mg PO every day for 2 weeks, then 50 mg/day PO for weeks 3 to 4; then the dose may be increased by 50 mg/day PO every 1 to 2 weeks until the maintenance dosage is achieved. The usual maintenance dose is 225 to 375 mg/day PO, given in two divided doses. If the patient is already receiving metabolism-inducing medications for seizure control, the dosage of lamotrigine should be approximately two times these dosages up to 400 mg daily in divided doses; see the manufacturer's recommendations. Therapeutic blood levels for lamotrigine are 3 to 14 mg/L.

Bipolar disorder. Adult: *PO:* Initial dosage depends on other medications that are being taken. Target dosage is 200 mg/daily of immediate-release medication.

◆ **Common adverse effects**

Gastrointestinal

Nausea, vomiting, indigestion. These effects are common during the initiation of therapy. Gradual increases in dosage and administration with food or milk will reduce gastric irritation.

Neurologic

Sedation, drowsiness, dizziness. These symptoms tend to disappear with continued therapy and possible dosage adjustment. Encourage the patient not to discontinue therapy without first consulting the healthcare provider. Provide for patient safety during episodes of drowsiness or dizziness. Patients must be warned not to work around machinery, operate motor vehicles, or perform other duties that require constant mental alertness until it is known how they are affected by this medication.

Sensory

Blurred vision. Caution the patient that blurred vision may occur, and make appropriate suggestions for the patient's personal safety.

◆ **Serious adverse effects**

Integumentary

Dermatologic reactions. Approximately 10% of patients who receive lamotrigine develop a skin rash and urticaria during the first 4 to 6 weeks of therapy. Slower increases in each dosage adjustment are thought to decrease the incidence of rash. In most cases, the rash resolves with continued therapy; however, the healthcare provider should be promptly informed because the rash could also be an early indicator of a more serious condition. Combination therapy with valproic acid appears to be more likely to precipitate a serious rash.

Encourage the patient not to discontinue the lamotrigine until alternative antiepileptic therapy can be considered to prevent renewed seizure activity.

Neurologic

Aseptic meningitis. Lamotrigine may cause aseptic meningitis. Patients should be advised to contact their healthcare provider immediately if they experience signs and symptoms of meningitis, such as headache, fever, stiff neck, nausea, vomiting, rash, and sensitivity to light. Patients should be evaluated for other causes of meningitis; if no other causes are found, the discontinuation of lamotrigine should be considered.

◆ **Drug interactions**

Drugs that enhance therapeutic and toxic effects. Valproic acid reduces the metabolism of lamotrigine by as much as 50%. Significant lamotrigine dosage reduction may be required.

Drugs that decrease therapeutic effects. Phenobarbital, phenytoin, primidone, carbamazepine, oxcarbazepine, ethosuximide, rifampin, acetaminophen, and progestin oral contraceptives enhance the metabolism of lamotrigine. Monitor the patient for the increased frequency of seizure activity. Monitoring changes in serum levels should help predict possible increased seizure activity. The twice-daily administration of lamotrigine may be necessary.

Enhanced sedation. Central nervous system depressants—including sleep aids, analgesics, tranquilizers, and alcohol—enhance the sedative effects of lamotrigine. Patients must be warned not to work around machinery, operate motor vehicles, or perform other duties that require constant mental alertness until it is known how they are affected by this medication. Provide for patient safety during episodes of drowsiness or dizziness.

---

levetiracetam (lĕ-vĕ-tĭr-ă-SĒ-tĕm)
Keppra (KĔP-ră)
⇄ *Do not confuse Keppra with Kaletra.*

Actions

Levetiracetam is classified as a pyrrolidine derivative chemically unrelated to other antiepileptic drugs available. Its mechanism of action is unknown. Unlike other antiepileptic agents, it does not appear to act on sodium, potassium, or calcium ion pathways or stimulate GABA.

Uses

Levetiracetam is approved for use in combination with other antiepileptic therapy to treat focal seizures, myoclonic seizures, and primary generalized tonic-clonic seizures in adults.

Therapeutic Outcomes

The primary therapeutic outcomes sought from levetiracetam are as follows:

1. Reduced frequency of seizures and reduced injury from seizure activity
2. Minimal adverse effects from therapy

❖ **Nursing Implications for Levetiracetam**

◆ **Premedication assessment**

1. Review the patient's medical record to document the frequency of seizure activity.
2. Perform a baseline assessment of the patient's speech patterns, degree of alertness, and orientation to name, place, and time before initiating therapy.

3. Review the patient's laboratory reports and report any abnormal renal function (e.g., BUN, creatinine, creatinine clearance).

◆ *Availability.* *PO:* 250-, 500-, 750-, and 1000-mg tablets; 250-, 500-, 750-, 1000-mg disintegrating tablets; 500- and 750-mg tablets, extended release (24 hr); 100 mg/mL oral solution.

   Injection: 100 mg/mL in 5-mL vials; 500 mg/mL; 1000 mg/100 mL; 1500 mg/100 mL.

◆ *Dosage and administration.* **Adult:** *PO:* Initial dose is 500 mg twice daily. Dosage may be increased every 2 weeks by 500 mg twice daily until a maximum dose of 3000 mg/day is attained.

   NOTE: Dosage adjustment is necessary in patients whose estimated creatinine clearance is less than 80 mL/min. See the package insert for additional instructions. The therapeutic blood levels for levetiracetam are 10 to 40 mg/L.

◆ *Common adverse effects*
   Neurologic
   Weakness, drowsiness, dizziness. These effects can be reduced by slowly increasing the dosage. They are usually mild, and they tend to resolve with continued therapy. Encourage the patient not to discontinue therapy without first consulting the healthcare provider. Provide for patient safety during episodes of weakness and dizziness. Patients must be warned not to work around machinery, operate motor vehicles, or perform other duties that require constant mental alertness until it is known how they are affected by this medication.

◆ *Serious adverse effects*
   Neurologic
   Confusion, disorientation. Make regularly scheduled assessments of the patient's speech patterns, degree of alertness, and orientation to name, place, and time and compare findings. Report any significant alterations to the healthcare provider.

◆ *Drug interactions*
   Enhanced sedation. Central nervous system depressants—including sleep aids, analgesics, tranquilizers, and alcohol—enhance the sedative effects of levetiracetam. Patients must be warned not to work around machinery, operate motor vehicles, or perform other duties that require constant mental alertness until it is known how they are affected by this medication.

---

oxcarbazepine (ŏks-kăr-BĂZ-ĕ-pēn)
   ⇄ *Do not confuse oxcarbazepine with olanzapine.*
Trileptal (trī-LĔP-tŏl)
   ⇄ *Do not confuse Trileptal with Tegretol.*

Actions
Oxcarbazepine is a prodrug that metabolizes into some of the active metabolites of carbamazepine. Oxcarbazepine interacts with sodium, potassium, and calcium ion channels, thereby stabilizing the neurons and preventing the repetitive firing and propagation of the electrical impulses that are thought to induce seizures.

Uses
Oxcarbazepine is used as monotherapy or combination therapy for the treatment of focal seizures in adults and as combination therapy for the treatment of focal seizures in children who are 4 to 16 years old.

Therapeutic Outcomes
The primary therapeutic outcomes expected from oxcarbazepine are as follows:
1. Reduced frequency of seizures and reduced injury from seizure activity
2. Minimal adverse effects from therapy

❖ **Nursing Implications for Oxcarbazepine**
◆ *Premedication assessment*
1. Because of this drug's potential to cause serious adverse reactions, the manufacturer recommends that serum electrolyte baseline levels be determined and then repeated periodically while the patient is receiving oxcarbazepine therapy.
2. Review the patient's medication history to ensure that the patient does not have an allergy to carbamazepine. If there is an allergy, inform the charge nurse and the healthcare provider immediately. Do not administer the medication without specific approval.
3. Perform a baseline assessment of the patient's speech patterns, degree of alertness, and orientation to name, place, and time before initiating therapy. Monitor the patient's behavioral responses to therapy.
4. Review the patient's medical record to document the frequency of seizure activity.

◆ *Availability.* *PO:* 150-, 300-, and 600-mg tablets; 150-, 300-, 600-mg tablets, extended release (24 hr); 300 mg/5 mL suspension.

◆ *Dosage and administration.* **Adult:** *PO:* Initial dosage is 300 mg twice daily for the first 3 days. The dosage may be increased by 300 mg/day every 3 days to 1200 mg/day. Dosages of 2400 mg/day have been found to be effective for patients converted from other anticonvulsant therapy to monotherapy with oxcarbazepine.

   Pediatric (4 to 16 years old): *PO:* Initial dosage is 4 to 5 mg/kg twice daily, not to exceed 600 mg/day. The dosage should be gradually increased over the next 2 weeks to a target maintenance level based on the patient's body weight:

20-24.9 kg	600-900 mg/day in two divided doses
25-34.9 kg	900-1200 mg/day in two divided doses
35-44.9 kg	900-1500 mg/day in two divided doses
45-49.9 kg	1200-1500 mg/day in two divided doses
50-59.9 kg	1200-1800 mg/day in two divided doses
60-69.9 kg	1200-2100 mg/day in two divided doses
>70 kg	1500-2100 mg/day in two divided doses

The therapeutic blood levels for oxcarbazepine are 3 to 40 mg/L.

◆ *Common adverse effects*
Neurologic
Confusion, poor coordination, drowsiness, dizziness. These effects can be reduced by slowly increasing the dosage; they are usually mild and tend to resolve with continued therapy. Encourage the patient not to discontinue therapy without first consulting the healthcare provider. Perform a baseline assessment of the patient's speech patterns, degree of alertness, and orientation to name, place, and time before initiating therapy. Make regularly scheduled subsequent evaluations of the patient's mental status, and compare findings; report any significant alterations. Provide for patient safety during episodes of drowsiness, confusion, or dizziness. Patients must be warned not to work around machinery, operate motor vehicles, or perform other duties that require constant mental alertness until it is known how they are affected by this medication.

◆ *Serious adverse effects*
Hematologic
Blood dyscrasias. Routine laboratory studies (i.e., RBC, WBC, and differential counts) should be scheduled. Monitor the patient for sore throat, fever, purpura, jaundice, or excessive and progressive weakness.

Nausea, headache, lethargy, confusion, obtundation, malaise. These are symptoms of hyponatremia. It is extremely important to notify the healthcare provider if the patient is exhibiting any of these conditions. Withhold additional doses of the drug until specific orders to administer the medication have been received.

◆ *Drug interactions*
Drugs that decrease therapeutic effects. Phenobarbital, primidone, phenytoin, valproic acid, carbamazepine, and verapamil may enhance the metabolism of oxcarbazepine. Monitor the patient for an increased frequency of seizure activity. Dosages of oxcarbazepine may need to be increased.

Estrogen- and progestin-containing contraceptives. Oxcarbazepine enhances the metabolism of estrogens and progestins. Spotting or bleeding may be an indication of reduced contraceptive activity. Recommend that the patient use other forms of birth control while taking oxcarbazepine.

---

phenobarbital (fē-nō-BĂR-bĭ-tŏl)

Actions
Phenobarbital, a long-acting barbiturate, elevates the seizure threshold and prevents the spread of electrical seizure activity by enhancing the inhibitory effect of GABA. The exact mechanism is unknown.

Uses
Phenobarbital is an effective antiepileptic agent. Because of its sedative effects, however, it is now used primarily as an alternative when single nonsedating antiepileptic drugs are unsuccessful for the control of seizures. Phenobarbital is most useful for treating focal and generalized tonic-clonic seizures and generalized myoclonic seizures, usually in combination with other antiepileptic drugs. The therapeutic blood levels for phenobarbital are 15 to 45 mg/L.

Therapeutic Outcomes
The primary therapeutic outcomes expected from phenobarbital are as follows:
1. Reduced frequency of seizures and reduced injury due to seizure activity
2. Minimal adverse effects from therapy

❖ **Nursing Implications for Phenobarbital**
◆ *Premedication assessment*
1. Perform a baseline assessment of the patient's speech patterns, degree of alertness, and orientation to name, place, and time before initiating therapy. Monitor the patient's behavioral responses to therapy.
2. Obtain the patient's vital signs (e.g., blood pressure, pulse, respirations).

◆ *Availability.* **PO:** tablets: 15, 16.2, 30, 32.4, 60, 64.8, 97.2, and 100 mg; elixir and solution: 20 mg/5 mL.
IV: 65 and 130 mg/mL.

◆ *Dosage and administration*
Seizure control. Adult: *PO:* 60 to 200 mg/day or 50 to 100 mg 2 to 3 times daily.
Status epilepticus. *IV:* 15 mg/kg as a single dose.
NOTE: Rapidly discontinuing phenobarbital after the long-term use of high dosages may result in symptoms that are similar to those of alcohol withdrawal. These may vary from weakness and anxiety to delirium and generalized seizures. Discontinuation of phenobarbital consists of cautious and gradual withdrawal over 2 to 4 weeks.

◆ *Common adverse effects.* General adverse effects of phenobarbital include drowsiness, lethargy, headache, muscle or joint pain, and mental depression.
Neurologic
Hangover, sedation, lethargy, diminished alertness. Patients may complain of "morning hangover," blurred vision, and transient hypotension on arising. Explain to the patient the need to first rise to a sitting position, stay sitting for several moments until any dizziness or lightheadedness passes, and then stand slowly. Assistance with ambulation may be required. If the hangover effect becomes troublesome, there should be a reduction in the dosage, a change in the medication, or both.

People who work around machinery, drive, administer medications, or perform other duties for which they must remain mentally alert should not take this medication while working.

◆ Serious adverse effects

Psychological

Excessive use or abuse. The habitual use of phenobarbital may result in physical dependence. Discuss the issue with the healthcare provider and make plans to cooperatively approach the gradual withdrawal of the medications being abused if seizure control is maintained.

Paradoxical response. Older patients may respond paradoxically to phenobarbital by demonstrating excitement, euphoria, restlessness, and confusion. Provide supportive physical care and safety during these responses.

Integumentary

Hypersensitivity. Reactions to phenobarbital are infrequent but may be serious. Report symptoms of hives, pruritus, rash, high fever, or the inflammation of the mucous membranes for evaluation by a healthcare provider.

Hematologic

Blood dyscrasias. Blood dyscrasias are rare; however, laboratory studies (e.g., RBC, WBC, differential, and platelet counts) should be scheduled when symptoms warrant. Stress the importance of the patient returning for this laboratory work. Monitor the patient for the development of sore throat, fever, purpura, jaundice, or excessive and progressive weakness.

◆ Drug interactions

Drugs that increase toxic effects. Antihistamines, alcohol, analgesics, anesthetics, tranquilizers, valproic acid, monoamine oxidase inhibitors, and other sedative-hypnotics increase the toxic effects of phenobarbital. Monitor the patient for excessive sedation, and reduce the dosage of phenobarbital or another medicine if necessary.

Phenytoin. The effects of phenobarbital on phenytoin are variable. Serum levels may be ordered, and a change in phenytoin dosage may be required. Observe patients for increased seizure activity and for signs of phenytoin toxicity (e.g., nystagmus, sedation, lethargy).

Reduced therapeutic effects. Phenobarbital reduces the effects of the following medicines:

- *Warfarin:* Monitor the patient's international normalized ratio and increase the dosage of warfarin, if necessary.
- *Estrogens:* This drug interaction may be critical in patients who are receiving contraceptives that contain estrogen. If patients develop spotting and breakthrough bleeding, a change in contraceptives and the use of alternative forms of contraception should be considered.
- *Corticosteroids, beta-adrenergic blockers, metronidazole, doxycycline, antidepressants, quinidine, and chlorpromazine:* The patient should be monitored for signs of increased activity of the illness for which the medication was prescribed. Dosage increases

may be necessary, or phenobarbital may have to be discontinued.

---

pregabalin (prĕ-GĂB-ă-lĭn)
Lyrica (LĬR-ĭ-kă)

Actions

The mechanism of action of pregabalin is unknown. It is chemically related to gabapentin. It does not appear to enhance GABA.

Uses

Pregabalin is an antiepileptic used in combination with other antiepileptic agents to control focal seizures. Pregabalin is also approved for the treatment of pain associated with fibromyalgia, diabetic neuropathy, and postherpetic neuralgia (a complication of acute herpes zoster activation, which is often described as unbearable itching, electric shock–like pain, or burning).

Pregabalin has the potential for abuse and dependence, and it has been designated as a Schedule V controlled substance. Symptoms suggestive of physical dependence (insomnia, nausea, headache, diarrhea) have been observed in some patients in clinical studies after the drug's abrupt discontinuation.

Therapeutic Outcomes

The primary therapeutic outcomes expected from pregabalin are as follows:

1. Reduced frequency of seizures and reduced injury from seizure activity
2. Symptomatic relief from pain associated with fibromyalgia, diabetic neuropathy, and postherpetic neuralgia
3. Minimal adverse effects from therapy

❖ Nursing Implications for Pregabalin

◆ Premedication assessment

1. Perform a baseline assessment of the patient's speech patterns, degree of alertness, and orientation to name, place, and time before initiating therapy. Monitor the patient's behavioral responses to therapy.
2. Obtain a baseline measurement of the patient's creatinine clearance for potential dosage adjustment.
3. Review the patient's medical record to document the frequency of seizure activity.
4. Review the patient's medical record for indications of a history of substance abuse.
5. When pregabalin is used as an analgesic, perform a pain assessment with the patient before administering it and at appropriate intervals during therapy. Report poor pain control and obtain a modification in the patient's orders.

◆ *Availability.* **PO:** capsules: 25, 50, 75, 100, 150, 200, 225, and 300 mg; tablets, 24-hr extended release: 82.5, 165, 330 mg; oral solution: 20 mg/mL.

◆ *Dosage and administration.* Dosages should be adjusted for patients with a creatinine clearance below 60 mL/min.

Seizure control. Adult: *PO:* 150 to 600 mg daily. Initially administer 50 mg three times daily or 75 mg twice daily. The daily dosage can be increased to a maximum of 600 mg daily in divided doses, depending on the patient's response and the development of any adverse effects.

Fibromyalgia. Adult: *PO:* 300 to 450 mg daily. Initially administer 75 mg twice daily and increase to 150 mg twice daily within 1 week. If there is a therapeutic benefit and the adverse effects are acceptable, the dosage may be increased to 225 mg twice daily for a total of 450 mg daily. The therapeutic blood levels for pregabalin have not been established.

Neuropathic pain associated with diabetic peripheral neuropathy. Adult: *PO:* Up to 300 mg daily. Initially administer 50 mg three times daily and increase to 100 mg three times daily within 1 week on the basis of the patient's tolerance.

Postherpetic neuralgia. Adult: *PO:* 150 to 600 mg daily. Initially administer 50 mg three times daily or 75 mg twice daily. For patients who do not experience sufficient pain relief after 2 to 4 weeks of treatment with 300 mg daily and who can tolerate adverse effects, the daily dosage can be increased to a maximum of 600 mg daily (i.e., 200 mg three times daily or 300 mg twice daily).

> **[!] Medication Safety Alert**
>
> Patients should be monitored for signs of pregabalin abuse, including dosage escalation, tolerance, and drug-seeking behavior. When discontinuing therapy, taper over at least 1 week to minimize the potential for withdrawal symptoms.

◆ **Common adverse effects**
Neurologic
Sedation, drowsiness, dizziness. These symptoms tend to disappear with continued therapy and possible dosage adjustment. Encourage the patient not to discontinue therapy without first consulting the healthcare provider. Provide for patient safety during episodes of drowsiness or dizziness. Patients must be warned not to work around machinery, operate motor vehicles, or perform other duties that require constant mental alertness until it is known how they are affected by this medication.
Sensory
Blurred vision. Caution the patient that blurred vision may occur, and make appropriate suggestions for the patient's personal safety.

◆ **Serious adverse effects**
Neurologic
Confusion, disorientation. Make regularly scheduled assessments of the patient's speech patterns, degree of alertness, and orientation to name, place, and time and compare findings. Report any significant alterations to the healthcare provider.
Psychological
Excessive use or abuse. Evaluate the patient's response to pregabalin as an analgesic. Identify his or her underlying needs and plan for the more appropriate management of those needs. Discuss the patient's case with the healthcare provider and make plans to cooperatively approach the gradual withdrawal of the medications that are being abused. Suggest a change to a milder analgesic when indicated.

Patients do not have to undergo the symptoms of withdrawal to be treated for addiction. They may be treated with the gradual reduction of daily opiate agonist doses. If withdrawal symptoms become severe, the patient may receive methadone. The temporary administration of tranquilizers and sedatives may help reduce both patient anxiety and the craving for the opiate agonist.

◆ **Drug interactions**
Enhanced sedation. Central nervous system depressants—including sleep aids, analgesics, tranquilizers, benzodiazepines, oxycodone, and alcohol—enhance the sedative effects of pregabalin. Patients must be warned not to work around machinery, operate motor vehicles, or perform other duties that require constant mental alertness until it is known how they are affected by this medication. Provide for patient safety during episodes of drowsiness or dizziness.

> **primidone** (PRĬ-mĭ-dōn)
> ***Do not confuse primidone with prednisone.***
> **Mysoline** (MĪ-sō-lēn)

Actions
Primidone is structurally related to the barbiturates. It is metabolized into phenobarbital and phenylethylmalonamide, both of which are active antiepileptic agents. The exact mechanism of its antiepileptic action is unknown.

Uses
Primidone is used in combination with other antiepileptic therapy to treat both focal seizures and generalized tonic-clonic seizures.

Therapeutic Outcomes
The primary therapeutic outcomes expected from primidone are as follows:
1. Reduced frequency of seizures and reduced injury from seizure activity
2. Minimal adverse effects from therapy

❖ **Nursing Implications for Primidone**
◆ *Premedication assessment*
1. Review the patient's routine blood studies to detect blood dyscrasias.

2. Perform a baseline assessment of the patient's speech patterns, degree of alertness, and orientation to name, place, and time before initiating therapy. Monitor the patient's behavioral responses to therapy. In children, assess the degree of excitability present.

3. Review the patient's medical record to document the frequency of seizure activity.

◆ *Availability. PO:* 50- and 250-mg tablets.

◆ *Dosage and administration.* **Adult:** *PO:* Initially 100 to 125 mg daily at bedtime for 3 days. On days 4 through 6, increase the dosage to 100 to 125 mg twice daily. On days 7 through 9, increase to 100 to 125 mg three times daily. Increase by 100 to 125 mg/day every 3 or 4 days until therapeutic response or intolerance develops. The typical dosage is 750 to 1500 mg/day. Do not exceed 2000 mg/day.

◆ *Common adverse effects.* These symptoms tend to disappear with continued therapy and possible dosage adjustment. Encourage the patient not to discontinue therapy without first consulting the healthcare provider.

Neurologic

Sedation, drowsiness, dizziness. People who work around machinery, operate motor vehicles, or perform other duties that require constant mental alertness should be particularly cautious until they know how this medication will affect them. Provide for patient safety during episodes of dizziness and report these patients to the healthcare provider for further evaluation.

Sensory

Blurred vision. Caution the patient that blurred vision may occur, and make appropriate suggestions for the patient's safety.

◆ *Serious adverse effects*

Hematologic

Blood dyscrasias. Blood dyscrasias have rarely been reported with the use of primidone. Routine laboratory studies (e.g., RBC, WBC, and differential counts) should be scheduled. Monitor the patient for sore throat, fever, purpura, jaundice, or excessive and progressive weakness.

Neurologic

Paradoxical excitability. Primidone may cause paradoxical excitability in children. During a period of excitement, protect patients from harm and provide for the physical channeling of energy (e.g., walk with them). Notify the healthcare provider of the need for a possible change in medication.

◆ *Drug interactions.* The drug interactions are the same as those associated with phenobarbital, because primidone is metabolized to phenobarbital.

Estrogen-containing   contraceptives. Phenobarbital enhances the metabolism of estrogens. Spotting or bleeding may be an indication of reduced estrogen levels and an indication of reduced contraceptive activity. Recommend that the patient use alternative forms of birth control while taking this medication.

Phenytoin. Phenytoin may increase phenobarbital serum levels when it is taken concurrently with primidone. Monitor patients for increased sedation.

---

tiagabine (tē-ĂG-ă-bēn)
⇌ *Do not confuse tiagabine with tizanidine.*
Gabitril (GĂB-ĭ-trĭl)
⇌ *Do not confuse Gabitril with gabapentin.*

Actions

The mechanism of action of tiagabine is unknown. It appears to prevent the reuptake of GABA into presynaptic neurons, thus permitting more GABA to be available to act as an inhibitory neurotransmitter.

Uses

Tiagabine is an antiepileptic usually used in combination with other antiepileptic agents to control focal seizures.

Therapeutic Outcomes

The primary therapeutic outcomes expected from tiagabine are as follows:

1. Reduced frequency of seizures and reduced injury from seizure activity
2. Minimal adverse effects from therapy

❖ **Nursing Implications for Tiagabine**

◆ *Premedication assessment*

1. Perform a baseline assessment of the patient's speech patterns, degree of alertness, and orientation to name, place, and time before initiating therapy. Monitor the patient's behavioral responses to therapy.
2. Review the patient's medical record to document the frequency of seizure activity.

◆ *Availability. PO:* 2-, 4-, 12-, and 16-mg tablets.

◆ *Dosage and administration.* **Adult:** *PO:* Initially 4 mg once daily. Increase daily dosage by 4 to 8 mg at weekly intervals until a clinical response is achieved or until a total daily dosage of 56 mg has been reached. A total daily dosage of 32 to 56 mg may be taken in two to four divided doses. The therapeutic blood levels for this drug have not been established.

◆ *Common adverse effects*

Neurologic

Sedation, drowsiness, dizziness. These symptoms tend to disappear with continued therapy and possible dosage adjustment. Encourage the patient not to discontinue therapy without first consulting the healthcare provider. People who work around machinery, operate motor vehicles, or perform other duties that require constant mental alertness should be particularly cautious until they know how this medication will affect them. Provide for patient safety during episodes of dizziness and report these patients to the healthcare provider for further evaluation.

◆ *Serious adverse effects*
Neurologic
Confusion, disorientation. Make regularly scheduled assessments of the patient's speech patterns, degree of alertness, and orientation to name, place, and time and compare findings. Report any significant alterations to the healthcare provider.

◆ *Drug interactions*
Drugs that decrease therapeutic effects. Phenobarbital, primidone, phenytoin, and carbamazepine may enhance the metabolism of tiagabine and thus decrease its therapeutic effect. Monitor the patient for the increased frequency of seizure activity. Monitoring changes in serum levels should help predict the potential for increased seizure activity.

Enhanced sedation. Central nervous system depressants—including sleep aids, analgesics, tranquilizers, and alcohol—may enhance the sedative effects of tiagabine. Patients must be warned not to work around machinery, operate motor vehicles, or perform other duties that require constant mental alertness until they know how they will be affected by this medication. Provide for patient safety during episodes of drowsiness or dizziness.

---

topiramate (tō-PĬR-ă-māt)
⇌ **Do not confuse topiramate with torsemide.**
Topamax (TŌ-pă-măks)

Actions
The mechanism of action of topiramate as an antiepileptic agent is unknown. Three potential mechanisms may support antiepileptic activity: (1) the prolonged blockade of sodium channels in the neuronal membrane, (2) the potentiation of the activity of the inhibitory neurotransmitter GABA, and (3) the antagonism of certain receptors of the excitatory neurotransmitter.

Uses
Topiramate is an antiepileptic used in combination with other antiepileptic agents to control focal and generalized tonic-clonic seizures. It is also used for patients 2 years old and older who have seizures associated with Lennox-Gastaut syndrome.

Topiramate has also been approved for adults for the prevention (but not treatment) of migraine headaches.

Therapeutic Outcomes
The primary therapeutic outcomes expected from topiramate are as follows:
1. Reduced frequency of seizures and reduced injury from seizure activity

2. Prevention of migraines
3. Minimal adverse effects from therapy

❖ **Nursing Implications for Topiramate**
◆ *Premedication assessment*
1. Perform a baseline assessment of the patient's speech patterns and degree of alertness, as well as orientation to name, place, and time before initiating therapy. Monitor the patient's behavioral responses to therapy.
2. Obtain the patient's baseline weight for future reference. Weight loss may be an adverse effect of topiramate therapy.
3. Assess the patient's baseline state of hydration. Rare cases of oligohidrosis (decreased sweating) and hyperthermia have been reported, particularly in children and in those patients who are taking other medications with anticholinergic activity. Proper hydration before and during activities such as exercise or exposure to warm temperatures is recommended.
4. Review the patient's medical record to document the frequency of seizure activity.
5. If this drug is used for migraine prevention, review the patient's medical record to document the frequency of migraine headaches.
6. Ask female patients if there is a possibility of pregnancy at this time. If so, notify the healthcare provider of this possibility before starting therapy.

◆ *Availability.* **PO:** 25-, 50-, 100-, and 200-mg tablets; 15- and 25-mg sprinkle capsules; 25-, 50-, 100-, 150-, and 200-mg sprinkle capsules, extended release (24 hr).

◆ *Dosage and administration*
Antiepileptic. **Adult:** *PO:* Initially 25 mg twice daily. Increase the daily dosage by 50 mg at weekly intervals until a clinical response is achieved. The usual recommended daily dosage is 400 mg in two divided doses. Topiramate may be taken with or without food. The tablets should not be broken because they taste bitter. The sprinkle capsules may be swallowed whole or administered by carefully opening the capsule and sprinkling the entire contents onto a small amount (e.g., 1 teaspoon) of soft food. Swallow this drug-food mixture immediately; do not chew. The therapeutic blood levels for topiramate are 5 to 25 mg/L.

Migraine prevention. **Adult:** *PO:* Use the tablets or sprinkle capsules. Dosage increase is as follows: week 1, 25 mg daily in the evening; week 2, 25 mg in the morning and 25 mg in the evening; week 3, 25 mg in the morning and 50 mg in the evening; week 4 and thereafter, 50 mg in the morning and 50 mg in the evening. Do not use topiramate to treat migraine headaches.

◆ *Common adverse effects*
Neurologic
Sedation, drowsiness, dizziness. These symptoms tend to disappear with continued therapy and possible dosage adjustment. Encourage the patient not to discontinue

therapy without first consulting the healthcare provider. People who work around machinery, operate motor vehicles, or perform other duties that require constant mental alertness should be particularly cautious until they know how the medication affects them. Provide for patient safety during episodes of dizziness and report these patients to the healthcare provider for further evaluation.

◆ *Serious adverse effects*

Neurologic

Confusion, disorientation. Make regularly scheduled assessments of the patient's speech patterns, degree of alertness, and orientation to name, place, and time and compare findings. Report any significant alterations to the healthcare provider.

Cleft palate in newborns. Topiramate increases the risk of development of cleft lip or cleft palate in infants born to women being treated with topiramate. Topiramate is classified as pregnancy category D; there is positive evidence of human fetal risk based on human data, but the potential benefits from the use of the drug in pregnant women may be acceptable in certain situations despite its risks.

Women taking topiramate should tell their healthcare providers immediately if they are planning to or have become pregnant. Patients should not stop taking topiramate unless told to do so by their healthcare provider.

Metabolic

Hydration status. Decreased sweating and overheating have been reported with the use of topiramate, primarily in children. Most cases occur in association with exposure to elevated environmental temperatures, vigorous activity, or both. Proper hydration before and during activities such as exercise or exposure to warm temperatures is recommended.

◆ *Drug interactions*

Drugs that decrease therapeutic effects. Phenobarbital, primidone, phenytoin, valproic acid, and carbamazepine may enhance the metabolism of topiramate. Monitor the patient for increased frequency of seizure activity.

Enhanced sedation. Central nervous system depressants—including sleep aids, analgesics, tranquilizers, and alcohol—enhance the sedative effects of topiramate. Patients must be warned not to work around machinery, operate motor vehicles, or perform other duties that require constant mental alertness until it is known how they are affected by this medication. Provide for patient safety during episodes of drowsiness or dizziness.

Estrogen-containing contraceptives. Topiramate enhances the metabolism of estrogens. Spotting or bleeding may be an indication of reduced estrogen levels and reduced contraceptive activity. Recommend that the patient use alternative forms of birth control while taking this medication.

---

valproic acid (văl-PRŌ-ĭk Ă-sĭd)
Depakene (DĔP-ă-kēn)

Actions

Valproic acid is an antiepileptic agent structurally unrelated to any other agent currently used to treat seizure disorders. Its mechanism of action is unknown; however, it appears to support GABA activity as an inhibitory neurotransmitter.

Uses

Valproic acid has broad activity against focal seizures and generalized tonic-clonic seizures. It is the only available agent that can be used as single-drug therapy for treating patients with a combination of generalized tonic-clonic, absence, or myoclonic seizures. Valproic acid is also being tested for use either alone or in combination with lithium or carbamazepine for treating acute mania associated with bipolar disorder in patients who do not respond to lithium therapy alone. It is also approved for the prevention of migraine headaches; it is not effective for the treatment of migraine headaches.

Therapeutic Outcomes

The primary therapeutic outcomes expected from valproic acid are as follows:
1. Reduced frequency of seizures and reduced injury from seizure activity
2. Treatment of acute mania in bipolar disorder
3. Prevention of migraines
4. Minimal adverse effects from therapy

❖ **Nursing Implications for Valproic Acid**

◆ *Premedication assessment*

1. The manufacturer recommends that the following baseline studies be completed before therapy is initiated and at regular intervals thereafter: liver function tests, bleeding time determination, and platelet count.
2. Review the patient's routine blood studies to detect blood dyscrasias and hepatotoxicity.
3. Perform a baseline assessment of the patient's speech patterns, degree of alertness, and orientation to name, place, and time before starting therapy. Monitor the patient's behavioral responses to therapy.
4. Ask female patients about the possibility of pregnancy.

◆ *Availability.* **PO:** 250-mg capsules; 125-mg capsules containing coated particles (sprinkles); 125-, 250-, and 500-mg tablets, sustained release (24 hr); 250 mg/5 mL solution.

Injection: 100 mg/mL in 5-mL vials.

◆ *Dosage and administration.* **Adult:** *PO:* 10 to 15 mg/kg daily, divided in two to three doses. Administer medication with food or milk to reduce gastric irritation. Increase by 5 to 10 mg/kg/day at weekly intervals. The maximum daily dosage is 60 mg/kg. The therapeutic blood levels are 40 to 100 mg/L. A capsule containing enteric-coated particles is available for patients who have persistent nausea and vomiting.

◆ *Common adverse effects*

Gastrointestinal

Nausea, vomiting, indigestion. These effects are common during initiation of therapy. Gradual increases in dosage and administration with food or milk reduce gastric irritation.

Neurologic

Sedation, drowsiness, dizziness. These symptoms tend to disappear with continued therapy and possible dosage adjustment. Encourage the patient not to discontinue therapy without first consulting the healthcare provider. People who work around machinery, operate motor vehicles, or perform other duties that require constant mental alertness should not take these medications while working. Provide for patient safety during episodes of dizziness and report these patients to the healthcare provider for further evaluation.

Sensory

Blurred vision. Caution the patient that blurred vision may occur, and make appropriate suggestions for the patient's personal safety.

◆ *Serious adverse effects*

Hematologic

Blood dyscrasias. Routine laboratory tests (e.g., RBC, WBC, differential, and platelet counts) should be scheduled. Monitor the patient for sore throat, fever, purpura, jaundice, or excessive and progressive weakness.

Neurologic

Birth defects. There is an increased risk of neural tube defects, craniofacial defects, and cardiovascular malformations in infants exposed to valproic acid during gestation. Women of childbearing age should use valproic acid only if it is essential to manage their medical conditions. Women who are not planning a pregnancy should use effective contraception. Women who become pregnant while taking valproic acid should not discontinue therapy without discussing it first with their healthcare providers.

Gastrointestinal

Hepatotoxicity. The symptoms of hepatotoxicity are anorexia, nausea, vomiting, jaundice, hepatomegaly, splenomegaly, and abnormal liver function test results (e.g., elevated bilirubin, AST, ALT, GGT, and alkaline phosphatase levels; increased PT).

Pancreatitis. The symptoms of pancreatitis are abdominal pain, nausea, vomiting, and anorexia. Report symptoms to the healthcare provider because of the potential for life-threatening complications.

◆ *Drug interactions*

Drugs that decrease therapeutic effects. Phenobarbital, primidone, phenytoin, topiramate, and carbamazepine may enhance the metabolism of valproic acid and thus decrease its therapeutic effect. Monitor the patient for the increased frequency of seizure activity. Monitoring changes in serum levels should help predict the potential for increased seizure activity.

Enhanced sedation. Central nervous system depressants—including sleep aids, analgesics, tranquilizers, and alcohol—enhance the sedative effects of valproic acid. Patients must be warned not to work around machinery, operate motor vehicles, or perform other duties that require constant mental alertness until it is known how they are affected by this medication. Provide for patient safety during episodes of drowsiness or dizziness.

---

zonisamide (zō-NĬS-ă-mīd)
Zonegran (Zō-nĕ-grăn)

Actions

Zonisamide is classified as a sulfonamide, and it is chemically unrelated to other antiepileptic agents. It acts by blocking sodium and calcium channels to stabilize the neuronal membranes, preventing propagation of a seizure stimulus. It does not affect GABA activity.

Uses

Zonisamide is approved for use in conjunction with other antiepileptic therapy for the treatment of focal seizures in adults.

Therapeutic Outcomes

The primary therapeutic outcomes sought from zonisamide are as follows:
1. Reduced frequency of seizures and reduced injury from seizure activity
2. Minimal adverse effects from therapy

❖ **Nursing Implications for Zonisamide**

◆ *Premedication assessment*

1. Review the patient's medication history to ensure that the patient does not have an allergy to sulfonamide medications (e.g., Bactrim, Septra). If the patient does have such an allergy, inform the charge nurse and the healthcare provider immediately. Do not administer the medication without specific approval.
2. Review the patient's medical record for a history of skin rashes. If the patient develops a rash, inform the charge nurse and the healthcare provider immediately. Do not administer the medication without specific approval.
3. Review the patient's medical record to document the frequency of seizure activity.
4. As a result of the potential for serious adverse reactions, the following baseline studies should be repeated at regular intervals: complete blood count, liver function tests, BUN, and serum creatinine.
5. Perform a baseline assessment of the patient's speech patterns, degree of alertness, and orientation to name, place, and time before starting therapy.
6. Obtain the patient's baseline vital signs.

◆ *Availability. PO:* 25-, 50-, and 100-mg capsules.

◆ *Dosage and administration.* **Adult:** *PO:* Initial dosage is 100 mg daily, taken with or without food. Because of sedative effects, the drug may be taken at bedtime. After 2 weeks, the dosage may be increased to 200 mg/day for at least 2 weeks. Both capsules may be taken at the same time. The dosage can be increased up to 600 mg/day, with at least 2 weeks between dosage changes to assess the therapeutic effects of therapy and to monitor for adverse effects. Encourage the patient to drink six to eight 8-ounce glasses of water daily while taking this medication. The therapeutic blood levels for zonisamide are 10 to 40 mg/L.

◆ *Common adverse effects*
Neurologic
Drowsiness, dizziness. These effects are usually mild and tend to resolve with continued therapy; they can be reduced by slowly increasing the dosage. Encourage the patient not to discontinue therapy without first consulting the healthcare provider. Provide for patient safety during episodes of dizziness. Patients must be warned not to work around machinery, operate motor vehicles, or perform other duties that require constant mental alertness until it is known how they are affected by this medication.

◆ *Serious adverse effects*
Neurologic
Confusion, disorientation. Make regularly scheduled assessments of the patient's speech patterns, degree of alertness, and orientation to name, place, and time and compare findings. Report any significant alterations to the healthcare provider.
Genitourinary
Nephrotoxicity. Monitor the patient's kidney function test results for abnormal findings. Report increasing BUN and creatinine levels; frank blood or smoky-colored urine; RBCs in excess of 0 to 3 on the urinalysis report; or back pain, abdominal pain, or pain on urination.
Hematologic
Blood dyscrasias. Routine laboratory studies (e.g., RBC, WBC, and differential counts) should be scheduled. Monitor the patient for sore throat, fever, purpura, jaundice, or excessive and progressive weakness.
Integumentary
Dermatologic reactions. Report a patient's rash or pruritus, with or without fever, immediately and withhold additional doses of the medication until approved by the healthcare provider.

◆ *Drug interactions*
Enhanced sedation. Central nervous system depressants—including sleep aids, analgesics, tranquilizers, and alcohol—enhance the sedative effects of zonisamide. Patients must be warned not to work around machinery, operate motor vehicles, or perform other duties that require constant mental alertness until it is known how they are affected by this medication.

See Table 18.2 for a listing of newer antiepileptic medications.

Table 18.2 Other Antiepileptic Drugs

GENERIC NAME	BRAND NAME	AVAILABILITY	ADULT DOSAGE RANGE	USE FOR SEIZURE
brivaracetam	Briviact Brivlera ♣	Intravenous: 50 mg/5 mL Oral solution: 10 mg/mL (300 mL) Tablets: 10, 25, 50, 75, 100 mg	50-200 mg/day	Focal-onset seizures (adjunct)
eslicarbazepine	Aptiom	Tablets: 200, 400, 600, 800 mg	Up to 1600 mg/day	Focal-onset seizures (adjunct)
lacosamide	Vimpat	Intravenous: 200 mg/20 mL Oral solution: 10 mg/mL (200, 465 mL) Tablets: 50, 100, 150, 200 mg	200-400 mg/day	Simple or complex focal seizures
perampanel	Fycompa	Oral suspension: 0.5 mg/mL (340 mL) Tablets: 2, 4, 6, 8, 10, 12 mg	2-12 mg/day	Focal onset seizures with or without secondary generalization (adjunct); primary generalized tonic-clonic seizures (adjunct)
rufinamide	Banzel	Oral suspension: 40 mg/mL (460 mL) Tablets: 200, 400 mg	400-3200 mg/day	Lennox-Gastaut syndrome (adjunct)

♣ Available in Canada.

Get Ready for the NCLEX® Examination!

Key Points

- Seizures are the result of the sudden excessive firing of a small number of neurons and the spread of electrical activity to adjacent neurons.
- There are several types and many causes of seizures. If the seizures are chronic and recurrent, then the patient is diagnosed as having epilepsy.
- Epilepsy is treated almost exclusively with antiepileptic medications.
- The effective treatment of epilepsy requires the cooperation of the patient and the healthcare provider.
- The desired therapeutic outcome of seizure treatment is to reduce the frequency of seizures while minimizing the adverse effects of drug therapy. To attain this, therapy must be individualized to consider the type of seizure activity and the age, gender, and concurrent medical conditions of the patient.
- Patients, as well as their families and caregivers, require education and support regarding their responsibilities with respect to the management of epilepsy.

Additional Learning Resources

SG Go to your Study Guide for additional Review Questions for the NCLEX® Examination, Critical Thinking Clinical Situations, and other learning activities to help you master this chapter content.

Go to your Evolve website (https://evolve.elsevier.com/Clayton) for additional online resources.

Review Questions for the NCLEX® Examination

1. The nurse witnesses a patient with a seizure disorder as he suddenly has spasms of his arms and legs, falling to the floor. He is initially unconscious and is quite groggy as he wakes up. Which type of seizure being demonstrated by this patient will be documented by the nurse?
   1. Tonic-clonic seizure
   2. Atonic seizure
   3. Focal simple motor seizure
   4. Absence seizure

2. An infant is brought to the emergency department with observable twitching of the extremities and a temperature of 104.2°F as reported by his parents. The nurse will take which of the following actions? *(Select all that apply.)*
   1. Take the infant's vital signs.
   2. Leave the infant and mother for a brief time to allow privacy.
   3. Assess the infant's airway.
   4. Restrain the infant and swaddle in blankets.
   5. Protect the infant from injury.

3. When caring for a patient with epilepsy who was hospitalized and was recovering from a seizure, what are the expected assessments/interventions by the nurse during the postictal time? *(Select all that apply.)*
   1. Place oxygen and suction equipment at the bedside.
   2. Determine whether any bodily harm occurred during the seizure.
   3. Evaluate the degree of weakness, speech pattern changes, and memory loss.
   4. Turn the patient on his or her side to allow secretions to drain out of the mouth.
   5. Encourage oral hygiene and ask the patient to brush his or her teeth.

4. The patient asked the nurse what to expect when taking the antiepileptic lamotrigine (Lamictal). What are appropriate responses by the nurse? *(Select all that apply.)*
   1. "As soon as you are started on lamotrigine, you can expect a decrease in the frequency of your seizures."
   2. "You will need frequent laboratory tests to check for the drug level so the dose can be adjusted."
   3. "Common side effects from this drug are nausea and gastrointestinal upset; this will decrease if you take the drug with food and as your body gets used to it."
   4. "You may feel drowsy or dizzy at first; these symptoms tend to disappear with continued therapy."
   5. "The drug dosage will need to be increased over several weeks before we get to the maintenance dose."

5. From the following medications ordered by the healthcare provider for patients with known seizure disorders, the nurse knows which medications are for the seizures? *(Select all that apply.)*
   1. Levetiracetam (Keppra) 500 mg PO
   2. Carbamazepine (Tegretol) 200 mg PO
   3. Terbinafine (Lamisil) 250 mg PO
   4. Gabapentin (Neurontin) 300 mg PO
   5. Phenytoin (Dilantin) 100 mg PO

6. The nurse was monitoring a patient recently started on pregabalin (Lyrica) for peripheral neuropathy for any adverse effects and notified the healthcare provider after the patient made which statement?
   1. "I keep having blurred vision, especially in the morning."
   2. "I have not noticed any significant change in my pain."
   3. "I find myself needing to take a nap after breakfast, I'm so sleepy."
   4. "I have a better appetite now since I have been started on this drug."

7. The nurse caring for a patient recently diagnosed with epilepsy remembered that the patient listed sulfa as an allergy. Which antiepileptic would the nurse recognize as being classified as a sulfonamide?
   1. Valproic acid (Depakene)
   2. Topiramate (Topamax)
   3. Zonisamide (Zonegran)
   4. Levetiracetam (Keppra)

19

Drugs Used for Pain Management

Objectives

1. Describe the pain assessment used for patients receiving opiate agonists.
2. Differentiate among the properties of opiate agonists, opiate partial agonists, and opiate antagonists.
3. Cite the common adverse effects of opiate agonists.
4. Identify opiate antagonists and expected therapeutic outcomes to monitor.
5. Describe the three pharmacologic effects of salicylates.
6. List the common and serious adverse effects and drug interactions associated with salicylates.

Key Terms

pain experience (PĀN ĕks-PĒR-ē-ĕns) (p. 292)
pain perception (pŭr-SĔP-shŭn) (p. 292)
pain threshold (THRĔSH-hōld) (p. 292)
pain tolerance (TŎL-ŭr-ĕns) (p. 292)
nociception (nō-sē-SĔP-shŭn) (p. 292)
acute pain (ă-KYŪT) (p. 292)
chronic pain (KRŎN-ĭk) (p. 293)
nociceptive pain (nō-sē-SĔP-tĭv) (p. 293)
somatic pain (sō-MĂ-tĭk) (p. 293)
visceral pain (VĬS-ŭr-ăl) (p. 293)
neuropathic pain (nyŭr-ō-PĂTH-ĭk) (p. 293)
idiopathic pain (ĭd-ē-ō-PĂTH-ĭk) (p. 293)
analgesics (ăn-ăl-JĒ-zĭks) (p. 293)
opiate agonists (Ō-pē-ăt ĂG-ŏ-nĭsts) (p. 294)

opiate partial agonists (Ō-pē-ăt PĂR-shŭl ĂG-ŏ-nĭsts) (p. 294)
opiate antagonists (Ō-pē-ăt ăn-TĂG-ŏ-nĭsts) (p. 294)
prostaglandin inhibitors (prŏs-tă-GLĂN-dĭn ĭn-HĬ-bĭ-tŭrz) (p. 294)
salicylates (săl-ĭ-SĬL-āts) (p. 294)
nonsteroidal antiinflammatory drugs (nŏn-stĕ-RŌY-dăl ĂN-tī-ĭn-FLĂ-mă-tō-rē) (p. 294)
nociceptors (nō-sē-SĔP-tŭrz) (p. 294)
opiate receptors (Ō-pē-ăt rē-SĔP-tŭrz) (p. 294)
range orders (RĀNJ ŌR-dŭrz) (p. 300)
drug tolerance (DRŬG TŎL-ŭr-ĕns) (p. 302)
ceiling effect (SĒ-lĭng ĕ-FĔKT) (p. 307)

PAIN

The International Association for the Study of Pain defines pain as "an unpleasant sensory and emotional experience associated with actual or potential tissue damage or described in terms of such damage." An unpleasant sensation that is part of a larger situation is called a *pain experience*. The pain experience is highly subjective and influenced by behavioral, physiologic, sensory, emotional (e.g., attention, anxiety, fatigue, suggestion, prior conditioning), and cultural factors for a particular person under a certain set of circumstances. This accounts for the wide variation in individual responses to the sensation of pain.

The three terms used in relationship to the pain experience are **pain perception**, **pain threshold**, and **pain tolerance**. *Pain perception* (also known as *nociception*) is an individual's awareness of the feeling or sensation of pain. *Pain threshold* is the point at which an individual first acknowledges or interprets a sensation as being painful. *Pain tolerance* is the individual's ability to endure pain.

Pain has physical and emotional components. Factors that decrease an individual's tolerance to pain include prolonged pain that is insufficiently relieved, fatigue accompanied by the inability to sleep, an increase in anxiety or fear, unresolved anger, depression, and isolation. Patients with severe intractable pain fear that the pain cannot be relieved, and patients with cancer fear that new or increasing pain means that the cancer is spreading or recurring.

Pain is usually described as acute or short term and as chronic or long term. **Acute pain** arises from sudden injury to the structures of the body (e.g., skin, muscles, viscera). The intensity of pain is usually proportional to the extent of tissue damage. The sympathetic nervous system is activated, resulting in an increase in the heart rate, pulse, respirations, and blood pressure. This sympathetic nervous system stimulation also causes nausea, diaphoresis, dilated pupils, and an elevated glucose level. Continuing or persistent pain results from ongoing tissue damage or from chemicals released by the surrounding cells during the initial trauma (e.g., a crushing injury). The intensity diminishes as the stimulus is removed or tissue repair and healing take place. Acute pain serves an important protective physiologic purpose that warns of potential or actual tissue damage.

Chronic pain has a slower onset and lasts longer than 3 months beyond the healing process. Chronic pain does not relate to an injury or provide physiologic value. Depending on the underlying cause, it is often subdivided into malignant (cancer) or nonmalignant (causes other than cancer) pain. It may arise from visceral organs, muscular and connective tissue, or neurologic factors such as diabetic neuropathy, trigeminal neuralgia, or amputation. As chronic pain progresses, especially poorly treated pain, other physical and emotional factors come into play, affecting almost every aspect of a patient's life—physical, mental, social, financial, and spiritual—and causing additional stress, anger, chronic fatigue, and depression. Although pain has always been viewed as a symptom of a disease or a condition, chronic pain and its harmful physiologic effects are now regarded as a disease itself.

Pain may also be classified by pathophysiology. **Nociceptive pain** is the result of a stimulus (e.g., chemical, thermal, mechanical) to pain receptors. Nociceptive pain is usually described by patients as dull and aching. It is called *somatic pain* if it originates from the skin, bones, joints, muscles, or connective tissue (e.g., arthritis pain) and *visceral pain* if it originates from the abdominal and thoracic organs. Nociception is the process whereby a person becomes aware of the presence of pain. There are four steps in nociception: (1) transduction, (2) transmission, (3) perception, and (4) modulation (Fig. 19.1).

Neuropathic pain results from injury to the peripheral or central nervous system (CNS) (e.g., trigeminal neuralgia). Patients describe neuropathic pain as stabbing and burning. Phantom limb pain is a neuropathic pain experienced by amputees in a body part that is no longer there. **Idiopathic pain** is a nonspecific pain of unknown origin. Anxiety, depression, and stress are often associated with this type of pain. Common areas associated with idiopathic pain are the pelvis, neck, shoulders, abdomen, and head.

PAIN MANAGEMENT

Analgesics are drugs that relieve pain without producing loss of consciousness or loss of reflexes. The search for an ideal analgesic continues. It is difficult to find one that meets this definition: it should be potent enough to provide maximum relief of pain; it should not cause dependence; it should cause a minimum of adverse effects (e.g., constipation, hallucinations, respiratory depression, nausea, vomiting); it should not cause tolerance; it should act promptly and over a long period with a minimum amount of sedation so that the patient is able to remain conscious and responsive; and it should be relatively inexpensive.

At present, no completely satisfactory classification of analgesics is available. Historically they have been

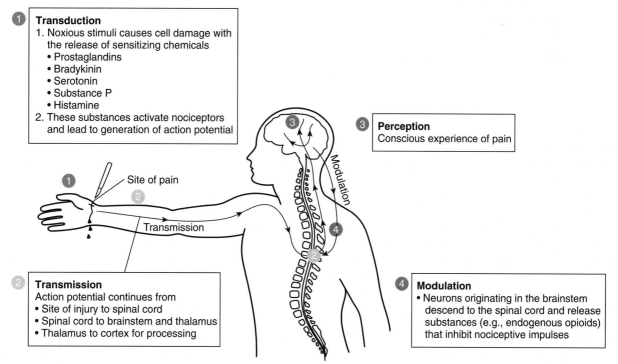

Fig. 19.1 Nociceptive pain originates when the tissue is injured. *1,* Transduction occurs when there is release of chemical mediators. *2,* Transmission involves the conduction of the action potential from the periphery (injury site) to the spinal cord and then to the brainstem, thalamus, and cerebral cortex. *3,* Perception is the conscious awareness of pain. *4,* Modulation involves signals from the brain going back down the spinal cord to modify incoming impulses. (Developed by M. McCaffery, C. Pasero, and J. A. Paice. From McCaffery M, Pasero C. *Pain: Clinical Manual.* 2nd ed. St. Louis: Mosby; 1999.)

categorized based on potency (mild, moderate, strong), origin (opium, synthetic, coal-tar derivative), or addictive properties (narcotic, nonnarcotic).

Research into the control of pain has recently given new insight into pathways of pain within the nervous system and a better understanding of precise mechanisms of action of analgesic agents. The current nomenclature for analgesics stems from these recent discoveries. In this chapter the medications have been divided into **opiate agonists, opiate partial agonists, opiate antagonists,** and **prostaglandin inhibitors** (acetaminophen, **salicylates,** and **nonsteroidal antiinflammatory drugs [NSAIDs]**). The commonly used term "opioid" refers broadly to all substances that bind to opiate receptors in the brain, including opiate agonists, opiate partial agonists, and opiate antagonists. Opioids, in general, are drugs from a variety of origins—opium (heroin, morphine, codeine) or synthetic (meperidine, fentanyl)—with varying degrees of analgesic potency, euphoric effect, and addictive properties.

ACTIONS

The pathways of the pain transmission signal from the site of injury to the brain for processing and reflexive action have not been fully identified. The first step leading to the sensation of pain is the stimulation of receptors known as *nociceptors* (see Fig. 19.1). These nerve endings are found in skin, blood vessels, joints, subcutaneous tissues, periosteum, viscera, and other tissues. The nociceptors are classified as thermal, chemical, and mechanical-thermal, based on the types of sensations that they transmit. The exact mechanism that causes stimulation of nociceptors is not fully understood; however, bradykinins, prostaglandins, leukotrienes, histamine, and serotonin sensitize these receptors. Receptor activation leads to action potentials that are transmitted along afferent nerve fibers to the spinal cord. A series of neurotransmitters (somatostatin, cholecystokinin, substance P) play roles in the transmission of nerve impulses from the site of damage to the spinal cord. Within the CNS, there may be at least four pain-transmitting pathways up the spinal cord to various areas of the brain for response.

The CNS contains a series of receptors that control pain. These are known as *opiate receptors* because stimulation of these receptors by the opiates blocks the pain sensation. These receptors are subdivided into four types: mu (μ), delta (δ), kappa (κ), and epsilon (ε) receptors. Sigma (σ) receptors are another type that react to opioid agonists and partial agonists. The receptors are located in different areas of the CNS. The κ receptors are found in greatest concentration in the cerebral cortex and in the substantia gelatinosa of the dorsal horn of the spinal cord. They are responsible for analgesia at the levels of the spinal cord and brain. Stimulation of κ receptors also produces sedation and dysphoria. The μ receptors are located in the pain-modulating centers of the CNS and induce central analgesia, euphoria, physical dependence,

miosis, and respiratory depression. The σ receptors are located in the limbic area of the brain and in the spinal cord and may play a role in the euphoria produced by selected opiates. The σ receptors are thought to produce the autonomic stimulation and psychotomimetic (e.g., hallucinations) and dysphoric effects of some opiate agonists and partial agonists. The functions of the σ receptors are under investigation. Research is focusing on developing synthetic chemicals that target specific receptors to maximize analgesia but minimize the potential for adverse effects, such as addiction.

As described, other chemicals—histamine, prostaglandins, serotonin, leukotrienes, substance P, and bradykinins—released during trauma also contribute to pain. Developing pharmaceuticals that block these chemicals is another effective way of stopping pain. Antihistamines (e.g., diphenhydramine), prostaglandin inhibitors (e.g., NSAIDs), substance P antagonists (e.g., capsaicin), and antidepressants that prolong norepinephrine and serotonin activity (e.g., tricyclic antidepressants, selective serotonin reuptake inhibitors) have analgesic properties.

Other pharmacologic agents can suppress pain by a variety of mechanisms. Adrenergic agents, such as norepinephrine and clonidine, and gamma-aminobutyric acid receptor stimulants (e.g., baclofen, gabapentin) produce significant analgesia by blocking nociceptor activity. Valproic acid, phenytoin, gabapentin, and carbamazepine act as analgesics by suppressing spontaneous neuronal firing, as occurs in trigeminal neuralgia. Tricyclic antidepressants inhibit the reuptake of serotonin and norepinephrine, causing the onset of analgesia to be more rapid as well as improving the outlook of the person with chronic pain and depression. Some antidepressants (e.g., amitriptyline) also block pain by antihistaminic and anticholinergic activity. Bisphosphonates (e.g., zoledronic acid) may be effective in treating cancer pain associated with bony metastases.

USES

The World Health Organization recommends a stepwise approach to pain management in relation to cancer pain (Fig. 19.2). Mild acute pain is effectively treated with analgesics such as aspirin, NSAIDs, or acetaminophen. Pain associated with inflammation responds well to NSAIDs. Unrelieved or moderate pain is generally treated with a moderate-potency opiate such as codeine or oxycodone, which is often used in combination with acetaminophen or aspirin (Tylenol with Codeine No. 3 and Percodan, respectively). Severe acute pain is treated with opiate agonists (e.g., morphine, hydromorphone, levorphanol). Morphine sulfate is usually the drug of choice for the treatment of severe chronic pain. Other agents such as antidepressants or anticonvulsants may be used as adjunctive therapy with analgesics, depending on the causes of pain.

The healthcare delivery system in the United States has an unfortunate, long-standing history of inadequate

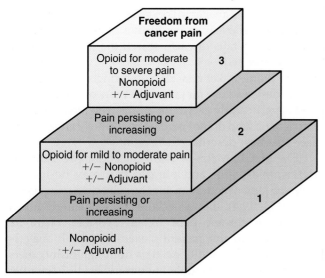

Fig. 19.2 World Health Organization's Pain Relief Ladder. (Adapted from World Health Organization, 2005. Retrieved from http://www.who.int/cancer/palliative/painladder/en.)

pain management. The Joint Commission's current standards for pain management therapy include the following primary therapeutic outcomes:

1. Relief of pain intensity and duration of pain complaint
2. Prevention of the conversion of persistent pain to chronic pain
3. Prevention of suffering and disability associated with pain
4. Prevention of psychological and socioeconomic consequences associated with inadequate pain management
5. Control of adverse effects associated with pain management
6. Optimization of the ability to perform activities of daily living (ADLs)

Although considered acceptable at one time, placebo therapy should never be used with pain management. One premise of pain management is that the patient should be believed when describing the presence of pain. The use of placebos implies a lack of belief in the patient's description and can seriously damage the patient-provider relationship. The American Pain Society has declared that the use of placebos is unethical and should be avoided.

A Note About Opioid Abuse

Opioids are commonly prescribed for pain. Evidence supports short-term efficacy (12 weeks or less) of opioid treatment for pain management. However, few studies have been conducted to assess the long-term benefits of opioids for chronic pain (pain lasting greater than 12 weeks) with outcomes examined at least 1 year later. Opioid pain medications present serious risks to health and wellness through debilitation and the potential for death from overdose. The Centers for Disease Control

and Prevention (CDC) reported 33,091 deaths from an overdose in the United States in 2015, a 2.8-fold increase from 2002. Over 59,000 deaths due to overdose were reported to the CDC in 2016. It is estimated that 2.1 million persons abuse or are dependent on prescription opioid pain medicine across the United States.

The CDC (Dowell et al, 2016) and Canada health authorities (Busse et al, 2017) have published guidelines for prescribing opioids for chronic noncancer pain. Both recommend nonpharmacologic therapy and nonopioid pharmacologic therapy for chronic pain. Opioids should only be considered if expected benefits for pain management and function are anticipated to outweigh risks to the health of the patient. If opioids are prescribed, they should be combined with nonpharmacologic therapy and nonopioid pharmacologic therapy (see Chapter 48).

❖ NURSING IMPLICATIONS FOR PAIN MANAGEMENT

The management of all types of pain is a major healthcare concern. Rating pain as the fifth vital sign means that the patient's pain should be assessed every time vital signs are taken and recorded. Taking the pain rating only when doing vital signs, however, is not sufficient. The nurse should also evaluate the pain level immediately before and after pain medications are given; at 1-, 2-, and 3-hour intervals for oral medications; and at 15- to 30-minute intervals after parenteral administration. Most assessment data sheets have a section on pain management that contains the following elements: rating before and after medication, nonpharmacologic measures initiated, patient teaching performed, and breakthrough pain measures implemented. The pain flow sheet provides the healthcare team members with a quick visual reference to evaluate the overall effectiveness of the pain management prescribed.

The American Pain Society has published "American Pain Society Recommendations for Improving the Quality of Acute and Cancer Pain Management" (Gordon et al, 2005). The American Pain Foundation developed the Pain Care Bill of Rights, which explains to the patient exactly what to expect and/or demand in the way of pain management (Box 19.1).

Nurses must assist the patient in managing pain. The first important step in this process is to believe the patient's description of the pain. Pain brings with it a variety of feelings, such as anxiety, anger, loneliness, frustration, and depression. Part of the patient's response is tied to past experiences, sociocultural factors, current emotional state, and beliefs regarding pain.

Psychological, physical, and environmental factors all must be considered in managing pain. Never overlook the value of general comfort measures such as a back rub, repositioning, and the use of hot or cold applications. A variety of relaxation techniques and diversional activities may prove psychologically beneficial. Decreasing environmental stimuli to ensure the patient gets successful periods of rest is essential.

The patient's pain must be evaluated in a consistent manner. A wide variety of assessment tools have been developed to enable healthcare providers to gain some degree of uniformity in interpreting and recording the patient's description of pain. Some of the pain assessment tools for use with infants and young children include the following:

- Riley Infant Pain Scale Assessment Tool
- Face, Legs, Activity, Cry, Consolability (FLACC) Scale, for use in nonverbal patients
- Pain Observation Scale for Young Children (POCIS), intended for children 1 to 4 years of age
- Modified Objective Pain Score (MOPS), intended for children 1 to 4 years of age after ear, nose, and throat surgery
- Toddler-Preschooler Postoperative Pain Scale (TPPPS), for use in evaluating pain in smaller children during and after medical or surgical procedures
- Postoperative Pain Score (POPS), for infants having surgical procedures
- Neonatal Infant Pain Scale (NIPS), for pain in preterm and full-term neonates; used to monitor pain before, during, and after a painful procedure

---

Box 19.1 Pain Care Bill of Rights

As a person with pain, you have the right to:
- Have your pain taken seriously and to be treated with dignity and respect by doctors, nurses, pharmacists, and other healthcare professionals.
- Have your pain thoroughly assessed and promptly treated.
- Be informed by your healthcare provider about the possible causes of your pain, and possible treatments, including the benefits, risks, and costs of each.
- Participate actively in decisions about how to manage your pain.
- Have your pain reassessed regularly and your treatment adjusted if your pain has not been eased.
- Be referred to a pain specialist if your pain persists.
- Get clear and prompt answers to your questions, take time to make decisions, and refuse a particular type of treatment if you choose.

Created by the American Pain Foundation. Retrieved from https://consumer. healthday.com/encyclopedia/pain-management-30/pain-health-news-520/ pain-care-bill-of-rights-646163.html.

The list of tools available is extensive, and the preceding is only a partial listing. For further information on pain scales and details of each, search the Internet to find the data needed.

The Wong-Baker FACES pain rating scale (Fig. 19.3) has widespread use for patients 3 years of age and older and is particularly useful for adults who have language barriers or who do not read because they can select the face that best describes their pain.

The McGill-Melzack Pain Questionnaire provides descriptive words and phrases that may be used to help the patient communicate the subjective pain experience (Fig. 19.4). It is especially useful for individuals who have chronic pain. When possible, chart the description in the patient's exact words. It may be necessary to seek additional data from significant others.

Scales such as the ones shown in Fig. 19.5 are often used to assess acute pain. The most common scale used asks the patient to rate the pain being experienced on a scale of 0 (no pain) to 10 (intense or excruciating). The degree of relief for the pain after an analgesic is given is again rated using the same 0-to-10 scale. When different potencies of analgesic agents are ordered for the same patient, the nurse can use these numerical rating data in combination with the other data gathered to determine whether a more or less potent analgesic agent should be administered. The color scale is similar to a slide rule. The patient selects the hue or depth of color that corresponds with the pain being experienced. The nurse turns the slide rule scale over, and a numerical value is identified that can be used to consistently record the patient's response.

Effective pain control depends on the degree of pain experienced. The previously described 0-to-10 scale is a useful way to determine the patient's level of pain. For a patient with mild to moderate acute pain, a non-narcotic agent may be successful, but a patient with severe chronic pain may need a potent analgesic such as morphine. The route of administration is chosen on the basis of several factors. One major consideration is how soon the action of the drug is needed. The oral and rectal routes have a longer onset of action than the parenteral route. It is sometimes erroneously believed that oral medications are inadequate to treat pain, but they can provide excellent pain relief if appropriate doses are provided. Generally the oral route is used initially to treat pain if no nausea and vomiting are

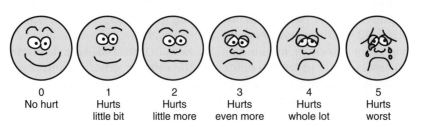

Fig. 19.3 Wong-Baker FACES pain rating scale. (From Hockenberry MJ, Wilson D. *Wong's Nursing Care of Infants and Children*. 10th ed. St. Louis: Mosby; 2015.)

McGill-Melzack
Pain Questionnaire

Patient's name _____ Age _____
File No._____ Date _____
Clinical category (e.g., cardiac, neurologic)
Diagnosis: _____
_____

Analgesic (if already administered):
1. Type_____
2. Dosage_____
3. Time given in relation to this test _____
Patient's intelligence: circle number that represents best estimate.

1 (low)   2   3   4   5 (high)

This questionnaire has been designed to tell us more about your pain. Four major questions we ask are:

1. Where is your pain?
2. What does it feel like?
3. How does it change with time?
4. How strong is it?

It is important that you tell us how your pain feels now. Please follow the instructions at the beginning of each part.

Part 1. Where Is Your Pain?

Please mark on the drawing below the areas where you feel pain. Put E if external, or I if internal, near the areas you mark. Put EI if both external and internal.

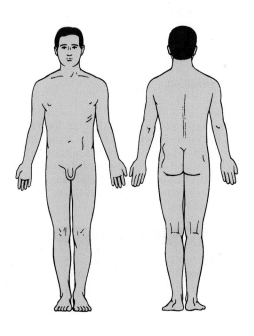

Part 2. What Does Your Pain Feel Like?

Some of the words below describe your present pain. Circle ONLY those words that best describe it. Leave out any category that is not suitable. Use only a single word in each appropriate category—the one that best applies.

1	6	11	16
Flickering	Tugging	Tiring	Annoying
Quivering	Pulling	Exhausting	Troublesome
Pulsing	Wrenching	12	Miserable
Throbbing	7	Sickening	Intense
Beating	Hot	Suffocating	Unbearable
Pounding	Burning	13	17
2	Scalding	Fearful	Spreading
Jumping	Searing	Frightful	Radiating
Flashing	8	Terrifying	Penetrating
Shooting	Tingling	14	Piercing
3	Itchy	Punishing	18
Pricking	Smarting	Grueling	Tight
Boring	Stinging	Cruel	Numb
Drilling	9	Vicious	Drawing
Stabbing	Dull	Killing	Squeezing
Lancinating	Sore	15	Tearing
4	Hurting	Wretched	19
Sharp	Aching	Blinding	Cool
Cutting	Heavy		Cold
Lacerating	10		Freezing
5	Tender		20
Pinching	Taut		Nagging
Pressing	Rasping		Nauseating
Gnawing	Splitting		Agonizing
Cramping			Dreadful
Crushing			Torturing

Part 3. How Does Your Pain Change with Time?

1. Which word or words would you use to describe the *pattern* of your pain?

1	2	3
Continuous	Rhythmic	Brief
Steady	Periodic	Momentary
Constant	Intermittent	Transient

2. What kind of things *relieve* your pain?

3. What kind of things *increase* your pain?

Part 4. How Strong Is Your Pain?

People agree that the following 5 words represent pain of increasing intensity. They are:

1	2	3	4	5
Mild	Discomforting	Distressing	Horrible	Excruciating

To answer each question below, write the number of the most appropriate word in the space beside the question.

1. Which word describes your pain right now? _____
2. Which word describes it at its worst? _____
3. Which word describes it when it is least? _____
4. Which word describes the worst toothache you ever had? _____
5. Which word describes the worst headache you ever had? _____
6. Which word describes the worst stomachache you ever had? _____

Fig. 19.4 McGill-Melzack Pain Questionnaire. (Copyright R. Melzack, 1970, 1975. Reprinted with permission from Dr. Melzack and Mapi Trust.)

A   PAIN INTENSITY SCALES

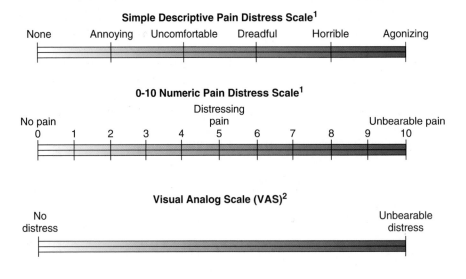

Simple Descriptive Pain Distress Scale[1]

None   Annoying   Uncomfortable   Dreadful   Horrible   Agonizing

0-10 Numeric Pain Distress Scale[1]

No pain   Distressing
                                    pain   Unbearable pain
0   1   2   3   4   5   6   7   8   9   10

Visual Analog Scale (VAS)[2]

No   Unbearable
distress   distress

B   PAIN RELIEF SCALES

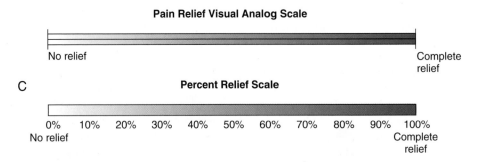

Pain Relief Visual Analog Scale

No relief   Complete
                                                  relief

C   Percent Relief Scale

0%   10%   20%   30%   40%   50%   60%   70%   80%   90%   100%
No relief   Complete
                                                  relief

[1]If used as a graphic rating scale, a 10-cm baseline is recommended.

[2]A 10-cm baseline is recommended for VAS scales.

Fig. 19.5 Pain rating scales. (A) Pain intensity scales. (B and C) Pain relief scales. (From Ignatavicius DD. Pain: the fifth vital sign. In Ignatavicius DD, Workman ML. *Medical-Surgical Nursing: Patient-Centered Collaborative Care.* 7th ed. St. Louis: Saunders; 2013:48. *A,* Redrawn from Agency for Health Care Policy and Research. *Acute Pain Management: Operative or Medical Procedures and Trauma.* AHCPR Publ. No. 92-0032. Rockville, MD: US Department of Health and Human Services; 1992. *B,* Redrawn from Fishman B, et al. The Memorial Pain Assessment Card: A valid instrument for the evaluation of cancer pain. *Cancer.* 1987;60(5):1151-1158. *C,* Redrawn from the Pain Research Group. Brief Pain Inventory. Madison, WI: Department of Neurology, University of Wisconsin-Madison.)

 Clinical Pitfall

All patients have a right to adequate management of pain. To help ensure appropriate analgesia, the rating of pain has been designated "the fifth vital sign." From a nursing standpoint, this means that pain should be assessed every time the vital signs are taken and recorded. Nurses should also evaluate the pain level immediately before administering a pain medication and afterward at 1-, 2-, and 3-hour intervals for oral medications and at 15- to 30-minute intervals after parenteral administration. Although pain assessment forms vary, the elements contained in each collect similar information about pain: rating before and after medication, nonpharmacologic measures initiated, patient teaching performed, and breakthrough pain measures implemented. The pain flow sheet provides the healthcare team members with a quick visual reference to evaluate the overall effectiveness of the pain management prescribed.

 Life Span Considerations
Analgesics

Maintaining a relatively steady blood level of analgesic is the best way to control pain. However, drug absorption, metabolism, and excretion are affected by the patient's age. Dosages and frequency of administration of analgesics may have to be increased in children, especially teenagers, because many medicines are more rapidly metabolized and excreted by patients in this age group. Conversely, an older adult may need a somewhat smaller dose of an analgesic given less frequently because of slower metabolism and excretion. In either situation, it is imperative that the nurse regularly assess the patient's pain level and contact the healthcare provider for adjustments in dosages and frequency based on the response to the analgesic.

present. The patient may initially be treated effectively with oral medications; however, the rectal, transdermal, subcutaneous, intramuscular, intraspinal, epidural, and intravenous (IV) routes may be required, depending on the patient and the course of the underlying disease.

Before initiating a pain assessment, assess the patient for hearing and visual impairment. If the person is unable to hear the questions or see the visual aids used to assess pain, any data collected may be invalid.

Nurses must evaluate and document the effectiveness of the pain medications given in the patient's medical record. Record and report all complaints of pain for analysis by the healthcare provider. The pattern of pain, particularly an increase in frequency or severity, may indicate new causes of pain. The main reasons for increased frequency or intensity of pain are pain from long-term immobility; pain from the treatment modalities used (e.g., surgery, chemotherapy, or radiation therapy); pain from direct extension of a tumor or metastasis into bone, nerve, or viscera; and pain unrelated to the original cause or the therapeutic treatments used.

◆ **Assessment**

History of pain experience

- *Medication history:* What medications are being prescribed, and how effective have they been? What dosage has been required to achieve adequate comfort? Has the patient had any adverse effects to the medications? If yes, get details of the adverse effects and the measures taken for management. What is the patient's attitude toward the use of pain medications (e.g., opioids, anxiolytics)? What are the family's or significant other's attitudes toward the use of medications to control the pain? Does the patient have any history of substance abuse?
- *Patient's perception of pain:* To identify the causes of the pain, have the patient describe his or her perception of it. What does the patient feel is the cause of the pain? In the older adult, multiple chronic and acute pain problems may be present, making it difficult to determine which problem is the most urgent or causing the most pain. Multiple pain complaints, combined with impaired hearing, vision, memory, and cognition, must be taken into consideration during the pain assessment. Evaluate the pain according to location, depth, quality, duration, and severity.
- Obtain baseline vital signs at least every shift or more often as dictated by the patient's condition and type of medications administered.
- Listen to the patient and *believe the pain experience* being described, regardless of whether the physical data substantiate the degree of discomfort described. *Do not* let personal biases or values interfere with establishing interventions that provide maximum pain relief for the individual. The myths that pain decreases with aging and that pain is expected with aging are *incorrect!*

- *Onset:* When was the pain first noticed? When was the most recent attack? Is the onset slow or abrupt? Is there any particular activity that starts the pain? Does the pain occur in response to eating certain foods?
- *Location:* What is the exact location of the pain? It may help to have the patient mark on a drawing of a human figure the areas where the pain is felt; this may be especially useful with pediatric patients, who can be given crayons to help identify different intensities in addition to the location. With acute pain, the site of the pain can be more easily identified; however, with chronic pain, this may be more difficult because the normal physiologic responses of the sympathetic nervous system are no longer present.
- *Depth:* What is the depth of the pain? Does it radiate, having the sensation of spreading out or diffusing over an area, or is it localized in a specific site? The lack of physical symptoms comparable with the pain described *does not* mean that the patient's complaints should be ignored.
- *Quality:* What is the actual sensation felt when the pain is present—stabbing, dull, cramping, sore, burning, or other? Is the pain always in the same place and of the same intensity?
- *Duration:* Is the pain continuous or intermittent? How often does it occur and, once felt, how long does it persist? Is there a cyclic pattern to the pain?
- *Severity:* Have the patient rate the pain using the pain scale methodology that is standard for the clinical setting. Self-reporting pain assessment tools are used for most children 3 years and older. After age 8, children understand numerical values, so one of the visual analog scales or word-graphic rating scales can be used.

Nonverbal observations. Note the patient's general body position during an episode of pain. Look for subtle clues such as facial grimaces, immobility of a particular part, and holding or resisting movement of an extremity. With pediatric patients, facial expressions, squinting, grimacing, and crying may also be used as indicators of pain level and pain relief.

Developmental differences influence the pain experience and how children in different age groups express pain. Infants may express pain through continual inconsolable crying, irritability, poor oral intake, and alterations in sleep pattern. Preschool children may verbalize pain; exhibit lack of cooperation; be "clingy" to parents, nurses, or significant others; and not want the site of the pain touched—they may actually push you away as you approach the painful area. Older children may deny pain in the presence of peers and display regressive behaviors in the presence of support personnel. In the older adult, it is useful to perform the Katz Index of Independence in Activities of Daily Living measurement and the "get up and go" test to determine the individual's functional status.

Pain relief. What specific measures relieve the pain? What has already been tried for pain relief, and what, if anything, has been beneficial?

Physical data. In the presence of pain, always examine the affected part for any alterations in appearance, change in sensation, or limitation in mobility or range of motion. In older adults, it is particularly important to evaluate the musculoskeletal and neurologic systems during the physical examination.

Behavioral responses. What coping mechanisms does the patient use to manage the pain experience—crying, anger, withdrawal, depression, anxiety, fear, or hopelessness? Is the individual introspective and self-focusing? Does the individual continue to perform ADLs despite the pain? Does the individual alter lifestyle patterns appropriately to enhance pain relief measures prescribed? Is the individual able to continue to work? Is the individual socially withdrawn? Is the person seeing more than one healthcare provider to try to obtain an answer about the origin of the pain or to obtain more pain medication from a different healthcare provider?

 Life Span Considerations

Pain in the Older Adult Patient

Pain assessment in the older adult patient must include more than a simple rating of pain using a pain scale. Many older adults suffer from more than one chronic illness, so obtain a nursing history and perform a physical and functional assessment to understand the effect of pain on the patient's ability to meet self-care needs.

◆ **Implementation**

Comfort measures
- Provide for the patient's basic hygiene and comfort. Use techniques such as back rubs, massage, hot and cold applications, or warm baths as ordered.
- Ask the patient what measures have been successful in the past in providing pain relief.
- Relieve pain by doing any or all of the following, as appropriate: (1) support an affected part during movement, provide appropriate assistance during movement or activities, or apply binders or splint an incisional area before initiating activities such as deep breathing and coughing; (2) give analgesics before starting painful activities and plan for the activity to take place during the medication's peak action; and/or (3) use hot or cold applications, massage, warm baths, pressure, and vibration as interventions for pain relief.

Exercise and activity. Unless contraindicated, moderate exercise should be encouraged. Often, pain causes the individual not to move the affected part or to position it in a manner that provides relief. Stress the need to prevent complications by using passive range of motion.

Regularly scheduled exercise is important to prevent further deterioration of the musculoskeletal system, especially in older patients who may also have diminished capacity.

Nonpharmacologic approaches. To enhance the effects of the medication therapy, use nonpharmacologic strategies such as relaxation techniques, visualization, meditation, biofeedback, and transcutaneous electrical nerve stimulation (TENS) units. (The patient will require instruction for using each of these prescribed techniques.) Assist with referral to a pain clinic for management of pain, especially chronic pain.

Goals should be established when initiating a treatment regimen. Prevention, reduction, or elimination of pain is an important therapeutic goal. The patient and caregiver(s) should be involved in the establishment of these goals so that outcomes important to the patient are incorporated into the treatment goals and so that they have realistic expectations. Pain, especially chronic pain, may not be completely eliminated but must be managed. Additional important goals include improving the patient's quality of life, functional capacity, and ability to retain independence. Specific therapeutic goals established may include the following:
- Pain at rest: <3 on pain scale
- Pain with movement: <5 on pain scale
- Able to have at least 6 hours of sleep uninterrupted by pain
- Able to work at a hobby (e.g., doing crafts, playing cards, gardening) for 1 hour

Medication. Even though pain medicine administration may be scheduled, encourage the patient to request pain medication before the pain escalates and becomes severe. Encourage open communication between the patient and the healthcare team regarding the effectiveness of the medications used. Although the smallest dose possible to control the pain is the goal of therapy, it is also important that the dose be sufficient to provide adequate relief. Therefore the patient must understand the importance of expressing the degree of relief being obtained so that appropriate dosage adjustments can be made.

The medication profile may list more than one analgesic order for the same patient. This requires the nurse to use judgment in choosing the correct medication for the patient based on pain assessment data collected.

The nurse must identify when the last dose of pain medication was administered by checking the patient's medication administration record. It is common practice for analgesics to be ordered intermittently on an "as-needed" (PRN) basis. Many clinical institutions have established policies for pain medications ordered on a PRN basis, referred to as *range orders*. Medication range order policies provide guidelines for the clinical staff to interpret the PRN ranges using the pain scale assessment as a guideline. However, in the case of chronic pain or intractable pain, it has been found that administering analgesics around the clock, such as every 3 to 4 hours, will maintain a more constant plasma level of the drug (steady state), resulting in more effective analgesia.

Patient-controlled analgesia (PCA) has gained acceptance in both the inpatient and ambulatory settings. Pumps are available for inpatient use and in ambulatory units for home or nursing home settings. The PCA method of administration allows the patient to control a small infusion pump containing an opiate agonist, usually morphine or fentanyl, which is connected to an indwelling IV catheter. When initiating the PCA pump procedure, a loading dose is often given to gain rapid blood levels necessary for analgesia. The patient then receives a slow continuous infusion from the infusion pump; this is referred to as a basal rate. Depending on the activity level and level of analgesia needed, the patient may push a button, self-administering a small bolus of analgesic to meet his or her immediate need. A timing device on the pump limits the amount and frequency of the dose that can be self-administered per hour. This approach allows the patient to have some control over the pain relief and eliminates the need for the patient to wait for a nurse to answer the call light, check the last dose of analgesics given, and prepare and administer the medication. When PCA is used, the nurse should explain the use of the PCA pump to the patient and observe the patient using it to validate understanding. Education includes allowing only the patient to use the control device, not the family. The degree of pain relief achieved should always be recorded. When pain relief is inadequate, assess for other causes and contact the prescriber to discuss a modification of the regimen.

PCA pumps are also used for chronic pain; however, the dose can be delivered intravenously or subcutaneously. For chronic pain treatment, the largest dose of the medication is given continuously with demand. Continuous subcutaneous opioid analgesia uses either a butterfly-type (25- to 27-gauge) needle or a special needle device placed subcutaneously into the subclavicular tissue or in the abdomen. The needle should be inserted in the body's trunk, usually the abdomen, because of diminished circulation in the extremities.

Epidural analgesia has long been used in obstetrics but is now recognized as an effective means for controlling acute pain in a variety of postoperative procedures. Epidural analgesia most commonly delivers morphine or fentanyl (sometimes combined with bupivacaine) into the subarachnoid space. It can be administered continuously with an infusion pump, intermittently by bolus administration, or via an implanted port. Nursing responsibilities during epidural analgesia involve the following:

- Check institutional policies for qualifications needed to administer and monitor the epidural analgesia.

- Use assessment tools to determine the degree of pain relief and assess the respiratory function, neurologic function, degree of sedation, and catheter status.
- Observe for narcotic-related adverse effects (i.e., respiratory depression, nausea and vomiting, pruritus, headaches) and catheter-related complications. Always have drugs and supplies in the immediate area to reverse a drug overdose.

Transdermal opioid analgesia uses fentanyl (Duragesic) for relief of chronic pain. It takes approximately 12 to 24 hours for the initial patch of medication to reach a steady blood level, so other analgesics must be used during this time. Once placed, the patch provides relief for up to 72 hours. Intermittent "rescue" dosing may still be needed during patch use. When the patch is terminated, the patient still needs to be monitored for an additional 24 hours because the drug may still be present in body tissues.

Pain control. Some patients will not ask for pain medication, so it is important to intervene and anticipate their needs. Ask the patient at what pain level is being perceived and then treat as appropriate.

Nutritional aspects. The patient should eat a well-balanced diet high in B-complex vitamins and limit or eliminate sugar, nicotine, caffeine, and alcohol intake. Drinking 8 to 10 eight-ounce glasses of water daily helps maintain normal elimination patterns. To minimize or avoid the constipating effects of opiates, the patient should increase intake of fiber and fluids. If long-term use of opiates is planned, stool softeners may be necessary.

◆ Patient Education

Teach the patient, family, and significant others the benefits of adequate pain control. Work with them to determine their perception of pain management, use of drug therapy, and nonpharmacologic approaches to pain management. If the patient is hesitant about these approaches, determine why. Stress that physical dependence is not a major factor with short-term use of analgesics and that during long-term use, such as with cancer, it is not the primary concern.

The major issues involved with long-term use of analgesics include obtaining sufficient pain control to provide comfort, ensuring that the patient has ample rest, and enhancing the patient's quality of life.

Inform the patient what medications are available for pain control and when and how to request them. Discuss the patient's expectations of pain management and how to rate the severity of pain honestly so that expectations can be met. Ask what level of exercise is attainable without severe pain. Is the pain control adequate for the individual to maintain ADLs or work?

Assist the patient to learn to cope effectively with the pain. Discuss changes in lifestyle needed to support adequate pain control. Include family members in discussions of pain management. Give praise when techniques are attempted, regardless of whether success is achieved.

Teach the patient how to self-administer the analgesics ordered on an outpatient basis. This will include transdermal, transmucosal, oral, and rectal routes of administration and care of infusion ports and central lines. Record the degree of understanding of the pre-scribed pain regimen.

Include social services information in the patient education process, especially how to connect with community resources available for the patient and family. Make sure that the patient and family understand how to obtain assistance with pain medication administration and patient care needs (e.g., visiting nurse, hospice).

Fostering health maintenance. Throughout the course of treatment, discuss medication information and how it will benefit the patient. Drug therapy for the manage-ment of pain should be coupled with comfort measures, relaxation techniques, meditation, stress management, and meeting the total care needs of the individual to ensure maintenance of ADLs. Provide the patient and significant others with important information contained in the specific drug monograph for the medicines prescribed. Additional health teaching and nursing interventions for adverse effects are described in the drug monographs that follow.

Seek cooperation and understanding of the following points so that medication adherence is increased: name of medications; dosage, route, and times of administra-tion; and common and serious adverse effects.

Patient self-assessment. Enlist the patient's aid in developing and maintaining a written record of monitor-ing parameters (e.g., frequency of pain attacks, activity performed when pain occurs, techniques used to control pain, degree of pain relief, exercise tolerance). See the Patient Self-Assessment Form for Analgesics on the Evolve website. Complete the Premedication Data column for use as a baseline to track response to drug therapy. Ensure that the patient understands how to use the form and instruct the patient to bring the completed form to follow-up visits. During follow-up visits, focus on issues that will foster adherence with the therapeutic interventions prescribed.

DRUG CLASS: OPIATE AGONISTS

The term *opiate* was once used to refer to drugs derived from opium, such as heroin and morphine. It has been found that many other analgesics not related to morphine act at the same sites within the brain. It is now under-stood that opiate agonists and opiate antagonists act at the same site as morphine to stimulate analgesic effects (opiate agonists) or block the effects of opiate agonists (opiate antagonists).

Another outdated term is *narcotic.* Originally, it referred to medications that induced a stupor or sleep. Over the past 80 years, it has gradually come to refer to addictive morphine-like analgesics. The Harrison Narcotic Act of 1914, which placed morphine-like products under governmental control, helped promote this association. The development of analgesics that are as potent as morphine but do not have its sedative or addictive properties makes the word *narcotic* outdated; the terms *opiate agonists* and *opiate partial agonists* should be used where appropriate.

Actions

Opiate agonists are a group of naturally occurring and synthetic substances that have the capability to relieve severe pain without the loss of consciousness. They act by stimulating the opiate receptors in the CNS. Most of these agents also produce physical dependence and are thus considered controlled substances under the federal Controlled Substances Act of 1970.

These agents can be subdivided into four groups: morphine and morphine-like derivatives, meperidine-like derivatives, methadone-like derivatives, and an "other" category (Table 19.1). Administration of these agents causes primary effects on the CNS (e.g., analgesia, suppression of the cough reflex, respiratory depression, drowsiness, sedation, mental clouding, euphoria, nausea and vomiting); there are also significant effects on the cardiovascular system and gastrointestinal (GI) and urinary tracts.

With continued, prolonged use, opiate agonists may produce tolerance and psychological and physical dependence. **Drug tolerance** occurs when a patient requires increases in dosing to receive the same analgesic relief. Development of tolerance seems to depend on the extent and duration of CNS depression. Patients who have prolonged depression by the continued use of opiate agonists have a higher incidence of developing tolerance. Patients who have developed tolerance to one opiate agonist usually require increased dosages of all opiate agonists to achieve the desired effect.

Patients who are physically dependent on opiate agonists remain asymptomatic as long as they are able to maintain their daily opiate agonist require-ment. Physical dependence may develop after 3 to 6 weeks of continual use of the opiate agonists if used for recreational purposes. Physical dependence after the use of opiates agonists for acute pain management is infrequent, but addiction has been reported after short courses of opiate agonist therapy. Early signs of withdrawal are restlessness, perspiration, gooseflesh, lacrimation, runny nose, and mydriasis. Over the next 24 hours, these symptoms intensify, and the patient develops muscular spasms; severe aches in the back, abdomen, and legs; abdominal and muscle cramps; hot and cold flashes; insomnia; nausea, vomiting, and diarrhea; severe sneezing; and increases in body

Table 19.1 Opiate Agonists

GENERIC NAME	BRAND NAME	AVAILABILITY	INITIAL ADULT DOSAGE RANGE	DURATION (HR)	DOSAGE EQUIVALENT TO MORPHINE (10 MG)	
					IM (MG)	ORAL (MG)
Morphine and Morphine-Like Derivatives						
codeine ❶	Codeine Sulfate, Codeine Phosphate	Tablets: 15, 30, 60 mg	*Analgesic:* PO: 15-60 mg q4-6h *Antitussive:* PO: 10-20 mg q4-6h	4-6	120	200
hydrocodone[a] ❶	Zohydro ER Hysingla ER	Capsule, extended release (12 hr): 10, 15, 20, 30, 40, 50 mg Tablet, extended-release (24-hr) abuse deterrent: 20, 30, 40, 60, 80, 100, 120 mg	—	—	—	30
hydromorphone ❶	Dilaudid	Tablets: 2, 4, 8 mg Liquid: 1 mg/mL Suppositories: 3 mg Injection: 1, 2, 4, 10 mg/mL; Tablets, extended-release (24-hr) abuse deterrent: 8, 12, 16, 32 mg	PO: 2 mg q4-6h Subcut, IM: 2 mg q4-6h IV: 1-2 mg q4-6h Rectal: 3 mg q6-8h	4-5	1.5	7.5
levorphanol ❶	—	Tablets: 2 mg	PO: 2 mg q6-8h	4-8	2	1 (chronic); 4 (acute)
morphine ❶	Morphine Sulfate Morphine Sulfate CR, MS-Contin Kadian Morphine Sulfate	Tablets: 15, 30 mg Tablets, sustained release (12 hr): 15, 30, 60, 100, 200 mg Capsules, extended release (24 hr): 10, 20, 30, 40, 50, 60, 80, 100, 200 mg Oral Solution: 10, 20, 100 mg/5 mL; 20 mg/mL Suppositories: 5, 10, 20, 30 mg Injection: 0.5, 1, 2, 4, 5, 8, 10, 15, 20, 25, 50 mg/mL; 150 mg/30 mL	PO: 10-30 mg q4h Subcut, IM: 10 mg/70 kg IV: 4-10 mg slowly Rectal: 10-20 mg q4h	4-5; 8-24 for sustained-release products	10	30 (chronic); 60 (acute)
morphine sulfate/naltrexone	Embeda[b]	Capsules, extended release: morphine (mg)/naltrexone (mg): 20/0.8, 30/1.2, 50/2, 60/2.4, 80/3.2, 100/4	PO: Start with lowest dosage; dose no more frequently than q12h. Requires individual patient adjustment.	12	—	—

Continued

Table 19.1 Opiate Agonists—cont'd

GENERIC NAME	BRAND NAME	AVAILABILITY	INITIAL ADULT DOSAGE RANGE	DURATION (HR)	DOSAGE EQUIVALENT TO MORPHINE (10 MG)	
					IM (MG)	ORAL (MG)
oxycodone ❶	Roxicodone	Tablets: 5, 10, 15, 20, 30 mg	PO: 5 mg q6h	4-5	15	20
	OxyContin	Tablets, controlled release (12-hr abuse deterrent): 10, 15, 20, 30, 40, 60, 80 mg	PO:10-160 mg q12h (controlled release)			
	Oxycodone	Capsules: 5 mg Oral solution: 5 mg/5 mL Oral Concentrate: 100 mg/5 mL				
	Xtampza ER	Capsules, extended release (12-hr), abuse deterrent, oral: 9, 13.5, 18, 27, 36 mg				
	Oxaydo	Tablets, abuse deterrent, oral: 5, 7.5 mg				
oxycodone with aspirin ❶	various	Tablets: 4.8 mg plus aspirin 325 mg	PO: 4.5 mg q6h	4-5	15	30
oxycodone with acetaminophen ❶	various	Tablets: 2.5, 5, 7.5, 10 mg plus acetaminophen 300 or 325 mg Solution: 5 mg plus acetaminophen 325 mg/5 mL	PO: 2.5-10 mg q4-6h	4-5	N/A	N/A
oxymorphone ❶	Opana, Opana ER 12 Hour Abuse-Deterrent	Tablets: 5, 10 mg Tablets, sustained release (12 hr): 5, 7.5, 10, 15, 20, 30, 40 mg Injection: 1 mg/mL	PO: 10-20 mg q4-6h PO: 5-10 mg q12h (sustained release) IV: 0.5 mg Subcut, IM: 1-1.5 mg q4-6h	3-6	1	10
Meperidine-Like Derivatives						
alfentanil ❶	Alfenta	Injection: 500 mcg/mL in 2-, 5-mL ampules	IV: Variable	>45 min	—	—
fentanyl ❶	–	Injection: 50 mcg/mL	IM: 50-100 mcg	1-2	0.1	—
	Fentora	Buccal lozenges: 100, 200, 400, 600, 800 mcg	Buccal: 200 mcg	1-2		
	Actiq	Oral transmucosal lollipop: 200, 400, 600, 800, 1200, 1600 mcg		Variable		
	Abstral	Sublingual tablets: 100, 200, 300, 400, 600, 800 mcg	Use for breakthrough pain; 100-200 mcg, adjust as needed			

Table 19.1 Opiate Agonists—cont'd

GENERIC NAME	BRAND NAME	AVAILABILITY	INITIAL ADULT DOSAGE RANGE	DURATION (HR)	DOSAGE EQUIVALENT TO MORPHINE (10 MG) IM (MG)	ORAL (MG)
	Subsys	Sublingual spray liquid: 100, 200, 400, 600, 800, 1200, 1600 mcg	Use for breakthrough pain; 100-200 mcg, adjust as needed			
	Lazanda ⇄ (*Do not confuse with Latuda*)	Nasal solution: 100, 300, and 400 mcg/actuation	Intranasal: 100 mcg (1 spray)			
	Duragesic (72 hr)	Transdermal patch: 12, 25, 37.5, 50, 62.5, 75, 87.5, 100 mcg	Upper torso: one patch q72h	72		
meperidine ❶	Demerol	Tablets: 50, 100 mg Oral Solution: 50 mg/5 mL Injection: 10, 25, 50, 75, 100 mg/1 mL	PO, subcut, IM: 50-150 mg q3-4h IV: 25-100 mg very slowly	2-4	50-100	300
sufentanil ❶	Sufenta	Injection: 50 mcg/mL in 1-, 2-, 5-mL ampules	IV: variable	2-3	—	—
Methadone-Like Derivatives						
methadone ❶	Methadone, Dolophine	Tablets: 5, 10 mg Tablets, orally disintegrating: 40 mg Oral Solution: 5, 10 mg/5 mL Injection: 10 mg/mL Oral concentrate: 10 mg/mL	*Analgesia:* PO, subcut, IM: 2.5-10 mg q8-12h *Maintenance:* PO: 20-40 mg; up to 120 mg daily	4-8 (may become substantially longer due to variable half-life)	5 (acute)	10 (acute)
Other Opiate Agonists						
tramadol ❶	Ultram ConZip	Tablets: 50 mg Tablets, extended release (24 hr): 100, 200, 300 mg Capsules, extended release (24 hr): 100, 150, 200, 300 mg	PO: 50-100 mg PO: 100 mg every 24 hours, adjust every 5 days as needed	4-6 —		100
tapentadol ❶	Nucynta Nucynta ER	Tablets: 50, 75, 100 mg Tablets, extended release (12 hr): 50, 100, 150, 200, 250 mg	PO: 50-100 mg	4-6	—	75-100

❶ High-alert medication.
aHydrocodone is available in combination with other ingredients for pain (e.g., acetaminophen, ibuprofen) (see Table 19.4).
bTablets contain naltrexone to prevent abuse.

temperature, blood pressure, and respiratory and heart rates. These symptoms reach a peak at 36 to 72 hours after discontinuation of the medication and disappear over the next 5 to 14 days.

Uses

Opiate agonists are used to relieve acute or chronic moderate to severe pain such as that associated with acute injury, postoperative pain, renal or biliary colic, myocardial infarction (MI), or cancer. These agents may be used to provide preoperative sedation and to supplement anesthesia. In patients with acute pulmonary edema, small doses of opiate agonists are used to reduce anxiety and produce positive cardiovascular hemodynamic effects to control edema. All opiate agonists are classified as Schedule II, Schedule III, or Schedule IV controlled substances because of the potential for abuse and dependence.

Tramadol is a synthetic opiate agonist that acts as an analgesic by selectively binding to the μ receptors and inhibiting the reuptake of norepinephrine and serotonin. It has some potential for abuse and dependence and is classified as a Schedule IV controlled substance.

Tapentadol is a newer synthetic opiate agonist that acts as an analgesic by selectively binding to the μ receptors and inhibiting the reuptake of norepinephrine. The opioid agonist action of tapentadol is stronger than that of tramadol, and tapentadol has a greater potential for dependence and abuse; thus it is classified as a Schedule II controlled substance.

Meperidine (Demerol), once a commonly prescribed opioid agonist in the management of pain, is much less frequently prescribed because of the adverse effects associated with its active metabolite, normeperidine. Use of meperidine for more than 1 to 2 days is not recommended. Patients receiving large oral doses of meperidine long term, those with renal impairment, and those with highly acidic urine are predisposed to accumulating normeperidine. Evidence of toxic levels of normeperidine includes excitation, tremors, and seizures.

Therapeutic Outcomes

The primary therapeutic outcomes from appropriate opiate agonist therapy are as follows:
1. Relief of pain intensity and reduced duration of pain complaint
2. Prevention of the conversion of persistent pain to chronic pain
3. Prevention of suffering and disability associated with pain
4. Prevention of psychological and socioeconomic consequences associated with inadequate pain management
5. Control of adverse effects associated with pain management
6. Optimization of the ability to perform ADLs

❖ Nursing Implications for Opiate Agonists
◆ Premedication assessment
1. Perform baseline neurologic assessment (e.g., orientation to date, time, and place; mental alertness; bilateral hand grip; and motor functioning).
2. Obtain vital signs; hold medication if respirations are below 12 breaths/min, or according to age-related respiratory parameters, and consult with healthcare provider.
3. Check bowel sounds and note consistency and frequency of passed stools. Review the voiding pattern and urine output.
4. Check prior use of analgesics.
5. Perform pain assessment before administration of an opiate agonist and at appropriate intervals during therapy. Report poor pain control promptly to the healthcare provider and obtain modification in orders.

◆ Availability, dosage, and administration. See Table 19.1.
Antidotes. Naloxone and naltrexone reverse the effects of opiate agonists.

◆ Common adverse effects
Neurologic
Lightheadedness, dizziness, sedation, sweating. These effects tend to occur most often with the initial dose. Symptoms can be reduced by keeping the patient supine. Provide for patient safety, reassurance, and comfort.

Confusion, disorientation. Perform a baseline assessment of the patient's degree of alertness and orientation to name, place, and time before initiating therapy. Make regularly scheduled evaluations of mental status and report alterations from baseline. Provide for patient safety during these episodes.

Cardiovascular
Orthostatic hypotension. Orthostatic hypotension, manifested by dizziness and weakness, occurs particularly when therapy is being initiated in a patient not in a supine position. Monitor blood pressure closely, especially if the patient complains of dizziness or faintness. Provide patient safety, assurance, and comfort.

Gastrointestinal
Nausea, vomiting. Symptoms can be reduced by keeping the patient supine.

Constipation. Continued use may cause constipation. Maintain the patient's state of hydration, and obtain an order for stool softeners or bulk-forming laxatives if necessary. Encourage the inclusion of sufficient roughage, fresh fruits, vegetables, and whole-grain products in the diet.

◆ Serious adverse effects
Respiratory
Respiratory depression. Opiate agonists make the respiratory centers less sensitive to carbon dioxide, causing respiratory depression. This may occur before the reduction in respiratory rate or tidal volume is

noticeable. Check the respiratory rate and depth often. Have equipment for respiratory assistance available.

Genitourinary

Urinary retention. Opiate agonists may produce spasms of the ureters and bladder, causing urinary retention. The patient may also have difficulty in starting the stream for urination. If the patient develops urinary hesitancy, assess for bladder distention. Report these adverse effects to the healthcare provider for further evaluation. Try to stimulate urination by running water or placing the patient's hands in water. If permitted, have male patients stand to void; female patients should sit on a bedpan or toilet with receptacle.

Psychological

Excessive use or abuse. Evaluate the patient's response to the analgesic. Identify underlying needs and plan for more appropriate management of those needs. Discuss the case with the healthcare provider and make plans to cooperatively approach gradual withdrawal of the medications being abused. Suggest a change to a milder analgesic when indicated.

Patients do not have to experience the symptoms of withdrawal to be treated for physical dependence. Patients may be treated by gradually reducing the daily dosage of the opiate agonist. If withdrawal symptoms become severe, the patient may receive methadone. Temporary administration of tranquilizers and sedatives may aid in reducing patient anxiety and craving for the opiate agonist.

◆ *Drug interactions*

> **Medication Safety Alert**
>
> A US Food and Drug Administration (FDA) review has found that the combined use of opioid medicines with benzodiazepines or other drugs that depress the CNS resulted in serious adverse reactions, including slowed or difficult breathing and deaths.

Central nervous system depressants. General anesthetics, phenothiazines, tranquilizers, sedative-hypnotics, tricyclic antidepressants, antihistamines, and alcohol enhance the depressant effects of opiate agonists. Respiratory depression, hypotension, and profound sedation or coma may result from this interaction unless the dosage of the opiate agonist has been reduced appropriately, usually by one-third to one-half the normal dosage.

Phenytoin. Phenytoin is an enzyme-inducing agent that may enhance the metabolism of meperidine to normeperidine. The dosage of meperidine may have to be increased for appropriate analgesia if used concurrently with phenytoin. Observe the patient closely and provide protection for the development of seizure activity secondary to increased normeperidine levels.

Carbamazepine. Carbamazepine may enhance the metabolism of tramadol, reducing its analgesic effect.

If used concurrently, the dosage of tramadol may need to be increased for appropriate analgesia.

Selective serotonin reuptake inhibitors, tricyclic antidepressants, monoamine oxidase inhibitors. All these agents increase serotonin levels, potentially causing serotonin syndrome when taken by a person receiving tramadol or tapentadol. These medicines should be used only under the supervision of the prescriber. There should be a 14-day washout period after discontinuation of monoamine oxidase inhibitors before starting tramadol or tapentadol therapy.

Warfarin. The oral anticoagulant effect of warfarin may be increased by tramadol. Carefully monitor the prothrombin time and international normalized ratio and adjust the dosage of warfarin as needed when tramadol is initiated or discontinued.

DRUG CLASS: OPIATE PARTIAL AGONISTS

Actions

Opiate partial agonists (e.g., buprenorphine, butorphanol, nalbuphine, pentazocine) are an interesting class of drugs because their pharmacologic actions depend on whether an opiate agonist has been administered previously and the extent to which physical dependence has developed to that opiate agonist. When used without prior administration of opiate agonists, the opiate partial agonists are effective analgesics. Their potency during the first few weeks of therapy is similar to that of morphine; however, after prolonged use, tolerance may develop. Increasing the dosage does not significantly increase the analgesia but definitely increases the incidence of adverse effects. This is called a *ceiling effect* because, contrary to the action of the opiate agonists, a larger dose does not produce a significantly greater analgesic effect.

If an opiate partial agonist is given to a patient with physical dependence on an opiate agonist such as morphine or meperidine, the opiate partial agonist will induce withdrawal symptoms. If the patient is not physically dependent on the opiate agonist, there is no interaction and the patient will be relieved of pain.

Uses

Opiate partial agonists may be used for the short-term relief (up to 3 weeks) of moderate to severe pain associated with cancer, burns, and renal colic, as well as for preoperative analgesia and obstetric and surgical analgesia. Nalbuphine has minimal physical dependence liability and is not a controlled substance. Because nalbuphine has a ceiling effect for analgesia and respiratory depression, it is often used as an analgesic for obstetric patients.

Therapeutic Outcomes

The primary therapeutic outcomes from opiate partial agonist therapy are as follows:
1. Relief of pain intensity and reduced duration of pain complaint

2. Prevention of the conversion of persistent pain to chronic pain
3. Prevention of suffering and disability associated with pain
4. Prevention of psychological and socioeconomic consequences associated with inadequate pain management
5. Control of adverse effects associated with pain management
6. Optimization of the ability to perform ADLs

❖ **Nursing Implications for Opiate Partial Agonists**
◆ *Premedication assessment*
1. Perform baseline neurologic assessment (e.g., orientation to date, time, and place; mental alertness; bilateral hand grip; and motor functioning).
2. Obtain vital signs; hold medication if respirations are below 12 breaths/min, or according to age-related respiratory parameters, and consult with healthcare provider.
3. Check bowel sounds and note consistency of stools. Review voiding pattern and urine output.
4. Check for prior use of opiate agonists.
5. Perform pain assessment before administration of the opiate agonist and at appropriate intervals during therapy. Report poor pain control promptly to the healthcare provider and obtain modification in orders.

◆ *Availability, dosage, and administration.* See Table 19.2.
Antidotes. Naloxone and naltrexone reverse the effects of opiate partial agonists.

◆ *Common adverse effects*
Neurologic
Clamminess, dizziness, sedation, sweating. These effects tend to occur most often with the initial dose. Symptoms can be reduced by keeping the patient supine. Provide patient safety, assurance, and comfort.
Gastrointestinal
Nausea, vomiting, dry mouth. These effects tend to occur most often with the initial dose. Symptoms can be reduced by keeping the patient supine. Provide patient safety, assurance, and comfort.
Constipation. Continued use may cause constipation. Maintain the patient's state of hydration and obtain an order for stool softeners or bulk-forming laxatives if necessary. Encourage the inclusion of sufficient roughage, fresh fruits, vegetables, and whole-grain products in the diet.

◆ *Serious adverse effects*
Neurologic
Confusion, disorientation, hallucinations. Butorphanol and pentazocine, and to a lesser degree nalbuphine, may produce hallucinations. Patients may complain of seeing multicolored flashing patterns or animals, with and without sound, or may have very vivid dreams. These adverse effects have been reported after only

one or two doses of medication and may occur in as many as one-third of patients taking butorphanol or pentazocine.
Perform a baseline assessment of the patient's degree of alertness and orientation to name, place, and time before initiating therapy. Make regularly scheduled subsequent evaluations of mental status, and report alterations from baseline. Provide for patient safety during these episodes. If recurring, seek a change in the medication order.
Respiratory
Respiratory depression. Opiate partial agonists make the respiratory centers less sensitive to carbon dioxide, causing respiratory depression. This may occur before the reduction in respiratory rate or tidal volume is noticeable. Check the respiratory rate and depth often.
Psychological
Excessive use or abuse. Repeated use may lead to tolerance and physical dependence. Evaluate the patient's response to the analgesic. Identify underlying needs and plan for more appropriate management of those needs. Discuss the case with the healthcare provider and make plans to approach gradual withdrawal of the medications being abused cooperatively. Suggest a change to a milder analgesic when indicated.
The patient does not have to experience symptoms of withdrawal to be treated for physical dependence, which is usually a gradual reduction of the daily opiate agonist dosage. If withdrawal symptoms become severe, the patient may receive methadone. Temporary administration of tranquilizers and sedatives may aid in reducing patient anxiety and craving for the opiate agonist.

◆ *Drug interactions*
Central nervous system depressants. General anesthetics, phenothiazines, tranquilizers, sedative-hypnotics, tricyclic antidepressants, antihistamines, and alcohol enhance the depressant effects of the opiate partial agonists. Respiratory depression, hypotension, and profound sedation or coma may result from this interaction unless the dosage of the opiate partial agonist has been reduced appropriately, usually by one-third to one-half the normal dosage.
Opiate agonists. Opiate partial agonists have weak antagonist activity. When administered to patients who have been receiving opiate agonists such as morphine or meperidine on a regular basis, it may precipitate withdrawal symptoms.

DRUG CLASS: OPIATE ANTAGONISTS

naloxone (năl-ŎKS-ōn)
Evzio (ev-zee' oh)

Actions
Naloxone is a so-called pure opiate antagonist because it has no other known effect than reversal of the CNS

Table 19.2 **Opiate Partial Agonists**

GENERIC NAME	BRAND NAME	AVAILABILITY	ADULT DOSAGE RANGE	DURATION (HR)	DOSAGE EQUIVALENT TO MORPHINE (10 MG)
buprenorphine	Buprenex	Tablets, sublingual: 2, 8 mg Injection: 0.3 mg/mL in 1-mL ampules	0.3 mg q 6-8h	6	IM/IV: 0.4 mg
	Butrans	Patch (weekly): 5, 7.5, 10, 15, 20 mcg/hr			
	Belbuca	Buccal Film: 75, 150, 300, 450, 600, 750, 900 mcg	75 mcg daily, may increase every 4 days		
	Probuphine Implant	Subcut Implant: 74.2 mg			
buprenorphine/ naloxone	Suboxone	Sublingual Film: 2/0.5, 4/1, 8/2, 12/3 mg buprenorphine/ naloxone	2/0.5 mg q2h		
	Bunavail	Buccal Film: 2.1/0.3, 4.2/0.7, 6.3/1 mg buprenorphine/ naloxone	2.1/0.3 mg q2h		
	Zubsolv	Tablets, sublingual: 0.7/0.18, 1.4/0.36, 2.9/0.71, 5.7/1.4, 8.6/2.1, 11.4/2.9 mg buprenorphine/ naloxone	1.4/0.36 mg q1.5-2h		
butorphanol	—	Injection: 1, 2 mg in 1-, 2-, 10-mL vials Nasal spray: 10 mg/mL	IM: 2 mg, repeat in 3-4 hr; maximum dosage, 4 mg IV: 1 mg, repeat in 3-4 hr Nasal: 1 spray in each nostril repeated in 3-4 hr	IM: 3-4	IM: 2 mg
nalbuphine	—	Injection: 10, 20 mg/mL in 1-, 10-mL vials	Subcut, IM, IV: 10 mg/70 kg, repeat q3-6h; maximum daily dosage, 160 mg	3-6	IM/IV/subcut: 10 mg
pentazocine	Talwin	Injection: 30 mg/mL in 1-, 10-mL vials Tablets (with naloxone 0.5 mg):[a] 50 mg	PO: 50-100 mg q3-4h; do not exceed 600 mg daily Subcut, IM, IV: 30 mg q3-4h; maximum daily dosage, 360 mg	4-5	30-60 mg

[a]Tablets contain naloxone to prevent abuse.

depressant effects of opiate agonists and opiate partial agonists. When administered to patients who have not recently received opiates, there is no respiratory depression, psychotomimetic effect, circulatory change, or other pharmacologic activity. If administered to a person addicted to opiate agonists or opiate partial agonists, withdrawal symptoms may be precipitated.

Uses

Naloxone is a drug of choice for treatment of respiratory depression when excessive doses of opiate agonists or opiate partial agonists have been administered, or when the causative agent is unknown. Naloxone is not effective in reversing CNS depression induced by tranquilizers or sedative-hypnotics. Naloxone has been added to pentazocine formulations to reduce its abuse by blocking the euphoric high associated with pentazocine.

Many emergency services (police, fire, ambulance) across the nation now carry prefilled syringes of naloxone (Evzio) to administer to patients emergently for potential overdoses of opiates (heroin, morphine, oxycodone, hydromorphone). This is similar to EpiPen or Auvi-Q use in acute anaphylaxis resulting from allergens (e.g., bee stings).

Therapeutic Outcomes

The primary therapeutic outcome expected from naloxone is reversal of respiratory depression secondary to opiate overdose.

❖ Nursing Implications for Naloxone

◆ Premedication assessment

1. Perform baseline neurologic assessment (e.g., orientation to date, time, and place; mental alertness; bilateral hand grip; and motor functioning).
2. Monitor vital signs; blood pressure, pulse, and respirations should be taken at frequent intervals until resolution of CNS depression. Then schedule vital signs to be taken at appropriate intervals because the duration of action of naloxone is short.
3. Check prior use of or dependence on opiate agonists or opiate partial agonists. Diagnostic testing for narcotic dependence may be performed in accordance with policies of the clinical site. Inform patient of risks involved.
4. Have supportive equipment available in immediate area to maintain respirations.
5. Check bowel sounds. Review voiding pattern and urine output.

◆ Availability.
Injection: 0.4 mg/mL in 1-mL prefilled syringes; 1 mg/mL in 2-mL prefilled syringes and 1- and 10-mL vials; 0.4, 2 mg in 0.4-mL prefilled autoinjector. *Nasal solution:* 4 mg/0.1 mL.

◆ Dosage and administration.
Adult: *IV: Postoperative opiate depression:* 0.1 to 0.2 mg every 2 to 3 minutes until the desired response is achieved.

Adult: *IM: Opiate overdose:* 0.4 to 2 mg every 2 to 3 minutes. If no response is seen after 10 minutes, the depressive condition may be caused by a drug or disease process not responsive to naloxone.

Adult: *Intranasal: Opiate overdose:* 4 mg (contents of 1 nasal spray) as a single dose in one nostril; may repeat every 2 to 3 minutes in alternating nostrils.

◆ Common adverse effects.
Naloxone rarely manifests any adverse effects. In rare cases when extremely high doses have been used, mental depression, apathy, inability to concentrate, sleepiness, irritability, anorexia, nausea, and vomiting have been reported. These adverse effects usually occurred in the first few days of treatment and dissipated rapidly with continued therapy.

Cardiovascular. Use with caution in patients with cardiovascular disease or in patients taking cardiovascular medicines (e.g., antihypertensives, antiarrhythmics). Abrupt reversal of opiate overdose by opioid antagonists may cause arrhythmias, pulmonary edema, and ventricular fibrillation.

Neurologic

Mental depression, apathy. Be aware of the potential for suicidal thoughts or suicide. Inform the healthcare provider immediately if the patient has any new or worsening symptoms of depression.

Gastrointestinal

Nausea, vomiting. Naloxone should be used with caution following the use of opiates during surgery because it may result in excitement, increased blood pressure, and a clinically important reversal of analgesia. The early reversal of opiate effects may induce nausea, vomiting, sweating, and tachycardia.

Naloxone should be given with caution to patients known or suspected to be physically dependent on opioids, including neonates born to women who are opiate dependent, because the drug may precipitate severe withdrawal symptoms. The severity of the symptoms depends on the dose of naloxone and the degree of dependence.

◆ Drug interactions.
There are no drug interactions other than that of the antagonist activity toward opiate agonists and opiate partial agonists.

---

naltrexone (năl-TRĔKS-ōn)
   Revia (rē-VĒ-ă) ♣ Available in Canada.
   Vivitrol (viv ih-trol')

Actions

Naltrexone is a pure opioid antagonist closely related to naloxone. It differs, however, in that it is active after oral administration and has a considerably longer duration of action. Naltrexone blocks the effects of opioids by competing for binding sites at opioid receptors. The mechanism of action of naltrexone in patients with alcoholism is not known.

Uses

Naltrexone is used clinically to block the pharmacologic effects of exogenously administered opiates in patients who are enrolled in drug abuse treatment programs. Naltrexone may diminish or eliminate opiate-seeking behavior by blocking the euphoric reinforcement produced by self-administration of opioids and by preventing the conditioned abstinence syndrome (i.e., opiate craving) that occurs after opiate withdrawal.

Naltrexone is also used as an adjunct in the treatment of alcoholism to support abstinence and reduce relapse rates and alcohol consumption. It must be used with other treatment forms such as group and behavior therapy; the expected effect of the drug treatment is a modest improvement in the outcome of conventional treatment.

Therapeutic Outcomes

The primary therapeutic outcomes expected from naltrexone are as follows:

1. Improved adherence with a substance abuse treatment program by reducing the craving for opioids
2. Improved adherence with an alcohol abuse treatment program by diminishing the craving for alcohol

❖ Nursing Implications for Naltrexone

◆ *Premedication assessment*

1. Perform baseline neurologic assessment (e.g., orientation to date, time, and place; mental alertness; bilateral hand grip; and motor functioning).
2. Monitor vital signs: temperature, blood pressure, pulse, and respirations.
3. Check laboratory values for hepatotoxicity; urine screen for opiate use.
4. Monitor for GI symptoms before and during therapy.
5. The manufacturer recommends that baseline determinations of liver function should be obtained in all patients before initiating therapy and repeated monthly for the next 6 months.
6. The manufacturer recommends a minimum of 7 to 10 days of abstinence from all opiates, a urinalysis to confirm the absence of opiates, and the use of a naloxone challenge test to ensure that the patient will not develop withdrawal symptoms.

◆ *Availability. PO:* 50-mg tablets.

IM: 380 mg/vial suspension, extended-release injection.

◆ *Dosage and administration*

Behavior modification. Naltrexone therapy in combination with behavior therapy is more effective than naltrexone or behavior therapy alone in prolonging opiate or alcohol cessation in patients formerly physically dependent on opiates or alcohol.

Treatment of opiate agonist dependence. *PO:* Induction dose of 25 mg. Observe for development of withdrawal symptoms. If none occur, administer 50 mg the next day. The maintenance regimen is 50 mg daily. Alternative regimens of 100 mg every other day or 150 mg every third day have been used to improve adherence during a behavior modification program (see Chapter 48).

Withdrawal symptoms. Naltrexone may precipitate acute and severe withdrawal symptoms in patients who are physically dependent on opioids. Addicts must be completely detoxified and opioid free before taking naltrexone. The manufacturer recommends a minimum of 7 to 10 days of abstinence from all opiates, a urinalysis to confirm the absence of opiates, and the use of a naloxone challenge test to ensure that the patient will not develop withdrawal symptoms.

Patients undergoing naltrexone therapy must be carefully instructed about the expectations of behavior modification associated with therapy. They should also

be advised that self-administration of small doses of opiates (e.g., heroin) during naltrexone therapy will not result in any euphoric effect and that large doses may result in serious adverse effects, including coma and death. Patients should also be given identification to notify medical personnel that they are taking a long-acting opiate antagonist.

Treatment of alcoholism. *PO:* 50 mg once daily (see also Chapter 48).

IM: 380 mg IM every 4 weeks as a gluteal injection, alternating buttocks.

◆ *Common adverse effects.* Many adverse effects have been associated with naltrexone therapy, but it is difficult to know exactly which ones are secondary to naltrexone alone because some patients may experience mild opiate withdrawal symptoms as well. The adverse effects of drug and alcohol abuse and poor nutritional states may contribute to the patient's discomfort.

Gastrointestinal

Nausea, vomiting, anorexia. Adverse effects are usually mild and tend to resolve with continued therapy. Encourage the patient not to discontinue therapy without first consulting the healthcare provider and treatment program.

Neurologic

Headache. Adverse effects are usually mild and tend to resolve with continued therapy. Encourage the patient not to discontinue therapy without first consulting the healthcare provider and treatment program.

◆ *Serious adverse effects*

Gastrointestinal

Hepatotoxicity. Hepatotoxicity has been reported after doses of 300 mg daily for 3 to 8 weeks. The symptoms of hepatotoxicity are jaundice, nausea, vomiting, anorexia, hepatomegaly, splenomegaly, and abnormal liver function test results (e.g., elevated bilirubin, aspartate aminotransferase [AST], alanine aminotransferase [ALT], and alkaline phosphatase levels; increased prothrombin time). Because many of these patients do not develop clinical symptoms but do develop abnormal liver function, strongly encourage patients to report for blood tests as scheduled. Report abnormal values to the appropriate healthcare provider.

◆ *Drug interactions*

Opioid-containing products. Patients taking naltrexone will probably not benefit from opioid-containing medicines such as analgesics, cough and cold preparations, and antidiarrheal preparations. These products should be avoided during naltrexone therapy when nonopiate therapy is available.

Clonidine. Clonidine may be administered in patients to reduce the severity of withdrawal symptoms precipitated or exacerbated by naltrexone.

DRUG CLASS: PROSTAGLANDIN INHIBITORS

acetaminophen (ă-sĕt-ă-MĬN-ō-fĕn)
    Tylenol (TĬ-lĕ-nŏl)

Actions

Acetaminophen is a synthetic nonopiate analgesic that works by prostaglandin inhibition in the CNS and blocks generation of pain impulses in the peripheral tissue. Control of elevated body temperature (antipyresis) results from inhibition of the heat-regulating center in the hypothalamus. Antipyretic effectiveness and analgesic potency are similar to those of aspirin in equal doses.

Uses

Acetaminophen is an effective analgesic-antipyretic for discomfort associated with bacterial and viral infections, headache, and musculoskeletal pain. It is a good substitute for patients who cannot take products containing aspirin because of allergic reactions; hypersensitivities; anticoagulant therapy; or possible bleeding problems from gastric or duodenal ulcers, gastritis, and hiatus hernia. This drug has no antiinflammatory activity and is therefore ineffective (other than as an analgesic) for the relief of symptoms of rheumatoid arthritis or other inflammation.

Therapeutic Outcomes

The primary therapeutic outcomes expected from acetaminophen are reduced pain and fever.

❖ Nursing Implications for Acetaminophen
◆ Premedication assessment

1. Take vital signs: temperature, blood pressure, pulse, and respirations.
2. Check laboratory data for hepatotoxicity or nephrotoxicity.
3. Monitor for GI symptoms before and during therapy.
4. Check bowel sounds and review voiding pattern and urine output.
5. When used as an analgesic, perform pain assessment before administering acetaminophen and at appropriate intervals during therapy. Report poor pain control promptly to the healthcare provider and obtain modification in orders.
6. When used as an antipyretic, take baseline temperature and continue monitoring temperature at appropriate intervals (e.g., every 2 to 4 hours, depending on severity of temperature elevation).

◆ Availability. PO: 325- and 500-mg caplets; 325- and 500-mg capsules and tablets; 80- and 160-mg chewable tablets; 650-mg extended-release tablets; 80- and 160-mg dispersible tablets; 80 mg/0.8 mL, 160 mg/5 mL, 500 mg/15 mL, and 650 mg/20.3 mL liquid.
Rectal: 80-, 120-, 325-, or 650-mg suppositories.
IV: 10 mg/mL solution in 100-mL vial.
To avoid toxicity, it is recommended that the adult receive no more than 4 g of acetaminophen daily. Patients who are chronic alcoholics should take no more than 2 g per day. The American Geriatrics Society guideline on the management of persistent pain recommends a prudent approach of less than 3 g per day.

◆ *Dosage and administration.* **Adult:** *PO:* 325 to 650 mg every 4 to 6 hours. Doses up to 1000 mg may be given four times daily for short-term therapy. Maximum dose is 3250 mg **daily** unless directed by healthcare provider; under healthcare provider supervision, do not exceed 4 g daily. *IV: Greater than 50 kg:* 1 g every 6 hours. Do not exceed 4 g in 24 hours. *Less than 50 kg:* 15 mg/kg (up to 750 mg) as a single dose and 75 mg/kg (up to 3750 mg) in 24 hours.

Pediatric: *PO:* 0 to 3 months, 40 mg; 4 to 11 months, 80 mg; 12 to 24 months, 120 mg; 2 to 3 years, 160 mg; 4 to 5 years, 240 mg; 6 to 8 years, 320 mg; 9 to 10 years, 400 mg; 11 to 12 years, 480 mg; older than 14 years, 650 mg. *Rectal:* 6 to 11 months: 80 mg every 6 hours, maximum daily dose: 320 mg; 12 to 36 months: 80 mg every 4 to 6 hours, maximum daily dose: 400 mg; 4 to 6 years: 120 mg every 4 to 6 hours, maximum daily dose: 600 mg; 7 up to 12 years: 325 mg every 4 to 6 hours, maximum daily dose: 1625 mg. *IV:* 15 mg/kg as a single dose and 75 mg/kg in 24 hours. *13 years of age and older, 50 kg or more:* 1000 mg every 6 hours or 650 mg every 4 hours. Do not exceed 1000 mg as a single dose and 4000 mg in 24 hours. *13 years and older, less than 50 kg:* 15 mg/kg every 6 hours or 12.5 mg/kg every 4 hours. Do not exceed 15 mg/kg (up to 750 mg) as a single dose and 75 mg/kg (up to 3750 mg) in 24 hours.

Antidote. The antidote is acetylcysteine.

◆ *Common adverse effects.* When used as directed, acetaminophen is extremely well tolerated.
Gastrointestinal
Gastric irritation. If gastric irritation occurs, administer medication with food, milk, antacids, or large amounts of water. If symptoms persist or increase in severity, report for healthcare provider evaluation.

◆ *Serious adverse effects*
Gastrointestinal
Hepatotoxicity. Overdosage caused by acute and chronic ingestion has risen dramatically in the past few years. Severe life-threatening hepatotoxicity has been reported in patients who ingest 5 to 8 g daily for several weeks or attempt suicide by consuming large quantities at one time. Hepatotoxicity is also more frequent with heavy alcohol use and ingestion of acetaminophen.

Early indications of toxicity include anorexia, nausea, vomiting, low blood pressure, drowsiness, confusion, and abdominal pain—symptoms often attributed to other causes. Within 2 to 4 days, symptoms of hepatotoxicity develop (jaundice and a rise in the AST and ALT levels and prothrombin time). If acetaminophen toxicity is suspected, consult the manufacturer, a university drug information center, or a poison control center for the most current recommendations for therapy.

◆ *Drug interactions*

Phenobarbital, carbamazepine, phenytoin, sulfinpyrazone. If acetaminophen is taken in large doses or over the long term, these agents may enhance hepatotoxicity.

Alcohol. Chronic excessive ingestion of alcohol may increase the potential for hepatotoxicity with therapeutic doses or overdoses of acetaminophen.

---

salicylates (săl-ĭ-SĬL-āts)

Actions

Salicylates are the most common analgesics used for the relief of slight to moderate pain. Salicylates were introduced into medicine in the late 19th century because of their three primary pharmacologic effects as analgesic, antipyretic, and antiinflammatory agents. Although the mechanisms of action are not fully known, most of the activity of salicylates comes from inhibiting prostaglandin synthesis. Salicylates inhibit the formation of prostaglandins that sensitize pain receptors to stimulation causing pain (analgesia), they inhibit the prostaglandins that produce the signs and symptoms of inflammation (e.g., redness, swelling, warmth), and they inhibit the synthesis and release of prostaglandins in the brain that cause the elevation of body temperature (antipyresis). A major benefit of salicylates is that they do not dull the consciousness level and do not cause mental sluggishness, memory disturbances, hallucinations, euphoria, or sedation.

A unique property of aspirin, compared with other salicylates, is inhibition of platelet aggregation and enhancement of bleeding time. The platelet loses its ability to aggregate and form clots for the duration of its lifetime (7 to 10 days). The mechanism of action is inhibition of the synthesis of thromboxane A_2, a potent vasoconstrictor and inducer of platelet aggregation.

Uses

The combination of pharmacologic effects makes salicylates the drug of choice for symptomatic relief of discomfort, pain, inflammation, or fever associated with bacterial and viral infections, headache, muscle aches, and rheumatoid arthritis. Salicylates can be taken to relieve pain on a long-term basis without causing drug dependence. The use of salicylates in children is not recommended because of the associated risk of Reye's syndrome.

Because of its antiplatelet activity, aspirin is also indicated for reducing the risk of recurrent transient ischemic attacks or stroke. Aspirin is also used to reduce the risk of MI in patients with previous MI or unstable angina pectoris. Aspirin is administered on arrival to the emergency room to those patients experiencing an acute MI.

Therapeutic Outcomes

The primary therapeutic outcomes expected from salicylates are reduced pain, reduced inflammation, and elimination of fever. The primary therapeutic outcomes expected from aspirin when used for antiplatelet therapy are reduced frequency of transient ischemic attack, stroke, or MI.

❖ **Nursing Implications for Salicylates**

◆ *Premedication assessment*

1. Perform baseline neurologic assessment (e.g., orientation to date, time, and place; mental alertness; bilateral hand grip; motor functioning).
2. Monitor vital signs (i.e., temperature, blood pressure, pulse, respirations).
3. Check laboratory values for hepatotoxicity, renal impairment, and clotting time.
4. Monitor for GI symptoms before and during therapy; conduct stool guaiac test if GI tract bleeding is suspected.
5. Check for concurrent use of anticoagulant agents.
6. If the patient is taking oral hypoglycemics, review baseline serum glucose level.
7. When used as an analgesic, perform pain assessment before administering salicylates and at appropriate intervals during therapy. Report poor pain control promptly to the healthcare provider and obtain modification in orders.

◆ *Availability.* See Tables 19.3 and 19.4.

◆ *Dosage and administration*

Treatment of pain, arthritis, acute rheumatic fever, and myocardial infarction prophylaxis. See Table 19.3.

Stroke prevention. See Table 19.3.

◆ *Common adverse effects.* As beneficial as salicylates are, they are not without adverse effects. In normal therapeutic dosages, they may produce GI irritation, occasional nausea, and gastric hemorrhage. Extreme caution should be used with administration to patients with a history of peptic ulcer, liver disease, or coagulation disorders.

Gastrointestinal

Gastric irritation. If gastric irritation occurs, give medication with food, milk, or antacids (1 hour later) or with large amounts of water. If symptoms persist or increase in severity, notify the healthcare provider. Aspirin is available in an enteric-coated form to reduce gastric irritation.

◆ *Serious adverse effects*

Gastrointestinal

Gastrointestinal bleeding. Dark, tarry stools and bright red or coffee-ground emesis may occur. Test any suspect stools or emesis for the presence of occult blood.

Toxicity

Salicylism. Patients receiving higher doses on a continuing basis are susceptible to developing salicylate intoxication (salicylism). Symptoms include tinnitus (ringing in the ears), impaired hearing, dimming of vision, sweating, fever, lethargy, dizziness, mental confusion, nausea, and vomiting. This condition is reversible on dosage reduction. Massive overdosage may lead to respiratory depression and coma. There is no antidote; primary treatment is discontinuing the drug, gastric lavage, forcing IV fluids, and alkalizing the urine with IV sodium bicarbonate.

Table 19.3 Nonsteroidal Antiinflammatory Drugs

GENERIC NAME	BRAND NAME	AVAILABILITY	USES AND DOSAGES	MAXIMUM DAILY DOSAGE (MG)
Salicylates				
aspirin	Ecotrin, St. Joseph	Tablets: 81, 325, 500 mg Tablets, sustained release: 81, 162, 325, 500 mg Tablets, chewable: 81 mg Suppositories: 60, 120, 200, 300, 600 mg	Minor aches and pains: 325-600 mg q4h Arthritis: 2.6-5.2 g/day in divided doses Acute rheumatic fever: 7.8 g/day Myocardial infarction prophylaxis: 75-325 mg daily Ischemic stroke and TIA: 50-325 mg daily	—
diflunisal		Tablets: 500 mg	Mild to moderate pain: Initially, 1000 mg, then 500 mg q8h Osteoarthritis and rheumatoid arthritis: 250-500 mg twice daily	1500
magnesium salicylate	Doan's	Tablets: 325, 580 mg	Mild aches and pains: 580-650 mg three or four times daily	4640
salsalate	—	Tablets: 500, 750 mg	Mild pain: 500-700 mg four to six times daily	3000
Nonsteroidal Antiinflammatory Drugs				
Cyclooxygenase-1 (COX-1) Inhibitors				
diclofenac	Cataflam, Voltaren Teva-Diclofenac 🍁	Tablets: 50 mg Tablets, delayed release (24 hr): 25, 50, 75, 100 mg Capsules: 18, 25, 35 mg	Rheumatoid and osteoarthritis, ankylosing spondylitis: 25-50 mg two or three times daily Primary dysmenorrhea: 50 mg three times daily	200
	Flector — Voltaren	Patch, transdermal: 1.3% Gel, transdermal: 3% Gel, transdermal: 1%	Apply to pain site twice daily. Do not apply to broken skin. For actinic keratoses: Apply twice daily. Avoid direct sun exposure. Osteoarthritis: Apply to affected arm, hand, foot, and knee joints four times daily. Do not apply to spine, hips, or shoulders.	
etodolac	—	Capsules: 200, 300 mg Tablets: 400, 500 mg Tablets, extended release: 400, 500, 600 mg	Osteoarthritis, pain: 300-400 mg three or four times daily	1200
fenoprofen	Nalfon	Capsules: 200, 400 mg Tablets: 600 mg	Rheumatoid and osteoarthritis: 300-600 mg three or four times daily Mild to moderate pain: 200 mg q4-6h	3200
flurbiprofen	—	Tablets: 50, 100 mg	Rheumatoid and osteoarthritis: 50-100 mg two or three times daily	300
ibuprofen	Motrin, Advil Apo-Ibuprofen 🍁	Tablets: 100, 200, 400, 600, 800 mg Tablets, chewable: 100, mg Capsules: 200 mg Suspension: 40 mg/mL, 50 mg/1.25 mL; 100 mg/5 mL IV: 10 mg/mL; 800 mg/8 mL	Rheumatoid and osteoarthritis: 300-600 mg three or four times daily Mild to moderate pain: 400 mg q4-6h Primary dysmenorrhea: 400 mg q4h Fever: Pediatric: 5-10 mg/kg three or four times daily	3200

Table 19.3   Nonsteroidal Antiinflammatory Drugs—cont'd

GENERIC NAME	BRAND NAME	AVAILABILITY	USES AND DOSAGES	MAXIMUM DAILY DOSAGE (MG)
indomethacin	Indocin Teva-Indomethacin ♣	Capsules: 25, 50 mg Capsules, sustained release: 75 mg Oral suspension: 25 mg/5 mL Suppository: 50 mg IV: 1 mg/mL/vial	Rheumatoid and osteoarthritis, ankylosing spondylitis: 25-50 mg three or four times daily Acute painful shoulder: 25-50 mg two or three times daily Acute gouty arthritis: 50 mg three times daily Closure of patent ductus arteriosus: IV, one to three doses at 12- to 24-hr intervals	200 for immediate release; 150 for sustained release
ketoprofen	Nu-Ketoprofen ♣	Capsules: 25, 50, 75 mg Capsules, extended release (24 hr): 200 mg	Rheumatoid and osteoarthritis: Initially, 75 mg three times daily or 50 mg four times daily; reduce initial dose by $\frac{1}{2}$ to $\frac{1}{3}$ in older patients or those with impaired renal function Mild pain, primary dysmenorrhea: 25-50 mg three or four times daily	300
ketorolac ❶	Apo-Ketorolac ♣	Tablets: 10 mg Injection 15 mg/mL in 1-mL vial and 30 mg/mL in vials and syringe; IM 60 mg/2 mL in 2-mL vials	Analgesic, antiinflammatory, antipyretic used for acute, short-term pain management: IM 60 mg or IV 30 mg, initially, 15-30 mg q6h PRN for pain; then PO, up to 40 mg/24 hr; do not exceed 5 days of therapy	120-150
meclofenamate	—	Capsules: 50, 100 mg	Rheumatoid and osteoarthritis: 200-400 mg daily in three or four equal doses Mild to moderate pain: 50-100 mg three or four times daily Primary dysmenorrhea: 100 mg three times daily	400
mefenamic acid	— PMS-Mefenamic acid ♣	Capsules: 250 mg	Moderate pain or primary dysmenorrhea: Initially 500 mg, then 250 mg q6h; do not exceed 7 days of therapy	1000
meloxicam	Mobic	Tablets: 7.5, 15 mg Capsules: 5, 10 mg	Osteoarthritis: 7.5-15 mg daily	15
nabumetone	—	Tablets: 500, 750 mg	Rheumatoid and osteoarthritis: 1000-1500 mg daily in one or two doses	2000
naproxen	Naprosyn, Aleve, Anaprox DS	Tablets: 220, 250, 275, 375, 500, 550 mg Tablets, extended release (24 hr): 375, 500, 750 mg Capsules: 220 mg Oral suspension: 125 mg/5 mL	Rheumatoid arthritis, osteoarthritis, ankylosing spondylitis: 250-375 mg twice daily Acute gout: 750-825 mg initially, followed by 250-275 mg q8h Moderate pain, primary dysmenorrhea, acute tendonitis, bursitis: 500-550 mg followed by 250-275 mg	1000
oxaprozin	Daypro	Caplets: 600 mg	Rheumatoid arthritis, osteoarthritis: 1200 mg once daily	1800

Table 19.3 Nonsteroidal Antiinflammatory Drugs—cont'd

GENERIC NAME	BRAND NAME	AVAILABILITY	USES AND DOSAGES	MAXIMUM DAILY DOSAGE (MG)
piroxicam	Feldene Teva-Pirocam ♣	Capsules: 10, 20 mg	Rheumatoid arthritis osteoarthritis: 20 mg once daily	200
sulindac	Apo-Sulin ♣	Tablets: 150, 200 mg	Rheumatoid arthritis, osteoarthritis, ankylosing spondylitis: 150 mg twice daily Acute painful shoulder: 200 mg twice daily	400
tolmetin	—	Tablets: 200, 600 mg Capsules: 400 mg	Rheumatoid arthritis, osteoarthritis: 400-600 mg three times daily	2000
Cyclooxygenase-2 (COX-2) Inhibitors				
celecoxib	Celebrex Apo-Celecoxib ♣	Capsules: 50, 100, 200, 400 mg	Rheumatoid arthritis, osteoarthritis: 100-200 mg twice daily Ankylosing spondylitis: 200-400 mg daily Acute pain and primary dysmenorrhea: 400 mg initially, followed by 200 mg on the first day, then 200 mg twice daily Familial adenomatous polyposis: 400 mg twice daily taken with food	—

♣ Available in Canada; ❶ High-alert medication.
TIA, Transient ischemic attack.

Table 19.4 Ingredients of Selected Analgesic Combination Products

PRODUCT	NONCONTROLLED SUBSTANCE			CONTROLLED SUBSTANCE	
	ASPIRIN (mg)	ACETAMINOPHEN[a] (mg)	OTHER (mg)	CODEINE (mg)	OTHER (mg)
Anacin caplets and tablets	400	—	Caffeine, 32	—	—
Anacin Maximum Strength	500	—	Caffeine, 32	—	—
BC Powder Arthritis Strength	742	—	Caffeine, 38 Salicylamide, 222	—	—
Excedrin Extra Strength	250	250	Caffeine, 65	—	—
Fioricet		300	Caffeine, 40	—	Butalbital, 50
Fiorinal	325	—	Caffeine, 40	—	Butalbital, 50
Fiorinal with Codeine	325	—	Caffeine, 40	30	Butalbital, 50
Lorcet HD	—	325	—	—	Hydrocodone, 10
Norco	—	325	—	—	Hydrocodone, 10
Percocet 7.5	—	325	—	—	Oxycodone, 7.5
Percogesic	—	325	Diphenhydramine, 12.5	—	—
Tylenol	—	325	—	—	—
with Codeine No. 3	—	300	—	30	—
with Codeine No. 4	—	300	—	60	—
Vicodin	—	300	—	—	Hydrocodone, 5
Vicodin ES	—	300	—	—	Hydrocodone, 7.5
Vicodin HP	—	300	—	—	Hydrocodone, 10 mg

[a]As of January 2014, acetaminophen content in combination products is limited to a maximum of 325 mg per tablet or capsule.

Patients who develop signs of salicylate toxicity should be reevaluated for other underlying diseases and the possibility that other medications would be more effective.

◆ *Drug interactions*

Nonsteroidal antiinflammatory drugs. It is possible that cyclooxygenase-1 (COX-1) inhibitors reduce the platelet-inhibiting effects of aspirin when administered at about the same time. The NSAID may block the receptor on platelets that aspirin would normally bind to, preventing the platelet inhibition caused by aspirin. One approach to avoid this interaction is to take aspirin several hours before the COX-1 NSAID. This might not be possible for a patient with severe rheumatoid arthritis who needs the analgesic effects around the clock.

Sulfinpyrazone, probenecid. Salicylates inhibit the excretion of uric acid by these agents. Although an occasional aspirin will not interfere with their effectiveness, regular use of salicylates or products containing salicylate should be discouraged. If analgesia is required, suggest acetaminophen.

Warfarin. Salicylates may enhance the anticoagulant effects of warfarin. Observe for petechiae; ecchymoses; nosebleeds; bleeding gums; dark, tarry stools; and bright red or coffee-ground emesis. Monitor prothrombin time and reduce the dosage of warfarin if necessary.

Valproic acid. Monitor the patient with concurrent therapy for signs of valproic acid toxicity, such as sedation or lethargy. Serum levels may be ordered, and the dosage of valproic acid may need to be reduced.

Oral hypoglycemic agents. Salicylates may enhance the hypoglycemic effects of these agents. Monitor for hypoglycemia, headache, weakness, decreased coordination, general apprehension, diaphoresis, hunger, or blurred or double vision. The dosage of the hypoglycemic agent may need to be reduced. Notify the healthcare provider if any of the previous symptoms appear.

Methotrexate. Monitor for signs of methotrexate toxicity: bone marrow suppression, decreased white blood cell (WBC) count, decreased red blood cell (RBC) count, sore throat, fever, or lethargy.

Corticosteroids. Although often used together, salicylates and corticosteroids may produce GI ulceration. Monitor for signs of GI bleeding; observe for the development of dark, tarry stools and bright red or coffee-ground emesis.

Ethanol. The patient should avoid aspirin within 8 to 10 hours of heavy alcohol use. Small amounts of GI bleeding often occur. If aspirin therapy is absolutely necessary, an enteric-coated product should be used.

DRUG CLASS: NONSTEROIDAL ANTIINFLAMMATORY DRUGS

Actions

Nonsteroidal antiinflammatory drugs are also known as *aspirin-like drugs*. They are chemically unrelated to salicylates but are prostaglandin inhibitors and share many of the same therapeutic actions and adverse effects. NSAIDs block COX-1 and cyclooxygenase-2 (COX-2). They all have varying degrees of analgesic, antipyretic, and antiinflammatory activity. Celecoxib is a COX-2 selective inhibitor, whereas all other NSAIDs are nonselective COX-1 and COX-2 inhibitors.

Uses

In clinical studies, all of these agents (see Table 19.3) are superior to placebos. Depending on the agent used, the dosage, and the patient, the adverse effects of therapy tend to be somewhat less than those associated with salicylate therapy. There is little difference between them in effectiveness or tolerance, but there is a difference in response among individuals, and switching to another NSAID for better therapeutic effect is appropriate. Longer-acting NSAIDs may be useful for patients who have difficulty remembering to take frequent doses. There is also substantial cost difference among NSAIDs, so it makes sense to try the lower-cost agents before moving to the more expensive agents. Many of these products are also available in generic form that will further reduce the expense of therapy.

These agents are used to relieve the pain and inflammation of rheumatoid arthritis, osteoarthritis, ankylosing spondylitis, and gout. Certain agents (e.g., ibuprofen, ketoprofen, naproxen, diclofenac, celecoxib) are also approved for use to control the discomfort of primary dysmenorrhea. Ibuprofen, naproxen, and ketoprofen are available over the counter to be used for the temporary relief of minor aches and pains associated with the common cold, headache, toothache, muscle aches, backaches, arthritis, and menstrual cramps, as well as to reduce fever. COX-2 inhibitors appear to have the advantage of causing fewer GI adverse effects, such as upper GI bleeding. This is significant because 7% to 8% of patients experience GI bleeding while using NSAIDs and it is a primary cause of hospitalizations caused by adverse effects of medications.

In April 2005, the FDA issued a warning about an increased risk of potentially fatal cardiovascular adverse effects (heart attack, stroke) that could be a class effect of NSAIDs. In 2015, the FDA strengthened the existing label warning that nonaspirin NSAIDs increase the potential of an MI or stroke. The prescription NSAID labels will be revised to reflect the following information:

- The risk of MI or stroke can occur in the first weeks of using an NSAID, and the risk may increase with longer use of the NSAID.
- The risk appears greater at higher doses.
- NSAIDs can increase the risk of MI or stroke in patients with or without heart disease or risk factors for heart disease.
- Patients treated with NSAIDs following a first MI were more likely to die in the first year after the

MI compared to patients who were not treated with NSAIDs after their first MI.

- NSAIDs increase the risk of heart failure.

Serious and potentially life-threatening GI bleeding are associated with NSAIDs. Nonsteroidal antiinflammatory drugs have also been associated with allergic reactions, including severe skin reactions and anaphylaxis, some of which occurred in patients without known prior exposure. If an NSAID is prescribed for chronic use, the lowest effective dose for the shortest duration should be used. Nonsteroidal antiinflammatory drugs should not be used in patients immediately after coronary artery bypass graft surgery.

Therapeutic Outcomes

The primary therapeutic outcomes expected from NSAIDs are reduced pain, reduced inflammation, and elimination of fever.

❖ Nursing Implications for NSAIDs

◆ Premedication assessment

1. Perform baseline neurologic assessment (e.g., orientation to date, time, and place; mental alertness; bilateral hand grip; motor functioning; peripheral sensations; and vision and hearing).
2. Monitor vital signs (i.e., temperature, blood pressure, pulse, and respirations).
3. Check laboratory data for hepatotoxicity, nephrotoxicity, bleeding time, and blood dyscrasias.
4. Monitor for GI symptoms before and during therapy; conduct a stool guaiac test if GI tract bleeding is suspected.
5. Check bowel sounds and note stool consistency. Review voiding pattern and urine output.
6. Check for concurrent use of anticoagulant agents.
7. When used as an analgesic, perform pain assessment before administering NSAIDs and at appropriate intervals during therapy. Report poor pain control promptly to the healthcare provider and obtain modification in orders.

◆ Availability, dosage, and administration. See Table 19.3.

 Medication Safety Alert

Do not administer NSAIDs to patients who are allergic to aspirin.

◆ Common adverse effects
Gastrointestinal

Gastric irritation, constipation. If gastric irritation occurs, give medication with food, milk, antacids, or large amounts of water. If symptoms persist or increase in severity, notify the healthcare provider. The use of stool softeners or bulk-forming laxatives may be necessary. Maintain the patient's state of hydration. Encourage the patient to include sufficient roughage, fresh fruits, vegetables, and whole-grain products in the diet.

◆ Serious adverse effects
Gastrointestinal

Gastrointestinal bleeding. Observe for the development of dark, tarry stools and bright red or coffee-ground emesis. Other factors for increased risk of bleeding include concurrent use of oral corticosteroids, anticoagulants, smoking, consuming more than three alcoholic drinks per day, age older than 60 years, and poor general health status. Special care should be taken in elderly or debilitated patients.

Hepatotoxicity. The symptoms of hepatotoxicity are anorexia, nausea, vomiting, jaundice, hepatomegaly, splenomegaly, and abnormal liver function tests (e.g., elevated bilirubin, AST, ALT, and alkaline phosphatase levels; increased prothrombin time).

Hypersensitivity

Hives, pruritus, rash, facial swelling. Report symptoms for further evaluation by the healthcare provider as soon as possible. This could become a medical emergency.

Genitourinary

Nephrotoxicity. Monitor urinalysis and kidney function tests for abnormal results. Report increasing blood urea nitrogen and creatinine levels, decreasing urine output or urine specific gravity despite amount of fluid intake, casts or protein in the urine, frank blood- or smoky-colored urine, or RBCs in excess of 0 to 3 on the urinalysis report.

Hematologic

Blood dyscrasias. Routine laboratory studies (e.g., RBC, WBC, and differential counts) should be scheduled. Monitor for sore throat, fever, purpura, jaundice, or excessive and progressive weakness.

◆ Drug interactions

Warfarin. Nonsteroidal antiinflammatory drugs increase bleeding risk through platelet inhibition. When used concurrently with warfarin, the patient may be at greater risk of bleeding even though the prothrombin time and international normalized ratio are within the therapeutic range. Observe for petechiae; ecchymoses; nosebleeds; bleeding gums; dark, tarry stools; and bright red or coffee-ground emesis. The dosage of warfarin may need to be reduced.

Phenytoin. Monitor the patient with concurrent therapy for signs of phenytoin toxicity, such as nystagmus, sedation, or lethargy. Serum levels may be ordered, and the dosage of phenytoin may need to be reduced.

Valproic acid. Aspirin inhibits valproic acid metabolism, increasing valproic acid blood levels. Monitor for valproic acid toxicity: sedation, drowsiness, dizziness, and blurred vision. Serum levels may be ordered, and the dosage of valproic acid may need to be reduced.

Oral hypoglycemic agents. Monitor for hypoglycemia: headache, weakness, decreased coordination, general apprehension, diaphoresis, hunger, and blurred or double vision. The dosage of the hypoglycemic agent may need to be reduced. Notify the healthcare provider if any of these symptoms appear.

Furosemide, thiazide diuretics. Nonsteroidal antiinflammatory drugs inhibit the diuretic activity of these agents. The dosage of the diuretic agents may need to be increased or NSAIDs discontinued. Maintain accurate intake and output and blood pressure records, and monitor for a decrease in diuretic and antihypertensive activity.

Probenecid. Probenecid inhibits the excretion of NSAIDs. Monitor for signs of toxicity: headache, drowsiness, and mental confusion.

Lithium. Nonsteroidal antiinflammatory drugs (except possibly sulindac and aspirin) may induce lithium toxicity. Monitor for lithium toxicity: nausea, anorexia, fine tremors, persistent vomiting, profuse diarrhea, hyperreflexia, lethargy, and weakness.

Aspirin. Cyclooxygenase-1 inhibitors may reduce the platelet-inhibiting effects of aspirin when administered at about the same time. An NSAID may block the receptor on platelets that aspirin would normally bind to, preventing the platelet inhibition caused by aspirin. To avoid this interaction, take the aspirin several hours before the COX-1 NSAID. This might not be possible for the person with severe rheumatoid arthritis who needs the analgesic effects around the clock.

Cholestyramine. Cholestyramine resins bind to NSAIDs in the gut, inhibiting absorption. Separate dosage administration by 2 hours. The NSAID dosage may need to be increased.

Get Ready for the NCLEX® Examination!

Key Points

- The pain experience is highly subjective and influenced by behavioral, physiologic, sensory, emotional (e.g., attention, anxiety, fatigue, suggestion, prior conditioning), and cultural factors for a particular person under a certain set of circumstances.
- Pain is usually described as acute or short term and as chronic or long term.
- Analgesics are drugs that relieve pain without producing loss of consciousness or reflex activity.
- Analgesic medications have been divided into opiate agonists, opiate partial agonists, opiate antagonists, and prostaglandin inhibitors (acetaminophen, salicylates, and nonsteroidal antiinflammatory drugs [NSAIDs]).
- Pain management has made significant progress, primarily because of better understanding of the pain experience; however, there is still a great deal to do in educating patients, family, and some healthcare providers about appropriate pain management.
- Nurses can play an important role in providing counseling and guidance to these groups in understanding pain and how to maintain an appropriate balance between daily activities and timing of analgesics to optimize quality of life.

Additional Learning Resources

SG Go to your Study Guide for additional Review Questions for the NCLEX® Examination, Critical Thinking Clinical Situations, and other learning activities to help you master this chapter content.

Go to your Evolve website (https://evolve.elsevier.com/Clayton) for additional online resources.

Review Questions for the NCLEX® Examination

1. Nurses working with patients in pain must recognize and avoid common misconceptions about pain. With regard to the pain experience, which statement is correct?
   1. The patient is the best authority on the pain experience.
   2. Chronic pain is mostly psychological in nature.
   3. Regular use of analgesics leads to drug dependence.
   4. The amount of tissue damage does not affect the perception of pain.
2. The nurse was reviewing an order for the pain medication tramadol (Ultram) for a postoperative patient and realized the drug is classified as what?
   1. Opiate partial agonist
   2. Opiate agonist
   3. Opiate antagonist
   4. Prostaglandin inhibitor
3. Nurses frequently assess a patient who is in pain. When assessing the pain, the nurse will do which of the following? *(Select all that apply.)*
   1. Request that the patient wait until the proper time to take pain medication.
   2. Question the patient about the location of the pain.
   3. Offer the patient a pain scale to quantify the pain.
   4. Use open-ended questions to find out about the pain.
   5. Ask about what has worked in the past to control the pain.

4. A patient will be receiving pain medication administered through a PCA system. To help family members understand how this therapy works, what does the nurse explain to the family?
   1. "It is important to allow the patient to have control over the frequency of administration of the pain medication."
   2. "This system of pain medication allows the patient to control the dose of the medication."
   3. "The patient is supposed to control the delivery of the medication, but you can push the button too if you see the patient in pain."
   4. "The types of medications that are commonly used in this PCA system are the nonsteroidal antiinflammatory drugs."

5. While preparing aspirin for the patient, the nurse reviewed which of the pharmacologic effects of salicylates? *(Select all that apply.)*
   1. Analgesic
   2. Antiepileptic
   3. Antipyretic
   4. Antiinflammatory
   5. Antiemetic

6. The patient who was taking aspirin for arthritis stated to the nurse that it was not working anymore and that she planned to stop taking it. What would be an appropriate response by the nurse?
   1. "I can see why you would want to stop taking it; you might be showing signs of physical dependence."
   2. "Okay, you have that right to refuse these drugs."
   3. "What prompted that? I'm sure the medication is working just fine."
   4. "I understand your frustration, but I think you need to talk this over with your healthcare provider first before making any decisions."

7. The nurse explains which of the many properties of diflunisal to the patient with osteoarthritis? *(Select all that apply.)*
   1. "This drug is classified as a prostaglandin inhibitor."
   2. "The adverse effects that need to be monitored include GI bleeding and liver function tests."
   3. "When taking salicylate therapy, you need to be careful with diuretic agents, because the diflunisal may increase the effectiveness of the diuretic."
   4. "This drug may require the monitoring of your kidney function so that adverse effects are identified."
   5. "If you need to take this long term, we will generally have you take the lowest effective dose to minimize adverse effects."

8. The nurse knows that the primary therapeutic outcomes for pain relief include which of these general considerations? *(Select all that apply.)*
   1. Optimize the patient's ability to perform ADLs.
   2. Control adverse effects of the pain medications.
   3. Prevent the conversion of acute pain to chronic pain.
   4. Control opioid dosing and consider placebo therapy instead.
   5. Prevent suffering and disability related to pain.

Introduction to Cardiovascular Disease and Metabolic Syndrome

20

https://evolve.elsevier.com/Clayton

Objectives

1. Identify the major risk factors for the development of metabolic syndrome.
2. Discuss the importance of lifestyle modification in the management of metabolic syndrome.
3. Explain the treatment goals for type 2 diabetes management, lipid management, and hypertension management.
4. Discuss the drug management of the underlying diseases in patients with metabolic syndrome.

Key Terms

cardiovascular disease (kăr-dē-ō-VĂS-kyū-lăr) (p. 321)
atherosclerotic cardiovascular disease (ăth-ĕr-ō-sklĕ-RŎ-tĭk) (p. 321)
coronary artery disease (KŎR-ō-năr-ē ĂR-tĕr-ē) (p. 321)
angina pectoris (ăn-JĪ-nă PĔK-tŏr-ĭs) (p. 321)
myocardial infarction (mī-ō-KĂR-dē-ăl ĭn-FĂRK-shŭn) (p. 321)
stroke (STRŌK) (p. 321)
hypertension (hī-pĕr-TĔN-shŭn) (p. 321)

dysrhythmias (dĭs-RĬTH-mē-ăz) (p. 321)
peripheral vascular disease (pĕ-RĬF-ĕr-ăl VĂS-kū-lăr) (p. 321)
peripheral arterial disease (pĕ-RĬF-ĕr-ăl ăr-TĔR-ē-ŭl) (p. 321)
heart failure (HĂRT FĀL-yŭr) (p. 321)
insulin resistance syndrome (ĬN-sŭl-ĭn rē-ZĬS-tĕns) (p. 322)
metabolic syndrome (mĕt-ĕ-BŎL-ĭk) (p. 322)
body mass index (BMI) (BŎ-dē MĂS ĬN-dĕks) (p. 322)

CARDIOVASCULAR DISEASES

Cardiovascular disease is a collective term used to refer to disorders of the circulatory system (heart, arteries, veins) of the body. The total direct and indirect costs of cardiovascular disease for 2013 were estimated to be $316.1 billion. This includes direct costs (e.g., professional personnel, hospital services, prescribed medications, home healthcare, and other medical durables) and lost productivity from indirect costs of premature death (Benjamin et al, 2017).

These diseases have been subdivided into the areas or organs of the body in which the pathology is most obvious, such as **atherosclerotic cardiovascular disease**, which refers to narrowing of arteries by atherosclerotic plaques caused by hypercholesterolemia, and **coronary artery disease** (see Chapter 21), which refers to narrowing or obstruction of the arteries of the heart, leading to **angina pectoris** and **myocardial infarction** (Chapter 24). **Stroke** (see Chapter 26) refers to either an obstruction (ischemic stroke) or rupture (hemorrhagic stroke) of blood vessels in the brain. An increase in the pressure with which blood circulates through the arteries and veins is referred to as **hypertension** (see Chapter 22).

Dysrhythmias (see Chapter 23) are abnormalities in the electrical conduction pathways of the heart that lead to inefficient pumping of blood through the circulatory system. **Peripheral vascular disease** involves disorders of the blood vessels of the arms and legs. It can be subdivided into two types, depending on whether it is arterial or venous in origin: **peripheral arterial disease** (see Chapter 25), such as obstructive arterial disease, or venous disorders, such as acute deep vein thrombosis (see Chapter 26). The long-term pathology of any one or a combination of these diseases affecting the circulatory system leads to **heart failure** (see Chapter 27) and eventual death.

METABOLIC SYNDROME

Many causative factors lead to cardiovascular disorders (Box 20.1). Lifestyle is recognized as the greatest contributor to a variety of diseases that reduce the quality of life and end lives prematurely. These diseases also cost the American economy billions of dollars that could be used in many more positive, beneficial ways. Since the 1920s, investigators have hypothesized about various factors that lead to cardiovascular disease. Research

Box 20.1 Cardiovascular Disorders

- Coronary artery disease
- Angina pectoris
- Acute myocardial infarction
- Congenital heart disease
- Pulmonary stenosis
- Coarctation of the aorta
- Atrial septal defect
- Ventricular septal defect
- Valvular heart disease
- Mitral stenosis and regurgitation
- Aortic stenosis and regurgitation
- Tricuspid stenosis and regurgitation
- Disorders of heart rate and rhythm (dysrhythmias)
- Cardiomyopathies
- Pericarditis
- Rheumatic heart disease
- Cancers of the heart
- Heart failure

Table 20.1 Definitions and Characteristics of Metabolic Syndrome[a]

Risk Factor Defining Limit	NATIONAL CHOLESTEROL EDUCATION PROGRAM (UNITED STATES)	
	Men	Women
Waist circumference (inches)[b]	>40	>35
High-density lipoprotein cholesterol (mg/dL)	<40	<50
Triglycerides (mg/dL)[c]	>150	>150
Blood pressure (mm Hg)	>130/85	>130/85
Fasting glucose (mg/dL)	>100	>100

Data from Alberti KG, Eckel RH, Grundy SM, et al; International Diabetes Federation Task Force on Epidemiology and Prevention; National Heart, Lung, and Blood Institute; American Heart Association; World Heart Federation; International Atherosclerosis Society; International Association for the Study of Obesity. Harmonizing the metabolic syndrome: a joint interim statement of the International Diabetes Federation Task Force on Epidemiology and Prevention; National Heart, Lung, and Blood Institute; American Heart Association; World Heart Federation; International Atherosclerosis Society; and International Association for the Study of Obesity. *Circulation.* 2009;120(16):1640-1645; and from International Diabetes Federation. *The IDF Consensus Worldwide Definition of the Metabolic Syndrome.* Brussels, Belgium: International Diabetes Federation; 2006. Available at https://www.idf.org/e-library/consensus-statements.html.
[a]People with central obesity and at least two of the remaining four factors are considered to have metabolic syndrome.
[b]There are specific circumferences for different ethnicities in the International Diabetes Federation document cited below.
[c]This also applies to those individuals with previously diagnosed type 2 diabetes.

during the 1960s indicated that persons with hypertension, diabetes mellitus, dyslipidemia, and obesity—alone or in combination—were at greater risk for progressive cardiovascular disease.

In 1988 a unifying pathway of insulin resistance, called *syndrome X*, was described. In 1998 the World Health Organization provided a working definition for this syndrome and renamed it *metabolic syndrome.* Insulin resistance leads to type 2 diabetes and induces atherosclerosis, which leads to coronary artery disease. Over the past 20 years, the hypothesis of insulin resistance has been studied in great depth, and the syndrome has been renamed to be more descriptive of the underlying causes. Other terms include *diabesity* and, more recently, **insulin resistance syndrome**.

Metabolic syndrome is still the most commonly used term worldwide. The key characteristics of metabolic syndrome are the presence of type 2 diabetes mellitus, abdominal obesity, hypertriglyceridemia, low levels of high-density lipoproteins (HDLs), and hypertension. Although metabolic syndrome occurs worldwide, an estimated 34.7% of adults (i.e., one in three) in the United States have metabolic syndrome. Hispanics have the highest rate (35.4%), followed by whites (33.4%) and blacks (32.7%). More than 4% of adolescents between the ages of 12 and 19 years also have metabolic syndrome.

Table 20.1 gives the definition of metabolic syndrome provided in a consensus statement by several international organizations that study atherosclerosis, obesity, cardiovascular disease, and diabetes (Alberti, 2009). People with central obesity and any two of the four other criteria are defined as having metabolic syndrome.

RESULTING CONDITIONS

People with metabolic syndrome are three times more likely to have (and twice as likely to die of) a heart attack or stroke than people without the syndrome.

People with metabolic syndrome have a fivefold greater risk of developing type 2 diabetes. On a global scale, up to 80% of the 200 million people with diabetes will die as a result of cardiovascular disease. This puts the prevalence of metabolic syndrome and diabetes substantially ahead of HIV/AIDS in terms of morbidity and mortality, yet the problem is not as well recognized. In addition to type 2 diabetes and heart disease, other factors associated with metabolic syndrome include renal disease, obstructive sleep apnea, polycystic ovary syndrome, cognitive decline in older adults, and dementia in older adults.

RISK FACTORS

Obesity and Sedentary Lifestyle

Risk factors for the development of metabolic syndrome include poor diet, sedentary lifestyle (lack of exercise), and genetic predisposition. The dietary habits of most Americans have changed significantly over the past 20 years, causing a dramatic increase in weight gain in the United States. Simply put, weight gain occurs when energy intake (food calories) exceeds energy expenditure (burning calories). The 1998 National Heart, Lung and Blood Institute expert report titled "Clinical Guidelines on the Identification, Evaluation and Treatment of Overweight and Obesity in Adults" described weight in proportion to height as the **body mass index (BMI)**. BMI is calculated the same way for both adults and children. The calculation is based on the following formulas:

KILOGRAMS AND METERS (OR CENTIMETERS)

$$BMI = \frac{Weight\ in\ kilograms\ (kg)}{(Height\ in\ meters\ [m])^2}$$

With the metric system, the formula for BMI is weight in kilograms divided by height in meters squared. Because height is commonly measured in centimeters, divide the height in centimeters by 100 to obtain the height in meters.

Example: Weight = 68 kg, Height = 165 cm (1.65 m)
Calculation: $68 \div (1.65)^2 = 24.98$

POUNDS AND INCHES

$$BMI = \frac{Weight\ in\ pounds\ (lb)}{(Height\ in\ inches\ [in])^2}\ 703$$

Calculate the BMI by dividing the weight in pounds (lb) by the height in inches (in) squared and multiplying by a conversion factor of 703.

Example: Weight = 150 lb, Height = 5'5" (65")
Calculation: $(150 \div 65^2) \times 703 = 24.96$

The National Heart, Blood and Lung Institute guidelines also describe overweight and obesity in terms of the BMI. Table 20.2 shows the relationship between BMI and weight (healthy weight, overweight, or obesity).

According to comparison data from the Centers for Disease Control and Prevention (2016), in 2010 no state had a prevalence of obesity less than 20%; 36 states had a prevalence of 25% to 30%; and 12 states had a prevalence of 30% or more. In 2015 no state had a prevalence of obesity less than 20%; 44 states had a prevalence of 25% to 30%; and 25 states had a prevalence of 30% or more. Fig. 20.1 presents a comparison of obesity rates by race/ethnicity and state.

A sedentary lifestyle contributes to overweight and obesity. New technologies such as labor-saving devices and remote-control devices, as well as the availability of entertainment through television and computers, have significantly reduced daily caloric expenditure. Today, despite common knowledge that regular exercise promotes health, more than 60% of Americans are not regularly physically active, and 32% do not engage in aerobic, leisure-time physical activity (Go, 2014).

Longer working hours that lead to less time to prepare food at home and larger portions of commercially prepared food aggravate the problem. The ease and convenience of food preparation (e.g., fast-food restaurants, drive-thrus, the use of a microwave versus a convection oven) and increases in portion sizes (e.g., "Supersize it, please!") have placed too many easily consumed calories on the table. Consequently, reduced physical activity and increased caloric intake have resulted in a national epidemic of obesity.

Alcohol and Smoking

Other negative lifestyle choices, such as excessive consumption of alcohol and cigarette smoking, aggravate metabolic syndrome. Excessive alcohol consumption causes fat accumulation in the liver, which is also associated with metabolic syndrome. Cigarette smoking is a major contributor to pulmonary disease (see Chapter 30) and hypertension (see Chapter 22). One study showed that employees with chronic work stress were more than twice as likely to have metabolic syndrome as those without work-related stress. Another study demonstrated that patients with job-related stress had a twofold increase in the risk of recurrent unstable angina and myocardial infarction.

Genetic Factors

Genetic factors influence each component of the syndrome as well as the syndrome itself. A family history of first-degree relatives (e.g., parents, siblings) that includes type 2 diabetes, hypertension, and early heart disease (e.g., angina, heart attack) greatly increases the likelihood that an individual will develop metabolic syndrome (Fig. 20.2).

TREATMENT

The variety of factors associated with the presence of metabolic syndrome requires an individualized approach to treatment that is based on a person's specific risk factors and diseases present. Lifestyle management is critical to prevent and treat the comorbidities that make up the metabolic syndrome. Research indicates that lifestyle changes alone may delay the onset of type 2 diabetes mellitus by more than 50%. The overall treatment goals for metabolic syndrome are listed in Box 20.2.

Weight loss and increased physical activity are usually the first steps of treatment. Reducing the number of calories consumed—while burning more calories—can have very positive effects in treating metabolic syndrome. Even a 10- to 15-pound weight loss can improve hypertension and hyperglycemia. Initial therapeutic goals are a 7% to 10% weight reduction during the first year of treatment, with an ongoing goal of a BMI less than 25 kg/m². Several dietary approaches can be used to lose weight. Adopting the DASH (*D*ietary *A*pproaches to *S*top *H*ypertension) diet may help patients who also have hypertension (see Chapter 22). The Mediterranean

Table 20.2	Relationship Between Body Mass Index and Categories of Obesity
Body Mass Index (kg/m²)	**Relationship to Weight**
<18.5	Underweight
18.5-24.9	Normal weight
25-29.9	Overweight
30-34.9	Obesity, class I
35-39.9	Obesity, class II
>40	Obesity, class III (extreme obesity)

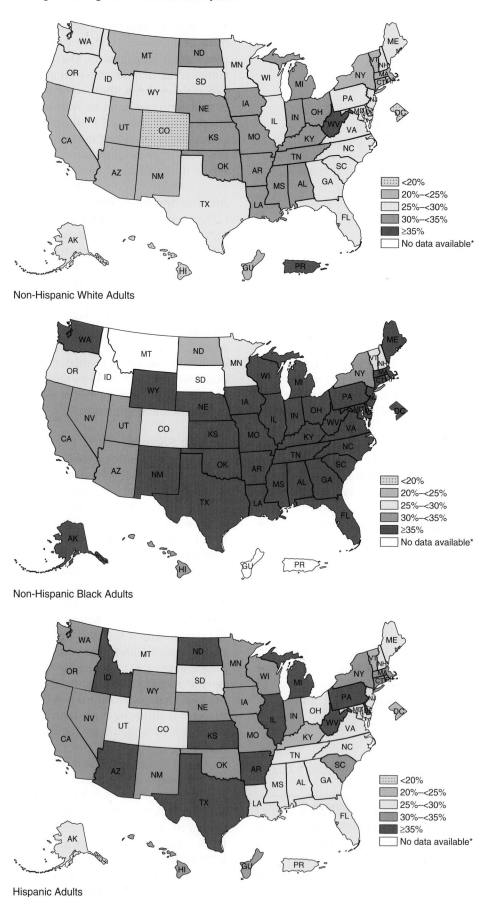

Fig. 20.1 Prevalence of self-reported obesity among US adults by race/ethnicity, state, and territory, BRFSS, 2014-2016. *Sample size <50 or the relative standard error (dividing the standard error by the prevalence) ≥ 30%. (From Behavioral Risk Factor Surveillance System [BRFSS], National Center for Chronic Disease Prevention and Health Promotion, Division of Population Health, Centers for Disease Control and Prevention; retrieved from https://www.cdc.gov/obesity/data/prevalence-maps.html.)

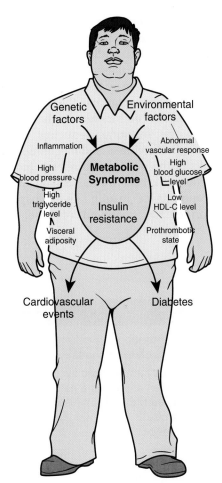

Fig. 20.2 Mechanisms of metabolic syndrome. *HDL-C*, High-density lipoprotein cholesterol.

Box 20.2	General Treatment Goals for Patients With Metabolic Syndrome

BLOOD PRESSURE GOALS
- <130/80 mm Hg
- Blood pressure should be measured at every visit

LIPID GOALS
- Low-density lipoproteins (LDLs)—individualized for each patient

BLOOD GLUCOSE GOALS
- Hemoglobin A_{1c} <7%
- Fasting plasma glucose <120 mg/dL
- Postprandial plasma glucose <180 mg/dL

diet—one rich in "good" fats (e.g., olive oil), containing a reasonable amount of carbohydrates, and with protein from fish and chicken—is frequently recommended. The diet should include reduced intake of saturated fat (<7% of total calories), lower cholesterol levels (<200 mg/day), and lower total fat intake (25% to 35% of total calories). Most dietary fat should be unsaturated, and the intake of simple sugars should be reduced. Non-pharmacologic therapy must include eliminating cigarette smoking, restricting alcohol intake, reducing stress, and controlling sodium (see Chapter 22). Other

appropriate diet plans are the US Department of Agriculture MyPlate Food Guide or the American College of Cardiology/American Heart Association diet recommendations (Eckel et al, 2014).

The American Association of Clinical Endocrinologists and the American College of Endocrinology recommend lifestyle therapy that includes a healthy meal plan (e.g., DASH diet, Mediterranean diets) and a physical activity program incorporating both aerobic and resistance exercise to maintain a BMI of 18 to 25 kg/m² (Garvey, 2016). Most patients with the metabolic syndrome are overweight, and weight reduction, which improves insulin sensitivity, is an important outcome goal of any diet. If the patient is overweight, a 10% weight loss is recommended. Physical activity should include aerobic and resistance training. The ultimate goal for aerobic exercise should be ≥150 min/week of moderate exercise (such as brisk walking) performed during three to five daily sessions per week. Resistance training should be done two to three times per week consisting of single-set exercises of the major muscle groups. Resistance training helps promote fat loss while preserving fat-free mass. Physical activity should be individualized based on the capabilities and preferences of the patient, taking into account health-related and physical limitations. A healthy meal plan and physical activity improves blood pressure, glucose levels, and triglycerides and increases HDL levels. The exercise sessions do not have to be completed at the same time; rather, they can be worked into a person's daily activities. More recent guidelines to reduce low-density lipoprotein (LDL) cholesterol and non-HDL cholesterol (see Chapter 21) and blood pressure (see Chapter 22) recommend exercise (Eckel et al, 2014).

If, after lifestyle modifications and diet and exercise, the patient is not able to meet the therapeutic goals for treating metabolic syndrome, then drug therapy may be necessary. Patient education is vitally important to make patients aware of and to treat metabolic syndrome. This education should be emphasized and reiterated frequently by the physician, the pharmacist, and the nurse.

The primary prevention of metabolic syndrome is becoming a common thread in the curriculum of children in the primary grades. This education focuses on the importance of moderate activity, dietary choices, and the prevention of alcohol consumption and smoking. Resources from the US Department of Agriculture, such as the MyPlate Food Guide (see Chapter 46), are often used as guidelines for this education; age- and gender-related activity and dietary information are also described.

Drug Therapy to Treat Underlying Conditions for Metabolic Syndrome

Hypertension. A combination of a thiazide diuretic plus an angiotensin-converting enzyme inhibitor, calcium channel blocker, or angiotensin receptor blocker will be necessary to treat hypertension in nonblack patients.

In the general black population, including those with diabetes, initial treatment should include a thiazide-type diuretic or calcium channel blocker. Other combinations of therapy may be used, depending on the person's race and the presence of other diseases. (See Chapter 22 for a discussion of the treatment of hypertension.)

Dyslipidemia. The treatment of dyslipidemia is generally to lower triglyceride and LDL cholesterol levels and to raise the HDL cholesterol level. After lifestyle changes, the medicines most commonly used are 3-hydroxymethylglutaryl coenzyme A reductase inhibitors (also known as statins) and fibric acid derivatives. (See Chapter 21 for a discussion of the treatment of dyslipidemias.)

Type 2 diabetes mellitus. Several different classes of medicines may be used to treat insulin resistance and type 2 diabetes. The thiazolidinediones reduce insulin resistance in the peripheral tissues. Metformin decreases the production of glucose by the liver; to a lesser extent it also reduces insulin resistance in the peripheral tissues. Alpha-glycosidase inhibitors reduce the absorption of glucose from the intestine, reducing postprandial hyperglycemia. Sulfonylureas and meglitinides stimulate the beta cells of the pancreas to release more insulin. Insulin injections also benefit patients who do not secrete adequate amounts of insulin. (See Chapter 35 for a discussion of the treatment of type 2 diabetes mellitus.)

Get Ready for the NCLEX® Examination!

Key Points

- Cardiovascular diseases are a major cause of premature death in the United States.
- More than 34% of the US adult population has metabolic syndrome; these individuals are at much greater risk for cardiovascular diseases. The key characteristics of metabolic syndrome are type 2 diabetes mellitus, abdominal obesity, hypertriglyceridemia, a low HDL cholesterol level, and hypertension.
- The most cost-effective and successful forms of treatment are smoking cessation, weight reduction, exercise, stress reduction, and dietary modifications. If changes in diet and exercise do not produce an acceptable decrease in blood lipid levels, blood glucose levels, and hypertension, then antilipemic agents, antihyperglycemic agents, and antihypertensive agents may be added to the patient's regimen.

Additional Learning Resources

SG Go to your Study Guide for additional Review Questions for the NCLEX® Examination, Critical Thinking Clinical Situations, and other learning activities to help you master this chapter content.

Go to your Evolve website (https://evolve.elsevier.com/Clayton) for additional online resources.

 Online Resources

Centers for Disease Control and Prevention, updated 2016 adult obesity prevalence maps and access to other illustrations and information: https://www.cdc.gov/obesity/data/prevalence-maps.html.

Review Questions for the NCLEX® Examination

1. Which risk factors for metabolic syndrome should the nurse include when assessing a patient who came into the clinic for a yearly checkup? *(Select all that apply.)*
   1. Regular exercise
   2. Being overweight
   3. Smoking
   4. Genetic predisposition
   5. Having high blood pressure

2. A nurse tells a 45-year-old male patient whose BMI was calculated to be 29 that this number means what?
   1. "This BMI indicates that you are underweight."
   2. "This means that you are within the expected normal weight."
   3. "A BMI over 25 indicates that you are considered overweight and close to obese."
   4. "According to the chart this BMI indicates that you are considered obese, class I."

3. A patient in the clinic asked the nurse for ways to reduce the risk of developing metabolic syndrome. Which statement by the nurse is appropriate?
   1. "You can't do anything to prevent metabolic syndrome because it is in your genes."
   2. "The best thing you can do to prevent metabolic syndrome is to not get diabetes."
   3. "Lifestyle modifications, including a heart-healthy diet and exercise, are important to practice to prevent the development of metabolic syndrome."
   4. "If you routinely get your blood checked for high cholesterol and eat a low-fat diet, you will not get metabolic syndrome."

4. Patients evaluated for metabolic syndrome should have which laboratory tests done? *(Select all that apply.)*
  1. Blood glucose
  2. Liver enzymes
  3. Thyroid hormone
  4. Lipid profile
  5. Hemoglobin A_{1c}

5. Recommendations for patients on how to manage their diabetes to prevent metabolic syndrome include which of the following? *(Select all that apply.)*
  1. Eating balanced meals
  2. Maintaining a hemoglobin A_{1c} of less than 8%
  3. Keeping the blood sugar less than 180 after meals
  4. Being physically active
  5. Having a BMI less than 25

6. A patient with metabolic syndrome who requires drug therapy after lifestyle changes were not effective was told by the nurse that which drugs may be used to manage the underlying diseases (hypertension, hyperlipidemia) causing the metabolic syndrome? *(Select all that apply.)*
  1. Thiazide diuretics
  2. Testosterone
  3. Statins
  4. Analgesics
  5. Angiotensin-converting enzyme inhibitors

7. A nurse is explaining to a patient the risk factors that are involved in developing metabolic syndrome. The nurse realized the patient needs further education after the patient made which statement?
  1. "I can control my diet, and get exercise routinely, to try to control my weight."
  2. "If I limit eating at restaurants to only three times a week instead of five, I should be able to control my weight."
  3. "I know that diabetes runs in my family, so I will control my diet and get my blood sugar checked every year."
  4. "I routinely check my blood pressure at home and have switched to the DASH diet to prevent hypertension."

21 Drugs Used to Treat Dyslipidemias

Objectives

1. Describe atherosclerosis and identify the four major types of lipoproteins.
2. Describe the primary approaches to treat lipid disorders.
3. Determine which antilipid medications are used for cholesterol control and which can be used for triglyceride control.
4. Differentiate between how statins work to control lipid levels and how the bile acid resins work to control lipid levels.

Key Terms

atherosclerotic cardiovascular disease (ASCVD) (ăth-ĕr-ō-sklĕ-RŌ-tĭk) (p. 328)
atherosclerosis (ăth-ĕr-ō-sklĕ-RŌ-sĭs) (p. 328)
hyperlipidemia (hī-pĕr-lĭp-ĭ-DĒ-mē-ă) (p. 328)
dyslipidemias (dĭs-lĭp-ĭ-DĒ-mē-ăz) (p. 328)

cholesterol (kō-LĔS-tĕ-rŏl) (p. 328)
triglycerides (trī-GLĬ-sĕ-rīdz) (p. 328)
lipoproteins (lī-pō-PRŌ-tēnz) (p. 328)
chylomicrons (kī-lō-MĪ-krŏnz) (p. 328)

ATHEROSCLEROTIC CARDIOVASCULAR DISEASE

For an introduction to cardiovascular diseases, see Chapter 20. Coronary artery disease (CAD) (also called *coronary heart disease*) is a major cause of premature death in the United States and most other industrialized nations. Almost one-third (31.9%) of the US population will die of a heart attack or stroke associated with atherosclerotic cardiovascular disease (ASCVD), one of every six deaths in the United States. Major treatable causes of ASCVD are cigarette smoking, sedentary lifestyle, and poor eating habits leading to obesity, hypertension, type 2 diabetes mellitus, and atherosclerosis (Benjamin et al, 2017). Atherosclerosis is characterized by the accumulation of fatty deposits on the inner walls of the arteries and arterioles throughout the body that reduces the blood supply to vital organs, resulting in strokes, angina pectoris, myocardial infarction, and peripheral vascular disease. A primary cause of atherosclerosis is the abnormal elevation of cholesterol and triglyceride levels in the blood. Hyperlipidemia is the broad term used to classify patients with high levels of blood fats (lipids). Dyslipidemias are further defined under hyperlipidemia as abnormalities that involve one or more of the blood lipids. Dyslipidemias can be the result of genetic abnormalities, secondary causes (e.g., lifestyle, drugs, underlying diseases), or both. A diet that is high in saturated fats, cholesterol, carbohydrates, total calories, and alcohol and a sedentary lifestyle contribute significantly to dyslipidemias.

TYPES OF LIPOPROTEINS

Cholesterol is a naturally occurring substance that is essential for synthesizing the body steroids that are used by the endocrine system, for synthesizing the bile acids that are needed for food absorption, and for cell membrane synthesis. The body is able to manufacture enough cholesterol to meet its metabolic needs. However, the body also converts excess dietary carbohydrates into triglycerides (a precursor of cholesterol), and it converts dietary fat into cholesterol. After being absorbed from the gastrointestinal (GI) tract, fats (lipids), triglycerides, and cholesterol are bound to circulating proteins called lipoproteins for transport through the body.

Lipoproteins are subdivided into five categories on the basis of their composition: chylomicrons, very-low-density lipoproteins (VLDLs), intermediate-density lipoproteins, low-density lipoproteins (LDLs), and high-density lipoproteins (HDLs). The five types differ in relative concentrations of triglycerides, cholesterol, and proteins. Clinically, the intermediate-density lipoproteins are included in the LDL measurement. Chylomicrons consist of about 90% triglycerides and 5% cholesterol; VLDLs represent about 15% to 20% of total serum cholesterol and most of the total blood triglyceride concentration, whereas HDLs contain about 20% to 30% cholesterol and 1% to 7% triglycerides.

The purpose of HDLs appears to be to transport cholesterol from peripheral cells to the liver for metabolism. HDLs are sometimes referred to as the "good" lipoproteins because high levels indicate that cholesterol is being removed from vascular tissue, where it may participate in the development of CAD. Low HDL levels are considered a positive risk factor for the development of CAD; high HDL levels are a negative risk factor for CAD.

LDLs account for 60% to 70% of total serum cholesterol and are the major contributor to atherosclerosis. The probability that atherosclerosis will develop is related directly to the concentration of LDL cholesterol (LDL-C) in the blood circulation. LDLs are the primary target of cholesterol-lowering therapy.

High triglyceride levels are also associated with an increased risk of CAD. Consequently, patient assessment and cholesterol-lowering treatment are based on the total cholesterol, LDL-C, HDL cholesterol (HDL-C), and triglyceride levels for individual patients. Other markers being tested to see whether they are better predictors of the risk for impending heart disease are the concentration of apolipoprotein A-I (the major protein component of HDL); apolipoprotein B (a measure of the total number of atherogenic particles); C-reactive protein (an indicator of inflammation); and non-HDL cholesterol, the sum of the cholesterol in both LDL-C and triglyceride-rich lipoproteins.

TREATMENT OF HYPERLIPIDEMIAS

An estimated 105 million American adults have total blood cholesterol levels of 200 mg/dL or more. Of these, about 32 million American adults have levels of 240 mg/dL or more (Go, 2014). Some of the most common hyperlipidemias of genetic origin are treatable with medicines. However, it is now recognized that lifestyle is the greatest contributor to the development of hyperlipidemia. A cluster of risk factors that relate directly to excesses in lifestyle is now recognized as metabolic syndrome (see Chapter 20).

In November 2013 the American College of Cardiology and the American Heart Association (ACC/AHA) published new guidelines to reduce the overall risk of ASCVD (Stone, 2014). Risk reduction is the cornerstone of the guidelines: maintaining a heart-healthy diet (see Chapter 46) for a healthy weight, regular exercise, and avoidance of tobacco products. The major changes in the guidelines are the elimination of LDL and non-LDL treatment goals, focus on the use of statins to treat hypercholesterolemia and the listing of four benefit groups (Table 21.1) with recommendations for the intensity of statin therapy (Table 21.2). Accompanying the guidelines is a new cardiovascular risk assessment calculator to estimate 10-year ASCVD risk and safety recommendations on the use of statin drugs. In 2017 the ACC published guidelines on the use of nonstatin therapies (bile acid-binding resins and ezetimibe) for lowering LDL in the management of ASCVD (Lloyd-Jones, 2017).

The nonstatins are reasonable to consider when the maximum tolerated statin dose is unsuccessful and additional LDL reduction is necessary.

DRUG THERAPY FOR HYPERLIPIDEMIAS

ACTIONS

See the individual drug monographs later in this chapter for information about the mechanisms of action of different antilipemic agents.

USES

Antilipemic agents may be used to treat hyperlipidemia only if diet, exercise, and weight reduction are not successful for adequately lowering LDL-C levels. The statins are the first line of therapy, but other antilipemic classes that lower LDL levels are the bile acid–binding resins (e.g., cholestyramine, colestipol, colesevelam) and niacin. The fibric acids (e.g., gemfibrozil, fenofibrate) are effective triglyceride-lowering agents but are not first-line drugs for the treatment of hyperlipidemias because they do not usually produce substantial reductions in LDL-C. Omega-3 fatty acids have been approved by the US Food and Drug Administration for treatment of very high triglyceride levels (>500 mg/dL) in adults. The fibrates raise HDL levels by 10% to 25%, and the statins raise HDL levels by 2% to 15%.

Selection of initial antilipemic therapy depends on the type of dyslipidemia present. Pharmacologic antilipemic therapy is often started with a statin because of their safety record and success in lowering cholesterol levels and reducing morbidity and mortality in ASCVD. The statins are the most potent and highly effective drugs for lowering LDL-C levels, and they appear to be relatively safe. However, they are substantially more expensive than other treatments. Prescription-strength niacin is effective for lowering total cholesterol and triglyceride levels and for raising HDL-C levels, but has serious adverse effects (vasomotor flushing, hepatotoxicity) in the higher doses needed for these antilipemic effects.

Before starting therapy, a lipid panel should be drawn and then repeated in 4 to 12 weeks after therapy is initiated. If the response to initial drug therapy is inadequate, it might be an indication that the patient is not compliant with therapy or that lifestyle changes are not being made. Have a discussion with the patient to assure that side effects are not limiting therapy. If the patient is compliant, the dosage of the statin should be increased or another drug should be added to the treatment regimen. The combination of a bile acid–binding resin with a statin can potentially lower LDL-C levels by greater than 50%. In rare cases of particularly high cholesterol levels, triple therapy with a statin, a bile acid–binding resin, *and* ezetimibe may be required. An alternative to be used in conjunction with the statins is a new class of drugs, the proprotein convertase subtilisin kexin type 9 (PCSK9) inhibitors (evolocumab,

Table 21.1 Statin Benefit Groups and Recommended Treatment

GROUP	DEFINITION	RECOMMENDATIONS
1	Patients who have already suffered a myocardial infarction, stable or unstable angina, stroke, transient ischemic attack, or peripheral arterial disease, or had a revascularization procedure. Even though these patients have had serious cardiovascular events, there is strong evidence that statins reduce mortality in patients with a history of ASCVD disease.	For adults age 75 yr or younger, high-intensity statins are first-line therapy unless contraindicated. Moderate-intensity statins are a second-line choice. For adults age >75 yr, first-line therapy with moderate-intensity dosage should be considered on a case-by-case basis. Nonstatin cholesterol-lowering agents may be prescribed on a risk-versus-benefit basis.
2	Adults age 21 yr or older with no clinical ASCVD but with LDL-C >190 mg/dL or triglycerides of 500 mg/dL.	Evaluate for secondary causes of hyperlipidemia (e.g., high-fat diet; hypothyroidism; obstructive liver disease; medicines such as diuretics, glucocorticoids, cyclosporine, amiodarone). Primary hypercholesterolemia should be treated with high-intensity statins unless contraindicated. Treat with highest dose tolerated. Once maximum statin dosage is achieved, addition of a nonstatin to further reduce LDL-C is indicated based on tolerance.
3	Adults age 40-75 yr with diabetes and LDL-C levels of 70-189 mg/dL but no clinical ASCVD. ASCVD is the main cause of illness and death in patients with diabetes.	Moderate-intensity statins should be started for patients with type 1 or type 2 diabetes. High-intensity statins are indicated in those with diabetes and an estimated 10-year ASCVD risk of 7.5% or greater. For adults age <40 or >75 yr, statins may be initiated taking into consideration risks, benefits, and drug interactions.
4	Adults without diabetes who have LDL-C levels of 70-189 mg/dL and an estimated 10-yr ASCVD risk of 7.5% or greater. The risk calculator is for men and women who are non-Hispanic Caucasian or African American, age 40-75 yr, with or without diabetes, with LDL-C levels of 70-189 mg/dL.	Start moderate- to high-intensity statin therapy in adults age 40-75, with no clinical ASCVD or diabetes, with an ASCVD risk of 7.5%. Start moderate-intensity statin therapy for those with an ASCVD risk of 5%-7.5%. Before starting therapy with the previous groups, clinicians should discuss risks/benefits and patient's preference.

ASCVD, Atherosclerotic cardiovascular disease; *LDL-C*, low-density lipoprotein cholesterol.

Table 21.2 Fixed Statin Dosage Recommendations Based on Intensity[a]

HIGH INTENSITY (LOWERS LDL BY >50%)	MODERATE INTENSITY (LOWERS LDL BY 30%-49%)	LOW INTENSITY (LOWERS LDL BY <30%)
Atorvastatin 40-80 mg Rosuvastatin 20-40 mg	Atorvastatin 10-20 mg Rosuvastatin 5-10 mg Simvastatin 20-40 mg Pravastatin 40-80 mg Lovastatin 40 mg Fluvastatin 80 mg Pitavastatin 2-4 mg	Simvastatin 10 mg Pravastatin 10-20 mg Lovastatin 20 mg Fluvastatin 20-40 mg Pitavastatin 1 mg

Adapted from Smith SC Jr, Grundy SM. 2013 ACC/AHA Guideline recommends fixed-dose strategies instead of targeted goals to lower blood cholesterol. *J Am Coll Cardiol.* 2014;64:601-612.
[a]See the Drug Class: HMG-CoA Reductase Inhibitors drug monograph later in this chapter for information on monitoring drug therapy.
LDL, Low-density lipoprotein.

alirocumab), are just coming available. Due to their current rarity of use and very high expense, their use will not be addressed in this edition. Drug therapy is likely to continue for many years or the patient's lifetime; plasma lipid levels return to pretreatment levels after 2 to 3 weeks if therapy is discontinued.

❖ NURSING IMPLICATIONS FOR HYPERLIPIDEMIA THERAPY

◆ Assessment

History of risk factors. Obtain the patient's age, note gender and race, and take a family history of the incidence of elevated cholesterol and lipid levels. Ask whether any first-generation family members have a history of or have died from ASCVD. Obtain the ages and details of individuals with a history of ASCVD. Are there any living relatives with elevated cholesterol or elevated triglyceride levels?

Hypertension. Ask whether the patient has ever been told that he or she has elevated blood pressure. If yes, obtain details. Ask about medications that have been prescribed. Are the medications being taken regularly? If not, why not? Take the patient's blood pressure in lying, sitting, and standing positions.

Smoking. Obtain a history of the number of cigarettes or cigars smoked daily. How long has the patient smoked? Has the patient ever tried to stop smoking? Determine the patient's knowledge of the effects of smoking on the vascular system. How does the individual feel about modifying his or her smoking habit?

Dietary habits

- Obtain a dietary history. Ask specific questions to obtain data related to foods eaten that are high in fat, cholesterol, refined carbohydrates, and sodium. Discuss the amount of fast foods and snack foods consumed, as well as the frequency of restaurant dining. Any of these factors tends to increase fat intake. Using a calorie counter, ask the person to estimate the number of calories eaten daily. How much meat, fish, and poultry is eaten daily (size and number of servings)? Estimate the percentage of total daily calories provided by fat.
- Discuss food preparation (e.g., baking, broiling, frying). How many servings of fruits and vegetables are eaten daily? What types of oils or fats are used in food preparation? See a nutrition text for additional dietary history questions.
- What are the frequency and volume of alcoholic beverages that are consumed?

Glucose intolerance. Ask specific questions regarding whether the individual has now or has ever had an elevated serum glucose (blood sugar) level. If yes, what dietary modifications have been made? How successful are they? What medications are being taken for the elevated serum glucose level (e.g., oral hypoglycemic agents, insulin)?

Elevated serum lipid levels. Find out whether the patient is aware of having elevated lipid, triglyceride, or cholesterol levels. If so, what measures has the patient tried for reduction, and what effect have the interventions had on the blood levels at subsequent examinations? Review available laboratory data (e.g., LDL, VLDL levels). A fasting lipoprotein profile that includes total cholesterol, LDL-C, HDL-C, and triglyceride levels is recommended for all adults 20 years old or older at least once every 5 years.

Obesity. Weigh the patient. Ask about any recent weight gain or loss and whether it was intentional or unintentional. Using the person's height and weight, determine the person's body mass index (see Chapter 20). If obesity is present, what strategies for weight reduction have been tried?

Psychomotor functions

- Type of lifestyle: Ask the patient to describe his or her exercise level in terms of amount (e.g., walking 3 miles), intensity (e.g., walking 3 mph), and frequency (e.g., walking every other day). Is the patient's job physically demanding or of a sedentary nature?
- Psychological stress: How much stress does the individual estimate having in his or her life? How does the patient cope with stressful situations at home and in the work setting?

◆ **Patient Education**

Nutrition. Patients who take bile acid–sequestering resins may require supplemental vitamins. (The fat-soluble vitamins—D, E, A, and K—may become deficient with long-term resin therapy.)

- Encourage the intake of high-bulk foods (e.g., whole grains, raw fruits and vegetables), as well as the intake of 8 to 10 eight-ounce glasses of water daily, to minimize the constipating effects of these resins.
- Arrange a dietary consultation with a nutritionist to address any dietary modifications needed (e.g., low fat, low cholesterol). Nurses should enhance and reinforce this teaching on a continuum. Stress the importance of attaining a normal weight as a major treatment goal of hyperlipidemia.

Vitamin K deficiency. If the patient is receiving a prescription for a bile acid–sequestering resin, teach the patient about the signs and symptoms of vitamin K deficiency, including bleeding gums; bruising; dark, tarry stools; and coffee-ground emesis. This interaction is rare, but if symptoms occur, they should be reported immediately to the healthcare provider.

Follow-up care. Stress the need for long-term regular assessment of the required serum levels (e.g., lipid profile values, liver studies, bleeding times) to track progress, identify the need for modifications in therapeutic interventions, and detect possible adverse effects of the medications. To obtain this information, blood studies and regular visits to the healthcare provider are necessary.

Relating to medication regimen. Examine the individual drug monographs for details about mixing drugs, scheduling medication administration, and techniques for improving compliance of patients taking these medications.

Fostering health maintenance

- Throughout the course of treatment, discuss medication information and how it will benefit the patient.
- Drug therapy is one component in the management of hyperlipidemia. Therapeutic lifestyle changes are as important as drug therapy; therefore the need to modify dietary habits and to control obesity, glucose

levels, serum cholesterol, lipids, and hypertension must be strongly emphasized. Teach the patient about which high-cholesterol and high-fat foods to avoid (e.g., liver, egg yolks, meats, fried foods, fatty desserts, nuts [cashews, macadamia, Brazil]). Cholesterol is an animal product and not found in plants. Encourage switching to skim or 1% fat milk, substituting egg whites, and increasing consumption of fruits (especially grapefruit) and vegetables. Discuss the use of unsaturated vegetable oils, such as corn, olive, and soybean. Cessation of smoking and an increase in daily exercise (30 minutes of moderate-intensity exercise most days of the week) are strongly recommended. People with metabolic syndrome must recognize the importance of weight reduction and increased exercise to modify the insulin resistance that can dramatically affect the management of the disorder.

- Provide the patient and significant others with the important information contained in the specific drug monographs for the drugs prescribed. Additional health teaching and nursing interventions for adverse effects are described in the drug monographs that follow.
- Seek the patient's cooperation and understanding of the following points so that medication compliance is increased: the name of the medication; its dosage, route, and times of administration; and its common and serious adverse effects.

Patient self-assessment. Enlist the patient's help with developing and maintaining a written record of monitoring parameters (e.g., daily serum glucose levels, blood pressure, weight) (see the Patient Self-Assessment Form for Cardiovascular Agents on the Evolve website). An individualized nutritional diary should also be kept while instituting and learning about diet modifications (e.g., a reduction in fats and refined carbohydrates, an increase in low-cholesterol foods). Complete the Premedication Data column for use as a baseline to track the patient's response to drug therapy. Ensure that the patient understands how to use the form and instruct the patient to bring the completed form to follow-up visits. During follow-up visits, focus on issues that will foster adherence with the therapeutic interventions prescribed.

DRUG CLASS: BILE ACID–BINDING RESINS

cholestyramine (co-les-ter-am-MEAN)
  Questran (QUEST-tran)
colestipol (co-LES-ti-pol)
  Colestid (co-LEST-tid)
colesevelam (cola-SEVA-lam)
  Welchol (WEL-coal)

Actions

Cholestyramine, colestipol, and colesevelam are resins that bind bile acids in the intestine. After oral administration, the resin forms a nonabsorbable complex with bile acids, preventing the enterohepatic recirculation of the bile acids. Removal of bile acids causes liver cells to compensate by increasing the metabolism of cholesterol to produce more bile acids, which results in a net reduction in the total cholesterol level. Bile acid–binding resins can reduce LDL-C levels by 15% to 30% and increase HDL levels by up to 5%. Some patients also have a 5% to 10% increase in their triglyceride levels.

Uses

Cholestyramine, colestipol, and colesevelam are used in conjunction with dietary therapy to decrease elevated cholesterol concentrations in patients with hyperlipidemia and to reduce the risks of atherosclerosis leading to ASCVD. These agents may also be used with statins to lower the LDL-C level even further. They are generally not used for patients who already have elevated triglyceride levels.

Other uses of the bile acid–binding resins include the treatment of pruritus secondary to partial biliary stasis, diarrhea secondary to excess fecal bile acids or pseudomembranous colitis, and digitalis glycoside toxicity.

Colesevelam has also received US Food and Drug Administration approval for reducing blood glucose and hemoglobin A_{1c} in adult patients with type 2 diabetes. It may be used alone or in combination with metformin, sulfonylureas, or insulin. Do not use this drug in patients with type 1 diabetes.

Therapeutic Outcomes

The primary therapeutic outcomes expected from bile acid–binding resin therapy are the reduction of the LDL and total cholesterol levels.

❖ **Nursing Implications for Bile Acid–Binding Resins**
◆ *Premedication assessment*
1. Serum triglyceride, lipoprotein, and cholesterol levels should be determined before the initiation of therapy and periodically thereafter.
2. Obtain patient data related to any GI alterations before the initiation of therapy (e.g., the presence of abdominal pain, nausea, flatus).

◆ *Availability*
  Cholestyramine. *PO:* 4-g powder packets.
  Colestipol. *PO:* 1-g tablets; granules in 5-g packets.
  Colesevelam. *PO:* 3.75-mg packets; 625-mg tablets.

◆ *Dosage and administration*
  Cholestyramine. *PO:* 4 g one to six times daily. Initial dosage is 4 g daily. Maintenance dosage is 8 to 16 g/day. Maximum daily dosage is 24 g.
  Colestipol. *PO: Granules:* 5 to 30 g/day in divided doses. Initial dosage is 5 g once or twice daily. *Tablets:* 2 to 16 g/day. Initial dosage is 2 g once or twice daily.
  Colesevelam. *PO:* 6 tablets once daily or in two divided doses with liquid at meals.

NOTES:
- The powder resin (cholestyramine) must be mixed with 2 to 6 ounces of water, juice, soup, applesauce, or crushed pineapple and should stand for a few minutes to allow absorption and dispersion. Do not attempt to swallow the dry powder. Follow administration with an additional glass of water.
- The recommended time of administration is with meals, but this may be modified to avoid interference with the absorption of other medications.
- Tablets should be swallowed whole; do not crush, chew, or cut them. Tablets should be taken with liquids.
- Taste may become a reason for noncompliance. Place the powder in a favorite beverage or opt for tablets to minimize the medication's objectionable taste.

◆ *Common adverse effects*
Gastrointestinal
Constipation, bloating, fullness, nausea, flatulence. These adverse effects can be minimized by starting with a low dose; mixing the drug with noncarbonated, pulpy juices or sauces; and swallowing it without gulping air. Maintain adequate fiber in the diet and drink sufficient water.

◆ *Drug interactions*
Digoxin, warfarin, thyroid hormones, thiazide diuretics, phenobarbital, nonsteroidal antiinflammatory agents, tetracycline, beta-blocking agents, gemfibrozil, glipizide, glyburide, oral contraceptives, phenytoin. The resins may bind with these medicines, which reduces absorption. The interaction can usually be minimized by administering these medicines 1 hour before or 4 hours after administration of resins.

Amiodarone. The resins significantly decrease the absorption of amiodarone. The resins also block the enterohepatic recirculation of amiodarone. Consequently, amiodarone and the resins should not be used concurrently.

Fat-soluble vitamins (D, E, A, and K), folic acid. High doses of resins may reduce the absorption of these agents, but this interaction is not usually significant in normally nourished patients.

DRUG CLASS: NIACIN

⇄ *Do not confuse niacin with Niaspan or Naprosyn.*

Actions
Niacin, also known as *nicotinic acid,* is a water-soluble B vitamin (also known as *vitamin B₃*). Its mechanisms of action as an antilipemic agent are not completely known, but they are not related to its effects as a vitamin.

Niacin inhibits VLDL synthesis by liver cells, which causes a decrease in LDL and triglyceride production. Triglyceride levels are reduced by 20% to 50%, and total cholesterol and LDL-C levels can be reduced by 5% to 25%. Niacin may also reduce the metabolism of HDL, thereby causing a 15% to 35% increase in HDL levels. Niacin also causes the release of histamine, causing peripheral vasodilation and increased blood flow (flushing of the skin).

Uses
Nicotinic acid is the only form of vitamin B₃ approved by the US Food and Drug Administration for the treatment of dyslipidemias. According to the 2017 American Association of Clinical Endocrinologists and the American College of Endocrinology guidelines for the management of dyslipidemia, niacin therapy is recommended principally as an adjunct for reducing triglycerides. Niacin therapy should not be used in individuals aggressively treated with a statin due to the absence of improved patient outcomes and safety concerns. In addition, the use of nicotinic acid is often limited by poor tolerability. Niacin should be used with caution in patients with diabetes because of their glucose intolerance.

Different forms of vitamin B₃ cannot be used interchangeably. Other forms of vitamin B₃ are niacinamide and inositol hexaniacinate, which do not lower elevated cholesterol levels. Immediate-release niacin products cause more facial and skin flushing, and the sustained-release products have a higher possibility of causing hepatotoxicity, than the immediate-release products. Dietary supplements of niacin should not be used to treat dyslipidemia. The recommended Dietary Reference Intake for nutritional supplementation is less than 20 mg/day. The dosage of niacin required to treat dyslipidemia is 1 to 6 g/day.

Therapeutic Outcomes
The primary therapeutic outcomes expected from niacin are reduction in LDL (5% to 25%) and total cholesterol levels, reduction in triglyceride levels (20% to 50%), and an increase in HDL levels (15% to 35%).

❖ **Nursing Implications for Niacin**
◆ *Premedication assessment*
1. Serum triglyceride and cholesterol levels should be determined before initiation of therapy and periodically thereafter.
2. Liver function tests (bilirubin, aspartate aminotransferase [AST], alanine aminotransferase [ALT], gamma-glutamyltransferase, and alkaline phosphatase levels; prothrombin time) should be determined before initiating therapy and every 6 to 8 weeks during the first year of therapy.
3. Baseline uric acid and blood glucose levels should be determined before initiating therapy. Niacin

therapy may induce hyperuricemia, gout, and hyperglycemia in susceptible patients.

4. Baseline blood pressure and heart rate should be determined before initiating therapy.

5. Obtain patient data related to any GI alterations before initiating therapy (e.g., the presence of abdominal pain, nausea, or flatus).

◆ *Availability.* *PO:* 50-, 100-, 250-, or 500-mg tablets; 250- or 500-mg timed-release capsules; 250- 500-, 750-, or 1000-mg timed-release tablets.

◆ *Dosage and administration.* *PO:* Weeks 1 to 4: 500 mg PO at bedtime. Weeks 5 to 8: 1000 mg PO at bedtime. After week 8, titrate to patient response and tolerance. If response to 1000 mg/day is inadequate, increase dose to 1500 mg/day PO at bedtime. If response to 1500 mg/day is inadequate, may subsequently increase dose to 2000 mg/day.

◆ *Common adverse effects*

Integumentary. Flushing, itching, and rash are common. Patients can reduce their symptoms by taking aspirin (325 mg) or ibuprofen (200 mg) 30 minutes before each dose of niacin.

Neurologic. Tingling and headache are frequently seen with these drugs.

Gastrointestinal

Nausea, gas, abdominal discomfort and pain. Gastrointestinal upset can be minimized by starting with low doses of these drugs and administering all doses with food.

The common adverse effects listed here usually occur at the beginning of therapy, especially with the immediate-release products. Tolerance develops quickly. Administer niacin with food.

Cardiovascular

Dizziness, faintness, hypotension. Niacin is a vasodilator, and it may cause hypotension, especially if a patient is receiving other antihypertensive agents. Anticipate the development of hypotension and take measures to prevent such an occurrence. Teach the patient to rise slowly from a supine or sitting position and to sit or lie down if he or she is feeling faint. Monitor blood pressure with the patient in both the supine and sitting positions.

◆ *Serious adverse effects*

Gastrointestinal

Hepatotoxicity. There appears to be a higher incidence of hepatotoxicity associated with the timed-release products. Some clinicians recommend limiting the timed-release products to 1500 mg daily to reduce the risk.

Fatigue, anorexia, nausea, malaise, jaundice. These are the early symptoms that are associated with hepatotoxicity. Report these to the healthcare provider for further evaluation.

Musculoskeletal

Myopathy. Symptoms of muscle aches, soreness, and weakness may be early signs of myopathy. Serum creatine phosphokinase levels that are more than 10 times the upper limit of normal confirm the diagnosis.

◆ *Drug interactions*

3-Hydroxy-3-methylglutaryl coenzyme A (HMG-CoA) reductase inhibitors. The potential of developing myopathy is increased when niacin is added to the treatment regimen. The incidence of this condition is less than 1%.

DRUG CLASS: HMG-COA REDUCTASE INHIBITORS

Actions

HMG-CoA reductase enzyme inhibitors (Table 21.3) are the most potent antilipemic agents available; they are also known as *statins.* The statins competitively inhibit the enzyme that is responsible for converting HMG-CoA to mevalonate in the biosynthetic pathway to cholesterol in the liver. The reduction in liver cholesterol increases the removal of LDLs from the circulating blood. Levels of LDL-C may be reduced by as much as 50%. The statins also cause reductions in VLDL and triglyceride levels (20% to 30%) and mild increases (5% to 15%) in HDL levels. These agents are more effective if administered at night because peak production of cholesterol occurs at this time. Statins also have other beneficial effects unrelated to their lipid-lowering capacity: they reduce inflammation, platelet aggregation, thrombin formation, and plasma viscosity, thereby reducing the factors that contribute to heart attacks and strokes.

Uses

Statins are used in conjunction with dietary therapy to decrease elevated cholesterol concentrations in patients with hyperlipidemia and to reduce the risks of atherosclerosis leading to ASCVD. The statins listed in Table 21.3 are similar in effectiveness at recommended starting doses and times, but they differ with regard to their potential for drug interactions. Other medicines also being taken by the patient may determine the most appropriate statin to be prescribed; this should be based on the avoidance of drug interactions. See Table 21.4 for combination products of atorvastatin and amlodipine (lipid-lowering agents with an antihypertensive agent; see Chapter 22 on calcium channel blockers) and simvastatin with ezetimibe-two lipid-lowering agents.

Therapeutic Outcomes

The primary therapeutic outcomes expected from HMG-CoA reductase inhibitors are reduction of LDL and total cholesterol levels.

Table 21.3   HMG-CoA Reductase Inhibitors (Statins)

GENERIC NAME	BRAND NAME	AVAILABILITY	DAILY DOSAGE RANGE	MAXIMUM DAILY DOSAGE RANGE
atorvastatin	Lipitor	Tablets: 10, 20, 40, 80 mg	10-40 mg daily at any time	Up to 80 mg daily
fluvastatin ⇄ *Do not confuse fluvastatin with fluoxetine.*	Lescol XL	Capsules: 20, 40 mg Tablets, extended release: 80 mg	20-80 mg at bedtime	Up to 80 mg at bedtime
lovastatin ⇄ *Do not confuse lovastatin with Lotensin or Lovenox.*	Altoprev Apo-Lovastatin ❧	Tablets: 10, 20, 40 mg Tablets, extended release: 20, 40, 60 mg	20-40 mg with evening meal *or* 10-60 mg daily at bedtime	80 mg daily (immediate release) *or* 60 mg daily at bedtime (extended release)
pitavastatin	Livalo	Tablets: 1, 2, 4 mg	2 mg once daily at any time, with or without food	Typical dosing range is 1-4 mg
pravastatin	Pravachol Nu-Pravastatin ❧ ⇄ *Do not confuse Pravachol with Prevacid, Prinivil, or propranolol.*	Tablets: 10, 20, 40, 80 mg	40 mg daily at any time	Up to 80 mg daily
rosuvastatin	Crestor	Tablets: 5, 10, 20, 40 mg	5-40 mg daily at any time	Up to 40 mg daily
simvastatin	Zocor ⇄ *Do not confuse Zocor with Cozaar, Zestril, Ziac, or Zoloft.*	Tablets: 5, 10, 20, 40, 80 mg Oral suspension: 20, 40 mg/5 mL in 150-mL bottles	5-40 mg daily at bedtime	Up to 40 mg at bedtime

❧ Available in Canada.

❖ Nursing Implications for HMG-CoA Reductase Inhibitors

◆ *Premedication assessment*

1. Serum triglyceride, lipoprotein, and cholesterol levels should be determined before initiating therapy, then at 4 to 12 weeks, and then annually after that.
2. Liver function tests (AST, ALT) should be obtained before initiating therapy and should be measured during therapy if symptoms suggestive of hepatotoxicity develop, but do not need to be measured routinely. Obtain data related to any GI alterations before initiating therapy (e.g., presence of abdominal pain, nausea, or flatus).
3. Confirm that the patient is not pregnant before initiating a statin. Instruct the female patient to notify her healthcare provider should she contemplate conception or become pregnant while receiving statin therapy.

◆ *Availability, dosage, and administration.* See Tables 21.3 and 21.4. Lovastatin should be administered with food at the evening meal to enhance absorption. The other statins may be administered without food.

◆ *Common adverse effects*

Neurologic

Headaches. This symptom is usually mild and disappears with continued therapy.

Gastrointestinal

Nausea, abdominal bloating, gas. These symptoms are usually mild and disappear with continued therapy.

◆ *Serious adverse effects*

Gastrointestinal

Hepatotoxicity. Liver function should be monitored as described previously. If the transaminases (AST, ALT) rise to three times the upper limit of normal

Table 21.4 HMG-CoA Reductase Inhibitor Combination Products

GENERIC NAME	BRAND NAME	AVAILABILITY	MAXIMUM DAILY DOSAGE RANGE
atorvastatin-amlodipine	Caduet	Tablets: 10 mg atorvastatin and 2.5 mg amlodipine 20 mg atorvastatin and 2.5 mg amlodipine 40 mg atorvastatin and 2.5 mg amlodipine 10 mg atorvastatin and 5 mg amlodipine 20 mg atorvastatin and 5 mg amlodipine 40 mg atorvastatin and 5 mg amlodipine 80 mg atorvastatin and 5 mg amlodipine 10 mg atorvastatin and 10 mg amlodipine 20 mg atorvastatin and 10 mg amlodipine 40 mg atorvastatin and 10 mg amlodipine 80 mg atorvastatin and 10 mg amlodipine	atorvastatin: 80 mg amlodipine: 10 mg
simvastatin-ezetimibe	Vytorin	Tablets: 10 mg simvastatin and 10 mg ezetimibe 20 mg simvastatin and 10 mg ezetimibe 40 mg simvastatin and 10 mg ezetimibe 80 mg simvastatin and 10 mg ezetimibe	simvastatin: 80 mg ezetimibe: 10 mg

and are persistent, then the medication should be discontinued.

Musculoskeletal

Myopathy, rhabdomyolysis. Symptoms of muscle aches, soreness, and weakness may be early signs of myopathy. Serum creatine phosphokinase levels more than 10 times the upper limit of normal confirm the diagnosis. Myopathy is most common with lovastatin (at <1%). Myopathy is more common (5%) if statins are used in combination with niacin, gemfibrozil, or cyclosporine. Rhabdomyolysis is a very serious condition in which kidney damage results from progressive myopathy. An early indication of rhabdomyolysis is pinkish or red-tinged urine secondary to myoglobin (muscle protein) passing through damaged glomeruli into the urine (myoglobinuria).

Cultural Considerations

Chinese patients and those with a Chinese ancestry should not be treated with doses of simvastatin greater than 20 mg when also taking niacin. These patients are more susceptible to developing myopathy. The cause of the increased frequency of myopathy is unknown.

◆ Drug interactions

Cyclosporine, itraconazole, ketoconazole, diltiazem, fluconazole, fibrates, niacin, nefazodone, verapamil, erythromycin, clarithromycin, ranolazine. The incidence of myopathy is increased when lovastatin, simvastatin, or atorvastatin is prescribed in conjunction with these medicines. These medicines inhibit the metabolism of the statins, inducing toxicity.

Cimetidine, ranitidine, omeprazole. Coadministration of these drugs with fluvastatin results in significantly increased fluvastatin levels. Dosage reductions of fluvastatin may be necessary.

Propranolol. Concurrent administration of propranolol and simvastatin results in a significantly lower serum level of simvastatin. Either increase the dosage of simvastatin or switch to another statin.

Rifampin. Concurrent administration of rifampin with fluvastatin, atorvastatin, or simvastatin results in significantly lower levels of the statin. Either increase the dosage of fluvastatin, atorvastatin, or simvastatin or switch to another statin. Monitor cholesterol levels 6 to 8 weeks after change of therapy. Do not discontinue the rifampin.

Warfarin. When lovastatin, simvastatin, rosuvastatin, or fluvastatin and warfarin are prescribed together, the prothrombin time (international normalized ratio [INR]) may be prolonged. Observe the patient for possible excessive anticoagulation and bleeding.

Grapefruit juice. Grapefruit juice inhibits the metabolism of atorvastatin, lovastatin, and simvastatin, thus increasing their plasma concentrations and resulting in a greater potential for myopathy. People who are taking these medications should avoid grapefruit juice.

DRUG CLASS: FIBRIC ACIDS

Actions

The mechanism of action of the fibric acids (e.g., gemfibrozil, fenofibrate) is unknown; however, they do lower triglyceride levels by 20% to 40%. In patients with hypertriglyceridemia, these drugs raise HDL levels by 20% to 25%. They also reduce LDL-C levels by 10% to 15% in patients with elevated cholesterol. Fenofibrate may lower LDL-C levels more effectively than gemfibrozil. However, in patients with concurrent hypertriglyceridemia, gemfibrozil may have no effect, or it may slightly increase LDL-C levels.

Uses

The fibrates are the most effective triglyceride-lowering agents. Gemfibrozil and fenofibrate are used in conjunction with dietary therapy to decrease elevated triglyceride levels in patients who are at risk for pancreatitis. Fibric acids must be used with caution in combination with statins because of the risk of myopathy and rhabdomyolysis.

Therapeutic Outcomes

The primary therapeutic outcomes expected from fibric acid therapy are a 20% to 40% reduction in triglyceride levels and a 20% to 25% increase in HDL levels.

❖ Nursing Implications for Fibric Acids

◆ Premedication assessment

1. Serum triglyceride, lipoprotein, and cholesterol levels should be measured before initiating therapy and periodically thereafter.
2. Liver function tests should be run before initiating therapy and then every 6 months thereafter.
3. Baseline blood glucose levels should be determined before gemfibrozil therapy. Gemfibrozil may cause moderate hyperglycemia.
4. Obtain patient data related to any GI alterations before initiating therapy (e.g., presence of abdominal pain, nausea, flatus).

◆ Availability

Gemfibrozil (lopid). *PO:* 600-mg tablets.

Fenofibrate. *PO:* Tablets: 35, 40, 48, 54, 105, 120, 145, and 160 mg; capsules: 30, 43, 50, 67, 90, 130, 134, 150, and 200 mg; delayed-release capsules: 45 and 135 mg.

◆ Dosage and administration

Gemfibrozil. *PO:* 1200 mg/day in two divided doses, 30 minutes before the morning and evening meals.

Fenofibrate. *PO:* Initially, 45 to 160 mg/day, given with meals. Increase dosage every 4 to 8 weeks up to 160 mg daily with a meal. Dosages of fenofibrate need to be reduced in older adult patients and in patients with renal insufficiency (see the manufacturer's recommendations).

◆ Common adverse effects

Gastrointestinal

Nausea, diarrhea, flatulence, bloating, abdominal distress. These are relatively common adverse effects. Starting with a lower dosage taken between meals can help to minimize these effects. If symptoms persist, notify the healthcare provider because potentially more serious complications may be developing.

◆ Serious adverse effects

Gastrointestinal

Fatigue, anorexia, nausea, malaise, jaundice. These are the early symptoms associated with gallbladder disease and hepatotoxicity. Report these symptoms to the healthcare provider for further evaluation.

Musculoskeletal

Myopathy. Symptoms of muscle aches, soreness, and weakness may be early signs of myopathy. Serum creatine phosphokinase levels of more than 10 times the upper limit of normal confirm the diagnosis. Myopathy is more common (5%) if statins are used in combination with gemfibrozil; it is most common with lovastatin and gemfibrozil.

◆ Drug interactions

Warfarin. The fibric acids may enhance the pharmacologic effects of warfarin. Reduce the dosage of warfarin using the prothrombin time (INR) as an indicator to prevent bleeding.

Sulfonylureas, insulin. Gemfibrozil may increase the pharmacologic effects of these agents. Monitor the patient for signs of hypoglycemia and reduce the dosage of the insulin or sulfonylurea as needed.

Bile acid–binding resins. These resins may bind to fenofibrate, reducing absorption. The interaction can usually be minimized by administering fenofibrate 1 hour before or 4 hours after administration of the resins.

HMG-CoA reductase inhibitors. The potential for developing myopathy is increased when fibric acids are added to the statin treatment regimen. The incidence is less than 5%.

DRUG CLASS: MISCELLANEOUS ANTILIPEMIC AGENTS

ezetimibe (ĕ-ZĔT-ĭ-mēb)
Zetia (ZĔ-tē-ă)

Actions

Ezetimibe is the first of a new class of agents used to reduce atherosclerosis. Ezetimibe acts by blocking the absorption of cholesterol from the small intestine. Unlike bile acid–binding resins, ezetimibe does not bind to cholesterol and reduce absorption. Instead, it acts on the small intestine to inhibit absorption of cholesterol derived from the cholesterol secreted in the bile and from the diet. Studies indicate that ezetimibe reduces levels of total cholesterol by about 12%, LDL-C by 18%, and triglycerides by 7%, and has a minimal effect on raising HDL levels.

Uses

Ezetimibe is used in conjunction with dietary therapy to decrease elevated cholesterol concentrations in patients with hyperlipidemia and to reduce the risks of atherosclerosis leading to ASCVD. This agent may also be used with the statins to lower cholesterol further (Vytorin; see Table 21.4). Combined therapy with fibric acid derivatives is not recommended. Ezetimibe may have an advantage over the bile acid–binding resins because it does not elevate triglyceride levels.

Therapeutic Outcomes

The primary therapeutic outcomes expected from ezetimibe therapy are reduction of LDL and total cholesterol levels.

❖ Nursing Implications for Ezetimibe

◆ *Premedication assessment*
1. Serum triglyceride, lipoprotein, and cholesterol levels should be determined before initiating therapy and periodically thereafter.
2. Obtain patient data related to any GI alterations before initiating therapy (e.g., presence of abdominal pain, nausea, flatus).

◆ *Availability. PO:* 10-mg tablets.

◆ *Dosage and administration.* **Adult:** *PO:* 10 mg once daily; may be taken with or without meals.

◆ *Common adverse effects*
   Gastrointestinal
   Abdominal pain, diarrhea.
These adverse effects are mild and generally do not require discontinuation of therapy.

◆ *Drug interactions*
   Bile acid–binding resins.
These resins may bind to ezetimibe, reducing absorption. The interaction can usually be minimized by administering ezetimibe 1 hour before or 4 hours after administering the resins.

---

omega-3 fatty acids
   Lovaza (lō-VĂ-ză)

Actions

Lovaza was the first of a new class of agents used to reduce atherosclerosis. Lovaza is a combination product that contains two omega-3 fatty acids: eicosapentaenoic acid and docosahexaenoic acid. Omega-3 fatty acids are sometimes referred to as *fish oils* because higher concentrations of these fatty acids are found in such oils. The mechanism of action is unknown, but the end result is that the omega-3 fatty acids reduce synthesis of triglycerides in the liver. Early studies indicate that Lovaza reduces triglyceride levels by 20% to 50%, with small increases in HDL-C levels also seen. In some cases, LDL-C levels are also increased.

Uses

Lovaza is used in conjunction with dietary therapy to decrease very elevated triglyceride levels (>500 mg/dL) in adult patients. This agent may also be used with statins to lower the cholesterol level even further. Lovaza may have an advantage over fibrates and niacin because it does not cause myositis or rhabdomyolysis, particularly when combined with statins. Lovaza should be used with caution in patients who are sensitive or allergic to fish. It should be discontinued in patients who have not shown an adequate response after 2 months of treatment.

Therapeutic Outcome

The primary therapeutic outcome expected from Lovaza therapy is the reduction of an elevated triglyceride level.

❖ Nursing Implications for Omega-3 Fatty Acids

◆ *Premedication assessment*
1. Serum triglyceride, total cholesterol, HDL-C, and LDL-C levels should be determined before initiating therapy and periodically thereafter.
2. Liver function tests (AST, ALT) should be completed before initiating therapy and periodically for the first year of therapy.
3. Obtain patient data related to any GI alterations before initiating therapy (e.g., presence of abdominal pain, nausea, flatus).

◆ *Availability. PO:* 1-g capsules.

◆ *Dosage and administration.* **Adult:** *PO:* 4 g once daily or 2 g twice daily.

◆ *Common and serious adverse effects.* If any of the following adverse effects occur, report them to the healthcare provider immediately: arm, back, or jaw pain; chest pain or discomfort; chest tightness or heaviness; difficult or labored breathing; fast or irregular heartbeat; nausea; shortness of breath; sweating; tightness in the chest; or wheezing.

Other minor adverse effects reported during clinical studies include back pain, unusual or unpleasant aftertaste, belching, a bloated and full feeling, a change in taste, chills, cough, diarrhea, excess air or gas in stomach, fever, a general feeling of discomfort or illness, headache, hoarseness, joint pain, loss of appetite, lower back or side pain, muscle aches and pains, pain, painful or difficult urination, rash, runny nose, shivering, sore throat, sweating, trouble sleeping, unusual tiredness or weakness, or vomiting. These symptoms should be reported to the healthcare provider if they persist.

◆ *Drug interactions.* No drug interactions have been reported to date.

Get Ready for the NCLEX® Examination!

Key Points

- Coronary artery disease is a major cause of premature death in the United States.
- Major treatable causes of ASCVD are hypertension, cigarette smoking, and atherosclerosis.
- A primary cause of atherosclerosis is the abnormal elevation of cholesterol and triglyceride levels in the blood in a disease known as *hyperlipidemia.* A diet high in saturated fats, cholesterol, carbohydrates, total calories, and alcohol—in combination with a sedentary lifestyle—comprise the most common and treatable causes of hyperlipidemia.
- The most cost-effective and successful forms of treatment are smoking cessation, weight reduction, exercise, and dietary modification. If changes in diet and exercise habits do not produce an acceptable decrease in blood lipid levels, an antilipemic agent may be added to the patient's regimen.
- Patients should be fully informed of the significance of hyperlipidemias, the potential complications involved with not modifying their lifestyles, and drug therapy. Drug therapy is likely to continue for many years or a lifetime.
- The primary medicines that are used to lower elevated cholesterol levels are the bile acid–binding resins, ezetimibe, and the statins. The fibric acid derivatives and omega-3 fatty acids lower triglyceride levels.

Additional Learning Resources

SG Go to your Study Guide for additional Review Questions for the NCLEX® Examination, Critical Thinking Clinical Situations, and other learning activities to help you master this chapter content.

Go to your Evolve website (https://evolve.elsevier.com/Clayton) for additional online resources.

Review Questions for the NCLEX® Examination

1. The nurse teaching a patient about lipoproteins realized further education was needed when the patient made which statement?
   1. "I understand that my body manufactures cholesterol and it is needed for normal functioning."
   2. "I need to watch my level of HDL and keep it low, while making sure my LDL level is higher."
   3. "If I overeat, my body converts the excess carbohydrates into triglycerides."
   4. "I need to watch my level of LDL and keep it low, while making sure my HDL level is higher."

2. Lifestyle modifications that can be implemented to reduce the risk of developing hyperlipidemia include which suggestions? *(Select all that apply.)*
   1. Maintaining a heart-healthy diet
   2. Daily dental hygiene
   3. Avoiding tobacco products
   4. Maintaining a healthy weight
   5. Getting regular exercise

3. A patient taking the fibric acid gemfibrozil asks the nurse what is the purpose of the drug. The nurse will respond with which appropriate statement?
   1. "The drug gemfibrozil is used to lower your triglyceride level."
   2. "Fibric acids are used to help lower your cholesterol level."
   3. "The doctor prescribed this drug to help lower the HDLs in your system."
   4. "This drug is useful for preventing insulin resistance."

4. A nurse teaching a patient who was prescribed niacin includes which of these common adverse effects? *(Select all that apply.)*
   1. Headache
   2. Nausea
   3. Diarrhea
   4. Flatulence
   5. Abdominal discomfort

5. A patient prescribed omega-3 fatty acids (Lovaza) asked the nurse what he should know about the drug. The nurse would respond with which appropriate statements? *(Select all that apply.)*
   1. "Lovaza is used to decrease very elevated triglyceride levels."
   2. "Lovaza is often used with statins to further lower cholesterol levels."
   3. "Lovaza may cause myositis or rhabdomyolysis."
   4. "Lovaza should be used with caution in patients who are allergic to fish."
   5. "Lovaza should be discontinued after 2 months of therapy if there is not an adequate response."

6. A patient recently diagnosed with dyslipidemia asks the nurse why she should take the newly prescribed statin. Which of these statements by the nurse is appropriate?
   1. "Your healthcare providers know what they are doing, and you have to take this drug."
   2. "The reason you need to take this prescribed statin is so you will have a decreased risk of developing cardiovascular diseases such as a heart attack or stroke."
   3. "The statin that has been ordered for you is because it has been shown to be the most effective drug to reducing your chances of developing metabolic syndrome."
   4. "I'm not really sure what this is for, but it is important for you to follow the recommendations we give you."

22

Drugs Used to Treat Hypertension

Objectives

1. Differentiate between primary and secondary hypertension.
2. Summarize nursing assessments and interventions used for the treatment of hypertension.
3. Identify recommended lifestyle modifications after a diagnosis of hypertension.
4. Identify initial options and progression of medicines used to treat hypertension.
5. Identify and summarize the action of five drug classes used to treat hypertension.

Key Terms

arterial blood pressure (ăr-TĔR-ē-ŭl BLŬD PRĔ-shŭr) (p. 340)
systolic blood pressure (sĭs-TŎL-ĭk) (p. 340)
diastolic blood pressure (dī-ă-STŎL-ĭk) (p. 340)
pulse pressure (PŬLS) (p. 340)
mean arterial pressure (MAP) (MĒN ăr-TĔR-ē-ŭl) (p. 340)

cardiac output (CO) (KĂR-dē-ăk ŎWT-pŭt) (p. 340)
hypertension (hī-pĕr-TĔN-shŭn) (p. 341)
primary hypertension (PRĪ-măr-ē) (p. 341)
secondary hypertension (SĔK-ŏn-dār-ē) (p. 341)
systolic hypertension (p. 341)

HYPERTENSION

See Chapter 20 for an introduction to cardiovascular diseases. A primary function of the heart is to circulate blood to the organs and tissues of the body. When the heart contracts (systole), blood is pumped from the right ventricle out through the pulmonary artery to the lungs, as well as from the left ventricle out through the aorta to the other organs and peripheral tissues. The pressure with which the blood is pumped from the heart is referred to as the arterial blood pressure or systolic blood pressure. When the heart muscle relaxes between contractions (diastole), the blood pressure drops to a lower level, the diastolic blood pressure. When recorded in the patient's chart, the systolic pressure is recorded first, followed by the diastolic pressure (e.g., 120/80 mm Hg). The difference between the systolic and diastolic pressures is called the pulse pressure, which is an indicator of the tone of the arterial blood vessel walls. The mean arterial pressure (MAP) is the average pressure throughout each cycle of the heartbeat and is significant because it is the pressure that actually pushes the blood through the circulatory system to perfuse organs and tissues. It is calculated by adding one-third of the pulse pressure to the diastolic pressure or by using the following equation, where DP is diastolic pressure and SP is systolic pressure:

$$MAP = DP + \frac{1}{3}(SP - DP)$$

Normal MAP readings generally fall between 70 and 110 mm Hg; however, the number 60 or higher has been targeted as enough pressure to adequately perfuse organs and tissues. Under normal conditions, the arterial blood pressure stays within narrow limits. It reaches its peak during high physical or emotional activity and is usually at its lowest level during sleep.

Arterial blood pressure (BP) can be defined as the product of cardiac output (CO) and peripheral vascular resistance (PVR):

$$BP = CO \times PVR$$

Cardiac output is the primary determinant of systolic pressure; peripheral vascular resistance determines the diastolic pressure. Cardiac output is determined by the stroke volume (the volume of blood ejected in a single contraction from the left ventricle), heart rate (controlled by the autonomic nervous system), and venous capacitance (elasticity of the blood vessel). Systolic blood pressure is thus increased by factors that increase heart rate or stroke volume. Venous capacitance affects the volume of blood (or preload) that is returned to the heart through the central venous circulation. Venous constriction decreases venous capacitance, increasing preload and systolic pressure, and venous dilation increases venous capacitance and decreases preload and systolic pressure. Peripheral vascular resistance is regulated primarily by contraction and dilation of arterioles. Arteriolar constriction increases peripheral vascular resistance and thus diastolic blood pressure. Other factors that affect vascular resistance include the elasticity of the blood vessel walls and the viscosity of the blood.

Hypertension is a disease characterized by an elevation of the systolic blood pressure, the diastolic blood pressure, or both. The likelihood of having a cardiovascular event (angina, myocardial infarction, heart failure, stroke, renal failure, retinopathy) increases as blood pressure increases. Studies have shown that a 20 mm Hg systolic blood pressure and a 10 mm Hg diastolic blood pressure above 115/75 mm Hg increases the risk of death from stroke, heart disease, and other vascular disease. **Primary hypertension** accounts for 90% of all clinical cases of high blood pressure. The cause of primary hypertension is unknown. At present, it is incurable but controllable. In the United States it is estimated that about 37% of the population —or greater than one-third of the population over age 20—have hypertension. The prevalence increases steadily with obesity and advancing age so that people who are normotensive at age 55 have a 90% lifetime risk of developing hypertension. In every age group, the incidence of hypertension is higher for African Americans than whites of both genders. Other major risk factors associated with high blood pressure are listed in Box 22.1. **Secondary hypertension** occurs after the development of another disorder within the body (Box 22.2).

The 2017 Guideline for the Prevention, Detection, Evaluation and Management of High Blood Pressure in Adults jointly published by the American College of Cardiology and the American Heart Association includes a new definition of hypertension and classification of blood pressure by stages that represent the degree of risk of nonfatal and fatal cardiovascular disease events and renal disease (Table 22.1).

The guidelines use elevation in both systolic and diastolic blood pressure readings above 115/75 mm Hg when making a diagnosis of hypertension. In an effort to get accurate blood pressure readings for diagnosis, the individual should be seated quietly for at least 5 minutes in a chair (rather than on an examination table), with feet on the floor and arm supported at heart level. An appropriately sized cuff (cuff bladder encircling at least 80% of the arm) should be used for accuracy. A person must have two or more elevated readings on two or more separate occasions after initial screening to be classified as having hypertension. When systolic and diastolic readings fall into two different stages, the higher of the two stages is used to classify the degree of hypertension present. Table 22.2 lists the blood pressure thresholds for classification of hypertension (elevated, stage 1 and stage 2 hypertension) and follow-up recommendations based on the initial set of blood pressure measurements.

The guidelines further urge health practitioners to use the systolic blood pressure as the major criterion for the diagnosis and management of hypertension in middle-aged and older Americans. Before this time, the diastolic blood pressure had been the major determinant for the control of blood pressure. Evidence indicates that **systolic hypertension** is the most common form of hypertension and is present in about two-thirds of hypertensive individuals older than 60 years.

When a person has been diagnosed with hypertension, further evaluation through medical history, physical examination, and laboratory tests should be completed to (1) identify causes of the high blood pressure; (2) assess the presence or absence of target organ damage

---

Box 22.1	Major Risk Factors Associated With Hypertension and Target Organ Damage

MAJOR RISK FACTORS
- Cigarette smoking
- Obesity (body mass index ≥30 kg/m²)
- Physical inactivity
- Dyslipidemia
- Diabetes mellitus
- Microalbuminuria or estimated glomerular filtration rate less than 60 mL/min
- Age (older than 55 for men, 65 for women)
- Family history of premature cardiovascular disease (men younger than age 55; women, age 65)

TARGET ORGAN DAMAGE
- Heart
  - Left ventricular hypertrophy
  - Angina or prior myocardial infarction
  - Prior coronary revascularization
  - Heart failure
- Brain
  - Stroke or transient ischemic attack
- Chronic kidney disease
  - Glomerular filtration rate
- Peripheral arterial disease
- Retinopathy
- Components of metabolic syndrome

Adapted from the Joint National Committee on Prevention, Detection, Evaluation, and Treatment of High Blood Pressure. *The Seventh Report of the Joint National Committee on Prevention, Detection, Evaluation, and Treatment of High Blood Pressure (JNC 7).* Bethesda, MD: National Institutes of Health; 2003. NIH publication 03-5233.

Box 22.2	Identifiable Causes of Hypertension

- Sleep apnea
- Drug-induced or related causes
- Chronic kidney disease
- Primary aldosteronism
- Renovascular disease
- Chronic steroid therapy and Cushing's syndrome
- Pheochromocytoma
- Coarctation of the aorta
- Thyroid or parathyroid disease

Adapted from the Joint National Committee on Prevention, Detection, Evaluation, and Treatment of High Blood Pressure. *The Seventh Report of the Joint National Committee on Prevention, Detection, Evaluation, and Treatment of High Blood Pressure (JNC 7).* Bethesda, MD: National Institutes of Health; 2003. NIH publication 03-5233.

Table 22.1	Classification and Management of Blood Pressure (BP) for Adults[a]				
BP CLASSIFICATION	BLOOD PRESSURE (MM HG)			LIFESTYLE MODIFICATION	INITIAL DRUG
	SYSTOLIC		DIASTOLIC		
Normal	<120	and	<80	Encourage	No treatment
Elevated	120-129	or	<80	Yes	Generally no treatment
Stage 1 hypertension	130-139	or	80-89	Yes	If risk is less than 10%, start with healthy lifestyle recommendation; if greater than 10%, start drug therapy with one of the following agents: ACEI or ARB, CCB or diuretic
Stage 2 hypertension	≥140	or	≥90	Yes	Two first-line drug combination from different classes

From Whelton PK, Carey RM, Aronow WS, et al. 2017 ACC/AHA/AAPA/ABC/ACPM/AGS/APhA/ASH/ASPC/NMA/PCNA Guideline for the Prevention, Detection, Evaluation, and Management of High Blood Pressure in Adults: A Report of the American College of Cardiology/American Heart Association Task Force on Clinical Practice Guidelines. *J Am Coll Cardiol.* Published online November 13, 2017. http://www.onlinejacc.org/content/early/2017/11/04/j.jacc.2017.11.005.
[a]Individuals with SBP and DBP in two categories should be designated to the higher BP category.
ACEI, Angiotensin-converting enzyme inhibitor; *ARB,* angiotensin-receptor blocker; *CCB,* calcium channel blocker.

Table 22.2	Recommended Follow-Up Schedule After Initial Blood Pressure Measurement	
INITIAL BLOOD PRESSURE (MM HG)		FOLLOW-UP RECOMMENDED
SYSTOLIC	DIASTOLIC	
< 120	< 80	Recheck in 1 yr
120-129	< 80	Recheck in 3 to 6 months [a]
130-139	80-89	Recheck in 3 to 6 months, if risk is less than 10% and following healthy lifestyle recommendations. Recheck in 1 month, if risk is greater than 10% receiving treatment
≥140	≥ 90	Recheck in 1 month. If goal met in 1 month, recheck in 3 to 6 months. If goal not met in month, consider different medication or titration. Continue rechecking monthly until control achieved
≥180	≥110	Evaluate or refer to source of care immediately or within 1 wk, depending on clinical situation

From Whelton PK, Carey RM, Aronow WS, et al. 2017 ACC/AHA/AAPA/ABC/ACPM/AGS/APhA/ASH/ASPC/NMA/PCNA Guideline for the Prevention, Detection, Evaluation, and Management of High Blood Pressure in Adults: A Report of the American College of Cardiology/American Heart Association Task Force on Clinical Practice Guidelines. *J Am Coll Cardiol.* Published online November 13, 2017. http://www.onlinejacc.org/content/early/2017/11/04/j.jacc.2017.11.005.
[a]Provide advice about lifestyle modifications.

and cardiovascular disease (see Box 22.1); and (3) identify other cardiovascular risk factors that may guide treatment (see Table 22.1).

TREATMENT OF HYPERTENSION

The primary purpose for controlling hypertension is to reduce the frequency of cardiovascular disease. To accomplish this goal, the 2017 guidelines recommend that blood pressure must be reduced and maintained below 130/80 mm Hg in adult patients. Noninstitutionalized ambulatory community-dwelling adult patients 65 years and older should maintain a systolic blood pressure of less than 130 mm Hg. For adults 65 years and older with hypertension and a high burden of comorbidity and limited life expectancy, clinical judgment, patient preference, and a team-based approach to assess risk/benefit are reasonable for decisions regarding intensity of BP lowering and choice of antihypertensive drugs. Major lifestyle modifications shown to lower blood pressure include weight reduction in those who are overweight or obese; adoption of the DASH (*D*ietary *A*pproaches to *S*top *H*ypertension) diet, the US Department of Agriculture (USDA) Food Patterns, or the American College of Cardiology/American Heart Association (ACC/AHA) diet recommendations; dietary sodium reduction; physical activity; and moderation of alcohol consumption (Table 22.3). Treatment schedules should interfere as little as possible with the patient's lifestyle; however, nonpharmacologic therapy must include elimination of smoking, weight control, routine activity, restriction of alcohol intake, stress reduction, a regular sleep pattern of at least 7 hours each night, and sodium control. If this therapy is successful in controlling high blood pressure, drug therapy is not necessary. Even if lifestyle changes are not adequate to control hypertension, they may reduce the number and doses of antihypertensive medications needed to manage the condition.

Table 22.3   Lifestyle Modifications to Manage Hypertension[a]

MODIFICATION	RECOMMENDATION	APPROXIMATE BLOOD PRESSURE REDUCTION (RANGE)
Weight reduction[b]	Maintain normal body weight (body mass index = 18.5-24.9 kg/m^2).	Systolic 5-20 mm Hg/10-kg weight loss
Adopt a healthy eating plan[c]	Consume a diet rich in fruits, whole grains, vegetables; includes low-fat dairy products, poultry, fish, legumes, nontropical vegetable oils, and nuts; limits intake of sweets, sugar-sweetened beverages, and red meats with a reduced content of saturated and total fat. Described in DASH diet, USDA Food Patterns, or AHA/ACC diet.	Systolic/diastolic 5-6/3 mm Hg
Dietary sodium reduction[c]	Reduce dietary sodium intake to no more than 2.4 g sodium or 6 g sodium chloride per day.	Systolic/diastolic 2-7/1-3 mm Hg
Physical activity[c]	Engage in regular aerobic physical activity three or four sessions per week, lasting an average of 40 minutes per session, involving moderate to vigorous intensity.[c]	Systolic 4-9 mm Hg
Moderation of alcohol[b] consumption	Limit consumption to no more than two drinks (1 oz or 30 mL ethanol [e.g., 24 oz beer, 10 oz wine, or 3 oz 80-proof whiskey])/day in most men and no more than one drink/day in women and lighter weight individuals.	Systolic 2-4 mm Hg

[a]The effects of implementing these modifications are dose and time dependent and could be greater for some individuals. For overall cardiovascular risk reduction, stop smoking.
[b]From the Joint National Committee on Prevention, Detection, Evaluation, and Treatment of High Blood Pressure. *The seventh report of the Joint National Committee on Prevention, Detection, Evaluation, and Treatment of High Blood Pressure (JNC 7)*. Bethesda, MD: National Institutes of Health; 2003. NIH publication 03-5233.
[c]From Eckel RH, Jakcic JM, Ard JD, et al. 2013 AHA/ACC Guideline on lifestyle management to reduce cardiovascular risk: a report of the American College of Cardiology/American Heart Association Task Force on Practice Guidelines. *Circulation*. 2014;129(25 suppl 2):S76-S99.
AHA, American Heart Association; *DASH*, Dietary Approaches to Stop Hypertension; *USDA*, US Department of Agriculture.

Patient education is vitally important in treating hypertension. This education should be emphasized and reiterated frequently by the physician, pharmacist, and nurse.

DRUG THERAPY FOR HYPERTENSION

ACTIONS

Drugs used in the treatment of hypertension can be subdivided into several categories of therapeutic agents based on site of action (Fig. 22.1). Pharmacologic classes of agents initially used to treat hypertension are angiotensin-converting enzyme (ACE) inhibitors or angiotensin II receptor blockers (ARBs), calcium channel blockers, and thiazide-type diuretics. Less frequently used agents are the beta-adrenergic blockers, direct renin inhibitors, aldosterone receptor antagonists, alpha-1 adrenergic blockers, central-acting alpha-2 agonists, and direct vasodilators. Agents may be used alone or in combination with other agents from different classes working by different mechanisms to optimize therapy while reducing adverse effects of the medicines.

USES

A key to long-term success with antihypertensive therapy is to individualize therapy for a patient based on demographic characteristics (e.g., age, gender, race), coexisting diseases and risk factors (e.g., migraine headaches, dysrhythmias, angina, diabetes mellitus),

previous therapy (what has or has not worked in the past), concurrent drug therapy for other illnesses, and cost. As outlined in Fig. 22.2, the 2017 guidelines stress the benefit of lifestyle changes to prevent and treat hypertension. Nonpharmacologic therapy is especially effective in managing hypertension in patients with elevated blood pressure and with stage 1 hypertension in adults with a 10-year cardiovascular risk less than 10%. Adult patients with a 10-year cardiovascular risk of 10% or greater treatment should be initiated with one of the four classes of medications recommended: an ACE inhibitor or ARB, a calcium channel blocker, and/or a diuretic and nonpharmacologic therapy. In adult patients with stage 1 hypertension it is reasonable to start with one first-line agent (such as a thiazide-like diuretic), especially in adults with a history of orthostatic hypotension. It is recommended to initiate two first-line agents of different classes (such as an ACE inhibitor and a thiazide-like diuretic or a calcium blocker with a thiazide-like diuretic) for adults with stage 2 hypertension and a blood pressure more than 20/10 mm Hg higher than their target (Fig. 22.3). Use of a combination product may simplify the regimen and enhance adherence. See Table 22.4 for a list of ingredients of antihypertensive combination products. Use caution in older adults because hypotension or orthostatic hypotension may develop. In black patients with hypertension but without heart failure and kidney disease, including those with diabetes, two or more antihypertensive agents are recommended, such as a thiazide-like diuretic and/

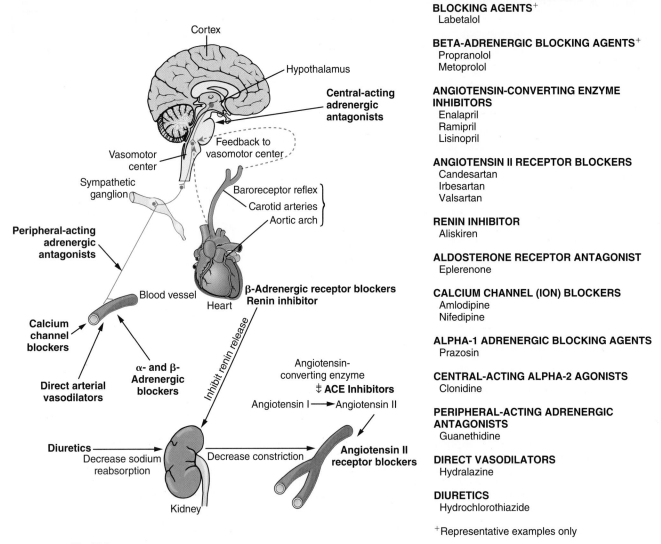

ALPHA- AND BETA-ADRENERGIC BLOCKING AGENTS$^+$
Labetalol

BETA-ADRENERGIC BLOCKING AGENTS$^+$
Propranolol
Metoprolol

ANGIOTENSIN-CONVERTING ENZYME INHIBITORS
Enalapril
Ramipril
Lisinopril

ANGIOTENSIN II RECEPTOR BLOCKERS
Candesartan
Irbesartan
Valsartan

RENIN INHIBITOR
Aliskiren

ALDOSTERONE RECEPTOR ANTAGONIST
Eplerenone

CALCIUM CHANNEL (ION) BLOCKERS
Amlodipine
Nifedipine

ALPHA-1 ADRENERGIC BLOCKING AGENTS
Prazosin

CENTRAL-ACTING ALPHA-2 AGONISTS
Clonidine

PERIPHERAL-ACTING ADRENERGIC ANTAGONISTS
Guanethidine

DIRECT VASODILATORS
Hydralazine

DIURETICS
Hydrochlorothiazide

$^+$Representative examples only

Fig. 22.1 Sites of action of antihypertensive agents. *ACE*, Angiotensin-converting enzyme. (Modified from US Department of Health and Human Services. *The Sixth Report of the Joint National Committee on Detection, Evaluation, and Treatment of High Blood Pressure [JNC-VI]*. Washington, DC: National Institutes of Health; 1997.)

or a calcium channel blocker. For all patients, a low dose should be selected to protect against adverse effects, although it may not immediately control the blood pressure. It must be recognized that it may take months to control hypertension adequately while avoiding adverse effects of therapy.

Because of many physiologic compensatory mechanisms that may aggravate lowering blood pressure, about 75% of hypertensive patients require a combination of medications that act by different pathways to achieve blood pressure goals (<130/80 mm Hg). If, after 1 month, the first drug is not effective, the dosage may be increased, or a second drug from another class with a different mechanism of action may be added (Fig. 22.3). After blood pressure is reduced to the goal level and maintenance doses of medicines are stabilized, it may be appropriate to change a patient's medication to a combination antihypertensive product to simplify the regimen and enhance compliance. See Table 22.4 for a list of the ingredients of antihypertensive combination products.

The guidelines also provide recommendations for specific groups of patients. For most patients with comorbidities, the blood pressure goal should be less than 130/80 mm Hg. For patients aged 65 years or older, a target systolic blood pressure of less than 130 mm Hg is recommended. In some patients with comorbidities, the goal may be a blood pressure of 140/90 mm Hg. For example, older patients with isolated systolic hypertension should first be treated with diuretics, with or without a beta blocker, or a dihydropyridine calcium channel blocker alone. Patients with high blood pressure and heart failure, and/or chronic kidney disease, should be treated with the ACE inhibitors or ARBs. Patients who have hypertension and have suffered a myocardial infarction should be treated with a beta-adrenergic blocking agent and, in most cases, an ACE inhibitor. Other studies have demonstrated that if a patient has

STATUS OF BLOOD PRESSURE

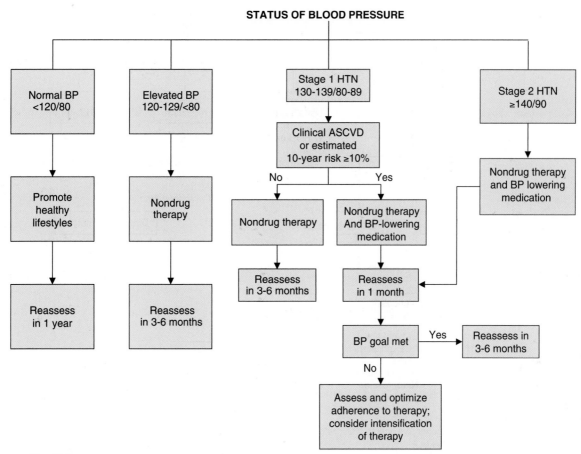

Fig. 22.2 Treatment algorithm for hypertension. *ASCVD,* Atherosclerotic cardiovascular disease; *BP,* blood pressure; *HTN,* hypertension. (From Whelton PK, Carey RM, Aronow WS, et al. 2017 ACC/AHA/AAPA/ABC/ACPM/AGS/APhA/ASH/ASPC/NMA/PCNA Guidelines for the Prevention, Detection, Evaluation, and Management of High Blood Pressure in Adults: A Report of the American College of Cardiology/American Heart Association Task Force on Clinical Practice Guidelines. *J Am Coll Cardiol.* Published online November 13, 2017. http://www.onlinejacc.org/content/early/2017/11/04/j.jacc.2017.11.005.)

heart failure, a diuretic, an ACE inhibitor, and an aldosterone receptor antagonist (e.g., spironolactone, eplerenone) may be beneficial. If a patient has angina pectoris, dihydropyridine calcium channel blockers (e.g., amlodipine, nifedipine) may be added to other therapy because they have been proven to relieve chest pain and reduce the incidence of stroke. Other combinations of therapy found to be particularly effective are an ACE inhibitor plus a diuretic or calcium channel blocker, or an ARB plus a diuretic. (See individual drug monographs for mechanisms of action of each class of antihypertensive agent.) Do not use an ACE inhibitor and ARB or direct renin inhibitor together in the same patient. There is generally little therapeutic gain compared with potential adverse effects that may develop.

Patients who have modified their lifestyles with appropriate exercise, diet, weight reduction, and control of hypertension for at least 1 year may be candidates for step-down therapy. The dosage of antihypertensive medications may be gradually reduced in a slow, deliberate manner. Most patients may still require some therapy, but occasionally the medicine can be discontinued.

Patients whose drugs have been discontinued should have regular follow-up examinations because blood pressure often rises again to hypertensive levels, sometimes months or years later, especially if lifestyle modifications are not continued.

❖ NURSING IMPLICATIONS FOR HYPERTENSIVE THERAPY

◆ Assessment

History of risk factors

- Make note of the patient's gender, age, and race. People who are older, male, and/or African American have a higher incidence of hypertension.
- Has the patient been told previously about the elevated blood pressure readings? If so, under what circumstances were the blood pressure readings taken?
- Is there a family history of hypertension, coronary heart disease, stroke, diabetes mellitus, or dyslipidemia?

Smoking. Obtain a history of the number of cigarettes or cigars smoked daily. How long has the person smoked? Has the person ever tried to stop smoking?

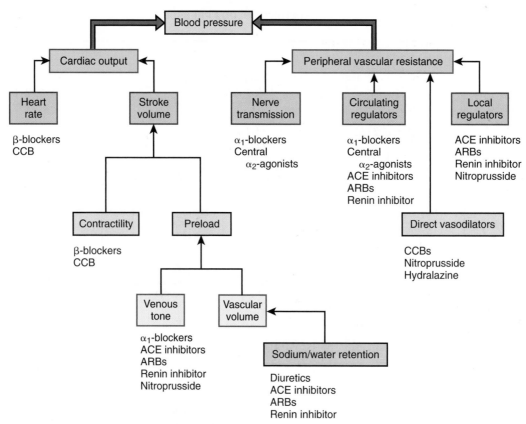

Fig. 22.3 Effects of antihypertensive agents. *ACE,* Angiotensin-converting enzyme; *ARB,* angiotensin II receptor blocker; *CCB,* calcium channel blocker.

Ask whether the person knows what effect smoking has on the vascular system. How does the individual feel about modifying the smoking habit?

Dietary habits. Obtain a dietary history. Ask specific questions to obtain data relating to the amount of salt used in cooking and at the table, as well as foods eaten that are high in fat, cholesterol, refined carbohydrates, and sodium. Using a calorie counter, ask the person to estimate the number of calories eaten daily. How much meat, fish, and poultry are eaten daily (size and number of servings)? Estimate the percentage of total daily calories provided by fats. Discuss food preparation (e.g., baked, broiled, fried foods). How many servings of fruits and vegetables are eaten daily? What types of oils or fats are used in food preparation? Consult a nutrition text for further dietary history questions. What is the frequency and volume of alcoholic beverages consumed?

Elevated serum lipids. Ask whether the patient is aware of having elevated lipid, triglyceride, or cholesterol levels. If elevated, what measures has the person tried for reduction and what effect have the interventions had on the blood levels at subsequent examinations? Review laboratory data available (e.g., cholesterol, triglyceride, low-density lipoprotein [LDL], very-low-density lipoprotein levels).

Renal function. Has the patient had any laboratory tests to evaluate renal function (e.g., urinalysis—microalbuminuria, proteinuria, microscopic hematuria) or had a blood analysis showing an elevated blood urea nitrogen (BUN) or serum creatinine level? Does the patient have nocturia?

Obesity. Ask about any recent weight gains or losses and whether intentional or unintentional. Note abnormal waist-to-hip ratio. Patients with more weight around their waist have a higher incidence of developing heart disease, hypertension, and diabetes (see Chapter 20).

Psychomotor functions
- Determine the patient's type of lifestyle. Have the patient describe exercise level in terms of amount (e.g., walking 3 miles), intensity (e.g., walking 3 mph), and frequency (e.g., walking every other day). Is the patient's job physically demanding or of a sedentary nature?
- Determine the patient's level of psychological stress. Ask the individual to estimate the amount of stress in his or her life. How does the person cope with stressful situations at home and in the workplace?
- Has the patient experienced any fatigue or reduction in activity level caused by intolerance or palpitations, angina, or dyspnea? When walking, do severe leg

Table 22.4 Combination Drugs for Hypertension

COMBINATION TYPE	FIXED-DOSE COMBINATION (mg)[a]	BRAND NAME
ACEIs and CCBs	amlodipine/benazepril (2.5/10, 5/10, 5/20, 5/40, 10/20, 10/40)	Lotrel
	enalapril/felodipine (5/2.5, 5/5)	Lexxel
	trandolapril/verapamil (2/180, 1/240, 2/240, 4/240)	Tarka
CCB and statin	amlodipine/atorvastatin (2.5/10 to 10/80)	Caduet
CCBs and ARBs	amlodipine/valsartan (5/160 to 10/320)	Exforge
	amlodipine/olmesartan (5/20 to 10/40)	Azor
	amlodipine/telmisartan (5/40, 5/80, 10/40, 10/80)	Twynsta
CCBs/diuretic/ARBs	amlodipine/hydrochlorothiazide/valsartan (5/12.5/160 to 10/25/320)	Exforge HCT
	amlodipine/hydrochlorothiazide/olmesartan (5/12.5/20 to 10/25/40)	Tribenzor
ACEIs and diuretics	benazepril/hydrochlorothiazide (5/6.25, 10/12.5, 20/12.5, 20/25)	Lotensin HCT
	captopril/hydrochlorothiazide (25/15, 25/25, 50/15, 50/25)	
	enalapril/hydrochlorothiazide (5/12.5, 10/25)	Vaseretic
	fosinopril/hydrochlorothiazide (10/12.5, 20/12.5)	
	lisinopril/hydrochlorothiazide (10/12.5, 20/12.5, 20/25)	Zestoretic
	moexipril/hydrochlorothiazide (7.5/12.5, 15/12.5, 15/25)	
	quinapril/hydrochlorothiazide (10/12.5, 20/12.5, 20/25)	Accuretic
ARBs and diuretics	azilsartan/chlorthalidone (40/12.5 to 40/25)	Edarbyclor
	candesartan/hydrochlorothiazide (16/12.5, 32/12.5, 32/25)	Atacand HCT
	irbesartan/hydrochlorothiazide (150/12.5, 300/12.5)	Avalide
	losartan potassium/hydrochlorothiazide (50/12.5, 100/12.5, 100/25)	Hyzaar
		⇄ Do not confuse Hyzaar with Cozaar.
	olmesartan/hydrochlorothiazide (20/12.5, 40/12.5, 40/25)	Benicar HCT
	telmisartan/hydrochlorothiazide (40/12.5, 80/12.5, 80/25)	Micardis HCT
	valsartan/hydrochlorothiazide (80/12.5, 160/12.5, 320/12.5, 160/25, 320/25)	Diovan HCT
BBs and diuretics	atenolol/chlorthalidone (50/25, 100/25)	Tenoretic
	bisoprolol/hydrochlorothiazide (2.5/6.25, 5/6.25, 10/6.25)	Ziac
		⇄ Do not confuse Ziac with Zocor or Tiazac.
	propranolol/hydrochlorothiazide (40/25, 80/25)	
	metoprolol/hydrochlorothiazide (25/12.5, 50/12.5, 100/12.5, 50/25, 100/25)	Lopressor HCT
	nadolol/bendroflumethiazide (40/5, 80/5)	Corzide
Direct renin inhibitor combination products	aliskiren/hydrochlorothiazide (150/12.5, 150/25, 300/12.5, 300/25)	Tekturna HCT
Diuretic and diuretic combination	amiloride HCl/hydrochlorothiazide (5/50)	
	spironolactone/hydrochlorothiazide (25/25, 50/50)	Aldactazide
	triamterene/hydrochlorothiazide (37.5/25, 50/25, 75/50)	Dyazide, Maxzide

[a]Some drug combinations are available in multiple fixed doses. Each drug dose is reported in milligrams.
ACEI, Angiotensin-converting enzyme inhibitor; *ARB,* angiotensin receptor blocker; *BB,* beta blocker; *CCB,* calcium channel blocker.

cramps (claudication) force him or her to stop and rest or severely limit ambulation?

Medication history

- Has the patient ever taken or is currently taking any medications for the treatment of high blood pressure? If blood pressure medications have been prescribed but are not being taken, why was the medicine discontinued? Were any adverse effects noticed while taking the medications, and how did the patient manage them?
- Obtain a list of all medications being taken, including prescribed drugs, over-the-counter drugs, herbal preparations, and street drugs. Research these medications in the drug monographs to determine potential drug-drug interactions that may affect the individual's blood pressure or the effectiveness of the medicines prescribed.
- If the patient is female, ask whether she is now or has been taking oral contraceptives or is receiving hormone replacement therapy.

Physical assessments

Blood pressure. Obtain two or more blood pressure measurements.

- The individual should be seated quietly for at least 5 minutes in a chair with a back support (rather than on an examination table), with feet on the floor and arm supported at heart level.
- An appropriately sized cuff (cuff bladder encircling at least 80% of the arm) should be used for accuracy.
- When measuring blood pressure, the cuff should be inflated to 30 mm Hg above the point at which the radial pulse disappears. The sphygmomanometer pressure should then be reduced at 2 to 3 mm/sec. Two readings should be taken at least 1 minute apart.
- Verify the readings in the opposite arm. A difference in blood pressure between the two arms can be expected in about 20% of patients. The higher value should be the one used in treatment decisions.
- People must have two or more elevated readings on two or more separate occasions after initial screening to be classified as having hypertension.
- Orthostatic hypotension is defined by a decrease in systolic blood pressure of 20 mm Hg or more, or diastolic blood pressure of 10 mm Hg or more, following rapid change of position from recumbent to standing or after 3 minutes of quiet standing. Food ingestion, time of day, age, and hydration can affect this form of hypotension, as can a history of parkinsonism, excessive blood loss, diabetes, or multiple myeloma.
- Ensure that the patient has not ingested caffeine within the past 2 to 3 hours.

Height and weight. Weigh and measure the patient. Measure the waste circumference 2 inches above the navel. What has the person's weight been? Ask about any recent weight gains or losses and whether intentional or unintentional. Calculate the body mass index (see Chapter 20 for more discussion and classification of body mass index).

Bruits. Check neck, abdomen, and extremities for the presence of bruits.

Peripheral pulses. Palpate and record femoral, popliteal, and pedal pulses bilaterally.

Eyes. As appropriate to the level of education, perform a funduscopic examination of the interior eye, noting arteriovenous nicking, hemorrhages, exudates, or papilledema.

◆ Implementation

- Perform nursing assessments on a scheduled basis.
- Make referrals as indicated for stress management, smoking cessation, and dietary counseling and for an exercise program appropriate for the individual's needs.
- When initiating antihypertensive therapy in a hospitalized patient, protect the patient from possible falls secondary to hypotension by assisting during ambulation and carefully assessing for faintness. Take blood pressure in supine, sitting, and standing positions to identify hypotensive responses.

◆ Patient Education

- Examine data to determine the individual's extent of understanding of hypertension and its control.
- Using the patient's history, analyze lifestyle elements to determine health teaching needs of the individual and significant others.

Baseline and diagnostic studies. Review the patient's chart and all reports available that are used to build baseline information (e.g., electrocardiogram; urinalysis; blood glucose, hematocrit, serum potassium, BUN, creatinine, and calcium levels; a lipid profile [total cholesterol, LDL cholesterol, high-density lipoprotein cholesterol, triglycerides] after a 9- to 12-hour fast).

Smoking

- Suggest that the patient stop smoking. Smoking causes vasoconstriction of the blood vessels; encourage a drastic reduction in—and preferably total abstinence from—smoking. Include information about smoking cessation and available support resources.
- Explain the increased risk of coronary artery disease if the habit is continued. It may be necessary to settle for a drastic decrease in smoking in some people, although abstinence should be the goal.

Nutritional status

- Dietary counseling is essential for the treatment of hypertension. Control of obesity alone may be sufficient to alter the hypertensive condition. Most patients are placed on a reduced-sodium diet (2.4 g sodium or <6 g table salt per day). The goal of dietary therapy is a reduction of cholesterol, lipids, saturated fat, and alcohol consumption. Foods high in potassium and calcium are encouraged to decrease blood pressure. See the DASH, USDA Food Patterns, or ACC/AHA diet for further information (see Table 22.3).

- Dietary planning should always involve the patient in menu planning so that personal preferences, availability of food products, and costs are discussed. Include the person who purchases food products and prepares the meals in the dietary counseling.
- Show the patient various food labels and explain what ingredients indicate a high sodium content (e.g., salt, sodium, sodium chloride, sodium bicarbonate, sodium aluminum sulfate). Suggest the use of a variety of spices as substitutes for sodium when cooking. Explain foods that should be avoided in large quantities (e.g., bacon, smoked meats, crab meat, tuna, crackers, processed cheeses, ham).
- Teach the individual to record weights in the same clothing, at the same time daily, and using the same scale. Generally, a weight gain or loss of more than 2 pounds is reported to a healthcare provider; however, specific parameters may vary and should be discussed during initiation of therapy.

Stress management

- Identify stress-producing situations in the patient's life and seek means to reduce these factors significantly. In some cases, referral for training in stress management, relaxation techniques, meditation, or biofeedback may be necessary. If stress is produced in the work setting, it may be appropriate to involve an industrial nurse.
- Stress within the family is often significant and may require professional counseling for the family and patient.

Exercise and activity. Develop a plan for moderate exercise to improve the patient's general condition. Consult a healthcare provider for any individual modifications deemed appropriate. Suggest including activities that the patient finds helpful in reducing stress. Nurses can help patients increase physical activity throughout the day by encouraging them to take part in the following:

- Play active games with their children.
- Engage in a sport.
- Find a friend with whom to walk or jog.
- Take a class in yoga or tai chi.
- Walk a dog.
- Garden on the weekends.
- Walk or bicycle to school or work.
- Take the stairs, avoiding the elevator.
- Park the car at the farthest point in the parking lot at work, school, or when shopping.

Blood pressure monitoring. Demonstrate the correct procedure for taking blood pressure. It is best to have the patient or family bring in the blood pressure equipment that will be used at home to perform the blood pressure measurement. Validate the patient's and family's understanding by having them perform this task on several occasions under supervision. Monitor blood pressure, pulse, and respirations at least every shift while the patient is hospitalized and stress the need for the patient to monitor blood pressure in accordance with a healthcare provider's orders after discharge (usually daily). The patient should be given some numerical guidelines, as established by a healthcare provider, for a desired goal of therapy and what to do if this is not being achieved. Normal home blood pressure should at least be lower than 140/90 mm Hg. Nighttime home blood pressure is usually lower than daytime pressure.

Medication regimen

- Caution the patient that for the first 2 weeks of antihypertensive therapy, drowsiness may occur. Patients should be told that this adverse effect is self-limiting. They should be cautious in operating power equipment and motor vehicles while this symptom occurs.
- A common adverse effect of antihypertensive medications is hypotension. Instruct the patient to rise slowly from a sitting or supine position. Tell the patient to avoid standing for long periods, especially within 2 hours of taking antihypertensive medication. Weakness, dizziness, or faintness can usually be relieved by increasing muscular activity or by sitting or lying down.
- Teach the person to perform exercises that prevent blood pooling in the extremities when sitting or standing for long periods. These exercises include flexing the calf muscles, wiggling the toes, rising on the toes, and then returning the feet to a flat position.
- Teach the person and significant others how to take and record blood pressure at prescribed intervals.
- The patient should always report a lack of response to the medication prescribed and/or a blood pressure that continues to rise after medications have been taken. (Ask a healthcare provider for specific parameters.)

Fostering health maintenance

- Throughout the course of treatment, discuss medication information and how it will benefit the patient.
- Drug therapy is one component in the management of hypertension. Lifestyle changes are equal in importance to drug therapy; therefore the need to maintain an exercise program and modify dietary habits to control obesity and serum cholesterol is crucial. Cessation of smoking and minimal alcoholic intake are strongly recommended.

- Provide the patient and significant others with the important information contained in the specific drug monographs for the drugs prescribed. Additional health teaching and nursing interventions for common and serious adverse effects will be found in each drug monograph.
- Seek cooperation and understanding of the following points so that medication compliance is increased: name of medication; dosage, routes, and times of administration; and common and serious adverse effects.
- The most effective therapy prescribed by a healthcare provider will control hypertension only if the patient is motivated. Motivation improves when the patient has a positive experience with and trust in healthcare providers. Empathy builds trust and is an excellent motivator.

Patient self-assessment. Enlist the patient's aid in developing and maintaining a written record of monitoring parameters (e.g., blood pressures, weight, exercise) (see the Patient Self-Assessment Form for Cardiovascular Agents on the Evolve website). Complete the Premedication Data column for use as a baseline to track response to drug therapy. Ensure that the patient understands how to use the form, and instruct the patient to bring the completed form to follow-up visits. During follow-up visits, focus on issues that will foster adherence with the therapeutic interventions prescribed.

DRUG CLASS: DIURETICS

Actions
The diuretics act as antihypertensive agents by causing volume depletion, sodium excretion, and vasodilation of peripheral arterioles. The mechanism of peripheral arteriolar vasodilation is unknown.

Uses
There are four classes of diuretic agents: carbonic anhydrase inhibitors, thiazide and thiazide-type agents, loop diuretics, and potassium-sparing diuretics (see Chapter 28). The carbonic anhydrase inhibitors are weak antihypertensive agents and therefore are not used for this purpose. The potassium-sparing diuretics are rarely used alone, but are commonly used in combination with thiazide and loop diuretics for added antihypertensive effect and to counteract the potassium-excreting effects of these more potent diuretic-antihypertensive agents.

The diuretics are the most commonly prescribed antihypertensive agents because they are a class of agents that have been shown to reduce cardiovascular morbidity and mortality associated with hypertension. The thiazides are most effective if the renal creatinine clearance is higher than 30 mL/min; however, as renal function deteriorates, the more potent loop diuretics are needed to continue excretion of sodium and water.

Diuretics are commonly prescribed in combination therapy. They potentiate the hypotensive activity of the nondiuretic antihypertensive agents, have a low incidence of adverse effects, and are often the least expensive of the antihypertensive agents.

Diuretics are used (often with other classes of antihypertensive therapy) to treat all stages of hypertension. The agents are discussed more extensively in Chapter 28.

❖ Nursing Implications for Diuretic Agents
◆ Premedication assessment
1. Obtain baseline blood pressure readings in supine and standing positions.
2. Obtain baseline weight and apical pulse.
3. Initiate laboratory studies as requested by a healthcare provider (e.g., electrolytes).
4. Obtain baseline assessment of patient's state of hydration.

◆ *Availability, dosage, and administration.* See Chapter 28.

DRUG CLASS: BETA-ADRENERGIC BLOCKING AGENTS

Actions
Beta-adrenergic blocking agents (beta blockers; see Table 12.3) inhibit cardiac response to sympathetic nerve stimulation by blocking the beta receptors. As a result, the heart rate, the cardiac output, and consequently the blood pressure are reduced. Beta blockers also inhibit renin release from the kidneys, diminishing the cascade of the renin-angiotensin-aldosterone system (RAAS) that would induce vasoconstriction and sodium reabsorption, aggravating hypertension.

Uses
Beta blockers reduce the morbidity and mortality associated with hypertension and are widely used as antihypertensive agents. The clinical advantages of beta blockers in treating hypertension include minimal postural or exercise hypotension, minimal effect on sexual function, blood pressure reduction in the supine position, and little or no slowing of the central nervous system (CNS).

The 2017 guidelines recommend beta blockers as alternative first-line therapy for stages 1 and 2 hypertension. However, beta blockers are not as effective in African-American patients and should be avoided in patients with asthma, type 1 diabetes mellitus, heart failure caused by systolic dysfunction, and peripheral vascular disease. Other studies now recommend thiazide diuretics and ACE inhibitors for initial therapy. Beta blocker therapy is still preferred for hypertensive patients with other strong indications, particularly those with symptomatic coronary heart disease (angina) or previous myocardial infarction.

❖ **Nursing Implications for Beta-Adrenergic Blocking Agents**

◆ *Premedication assessment*

1. Check the patient's history for respiratory conditions that could be aggravated by bronchoconstriction, type 1 diabetes mellitus, heart failure, or peripheral vascular disease. If any of these conditions are present, contact the healthcare provider to discuss the situation before initiating beta blocker therapy.

2. Obtain baseline blood pressure readings in supine and standing positions and apical pulse. Hold medication if systolic blood pressure is less than 100 mm Hg or the heart rate is less than 50 beats/min, and contact the prescriber.

◆ *Availability, dosage, and administration.* See Table 12.3.

Individualization of dosage. Although the onset of activity of beta blockers is rapid, it may often take several days to weeks for a patient to show optimal improvement and become stabilized on an adequate maintenance dosage. Patients must be periodically reevaluated to determine the lowest effective dosage necessary to control the disorder being treated.

Sudden discontinuation. Patients must be counseled against poor compliance or sudden discontinuation of therapy without a healthcare provider's advice. Sudden discontinuation of therapy has resulted in an exacerbation of anginal symptoms, followed in some cases by myocardial infarction. When discontinuing long-term treatment with beta blockers, the dosage should be gradually reduced over a period of 1 to 2 weeks with careful monitoring of the patient. If anginal symptoms develop or become more frequent, beta blocker therapy should be restarted, at least temporarily. Most of the adverse effects associated with beta blockers are dosage related. Response by individual patients is highly variable. Many of these adverse effects may occur but might be transient. Strongly encourage patients to see their healthcare provider before discontinuing therapy. Minor dosage adjustment may be all that is required for most adverse effects.

◆ *Common adverse effects*

Cardiovascular

Bradycardia, peripheral vasoconstriction (purple, mottled skin). Withhold additional doses until the patient is evaluated by a healthcare provider.

Heart failure. Monitor the patient for an increase in edema, dyspnea, crackles, bradycardia, and orthopnea. Notify a healthcare provider if these symptoms develop.

Respiratory

Bronchospasm, wheezing. Withhold additional doses until the patient has been evaluated by a healthcare provider.

Endocrine

Patients with diabetes. Monitor the patient for symptoms of hypoglycemia: headache, weakness, decreased coordination, general apprehension, diaphoresis, hunger, or blurred or double vision. Many of these symptoms may be masked by the beta blockers. Notify a healthcare provider if any of these symptoms appear intermittently.

◆ *Drug interactions*

Antihypertensive agents. All beta blockers have hypotensive properties that are additive with antihypertensive agents (e.g., methyldopa, hydralazine, clonidine, prazosin, minoxidil, captopril, diltiazem, verapamil, reserpine). If it is decided to discontinue therapy in a patient receiving beta blockers and clonidine concurrently, the beta blocker should be withdrawn gradually and discontinued several days before the gradual withdrawal of the clonidine. Severe rebound hypertension may occur if the beta blocker is not gradually discontinued first.

Beta-adrenergic agents. Depending on the dosages used, the beta stimulants (e.g., isoproterenol, metaproterenol, terbutaline, albuterol; see Table 12.2) may inhibit the action of the beta blockers, and vice versa.

Lidocaine, procainamide, phenytoin, disopyramide, digoxin. Although these drugs are occasionally used concurrently, monitor the patient carefully for additional dysrhythmias, bradycardia, and signs of heart failure.

Enzyme-inducing agents. Enzyme-inducing agents such as cimetidine, phenobarbital, and phenytoin enhance the metabolism of propranolol, metoprolol, pindolol, and timolol. This reaction probably does not occur with nadolol or atenolol because they are not metabolized but are excreted unchanged. The dosage of the beta blocker may have to be increased to provide therapeutic activity. If the enzyme-inducing agent is discontinued, the dosage of the beta-blocking agent will also require reduction.

Nonsteroidal antiinflammatory drugs. Indomethacin, and possibly other prostaglandin inhibitors, may inhibit the antihypertensive activity of beta blockers, resulting in loss of hypertensive control. The dosage of the beta blocker may have to be increased to compensate for the antihypertensive inhibitory effect of nonsteroidal antiinflammatory drugs (NSAIDs).

DRUG CLASS: ANGIOTENSIN-CONVERTING ENZYME INHIBITORS

Actions

Angiotensin-converting enzyme inhibitors (Table 22.5) represent a major breakthrough in the treatment of hypertension. The RAAS plays a major role in the regulation of blood pressure. When there is a reduction in blood pressure, sodium concentration, or renal blood flow, renin is secreted by the kidneys. The renin converts angiotensinogen, which is secreted by the liver, to angiotensin I. Angiotensin I is then converted by angiotensin I–converting enzyme to angiotensin II. Angiotensin II produces potent vasoconstriction by

Table 22.5   Angiotensin-Converting Enzyme (ACE) Inhibitors

GENERIC NAME	BRAND NAME	AVAILABILITY	APPROVED USES	DOSAGE RANGE
benazepril ⇄ *Do not confuse benazepril with Benadryl allergy, Benzonatate, or donepezil.*	Lotensin ⇄ *Do not confuse Lotensin with Lioresal, Loniten♣, or Lovastatin.*	Tablets: 5, 10, 20, 40 mg	Hypertension	PO: Initial: 10 mg once daily Maintenance: 20-40 mg daily Maximum: 80 mg/day
captopril ⇄ *Do not confuse captopril with carvedilol.*	—	Tablets: 12.5, 25, 50, 100 mg	Hypertension, heart failure, diabetic nephropathy	PO: Initial: 12.5-25 mg two or three times daily 1 hr before meals Maintenance: 50-450 mg daily 1 hr before meals in two or three divided doses
enalapril ⇄ *Do not confuse enalapril with Eldepryl.*	Vasotec ⇄ *Do not confuse Vasotec with Norvasc.*	Tablets: 2.5, 5, 10, 20 mg Oral solution: 1 m/mL in 150 mL bottle	Hypertension, heart failure	PO: Initial: 2.5-5 mg once daily Maintenance: 10-40 mg daily
enalaprilat	Vasotec IV ♣	Injection: 1.25 mg/mL	Hypertension	IV: 0.625-1.25 mg over 5 min every 6 hr
fosinopril ⇄ *Do not confuse fosinopril with bisoprolol or furosemide*	–	Tablets: 10, 20, 40 mg	Hypertension, heart failure	PO: Initial: 10 mg once daily Maintenance: 20-40 mg daily Maximum: 80 mg/day
lisinopril	Prinivil ⇄ *Do not confuse Prinivil with, Pravachol, Prevacid, Prilosec, or Zestril.* ⇄ *Do not confuse Zestril with Vistaril, Zerit, Zocor, or Zyrtec.*	Tablets: 2.5, 5, 10, 20, 30, 40 mg Oral solution: 1 mg/mL in 150-mL bottle	Hypertension, heart failure, post–myocardial infarction	PO: Initial: 5-10 mg once daily Maintenance: 20-40 mg daily Maximum: 80 mg/day
moexipril	–	Tablets: 7.5, 15 mg	Hypertension	PO: Initial: with diuretic, 3.75 mg; without diuretic, 7.5 mg Maintenance: 7.5-30 mg in one or two divided doses 1 hr before meals
perindopril	–	Tablets: 2, 4, 8 mg	Hypertension	PO: Initial: 4 mg daily Maintenance: 4-8 mg daily Maximum: 16 mg/day
quinapril	Accupril ⇄ *Do not confuse Accupril with AcipHex, Accolate, Altace, or Aricept.*	Tablets: 5, 10, 20, 40 mg	Hypertension, heart failure	PO: Initial: 10-20 mg daily without diuretic; 5 mg daily with diuretic Maintenance: 20-80 mg daily
ramipril ⇄ *Do not confuse ramipril with rifampin.*	Altace ⇄ *Do not confuse Altace with Accupril, Amaryl, or Norvasc.*	Capsules: 1.25, 2.5, 5, 10 mg	Hypertension, heart failure	PO: Initial: 1.25-2.5 mg daily Maintenance: 2.5-20 mg daily
trandolapril ⇄ *Do not confuse trandolapril with tramadol.*		Tablets: 1, 2, 4 mg	Hypertension, heart failure	PO: Initial: 1 mg daily Maintenance: 2-4 mg daily

♣ Available in Canada.

acting on receptors within blood vessels. It also promotes aldosterone secretion, which causes sodium retention by stimulation of mineralocorticoid receptors in the adrenal cortex. These actions result in increased blood pressure secondary to the vasoconstriction and enhanced cardiac output secondary to sodium retention. The ACE inhibitors inhibit angiotensin I–converting enzyme, the enzyme responsible for the conversion of angiotensin I to angiotensin II, thus reducing serum levels of this potent vasoconstrictor and aldosterone stimulant.

Uses

Angiotensin-converting enzyme inhibitors reduce blood pressure, preserve cardiac output, and increase renal blood flow. They are effective as single therapy for stage 1 or 2 hypertension, severe accelerated hypertension, and renal hypertension. Although they may be used alone, they tend to be more effective when combined with diuretic therapy. They are not as effective in lowering blood pressure in African Americans unless used with a diuretic. Advantages of ACE inhibitors are the infrequency of orthostatic hypotension; lack of CNS depression and sexual dysfunction adverse effects; lack of aggravation of asthma, obstructive pulmonary disease, gout, cholesterol levels, or diabetes; and an additive effect with diuretics. The ACE inhibitors are also effective in the treatment of heart failure and following myocardial infarction and are routinely used to slow the progression of diabetic nephropathy. Angiotensin-converting enzyme inhibitors should not be administered as cotherapy with ARBs or direct renin inhibitors.

Therapeutic Outcome

The primary therapeutic outcome expected from the ACE inhibitors is reduction in blood pressure.

❖ Nursing Implications for Angiotensin-Converting Enzyme Inhibitors

◆ *Premedication assessment*

1. Obtain baseline blood pressure readings in supine and standing positions and apical pulse. Hold medication if systolic blood pressure is less than 100 mm Hg or the heart rate is less than 50 beats/min, and contact the prescriber.
2. Obtain a history of bowel elimination patterns.
3. Initiate laboratory studies as requested by a healthcare provider (e.g., renal function tests such as BUN, serum creatinine, and electrolyte levels and complete blood count [CBC]) to serve as a baseline for future comparison.
4. Ask whether the patient is pregnant or likely to become pregnant. If so, discuss with a healthcare provider before initiating ACE inhibitor therapy.
5. Ask if the patient has a persistent cough.

◆ *Availability, dosage, and administration.* See Table 22.5. Captopril should be administered without food and requires two- to three-times-daily dosing. All the

other agents may be administered one or two times daily.

NOTE: The initial doses of ACE inhibitors may cause hypotension with dizziness, tachycardia, and fainting; these adverse effects occur more commonly in patients also receiving diuretics. Symptoms occur within 3 hours after the first several doses. This effect may be minimized by discontinuing the diuretic 1 week before initiating ACE inhibitor therapy. Patients should be warned that this adverse effect may occur, that it is transient, and that they should lie down immediately if symptoms develop.

◆ *Common adverse effects*
Gastrointestinal
Nausea, diarrhea. These adverse effects are usually mild and tend to resolve with continued therapy. Encourage the patient not to discontinue therapy without first consulting a healthcare provider.
Neurologic
Fatigue, headache. These adverse effects are usually mild and tend to resolve with continued therapy. Encourage the patient not to discontinue therapy without first consulting a healthcare provider.
Cardiovascular
Orthostatic hypotension (dizziness, weakness, faintness). Although these adverse effects are infrequent and usually mild, certain patients, particularly those also receiving diuretics, may suffer some degree of orthostatic hypotension, especially when therapy is initiated. Observe the patient closely for at least 2 hours after the initial dose is given and for at least an additional hour until blood pressure has stabilized.

Monitor the blood pressure in both the supine and standing positions. Anticipate the development of postural hypotension and take measures to prevent an occurrence. Teach the patient to rise slowly from a supine or sitting position and to sit or lie down if feeling faint.
Inflammatory
Chronic cough. As many as one-third of patients receiving ACE inhibitors may develop a chronic, dry, nonproductive, persistent cough. This is thought to be caused by an accumulation of bradykinin. It may appear from 1 week to 6 months after initiation of ACE inhibitor therapy. Women appear to be more susceptible than men. Patients should be told to contact their healthcare provider if the cough becomes troublesome. The cough resolves within 1 to 30 days after discontinuation of therapy. An ARB agent may be substituted for the ACE inhibitor if the frequency of cough is excessive.

◆ *Serious adverse effects*
Pregnancy. Medications that act directly on the RAAS can cause fetal and neonatal harm. There is concern about the potential for birth defects in neonates whose mothers received ACE inhibitors, especially during the second and third trimesters of pregnancy. Women who wish to become pregnant or who become pregnant while

receiving ACE inhibitors should discuss alternative therapies with their healthcare provider as soon as possible.

Hypersensitivity

Swelling of the face, eyes, lips, and tongue; difficulty breathing. Angioedema has been reported to occur in a small number of patients, especially after the first dose. The patient should be cautioned to discontinue further therapy and seek medical attention immediately.

Life Span Considerations

Antihypertensive Therapy

Older adults are more likely to develop orthostatic hypotension with antihypertensive therapy. The patient's blood pressure should be monitored in the supine and sitting positions during the initiation of antihypertensive therapy or when the drug dosage is adjusted. Safety precautions should be initiated to prevent accidental injury. Teach the patient to rise slowly from a supine to a sitting and then a standing position.

Medication Safety Alert

Hypotension With ACE Inhibitors

The initial doses of ACE inhibitors may cause hypotension with dizziness, tachycardia, and fainting; these adverse effects occur more commonly in patients also receiving diuretics. Symptoms occur within 3 hours after the first several doses. This effect may be minimized by discontinuing the diuretic 1 week before initiating ACE inhibitor therapy. Patients should be warned that this adverse effect may occur, that it is transient, and that they should lie down immediately if symptoms develop.

Hematologic

Neutropenia. Neutropenia (300 neutrophils/mm^3) and agranulocytosis (drug-induced bone marrow suppression) have rarely been observed in patients receiving ACE inhibitors. The neutropenia appears within the first 3 to 12 weeks of therapy and develops slowly; the white blood cell count falls to its nadir in 10 to 30 days. The white blood cell count returns to normal about 2 weeks after discontinuation of ACE inhibitor therapy.

The patients most susceptible are those receiving captopril who also have impaired renal function or serious autoimmune diseases, such as lupus erythematosus, or who are exposed to drugs known to affect the white cells or immune response, such as corticosteroids.

Patients at risk should have differential and total white blood cell counts determined before initiation of therapy and then every 2 weeks thereafter for the first 3 months of therapy. Stress the importance of returning for this laboratory work. Patients should be told to notify their healthcare provider promptly if any evidence of infection such as sore throat or fever, which may be an indicator of neutropenia, develops.

Renal

Hyperkalemia. Because ACE inhibitors inhibit aldosterone, patients may develop slight increases in serum potassium levels. Approximately 1% of patients may develop hyperkalemia (potassium higher than 5.7 mEq/L). Most cases resolve without discontinuation of therapy. Patients most susceptible to the development of hyperkalemia are those with renal impairment or diabetes mellitus and those already receiving a potassium supplement or a potassium-sparing diuretic. Many symptoms associated with altered fluid and electrolyte balance are subtle and interspersed with general symptoms of drug toxicity or the disease process itself.

Gather data relative to changes in the patient's mental status (e.g., alertness, orientation, and confusion), muscle strength, muscle cramps, tremors, nausea, and general appearance (e.g., drowsy, anxious, or lethargic).

Always check the electrolyte reports for early indications of electrolyte imbalance. Keep accurate records of intake and output, daily weights, and vital signs.

Nephrotoxicity. A small number of hypertensive patients who are receiving ACE inhibitors, particularly those with preexisting renal impairment and those also taking NSAIDs, have developed increased BUN and serum creatinine levels. These elevations have usually been minor and transient, especially when the ACE inhibitor was administered concomitantly with a diuretic. Renal function should be monitored during the first few weeks of therapy. Report increasing BUN and creatinine levels. Dosage reduction of the ACE inhibitor or possible discontinuation of the NSAID or diuretic may be required.

◆ Drug interactions

Drugs that enhance therapeutic and toxic effects. These include diuretics, phenothiazines, alcohol, beta-adrenergic blocking agents (e.g., metoprolol, carvedilol), and other antihypertensive agents. Monitor the blood pressure response to the cumulative effects of antihypertensive agents. Obtain blood pressure readings in supine and standing positions.

Drugs that reduce therapeutic effects. Antacids may diminish absorption of ACE inhibitors. Separate the administration times by 2 hours. Nonsteroidal antiinflammatory drugs may reduce the antihypertensive effects of the ACE inhibitors. Rifampin may decrease the antihypertensive effects of enalapril. Monitor carefully for poor blood pressure control or a gradually increasing blood pressure.

Digoxin. Angiotensin-converting enzyme inhibitors may increase or decrease the serum levels of digoxin. Monitor for symptoms of anorexia, nausea, vomiting, headaches, blurred or colored vision, bradycardia, heart failure, or arrhythmias. A digoxin serum level may be ordered by a healthcare provider.

Lithium. Angiotensin-converting enzyme inhibitors may induce lithium toxicity. Monitor for lithium toxicity manifested by nausea, anorexia, fine tremors, persistent vomiting, profuse diarrhea, hyperreflexia, lethargy, and weakness.

Hyperkalemia. Angiotensin-converting enzyme inhibitors may cause small increases in potassium levels by inhibiting aldosterone secretion. Patients should not take dietary supplements of potassium or potassium-sparing diuretics (e.g., triamterene, spironolactone, amiloride) without specific approval from the healthcare provider. If a patient has received spironolactone or eplerenone up to several months before ACE inhibitor therapy, the serum potassium level should be monitored closely because the potassium-sparing effect of spironolactone or eplerenone may persist. Serum potassium levels should be monitored when the antibiotic trimethoprim is used with ACE inhibitors.

Capsaicin. Capsaicin may cause or aggravate coughing associated with ACE inhibitor therapy. Monitor for increased frequency of dry, persistent cough. Report to the healthcare provider.

DRUG CLASS: ANGIOTENSIN II RECEPTOR BLOCKERS

Actions

Angiotensin II receptor blockers (Table 22.6) are a class of antihypertensive agents that act by binding to angiotensin II receptor sites, blocking the very potent vasoconstrictor from binding to the angiotensin II type 1 receptor (AT_1 receptor) sites in the vascular smooth muscle, brain, heart, kidneys, and adrenal glands. The blood pressure–elevating and sodium-retaining effects of angiotensin II are thus blocked. The angiotensin II receptor blockers have no effect on renal function, prostaglandin levels, triglycerides, cholesterol, or blood glucose levels. These agents do not affect bradykinin and therefore do not cause a dry cough.

Uses

Angiotensin II receptor blockers are as effective in lowering blood pressure as ACE inhibitors and beta blockers. Men and women usually have similar responses; however, African-American patients do not respond as well to monotherapy. Angiotensin II receptor blockers are indicated for the treatment of hypertension and may be used alone or in combination with other antihypertensive agents, particularly thiazide-type diuretics. The blood pressure–lowering effect is seen within 1 week, but it may take 3 to 6 weeks to achieve the full therapeutic effect. If the antihypertensive effect is not controlled by ARBs alone, a low dosage of a diuretic, usually hydrochlorothiazide, may be added. Angiotensin II receptor blockers should not be administered as cotherapy with ACE inhibitors or direct renin inhibitors.

Table 22.6   Angiotensin II Receptor Blockers (ARBs)

GENERIC NAME	BRAND NAME	AVAILABILITY	DOSAGE RANGE
azilsartan	Edarbi	Tablets: 40, 80 mg	PO: 80 mg once daily; 40 mg once daily with high-dose diuretic therapy
candesartan	Atacand ⇄ Do not confuse Atacand with antacid or Avandia.	Tablets: 4, 8, 16, 32 mg	PO: Initial: 16 mg once daily; adjust over 4-6 wk with total daily dosage from 8-32 mg Dose may be administered once or twice daily for optimal control
eprosartan	Teveten	Tablets: 600 mg	PO: Initial: 600 mg once daily Maximum: 800 mg/day Dose may be administered once or twice daily for optimal control
irbesartan	Avapro ⇄ Do not confuse Avapro with Anaprox or Avelox.	Tablets: 75, 150, 300 mg	PO: Initial: 150 mg once daily; adjust over 3-4 wk with a total daily dosage of 300 mg daily
losartan ⇄ Do not confuse losartan with loratadine.	Cozaar ⇄ Do not confuse Cozaar with Corgard, Hyzaar, or Zocor.	Tablets: 25, 50, 100 mg	PO: 50 mg once daily; adjust over 4-6 wk with a total daily dosage from 25-100 mg administered once or twice daily for optimal control
olmesartan	Benicar	Tablets: 5, 20, 40 mg	PO: Initial: 20 mg once daily; adjust over 2 wk with total daily dosage of 20-40 mg Twice-daily dosing offers no benefit
telmisartan	Micardis	Tablets: 20, 40, 80 mg	PO: Initial: 40 mg once daily; adjust over 4-6 wk with total daily dosage from 20-80 mg
valsartan	Diovan ⇄ Do not confuse Diovan with Zyban.	Tablets: 40, 80, 160, 320 mg	PO: Initial: 80 mg once daily; adjust over 4-6 wk with total daily dosage from 80-320 mg

Therapeutic Outcome

The primary therapeutic outcome expected from ARBs is reduction in blood pressure.

❖ **Nursing Implications for Angiotensin II Receptor Blockers**

◆ *Premedication assessment*

1. Obtain baseline blood pressure readings in supine and standing positions and apical pulse. Hold medication if systolic blood pressure is less than 100 mm Hg or the heart rate is less than 50 beats/min, and contact the prescriber.
2. Initiate laboratory studies as requested by the healthcare provider (e.g., renal function tests such as BUN, serum creatinine, electrolyte levels, and CBC) to serve as a baseline for future comparison.
3. Ask whether the patient is pregnant or likely to become pregnant. If so, discuss with the healthcare provider before initiating ARB therapy.
4. Obtain a history of bowel elimination patterns and any gastrointestinal symptoms.

◆ *Availability, dosage, and administration.* See Table 22.6.

◆ *Common adverse effects*

Gastrointestinal

Dyspepsia, cramps, diarrhea. These adverse effects are usually mild and tend to resolve with continued therapy. Encourage the patient not to discontinue therapy without first consulting the healthcare provider.

Neurologic

Headache. This adverse effect is usually mild and tends to resolve with continued therapy. Encourage the patient not to discontinue therapy without first consulting the healthcare provider.

Cardiovascular

Orthostatic hypotension (dizziness, weakness, faintness). Although these adverse effects are infrequent and usually mild, certain patients, particularly those also receiving diuretics, may suffer some degree of orthostatic hypotension, especially when therapy is initiated. Observe the patient closely for at least 2 hours after the initial dose and for at least 1 additional hour until blood pressure has stabilized.

Monitor the blood pressure in both the supine and standing positions. Anticipate the development of postural hypotension and take measures to prevent an occurrence. Teach the patient to rise slowly from a supine or sitting position and to sit or lie down if feeling faint.

◆ *Serious adverse effects*

Pregnancy. Medications that act directly on the RAAS can cause fetal and neonatal harm. There is potential for birth defects in neonates whose mothers have received ARBs, especially during the second and third trimesters of pregnancy. Women who wish to become pregnant or who become pregnant while receiving ARBs

should discuss alternative therapies with their healthcare provider as soon as possible.

Renal

Hyperkalemia. Because ARBs inhibit aldosterone secretion, patients may develop slight increases in serum potassium levels. Most cases resolve without discontinuation of therapy. Patients most susceptible to the development of hyperkalemia are those with renal impairment or diabetes mellitus and those already receiving a potassium supplement, eplerenone, or a potassium-sparing diuretic. Many symptoms associated with altered fluid and electrolyte balance are subtle and interspersed with general symptoms of drug toxicity or the disease process itself.

Gather data relative to changes in the patient's mental status (e.g., alertness, orientation, confusion), muscle strength, muscle cramps, tremors, nausea, and general appearance (e.g., being drowsy, anxious, lethargic).

Always check the electrolyte reports for early indications of electrolyte imbalance. Keep accurate records of intake and output, daily weights, and vital signs.

◆ *Drug interactions*

Drugs that enhance therapeutic and toxic effects. These include diuretics, phenothiazines, alcohol, beta-adrenergic blocking agents (e.g., metoprolol, carvedilol), and other antihypertensive agents. Cimetidine and fluconazole inhibit the metabolism of losartan, causing an increased antihypertensive effect. Monitor the blood pressure response to the cumulative effects of antihypertensive agents. Obtain blood pressure readings in supine and standing positions.

Drugs that reduce therapeutic effects. Rifampin increases the metabolism of losartan, reducing its antihypertensive effects. The dosage of losartan may need to be increased, or the patient may be switched to another ARB.

Hyperkalemia. Angiotensin II receptor blockers may cause small increases in potassium levels by reducing aldosterone secretion. Patients should not take dietary supplements of potassium or potassium-sparing diuretics (e.g., triamterene, spironolactone, amiloride) without specific approval from the healthcare provider. If a patient has received spironolactone or eplerenone up to several months before ARB therapy, the serum potassium level should be monitored closely because the potassium-sparing effect of spironolactone and eplerenone may persist. Serum potassium levels should be monitored when the antibiotic trimethoprim is used with ARB therapy.

DRUG CLASS: DIRECT RENIN INHIBITOR

aliskiren (ă-lĭs-KĬR-ĕn)
⇄ Do not confuse aliskiren with Azilect.
Tekturna (TĔK-tŭrn-ă)

Actions

Renin is secreted by the kidneys in response to decreases in blood volume and renal perfusion. It is the first step in the RAAS. By regulating electrolyte and fluid balance in the body, this system plays an important role in the development of hypertension and atherosclerosis. Renin is responsible for the eventual conversion of angiotensinogen to the potent vasoconstrictor angiotensin II. Aliskiren, a direct renin inhibitor, blocks the first step in the RAAS cascade, preventing angiotensin II from activating its receptors and thus preventing the release of catecholamines, aldosterone secretion, and sodium reabsorption that would otherwise result in hypertension.

Uses

Aliskiren, a direct renin inhibitor, lowers blood pressure similar to the ACE inhibitors and ARBs. It does not cause reflex tachycardia as direct vasodilator antihypertensive agents (e.g., hydralazine) do. Men and women usually have similar responses. African-American patients and older patients do not respond as well to monotherapy as do younger patients. Aliskiren is indicated for the treatment of hypertension and may be used alone or in combination with other antihypertensive agents. The blood pressure–lowering effect is seen within 2 weeks, but it may take 3 to 6 weeks to achieve the full therapeutic effect. Aliskiren should be reserved for those patients who do not respond adequately to ACE inhibitors or ARBs because they have been proved to be effective antihypertensive agents and should be tried first. In general, aliskiren should not be used concurrently with ACE inhibitor or ARB therapy.

Therapeutic Outcome

The primary therapeutic outcome expected from renin inhibitors is reduction in blood pressure.

❖ Nursing Implications for Aliskiren

◆ *Premedication assessment*

1. Obtain baseline blood pressure readings in supine and standing positions and apical pulse. Hold medication if systolic blood pressure is less than 100 mm Hg or the heart rate is less than 50 beats/min, and contact the prescriber.
2. Initiate laboratory studies as requested by the healthcare provider (e.g., renal function tests such as BUN, serum creatinine, and electrolyte levels and CBC) to serve as a baseline for future comparison.
3. Ask whether the patient is pregnant or likely to become pregnant. If so, discuss with the healthcare provider before initiating renin inhibitor therapy.
4. Obtain a history of bowel elimination patterns and any gastrointestinal symptoms, frequency of headaches, dizziness, and fatigue.

◆ *Availability. PO:* 150- and 300-mg tablets.

◆ *Dosage and administration. PO:* Initially, 150 mg once daily. After a few weeks, if the blood pressure is not adequately controlled, increase to 300 mg once daily.

◆ *Common adverse effects*

Gastrointestinal

Dyspepsia, cramps, diarrhea. These adverse effects are usually mild and tend to resolve with continued therapy. Encourage the patient not to discontinue therapy without first consulting the healthcare provider.

Neurologic

Headache. This adverse effect is usually mild and tends to resolve with continued therapy. Encourage the patient not to discontinue therapy without first consulting the healthcare provider.

Cardiovascular

Orthostatic hypotension (dizziness, fatigue, faintness). Although these adverse effects are infrequent and usually mild, certain patients, particularly those also receiving diuretics, may suffer some degree of orthostatic hypotension, especially when therapy is initiated. Observe the patient closely for at least 2 hours after the initial dose and for at least 1 additional hour until blood pressure has stabilized.

Monitor the blood pressure in both the supine and standing positions. Anticipate the development of postural hypotension and take measures to prevent an occurrence. Teach the patient to rise slowly from a supine or sitting position and to sit or lie down if feeling faint.

◆ *Serious adverse effects*

Pregnancy. Medications that act directly on the RAAS can cause fetal and neonatal harm. There is potential for birth defects in neonates whose mothers have received renin inhibitors, especially during the second and third trimesters of pregnancy. Women who wish to become pregnant or who become pregnant while receiving renin inhibitors should discuss alternative therapies with their healthcare provider as soon as possible.

Renal

Serum electrolytes. Renin inhibitors block aldosterone secretion and patients may develop slight increases in serum potassium. Most cases resolve without discontinuation of therapy. Patients most susceptible to the development of hyperkalemia are those with renal impairment or diabetes mellitus and those already receiving a potassium supplement, eplerenone, or a potassium-sparing diuretic. Many symptoms associated with altered fluid and electrolyte balance are subtle and interspersed with general symptoms of drug toxicity or the disease process itself. Gather data relative to changes in the patient's mental status (e.g., alertness, orientation, confusion), muscle strength, muscle cramps, tremors, nausea, and general appearance (e.g., being drowsy, anxious, lethargic). Check the electrolyte reports for early indications of electrolyte imbalance. Keep accurate records of intake and output, daily weights, and vital signs.

◆ *Drug interactions*

Drugs that enhance therapeutic and toxic effects. These include diuretics, phenothiazines, alcohol, beta blockers (e.g., metoprolol, carvedilol), and other antihypertensive agents. Ketoconazole, itraconazole, and atorvastatin increase serum concentrations of aliskiren, causing an increased antihypertensive effect. Monitor the patient's blood pressure response to the cumulative effects of antihypertensive agents. Obtain blood pressure readings in supine and standing positions.

Drugs that reduce therapeutic effects. Valsartan, irbesartan, and hydrochlorothiazide reduce serum levels of aliskiren, reducing its antihypertensive effects. The dosage of aliskiren may need to be increased, or the patient may be switched to other therapy.

Hyperkalemia. Renin inhibitors may cause small increases in potassium levels by reducing aldosterone secretion. Patients should not take dietary supplements of potassium or potassium-sparing diuretics (e.g., triamterene, spironolactone, amiloride), ARBs, or ACE inhibitors without specific approval from a healthcare provider. If a patient has received spironolactone or eplerenone up to several months before renin inhibitor therapy, the serum potassium level should be monitored closely because the potassium-sparing effects of spironolactone and eplerenone may persist.

The antibacterial trimethoprim may enhance the hyperkalemic effect of aliskiren, ACE inhibitors, and ARBs. Monitor serum potassium levels.

DRUG CLASS: ALDOSTERONE RECEPTOR ANTAGONIST

eplerenone (ĕp-LĔR-ĕ-nōn)
Inspra (ĬN-spră)

Actions

Eplerenone represents the first of a new class of antihypertensive agents known as *aldosterone receptor blocking agents.* The RAAS plays a major role in the regulation of blood pressure. When there is a reduction in blood pressure, sodium concentration, or renal blood flow, renin is secreted by the kidneys. The renin converts angiotensinogen, which is secreted by the liver, to angiotensin I. Angiotensin I is converted by angiotensin I–converting enzyme to angiotensin II. Angiotensin II produces potent vasoconstriction by acting on receptors within blood vessels. It also promotes aldosterone secretion, which causes sodium retention by stimulation of mineralocorticoid receptors in the adrenal cortex, blood vessels, and brain. These actions result in increased blood pressure secondary to the vasoconstriction and enhanced cardiac output secondary to sodium retention. Eplerenone, the aldosterone receptor blocking agent, blocks stimulation of the mineralocorticoid receptors by aldosterone, thus preventing sodium reabsorption.

Uses

Eplerenone is used in treating hypertension and heart failure, either alone or in combination with other antihypertensive agents.

Therapeutic Outcome

The primary therapeutic outcome expected from eplerenone is reduction in blood pressure.

❖ **Nursing Implications for Eplerenone**
◆ *Premedication assessment*

1. Obtain baseline blood pressure readings in supine and standing positions. Hold medication if systolic blood pressure is less than 100 mm Hg or the heart rate is less than 50 beats/min, and contact the prescriber.
2. Obtain a history of bowel elimination patterns.
3. Initiate laboratory studies as requested by the healthcare provider—including renal function tests such as BUN and serum creatinine; electrolyte, triglyceride, and cholesterol levels; liver function tests (e.g., bilirubin, aspartate aminotransferase, alanine aminotransferase, gamma-glutamyltransferase, and alkaline phosphatase levels; prothrombin time); and uric acid—that will serve as a baseline for future comparison.
4. Ask whether the patient is pregnant or likely to become pregnant. If so, discuss with a healthcare provider before initiating eplerenone therapy.

◆ *Availability.* **PO:** 25- and 50-mg tablets.

◆ *Dosage and administration.* **PO:** Initially, 50 mg once daily, with or without food. The full therapeutic effect should be apparent within 4 weeks. For patients with an inadequate blood pressure response, the dosage may be increased to 50 mg twice daily.

> [!] **Medication Safety Alert**
>
> Eplerenone therapy is contraindicated in patients with the following:
> - Serum potassium level higher than 5.5 mEq/L.
> - Type 2 diabetes with microalbuminuria.
> - Serum creatinine level higher than 2 mg/dL in men or 1.8 mg/dL in women.
> - Creatinine clearance lower than 50 mL/min.
> - Patients taking potassium-sparing diuretics (e.g., amiloride, spironolactone, or triamterene).
> - Patients taking strong metabolic inhibitors (e.g., ketoconazole, itraconazole).
>
> For patients older than 65 years, or patients with mild to moderate hepatic failure, dosages higher than 50 mg daily are not recommended. For patients taking metabolism inhibitors such as cimetidine, erythromycin, saquinavir, verapamil, diltiazem, or fluconazole, the starting dosage should be reduced to 25 mg once daily.

◆ *Common adverse effects*

Gastrointestinal

Nausea, diarrhea. These adverse effects are usually mild and tend to resolve with continued therapy. Encourage the patient not to discontinue therapy without first consulting a healthcare provider.

Neurologic

Fatigue, headache. These adverse effects are usually mild and tend to resolve with continued therapy. Encourage the patient not to discontinue therapy without first consulting a healthcare provider.

Cardiovascular

Orthostatic hypotension (dizziness, weakness, faintness). Although these adverse effects are infrequent and usually mild, certain patients, particularly those who are also receiving diuretics, may suffer some degree of orthostatic hypotension, especially when therapy is initiated.

Monitor the blood pressure in both the supine and standing positions. Anticipate the development of postural hypotension and take measures to prevent an occurrence. Teach the patient to rise slowly from a supine or sitting position and to sit or lie down if feeling faint.

◆ *Serious adverse effects*

Gynecomastia, vaginal bleeding. A small number of men have developed gynecomastia and a small number of women have developed vaginal bleeding while receiving eplerenone therapy. Report these conditions to a healthcare provider.

Renal

Nephrotoxicity. A small number of hypertensive patients who are receiving eplerenone, particularly those with preexisting renal impairment, have developed increases in BUN and serum creatinine levels. Renal function should be monitored during the first few weeks of therapy. Report increasing BUN and creatinine levels. Dosage reduction or discontinuation of eplerenone may be required. Eplerenone therapy is not recommended in patients with creatinine clearances lower than 50 mL/min.

Hyperkalemia. Because eplerenone inhibits aldosterone, patients may develop slight increases in serum potassium levels. Patients most susceptible to the development of hyperkalemia (potassium higher than 5.5 mEq/L) are those with renal impairment or diabetes mellitus. Many symptoms associated with altered fluid and electrolyte balance are subtle and interspersed with general symptoms of drug toxicity or the disease process itself.

Gather data relative to changes in the patient's mental status (e.g., alertness, orientation, confusion), muscle strength, muscle cramps, heart rate and rhythm, tremors, nausea, and general appearance (e.g., drowsy, anxious, lethargic).

Always check the electrolyte reports for early indications of electrolyte imbalance. Keep accurate records of intake and output, daily weights, and vital signs.

Metabolic

Hypertriglyceridemia, hypercholesterolemia, hyperuricemia. Increases in serum triglyceride, cholesterol, and uric acid levels have been reported during eplerenone therapy. Report rising levels to a healthcare provider.

Gastrointestinal

Hepatotoxicity. The symptoms of hepatotoxicity are anorexia, nausea, vomiting, jaundice, hepatomegaly, splenomegaly, and abnormal liver function test results (e.g., elevated bilirubin, aspartate aminotransferase, alanine aminotransferase, gamma-glutamyltransferase, and alkaline phosphatase levels; increased prothrombin time).

◆ *Drug interactions*

Drugs that enhance therapeutic and toxic effects. These include diuretics, phenothiazines, ketoconazole, alcohol, beta blockers (e.g., metoprolol, carvedilol), and other antihypertensive agents. Monitor the blood pressure response to the cumulative effects of antihypertensive agents. Obtain blood pressure readings in supine and standing positions. Assess the patient for hypotension, lightheadedness, dizziness, and bradycardia. Provide for patient safety; prevent falls.

Drugs that may induce hyperkalemia. Concurrent use of eplerenone and the following agents may induce hyperkalemia: ACE inhibitors (e.g., lisinopril, captopril, enalapril, ramipril), ARBs (e.g., losartan, candesartan, valsartan), potassium-sparing diuretics (e.g., triamterene, amiloride, spironolactone), salt substitutes (which often contain higher concentrations of potassium for flavoring), and foods marketed as "low sodium," which often have higher concentrations of potassium for flavoring.

The antibacterial trimethoprim may enhance the hyperkalemic effect of eplerenone. Monitor serum potassium levels.

Lithium. Eplerenone may induce lithium toxicity. Monitor for lithium toxicity manifested by nausea, anorexia, fine tremors, persistent vomiting, profuse diarrhea, hyperreflexia, lethargy, and weakness.

Grapefruit juice. Grapefruit juice slows the metabolism of eplerenone in a minor way. If the patient develops orthostatic hypotension, a dosage reduction in eplerenone may be required.

St. John's wort. St. John's wort stimulates the metabolism of eplerenone. A dosage increase in eplerenone may be necessary.

DRUG CLASS: CALCIUM CHANNEL BLOCKERS

Actions

Calcium channel blockers are also known variously as *calcium antagonists, calcium ion antagonists, slow channel blockers,* and *calcium ion influx inhibitors.* These agents inhibit the movement of calcium ions across a cell membrane. This results in fewer dysrhythmias, a slower rate of contraction of the heart, and relaxation of smooth muscle of blood vessels, causing vasodilation and reduced blood pressure. The calcium channel blockers are classified by structure: benzothiazepine (diltiazem), diphenylalkylamine (verapamil), and dihydropyridines (amlodipine, clevidipine, felodipine, isradipine, nicardipine, nifedipine, nimodipine, and nisoldipine).

Uses

Although each of these agents acts by calcium ion inhibition, there are significant differences in clinical use because they act somewhat differently on coronary blood vessels, systemic blood vessels, pacemaker cells of the heart, and conducting tissue of the heart. Their clinical effects are also dependent on the type and severity of the patient's disease. All the available calcium channel blockers are effective antihypertensive agents, but clinicians tend to use those in the dihydropyridine group more often because they have better peripheral vasodilating effects, reducing afterload. Calcium channel blockers are more effective in patients with higher pretreatment blood pressure. They increase renal sodium excretion and are usually well tolerated. Calcium channel blockers are ideal as first- or second-line medicines in patients with hypertension and coexisting angina and are an alternative to the use of beta blockers in patients with asthma or diabetes mellitus. They are particularly effective in African Americans and older patients with hypertension, who are more likely to have low-renin hypertension. The calcium channel blockers also do not affect gout or peripheral vascular disease. Verapamil and diltiazem are also effective antidysrhythmic agents (see Chapter 23).

Therapeutic Outcome

The primary therapeutic outcome expected from calcium channel blocker therapy is reduction in blood pressure.

❖ Nursing Implications for Calcium Channel Blockers

◆ *Premedication assessment*
1. Obtain baseline blood pressure readings in the supine and standing positions and apical pulse. Hold medication if systolic blood pressure is less than 100 mm Hg or the heart rate is less than 50 beats/min, and contact the prescriber.
2. Obtain baseline weight.
3. If the patient is taking digoxin concurrently, initiate close monitoring for potential digitalis toxicity.

◆ *Availability, dosage, and administration.* See Table 22.7.

Dosage adjustments. See individual drug monographs for dosage parameters. Adjustments are made based on the individual patient's response to therapy.

◆ *Serious adverse effects*
Cardiovascular, circulatory
Hypotension and syncope. Caution the patient that hypotension and syncope may occur during the first

week of therapy. These adverse effects decline once the dosage is stabilized. Take blood pressure readings every shift in the hospitalized patient and stress the need for the patient to monitor blood pressure after discharge. Prevent hypotensive episodes by instructing the patient to rise slowly from a supine or sitting position and perform exercises to prevent blood pooling when standing or sitting in one position for a prolonged period. If faintness occurs, instruct the patient to sit or lie down.

Edema. Assess the patient for development of edema. Perform daily weights at the same time, in similar clothing, and on the same scale. Report increases in weight to a healthcare provider for further evaluation. Edema is more common with diltiazem and the dihydropyridine calcium channel blockers.

◆ *Drug interactions*
Drugs that enhance therapeutic and toxic effects. These include diuretics, phenothiazines, alcohol, beta blockers (e.g., metoprolol, carvedilol), histamine-2 antagonists (e.g., cimetidine, ranitidine), and other antihypertensive agents. Monitor the blood pressure response to the cumulative effects of antihypertensive agents. Obtain blood pressure readings in supine and standing positions. Assess the patient for hypotension, lightheadedness, dizziness, and bradycardia. Provide for patient safety; prevent falls.

Grapefruit juice. Grapefruit juice (approximately 200 mL) may elevate serum concentrations of felodipine, verapamil, nisoldipine, nifedipine, nicardipine, and possibly amlodipine, potentially causing hypotension. Grapefruit juice should not be consumed within 2 hours before or 4 hours after administration of affected calcium channel blockers.

Digoxin. Calcium channel blockers may increase serum levels of digoxin. Monitor the patient for symptoms of anorexia, nausea, vomiting, headaches, blurred or colored vision, and bradycardia. The healthcare provider may order a digoxin serum level.

DRUG CLASS: ALPHA-1 ADRENERGIC BLOCKING AGENTS

Actions

Alpha-1 blockers—doxazosin, prazosin, and terazosin—act by blocking postsynaptic alpha-1 adrenergic receptors to produce arteriolar and venous vasodilation, reducing peripheral vascular resistance without reducing cardiac output or inducing a reflex tachycardia. They produce a decrease in standing blood pressure slightly greater than in supine blood pressure. These agents also have a modest positive effect on serum lipid levels, increasing high-density lipoprotein cholesterol and reducing LDL cholesterol, total cholesterol, and triglyceride concentrations.

Alpha-1 blockers do not increase catecholamines; therefore there is no increase in heart rate or myocardial

Table 22.7 **Calcium Channel Blockers Used to Treat Hypertension**

GENERIC NAME	BRAND NAME	AVAILABILITY	DOSAGE RANGE
amlodipine ⇄ *Do not confuse amlodipine with amiloride or amiodarone.*	Norvasc ⇄ *Do not confuse Norvasc with Altace or Vasotec.*	Tablets: 2.5, 5, 10 mg	PO: Initial: 5 mg once daily; adjust over 7-14 days to a maximum of 10 mg/day
diltiazem	Cardizem ⇄ *Do not confuse Cardizem with Cardene or clonidine.* Cardizem LA Cardizem CD	Tablets: 30, 60, 90, 120 mg Tablets, extended release (24 hr): 120, 180, 240, 300, 360, 420 mg Capsules, sustained release (24 hr): 120, 180, 240, 300, 360, 420 mg IV: 5 mg/mL in 5-, 10-, 25-mL vials Powder for injection: 100 mg	PO: Initial: 60- to 120-mg sustained-release capsule twice daily; adjust as needed after 14 days Maintenance: 240-360 mg daily Maximum: 480 mg once daily
felodipine	–	Tablets, extended release (24 hr): 2.5, 5, 10 mg	PO: Initial: 5 mg daily; adjust after 14 days Maintenance: 2.5-10 mg daily Maximum:10 mg daily
isradipine	–	Capsules: 2.5, 5 mg	PO: Initial: 2.5 mg twice daily Maximal response may require 2-4 wk Maintenance: 10 mg daily Maximum: 20 mg daily
nicardipine	Cardene ⇄ *Do not confuse Cardene with Cardizem, Cardura, or codeine.*	Capsules: 20, 30 mg IV: 2.5 mg/mL in 10-mL vial; 0.1 and 0.2 mg/mL in 200-, 250-mL premixed containers	PO: Immediate release: Initial: 20 mg three times daily Maximal response may require 2 wk of therapy Adjust dosage by measuring blood pressure about 8 hr after last dose Peak effect is determined by measuring blood pressure 1-2 hr after dose administration Maintenance: 20-40 mg three times daily Maximum: 120 mg daily Extended release: Initial: 30 mg twice daily Maximum: 120 mg daily IV: 5 mg/hr by continuous infusion May titrate by 2.5 mg/hr every 15 min Maximum: 15 mg/hr
nifedipine	Procardia ⇄ *Do not confuse Procardia with Provera or Peri-Colace.*	Capsules: 10, 20 mg Tablets, sustained release (24 hr): 30, 60, 90 mg	PO: Initial: 30-60 mg once daily of extended-release formulation. Immediate-release (IR) formulation not indicated for hypertension management Maximum: sustained-release tablets, 120 mg daily
nisoldipine	Sular – Geometrix delivery system Generic version – Extended release original formulation (not equivalent to Sular)	Tablets, sustained release (24 hr): 8.5, 17, 25.5, 34 mg Tablets, extended release (24 hr): 10, 20, 30, 40 mg	Sular, PO: Initial: 17 mg once daily; Maintenance: 17-34 mg once daily Sular, Maximum dose 34 mg/day Nisoldipine ER tablet (original formulation), PO: Initial 20 mg once a day Maintenance: 20-40 mg once daily; Maximum dose 60 mg/day
verapamil	Calan ⇄ *Do not confuse Calan with Colace.*	Tablets: 40, 80, 120 mg Tablets, sustained release (24 hr): 120, 180, 240 mg Capsules, sustained release (24 hr): 100, 120, 180, 200, 240, 300, 360 mg IV: 2.5 mg/mL in 2- and 4-mL ampules and syringes	PO: Initial: 80 mg three or four times daily Sustained-release tablets and capsules: 120-240 mg once daily in the morning Maintenance: 240-480 mg daily Administer with food

oxygen consumption. They also have no effect on uric acid concentrations.

Because of the presence of alpha-1 receptors on the prostate gland and certain areas of the bladder, terazosin and doxazosin are also able to reduce urinary outflow resistance in men with enlarged prostate glands.

Uses

Alpha-1 blockers may be used alone or in combination with other antihypertensive agents in the treatment of stage 1 or 2 hypertension, particularly in men with benign prostatic hyperplasia. They have additive effects with beta blockers and diuretics. Blood pressure response with alpha-1 blockers appears to be similar in African-American and white patients. These agents can be used safely in patients with angina, gout, and hyperlipidemia. The three alpha-1 blockers have similar antihypertensive effects and adverse effects. Doxazosin and terazosin have a longer duration of action and can be administered once daily. Prazosin is often used with diuretic therapy because of its tendency to cause sodium and water retention.

Doxazosin and terazosin are also used to reduce mild to moderate urinary obstruction manifestations (e.g., hesitancy, terminal dribbling of urine, interrupted stream, impaired size and force of stream, sensation of incomplete bladder emptying) in men with benign prostatic hyperplasia (see Chapter 40).

Therapeutic Outcomes

The primary therapeutic outcomes expected from alpha-1 blocker therapy are reduction of blood pressure and reduction of symptoms of benign prostatic hyperplasia with improvement in urine flow.

❖ Nursing Implications for Alpha-1 Adrenergic Blocking Agents

◆ *Premedication assessment*

1. Obtain baseline blood pressure readings in supine and standing positions and apical pulse. Hold medication if systolic blood pressure is less than 100 mm Hg or the heart rate is less than 50 beats/min, and contact the prescriber.
2. Check if patient is pregnant or has a history of severe cerebral or coronary arteriosclerosis, gastritis, or peptic ulcer disease. (Reduction of blood pressure may diminish blood flow to these regions, which causes therapy to worsen the condition.)

◆ *Availability, dosage, and administration.* See Table 22.8.

◆ **Common adverse effects**
Neurologic

Drowsiness, headache, dizziness, weakness, lethargy. Tell the patient that these adverse effects may occur but that they tend to be self-limiting. Tell the patient not to stop taking the medication and to

 Medication Safety Alert

The initial doses of doxazosin, prazosin, and terazosin may cause hypotension with dizziness, tachycardia, and fainting; these adverse effects occur in less than 1% of patients starting therapy. Symptoms occur 15 to 90 minutes after administration of the initial dose and occur most often in patients who are already receiving propranolol and presumably other beta blockers. These effects may be minimized by giving the first doses with food and limiting the initial dose to 1 mg. Patients should be warned that these adverse effects may occur, that they are transient, and that the patient should lie down immediately if symptoms develop.

consult a healthcare provider if the problem becomes unacceptable.

Cardiovascular

Dizziness, tachycardia, fainting. These adverse effects occur in about 1% of patients when therapy is initiated. Symptoms develop 15 to 90 minutes after the first few doses are taken. To decrease the incidence, give the first few doses with food and limit the initial dose to 1 mg. Instruct the patient to lie down immediately if these symptoms start to occur, and provide for the patient's safety.

◆ *Drug interactions*

Drugs that enhance therapeutic and toxic effects. These include diuretics, alcohol, beta blockers (e.g., metoprolol, carvedilol), and other antihypertensive agents. Monitor the blood pressure response to the cumulative effects of antihypertensive agents. Obtain blood pressure readings in supine and standing positions. Monitor for an increase in severity of adverse effects such as sedation, hypotension, and bradycardia or tachycardia.

DRUG CLASS: CENTRAL-ACTING ALPHA-2 AGONISTS

Actions

Central-acting alpha-2 agonists (e.g., clonidine, guanfacine, methyldopa) act by stimulating the alpha-adrenergic receptors in the brainstem, resulting in reduced sympathetic outflow from the CNS and decreased heart rate and peripheral vascular resistance, causing a drop in both systolic and diastolic blood pressures.

Uses

Alpha-2 agonists are considered adjunctive antihypertensive agents and are recommended for use only in combination with preferred or alternative antihypertensive agents. Clonidine is available as a transdermal therapeutic system (TTS) that is applied once weekly. These drugs cause more frequent adverse effects such as sedation, dizziness, dry mouth, fatigue, and sexual dysfunction. When used alone, methyldopa often causes fluid retention. They can safely be used in combination

Table 22.8 Alpha-1 Adrenergic Blocking Agents

GENERIC NAME	BRAND NAME	AVAILABILITY	DOSAGE RANGE
doxazosin ⇄ Do not confuse doxazosin with donepezil.	Cardura ⇄ Do not confuse Cardura with K-Dur, Ridaura, Cardene, or Coumadin.	Tablets: 1, 2, 4, 8 mg Tablets, extended release (24 hr): 4, 8 mg	**Hypertension:** PO: Initial: 1 mg daily AM or PM; hypotensive effects are most likely within 2-6 hr; monitor standing blood pressure Maintenance: increase to 2 mg; then, if needed, to 4, 8, and 16 mg to achieve desired reduction in blood pressure **Benign prostatic hyperplasia:** PO: Initial: as for hypertension; increase dosage at weekly intervals to 2 mg, then 4 and 8 mg once daily Maintenance: 8 mg daily; monitor blood pressure Maximum: 8 mg daily
prazosin	Minipress	Capsules: 1, 2, 5 mg	**Hypertension:** PO: Initial: 1 mg two or three times daily, with first dose at bedtime to reduce syncopal episodes. Maintenance: 6-15 mg/day in two or three divided doses Maximum dosage: 40 mg/day
terazosin		Capsules: 1, 2, 5, 10 mg	**Hypertension:** PO: Initial: 1 mg at bedtime; measure blood pressure 2-3 hr after dosing and evaluate for symptoms of dizziness or tachycardia; if response is substantially diminished at 24 hr, increase dosage Maintenance: 1-5 mg daily Maximum dose: 20 mg/day **Benign prostatic hyperplasia:** PO: Initial: as for hypertension; gradually increase dosage in stepwise fashion to 2, 5, or 10 mg daily for acceptable urinary output Maintenance: 10 mg daily for 4-6 wk to assess urinary response Maximum dose: 20 mg/day

with other agents such as diuretics, vasodilators, and beta blockers.

Therapeutic Outcome

The primary therapeutic outcome expected from the alpha-2 agonists is reduction in blood pressure.

❖ Nursing Implications for Central-Acting Alpha-2 Agonists

◆ *Premedication assessment*

1. Obtain baseline blood pressure readings in supine and standing positions and apical pulse. Hold medication if systolic blood pressure is less than 100 mm Hg or the heart rate is less than 50 beats/min, and contact the prescriber.
2. Assess the patient's mental status; affective and cognitive behaviors should be used as a baseline for subsequent comparison. If depression is suspected, report to a healthcare provider.
3. Obtain baseline data relating to usual sleep pattern.

◆ *Availability, dosage, and administration.* See Table 22.9.

Sudden discontinuation. Never suddenly discontinue clonidine because it could cause a rebound effect with

a rapid increase in blood pressure, manifested by nervousness, agitation, restlessness, tremors, headache, nausea, and increased salivation. Rebound symptoms are most pronounced after 1 to 2 months of therapy and may begin to appear within a few hours of a missed dose. Within 8 to 24 hours, severe symptoms may develop.

When therapy is to be discontinued, a gradual reduction in dosage is necessary over 2 to 4 days, during which blood pressure must be carefully monitored.

If the clonidine TTS patch becomes loose, the adhesive overlay should be applied directly over the TTS patch to ensure good adhesion.

◆ *Common adverse effects*

Neurologic

Drowsiness, dizziness. These symptoms may occur, but they tend to be self-limiting. Tell the patient not to discontinue the medication and to consult a healthcare provider if the adverse effects become an unacceptable problem.

Gastrointestinal

Dry mouth. These symptoms may occur, but they tend to be self-limiting. Tell the patient not to discontinue the medication and to consult a healthcare provider if the adverse effects become an unacceptable problem.

Table 22.9 Central-Acting Alpha-2 Agonists

GENERIC NAME	BRAND NAME	AVAILABILITY	DOSAGE RANGE
clonidine ⇄ *Do not confuse clonidine with colchicine, Cardizem, Klonopin, or clonazepam.*	Catapres, Catapres-TTS	Tablets: 0.1, 0.2, 0.3 mg Transdermal patch: 　TTS-1 = 0.1 mg/day 　TTS-2 = 0.2 mg/day 　TTS-3 = 0.3 mg/day	PO: Initial: 0.1 mg twice daily Maintenance: 0.2-0.8 mg daily in two or three divided doses Maximum: 2.4 mg daily Transdermal: Apply to hairless area of intact skin on upper arm or torso once every 7 days; use a different site each wk Initial: Start with 0.1-mg patch; after second wk, add another 0.1-mg patch or use a larger system Maximum: Two 0.3-mg patches/wk Note: Antihypertensive effect starts 2-3 days after initiation of therapy
	Kapvay	Tablets extended release (12 hr): 0.1 m	Attention-deficit/hyperactivity disorder (ADHD): PO: Initial: 0.4 mg daily for children over 6 years and older
guanfacine	–	Tablets: 1, 2 mg	**Hypertension (IR only):** PO: Initial: 1 mg daily at bedtime Maintenance: 1-2 mg Maximum: 3 mg daily
	Intuniv	Tablets, extended release: 1, 2, 3, 4 mg (for ADHD)	See guanfacine tablets for dosage range for hypertension **Attention-deficit/hyperactivity disorder (ADHD):** PO: Initial: 1 mg daily Maintenance: 1-4 mg daily When discontinuing, taper the dose no more rapidly than 1 mg every 3-7 days
methyldopa ⇄ *Do not confuse methyldopa with levodopa or L-dopa.*	—	Tablets: 250, 500 mg IV: 50 mg/mL	PO: Initial: 250 mg two or three times daily Maintenance: 500 mg to 3 g daily in two to four doses

TTS, Transdermal therapeutic system.

Genitourinary

Altered urine color. Methyldopa or its metabolites may discolor the urine, causing it to darken on exposure to air. It is to be expected and is not harmful.

Altered test reactions. Methyldopa may cause up to 20% of patients to develop a positive reaction to the direct Coombs test. However, less than 0.2% of these patients will develop hemolytic anemia. Blood counts should be determined annually during therapy to detect hemolytic anemia.

◆ **Serious adverse effects**

Psychological

Depression. Assess the patient's affect (e.g., loneliness, sadness, anxiety, anger), cognition (e.g., confusion, ambivalence, loss of interest), and other behavioral responses (e.g., agitation, irritability, altered activity level, withdrawal) before starting therapy. After starting therapy with clonidine, carefully monitor the patient for changes in usual response patterns. Assess otherwise normal emotions for an increase in duration or intensity.

Note the patient's degree of socialization, response to stimulation, and changes in interactions with others. All individuals taking this drug should be monitored for development of depression, especially those with a history of depression.

Integumentary

Rash. About 10% to 15% of patients using the clonidine TTS patch develop contact dermatitis. Patients who develop moderate or severe erythema or vesicle formation at the site of application of clonidine TTS patches should consult a healthcare provider about the possible need to remove the TTS patch and use alternative therapy.

◆ **Drug interactions**

Drugs that enhance therapeutic and toxic effects. These include digoxin, alcohol, beta blockers (e.g., metoprolol, carvedilol), verapamil, and other antihypertensive agents. Monitor the blood pressure response to the cumulative effects of antihypertensive agents. Obtain blood pressure readings in supine and standing positions. Monitor for an increase in severity of adverse effects such as sedation, hypotension, and bradycardia or tachycardia.

Drugs that reduce therapeutic effects. Tricyclic antidepressants (e.g., amitriptyline, imipramine, desipramine), trazodone, and prazosin may block the antihypertensive effects of clonidine and methyldopa. Beta blockers (e.g., propranolol, atenolol, pindolol) may cause potentially life-threatening increases in blood pressure when taken with clonidine. Monitor carefully for poor blood pressure control or a gradually increasing blood pressure.

Sedative effects. Alcohol, phenobarbital, phenothiazines, benzodiazepines, tricyclic antidepressants, antihistamines, and any other drugs that cause sedation or drowsiness all potentiate the sedative effects of clonidine and methyldopa. Patients should be warned that their tolerance to alcohol and other depressants may be diminished.

Haloperidol. Methyldopa used concurrently with haloperidol may produce irritability, aggressiveness, abusive behavior, and dementia. Concurrent use is usually not recommended.

DRUG CLASS: DIRECT VASODILATORS

---

hydralazine (hī-DRĂL-ă-zēn)

Actions

Hydralazine causes direct arteriolar smooth muscle relaxation, resulting in reduced peripheral vascular resistance. The reduction in peripheral resistance causes a reflex increase in heart rate, cardiac output, and renin release with sodium and water retention. Consequently, the hypotensive effectiveness is reduced unless the patient is also taking a sympathetic inhibitor (e.g., beta blocker) and a diuretic.

Uses

Hydralazine is used to treat stage 2 hypertension and hypertension associated with renal disease and toxemia of pregnancy. It may also be used to provide symptomatic relief in patients with heart failure by reducing resistance (afterload) to left ventricular output. Because of the reflex increase in cardiac rate, hydralazine is often used in combination with a drug that inhibits tachycardia (e.g., beta blockers, clonidine, methyldopa).

A combination product (BiDil) containing hydralazine and isosorbide dinitrate has been approved by the US Food and Drug Administration. This combination has been shown to reduce hospitalizations, improve quality of life, and reduce mortality in African Americans with hypertension and heart failure.

Therapeutic Outcome

The primary therapeutic outcome of hydralazine is reduction in blood pressure.

❖ **Nursing Implications for Hydralazine**
◆ *Premedication assessment*
1. Obtain baseline blood pressure readings in the supine and standing positions and apical pulse. Hold medication if systolic blood pressure is less than 100 mm Hg or the heart rate is less than 50 beats/min, and contact the prescriber.

◆ *Availability.* **PO:** 10-, 25-, 50-, and 100-mg tablets.
Intramuscular (IM), intravenous (IV): 20 mg/mL in 1-mL vials.

◆ *Dosage and administration.* **Adult:** *PO:* Initially, 10 mg four times daily for the first 2 to 4 days, then 25 mg four times daily. The second week, increase the dosage to 50 mg four times daily as the patient tolerates the dosage and the blood pressure is brought under control. Maximum daily dosage is 300 mg.

IM, IV: 10- to 20-mg IV bolus or 10 to 50 mg IM, repeated as necessary, usually every 4 to 6 hours. Monitor blood pressure often. Results usually become evident within 10 to 20 minutes.

◆ *Common adverse effects*
Neurologic
Dizziness, numbness, tingling in the legs. Although these symptoms may be anticipated, they require monitoring. If severe, they should be reported so that the dosage can be adjusted appropriately.

Nausea. This symptom may be anticipated; monitoring is required. If severe, report to a healthcare provider so that the dosage can be adjusted.
Cardiovascular
Orthostatic hypotension. This may occur, particularly during initiation of therapy. Patients can usually avoid this complication by rising slowly from supine and sitting positions.

Palpitations, tachycardia. Although these symptoms may be anticipated, they require monitoring. If severe, they should be reported so that the dosage can be adjusted appropriately.
Respiratory
Nasal congestion. Nasal congestion can be treated with an antihistamine such as chlorpheniramine.

◆ *Serious adverse effects*
Immunologic, inflammatory
Fever, chills, joint and muscle pain, skin eruptions. Tell patients to report the development of these symptoms to a healthcare provider. Monitor laboratory reports for leukocyte counts and antinuclear antibody titer.

◆ *Drug interactions*
Drugs that enhance therapeutic and toxic effects. These include diuretics, alcohol, beta blockers (e.g., propranolol, atenolol, pindolol), and other antihypertensive agents. Monitor the blood pressure response to the cumulative effects of antihypertensive agents. Obtain blood pressure

readings in supine and standing positions. Monitor for an increase in severity of adverse effects, such as sedation, hypotension, and bradycardia or tachycardia.

---

nitroprusside sodium (nī-trō-PRŬS-īd)
  Nitropress (NĪ-trō-prĕs)

Actions

Nitroprusside is a potent vasodilator that acts directly on the smooth muscle of blood vessels. It produces both arterial and venous vasodilation, thus reducing both preload and afterload on the heart.

Uses

Nitroprusside is used in patients with sudden severe hypertensive crisis and in those with refractory heart failure.

Therapeutic Outcomes

The primary therapeutic outcomes of nitroprusside are reduction in blood pressure and improvement in symptoms associated with heart failure.

◆ *Availability. IV:* 25 mg/mL in 2-mL vials.

Get Ready for the NCLEX® Examination!

Key Points

- The public has made significant strides in recognizing the risk factors associated with cardiovascular disease. This awareness has led to a reduced incidence of heart attacks and strokes. Hypertension, however, is still a national health problem. Nurses can play a significant role in public education efforts, monitor for nonadherence, monitor blood pressure response to therapy, and encourage patients to make changes in lifestyle to reduce the severity of hypertension.
- Nonadherence to hypertensive therapy is a major problem, and nurses need to understand that educating the patient regarding the consequences of discontinuing therapy is not enough. Rather, the nurse must investigate the "whys" for discontinuing the therapy. Many of the reasons the patient gives may be overcome or reduced by proper interventions or a change in the type of antihypertensive agents prescribed.
- Because hypertension is a silent killer, it is important that nurses and other health professionals extend public screening programs to the community.
- Current guidelines use the systolic blood pressure as the major criterion for the diagnosis and management of hypertension in middle-aged and older Americans.
- The primary purpose for controlling hypertension is to reduce the frequency of cardiovascular disease (angina, myocardial infarction, heart failure, stroke) as well as renal failure and retinopathy. To accomplish this goal, the ASH/ISH guidelines recommend that blood pressure must be reduced and maintained below 140/90 mm Hg in patients under the age of 80, including those with diabetes mellitus or chronic kidney disease, if possible. The goal for those patients 80 years of age or older is below 150/90 mm Hg. The target for patients with diabetes or chronic kidney disease should still be under 140/90 mm Hg.

Additional Learning Resources

SG Go to your Study Guide for additional *Review Questions* for the NCLEX® Examination, *Critical Thinking Clinical Situations,* and other learning activities to help you master this chapter content.

Go to your Evolve website (https://evolve.elsevier.com/Clayton) for additional online resources.

Review Questions for the NCLEX® Examination

1. A patient asked the nurse about the difference between primary and secondary hypertension. Which statement by the nurse accurately answers the question?
   1. "Primary hypertension accounts for 90% of all clinical cases of high blood pressure."
   2. "It does not matter whether you have primary or secondary hypertension; your treatment plan will be the same."
   3. "Primary hypertension has no identifiable cause, and secondary hypertension is caused by some other conditions."
   4. "Primary hypertension is curable, and secondary hypertension is only controllable."

2. The nurse reviewing the assessments and interventions for patients with hypertension knows that which of the following are key components? *(Select all that apply.)*
   1. Monitoring blood pressure
   2. Listening for bowel sounds
   3. Reviewing diet history
   4. Checking laboratory values for kidney function
   5. Determining the physical activity level of the patient

3. After discussing lifestyle modifications with the patient who is hypertensive, the nurse will reinforce teaching after the patient makes which statement?
   1. "I can eat tuna and crackers for a midafternoon snack."
   2. "I will walk every day at least 20 minutes."
   3. "I will weigh myself at the same time every day and report a weight gain of more than 2 pounds."
   4. "I think that I can keep track of my blood pressure using a journal to record it."

4. The nurse was discussing the various drug classifications used for hypertension with a new nurse during orientation and reviewed which drug classifications in the discussion? *(Select all that apply.)*
   1. Alpha-1 adrenergic blockers
   2. Antihistamines
   3. Anticholinergic agents
   4. Angiotensin II receptor blockers
   5. Angiotensin-converting enzyme inhibitors

5. The nurse explains to a patient with newly diagnosed hypertension the initial therapy, which may include what drug classes? *(Select all that apply.)*
   1. Diuretics
   2. Beta blockers
   3. Aldosterone receptor antagonists
   4. Angiotensin II receptor blockers
   5. Calcium channel blockers

6. The nurse preparing the drug irbesartan (Avapro) from the drug class angiotensin II receptor blockers knows that this drug works by which mechanism?
   1. Inhibiting the conversion of angiotensin I to angiotensin II.
   2. Binding to and blocking angiotensin II receptor sites.
   3. Preventing the release of catecholamines.
   4. Blocking the stimulation of mineralocorticoid receptors.

7. The nurse is administering amlodipine (Norvasc) to a patient who asked how the drug works. Which statement is an appropriate response by the nurse?
   1. "This drug blocks the receptors that stimulate the release of renin from the kidneys."
   2. "This drug helps relax your blood vessels and slows your heart rate, which lowers your blood pressure."
   3. "This drug will help you get rid of excess water, which will lower your blood pressure."
   4. "This drug is designed to dilate your blood vessels, which in turn will lower your blood pressure."

8. The nurse is reviewing an order for the drug hydralazine that will be administered to a patient with persistent high blood pressure. The nurse recognizes this drug as which type of antihypertensive?
   1. Calcium channel blocker
   2. Beta blocker
   3. Central-acting alpha-2 agonist
   4. Direct vasodilator

9. While reviewing the drug hydrochlorothiazide for a patient with hypertension, the nurse also checked which laboratory values before administration? *(Select all that apply.)*
   1. Potassium
   2. Chloride
   3. Sodium
   4. Creatinine clearance
   5. Alkaline phosphatase

10. After teaching the patient about the new prescription drug captopril, an ACE inhibitor, the nurse knew that further education was needed after the patient responded with which statement?
    1. "If I start to develop a cough after taking captopril, I will notify my physician."
    2. "As I understand it, I will have to get out of bed slowly to let my blood pressure stabilize."
    3. "I should take captopril with food so it will not upset my stomach."
    4. "This drug will help control my blood pressure and treat my heart failure."

23

Drugs Used to Treat Dysrhythmias

Objectives

1. Describe the anatomic structures and conduction system of the heart.
2. Identify the classification of drugs used to treat dysrhythmias.
3. Identify baseline nursing assessments that should be implemented during the treatment of dysrhythmias.
4. Cite common adverse effects that may be observed with the administration of antidysrhythmic drugs.
5. List the six cardinal signs of cardiovascular disease.

Key Terms

conduction system (kŭn-DŬK-shŭn SĬS-tĕm) (p. 368)
dysrhythmia (dĭs-RĬTH-mē-ă) (p. 368)
atrial flutter (Ā-trē-ŭl FLŬ-tĕr) (p. 369)
atrial fibrillation (Ā-trē-ŭl fĭb-rĭ-LĀ-shŭn) (p. 369)

paroxysmal supraventricular tachycardia (PSVT) (păr-ŏk-SĬZ-măl sū-pră-věn-TRĬK-yū-lăr tăk-ĕ-KĂR-dē-ă) (p. 369)
atrioventricular blocks (ā-trē-ō-věn-TRĬK-yū-lăr BLŎKS) (p. 369)
tinnitus (TĬ-nĭ-tŭs; tĭ-NĪ-tĭs) (p. 373)

DYSRHYTHMIAS

The function of the heart is to sustain life by rhythmically pumping blood to all the vital organs and the rest of the body's tissues. The conduction system, or electrical system, of the heart is the anatomic structure that controls the sequence of muscle contractions so that an optimal volume of blood is pumped from the heart with each beat (Fig. 23.1). The conduction system is composed of nerve fibers that carry the electrical impulses to the cardiac muscle, causing it to contract.

In the normal heart, a contraction of the heart muscle begins in the pacemaker cells of the sinoatrial (SA) node. The electrical wave passes through the conduction system in the atrial muscle and causes it to contract, forcing blood from the atrial chambers into the ventricles below. The electrical current then enters the atrioventricular (AV) node, which focuses and conducts an electrical current through the bundle of His and Purkinje fibers to the ventricular muscle tissue. The muscle contracts from the apex upward, causing blood to be pumped from the right ventricle into the pulmonary artery to the lungs and from the left ventricle into the aorta to the rest of the body.

A dysrhythmia (sometimes called an *arrhythmia*) occurs when there is a disturbance of the normal electrical conduction, resulting in an abnormal heart muscle contraction or heart rate. All people have an occasional irregular contraction of the heart. The danger is the frequency with which the dysrhythmia occurs because the heart muscle loses its efficiency in pumping an adequate volume of blood. Thus certain types of dysrhythmias can produce additional dysrhythmias that can stop the heart from pumping even though it continues to beat for a short time (fibrillation). A person may sense an abnormal contraction (dysrhythmia) because of a "flip-flop" or racing of the heart. A nurse may also suspect that a patient is having dysrhythmia because of an irregular pulse. Dysrhythmias, however, must be identified with the aid of an electrocardiogram (ECG), which provides a tracing of the electrical activity of the heart.

Dysrhythmias are caused by the firing of abnormal pacemaker cells, blockage of normal electrical pathways, or a combination of both. Normally, the rate and rhythm of electrical activity and muscle contraction are regulated by the pacemaker cells of the SA node. High emotional stress, ischemia (see Chapter 24), or heart failure (see Chapter 27) may trigger normally quiet pacemaker cells in areas of the heart other than the SA or AV nodes to fire. This sends an electrical impulse out of sequence with those from the normal pacemaker cells, causing an irregular muscular contraction, sometimes sensed as a flip-flop of the heart. The second cause of a dysrhythmia is a partial obstruction of the normal conduction pathway, causing an irregular flow of electrical impulses that results in an irregular pattern of muscle contractions. This is sometimes called a *reentrant dysrhythmia*. Normally, healthy heart tissue has mechanisms that protect against reentrant dysrhythmias. Various forms of heart disease cause changes in the conduction pathways that allow continuous reentrant dysrhythmias.

Dysrhythmias are most commonly classified by origin within the heart tissues. Those that develop above the bundle of His (see Fig. 23.1) are called *supraventricular*. Examples of supraventricular dysrhythmias are **atrial flutter**, **atrial fibrillation**, premature atrial contractions, sinus tachycardia, sinus bradycardia, and **paroxysmal supraventricular tachycardia (PSVT)**. Junctional dysrhythmias are those developing near or within the AV node. Dysrhythmias developing below the bundle of His are referred to as *ventricular dysrhythmias*. These include premature ventricular contractions (PVCs), ventricular tachycardia (VT), and ventricular fibrillation. Dysrhythmias that result from obstruction of conduction pathways are described by location (e.g., supraventricular or ventricular, left or right bundle branches). **Atrioventricular blocks** can be subclassified by degree of block: first degree = partial block, delayed AV conduction; second degree = partial block, with occasional blocked beats; and third degree = complete block, in which the atria and ventricles function independently of each other. (It is beyond the scope of this text to describe each type of arrhythmia.) Another method of classification is based on heartbeat rate: bradyarrhythmia (less than 60 beats/min) or tachyarrhythmia (more than 100 beats/min).

The tissues of the electrical system can be classified by conduction rate, depending on whether calcium or sodium ions create the stimulus for muscle contraction. The SA and AV nodes depend on calcium ions for electrical conduction and are referred to as *slow conduction fibers*. The atrial muscle, His-Purkinje system, and ventricular muscle depend on sodium for contraction and are sometimes referred to as *fast conduction fibers*.

TREATMENT FOR DYSRHYTHMIAS

When a dysrhythmia is suspected, a patient is often admitted to a monitored floor in an acute care setting, where wire leads are placed in appropriate locations to provide continuous electrocardiographic monitoring (telemetry). A combination of the physical examination, patient history, and electrocardiographic pattern is used to diagnose the underlying cause of the dysrhythmia. The goal of treatment is to restore normal sinus rhythm and normal cardiac function and prevent recurrence of life-threatening dysrhythmias.

DRUG THERAPY FOR DYSRHYTHMIAS

ACTIONS

Antidysrhythmic agents are complex agents with multiple mechanisms of action. They are classified using the Vaughan Williams classification system according to their effects on the electrical conduction system of the heart (Table 23.1). Class I agents act as myocardial depressants by inhibiting sodium ion movement. The Class Ia agents prolong the duration of the electrical stimulation on cells and the refractory time between

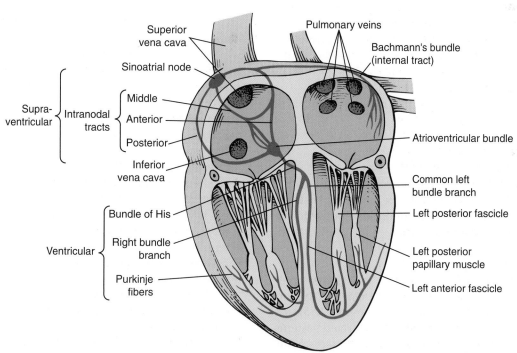

Fig. 23.1 Schematic diagram of the heart, illustrating the conduction system. (Modified from Monahan FD, Sands JK, Neighbors M, et al. *Phipps' Medical-Surgical Nursing: Health and Illness Perspectives.* 8th ed. St. Louis: Mosby; 2007.)

Table 23.1 Classification of Antidysrhythmic Agents

CLASS[a]	DRUGS	MECHANISM	EFFECT CV	EFFECT RP	EFFECT AM
Ia	quinidine	Na channel blockers (intermediate-acting)	↓	—	↓
Ib	lidocaine (Xylocaine) mexiletine	Na channel blockers (quick-acting)	↓/↔	↓	↓
Ic	flecainide propafenone (Rythmol)	Na channel blockers (slow-acting)	↓	↔	↓
II	propranolol (Inderal) esmolol (Brevibloc) metoprolol (Lopressor)	Beta blockers	↓	—	↓
III	amiodarone (Cordarone) sotalol (Betapace) ibutilide (Corvert) dofetilide (Tikosyn)	K channel blockers	↓/↔	—	↔
IV	verapamil (Calan) diltiazem (Cardizem)	Ca channel blockers	↓	—	↓
Miscellaneous	digoxin (Lanoxin) adenosine (Adenocard)	Vagal stimulation Slows conduction	↓	↓/↔	↓

[a]Vaughan Williams classification system.
AM, Automaticity; *Ca*, calcium; *CV*, conduction velocity; *Na*, sodium; *RP*, refractory period.

electrical impulses. Class Ib agents shorten the duration of the electrical stimulation and the time between the electrical impulses. Class Ic antidysrhythmics are the most potent myocardial depressants and slow the conduction rate through the atria and the ventricles.

Class II agents are beta-adrenergic blocking agents (beta blockers). Many dysrhythmias are caused by stimulation of the beta cells of the sympathetic nervous system of the heart. Class III agents slow the rate of electrical conduction and prolong the time interval between contractions by blocking potassium channels. Class IV agents block calcium ion flow, prolonging duration of the electrical stimulation and slowing AV node conduction.

USES

See individual drug monographs for uses of antidysrhythmic agents.

❖ NURSING IMPLICATIONS FOR ANTIDYSRHYTHMIC AGENTS

The information that nurses assess relative to the cardinal signs of cardiovascular disease can provide a basis for subsequent evaluation of the patient's response to the therapeutic modalities prescribed.

◆ Assessment

Dysrhythmias are initially assessed by electrocardiographic monitoring. Various types of telemetry monitoring equipment are available. It is vitally important for the nurse not to rely completely on computerized systems but rather to perform frequent patient assessments while viewing the telemetry system as an adjunct to astute nursing observations. A 24-hour ambulatory ECG

(Holter monitor), electrophysiologic studies, exercise electrocardiography, and laboratory values are used to analyze and diagnose the patient's myocardial status.

Patients may be admitted to the coronary care unit, where specialized monitoring equipment is available for continuous surveillance of the patient. The nurses in this care unit have advanced education in cardiac physiology and the nursing care of these individuals. (See a general medical-surgical nursing text or critical care textbook for an in-depth explanation of care of the patient with a dysrhythmia.)

Medication history. Obtain details of all medications prescribed and being taken. Tactfully find out if the prescribed medications are being taken regularly and, if not, why.

History of six cardinal signs of cardiovascular disease
1. *Dyspnea (difficulty in breathing):* Record if dyspnea occurs while resting or during exertion. Is the patient affected by position, such as lying down? Does he or she awaken from sleep at night?
2. *Chest pain:* Record data as to the time of onset, frequency, duration, and quality of the chest pain. Note any conditions that the patient has found that either aggravate or relieve the chest pain. Are there any associated symptoms with the pain, such as sweating, ashen gray or pale skin, heart skipping a beat, shortness of breath, nausea or vomiting, or racing of the heart? (Not all patients with a dysrhythmia have chest pain.)
3. *Fatigue:* Determine whether fatigue occurs only at specific times of the day, such as evening. Ask the patient if fatigue decreases in relation to a decrease

in activity level or if it is present at about the same time daily. Can he or she keep up with family and coworkers?

4. *Edema:* Record the presence or absence of edema. If present, record location of edema, assessment data (e.g., degree of pitting present; ankle, midcalf, or thigh circumference), and any measures that the patient has used to eliminate edema. Chart the time of day that the edema is present (e.g., when rising in the morning, later in the evening) and the specific parts where it is present on the body. When performing daily weights, use the same scale, at the same time of day, with the patient in a similar type of clothing.

5. *Syncope:* Ask the patient about conditions surrounding any episodes of syncope (faintness or dizziness). Record the degree of symptoms such as general muscle weakness, inability to stand upright, feeling of faintness, or loss of consciousness. Record what activities, if any, bring on these syncopal episodes.

6. *Palpitations:* Record the patient's description of palpitations, such as "my heart skips some beats" or "it began to feel as if it were racing." Ask if these conditions are preceded by mild or strenuous exercise and how long the palpitations last.

Basic mental status. Identify the person's level of consciousness and clarity of thought. Both of these factors are indicators of adequate or inadequate cerebral perfusion. Subsequent regular observations for these data should be made so that apparent improvement or deterioration can be assessed. Schedule basic neurologic assessments at least once per shift.

Vital signs. Vital signs should be taken as often as necessary to monitor the patient's status.

- *Blood pressure:* Blood pressure readings should be performed at least twice daily in stable cardiac patients and more often if indicated by the patient's symptoms or the healthcare provider's orders. Be sure to use the proper-sized blood pressure cuff and have the patient's arm at heart level.
- *Record the blood pressure in both arms:* A systolic pressure variance of 5 to 10 mm Hg is normal; readings reflecting a variance of more than 10 mm Hg should be reported for further evaluation. Always report a narrowing pulse pressure (difference between systolic and diastolic readings).
- *Pulse:* Assess bilaterally the rhythm, quality, equality, and strength of the pulses (carotid, brachial, radial, femoral, popliteal, posterior tibial, and dorsalis pedis). If any pulse is diminished or absent, record the level at which initial changes are noted. The usual words to describe the pulse are *absent, weak, normal, increased,* or *bounding.* Report irregular rate, rhythm, and patient-reported palpitations. Check for delayed capillary refill.
- *Respirations:* Observe and chart the rate and depth of respirations. Check breath sounds at least every shift, making specific notations regarding the presence of abnormal breath sounds such as crackles or wheezes. Observe the degree of dyspnea that occurs and whether it happens with or without exertion.
- *Temperature:* Record the patient's temperature at least every shift.
- *Oxygen saturation:* Record the patient's O_2 saturation using a pulse oximeter with each vital sign measurement.

Auscultation and percussion. Nurses with advanced skills can perform auscultation and percussion to note changes in heart size and heart and lung sounds. (See a medical-surgical nursing text for details about performing these skills.) As appropriate to nursing skills, note changes in cardiac rhythm, heart rate, changes in heart sounds, or murmurs.

Laboratory and diagnostic tests. Review laboratory tests and report abnormal results to the healthcare provider promptly. Such tests may include levels of serum electrolytes, especially potassium, calcium, magnesium, and sodium; arterial blood gases such as pH, partial pressures of oxygen (Po_2) and carbon dioxide (Pco_2), and bicarbonate (HCO_3^-) level; coagulation studies to evaluate the blood clotting; serum enzyme levels, including aspartate aminotransferase (AST), creatine kinase-MB, (CK-MB), troponin, D-dimer, and lactate dehydrogenase (LDH); serum lipid levels (e.g., cholesterol, triglycerides); electrocardiography; chest radiography; nuclear cardiography; cardiac catheterization; electrophysiologic studies; and exercise treadmill.

Examine urinalysis reports and perform hourly monitoring of intake and output as ordered. Report output that is less than intake or below 30 to 50 mL per hour for an adult patient. Monitor other renal function tests such as the blood urea nitrogen and serum creatinine. Abnormalities of these tests or insufficient hourly output may indicate inadequate renal perfusion.

◆ **Implementation**
- Monitor ECG tracings on a continuum (telemetry).
- Perform physical assessments of the patient in accordance with the clinical setting's policies (e.g., every 4 to 8 hours, depending on the patient's status).
- Assist the patient, as needed, to perform activities of daily living. Make note of the degree of impairment or dyspnea seen with and without exertion.
- Administer oxygen as ordered and as necessary (PRN).
- Be aware of the policy for calling "codes," location of the emergency cart, and procedures used to check the emergency cart supplies. Know the procedure for defibrillation and cardioversion.
- Administer prescribed medications and treatments per the Advanced Cardiac Life Support protocol that

can best alleviate the patient's symptoms and provide the maximum level of comfort.

- Encourage physical activity as prescribed. Do not allow the patient to overexert or become fatigued.
- Institute measures to reduce anxiety. Support the patient in a calm manner, even if he or she responds in a hostile or confrontational way.

◆ **Patient Education**

- Review the patient's history to identify modifiable coronary artery disease factors. Design an individualized approach to help the patient modify factors that are within his or her control.
- Cooperatively discuss and practice using coping mechanisms to handle the individual's anxiety.
- Teach the patient to take his or her own pulse and blood pressure, and emphasize signs and symptoms that should be reported. The use of technology to monitor pulse and blood pressure in the form of activities trackers, such as Fitbits and smart watches, can assist the patient in keeping track of these vital signs.

Fostering health maintenance

- Throughout the course of treatment, discuss medication information and how it will benefit the patient.
- Drug therapy is one component of the treatment of dysrhythmias, and it is critical that the medications be taken as prescribed. Provide the patient and significant others with the important information contained in the specific drug monographs for the drugs prescribed. Additional health teaching and nursing interventions for drug adverse effects to expect and report will be found in each drug monograph.
- Seek cooperation and understanding of the following points so that medication compliance is increased: name of medication; dosage, route, and times of administration; and common and serious adverse effects.

Patient self-assessment. Enlist the patient's aid in developing and maintaining a written record of monitoring parameters (e.g., pulse rate, blood pressure, degree of dyspnea and precipitating causes, chest pain, edema). See the Patient Self-Assessment Form for Cardiovascular Agents on the Evolve website. Complete the Premedication Data column for use as a baseline to track response to drug therapy. Ensure that the patient understands how to use the form, and instruct the patient to bring the completed form to follow-up visits. During follow-up visits, focus on issues that will foster adherence to the therapeutic interventions prescribed.

DRUG CLASS: CLASS IA ANTIDYSRHYTHMIC AGENTS

quinidine (KWĬN-ĭ-dēn)
⮀ *Do not confuse quinidine with quinacrine or quinine.*

Actions

Quinidine, originally obtained from cinchona bark, has been used as an antidysrhythmic agent for several decades. It is classified as a class Ia antidysrhythmic agent, working on the muscle of the heart and stabilizing the rate of conduction of impulses. It slows the heart and changes a rapid, irregular pulse to a slow, regular pulse.

Uses

Quinidine is used most often to suppress atrial fibrillation, atrial flutter, PSVT and VT, and life-threatening PVCs. Use with extreme caution in patients with digitalis intoxication or heart block.

Therapeutic Outcome

The primary therapeutic outcome expected from quinidine therapy is conversion of a dysrhythmia to normal sinus rhythm.

❖ **Nursing Implications for Quinidine**

◆ *Premedication assessment*

1. Obtain data relating to the six cardinal signs of cardiovascular disease, vital signs, and pulse oximetry level to be used as a baseline for subsequent evaluation of response to therapy.
2. Assess and record data relating to the patient's usual pattern of bowel elimination.

◆ *Availability*

Quinidine sulfate. *PO:* 200- and 300-mg tablets.
Quinidine gluconate. *PO:* 324-mg tablets, sustained release.
IM, IV: 80 mg/mL quinidine in 10-mL vials.

 Medication Safety Alert

Do not confuse quinidine and quinine. They are both administered in dosages of 300 mg.

◆ *Dosage and administration*

Quinidine sulfate. Adult: *PO:* 200 to 300 mg every 6 to 8 hours. Higher doses may be used, but the maximum single dose should not exceed 600 mg. Administer with food or milk if gastric irritation develops.

 Medication Safety Alert

Intravenous administration of quinidine is extremely hazardous. Blood pressure and ECG readings should be monitored continuously because hypotension and dysrhythmia may occur. Therapeutic blood levels are 2 to 6 mg/L.

Serum levels of quinidine are determined to measure the amount in the bloodstream. Blood should be drawn before the daily dose of medication is given or at least 6 hours after administration. It is important to be consistent in the time of drawing the blood and administering the dose if more than one serum level is to be drawn from the same patient.

Quinidine gluconate. Adult: *PO:* 648 mg every 8 hours; increase cautiously to desired effect. Administer with food or milk if gastric irritation develops.

Adult: *IM:* not recommended.

IV: 0.25 mg/kg/min until sinus rhythm is achieved. Maximum is 10 mg/kg.

◆ Common Adverse Effects

Gastrointestinal

Diarrhea. Diarrhea is common during initiation of therapy. It usually subsides, but occasionally a different medication may need to be administered because of this adverse effect. Chart the frequency and consistency of the diarrhea and monitor the patient for dehydration and electrolyte imbalance.

Neurologic

Dizziness, faintness. Dizziness or faintness may occur, particularly during initiation of therapy. These effects usually subside within a few days. Instruct the patient to rise slowly from a supine position. Monitor the patient's blood pressure.

◆ Serious Adverse Effects

Hypersensitivity

Cinchonism. Monitor patients for signs of cinchonism and report the development of rash, chills, fever, **tinnitus** (ringing in the ears), and increasing mental confusion.

Cardiovascular

Hypotension with diuretics and antihypertensive agents. Instruct the patient to rise slowly from a supine position. If symptoms become excessive (e.g., the systolic blood pressure remains below 100 mm Hg), report to the healthcare provider.

◆ Drug Interactions

Drugs that enhance therapeutic and toxic effects. These include cimetidine, diltiazem, phenothiazines, procainamide, digoxin, verapamil, amiodarone, ketoconazole, fluoroquinolones (e.g., ciprofloxacin), ziprasidone, and beta-adrenergic blocking agents (e.g., propranolol, atenolol). Monitor for increases in severity of drug effects such as bradycardia, tachycardia, and hypotension.

Drugs that reduce therapeutic effects. These include rifampin, phenobarbital, nifedipine, phenytoin, and sucralfate. Monitor for an increase in the frequency of dysrhythmia.

Neuromuscular blockade, respiratory depression. Quinidine may prolong the effects of the surgical muscle relaxants (e.g., succinylcholine) and aminoglycoside antibiotics (e.g., gentamicin, tobramycin). Monitor the patient's respiratory rate and depth. Observe for signs of cyanosis and additional dysrhythmias. Patients who are on respirators may require additional time to be weaned from ventilatory assistance.

Digoxin. Quinidine may increase the effects of digoxin. Monitor the patient for symptoms of anorexia, nausea, vomiting, headaches, blurred or colored vision, and bradycardia. A digoxin serum level and quinidine serum level may be ordered by the healthcare provider.

Warfarin. Quinidine may increase the anticoagulant effects of warfarin. Monitor for signs of increased bleeding: bleeding gums, increased menstrual flow, petechiae, and bruises. Monitor the laboratory report and notify the physician immediately if the prothrombin time or the international normalized ratio (INR) is abnormally high.

DRUG CLASS: CLASS IB ANTIDYSRHYTHMIC AGENTS

lidocaine (LĬ-dō-kān)
Xylocaine (ZĬ-lō-kān)

Actions

Lidocaine is a class Ib antidysrhythmic agent.

Uses

Lidocaine is used in the treatment of life-threatening PVCs, VT, and ventricular fibrillation.

Therapeutic Outcome

The primary therapeutic outcome expected from lidocaine therapy is conversion of dysrhythmia to normal sinus rhythm. Due to infrequency of use, no additional information is presented here on lidocaine.

 Life Span Considerations: Lidocaine

Lidocaine for IV use to treat dysrhythmias, often used for older adults, is different from lidocaine used as a local anesthetic. For use with dysrhythmias, check the label carefully to ensure that it says "lidocaine (or Xylocaine) for cardiac dysrhythmia." Serious dysrhythmias may result if lidocaine with preservatives or lidocaine with epinephrine is administered intravenously to the patient.

DRUG CLASS: CLASS IC ANTIDYSRHYTHMIC AGENTS

flecainide acetate (flĕ-KĀ-nīd ĂS-ĭ-tāt)
Apo-Flecainide (ĂP-ō flĕ-KĀ-nīd) ◆

Actions

Flecainide acetate is a class Ic antidysrhythmic agent that may be taken orally.

Uses

Flecainide may be used in the prevention of paroxysmal atrial fibrillation/flutter (PAF) associated with disabling symptoms, PSVTs, and prevention of life-threatening ventricular dysrhythmias such as sustained VT. Flecainide is usually used for more serious ventricular dysrhythmias that have not responded to more traditional therapy. In addition to its therapeutic activity, a particular advantage is its twice-daily dosing schedule. Flecainide has a negative inotropic effect and may cause or worsen heart failure, particularly in patients with preexisting severe heart failure. This adverse effect may take hours to months to develop. New or worsened heart failure occurs in approximately 5% of patients. Flecainide may also aggravate an existing dysrhythmia and precipitate new ones, especially in patients with underlying heart disease.

Therapeutic Outcome

The primary therapeutic outcome expected from flecainide therapy is conversion of dysrhythmia to normal sinus rhythm.

❖ Nursing Implications for Flecainide

◆ *Premedication assessment*

1. Obtain data relating to the six cardinal signs of cardiovascular disease, vital signs, and pulse oximetry levels to be used as a baseline for subsequent evaluation of response to therapy.
2. If any symptoms of heart failure are present, notify the healthcare provider before starting therapy.

◆ *Availability. PO:* 50-, 100-, and 150-mg tablets.

◆ *Dosage and administration*

PSVT, PAF. Adult: *PO:* Initially, 50 mg every 12 hours, increasing 50 mg twice daily every 4 days. Maximum daily dosage is 300 mg.

Sustained VT. Adult: *PO:* Initially, 100 mg every 12 hours; increase in 50-mg increments twice daily every 4 days. Most patients respond at 150 mg twice daily. Maximum daily dosage is 400 mg.

> **⚠ Medication Safety Alert**
>
> Reduce dose of flecainide 50% when administered with amiodarone.
>
> Flecainide should not be used in patients with second- or third-degree AV block in the absence of an artificial ventricular pacemaker and must be used with caution in patients with known heart failure. Monitor the ECG before and during initiation of therapy.

◆ *Common adverse effects.* The more frequent adverse effects that occur with flecainide therapy are dizziness, lightheadedness, faintness, and unsteadiness (19%); visual disturbances, such as blurred vision, difficulty in focusing, and spots before the eyes (16%); dyspnea (1%); headache (10%); nausea (9%); fatigue (8%); constipation (5%); edema (3%); and abdominal pain (3%).

Neurologic

Dizziness, headache. These adverse effects are usually mild and tend to resolve with continued therapy. Encourage the patient not to discontinue therapy without first consulting the healthcare provider.

Gastrointestinal

Constipation, nausea. These adverse effects are usually mild and tend to resolve with continued therapy. Encourage the patient not to discontinue therapy without first consulting the healthcare provider.

◆ *Serious adverse effects*

Sensory

Visual disturbances. Provide for patient safety during temporary visual impairment. Caution the patient to avoid temporarily any tasks that require visual acuity, such as driving or operating power machinery. Instruct the patient not to rub the eyes with force when tearing.

These adverse effects are usually mild and tend to resolve with continued therapy. Encourage the patient not to discontinue therapy without first consulting the healthcare provider.

Cardiovascular

Increasing dyspnea, exercise intolerance, edema. Flecainide may induce or aggravate preexisting heart failure. If these symptoms become more pronounced, the patient should be instructed to contact the healthcare provider for further evaluation.

Dysrhythmias. Flecainide may induce or aggravate preexisting dysrhythmias. The patient should be instructed to contact the healthcare provider for further evaluation if sensations of a jumping or racing heart develop.

◆ *Drug interactions*

Drugs that enhance therapeutic and toxic effects. These include amiodarone, cimetidine, verapamil, and protease inhibitors (e.g., ritonavir). Monitor for increases of drug effects such as dysrhythmias, heart failure, and bradycardia.

Digoxin. When multiple doses of flecainide are administered to patients stabilized on a dose of digoxin, there is a 10% to 20% increase in serum digoxin concentrations. This increase may result in signs of digitalis toxicity, such as anorexia, nausea, fatigue, blurred or colored vision, bradycardia, and dysrhythmias. Monitor serum digoxin levels, ECG readings, and the clinical course of the patient closely.

Propranolol. When flecainide and propranolol are administered concurrently, there is a 20% increase in serum flecainide levels and a 30% increase in propranolol levels, with additive pharmacologic effects from each. Monitor serum levels, ECG readings, and the clinical course of the patient closely. Dosage reductions of either one or both agents may be required.

Urinary acidifiers. These agents (e.g., ascorbic acid, ammonium chloride) may lower the urine pH, causing an increase in the urinary excretion of flecainide. Patients should be observed for redevelopment of dysrhythmias, which may require an increase in dosage of flecainide.

---

propafenone (prō-PĂ-fĕ-nōn)
    Rythmol (RĬTH-mŏl)

Actions

Propafenone is a class Ic antidysrhythmic agent. It also has weak beta-blocking and calcium channel blocking effects.

Uses

Propafenone is used for the treatment of paroxysmal atrial fibrillation and life-threatening ventricular dysrhythmias such as VT. Because propafenone can cause additional dysrhythmias, it is used only with patients in whom the benefits outweigh the potential risks.

Therapeutic Outcome

The primary therapeutic outcome expected from propafenone therapy is conversion of dysrhythmia to normal sinus rhythm.

❖ Nursing Implications for Propafenone

◆ *Premedication assessment*

1. Obtain data relating to the six cardinal signs of cardiovascular disease, vital signs, and continuous pulse oximetry and electrocardiographic monitoring to be used as a baseline for subsequent evaluation of response to therapy.
2. Record data relating to any gastrointestinal symptoms present before initiation of therapy.

◆ *Availability*

PO: 150-, 225-, and 300-mg tablets; 225-, 325-, and 425-mg capsules, extended release (12 hr).

◆ *Dosage and administration. PO:* Initially, 150 mg every 8 hours. At 3- or 4-day intervals, the dosage may be increased to 225 mg every 8 hours and then 300 mg every 8 hours (900 mg/day).

> **Medication Safety Alert**
>
> Because propafenone has mild beta-adrenergic blocking properties, it should not be used in patients with asthma.
> Administer in divided doses around the clock. If a patient misses a dose of propafenone, the next dose should not be doubled because of an increased risk of adverse reactions.

◆ *Common adverse effects*

Neurologic

Dizziness. This may occur, particularly during the initiation of therapy. Dizziness usually subsides within a few days. Instruct the patient to rise slowly from a supine position. Monitor the patient's blood pressure.

Gastrointestinal

Nausea, vomiting, constipation. Gastrointestinal complaints occur in approximately 11% of patients, but discontinuation of therapy is rarely required. Administer with food or milk to alleviate nausea. Encourage the patient not to discontinue therapy without first consulting the healthcare provider.

◆ *Serious adverse effects*

Cardiovascular

Dysrhythmias. Propafenone may induce or aggravate dysrhythmias. Patients with more serious dysrhythmias

such as sustained VT are more susceptible to myocardial toxicity. The patient should be instructed to contact the healthcare provider for further evaluation if sensations of a jumping or racing heart develop.

◆ *Drug interactions*

Drugs that enhance therapeutic and toxic effects. These include quinidine, cimetidine, protease inhibitors (e.g., ritonavir), ziprasidone, fluoxetine, and fluoroquinolones (e.g., ciprofloxacin). Monitor for an increase in severity of adverse effects from propafenone, such as hypotension, somnolence, bradycardia, and dysrhythmias.

Drugs that decrease therapeutic effects

Rifampin. Monitor patients with concurrent therapy for increased frequency of dysrhythmias.

Digoxin. Propafenone produces dose-related increases in serum digoxin levels. Measure plasma digoxin levels and reduce digoxin dosage when propafenone is started.

Propranolol, metoprolol. Propafenone appears to inhibit the metabolism of these beta blockers. A reduction in beta blocker dosage may be necessary during concurrent therapy with propafenone.

Warfarin. Propafenone increases plasma warfarin concentrations by inhibiting warfarin metabolism, thus prolonging prothrombin time. Observe for the development of petechiae; ecchymoses; nosebleeds; bleeding gums; dark, tarry stools; and bright red or coffee-ground emesis. Monitor the prothrombin time (INR) and reduce the dosage of warfarin if necessary.

DRUG CLASS: CLASS II ANTIDYSRHYTHMIC AGENTS: BETA-ADRENERGIC BLOCKING AGENTS

Actions

The beta-adrenergic blocking agents (e.g., esmolol, metoprolol) are used widely as antidysrhythmic agents. These agents inhibit cardiac response to sympathetic nerve stimulation by blocking the beta receptors. As a result, the heart rate, systolic blood pressure, and cardiac output are reduced.

Uses

These agents are effective in the treatment of various ventricular dysrhythmias, sinus tachycardia, PSVT, PVCs, and tachycardia associated with atrial flutter or fibrillation because AV conduction is diminished.

Therapeutic Outcome

The primary therapeutic outcome expected from beta blocker therapy is conversion to, and maintenance of, normal sinus rhythm.

❖ Nursing Implications for Beta-Adrenergic Blocking Agents

See Chapter 12 for further discussion of the nursing implications associated with beta-adrenergic inhibition.

DRUG CLASS: CLASS III ANTIDYSRHYTHMIC AGENTS

---

amiodarone hydrochloride (ăm-ē-Ō-dă-rŏn hī-drō-KLŌR-īd)
⇄ *Do not confuse amiodarone with trazodone, amantadine, or amlodipine.*
Pacerone (pace' er own)

Actions

Although its mechanism of action is unknown, amiodarone is a class III antidysrhythmic agent that prolongs the action potential of atrial and ventricular tissue and increases the refractory period without altering the resting membrane potential, thus delaying repolarization. In addition, amiodarone has been shown to antagonize noncompetitively both alpha- and beta-adrenergic receptors, causing systemic and coronary vasodilation.

Uses

Amiodarone is being used in the management of life-threatening supraventricular tachydysrhythmias, atrial fibrillation and flutter, bradycardia-tachycardia syndromes, ventricular tachycardia and fibrillation, and hypertrophic cardiomyopathy resistant to currently available therapy.

Adverse Effects

Adverse reactions are very common with the use of amiodarone, particularly in patients receiving more than 400 mg/day. Approximately 15% to 20% of patients discontinue therapy because of adverse effects.

Therapeutic Outcome

The primary therapeutic outcome expected from amiodarone therapy is conversion to, and maintenance of, normal sinus rhythm.

❖ Nursing Implications for Amiodarone

◆ Premedication assessment

1. Obtain data relating to the six cardinal signs of cardiovascular disease, vital signs, pulse oximetry, and electrocardiographic tracings to be used as a baseline for subsequent evaluation of response to therapy.
2. Initiate requested laboratory tests to be used for evaluation of pulmonary, ophthalmic, thyroid, and liver function.
3. Record data relating to the patient's usual sleep pattern and any gastrointestinal symptoms present before initiation of therapy.

◆ Availability. *PO:* 100-, 200-, and 400-mg tablets.

IV: 50 mg/mL in 3-, 9-, and 18-mL ampules; 1.5 mg/mL in 100-mL and 1.8 mg/mL in 200-mL and 1.8 mg/mL in 250-mL dextrose IV solutions.

◆ *Dosage and administration.* The difficulty of using amiodarone effectively and safely is that it poses a significant risk to patients. Patients must be hospitalized while the loading dose is given, and the response often requires 2 weeks or more. Because absorption and elimination are variable, maintenance dose selection is difficult, and it is not unusual for a reduction in dosage or discontinuation of treatment to be required. The time at which a previously controlled life-threatening dysrhythmia will recur after discontinuation or dosage adjustment is unpredictable, ranging from weeks to months. Attempts to substitute other antidysrhythmic agents when amiodarone is discontinued are made difficult by the gradually but unpredictably changing amiodarone body store. A similar problem exists when amiodarone is not effective; it still poses the risk of a drug interaction with whatever subsequent treatment is tried.

PO: Loading dose: 800 to 1600 mg daily in divided doses for 1 to 3 weeks until an initial therapeutic response occurs. After the loading dose, a dosage of 600 to 800 mg daily is given for approximately 1 month. *Maintenance:* The lowest effective dosage should be used, generally 400 mg daily.

IV: 150 mg intravenous piggyback over 10 minutes, followed by an infusion of 60 mg/hr for 6 hours, then 30 mg/hr for the next 18 hours.

⚠ Medication Safety Alert

Amiodarone is contraindicated in patients with severe sinus node dysfunction that causes sinus bradycardia, with second- and third-degree AV block, and when episodes of bradycardia have caused syncope (except in the presence of a pacemaker).

Baseline tests. Before the start of therapy, baseline pulmonary, ophthalmic, thyroid, and liver function tests should be completed.

Gastric irritation. If gastric irritation occurs, administer with food or milk. If symptoms persist or increase in severity, report this to the healthcare provider for evaluation.

◆ *Serious adverse effects*

Neurologic

Fatigue, tremors, involuntary movements, sleep disturbances, numbness and tingling, dizziness, ataxia, confusion. Many of these symptoms are dose related and resolve with reduction of dosage or discontinuation of therapy. Peripheral neuropathy may be associated with long-term therapy, although the onset and presentation of symptoms are variable. Symptoms usually resolve 1 to 4 months after the discontinuation of therapy. Teach the patient to rise slowly from a supine or sitting position, and encourage the patient to sit or lie down if feeling faint.

Perform a baseline assessment of the patient's degree of alertness and orientation to name, place, and time before starting therapy. Make regularly scheduled subsequent mental status evaluations and compare findings. Report development of mental status changes. Provide for patient safety during episodes of dizziness.

Respiratory

Exertional dyspnea, nonproductive cough, pleuritic chest pain. Pulmonary interstitial pneumonitis or alveolitis has been reported in 10% to 15% of patients. Particular care should be taken not to assume that such symptoms are related to cardiac failure. Tests for diffusion capacity are most likely to show an abnormality. Symptoms gradually resolve after discontinuation of therapy. Periodic chest radiographs and clinical evaluation are recommended every 3 to 6 months.

Endocrine

Thyroid disorders. Administration of amiodarone has been associated with the development of hypothyroidism (2% to 10%) and hyperthyroidism (1% to 3%). Patients with a history of thyroid disorders appear to be more susceptible to this complication. Baseline and periodic thyroid function tests should be completed in all patients.

Sensory

Yellow-brown pigmentations in the cornea, blurred vision, halos. Corneal microdeposits have been observed by slit-lamp examination as early as 2 weeks after the initiation of therapy. Symptoms of blurred vision, narrowing peripheral vision, or visual halos develop in about 10% of patients. This complication is reversible after drug withdrawal. Use of methylcellulose ophthalmic solution and a minimization of the maintenance doses may limit this complication. Provide for patient safety during temporary visual impairment. Instruct the patient not to rub the eyes with force when tearing.

Gastrointestinal

Nausea, vomiting, constipation, abdominal pain, anorexia. Gastrointestinal complaints occur in about 25% of patients but rarely require discontinuation of therapy. These adverse effects commonly occur during high-dosage administration and usually respond to a dosage reduction or divided dosages.

Hepatotoxicity. Abnormal liver function test results (e.g., AST, alanine aminotransferase) occur in 4% to 9% of patients. Liver enzyme levels in patients on relatively high maintenance doses should be monitored on a regular basis. Persistent significant elevations in the liver enzymes or hepatomegaly are indications for considering a reduction in dosage or discontinuation of therapy. Hepatitis and other liver abnormalities may develop in 1% to 3% of patients. The symptoms of hepatotoxicity are anorexia, nausea, vomiting, jaundice, hepatomegaly, splenomegaly, and abnormal liver function tests.

Cardiovascular

Dysrhythmias. Amiodarone can cause an exacerbation of the preexisting dysrhythmia, and in 2% to 4% of patients induce other new dysrhythmias as well.

Integumentary

Photosensitivity. Amiodarone has produced photosensitivity resulting in a rash in approximately 10% of patients. The severity of the rash may depend on the degree of sun exposure. Symptoms such as burning, tingling, erythema, and blistering may occur as early as 2 hours after exposure to the sun. The use of sunscreens may minimize this adverse effect. Patients should be encouraged to wear long-sleeved shirts and to avoid wearing shorts outdoors. Photosensitivity may persist for up to 4 months after discontinuation of therapy. With long-term treatment, a blue-gray discoloration of the exposed skin may occur. The risk is increased in patients of fair complexion and those with excessive sun exposure, and may be related to cumulative dose and duration of therapy. This effect gradually subsides after discontinuation of therapy. The patient should also be instructed not to use artificial tanning lamps.

◆ Drug interactions

Cimetidine, fluoroquinolones, azole-type antifungal agents, protease inhibitors, macrolide antibiotics. Administration of these drugs concurrently with amiodarone significantly increases serum levels of amiodarone. Reduce the dosage of amiodarone and monitor closely for dysrhythmias if administered concurrently.

Rifampin. Rifampin significantly reduces the serum levels of amiodarone. The dose of amiodarone may need to be increased for therapeutic effect.

Cholestyramine. Cholestyramine significantly reduces the serum levels of amiodarone. The dose of amiodarone may need to be increased for therapeutic effect.

Fentanyl. When used concurrently, fentanyl and amiodarone may cause hypotension, bradycardia, decreased cardiac output, and sinus arrest. Monitor heart rate, ECG, and pulmonary function closely.

Digoxin. Administration of amiodarone to patients receiving digoxin therapy regularly results in an increase in the serum digoxin concentration. The dose of digoxin should be reduced by 50% or discontinued. Digoxin serum levels should be closely monitored and patients observed for clinical evidence of toxicity (e.g., anorexia, nausea, fatigue, blurred or colored vision, bradycardia, dysrhythmia).

Warfarin. Potentiation of warfarin is almost always seen within 3 to 4 days in patients receiving concomitant therapy. The dose of the anticoagulant should be reduced by one-third to one-half, and prothrombin times (INR) should be monitored closely. Observe for the development of petechiae; ecchymoses; nosebleeds; bleeding gums; dark, tarry stools; and bright red or coffee-ground emesis.

Quinidine. Elevation of quinidine serum levels by 32% to 50% is often observed within 2 to 3 days. The dosage of quinidine should be reduced by one-third to one-half or discontinued.

Phenytoin. Elevation of phenytoin serum levels by 200% to 300% is observed over several weeks. The dosage of phenytoin must be gradually reduced, based on patient response. Monitor patients undergoing concurrent therapy for signs of phenytoin toxicity: nystagmus, sedation, and lethargy. Serum levels should be monitored periodically. Phenytoin may also reduce amiodarone levels. Monitor closely for loss of therapeutic effects.

Beta blockers, calcium channel blockers. Amiodarone should be used with caution in patients receiving beta-adrenergic blocking agents (e.g., propranolol, timolol, nadolol, pindolol) or calcium channel blockers (e.g., diltiazem, verapamil, nifedipine) because of the possible potentiation of bradycardia, sinus arrest, and AV block. If necessary, amiodarone can be used after insertion of a pacemaker in patients with severe bradycardia or sinus arrest.

Theophylline. Amiodarone may increase theophylline serum levels, resulting in toxicity. Effects may not be observed until after at least 1 week of concurrent therapy. Toxicity may persist for more than 1 week after amiodarone has been discontinued.

---

dofetilide (dō-FĚT-ĭ-līd)
Tikosyn (TIK-o-sin)

Actions

Dofetilide is a class III antidysrhythmic agent. It acts by blocking the cardiac potassium ion channels, delaying repolarization and thus prolonging the refractory period in the atria and ventricles. On an ECG rhythm strip, the Q–T interval will be prolonged. In clinically useful doses, dofetilide has no effect on sodium channels or alpha- and beta-adrenergic receptors.

Uses

Dofetilide blocks reentrant dysrhythmias such as atrial fibrillation/flutter and VT and prevents their reformation. Thus it is used to convert atrial fibrillation/flutter to normal sinus rhythm and maintain sinus rhythm after conversion.

Adverse Effects

Prolongation of the Q–T interval may induce ventricular dysrhythmias, particularly torsades de pointes (a ventricular dysrhythmia associated with prolongation of the Q–Tc interval on the ECG), syncope, and sudden death. Using only the minimal dose necessary for maintenance of normal sinus rhythm is important because the frequency of dysrhythmias is directly correlated to increase in dose and further prolongation of the Q–T interval.

Therapeutic Outcome

The primary therapeutic outcome expected from dofetilide therapy is conversion to, and maintenance of, normal sinus rhythm.

❖ Nursing Implications for Dofetilide
◆ Premedication assessment
1. Obtain baseline blood pressure readings in supine and standing positions and apical pulse.

2. Initiate laboratory studies requested by the healthcare provider (e.g., renal function tests such as blood urea nitrogen, serum creatinine, and electrolyte levels) to be used as a baseline for future comparison.

◆ **Availability.** *PO:* 125-, 250-, and 500-mcg capsules.

◆ **Dosage and administration.** Before dofetilide is initiated:
- Patients must be admitted to a unit with continuous ECG monitoring available and personnel trained in the treatment of serious ventricular dysrhythmias and the initiation of dofetilide. Therapy must be continuously monitored for at least 3 days.
- Patients with atrial fibrillation must be anticoagulated before electrical or pharmacologic cardioversion to normal sinus rhythm.
- Hypokalemia must be corrected before initiation of dofetilide therapy.
- The Q–Tc interval must be assessed. If the interval is more than 440 to 500 milliseconds, dofetilide is contraindicated.
- The creatinine clearance must be calculated.

PO: Initial: Based on calculated creatinine clearance with continuous ECG monitoring, give the following doses:

CALCULATED CREATININE CLEARANCE	DOFETILIDE DOSE
>60 mL/min	500 mcg twice daily
40 to 60 mL/min	250 mcg twice daily
20 to <40 mL/min	125 mcg twice daily
<20 mL/min	dofetilide contraindicated

Dosage adjustment: 2 to 3 hours after administration of the first dose, reassess the Q–Tc interval. If the Q–Tc interval has increased 15% or more compared with baseline, or is >500 msec, then adjust the dose as follows:

IF THE STARTING DOSE BASED ON CREATININE CLEARANCE IS:	THEN THE NEW DOSE BASED ON Q–TC INTERVAL IS:
500 mcg twice daily	250 mcg twice daily
250 mcg twice daily	125 mcg twice daily
125 mcg twice daily	125 mcg daily
<20 mL/min	dofetilide contraindicated

If, after the second dose, the Q–Tc interval is more than 500 to 550 milliseconds, dofetilide should be discontinued.

Renal function and Q–Tc interval should be recalculated every 3 months. If creatinine clearance falls, adjust the dofetilide dose according to the initial dose. If the Q–Tc interval is more than 500 to 550 milliseconds, dofetilide should be discontinued and patients should be monitored by ECG until the Q–Tc returns to baseline.

If a patient misses a dose, the dose should not be doubled at the next dose. The next dose should be taken at the scheduled time.

◆ *Common adverse effects*

Cardiovascular

Dysrhythmias. Various dysrhythmias (e.g., ventricular fibrillation, VT, torsades de pointes, AV block, heart block) have been reported in up to 15% of patients receiving dofetilide. Continuous ECG monitoring is crucial until the patient is stable.

Chest pain. Occurs in 10% of patients.

Gastrointestinal

Nausea, abdominal pain, diarrhea. Nausea occurs in 5% of patients, abdominal pain in 3% of patients, and diarrhea in 3% of patients. These adverse effects are usually mild and tend to resolve with continued therapy. Encourage the patient not to discontinue therapy without first consulting the healthcare provider.

Neurologic

Headache. Headache occurs in 11% of patients taking dofetilide. The headaches are usually mild and tend to resolve with continued therapy. Encourage the patient not to discontinue therapy without first consulting the healthcare provider.

Other

Dizziness, insomnia, rash. Dizziness occurs in 8% of patients, insomnia in 4%, and rash in 3%.

◆ *Drug interactions*

Drugs that enhance toxic effects. Cimetidine, trimethoprim, and ketoconazole inhibit urinary excretion of dofetilide, potentially causing an increase in plasma concentrations and prolongation of the Q–Tc interval.

Other medicines that prolong the Q–Tc interval may cause serious toxicity when used concurrently with dofetilide. These include some other antidysrhythmic agents (amiodarone, quinidine, sotalol) chlorpromazine, dolasetron, droperidol, moxifloxacin, and ziprasidone.

 Medication Safety Alert

Dofetilide must be discontinued at least 48 hours before the initiation of other medicines that may enhance toxic effects from dofetilide.

DRUG CLASS: CLASS IV ANTIDYSRHYTHMIC AGENTS: CALCIUM CHANNEL BLOCKING AGENTS

Actions

The calcium channel blockers (e.g., verapamil, diltiazem) are used widely as antidysrhythmic agents. These agents inhibit cardiac response by blocking the L-type calcium channels in the SA and AV nodal tissue. This slows AV conduction, prolongs refractoriness, and decreases automaticity.

Uses

These agents are effective in the treatment of automatic and reentrant tachycardias. They are contraindicated in systolic heart failure.

Therapeutic Outcome

The primary therapeutic outcome expected from calcium channel blocker therapy is conversion to, and maintenance of, normal sinus rhythm.

❖ **Nursing Implications for Calcium Channel Blocking Agents**

See Chapter 22 for further discussion of nursing implications associated with calcium channel blocking agents.

DRUG CLASS: MISCELLANEOUS ANTIDYSRHYTHMIC AGENTS

adenosine (ă-DĔN-ō-sēn)
Adenocard (ă-DĔN-ō-kărd)

Actions

Adenosine is a naturally occurring chemical found in every cell within the body. It is not related to other antidysrhythmic agents. It has a variety of physiologic roles, including energy transfer, promotion of prostaglandin release, inhibition of platelet aggregation, antiadrenergic effects, coronary vasodilation, and suppression of heart rate.

Uses

Because of its strong depressant effects on the SA and AV nodes, adenosine is recommended for the treatment of PSVT that involves conduction in the SA node, atrium, or AV node. Adenosine does not convert atrial flutter, atrial fibrillation, or VT to normal sinus rhythm.

Therapeutic Outcome

The primary therapeutic outcome expected from adenosine therapy is conversion of PVSTs to normal sinus rhythm.

❖ **Nursing Implications for Adenosine**

◆ *Premedication assessment.*

1. Obtain data relating to the six cardinal signs of cardiovascular disease, vital signs, pulse oximetry, and continuous electrocardiographic monitoring to be used as a baseline for subsequent evaluation of response to therapy.

◆ *Availability.* **IV:** 3 mg/mL in 2-, 4-, 20-, and 30-mL vials.

◆ *Dosage and administration.* **IV:** 6 mg administered by rapid IV bolus injection (over 1 to 2 seconds) followed by a saline flush. A follow-up dose of 12 mg by rapid IV bolus is recommended if the initial dose is unsuccessful in restoring a normal heart rate. The 12-mg dose may be repeated once if required. Normal saline (0.9% sodium chloride) is the diluent.

◆ *Common adverse effects.* The most commonly reported adverse reactions with adenosine include flushing of the face (18%), shortness of breath (12%), chest pressure

(7%), nausea (3%), and headache and lightheadedness (2%). Because the half-life of adenosine is less than 10 seconds, adverse effects are very short-lived. Treatment of any prolonged adverse effect would include oxygen and possibly other antidysrhythmic agents.

◆ *Drug interactions*

Drugs that enhance therapeutic and toxic effects. Dipyridamole and carbamazepine potentiate the effects of adenosine. Smaller doses of adenosine should be used if therapy is required.

Drugs that reduce therapeutic effects. Theophylline, aminophylline, and caffeine competitively antagonize adenosine; thus larger doses of adenosine are required with concurrent use.

digoxin (dǐ-JŎKS-ǐn)
   Lanoxin (lǎ-NŎKS-ǐn)

Actions

Digoxin slows conduction through the AV node, reducing conduction velocity and automaticity. It has a positive inotropic effect, increasing cardiac output.

Uses

As an antidysrhythmic agent, digoxin may be used to treat atrial fibrillation, atrial flutter, and paroxysmal supraventricular tachycardia.

Therapeutic Outcome

The primary therapeutic outcome expected from digoxin therapy is conversion of supraventricular tachycardias to normal sinus rhythm and increased cardiac output.

❖ **Nursing Implications for Digoxin**
See Chapter 27 for further discussion of nursing implications associated with digoxin therapy.

Get Ready for the NCLEX® Examination!

Key Points

- Dysrhythmias are complex in origin, severity, and treatment for control.
- Many of the agents used to treat dysrhythmias have serious adverse effects and must be monitored closely.
- Nurses need to check references carefully in advance of administering these drugs for the correct method of preparation, preadministration assessments needed, rate of administration of IV drugs, and monitoring parameters essential during drug administration. If any monitoring parameter (e.g., blood pressure) is not within desired limits, hold the medication and notify the healthcare provider.
- Nurses can play a significant role in public education efforts, monitoring patient response to therapy, monitoring for noncompliance, and encouraging patients to participate in their own therapy.

Additional Learning Resources

SG Go to your Study Guide for additional Review Questions for the NCLEX® Examination, Critical Thinking Clinical Situations, and other learning activities to help you master this chapter content.

Go to your Evolve website (https://evolve.elsevier.com/Clayton) for additional online resources.

Review Questions for the NCLEX® Examination

1. Identify the correct order that the electrical impulse travels in the normal conduction pathway of the heart.
   1. The Purkinje fibers
   2. The AV node
   3. The bundle of His
   4. The SA node

2. The nurse reviewed the classifications of drugs that can be used to treat dysrhythmias, and knows they include which mechanism of action? *(Select all that apply.)*
   1. Beta-adrenergic blockers
   2. Calcium channel blockers
   3. Chloride channel blockers
   4. Sodium channel blockers
   5. Potassium channel blockers

3. The nurse reviewing the laboratory results of a 68-year-old female patient on propafenone for paroxysmal atrial fibrillation knows which of the following laboratory tests are monitored for patients on antidysrhythmic agents? *(Select all that apply.)*
   1. PSA
   2. CK-MB
   3. AST
   4. TSH
   5. LDH

4. The nurse administering a class III antidysrhythmic agent to a 57-year-old male patient with a history of ventricular tachycardia knows that it is important to observe for which of these adverse effects? *(Select all that apply.)*
   1. Thyroid disorders
   2. Photosensitivity
   3. Exertional dyspnea
   4. Sinus rhythm
   5. Nausea and constipation

5. A nurse assessing a 48-year-old male patient for signs of cardiovascular disease looks for which of these symptoms? *(Select all that apply.)*
   1. Palpitations
   2. Shortness of breath
   3. Syncope
   4. Fatigue
   5. Confusion

6. A patient starting on the antidysrhythmic flecainide asks the nurse what is meant by the term *dysrhythmia*. What is an appropriate response by the nurse?
   1. "A dysrhythmia is any life-threatening heart rhythm."
   2. "A dysrhythmia is when your heart beats too fast and we need to slow it down."
   3. "You have an irregular heart rate and rhythm, and this medication is helping to convert your heart to a more normal rate and rhythm."
   4. "Dysrhythmias are signs of heart failure, and you need to be on these medications to prevent any further progression of the problem."

Objectives

1. Define *angina pectoris* and identify assessment data needed to evaluate an anginal attack.
2. Differentiate between *chronic stable angina* and *unstable angina* and the drug therapy used for each type.
3. Describe the actions of the drug classifications used to treat angina and the effect on the myocardial tissue of the heart.
4. Identify risk factor management and healthy lifestyle changes that are taught to prevent disease progression and myocardial infarction or death.

Key Terms

angina pectoris (ăn-JĬ-nă PĔK-tŏr-ĭs) (p. 382)
ischemia (ĭs-KĒ-mē-ă) (p. 382)
chronic stable angina (KRŎN-ĭk STĀ-bŭl) (p. 382)

unstable angina (ŭn-STĀ-bŭl) (p. 382)
variant angina (VĂR-ē-ĕnt) (p. 382)

ANGINA PECTORIS

Coronary artery disease (CAD) is the leading cause of disability, socioeconomic loss, and death in the United States, and angina pectoris is the first clinical indication of underlying CAD in many patients. **Angina pectoris** is the name given to a feeling of chest discomfort arising from the heart because of lack of oxygen getting to the heart cells. It is a symptom of CAD and is also called *ischemic heart disease.* **Ischemia** develops when the supply of oxygen needed by the heart cells is inadequate. The lack of oxygen occurs when blood flow through the coronary arteries is reduced by atherosclerosis or spasm of the arteries. Atherosclerosis can develop as localized plaques or as a generalized narrowing of the coronary arteries. Patients are usually asymptomatic until there is at least 50% narrowing of the artery. Coronary artery disease caused by atherosclerosis is a progressive disease; however, progression can be slowed with diet control and with the use of cholesterol-lowering agents (see Chapter 21).

The presentation of angina pectoris is highly variable. The sensation of discomfort is often described variously as squeezing, tightness, choking, pressure, burning, or heaviness. This discomfort may radiate to the neck, lower jaw, shoulder, and arm. The usual anginal attack begins gradually, reaches its peak intensity over the next several minutes, and then gradually subsides after the person stops activity and rests. Attacks can last from 30 seconds to 30 minutes. Anginal episodes are usually precipitated by factors that require an increased oxygen supply (e.g., physical activity, such as climbing a flight of stairs or lifting). Other precipitating factors include exposure to cold temperatures, emotional stress, sexual intercourse, and eating a large meal.

Angina pectoris is classified as chronic stable, unstable, or variant angina. **Chronic stable angina** is precipitated by physical exertion or stress, lasts only a few minutes, and is relieved by rest or nitroglycerin. It is usually caused by fixed atherosclerotic obstruction in the coronary arteries. **Unstable angina** is unpredictable; it changes in ease of onset, frequency, duration, and intensity. It is probably caused by a combination of atherosclerotic narrowing, vasospasm, and thrombus formation. **Variant angina** occurs while the patient is at rest; it is characterized by specific electrocardiographic changes, and it is caused by vasospasm of a coronary artery reducing blood flow. The type of angina pectoris is diagnosed by a combination of history, electrocardiographic changes during an anginal attack, and exercise tolerance testing, with or without thallium-201 scintigraphy.

TREATMENT OF ANGINA PECTORIS

The goals for the treatment of angina pectoris are to prevent myocardial infarction and death (thereby prolonging life) and to relieve anginal pain symptoms (thereby improving the quality of life). In many cases, coronary angioplasty or coronary artery bypass surgery will be considered first because these treatments have been proven to save lives over time. The choice of therapy often depends on the patient's clinical response to initial medical therapy.

All patients should receive extensive patient education to help them reduce their risks related to CAD. The avoidance of activities that can precipitate attacks (e.g., strenuous exercise, exposure to cold weather, drinking caffeine-containing beverages, cigarette smoking, eating heavy meals, emotional stress) should be attempted. Risk factors (e.g., diabetes mellitus, hypertension, dyslipidemia) must also be treated. A structured exercise program designed for each patient can be successful for weight reduction among overweight patients, and it can also improve cardiovascular health. Healthy muscle tissue requires less oxygen. Medications, in combination with risk reduction and exercise, are effective in preventing ischemic attacks and myocardial infarction.

DRUG THERAPY FOR ANGINA PECTORIS

ACTIONS

The underlying pathophysiology of ischemic heart disease is an imbalance between the oxygen demands of the heart and the ability of coronary arteries to deliver the needed oxygen, the spasticity of the coronary arteries, platelet aggregation, and thrombus formation. The oxygen demand of the heart is determined by the heart rate, contractility, and ventricular volume. Therefore the pharmacologic treatment of angina is aimed at decreasing oxygen demand by decreasing heart rate, myocardial contractility, and ventricular volume without inducing heart failure. Because platelet aggregation, blood flow turbulence, and blood viscosity also play certain roles—especially with unstable angina—platelet inhibitors are also prescribed to prevent anginal attacks (see Chapter 26). Because atherosclerosis causes narrowing and closure of the coronary arteries, inducing angina and myocardial infarction, the use of the 3-hydroxy-3-methylglutaryl coenzyme A (HMG-CoA) reductase inhibitors (i.e., the statins) has also become standard therapy in preventing and treating angina pectoris (see Chapter 21).

USES

Seven groups of drugs may be used to treat angina pectoris: nitrates, beta-adrenergic blockers, angiotensin-converting enzyme (ACE) inhibitors, calcium channel blockers, statins, platelet-active agents, and myocardial cell sodium channel blocker. Combination therapy is beneficial for many patients. Beta blockers, calcium channel blockers, statins, long-acting nitrates, and ranolazine can prevent anginal episodes. Risk factor management, healthy lifestyle changes, antiplatelet agents, and ACE inhibitors can prevent disease progression and myocardial infarction or death.

Drug therapy for patients with angina must be individualized. Most patients will be given prescriptions for medication (e.g., nitroglycerin in the form of sublingual tablets or translingual spray) to treat acute attacks and prescriptions for therapy to prevent further ischemia and myocardial infarction (and possible death). Therapy to prevent myocardial infarction consists of statins to lower the low-density lipoprotein cholesterol level and to reduce inflammation; platelet inhibitors to prevent platelet aggregation and thrombus formation; and ACE inhibitors to help dilate coronary blood vessels and to reduce the potential for thrombus formation.

The most effective agents for relieving ischemia and angina are beta blockers, calcium channel blockers, and nitrates. The drug ranolazine modifies metabolism in the myocardial cells to reduce the oxygen demand of the contracting heart muscles, thereby reducing symptoms of angina.

Deciding which medicine to use depends on other conditions that the patient may have and the expected adverse effects of therapy. Aspirin or clopidogrel (see Chapter 26), which are platelet-active agents, may also be considered to slow platelet aggregation. Many patients will have revascularization procedures (e.g., stent placement, coronary artery bypass grafting) to restore blood flow and to reduce symptomatology. Even after revascularization, patients will still require antianginal drug therapy.

❖ NURSING IMPLICATIONS FOR ANGINAL THERAPY

◆ Assessment

History of anginal attacks. Ask the patient specific questions to identify the onset, duration, and intensity of the pain. Ask the patient to describe the chest sensation and the pattern of occurrence (e.g., under the sternum; in the jaw, neck, and shoulder; radiation down the left arm, the right arm, or both; into the wrist, hand, and fingers). What activities precipitate an attack? Does the pain occur with or without exertion? Is the pain relieved by rest? Does the chest pain occur shortly after eating? Does the individual experience fatigue, shortness of breath, indigestion, or nausea in relation to the anginal attack? Work with the patient to plan interventions that will minimize the factors that trigger attacks. Mutually establish goals with the patient to alter risk factors that are modifiable.

Medication history
- What medications—both prescription and nonprescription—are being taken?
- Does the patient take any herbal or dietary supplements?

- What medications are being used for the treatment of the angina?
- What effect does taking nitroglycerin have on the anginal pain? How many nitroglycerin tablets are required for the patient to obtain pain relief during an attack? How many nitroglycerin tablets are being taken daily? How old is the nitroglycerin that is being used sublingually? Is it stored properly?
- Have the prescribed medications been taken regularly? If not, determine the reasons for the patient's nonadherence. Analyze nonadherence issues, and plan interventions with the patient. Plan to review drug administration, as needed.

Central nervous system

- *Mental status:* Determine the individual's level of consciousness and clarity of thought. Check for orientation to date, time, and place, as well as level of confusion, restlessness, or irritability. Ask the patient whether he or she has noticed any changes in memory or level of awareness; these factors are indicators of cerebral perfusion.
- *Syncope:* Ask the patient to describe the conditions surrounding any episodes of syncope. Record the degree of presenting symptoms, such as general mental weakness, inability to stand upright, feeling faint, or loss of consciousness. Record what activities, if any, bring on these episodes.
- *Anxiety:* What degree of apprehension is present? Did a stressful event precipitate the attack? Plan for stress reduction education and a discussion of effective means of coping with stressful events.

Cardiovascular system

- *Palpitations:* Record the patient's description of palpitations, such as "my heart skips some beats" or "it began to feel as if it were racing." Ask if these conditions are preceded by mild or strenuous exercise and how long the palpitations last.
- *Heart rate:* Count and record the rate, rhythm, and quality of the pulse.
- *Blood pressure:* Record the blood pressure. It may be increased or decreased during an attack. Compare with previous baseline readings.
- *Respirations:* The patient may be dyspneic. Ask whether the attack occurred while the patient was at rest or during exertion.
- *Cardiovascular history:* What concurrent cardiovascular disease does the patient have (e.g., hypertension, dyslipidemia)?
- *Peripheral perfusion:* Determine the patient's peripheral perfusion by checking the pedal pulses in the lower extremities and the skin color and temperature. Note any loss of hair on the lower legs, which denotes decreased circulation.
- *Smoking:* Does the patient smoke? How much? Does the patient understand the effects of smoking on the cardiovascular system?

- Ask what, if any, activities of daily living have been altered to cope with the patient's symptoms.

Nutritional history

- *Diet:* Is the patient on a special diet (e.g., low-sodium diet, low-fat diet)? Is the patient being treated for high cholesterol? Does eating cause fatigue or shortness of breath?
- *Fluids:* Does the patient have any edema, especially in the ankles? Examine the dietary history to establish whether a referral to a nutritionist would benefit the individual's understanding of the diet regimen.

◆ Implementation

Obtain the patient's vital signs, and include an assessment of the individual's pain rating.

- Adequate tissue perfusion is essential. Instruct the patient to take measures to avoid fatigue and cold weather, which can cause vasoconstriction, and provide for the patient's personal safety when symptoms of hypoxia are present (e.g., lightheadedness, dyspnea, chest pain).
- When pain is present, comfort measures and prescribed pain medications must be implemented to allow the individual to decrease the pain. Fatigue may increase the perception of pain; spacing activities so that fatigue does not occur is recommended. Administer oxygen as prescribed and check the patient's oxygen saturation.
- For information about medication administration, see the individual drug monographs.

◆ Patient Education

Medications

- Teach the patient about the signs and symptoms of hypotension, which may occur when nitrates are taken. Weakness, dizziness, or faintness can usually be relieved by increasing muscular activity (i.e., alternating flexing and relaxing the muscles in the legs) or by sitting or lying down. Resting for 10 to 15 minutes after taking medication may also assist the patient with the management of hypotension. Because lightheadedness or fainting is a possibility when taking nitroglycerin, safety measures to prevent injury from transient orthostatic hypotension must be stressed.
- Explain that a headache may occur with the use of nitroglycerin but that it should subside within 20 to 30 minutes.
- Teach specific administration techniques to the patient for the type of medication prescribed (e.g., sublingual or transmucosal tablets, translingual spray, topical ointment, transdermal patches). Refer to Chapter 7, Figs. 7.2, 7.3, and 7.4, for further description of percutaneous administration of nitroglycerin.

Lifestyle modifications. Lifestyle modifications are essential for many individuals with angina. Teach the patient about appropriate behavioral changes, such as stress management (e.g., relaxation techniques, meditation, three-part breathing).

- The patient must resume activities of daily living within the boundaries set by the healthcare provider. Encourage activities such as regular moderate exercise, meal preparation, the resumption of usual sexual activity, and social interactions.
- Individuals who are unable to attain the degree of activity hoped for through drug therapy may become frustrated. Allow for the verbalization of feelings and then implement actions that are appropriate to the circumstances.
- Participation in regular exercise is essential. Follow the guidelines of the American Heart Association regarding an exercise program. Increase the patient's exercise demands gradually and monitor the effects on his or her cardiovascular system. Changes in the level of exercise may require participation in a supervised program (e.g., cardiac rehabilitation). Tell the patient to avoid overexertion. Anginal pain may occur with exercise, and taking nitroglycerin before exercise or before performing certain activities may be recommended. Instruct the patient to always stop exercising or performing any activity when chest pain is present.
- Discuss the need for smoking cessation and make referrals to available self-help programs in the area. Smoking causes vasoconstriction; encourage a drastic reduction in smoking and preferably complete elimination of smoking. Encourage the patient to set a date to stop smoking.
- Dietary modifications aimed at decreasing the cholesterol level and a reducing program to maintain the ideal weight are usually prescribed by the physician. Depending on coexisting conditions, other dietary modifications (e.g., a low-sodium diet) may be suggested. Discourage the use of caffeine-containing products, because they may precipitate an anginal attack when they are taken in excess.
- If hypertension accompanies the angina, stress the importance of following prescribed dietary and medicinal regimens to control the disease.
- Instruct the patient not to ingest alcohol while receiving nitroglycerin therapy. Alcohol causes vasodilation, which potentially results in postural hypotension.
- Teach the patient about the proper storage of medication (especially sublingual nitroglycerin) in a dark, airtight container. Show the patient the medication's expiration date and stress the importance of having the prescription refilled before the expiration date.
- Always report poor pain control to the healthcare provider.

Fostering health maintenance

- Throughout the course of treatment, discuss medication information and how it will benefit the patient.

- Drug therapy is essential to maintain the adequate oxygenation of the myocardial cells and body tissues. Although medications can control the anginal attacks, lifestyle changes to deal with the management of precipitating factors must also occur.
- Provide the patient and his or her significant others with the important information contained in the specific drug monographs for the drugs prescribed. Additional health teaching and nursing interventions for common and serious adverse effects are described in the drug monographs later in this chapter.
- Seek cooperation and understanding with regard to the following points so that medication adherence is increased: the name of the medication; its dosage, route, and times of administration; and its common and serious adverse effects.

Patient self-assessment. Enlist the patient's help with developing and maintaining a written record of monitoring parameters (e.g., blood pressure, pulse, degree of pain relief, exercise tolerance, adverse effects experienced). See the Patient Self-Assessment Form for Cardiovascular Agents on the Evolve website. Complete the Premedication Data column for use as a baseline to track the patient's response to drug therapy. Ensure that the patient understands how to use the form, and instruct the patient to bring the completed form to follow-up visits. During follow-up visits, focus on issues that will foster the patient's adherence with the therapeutic interventions prescribed.

DRUG CLASS: NITRATES

Actions

The nitrates are the oldest effective therapy for angina pectoris. Although they have also been called *coronary vasodilators*, these agents do not increase total coronary blood flow. First, nitrates relieve angina pectoris by inducing the relaxation of the peripheral vascular smooth muscles, which results in the dilation of the arteries and veins. This reduces venous blood return (i.e., reduced preload) to the heart, which in turn leads to decreased oxygen demands on the heart. Second, nitrates increase the myocardial oxygen supply by dilating the large coronary arteries and redistributing blood flow, thereby enhancing oxygen supply to ischemic areas.

Uses

Nitroglycerin is the drug of choice for the treatment of angina pectoris. It is available in different dosages so that it can be adjusted to patient needs. Sublingual tablets dissolve quite rapidly and are used primarily for acute attacks of angina. The sustained-release tablets and capsules, ointments, and transdermal patches are used prophylactically to prevent anginal attacks. All long-acting nitrates, including isosorbide dinitrate and mononitrate, appear to be equally effective when a sufficient nitrate-free interval (as discussed under Topical

Ointment Administration and Transdermal Patch Administration later in this section) is incorporated into the medicine regimen. The translingual spray may be used for both the prophylaxis and acute treatment of anginal attacks.

Continued use of transdermal nitroglycerin patches and frequent doses of oral nitrates and sustained-release nitrates causes the development of tolerance and the loss of the antianginal response. The best way to avoid tolerance is to have periodic 8- to 12-hour nitrate-free periods. Depending on the type of angina, patients will be told when not to use nitrates (e.g., bedtime), unless they have an acute attack. When used with beta blockers or calcium antagonists, nitrates produce greater anti-anginal and antiischemic effects than when they are used alone. These agents also help provide prophylaxis against attacks during nitrate-free periods.

Therapeutic Outcomes

The primary therapeutic outcomes from nitrate therapy are as follows:

1. Relief of anginal pain during an attack
2. Reduced frequency and severity of anginal attacks
3. Increased tolerance of activities

❖ Nursing Implications for Nitrates

◆ Premedication assessment

1. Assess the level, location, duration, intensity, and pattern of the patient's pain.
2. Ask the patient when the last dose of nitrates was taken and what degree of relief was obtained.

◆ Availability, dosage, and administration. See Table 24.1.

Sublingual administration

1. Instruct the patient to sit or lie down at the first sign of an oncoming anginal attack.
2. Instruct the patient to place a tablet under the tongue and allow it to dissolve; encourage the patient not to swallow the saliva immediately.
3. The American Heart Association (O'Gara et al, 2013) recommends that if chest pain is not relieved with one sublingual nitroglycerin tablet within 5 minutes, the patient should seek emergency medical attention (i.e., call 911). While waiting for emergency care, the patient can take one more tablet and then take a third tablet 5 minutes later if the pain is not relieved.
4. One or two tablets may be taken prophylactically a few minutes before engaging in activities that may trigger an anginal attack.
5. Chart the patient's ability to place the sublingual medication under the tongue correctly.

Medication deterioration. Every 6 months, the nitroglycerin prescription should be refilled and the old tablets safely discarded. (Be sure that the patient knows how to read the expiration date and have the prescription refilled.)

Medication storage. Store nitroglycerin in its original dark-colored glass container with a tight lid.

Medication accessibility. Nonhospitalized patients should carry nitroglycerin at all times, but not in a pocket directly next to the body, because heat hastens the deterioration of the medication. When taken, the drug should produce a slight stinging or burning sensation in the mouth, which usually indicates that it is still potent.

Allow the hospitalized patient to keep the nitroglycerin at the bedside or on his or her person, if ambulatory. Check the hospital policy to see if a fresh supply of medicine should be issued rather than using the agents that the patient brought from home. (Remember that the nurse is still responsible for gathering and charting relevant data regarding all medication taken by the patient when the medication is left at the bedside.)

Sustained-release tablet administration. Sustained-release nitroglycerin is usually taken on an empty stomach every 8 to 12 hours. If gastritis develops, the sustained-release tablet may be taken with food.

Translingual spray administration. Patients should familiarize themselves with the position of the spray orifice, which can be identified by the finger rest on top of the valve. This can be particularly helpful for administration at night. The spray is highly flammable; instruct the patient not to use the spray where it may be ignited.

1. At the time of administration, the patient should preferably be in a sitting position.
2. The canister should be held vertically, with the valve head uppermost and the spray orifice as close to the mouth as possible. Do not shake the container, because any bubbles formed may slow the release of nitroglycerin.
3. The dose should be sprayed onto or under the tongue by pressing the button firmly.
4. The patient's mouth should be closed immediately after each dose. The spray should not be swallowed or inhaled.

> **⚠ Medication Safety Alert**
>
> The American Heart Association (O'Gara et al, 2013) now recommends that if chest pain is not relieved by one sublingual nitroglycerin dose within 5 minutes, the patient should seek emergency medical attention (i.e., call 911).

Topical ointment administration. See Chapter 7, Fig. 7.3. Nitroglycerin ointment is usually applied on arising in the morning; 6 hours later the first dose is removed and a second dose is applied. The second dose of the ointment is removed after 6 hours, giving a nitrate-free period of 10 to 12 hours until the next morning.

1. Apply clean gloves before administering the ointment to prevent absorbing the drug through your skin.
2. Position the dose-measuring applicator paper with the printed side down.
3. Squeeze the proper amount (usually 1 to 2 inches) of ointment onto the applicator paper.

Table **24.1** **Nitrates**

GENERIC NAME	BRAND NAME	AVAILABILITY	ONSET	DURATION	DOSAGE RANGE
isosorbide dinitrate ⇄ *Do not confuse isosorbide dinitrate with isosorbide mononitrate.*	Isordil	Tablets, oral: 5, 10, 20, 30, 40 mg	30-60 min	4-6 hr	PO: 5-40 mg two to three times daily on empty stomach
		Tablets and capsules, sustained release: 40 mg	30-60 min	6-8 hr	PO: 40-160 mg/day (a nitrate free interval of >18 hr is recommended; however, an interval has not been clearly established) Maximum: 160 mg/day
isosorbide mononitrate ⇄ *Do not confuse isosorbide mononitrate with isosorbide dinitrate.*	—.	Tablets, oral: 10, 20 mg	30-60 min	N/A	PO: 20 mg twice daily, 7 hr apart
	—	Tablets, sustained release (24 hr): 30, 60, 120 mg	3-4 hr	8-12 hr	PO: 30-240 mg once daily; do not crush or chew tablets
nitroglycerin ⇄ *Do not confuse nitroglycerin with glycerin.*	Nitrostat	Tablets, sublingual: 0.3, 0.4, 0.6 mg	1-2 min	>30 min	Sublingual: 0.3-0.6 mg for prophylactic use before activity that may induce angina pectoris or at time of acute attack
		Capsules, oral, sustained release: 2.5, 6.5, 9 mg	30-45 min	3-8 hr	PO: 2.5-6.5 mg two to four times daily for prophylaxis
	Nitro-Bid	Ointment: 2%	30 min	3 hr	Topical: 0.5-2 inches of ointment using special applicator every 6 hr for two doses, then no dose for 12 hr, followed by two doses for 6 hr each
	Nitro-Dur	Patch, transmucosal: 0.1, 0.2, 0.3, 0.4, 0.6, 0.8 mg/hr	30-60 min	Less than 24 hr	Topical: Initial 0.2 to 0.4 mg/hr for 12 hr daily; Titrate dose to response; patient should wait 12 hr after removing old patch before applying new patch
	Nitrolingual Pumpspray	Spray, translingual metered: 0.4 mg	2 min	30-60 min	Spray: One or two sprays onto or under tongue for acute attack; repeat if needed in 3-5 min; may be used prophylactically 5-10 min before exercise
	Nitroglycerin IV ❶	IV: 5 mg/mL in 10-mL vials; 100, 200, 400 mcg in 250 and 500 mL	1-2 min	3-5 min	IV: Initial: 5 mcg/min through an infusion pump; adjust dosage as needed

❶ High-alert medication.

4. Place the measuring applicator paper on the skin, ointment-side down, and spread the ointment in a thin, uniform layer under the paper. Do not spread beyond the paper margins. Do not massage the ointment or rub it in. Any area without hair may be used; however, many people prefer the chest, the flank, or the upper arm. The lower extremities are not used, especially if there is reduced peripheral perfusion. (Because of the potential for skin irritation, do not shave an area to apply the medication; instead use scissors to clip hair if needed.)

5. Help the patient to develop a site rotation schedule to prevent skin irritation. Tell the patient not to apply the ointment to an area that still shows signs of irritation. Use of the applicator allows measuring of the proper dose and prevents absorption through the fingertips.

6. Cover the area where the patch is placed with a clear plastic wrap and then tape the plastic wrap in place. (Alert the patient that the medication may discolor clothing.)

7. Perform hand hygiene before applying and after removing gloves.

8. Close the tube tightly and store it in a cool place.
9. When terminating the use of the topical ointment, gradually reduce the dose and frequency of application over the course of 4 to 6 weeks.
10. When removing the ointment paper, apply clean gloves, wipe the area with tissue to remove the ointment, and then reapply the ointment to a different area at the appropriate time interval for rotating sites.

Transdermal patch administration. See Chapter 7, Fig. 7.4. The transdermal patch provides a controlled release of nitroglycerin through a semipermeable membrane for 24 hours when it is applied to intact skin. The dosage released depends on the surface area of the patch. The therapeutic effect can be observed about 30 minutes after attachment, and it continues for about 30 minutes after removal. Current recommendations are to apply the patch and leave it in place for 12 to 14 hours, followed by a 10- to 12-hour patch-free (nitrate-free) interval. The patch is then reapplied for another 12 to 14 hours.

1. Apply clean gloves.
2. The patch should be applied to a clean, dry, hairless area of skin. Do not apply the patch to shaved areas, because skin irritation may alter drug absorption. If hair is likely to interfere with patch adhesion or removal, then trim the hair but do not shave it. Optimal locations for patch placement are the upper chest or side; the pelvis; and the inner, upper arm. Avoid scars, skinfolds, and wounds. Rotate the skin sites daily. (Help the patient develop a rotation chart.)
3. Perform hand hygiene before applying and after removing gloves.
4. See individual product information to determine whether the patient's patch can be worn while swimming, bathing, or showering.
5. If the patch becomes partially dislodged, discard it and replace it with a new patch.
6. Sublingual nitroglycerin may be necessary for anginal attacks, especially while the dosage is being adjusted.
7. Dispose of used patches in a place that is out of reach of children. Discarded patches still contain enough of the active ingredient to be dangerous to children.

Intravenous nitroglycerin administration. Intravenous nitroglycerin is used in an acute inpatient setting (e.g., intensive care unit, cardiac telemetry unit), and it requires continuous monitoring of vital signs (i.e., blood pressure, pulse, respirations, oxygen saturation levels, and central venous pressure).

An infusion pump must be used to monitor the precise delivery of the infusion. The dose is titrated to achieve the desired clinical response. Gradual weaning is needed under controlled conditions to prevent a rebound action.

This medication is never mixed with other medications and is administered only with intravenous administration sets known as "nitro tubing," which are made specifically for use with nitroglycerin. Most other plastic administration sets absorb the drug. See the manufacturer's literature for exact directions for preparation and administration of the drug.

◆ *Common adverse effects*

Cardiovascular

Excessive hypotension. Excessive hypotension is an extension of the nitrate's pharmacologic activity. Other possible adverse effects include dizziness, nausea, flushing, and (rarely) syncope. Report these adverse effects so that a more appropriate dosage adjustment may be made.

Neurologic

Prolonged headache. The most common adverse effect of nitrate therapy is headache. This can range from a mild sensation of fullness in the head to an intense and severe generalized headache. Most patients develop a tolerance within a few weeks of starting therapy. Analgesics (e.g., acetaminophen) may be used, if needed. Report these adverse effects so that a more appropriate dosage adjustment may be made.

Tolerance (increasing dosage to attain relief). Tolerance to the nitrate dosages can develop rapidly, particularly if large doses are administered frequently. Tolerance can appear within a few days, and it may be well established within a few weeks. The smallest dose needed to obtain satisfactory results should be used to minimize the development of tolerance. Tolerance is broken by withdrawing the drug for a short period of time.

◆ *Drug interactions*

Alcohol. Alcohol accentuates the vasodilation and postural hypotension caused by the nitrates. Patients should be warned that drinking alcohol while taking nitrates may cause hypotension.

Calcium channel blockers and beta-adrenergic blockers. Calcium channel blockers and beta-adrenergic blockers may significantly lower blood pressure. Dosage adjustments may be necessary.

Avanafil, sildenafil, tadalafil, and vardenafil. The concurrent use of nitrates and these agents used for erectile dysfunction is contraindicated. These agents potentiate the vasodilatory effects of the nitrates, which results in a significant drop in blood pressure that may be fatal.

DRUG CLASS: BETA-ADRENERGIC BLOCKERS

Actions

The beta-adrenergic blockers (i.e., beta blockers) (see Table 12.3) reduce myocardial oxygen demand by blocking the beta-adrenergic receptors in the heart, thereby preventing stimulation from norepinephrine and epinephrine that would normally cause an increased heart rate. Beta blockers also reduce blood pressure (see Chapter 22).

Uses

The goals of beta blocker therapy are to reduce the number of anginal attacks, reduce nitroglycerin use, and improve exercise tolerance while minimizing adverse effects. It is recommended that a patient who is admitted to the hospital with an acute myocardial infarction receive a beta blocker on arrival and be prescribed a beta blocker on discharge.

All beta blockers are effective for the treatment of angina pectoris, so product selection should be based on other conditions that the patient may have (e.g., diabetes, chronic obstructive airway disease, peripheral vascular disease) and adherence issues. The cardioselective agents (see Chapter 12) will have less effect on the beta-2 receptors of the lungs and the peripheral vasculature, thereby minimizing the adverse effects involving these body systems. Atenolol, betaxolol, and metoprolol are examples of beta blockers that can be administered once daily to minimize anginal attacks if adherence is a problem.

Dosages of beta blockers needed to control angina are extremely patient specific; therefore therapy should start at low doses and be increased, depending on the patient's needs. Optimally, exercise stress tests should be used to determine the most appropriate dosage. Combination therapy with nitrates and beta blockers appears to be more effective than nitrates or beta blockers alone. Beta blockers may also be combined with calcium channel blockers (e.g., verapamil, diltiazem, or the long-acting dihydropyridines; see the discussion of these drugs in the next section of this chapter).

Therapeutic Outcomes

The primary therapeutic outcomes expected from beta blocker therapy are as follows:

1. Decreased frequency and severity of anginal attacks
2. Increased tolerance of activities
3. Reduced use of nitroglycerin for acute anginal attacks

❖ **Nursing Implications for Beta-Adrenergic Blockers**

◆ *Premedication assessment*

1. Obtain baseline blood pressure readings with the patient in both the supine and standing positions; assess the pulse rate.
2. Check the patient's history for respiratory disorders such as bronchospasm, chronic bronchitis, emphysema, and asthma.
3. Check the patient for a history of diabetes. If diabetes is present, determine the patient's baseline serum glucose level before starting therapy.

See Chapter 12 for further discussion of patient education and the nursing process associated with beta-adrenergic blockers.

DRUG CLASS: CALCIUM CHANNEL BLOCKERS

Actions

These agents are known variously as *calcium antagonists, calcium ion antagonists, slow channel blockers,* and *calcium ion influx inhibitors.* Regardless of what they are called, they all share the ability to inhibit the movement of calcium ions across a cell membrane.

Calcium channel blockers (Table 24.2) may be used to treat angina pectoris by decreasing myocardial oxygen demand (i.e., decreasing workload) and increasing myocardial blood supply by dilating the coronary arteries. By inhibiting smooth muscle contraction, calcium channel blockers dilate blood vessels and decrease their resistance to blood flow. The dilation of the peripheral vessels reduces the workload of the heart. Coronary artery dilation improves coronary blood flow.

Uses

Although each of these agents acts by calcium ion inhibition, there are significant differences in clinical use. Their clinical effects also depend on the type and severity of the patient's disease. The primary calcium channel blockers used to treat angina are the long-acting dihydropyridines (e.g., amlodipine, nicardipine, nifedipine), as well as diltiazem (benzothiazepine) and verapamil (diphenylalkylamine). The overall effect of calcium channel blockers will be the combined effects of vasodilator and myocardial actions with reflex-mediated adrenergic activity. Nifedipine, a potent peripheral arterial vasodilator, reduces peripheral vascular resistance; this may cause a reflex tachycardia. Verapamil and diltiazem also have myocardial depressant effects that prevent tachycardia. However, they must be used with extreme caution in patients who may be developing heart failure.

Therapeutic Outcomes

The primary therapeutic outcomes expected from the calcium channel blockers are as follows:

1. Decreased frequency and severity of anginal attacks
2. Increased tolerance of activities

❖ **Nursing Implications for Calcium Channel Blockers**

◆ *Premedication assessment*

1. Obtain baseline blood pressure readings with the patient in both the supine and standing positions.
2. Check the patient for a history of heart failure; withhold the drug and consult the healthcare provider if heart failure is present.
3. Check the patient's laboratory values for hepatotoxicity.

◆ *Availability, dosage, and administration.* See Table 24.2. See Chapter 22 for a further discussion of patient education and the nursing process associated with calcium channel blocker therapy.

DRUG CLASS: ANGIOTENSIN-CONVERTING ENZYME INHIBITORS

Actions

Angiotensin-converting enzyme inhibitors represent a major breakthrough in the treatment of cardiovascular disease. Their action is more completely described on pp. 351-354. By inhibiting ACE, these drugs have significant

Table 24.2   Calcium Channel Blockers Used to Treat Angina Pectoris

GENERIC NAME	BRAND NAME	AVAILABILITY	DOSAGE RANGE
amlodipine ⇌ Do not confuse amlodipine with amiloride or amiodarone.	Norvasc ⇌ Do not confuse Norvasc with Altace or Vasotec.	Tablets: 2.5, 5, 10 mg Oral suspension: 1 mg/mL in 120-mL bottle	PO: Initial: 5 mg once daily; adjust over 7-14 days to maximum of 10 mg/day
diltiazem	Cardizem ⇌ Do not confuse Cardizem with clonidine.	Tablets: 30, 60, 90, 120 mg	PO: Initial: 30 mg four times daily, gradually increase to 180-320 mg in three or four divided doses
	Cardizem LA, Cardizem CD	Tablets, sustained release (24 hr), and capsules (24 hr): 120, 180, 240, 300, 360, 420 mg	PO: Initial: 120-180 mg sustained-release capsule once daily; adjust as needed after 14 days. Maximum dose: 480 mg daily
nicardipine	—	Capsules: 20, 30 mg	PO: Initial: 20 mg three times daily. Maximal response may require 2 wk of therapy. Allow at least 3 days between dosage adjustments. Maintenance: 20-40 mg three times daily
nifedipine	Procardia ⇌ Do not confuse Procardia with Provera or Peri-Colace.	Capsules: 10, 20 mg	PO: Initial: 10 mg three times daily; adjust over 7-14 days to balance antianginal and hypotensive activity. Maximum dose: 180 mg/day
	Adalat CC Procardia XL	Tablets, extended release (24 hr): 30, 60, 90 mg	Extended-release tablets: 30-60 mg once daily. Maximum; extended-release tablets: 120 mg daily
verapamil	Calan ⇌ Do not confuse Calan with Colace.	Tablets: 40, 80, 120 mg	PO: Initial, immediate release: 40-120 mg three times daily
	Calan SR	Tablets and capsules, sustained release (24 hr): 100, 120, 180, 200, 240, 300, 360 mg	PO: Initial: 180 mg once daily at bedtime. Maintenance: 120-480 mg daily. Administer with food

actions on the endothelial walls of coronary arteries; they promote vasodilation and minimize platelet cell aggregation, thereby preventing thrombus formation.

Uses

Angiotensin-converting enzyme inhibitors have been proven to reduce the incidence of myocardial infarction, and they should be used as routine secondary prevention for patients with known CAD, particularly for patients with diabetes mellitus without renal failure. Angiotensin-converting enzyme inhibitors are recommended for the treatment of patients with an acute myocardial infarction or heart failure with left ventricular systolic dysfunction.

Therapeutic Outcome

The primary therapeutic outcome expected from the ACE inhibitors is a reduction in the frequency of recurrent myocardial infarction.

❖ **Nursing Implications for Angiotensin-Converting Enzyme Inhibitors**

◆ *Premedication assessment*

1. Obtain baseline blood pressure readings with the patient in both the supine and standing positions; assess the apical pulse.
2. Obtain a history of the patient's bowel elimination patterns.
3. Initiate laboratory studies as requested by the healthcare provider (e.g., electrocardiography; renal function tests such as blood urea nitrogen, serum creatinine, and electrolyte levels; and complete blood count) to serve as a baseline for future comparison.
4. Ask if the patient has a persistent cough.

◆ *Availability, dosage, and administration.* See Table 22.5 and Chapter 22 for further discussion of patient education and the nursing process associated with ACE inhibitor therapy.

 Medication Safety Alert

The initial doses of ACE inhibitors may cause hypotension with dizziness, tachycardia, and fainting; these adverse effects occur more commonly in patients who are also receiving diuretics. Symptoms occur within 3 hours after the first several doses. This effect may be minimized by discontinuing the diuretic 1 week before initiating ACE inhibitor therapy. Patients should be warned that this adverse effect may occur, that it is transient, and that they should lie down immediately if symptoms develop.

DRUG CLASS: MYOCARDIAL CELL SODIUM CHANNEL BLOCKER

ranolazine (răn-Ō-lă-zēn)
Ranexa (răn-ĔKS-ă)

Actions

Ranolazine is a myocardial cell sodium channel blocker. It is thought that ranolazine produces myocardial relaxation reducing anginal symptoms through this mechanism although this is uncertain. As the demand for oxygen is reduced, the imbalance between the oxygen supply and demand diminishes, thereby reducing myocardial ischemia and angina symptoms.

Uses

Ranolazine is the first new agent in more than 20 years to be used to treat chronic stable angina. It is used in combination with a dihydropyridine calcium channel blocker (e.g., amlodipine), beta blockers, and nitrates. Unlike other antianginal medicines, ranolazine does not affect the blood pressure or heart rate. Because ranolazine prolongs the Q–T interval (i.e., a potentially life-threatening event), it should only be used to treat angina in patients who have not achieved an antianginal response with other agents or in those who cannot tolerate the adverse effects of the other medicines. Ranolazine will not reduce the symptoms of an acute anginal episode.

Therapeutic Outcomes

The primary therapeutic outcomes expected from ranolazine therapy are as follows:
1. Reduced frequency and severity of anginal attacks
2. Increased tolerance of activities
3. Reduced use of nitroglycerin during acute anginal attacks

❖ Nursing Implications for Ranolazine

◆ *Premedication assessment.* Initiate laboratory studies as requested by the healthcare provider (e.g., electrocardiography; renal function tests such as blood urea nitrogen, serum creatinine, and electrolyte levels; and complete blood count) to serve as a baseline for future comparison.

◆ *Availability*
PO: 500- and 1000-mg tablets, extended release (12 hr).

 Medication Safety Alert

It is recommended that ranolazine *not* be taken concurrently with other medicines that are known to prolong the Q–T interval, such as quinidine, dofetilide, sotalol, erythromycin, and antipsychotics (e.g., thioridazine, ziprasidone). Baseline and follow-up electrocardiograms should be obtained to evaluate the effects of these drugs on the patient's Q–T interval.

◆ *Dosage and administration. PO:* 500 mg twice daily; dosage may be increased to 1000 mg twice daily. Ranolazine may be taken with or without food. Tablets should be swallowed whole: *do not* crush, break, or chew tablets.

◆ *Common adverse effects*
  Neurologic
  Dizziness and headache. These adverse effects are usually mild, occurring in fewer than 5% of patients. Patients should not operate an automobile or machinery or engage in activities that require mental alertness until it is known how they will react to the medicine. Patients should withhold medicine and contact their healthcare provider if they experience palpitations or fainting spells while taking ranolazine.
  Gastrointestinal
  Constipation, nausea. These adverse effects are usually mild, occurring in fewer than 6% of patients.

◆ *Drug interactions*
  Drugs that enhance therapeutic and toxic effects. Azole-type antifungals (e.g., ketoconazole, fluconazole), macrolide antibiotics (e.g., erythromycin, clarithromycin), grapefruit juice, verapamil, diltiazem, and protease inhibitors (e.g., ritonavir) significantly increase the serum levels and potential toxicity of ranolazine. In general, these agents should not be used concurrently with ranolazine. If they are used concurrently, monitor patients closely for the development of dizziness, nausea, weakness, loss of muscle strength, constipation, and headache.
  Statins, tacrolimus, sirolimus. Ranolazine inhibits the metabolism of HMG-CoA inhibitors (statins), tacrolimus, and sirolimus. Reduce the dosage of these agents per manufacturers' recommendations.

Get Ready for the NCLEX® Examination!

Key Points

- Coronary artery disease is the leading cause of disability, socioeconomic loss, and death in the United States.
- Angina pectoris is the first clinical indication of underlying CAD in many patients.
- The frequency of anginal attacks can be reduced by controlling risk factors and avoiding precipitating causes (e.g., stress).
- Medicines such as nitrates, beta blockers, ACE inhibitors, statins, platelet inhibitors, and calcium channel blockers can help to control symptoms.
- Nurses can play a significant role in public education efforts, monitoring for noncompliance, monitoring patients' responses to therapy, and encouraging patients to make changes in their lifestyles to reduce the severity of angina pectoris.

Additional Learning Resources

SG Go to your Study Guide for additional Review Questions for the NCLEX® Examination, Critical Thinking Clinical Situations, and other learning activities to help you master this chapter content.

Go to your Evolve website (https://evolve.elsevier.com/Clayton) for additional online resources.

Review Questions for the NCLEX® Examination

1. The nurse is teaching a 73-year-old female patient about precipitating factors of angina and recognizes that further teaching is needed when the patient makes which statement?
   1. "I now know that it is okay for me to be intimate with my husband."
   2. "I understand that I need to rest for 1 to 2 hours after every meal."
   3. "I should avoid being outside when it gets really cold."
   4. "I will cut back on my coffee intake, but I can still have regular Coke."

2. A nurse was caring for a 65-year-old male patient who was diagnosed with chronic stable angina and knows which is the difference between chronic stable angina and unstable angina?
   1. Unstable angina is easily treated with rest.
   2. Unstable angina is treated with nitrates.
   3. Chronic stable angina lasts for more than 30 minutes.
   4. Chronic stable angina occurs at unpredictable times.

3. The nurse is preparing to administer a calcium channel blocker to a patient with angina and will need to assess for which of the following? (Select all that apply.)
   1. Frequent cough
   2. Laboratory values for nephrotoxicity
   3. Baseline supine and standing blood pressure
   4. Laboratory values for hepatotoxicity
   5. History of heart failure

4. After the administration of a nitrate to a patient with angina, the nurse explained to the patient that which of the following effects may be experienced? (Select all that apply.)
   1. Chronic cough
   2. Earache
   3. Hypotension
   4. Prolonged palpitations
   5. Headache

5. For the patient experiencing angina and ischemia, the most effective agents for relieving these conditions include which classification of drugs? (Select all that apply.)
   1. Nitrates
   2. Beta blockers
   3. Calcium channel blockers
   4. Platelet active agents
   5. HMG-CoA reductase inhibitors

6. The nurse was discussing risk factor management with a 58-year-old male patient who was admitted with chest pain and realized that the patient needed further education after he made which statement?
   1. "I know that I should quit smoking. I have been meaning to for a while, but this really hits home that I need to."
   2. "I think maybe I should learn to cook because my wife always insists on meat and potatoes and gravy; we have such heavy meals."
   3. "I walk every day with my dog for at least 20 minutes and longer in nice weather."
   4. "I figure I don't need to do anything different; I can just take my pills for this."

7. The nurse administering the calcium channel blocker amlodipine (Norvasc) explained to the patient what effect the drug has on the heart. Which statement is appropriate for the nurse to make?
   1. "This drug will prevent angina by dilating the coronary vessels."
   2. "This drug will prevent angina by blocking the receptors in the heart that increase the heart rate."
   3. "This drug will prevent angina by blocking the movement of calcium ions, which in turn decreases oxygen demand on the heart."
   4. "This drug will prevent angina by blocking the conversion of angiotensin I to angiotensin II, which is a potent vasoconstrictor."

Drugs Used to Treat Peripheral Vascular Disease

25

Objectives

1. Describe the baseline assessments needed to evaluate a patient with peripheral vascular disease.
2. Identify specific measures that the patient can use to improve peripheral circulation and prevent the complications of peripheral vascular disease.
3. Identify the systemic effects to expect when peripheral vasodilating agents are administered.
4. Explain why hypotension and tachycardia occur frequently with the use of pentoxifylline and cilostazol.
5. Cite both pharmacologic and nonpharmacologic goals of the treatment for peripheral vascular disease.

Key Terms

peripheral arterial disease (p. 393)
arteriosclerosis obliterans (ăr-tē-rē-ō-sklĕ-RŌ-sĭs ŏ-BLĬ-tĕr-ănz) (p. 393)
intermittent claudication (ĭn-tĕr-MĬT-ĕnt klaw-dĭ-KĀ-shŭn) (p. 393)

paresthesias (păr-ĕs-THĒ-zē-ăz) (p. 393)
Raynaud's disease (rā-NŌZ) (p. 393)
vasospasm (VĂ-zō-spă-zĭm) (p. 394)

PERIPHERAL VASCULAR DISEASE

The term *peripheral vascular disease* can be applied to a variety of illnesses associated with blood vessels outside the heart, but it generally refers to diseases of the blood vessels of the arms and legs (the extremities). These illnesses can be subdivided into two types based on arterial or venous origin: (1) peripheral arterial disease and (2) venous disorders, such as acute deep vein thrombosis (see Chapter 26). The arterial disorders are subdivided into those that result from arterial narrowing and occlusion (obstructive) and those caused by arterial spasm (vasospastic).

The most common form of obstructive arterial disease is arteriosclerosis obliterans, also called *atherosclerosis obliterans*. It results from atherosclerotic plaque formation, with narrowing of the lower aorta and the major arteries that provide circulation to the legs. As with atherosclerosis of the coronary arteries, the risk factors that play an important role in the development of this disease are high levels of low-density lipoprotein (LDL) cholesterol, hypertension, cigarette smoking, low levels of high-density lipoprotein cholesterol, and diabetes mellitus.

Patients tend to remain free of symptoms until there is significant narrowing (75% to 90%) in key locations of the major arteries and arterioles of the legs. The typical pain pattern described is one of aching, cramping, tightness, or weakness that occurs during exercise.

The primary pathophysiology is obstruction of blood flow through the arteries, resulting in ischemia to the tissues supplied by those arteries. A term commonly applied to this condition is *intermittent claudication*; it manifests as pain secondary to lack of oxygen to the muscles during exercise. During the early stages of symptoms, the patient finds relief by stopping the exercise for a few minutes. Without treatment, as the disease progresses over time, the arteries become obstructed, resulting in thrombosis and the potential for gangrene. Additional symptoms that develop are pain at rest, numbness, and paresthesias (numbness with a tingling sensation). The disease is often accompanied by increased blood viscosity. Physical findings on the lower extremities are reduced arterial pulsations on palpation; systolic bruits over the involved arteries; waxy, pale, and dry skin; a lower temperature of the skin of the extremity; edema; and numbness to sensation.

Peripheral vascular disease caused by arterial vasospasm is known as Raynaud's disease, named after the man who first described the illness in 1862. It is unfortunate that, more than 150 years later, the pathophysiology and treatment of this condition are still not well defined. Raynaud's disease is classified as either primary, in which the cause is unknown, or as secondary, in which other conditions contribute to the symptoms. Secondary causes are frequent exposure to cold weather, obstructive arterial disease, occupational trauma (e.g., pneumatic hammer users, pianists), and certain drugs (e.g., beta blockers, imipramine, nicotine, bromocriptine, vinblastine, clonidine). Heredity may also play a role. The onset of Raynaud's disease is usually during the teenage years to the 40s, and it occurs four times more frequently in women.

Raynaud's disease is thought to be caused by **vasospasm** (vasoconstriction of blood vessels) and subsequent ischemia of the arteries of the skin of the hands, fingers, and sometimes toes. The physiologic mechanisms that trigger the vasospasm are unknown. Sudden coldness applied to the extremity, such as cold water, can induce an attack. The signs and symptoms associated with Raynaud's disease are numbness, tingling, a sense of skin tightness in the affected area, and blanching of the skin because of sudden vasoconstriction followed by cyanosis. As the attack subsides, vasodilation causes a redness, or rubor, to the pale skin. The skin appears normal except during spasm. During the early years of the illness, only the fingertips of both hands are involved. However, as the disease progresses, the skin on the hands is also affected by the arteriospasm.

TREATMENT OF PERIPHERAL VASCULAR DISEASE

The goals of treatment of arteriosclerosis obliterans are reversal of the progression of the atherosclerosis, improved blood flow, pain relief, and prevention of skin ulceration and gangrene. An important concept that must be stressed to most patients is that other diseases that they may have (e.g., diabetes, hypertension, angina, dyslipidemia) are all interrelated. Control of diet, high blood pressure, smoking, weight, and diabetes will significantly help all these diseases.

Implementation of the American Heart Association's diet—an eating plan for healthy Americans—can arrest the progression of atherosclerosis. Lipid-lowering agents can be started if diet modifications do not successfully treat the hypercholesterolemia. A daily exercise program (usually walking) can significantly improve collateral blood circulation around areas of obstruction and reduce the frequency of intermittent claudication. Proper foot care (e.g., keeping feet warm and dry, wearing properly fitting shoes), especially if the patient has diabetes, is also extremely important to prevent ulcerative complications. Other nonpharmacologic treatments for improving blood flow to the extremities include avoiding cold, elevating the head of the bed by 12 to 16 inches, and arterial angioplasty and surgery.

Most vasospastic attacks of Raynaud's disease can be stopped by avoiding cold temperatures, emotional stress, tobacco, and drugs that are known to induce attacks. Keeping the hands and feet warm with gloves and socks and using foam wraparounds when handling iced beverages can reduce exposure to cold.

DRUG THERAPY FOR PERIPHERAL VASCULAR DISEASE

ACTIONS

As the causes of peripheral vascular disease have come to be better understood, clinical studies have defined which pharmacologic therapies are truly successful. It has been shown that nonpharmacologic treatment of arteriosclerosis obliterans is substantially more successful in treating the underlying pathologic condition. Pentoxifylline has had limited success; it is classified as a hemorheologic agent. It acts by enhancing red blood cell flexibility, which reduces blood viscosity, thus providing better oxygenation to muscle tissue to stop intermittent claudication. Vasodilator therapy, the mainstay of treatment until the 1980s, has little long-term benefit in most cases. A new approach to treatment became available in the form of the platelet aggregation inhibitor cilostazol. Clopidogrel and vorapaxar, newer platelet aggregation inhibitors, are also approved for the treatment of peripheral arterial disease (see Chapter 26). When drug therapy for Raynaud's disease is required, such as when the disease interferes with an individual's ability to work, agents with a vasodilating effect are used.

USES

Pentoxifylline and cilostazol are the only agents approved by the US Food and Drug Administration that are specifically indicated for the treatment of intermittent claudication caused by chronic occlusive arterial disease of the limbs. Although approved, pentoxifylline is not effective for treatment of claudication (Gerhard-Herman et al, 2016). Classes of drugs that have been somewhat successful in treating Raynaud's disease are calcium channel blockers, adrenergic antagonists, angiotensin-converting enzyme (ACE) inhibitors, and direct vasodilators.

The three calcium ion antagonists studied for the treatment of Raynaud's disease are diltiazem, verapamil, and nifedipine. Of the three, nifedipine has had the greatest success in reducing the frequency of vasospastic attack in about two-thirds of patients.

Adrenergic antagonists (e.g., prazosin, reserpine, methyldopa) have been used for many years for the treatment of Raynaud's disease. Unfortunately, treatment has been only moderately successful, and many adverse effects are associated with the use of these drugs.

The ACE inhibitors cause an increase in bradykinin, a potent vasodilator. Captopril has been the most extensively tested, and it has been shown to reduce the frequency and severity of attacks.

For more than 50 years, nitroglycerin, a direct vasodilator, has been applied as an ointment base to the hands of patients with Raynaud's disease. The treatment reduces the frequency and severity of attacks, but the adverse effects of dizziness, headache, and postural hypotension limit its use.

❖ NURSING IMPLICATIONS FOR PERIPHERAL VASCULAR DISEASE THERAPY

◆ Assessment

A baseline assessment of the patient should be completed that includes the following elements for evaluating the history and degree of oxygenation existing in the extremities. Subsequent regular assessments should be performed for comparison and analysis of therapeutic effectiveness or lack of response to any treatments initiated.

History of risk factors. Determine the patient's age, gender, and race and obtain a family history of the incidence of symptoms of peripheral vascular disease, hypertension, and cardiac disease.

Impotence. If the patient is male, has he experienced impotence?

Hypertension. Take the patient's blood pressure in sitting and supine positions daily. Ask about medications that have been prescribed. Are the medications being taken regularly? If not, why not?

Smoking. Obtain a history of the number of cigarettes or cigars that the patient smokes daily; include other sources of nicotine, such as chewing tobacco and replacement therapy. How long has the person smoked? Has the person ever tried to stop smoking? Ask if the patient understands the effect of smoking on the vascular system. How does the individual feel about modifying his or her smoking habit?

Dietary habits

- Obtain the patient's dietary history. Ask specific questions to obtain information about foods eaten that are high in fat, cholesterol, refined carbohydrates, and sodium. Using a calorie counter, ask the person to estimate the number of calories eaten per day. How much meat, fish, and poultry is eaten daily (size and number of servings)? Estimate the percentage of total daily calories provided by fats.
- Discuss food preparation (e.g., baked, broiled, fried). How many servings of fruits and vegetables are eaten daily? What types of oils and fats are used in food preparation? See a nutrition text for further dietary history questions.
- What is the frequency and volume of alcoholic beverages consumed?

Glucose intolerance. Ask specific questions about whether the individual currently has or has ever had an elevated serum glucose (blood sugar) level. If yes, what dietary modifications have been made? How successful have they been? What medications are being taken for the elevated serum glucose level (e.g., oral hypoglycemic agents, insulin)?

Elevated serum lipid levels. Find out whether the patient is aware of having elevated lipid, triglyceride, or cholesterol levels. If any of these levels are elevated, what measures has the patient tried for reduction and what effect have the interventions had on the blood levels during subsequent examinations? Review any laboratory data available (e.g., LDL, very-low-density lipoprotein, liver function tests, clotting time).

Leg ulcers. Has the individual developed any slow-to-heal or nonhealing sores? This would indicate poor circulation.

Obesity. Weigh the patient. Ask about any recent weight gains or losses and whether it was intentional or unintentional.

Psychomotor functions

Type of lifestyle. Ask the patient to describe his or her exercise level in terms of amount (e.g., walking three blocks), intensity (e.g., how long does it take to walk three blocks?), and frequency (e.g., walking every other day). Is the patient's job physically demanding or sedentary?

Psychological stress. How much stress does the individual estimate having in his or her life? How does the individual cope with stressful situations at home and at work?

Assessment of tissue

Oxygenation. Observe the color of each hand, finger, leg, and foot; report cyanosis or reddish-blue areas. Does the patient have dependent cyanosis (cyanosis when the legs are in the dependent position)? Examine the skin of the extremities for any signs of ulceration.

Temperature. Feel the temperature in each hand, finger, leg, and foot. Report any paleness or coldness. (NOTE: These symptoms of poor circulation will be increased if the limb is elevated above the level of the heart.)

Edema. Assess, record, and report edema and its extent, and determine whether it is relieved or unchanged when the limb is dependent.

Peripheral pulses. Record the pedal and/or radial pulses (Fig. 25.1) at least every 4 hours in any limb in which circulatory impairment is found. Compare findings among the extremities and report diminished or absent pulses immediately. When pulses are difficult to palpate or absent, a Doppler ultrasound device may help determine peripheral blood flow.

Limb pain. Assess pain in the patient carefully. Pain during exercise that is relieved by rest may be caused by claudication. Conversely, pain when the patient is at rest may result from sudden obstruction by a thrombus or an embolus. Check the apprehension level of the patient, pedal and radial pulses, details of onset and location of pain, and vital signs. Until the status of the patient's limb pain is established, have the patient remain on bed rest and administer an analgesic if ordered. Notify the patient's healthcare provider of any pertinent findings.

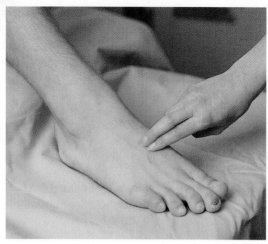

Fig. 25.1 Assessing for a peripheral pulse. (From Perry AG, Potter PA, Ostendorf W. *Nursing Interventions and Clinical Skills.* 6th ed. St. Louis: Mosby; 2016.)

◆ Implementation

- Prepare the patient for diagnostic tests (e.g., ultrasonography, pulse volume recordings, segmental limb pressure, exercise testing) and possible invasive procedures, such as arteriography.
- Do not place pillows in the popliteal space or flex the knee rest on the patient's bed. Use a cradle or footboard to prevent the bed sheets from constricting the patient's circulation.
- Always check with the healthcare provider before initiating any elevation of the patient's extremities. This action is contraindicated in patients with arterial insufficiency.
- Perform baseline assessments of tissue perfusion (e.g., skin temperature, peripheral pulses) at intervals appropriate to the patient's status (at least every 4 hours).
- Implement pain management measures.

◆ Patient Education

Promoting tissue perfusion

- Teach the patient self-care measures that promote peripheral circulation.
- Smoking causes vasoconstriction of the blood vessels. Therefore encourage a drastic reduction in—and preferably total abstinence from—smoking. Include information about smoking cessation and available support resources.
- Encourage patients to wear nothing that constricts peripheral blood flow (e.g., tight-fitting anklets, socks, garters). Tell the patient not to elevate the extremities above the level of the heart without specific orders from the healthcare provider to do so. The healthcare provider may order the patient's head of bed to be elevated at night.

- Meticulous foot and hand care is essential. Teach the patient proper self-care of the limbs, including visual inspection techniques, and explain how to take femoral, popliteal, and pedal pulses.
- Stress the need for the patient to inspect the extremities for possible skin breakdown or signs of infection. The patient should notify the healthcare provider immediately of sudden changes in color, such as mottling or a more purplish color.
- Areas of discoloration in nails, cracking of the skin, and calluses or blisters on the extremities require complete follow-up. Listen to the patient's description of any changes that have been noted. Tell the patient that going barefoot can be dangerous because of the potential for injuries to the feet.
- Cold temperatures will increase pain or decrease sensations in the extremities. Hot tubs or hot showers may cause additional vasodilation that adds to the effects of any vasodilators the patient is taking. Because of the possible decrease in sensation in the extremities, encourage the patient to test the water temperature before immersing the hands or feet. After bathing, gently pat (i.e., do not vigorously rub) the feet and hands to dry them.
- To avoid skin breakdown, the patient should alternate pairs of shoes to allow for thorough drying between wearings, change socks or hose daily, and avoid rubber-soled shoes.
- The patient should avoid standing or sitting for prolonged periods. Patients who must sit for extended periods must have a properly fitting chair. The seat should be of the correct depth so that no pressure is exerted on the popliteal space. Encourage the patient not to sit with knees or ankles crossed and to take frequent short breaks for walks. Furthermore, those who must stand for long periods should seek out tasks of the job that can be performed while sitting in a properly fitting chair or other alternatives.

Psychomotor functions

- Maximum mobility should be maintained. Devise a daily activity plan that includes walks and usual activities of daily living, such as shopping and housework.
- Pain management and the psychological aspects of dealing with a prolonged illness with persistent symptoms are major challenges for both the patient and the nurse (see Chapter 19).

Environment. During periods of exposure to cold temperature, the patient should wear several layers of lightweight clothing. Caution should be exercised during exposure to the cold to avoid frostbite. Because of decreased sensation in the extremities, frostbite can occur without the patient's awareness.

Nutritional aspects

- Dietary education is strongly indicated for the treatment of peripheral vascular disease. It is particularly important to control obesity and cholesterol and triglyceride levels.
- When ulcerations are present, encourage a high-protein diet with adequate intake of vitamins to promote the healing process.
- Unless other medical conditions contraindicate, instruct the patient to drink eight 8-ounce glasses of water daily to promote adequate hydration of body tissues. Maintaining blood volume will help reduce peripheral vasoconstriction. Check with the healthcare provider regarding recommendations for fluid or caffeine restriction.

Medication regimen

- Certain medications for the treatment of peripheral vascular disease cause dilation of blood vessels. As a result, orthostatic hypotension may occur. Teach the patient to rise slowly from sitting or lying positions, adjust balance for stability, flex the leg muscles, and then proceed with movement.
- Teach the patient to take and record his or her own blood pressure.
- Administer prescribed medications, and consult a healthcare provider before discontinuing any medications.

Fostering health maintenance

- Throughout the course of treatment, discuss medication information and explain how the medication will benefit the patient.
- Drug therapy is not a total solution for atherosclerosis. The patient may not be committed to the lifestyle changes needed to control the modifiable aspects of the disease. Often, setting short-term goals to control the pain and finding other interventions that will allow the patient to view efforts positively will help encourage permanent adoption of the needed changes.
- Patients who are unresponsive to lifestyle modifications and drug therapy may require surgical interventions to reestablish blood flow to the affected area. Procedures such as bypass grafting, endarterectomy, or angioplasty may be appropriate. Failure to reestablish blood flow to an extremity may result in amputation.
- Provide the patient and significant others with important information contained in the specific drug monographs for the drugs prescribed. Additional health teaching and nursing interventions for common and serious adverse effects are described in each drug monograph.
- Seek cooperation and understanding of the following points so that medication compliance is increased: name of medication; dosage, route, and times of administration; and common and serious adverse effects.

Patient self-assessment. Enlist the patient's help with developing and maintaining a written record of monitoring parameters (e.g., color of limb, pain in limb, temperature and pulses in limb, amount of edema present). See the Patient Self-Assessment Form for Cardiovascular Agents on the Evolve website. Complete the Premedication Data column for use as a baseline to track the patient's response to drug therapy. Ensure that the patient understands how to use the form, and instruct the patient to bring the completed form to follow-up visits. During follow-up visits, focus on issues that will foster adherence to the therapeutic interventions prescribed.

DRUG CLASS: HEMORHEOLOGIC AGENTS

---

pentoxifylline (pĕn-tŏk-ĭ-FĬ-lēn)

Actions

Pentoxifylline is not an anticoagulant, but it is thought to increase erythrocyte flexibility, decrease the concentration of fibrinogen in blood, and prevent aggregation of red blood cells and platelets. These actions decrease the viscosity of blood and improve its flow properties, resulting in increased blood flow to the affected microcirculation to enhance tissue oxygenation.

Uses

Pentoxifylline is the agent approved for the treatment of intermittent claudication. Pentoxifylline therapy should be considered an adjunct to—not a replacement for—smoking cessation, weight loss, exercise therapy, surgical bypass, or removal of arterial obstructions in the treatment of peripheral vascular disease.

Therapeutic Outcome

The primary therapeutic outcome expected from pentoxifylline is improved tissue perfusion with a reduced frequency of pain, improved tolerance to exercise, and improved peripheral pulses.

❖ Nursing Implications for Pentoxifylline

◆ *Premedication assessment*

1. Perform baseline gastrointestinal assessments to determine whether nausea, vomiting, dyspepsia, or intolerance to caffeine products exists.
2. Assess the patient for the presence of dizziness or headache.
3. Ask specifically about any cardiac symptoms. Report these to the healthcare provider if they are present.
4. Obtain baseline data regarding the degree of pain present.
5. Inquire about a history of stroke, bleeding in the eyes, kidney problems, recent surgery, and peptic ulcer disease.

◆ *Availability. PO:* 400-mg tablets, extended release.

◆ *Dosage and administration. PO:* 400 mg three times daily. If adverse gastrointestinal or central nervous system effects develop, the dosage should be reduced to 400 mg twice daily. If adverse effects persist, therapy should be discontinued. Symptomatic relief may start within 2 to 4 weeks, but treatment should be continued for at least 8 weeks to achieve maximal efficacy.

◆ *Common adverse effects*
Gastrointestinal
Nausea, vomiting, dyspepsia. Dyspepsia, nausea, and vomiting occur in about 1% to 3% of patients. Belching and flatus occur in less than 1% of patients. These adverse effects are usually mild, and they tend to resolve with continued therapy. Administration with food or milk may help minimize the patient's discomfort. Encourage the patient not to discontinue therapy without first consulting the healthcare provider.

Neurologic
Dizziness, headache. Central nervous system disturbances characterized by dizziness occur in about 2% of patients, and headache and tremor occur less frequently. These adverse effects are usually mild, and they tend to resolve with continued therapy. Provide for the patient's safety during episodes of dizziness, and encourage the patient to sit or lie down if feeling faint. Encourage the patient not to discontinue therapy without first consulting the healthcare provider.

◆ *Serious adverse effects*
Cardiovascular
Chest pain, dysrhythmias, shortness of breath. Without causing undue alarm, strongly encourage the patient to seek the healthcare provider's attention for further evaluation.

◆ *Pharmacodynamics*
Intolerance to caffeine, theophylline, theobromine. Pentoxifylline is a xanthine derivative. The patient should be asked specifically about any intolerance to xanthine derivatives before starting therapy.

◆ *Drug interactions*
Antihypertensive agents. Although pentoxifylline is not an antihypertensive agent, patients receiving pentoxifylline therapy frequently display a small reduction in systemic blood pressure. Blood pressure should be monitored to observe for hypotension. The dosage of antihypertensive therapy may have to be reduced to minimize adverse effects.

Theophylline. Concurrent use of pentoxifylline and theophylline-containing drugs leads to increased theophylline levels and theophylline toxicity in some individuals. Monitor patients closely for signs of toxicity (e.g., nausea, tachycardia), and adjust the theophylline dosage as necessary.

DRUG CLASS: PLATELET AGGREGATION INHIBITOR

cilostazol (sī-LŌ-stă-zŏl)

Actions
Cilostazol is a selective inhibitor of cellular cyclic adenosine monophosphate (cAMP) phosphodiesterase 3. Suppression of this enzyme causes increased levels of cAMP, resulting in vasodilation and inhibition of platelet aggregation. Other mechanisms in addition to vasodilation are thought to play a role but are not fully known at this time.

Uses
Cilostazol is approved for the treatment of intermittent claudication. Cilostazol therapy should be considered an adjunct to—not a replacement for—smoking cessation, weight loss, exercise therapy, surgical bypass, or removal of arterial obstructions in the treatment of peripheral vascular disease.

> **Medication Safety Alert**
>
> Cilostazol should not be used to treat patients with heart failure of any severity.

Therapeutic Outcome
The primary therapeutic outcome expected from cilostazol is singular improved tissue perfusion with a reduced frequency of pain, improved tolerance to exercise, and improved peripheral pulses.

❖ **Nursing Implications for Cilostazol**
◆ *Premedication assessment*
1. Assess the patient for the presence of dizziness or headache.
2. Obtain a baseline assessment of the degree of pain present and any symptoms of peripheral vascular disease.
3. Ask the patient specifically about any cardiac symptoms, peptic ulcer disease, or heart failure. Report these to the healthcare provider if they are present.

◆ *Availability. PO:* 50- and 100-mg tablets.

◆ *Dosage and administration. PO:* 100 mg twice daily taken 30 minutes before or 2 hours after breakfast and dinner. Symptomatic relief may start within 2 to 4 weeks, but treatment should be continued for at least 12 weeks to achieve maximum efficacy.

> **Medication Safety Alert**
>
> Do not administer cilostazol to patients with heart failure. Phosphodiesterase inhibitors have been reported to significantly worsen heart failure.

◆ *Common adverse effects*

Gastrointestinal

Dyspepsia, diarrhea. Dyspepsia occurs in 6% of patients and diarrhea occurs in 19% of patients. These adverse effects are usually mild, and they tend to resolve with continued therapy. Encourage the patient not to discontinue therapy without first consulting the healthcare provider.

Neurologic

Dizziness, headache. Central nervous system disturbances characterized by dizziness occur in about 10% of patients. Headache may occur in 34% of patients, and it may be severe enough to cause the discontinuation of therapy. These adverse effects are usually mild, and they tend to resolve with continued therapy. Provide for patient safety during episodes of dizziness. Encourage the patient to sit or lie down if feeling faint. Encourage the patient not to discontinue therapy without first consulting the healthcare provider.

◆ *Serious adverse effects*

Cardiovascular

Chest pain, palpitations, dysrhythmias, shortness of breath. Without causing undue alarm, strongly encourage the patient to seek the healthcare provider's attention for further evaluation.

◆ *Drug interactions*

Diltiazem, erythromycin, omeprazole, fluconazole, fluvoxamine, fluoxetine, sertraline, ketoconazole, grapefruit juice. These substances will inhibit the metabolism of cilostazol. If cilostazol therapy is necessary for patients who are already receiving any of the preceding drugs, the starting dose of cilostazol should be half of the normal starting dose. Monitor patients closely for an increased incidence of adverse effects.

Get Ready for the NCLEX® Examination!

Key Points

- Peripheral vascular disease is a cause of significant morbidity in the United States. Major treatable causes of peripheral vascular disease are hypertension, cigarette smoking, and atherosclerosis.
- The most cost-effective and successful forms of treatment are smoking cessation, weight reduction, exercise, and dietary modification.
- Patients should be fully informed about the significance of peripheral vascular disease, the potential complications of not participating in lifestyle modification, and the use of drug therapy.

Additional Learning Resources

SG Go to your Study Guide for additional Review Questions for the NCLEX® Examination, Critical Thinking Clinical Situations, and other learning activities to help you master this chapter content.

Go to your Evolve website (https://evolve.elsevier.com/Clayton) for additional online resources.

Review Questions for the NCLEX® Examination

1. The premedication assessments that the nurse performs on patients with peripheral vascular disease include which of the following? *(Select all that apply.)*
   1. Checking for renal disease
   2. Obtaining a pain rating
   3. Evaluating the peripheral pulses
   4. Checking the temperature of extremities
   5. Evaluating the level of psychological stress

2. The nurse knows that the most significant risk factors for developing peripheral vascular disease include which conditions?
   1. Hypertension, low LDL levels, poor peripheral circulation
   2. Smoking, hypertension, high LDL levels
   3. Poor peripheral circulation, low LDL levels, smoking
   4. Poor peripheral circulation, high LDL levels, hypothyroidism

3. The nurse was explaining to a 52-year-old male patient the meaning of his new diagnosis of "claudication." Which is an appropriate statement by the nurse?
   1. "This condition is from poor circulation resulting in a lack of oxygen to the muscles during exercise."
   2. "When patients get this, there usually is also a deep vein thrombus in the leg."
   3. "The pain you have when walking is from a vasospasm, which will cause your skin to blanch."
   4. "Generally, you do not have to treat this condition until you get pain at rest, along with numbness and tingling in your legs."

4. The nurse teaching a patient about ways to prevent vasospasms associated with Raynaud's disease includes which of these instructions? *(Select all that apply.)*
   1. Avoid holding cold beverages
   2. Avoid handling hot beverages
   3. Keep hands and feet warm with gloves and socks
   4. Limiting the amount of fluids and calories daily
   5. Exercise vigorously three times a day

5. The nurse who is reviewing the common adverse effects of cilostazol (Pletal) with the patient who has peripheral vascular disease includes which of these effects in the teaching? *(Select all that apply.)*
   1. Dizziness
   2. Rhinorrhea
   3. Diarrhea
   4. Headache
   5. Dryness of the mouth

6. The nurse teaches a patient with any venous circulation disorder that the best way to prevent venous stasis and increase venous return would be to what?
   1. Ambulate
   2. Sit with the legs elevated
   3. Frequently rotate the ankles
   4. Continuously wear compression-gradient stockings

7. The patient who was started on pentoxifylline asked the nurse how the drug works. Which statement is an appropriate response by the nurse?
   1. "Pentoxifylline acts as an anticoagulant so you will not develop clots in your legs."
   2. "Pentoxifylline works by increasing the flexibility of your red blood cells so clotting does not happen so easily."
   3. "Pentoxifylline increases the viscosity of blood, which means it makes your blood thicker."
   4. "Pentoxifylline breaks down the plaque in your blood vessels so that you will not have any blood clots develop."

8. The nurse educating a patient with peripheral vascular disease on the goals of therapy recognizes the need for further education after the patient makes which statement?
   1. "I understand that I will need to keep walking to help maintain my circulation."
   2. "I realize I will have to eat more baked foods and eliminate the fried foods to decrease calories provided by fats."
   3. "I already have poor circulation, so there really is nothing I can do to stop the process."
   4. "If I could keep my weight down and manage my blood sugars better, I hope to reduce the need to be on any drugs for this."

Drugs Used to Treat Thromboembolic Disorders

26

Objectives

1. Explain the primary purposes of anticoagulant therapy.
2. Describe conditions that place an individual at risk for developing blood clots and nursing interventions used to prevent these conditions.
3. Identify the actions of platelet inhibitors, anticoagulants, thrombin inhibitors, glycoprotein IIb/IIIa inhibitors, and fibrinolytic agents.

4. Describe specific monitoring procedures and laboratory data used to detect hemorrhage in the patient taking anticoagulants.
5. Describe the nursing assessments needed to monitor therapeutic response and adverse effects from anticoagulant therapy.

Key Terms

thromboembolic diseases (thrŏm-bō-ĕm-BŎL-ĭk) (p. 401)
thrombosis (thrŏm-BŌ-sĭs) (p. 401)
thrombus (THRŎM-bŭs) (p. 401)
embolus (ĔM-bō-lŭs) (p. 401)
intrinsic clotting pathway (ĭn-TRĬN-zĭk KLŎT-ĭng PĂTH-wā) (p. 401)
extrinsic clotting pathway (ĕks-TRĬN-zĭk) (p. 401)

fibrinolytic agents (fī-brĭn-ō-LĬT-ĭk Ā-gĕntz) (p. 402)
platelet inhibitors (PLĀT-lĕt ĭn-HĬB-ĭ-tĕrz) (p. 403)
factor Xa inhibitor (fact-tor TEN a in-HIB-i-terz)
anticoagulants (ăn-tī-kō-ĂG-yū-lănts) (p. 403)
thrombin inhibitors (THRŎM-bĭn) (p. 403)
glycoprotein IIb/IIIa inhibitors (glī-cō-PRŌ-tēn ĭn-HĬ-bĭ-tĕrz) (p. 403)

THROMBOEMBOLIC DISEASES

Diseases associated with abnormal clotting within blood vessels are known as **thromboembolic diseases** and are major causes of morbidity and mortality. **Thrombosis** is the process of formation of a fibrin blood clot (**thrombus**). An **embolus** is a small fragment of a thrombus that breaks off and circulates until it becomes trapped in a capillary, causing ischemia or infarction to the area distal to the obstruction (e.g., cerebral embolism, pulmonary embolism [PE]).

Major causes of thrombus formation are immobilization with venous stasis; surgery and the postoperative period; trauma to lower limbs; certain illnesses (e.g., heart failure, vasospasm, ulcerative colitis); cancers of the lung, prostate, stomach, and pancreas; pregnancy and oral contraceptives; and heredity.

Normally, blood clot formation and dissolution constitute a fine balance within the cardiovascular system. The clotting proteins normally circulate in an inactive state and must be activated to form a fibrin clot. When there is a trigger, such as increased blood viscosity from bed rest and stasis or damage to a blood vessel wall, the clotting cascade is activated. For example, if a blood vessel is injured and collagen in the vessel wall is exposed, platelets first adhere to the site of injury and release adenosine diphosphate (ADP), leading to additional platelet aggregation that forms a "platelet plug." At the same time platelets are forming a plug, the intrinsic clotting pathway is triggered by the presence of collagen activating factor XII. Activated factor XIIa activates factor XI to XIa, which activates factor IX to IXa. Factor IXa, in the presence of calcium, platelet factor 3, and factor VIII, activates factor X. Activated factor Xa, in the presence of calcium, platelet factor 3, and factor V, stimulates the conversion of prothrombin to thrombin (Fig. 26.1).

Sources outside the blood vessels, such as tissue extract or thromboplastin (tissue factor), can trigger the extrinsic clotting pathway by activating factors VII to VIIa. Factor VIIa can also activate factor X, which results in the formation of thrombin. After stimulation from the intrinsic or extrinsic pathway, thrombin, in the presence of calcium, activates fibrinogen to soluble fibrin. With time and the presence of factor XIII, the loose fibrin mesh is converted to a tight, insoluble fibrin mesh clot. Thrombin also stimulates platelet aggregation and stimulates further activity of factors V, VIIa, VII, and Xa. As the fibrin clot is being formed, it also triggers the release of fibrinolysin, an enzyme that dissolves fibrin, preventing the clot from spreading.

Intrinsic Clotting Pathway   **Extrinsic Clotting Pathway**

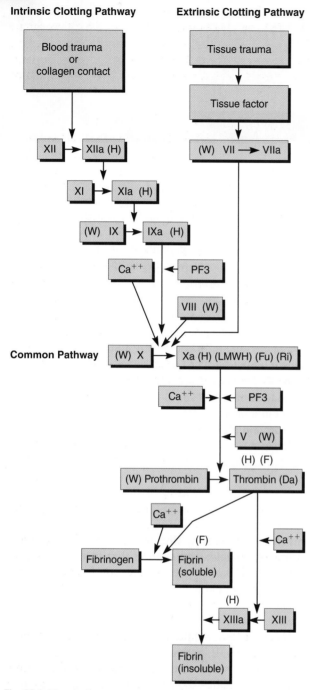

Common Pathway

Fig. 26.1 The clotting cascade. *Da*, Site of direct thrombin inhibitors; *F*, site of fibrinolytic action; *Fu*, fondaparinux; *H*, site of heparin action; *LMWH*, site of low-molecular-weight heparins; *PF3*, platelet factor 3; *Ri*, rivaroxaban; *W*, site of warfarin action.

Historically, thrombi have been classified into red and white blood clots. A red thrombus is actually a venous thrombus and is composed almost entirely of fibrin and erythrocytes (red blood cells), with a few platelets. Venous thrombi generally form in response to venous stasis after immobility or surgery. The poor circulation prevents the dilution of activated coagulation factors that normally occurs by rapidly circulating blood. The most common location of red thrombus formation is deep vein thrombosis (DVT) of the lower extremities.

These thrombi may extend upward into the veins of the thigh and have the potential of fragmenting, subsequently causing life-threatening pulmonary emboli. White thrombi develop in arteries and are composed of platelets and fibrin. This type of thrombus forms in areas of high blood flow in response to injured vessel walls. Coronary artery occlusion leading to myocardial infarction (MI) is an example of a white thrombus.

TREATMENT OF THROMBOEMBOLIC DISEASES

Diseases caused by intravascular clotting (e.g., DVT, MI, dysrhythmias with clot formation, coronary vasospasm leading to thrombus formation) are major causes of death. When thrombosis is suspected, patients are admitted to the hospital where they can be closely observed for further signs and symptoms of thrombosis formation and progression, and anticoagulant or fibrinolytic therapy can be started. A combination of physical examination, patient history, Doppler ultrasound, phlebography, radiolabeled fibrinogen studies, and angiography is used to diagnose the presence and cause of a thrombus and embolism. Routine laboratory tests that are run to assess the clotting process and ensure that occult bleeding is not present are platelet count, hematocrit, prothrombin time (PT) (reported as the international normalized ratio [INR]), activated partial thromboplastin time (aPTT), activated clotting time (ACT), urinalysis, and stool guaiac test.

Nonpharmacologic prevention and treatment of thromboembolic disease (TED) include patient education on how to prevent venous stasis (e.g., leg exercises, leg elevation) and clinical use of sequential compression devices (SCDs). If a patient having a heart attack (MI, acute coronary syndrome) can be transported to a cardiac intensive care facility soon after symptoms develop, revascularization treatment to reopen the coronary arteries may be performed. **Fibrinolytic agents** may be used to dissolve the arterial clot before it is permanently attached to vessel walls, causing complete obstruction. Revascularization procedures used may be a percutaneous coronary intervention (PCI) or coronary artery bypass graft (CABG). In PCI, also known as angioplasty, a catheter is inserted into the femoral artery and advanced up the aorta into the site of the coronary artery obstruction. The tip of the catheter can be equipped with different types of devices, such as a balloon to dilate the artery obstruction, or blades or lasers to reduce or remove the obstruction. A vascular stent is then often placed in the artery to keep the formerly obstructed area open. If a patient has multiple narrowed or obstructed arteries, a CABG procedure is performed, wherein a segment of the saphenous vein from the leg is harvested and attached to the coronary artery above and below the obstruction, forming a bypass for perfusion to the myocardial tissues below. The internal mammary artery can also be used in this procedure. The major pharmacologic treatments used in the prevention and treatment of TEDs are discussed in the next section.

DRUG THERAPY FOR THROMBOEMBOLIC DISEASES

ACTIONS

The pharmacologic agents used to treat TED act either to prevent platelet aggregation or inhibit a variety of steps in the fibrin clot formation cascade (see Fig. 26.1). See individual drug monographs later in this chapter for a more detailed discussion of mechanisms of action.

USES

Agents used in the prevention and treatment of TED can be divided into **platelet inhibitors, factor Xa inhibitors, anticoagulants, thrombin inhibitors, glycoprotein IIb/IIIa inhibitors**, and fibrinolytic agents. Antiplatelet agents (e.g., aspirin, clopidogrel, prasugrel, ticagrelor, cangrelor) are used preventively to reduce arterial clot formation (white thrombi) by inhibiting platelet aggregation. Anticoagulants (e.g., apixaban, dabigatran, warfarin, fondaparinux, rivaroxaban, heparin, heparin derivatives [enoxaparin, dalteparin]) are also used prophylactically to prevent the formation of arterial and venous thrombi in predisposed patients. The heparin derivatives are also known as low-molecular-weight heparins (LMWHs). The primary purpose of anticoagulants is to prevent the formation of new clots or the extension of existing clots. They cannot dissolve an existing (white or red) clot. The glycoprotein IIb/IIIa inhibitors (e.g., abciximab, eptifibatide, tirofiban) are used to prevent clot formation during PCI procedures. Fibrinolytic agents (e.g., streptokinase, alteplase) are used to dissolve arterial (fibrin-rich, white) thromboemboli once formed.

LABORATORY TESTS FOR MONITORING ANTICOAGULANT THERAPY

While receiving anticoagulant therapy, the patient will undergo regular monitoring of coagulation studies, including monitoring of the PT (reported as the INR), ecarin clotting time (ECT), thrombin time (TT), ACT, aPTT, and platelet counts. These laboratory studies monitor the time it takes for the blood to clot. Results of these studies may be used as guidelines for drug dosing by the prescriber.

❖ NURSING IMPLICATIONS FOR ANTICOAGULANT THERAPY

◆ Assessment

History. Ask specific questions to determine whether the patient or family members have a history of any type of vascular difficulty. Patients at greater risk for clot formation are those with a history of clot formation; those who have recently undergone abdominal, thoracic, or orthopedic surgery; and those on prolonged bed rest or inadequately controlled anticoagulant therapy. Does the patient have any disease processes that could potentially increase the risk of bleeding (e.g., ulcer disease, concurrent chemotherapy, or radiation therapy)?

Current symptoms
- Ask the patient to describe the symptoms. Is the patient currently taking, or has the patient recently taken, anticoagulants? Individualize further questioning to obtain data that would support or rule out thrombosis formation or progression of thrombosis.
- Collect data about reduced tissue perfusion (e.g., symptoms relating to cerebral, cardiopulmonary, or peripheral vascular disease, depending on the underlying pathophysiology). Perform a focused assessment at appropriate intervals that are consistent with the patient's status to detect further signs and symptoms of thrombosis formation or progression.
- To prevent thrombus extension or progression, SCDs are used. These devices inflate and deflate to promote venous return from the legs. SCDs are removed when ambulating and discontinued when the patient resumes full activity.

Medications
- Obtain a thorough medication history of both prescribed and over-the-counter medications being taken.
- Ask specific questions relating to medicines being taken that affect clotting.
- Ask whether the patient has been complying with medication regimens and if any dosage adjustment has taken place. If anticoagulants are being taken, has the patient reported for scheduled laboratory studies? Has the patient had any reactions to the medication?

Basic assessment
- Obtain vital signs and auscultation of breath sounds. Observe for dyspnea at rest or with exertion.
- Check mental status (e.g., orientation to date, time, and place; alertness; confusion). Use as a baseline for future comparison.
- Assess for specific signs of reduced tissue perfusion. Perform a focused assessment depending on the underlying pathologic condition (e.g., cardiopulmonary, cerebral, or peripheral vascular disease). If the presence of a thrombus is suspected in an extremity, complete a comparative assessment of the unaffected extremity.
- Collect data about any pain experienced.
- Ask specific questions about the patient's state of hydration. Review intake and output.

Diagnostic studies. Review completed diagnostic studies and laboratory data (e.g., PT, aPTT, INR), hematocrit, platelet count, Doppler studies, exercise testing, serum triglyceride levels, arteriogram, and cardiac enzyme studies.

Implementation

Techniques for preventing clot formation

- Provide early, regular ambulation after surgery. Use active or passive leg exercises for patients on bed rest or restricted activity.
- Develop and follow a specific turning schedule for patients on complete bed rest to prevent tissue breakdown and blood stasis. Implement regular back care and deep breathing and coughing exercises as part of general nursing care.
- Do not flex the patient's knees or place pressure against the popliteal space with pillows.
- Do not allow the patient to stand or sit motionless for prolonged periods.
- Use properly fitted TED deterrent stockings only when ordered. Remove stockings and inspect the skin on every shift. Make sure that they are being worn properly and remain wrinkle-free.
- Apply SCDs as ordered and indicated. Make sure that they are applied properly.

Patient assessment. Monitor vital signs and mental status every 4 to 8 hours or more frequently, depending on the patient's status. Observe for signs and symptoms of bleeding caused by medications (e.g., blurred vision, hematuria, ecchymosis, occult blood in the stools, change in mentation).

Nutritional status

- The dietary regimen will depend on the patient's diagnosis and clinical status.
- Adequate hydration to promote fluidity of the blood is important. Unless coexisting diagnoses prohibit, give at least six to eight 8-ounce glasses of liquid daily.

Laboratory and diagnostic data. Monitoring and reporting laboratory results to the prescriber are essential during anticoagulant therapy. Coagulation tests that might be ordered include the following: whole blood clotting time, ECT, TT, PT, aPTT, and ACT. The PT, reported as the INR, is routinely used to monitor warfarin therapy, and the aPTT and anti–factor Xa levels are most commonly used to monitor heparin therapy. The ECT and TT are used to monitor dabigatran therapy.

Medication administration. Never administer an anticoagulant without first checking the patient's chart for the most recent laboratory results. Be certain that the anticoagulant to be administered is ordered after the most recent results have been reported to the healthcare provider. Follow policy statements regarding checking of anticoagulant doses with other qualified professionals. Reduce localized bleeding at the injection site by using the smallest needle possible for injections, and rotate injection sites. See individual drug monographs later in this chapter for specific administration techniques related to a particular medicine.

Patient Education

Nutritional status

- While receiving anticoagulant therapy, patients should maintain their normal intake of green leafy vegetables that contain vitamin K. (Vitamin K inhibits the action of warfarin.) Patients should not start a major change in diet without discussing it with their healthcare provider, pharmacist, and nutritionist.
- Unless comorbidities prohibit, instruct the patient to drink six to eight 8-ounce glasses of liquid daily.

Exercise and activity

- Discuss the level of exercise prescribed by the healthcare provider. Walking may be prescribed to promote venous blood flow. Elevation of the legs when seated may be encouraged to promote venous blood flow.
- Stress the need to prevent body injury while taking anticoagulants. Tell the patient to avoid using power equipment, use care in stepping up onto or down from curbs, not participate in contact sports, use only an electric razor, and brush teeth gently with a soft-bristled toothbrush.

Medication regimen

- Instruct the patient to take the dosage of the medication exactly as prescribed. Explain the importance of returning for laboratory blood tests to determine its effectiveness and the need to adjust medicine dosages. Tell the patient to resume a regular schedule if one dose of warfarin is missed. If two or more doses are missed, the patient should consult the healthcare provider.
- Tell the patient to wear a medical alert bracelet.
- Explain symptoms that the patient should report, such as nosebleeds, tarry stools, coffee-ground or blood-tinged vomitus, petechiae (tiny purple or red spots occurring in various sites on the skin), ecchymoses (bruises), hematuria (blood in the urine), bleeding from the gums or any other body opening, or cuts or injuries from which the bleeding is difficult to control. Check dressings periodically for bleeding. Report excessive menstrual flow.
- In some cases, the healthcare provider may want the patient to perform guaiac testing to detect occult blood in the stool. If ordered, specific patient education should be done to teach the patient or support person how to perform the test.
- Tell patients that because not all bleeding is clearly visible, they should report immediately a rapid weak pulse, deep rapid respirations, moist clammy skin, and a general feeling of weakness or faintness.

- Tell the patient *not* to take any medication, including over-the-counter medications, without first consulting the healthcare provider because many drugs interact with warfarin to increase or decrease its effectiveness. Tell the patient to never discontinue anticoagulant therapy without healthcare provider agreement.
- Patients should always inform any healthcare provider (e.g., prescriber, home healthcare provider, dentist) that anticoagulant therapy is being taken whenever seeking care.

Fostering health maintenance

- Throughout the course of treatment, discuss medication information and how it will benefit the patient.
- Provide the patient and significant others with important information contained in the specific drug monographs for the medicines prescribed. Additional health teaching and nursing interventions for common and serious adverse effects are described in the drug monographs in this chapter. Urge the patient to use caution in cutting with a knife or using any other sharp objects.
- Seek cooperation and understanding of the following points so that medication compliance is increased: name of medication; dosage, route, and times of administration; and common and serious adverse effects.

Patient self-assessment. Enlist the patient's aid in developing and maintaining a written record of monitoring parameters. See the Patient Self-Assessment Form for Anticoagulants on the Evolve website. Complete the Premedication Data column for use as a baseline to track response to drug therapy. Ensure that the patient understands how to use the form, and instruct the patient to bring the completed form to follow-up visits. During follow-up visits, focus on issues that will foster adherence with the therapeutic interventions prescribed.

DRUG CLASS: PLATELET INHIBITORS

aspirin (ĂS-prĭn)

Actions

Aspirin is well known as a salicylate and a nonsteroidal antiinflammatory drug (NSAID). A unique property of aspirin, compared with other salicylates, is platelet aggregation inhibition with prolongation of bleeding time. The platelet loses its ability to aggregate and form clots for the duration of its lifetime (7 to 10 days). The mechanism of action is acetylation of the cyclooxygenase enzyme, which inhibits the synthesis of thromboxane A_2, a potent vasoconstrictor and inducer of platelet aggregation.

Uses

There is controversy in the literature as to whether aspirin is equally effective for men and women. When used as primary prevention, aspirin therapy was associated with a significant reduction in MI among men older than 45 years but had no effect on the incidence of stroke. Conversely, women taking aspirin had a lower rate of stroke, but no effect was found in relation to MI. Nevertheless, aspirin is administered to both men and women at the onset of an acute MI.

Therapeutic Outcomes

The primary therapeutic outcomes expected from aspirin therapy when used for antiplatelet therapy are reduced frequencies of transient ischemic attacks (TIAs), stroke, or MI.

❖ **Nursing Implications for Aspirin Therapy**
◆ *Premedication assessment*
1. Perform baseline neurologic assessment: orientation to date, time, and place; mental alertness; bilateral hand grip; motor functioning (balance and hearing).
2. Monitor for gastrointestinal (GI) symptoms before and during therapy. Stool guaiac testing may be ordered if GI tract bleeding is suspected.
3. Check on concurrent use of anticoagulant agents.
4. If the patient is receiving oral hypoglycemic agents, review baseline serum glucose levels.

◆ *Availability, dosage, and administration.* See Chapter 19, specifically Tables 19.3 and 19.4.
   Prevention of transient ischemic attacks and stroke. Adult: *PO:* 50 to 325 mg daily.
   Treatment of suspected myocardial infarction. Adult: *PO:* 160 to 325 mg as soon as possible. Continue 160 to 325 mg daily for at least 30 days.
   Prevention of myocardial infarction. Adult: *PO:* 75 to 162 mg daily. Current literature mostly supports the use of 81 mg daily for prevention.

---

clopidogrel (klō-PĬD-ō-grĕl)
   Plavix (PLĂ-vĭks)
   ⇌ *Do not confuse Plavix with Paxil.*

Actions

Clopidogrel is a second-generation thienopyridine chemically related to prasugrel. Clopidogrel is a prodrug; one of its metabolites, as yet unknown, is thought to act by inhibiting the ADP pathway required for platelet aggregation. The full antiplatelet activity is seen after 3 to 7 days of continuous therapy. The antiaggregatory effect persists for approximately 5 days after discontinuation of therapy. Clopidogrel also prolongs bleeding time.

Uses

Clopidogrel is used to reduce the risk of additional atherosclerotic events (e.g., MI, stroke, vascular death) in patients who have had a recent stroke, a recent MI, or coronary bypass grafting or have established peripheral arterial disease. The medical histories of patients at greatest risk include TIAs, atrial fibrillation, angina pectoris, and carotid artery stenosis. Because clopidogrel has a different mechanism of action from aspirin, it is anticipated that healthcare providers may use both drugs concurrently. The overall safety profile of clopidogrel appears to be at least as good as that of medium-dose aspirin.

Therapeutic Outcomes

The primary therapeutic outcomes expected from clopidogrel therapy are reduced frequency of TIAs, stroke, MI, or complications from peripheral vascular disease.

❖ Nursing Implications for Clopidogrel

◆ Premedication assessment

1. Obtain baseline vital signs.
2. Order baseline laboratory studies as requested by the healthcare provider (e.g., complete blood count [CBC] with differential count).
3. Assess and record any GI symptoms.

◆ Availability. PO: 75- and 300-mg tablets.

◆ Dosage and administration. **Adult:** *PO: Initial:* 300 or 600 mg for acute MI and PCI; otherwise, 75 mg. *Maintenance:* 75 mg once daily with food or on an empty stomach. (Aspirin may be concurrently prescribed.)

◆ Common adverse effects

Gastrointestinal

Nausea, vomiting, anorexia, diarrhea. These effects tend to occur most frequently with early dosages and tend to resolve with continued therapy over the next 2 weeks. They can also be minimized by taking the medication with food. Encourage the patient not to discontinue therapy without first consulting the healthcare provider.

◆ Serious adverse effects

Hematologic

Thrombotic thrombocytopenic purpura. Thrombotic thrombocytopenic purpura is a very rare but potentially life-threatening condition that may occur within 2 weeks of the initiation of therapy. Early indications are abnormal neurologic findings and fever, followed by renal impairment. If suspected, contact the healthcare provider immediately.

Neutropenia, agranulocytosis. Neutropenia (absolute neutrophil count below 1200 neutrophils/mm^3) was discovered in 0.4% of patients in clinical trials. While neutropenic, patients are very susceptible to infection. Encourage the patient to report symptoms of infection (e.g., sore throat, fever, excessive fatigue) to the healthcare provider as soon as possible.

Bleeding. A normal physiologic effect of clopidogrel is prolongation of bleeding time. Patients should report any incidents of bleeding as soon as possible. Incidents to be reported include nosebleeds; easy bruising; bright red or coffee-ground emesis; hematuria; and dark, tarry stools.

Patients should inform other healthcare practitioners (e.g., other physicians, dentist) that they are receiving platelet inhibitor therapy.

◆ Drug interactions

Drugs that increase therapeutic and toxic effects. Heparin, LMWHs, warfarin, aspirin, NSAIDs, fondaparinux, and direct thrombin inhibitors (e.g., argatroban, bivalirudin, dabigatran) will have an additive bleeding effect on the patient. Monitor very closely for indications of bleeding. Caution should be used when any of these drugs are coadministered with clopidogrel.

---

prasugrel (PRĂ-sū-grĕl)
⇌ *Do not confuse prasugrel with Pravachol.*
Effient (ĔF-ē-ĕnt)

Actions

Prasugrel is a third-generation thienopyridine that is similar to clopidogrel. Prasugrel is a prodrug that must be metabolized to the active drug, which then irreversibly binds to the platelet P2Y12 receptors, inhibiting the ADP pathway required for platelet aggregation. The antiplatelet activity is seen after 1 to 2 hours and continues for 24 hours. The antiaggregatory effect persists for 5 to 9 days after discontinuation of therapy with new platelet production. Prasugrel also prolongs bleeding time. The steady-state effect is seen after 3 days of continuous therapy.

Uses

Compared with clopidogrel, prasugrel shows a greater platelet inhibitory effect and has a more rapid onset of action, but it also has an increased risk of major bleeding. Prasugrel is approved for use in the prevention of blood clot formation in patients suffering an MI who are undergoing a PCI with or without stent placement. Although not recommended in patients older than 75 years of age, prasugrel appears to be more effective and should be considered in patients over 75 with a history of MI or with diabetes. Clopidogrel remains the first-line thienopyridine in treatment of patients with an MI who have a history of TIA or stroke, in those patients being treated with CABG, and in those patients over 75 years (with the exception of those over 75 years with diabetes or prior MI). Aspirin therapy should be continued with prasugrel therapy.

Therapeutic Outcome

The primary therapeutic outcome expected from prasugrel is reduced blood clot formation in the treatment of an MI with a PCI procedure.

❖ **Nursing Implications for Prasugrel**
◆ *Premedication assessment*
  1. Obtain baseline vital signs.
  2. Order baseline laboratory studies as requested by the healthcare provider (e.g., CBC).
  3. Ask the patient about a history of active bleeding, TIA, stroke, or hypersensitivity to prasugrel. Notify the healthcare provider of these findings.

◆ *Availability.* *PO:* 5- and 10-mg tablets.

◆ *Dosage and administration.* **Adult:** *PO:* Initially, 60-mg loading dose followed by a daily maintenance dose of 10 mg. If the patient weighs less than 60 kg, 5 mg daily is recommended. Patients should also continue to take aspirin, 75 to 325 mg once daily.

◆ *Common adverse effects*
  Hematologic
  Bleeding. The normal physiologic effect of prasugrel is prolongation of bleeding time. Patients should report any incidents of bleeding as soon as possible. Incidents to be reported include nosebleeds; easy bruising; bright red or coffee-ground emesis; hematuria; and dark, tarry stools.
  Patients should inform other healthcare practitioners (e.g., another physician, dentist) that they are receiving platelet inhibitor therapy.

◆ *Serious adverse effects*
  Hematologic
  Thrombotic thrombocytopenic purpura. Thrombotic thrombocytopenic purpura is a very rare but potentially life-threatening condition that may occur within the first 3 months of the initiation of therapy. Early indications are abnormal neurologic findings and fever, followed by renal impairment. If suspected, contact the healthcare provider immediately.

◆ *Drug interactions*
  Drugs that increase therapeutic and toxic effects. Heparin, LMWHs, warfarin, aspirin, NSAIDs, fondaparinux, and direct thrombin inhibitors (e.g., argatroban, dabigatran, bivalirudin) will have an additive bleeding effect in the patient. Monitor very closely for indications of bleeding. Caution should be used when any of these drugs are coadministered with prasugrel.

ticagrelor (tī-KĂ-grĕ-lŏr)
Brilinta (brĭ-LĬN-tă)

Actions
Ticagrelor is a platelet aggregation inhibitor that binds to the platelet P2Y12 receptors, inhibiting the ADP pathway required for platelet aggregation. It is not chemically related to clopidogrel or prasugrel, is not a prodrug requiring metabolism for action, and is the first platelet inhibitor to have direct, reversible binding to the receptor site. The maximum antiplatelet activity is seen at about 2 hours and continues for 8 hours. The antiaggregatory effect persists for 5 days after discontinuation of therapy.

Uses
Ticagrelor is indicated to reduce the rate of cardiovascular death, MI, and stroke in patients with acute coronary syndrome or a history of MI. It also reduces the rate of stent thrombosis in those patients who have received a stent for treatment of acute coronary syndrome. Patients should continue low-dose aspirin therapy with ticagrelor.

Therapeutic Outcome
The primary therapeutic outcome expected from ticagrelor is lower frequency of blood clots associated with MI.

❖ **Nursing Implications for Ticagrelor**
◆ *Premedication assessment*
  1. Obtain baseline vital signs.
  2. Order baseline laboratory studies requested by the healthcare provider (e.g., CBC).

◆ *Availability.* *PO:* 60- and 90-mg tablets.

◆ *Dosage and administration.* *PO:* Loading dose, 180 mg of ticagrelor with 325 mg of aspirin, followed by 90 mg ticagrelor with 75 to 100 mg aspirin daily for 1 year. After 1 year, ticagrelor 60 mg twice a day with 75 to 100 mg of aspirin.

> **! Medication Safety Alert**
> - Do not exceed 100 mg of aspirin daily. Larger doses reduce the effectiveness of ticagrelor.
> - Ticagrelor is contraindicated in patients who have a history of intracranial hemorrhage (hemorrhagic stroke).
> - Ticagrelor is contraindicated in moderate to severe liver failure. Ticagrelor is normally metabolized by enzymes in the liver, so metabolism may be diminished, causing higher circulating levels of ticagrelor. Furthermore, production of clotting factors is reduced in patients with liver failure, making patients more susceptible to hemorrhage.

◆ *Common adverse effects*
  Hematologic
  Bleeding. A normal physiologic effect of ticagrelor is prolongation of bleeding time. Patients should report any incidents of bleeding as soon as possible. Incidents to be reported include nosebleeds; easy bruising; bright red or coffee-ground emesis; hematuria; and dark, tarry stools.
  Patients should inform other healthcare practitioners (e.g., another physician, dentist) that they are receiving platelet inhibitor therapy.

Respiratory

Dyspnea. Fourteen percent of patients receiving ticagrelor develop mild to moderate dyspnea, which resolves with continued therapy. If the patient develops new, prolonged, or worsened dyspnea, notify the healthcare provider. Seek underlying causes of dyspnea. If ticagrelor is determined to be the cause of the dyspnea, there is no need to discontinue therapy; continue ticagrelor without interruption.

◆ *Drug interactions*

Drugs that increase therapeutic and toxic effects

Combined pharmacologic effect. Anticoagulants/platelet inhibitors that have an additive bleeding effect in the patient include heparin, LMWHs, warfarin, aspirin, NSAIDs, fondaparinux, and direct thrombin inhibitors (e.g., argatroban, dabigatran, desirudin). Monitor very closely for indications of bleeding. Caution should be used when any of these drugs are coadministered with ticagrelor.

Reduced metabolism. Drugs that inhibit the metabolism of ticagrelor, increasing the likelihood of bleeding, include ketoconazole, itraconazole, voriconazole, clarithromycin, and ritonavir. Monitor very closely for indications of bleeding. Caution should be used when any of these drugs are coadministered with ticagrelor.

Drugs that decrease therapeutic effects. Drugs that may decrease the therapeutic activity of ticagrelor by increasing its rate of metabolism include carbamazepine, dexamethasone, phenobarbital, phenytoin, and rifampin.

DRUG CLASS: FACTOR XA INHIBITORS

Actions

Apixaban, betrixaban, edoxaban, and rivaroxaban are reversible and selective factor Xa inhibitors that reduce thrombus formation. They do not affect platelet activity and do prolong PT (INR) and aPTT.

Uses

Apixaban is used to:
- Reduce the risk of stroke and systemic embolism in patients with nonvalvular atrial fibrillation.
- Treat DVT and PE.
- Reduce the risk of recurrence of DVT and PE after treatment.
- Prevent (prophylaxis) DVT, which may lead to PE, in patients undergoing hip or knee replacement surgery.

Betrixaban is used to:
- Prevent (prophylaxis) DVT and PE in adult patients hospitalized for an acute medical illness who are at risk for thromboembolic complications due to moderate or severe restricted mobility.

Edoxaban is used to:
- Reduce the risk of stroke and systemic embolism in patients with nonvalvular atrial fibrillation.
- Treat DVT and PE.

Rivaroxaban is used to:
- Reduce the risk of stroke and systemic embolism in patients with nonvalvular atrial fibrillation.
- Treat DVT and PE.
- Reduce the risk of recurrence of DVT and PE after treatment.
- Prevent (prophylaxis) DVT, which may lead to PE, in patients undergoing hip or knee replacement surgery.

The factor Xa inhibitors do not need to be monitored with anticoagulation tests (PT [INR] and aPTT).

Some of the factor Xa inhibitors may need a dose reduction due to renal function, age, weight, and drug interactions. Their greatest drawback in clinical use is that there is no antidote for the factor Xa inhibitors should hemorrhage occur.

Therapeutic Outcome

The primary therapeutic outcomes expected from factor Xa inhibitors are prevention of DVT and PE and reduction of the risk of thromboembolism in patients with atrial fibrillation. They are also used for the treatment of DVT and PE.

❖ **Nursing Implications for Factor Xa Inhibitors**

◆ *Premedication assessment*

1. Obtain baseline vital signs.
2. Initiate laboratory studies as requested by the healthcare provider (e.g., renal function tests such as blood urea nitrogen, serum creatinine, stool occult blood, and CBC) to serve as a baseline for future comparison.
3. Inspect the skin and mucous membranes for petechiae, ecchymoses, or hematomas. Also, monitor for hematuria, bleeding gums, and melena before administering each dose of medicine.

◆ *Availability, dosage, and administration.* See Table 26.1.

! Medication Safety Alert

- Do not administer to patients who have active major bleeding or a hypersensitivity to the factor Xa inhibitors.
- Premature discontinuation of the factor Xa inhibitors increases the risk of thrombosis. If anticoagulation is discontinued for a reason other than pathologic bleeding or completion of a course of therapy, coverage with another anticoagulant should be considered.
- Do not administer apixaban or rivaroxaban to patients with moderate to severe hepatic impairment or a creatinine clearance less than 30 mL/min.
- Do not administer edoxaban to patients with creatinine clearance greater than 95 mL/min.
- Administer extremely cautiously to patients who have been given spinal/epidural anesthesia or who have undergone spinal puncture. These patients are at increased risk of developing an epidural or spinal hematoma, which may cause paralysis.

Table 26.1   Factor Xa Inhibitors

GENERIC NAME	BRAND NAME	AVAILABILITY	DOSAGE
apixaban	Eliquis	Tablets: 2.5, 5 mg	*DVT and PE:* *Treatment:* 10 mg twice daily for 7 days followed by 5 mg twice daily *Reduction in the risk of recurrence:* 2.5 mg twice daily after at least 6 mo of treatment for DVT or PE *Nonvalvular atrial fibrillation (to prevent stroke and systemic embolism):* 5 mg twice daily unless patient has any 2 of the following: Age ≥80 years, body weight ≤60 kg, or serum creatinine ≥1.5 mg/dL; then reduce dose to 2.5 mg twice daily *Prophylaxis of DVT and PE:* *Hip replacement surgery:* 2.5 mg twice daily beginning 12-24 hr postoperatively; duration: 35 days *Knee replacement surgery:* 2.5 mg twice daily beginning 12-24 hr postoperatively; duration: 12 days
betrixaban	Bevyxxa	Capsules: 40, 80 mg	Initially 160 mg, followed by 80 mg once daily, taken with food for 35-42 days
edoxaban	Savaysa	Tablets: 15, 30, 60 mg	*Treatment for DVT and PE:* 60 mg once daily after 5-10 days of initial therapy with a parenteral anticoagulant *Nonvalvular atrial fibrillation (to prevent stroke and systemic embolism):* 60 mg once daily
rivaroxaban	Xarelto	Tablets: 10, 15, 20 mg	*DVT and PE:* *Treatment:* 15 mg twice daily with food for the first 21 days *Reduction in the risk of recurrence:* 10 mg orally once daily with or without food, after at least 6 months of standard anticoagulant therapy *Nonvalvular atrial fibrillation (to prevent stroke and systemic embolism):* 20 mg once daily with the evening meal *Prophylaxis of DVT and PE:* *Hip replacement surgery:* 10 mg once daily beginning at least 6 to 10 hours after surgery; total duration of therapy: 35 days *Knee replacement surgery:* 10 mg once daily beginning at least 6 to 10 hours after surgery; recommended total duration of therapy: 12 days

◆ *Common adverse effects*

Hematologic

Bleeding. A normal physiologic effect of factor Xa inhibitors is prolongation of bleeding time. Patients should report any incidents of bleeding as soon as possible. Incidents to be reported include nosebleeds; easy bruising; bright red or coffee-ground emesis; hematuria; and dark, tarry stools.

Patients should inform other healthcare practitioners (e.g., another physician, dentist) that they are receiving factor Xa inhibitor therapy.

◆ *Drug interactions*

Drugs that increase therapeutic and toxic effects

Increased pharmacologic effect. Heparin, LMWHs, warfarin, aspirin, NSAIDs, fondaparinux, vorapaxar, selective serotonin reuptake inhibitors, omega-3 fatty acids, and direct thrombin inhibitors (e.g., desirudin, argatroban, bivalirudin) will have an additive bleeding effect in the patient. Monitor very closely for indications of bleeding. Caution should be used when any of these drugs is coadministered with factor Xa inhibitors.

Reduced metabolism. Ketoconazole, itraconazole, voriconazole, clarithromycin, and ritonavir inhibit the metabolism of apixaban, betrixaban, and rivaroxaban, increasing the likelihood of bleeding. Monitor very closely for indications of bleeding. Caution should be used when any of these drugs is coadministered with factor Xa inhibitors.

Drugs that decrease therapeutic effects. When used concurrently with factor Xa inhibitors, estrogens, progestins, carbamazepine, dexamethasone, phenobarbital, phenytoin, rifampin, and St. John's wort may decrease their therapeutic activity by increasing their rate of metabolism.

DRUG CLASS: ANTICOAGULANTS

dalteparin (dăl-TĔ-păr-ĭn)
Fragmin (FRĂG-mĭn)

Actions

Dalteparin is the second (after enoxaparin) of the LMWHs that are essentially the active components of the heparin protein molecule. The LMWHs have the advantage of specific action at certain steps of the coagulation pathway, resulting in less potential for hemorrhage and longer duration of action. Dalteparin enhances antithrombin activity primarily against factor Xa, which prevents completion of the coagulation cascade. Dalteparin has no antiplatelet activity. Because it has no effect on thrombin, there is no effect on the aPTT.

Uses

Dalteparin is used to prevent and treat DVT after hip replacement surgery or abdominal surgery and in any medically ill patients. It may also be used for systemic anticoagulation and in combination with aspirin to prevent clot formation in patients with unstable angina pectoris and non–ST segment elevation MI (NSTEMI). Dalteparin may also be used during hemodialysis in connection with acute and chronic renal failure and in the prevention and treatment of venous thromboembolism in patients with cancer. Dalteparin is manufactured from heparin derived from pigs and should not be used in patients allergic to pork by-products.

Therapeutic Outcomes

The primary therapeutic outcomes from dalteparin therapy are treatment and prevention of DVT after abdominal or hip replacement surgery and prevention of clot formation in patients with angina pectoris and NSTEMI.

❖ Nursing Implications for Dalteparin
◆ Premedication assessment
1. Perform scheduled laboratory tests, including CBC, platelet count, and stool occult blood tests, before starting dalteparin therapy.
2. Obtain baseline vital signs.

◆ Availability. Subcutaneous: anti–factor Xa: 2500, 5000, 7500, 10,000, 12,500, 15,000, and 18,000 units in prefilled syringes with a 27-gauge, ½-inch needle (preservative free); 25,000 units/mL multidose vial that also contains benzyl alcohol preservative.

◆ Dosage and administration. Adult: *Subcutaneous:* Administer by deep subcutaneous injection into a U-shaped area around the navel, upper outer side of the thigh, or upper outer quadrangle of the buttock. When the area around the navel or the thigh is used, lift up a fold of skin with the thumb and forefinger while giving the injection. Insert the entire length of the needle at a 45- to 90-degree angle. The skinfold should be held throughout the injection. Inject the drug slowly, leaving the needle in place for 10 seconds after injection. To minimize bruising, do not rub the injection site after completion of the injection. Alternate injection sites every 24 hours.

Periodic CBCs (including platelet count) and stool occult blood tests are recommended during the course of treatment with dalteparin. No special monitoring of clotting times (e.g., aPTT) is required.

 Medication Safety Alert

Do not inject dalteparin intramuscularly! To prevent loss of drug, do not expel air bubble from prefilled syringe before injection.

Dosage range
Angina, myocardial infarction: clot formation prophylaxis. *Subcutaneous:* 120 units/kg (but no more than 10,000 units) every 12 hours with concurrent oral aspirin (75 to 165 mg/day) therapy.

Hip replacement surgery: DVT prophylaxis. *Subcutaneous:* 2500 to 5000 units before surgery. At 4 to 8 hours after surgery, 2500 units. Postoperative days: 5000 units daily. The usual duration of administration is 5 to 10 days after surgery.

Abdominal surgery: DVT prophylaxis. *Subcutaneous:* 2500 units once daily, starting 1 to 2 hours before surgery and repeating for 5 to 10 days postoperatively. *High-risk patients:* In abdominal surgery patients at high risk for thromboembolic complications (e.g., malignancy), administer 5000 units the evening before surgery and repeat once daily for 5 to 10 days postoperatively. Alternatively, in patients with malignancy, administer 2500 units 1 to 2 hours before surgery with an additional 2500 units 12 hours later, and then 5000 units once daily for 5 to 10 days postoperatively. In medical patients with severely restricted mobility during acute illness, 5000 units administered once daily.

Treatment of symptomatic venous thromboembolism. *Subcutaneous:* In patients with cancer and symptomatic venous thromboembolism, the recommended dosage of dalteparin for the first 30 days of treatment is 200 units/kg total body weight once daily. Therapy of 150 mg/kg daily may be continued for 2 to 6 months. The total daily dose should not exceed 18,000 units.

◆ Common adverse effects
Hematologic
Hematoma formation and bleeding at injection site. Inappropriate administration techniques lead to hematoma formation at the site of injection. **Use proper technique!**

◆ Serious adverse effects
Hematologic
Bleeding. Inspect the skin and mucous membranes for petechiae, ecchymoses, or hematomas; also monitor for bleeding gums. Assess and record vital signs at regular intervals. Monitor and report signs and symptoms of internal bleeding.

 Medication Safety Alert

Signs and symptoms of internal bleeding include decreasing blood pressure; increasing pulse; cold, clammy skin; feeling faint; and disoriented sensorium.

Check urine and stools for blood. Urine may appear red, smoke colored, or brownish. Stools may appear to be dark and tarry. Perform an occult blood test on the stool if necessary. Vomitus may contain bright red blood or may have a coffee-ground appearance.

Assessment of dressings or drainage tubes for any signs of bleeding is necessary for postoperative patients.

Thrombocytopenia. Dalteparin may cause type I or II heparin-induced thrombocytopenia (HIT) (see monograph on Heparin later in this chapter). Monitor platelet counts daily.

Thrombotic thrombocytopenic purpura. Thrombotic thrombocytopenic purpura is a very rare but potentially life-threatening condition that may occur within the first 3 months of the initiation of therapy. Early indications are abnormal neurologic findings and fever, followed by renal impairment. If suspected, contact the healthcare provider immediately.

◆ *Drug interactions.* No clinically significant drug interactions have been reported, but dalteparin should be used cautiously in patients receiving antiplatelet or warfarin therapy.

---

enoxaparin (ĕ-nŏks-ă-PĂR-ĭn)
⇄ *Do not confuse enoxaparin with enoxacin.*
Lovenox (LŌ-vĕn-ŏks)
⇄ *Do not confuse Lovenox with Avonex, Lanoxin, Lotronex, Protonix, or Luvox.*

Actions
Enoxaparin is the first of the LMWHs that are essentially the active components of the heparin protein molecule. The LMWHs have the advantage of specific action at certain steps of the coagulation pathway, resulting in less potential for hemorrhage and longer duration of action. Enoxaparin is specifically active against factor Xa and thrombin; it prevents completion of the coagulation cascade. Enoxaparin has no antiplatelet activity and does not affect the PT or aPTT.

Uses
Enoxaparin is used to prevent DVT after hip replacement surgery, knee replacement surgery, or abdominal surgery. It is also approved for use with warfarin to treat acute DVT, with or without PE, and for treatment of ST segment elevation MI. It is also used to prevent ischemic complications of unstable angina and NSTEMI when coadministered with aspirin. Enoxaparin is manufactured from heparin derived from pigs and should not be used in patients allergic to pork by-products.

Therapeutic Outcome
The primary therapeutic outcome from enoxaparin therapy is prevention of DVT after hip or knee replacement surgery and ischemic complications of angina and MI.

❖ **Nursing Implications for Enoxaparin**
◆ *Premedication assessment*
1. Perform scheduled laboratory tests, including CBC, platelet count, and stool occult blood tests, before starting enoxaparin therapy.
2. Obtain baseline vital signs.

◆ *Availability. Subcutaneous:* 30 mg in 0.3 mL, 40 mg in 0.4 mL, 60 mg in 0.6 mL, 80 mg in 0.8 mL, 100 mg in 1 mL, 120 mg in 0.8 mL, and 150 mg in 1 mL. Each concentration is packaged in a prefilled syringe (preservative free) with a 27-gauge, ½-inch needle. A 300-mg/3-mL multidose vial is available and contains benzyl alcohol preservative.

◆ *Dosage and administration.* **Adult:** *Subcutaneous:* Do not expel the air bubble from the prefilled syringe before administration. Administer by deep subcutaneous injection into the anterolateral or posterolateral abdominal wall every 12 to 24 hours. The entire length of the needle should be introduced into a skinfold held between the thumb and forefinger; the skinfold should be held throughout the injection. Inject the drug slowly, leaving the needle in place for 10 seconds after injection. To minimize bruising, do not rub the injection site after completion of the injection. Rotate sites every 12 hours.

Periodic CBCs (including platelet count) and stool occult blood tests are recommended during the course of treatment with enoxaparin. No special monitoring of clotting times is required.

⚠ Medication Safety Alert

- **Do not inject enoxaparin intramuscularly.** To prevent loss of drug, do not expel air bubble from syringe before injection.
- Dosage adjustment is required in patients with a creatinine clearance lower than 30 mL/min.
- Men less than 57 kg (125 lb) and women less than 45 kg (99 lb) who receive standard doses of enoxaparin of 30 to 40 mg one or two times daily should be more carefully observed for signs and symptoms of bleeding.

Dosage range. *Subcutaneous: Prophylaxis:* 30 mg twice daily or 40 mg once daily, depending on the medical and surgical condition.

Therapeutic: 1 mg/kg every 12 hours or 1.5 mg/kg every 24 hours, administered at the same time daily. Dosage adjustment is recommended for patients older than 75 years.

◆ *Common adverse effects*
Hematologic
Hematoma formation and bleeding at injection site. Inappropriate administration techniques lead to hematoma formation at the site of injection. **Use proper technique!**

◆ *Serious adverse effects*

Hematologic

Bleeding. Inspect the skin and mucous membranes for petechiae, ecchymoses, or hematomas; also monitor for bleeding gums. Assess and record vital signs at regular intervals. Watch for and report signs and symptoms of internal bleeding (e.g., decreasing blood pressure; increasing pulse; cold, clammy skin; feeling faint; disoriented sensorium).

Check urine and stools for blood. Urine may appear red, smoke colored, or brownish. Stools may appear to be dark and tarry. Perform an occult blood test on the stool if necessary. Vomitus may contain bright red blood or may have a coffee-ground appearance.

Assessment of dressings or drainage tubes for any signs of bleeding is necessary for postoperative patients.

Thrombocytopenia. Enoxaparin may induce type I or type II HIT (see monograph on Heparin later in this chapter). Monitor platelet counts on a daily basis.

Thrombotic thrombocytopenic purpura. Thrombotic thrombocytopenic purpura is a very rare but potentially life-threatening condition that may occur within the first 3 months after the initiation of therapy. Early indications are abnormal neurologic findings and fever, followed by renal impairment. If suspected, contact the healthcare provider immediately.

◆ *Drug interactions.* No clinically significant drug interactions have been reported, but enoxaparin should be used cautiously in patients receiving antiplatelet or warfarin therapy.

---

fondaparinux (fŏn-dĕ-PĂR-ĭn-ŭks)
Arixtra (ăr-ĬKS-tră)

Actions

Fondaparinux is a selective factor Xa inhibitor. Fondaparinux binds to antithrombin III, potentiating its action against factor Xa, preventing completion of the coagulation cascade. Fondaparinux has no antiplatelet activity and has no effect on the PT and aPTT.

Uses

Fondaparinux is used to prevent DVT in patients undergoing hip fracture or hip replacement surgery, knee replacement surgery, or abdominal surgery and, in combination with warfarin, to treat patients with acute DVT. It is also used to treat acute pulmonary embolism in conjunction with warfarin. When discontinued, fondaparinux-mediated anticoagulation remains for 2 to 4 days in patients with normal renal function and longer in patients with renal impairment. Fondaparinux cannot be used interchangeably (unit for unit) with heparin or LMWHs because they differ in manufacturing process, anti–factor Xa and anti–factor IIa activity, units, and dosage. Although they have similar mechanisms of action, fondaparinux is not an LMWH product.

Therapeutic Outcomes

The primary therapeutic outcomes from fondaparinux therapy are prevention of DVT in patients after hip, knee, or abdominal surgery and treatment of acute DVT.

❖ **Nursing Implications for Fondaparinux**
◆ *Premedication assessment*

1. Perform scheduled laboratory tests, including serum creatinine, CBC, platelet count, and stool occult blood tests, before starting fondaparinux therapy.
2. Obtain baseline vital signs.
3. Inspect the skin and mucous membranes for petechiae, ecchymoses, or hematomas. Also monitor for hematuria, bleeding gums, and melena before administering each dose of medication.

◆ *Availability.* **Subcutaneous:** 2.5 mg in 0.5 mL, 5 mg in 0.4 mL, 7.5 mg in 0.6 mL, and 10 mg in 0.8 mL single-dose prefilled syringes (preservative free) with 27-gauge, ½-inch needles.

◆ *Dosage and administration.* **Adult:** *Subcutaneous:* Do not expel the air bubble from the prefilled syringe before administration. Administer by deep subcutaneous injection, rotating the injection sites. The administration site should vary with each injection. Using the thumb and forefinger, a fold of skin must be lifted for giving the injection. Insert the entire length of the needle at a 45- to 90-degree angle. The skinfold should be held throughout the injection. Inject the drug slowly. When all contents have been injected from the syringe, the plunger should be released, allowing it to rise automatically while the needle withdraws from the skin and retracts into the security sleeve. Discard into a sharps container. To minimize bruising, do not rub the injection site after completion of the injection.

Periodic serum creatinine, CBC (including platelet count), and stool occult blood tests are recommended during the course of treatment with fondaparinux. No special monitoring of clotting times (aPTT) is required.

! Medication Safety Alert

- Do not inject fondaparinux intramuscularly!
- Use with caution in patients with a creatinine clearance of 30 to 50 mL/min.
- Do not use in patients with a creatinine clearance less than 30 mL/min.

Dosage range

DVT prophylaxis. *Subcutaneous:* 2.5 mg daily at least 6 to 8 hours after hip fracture, hip replacement, or knee replacement surgery. The usual duration of once daily administration is 5 to 9 days, and up to 11 days of administration has been tolerated. In patients undergoing hip fracture surgery, an extended prophylaxis course of up to 24 additional days is recommended. After abdominal surgery in patients weighing at least 50 kg, administer 2.5 mg subcutaneously 6 to 8 hours after surgery. Usual once-daily administration is 5 to 9 days, up to 10 days. Do not administer to patients weighing less than 50 kg.

Acute DVT and PE treatment. *Subcutaneous:* 5 mg (body weight <50 kg), 7.5 mg (body weight = 50 to 100 kg), or 10 mg (body weight >100 kg) once daily. Continue treatment for at least 5 days until a therapeutic oral anticoagulant effect becomes established (INR 2 to 3). Initiate concomitant treatment with warfarin as soon as possible, usually within 72 hours. The usual duration of administration of fondaparinux is 5 to 9 days (up to 26 days).

◆ *Common adverse effects*

Hematologic

Hematoma formation and bleeding at injection site. Inappropriate administration techniques lead to hematoma formation at the site of injection. **Use proper technique!**

◆ *Serious adverse effects*

Hematologic

Bleeding. Inspect the skin and mucous membranes for petechiae, ecchymoses, or hematomas; also monitor for bleeding gums. Assess and record vital signs at regular intervals. Monitor and report signs and symptoms of internal bleeding (e.g., decreasing blood pressure; increasing pulse; cold, clammy skin; feeling faint; disoriented sensorium).

Check urine and stools for blood. Urine may appear red, smoke colored, or brownish. Stools may appear to be dark and tarry. Perform an occult blood test on the stool if necessary. Vomitus may contain bright red blood or may have a coffee-ground appearance.

Assessment of dressings or drainage tubes for any signs of bleeding is necessary for postoperative patients.

Thrombocytopenia. Fondaparinux may cause thrombocytopenia. Monitor platelet counts on a daily basis. It is recommended that fondaparinux therapy be discontinued if platelet counts drop below 100,000/mm^3.

◆ *Drug interactions.* No clinically significant drug interactions have been reported, but fondaparinux should be used cautiously in patients receiving antiplatelet or warfarin therapy.

---

heparin (HĔP-rĭn)
⇌ *Do not confuse heparin with Hespan.*

Actions

Heparin is a natural substance extracted from gut and lung tissue of pigs and cows. In full therapeutic doses, heparin acts as a catalyst to accelerate the rate of action of a naturally occurring inhibitor of thrombin, antithrombin III (sometimes called the heparin cofactor). In the presence of heparin, antithrombin III rapidly neutralizes factor IIa; activated factors IX, X, XI, and XII; and plasmin. Heparin also inhibits activation of factor VIII, the fibrin stabilizing factor, preventing soluble fibrin clots from becoming insoluble clots (see Fig. 26.1). Heparin has no fibrinolytic activity and cannot lyse established fibrin clots.

In low doses, heparin causes the neutralization of only factor Xa, preventing the conversion of prothrombin to thrombin, which allows lower dosages to be used with fewer complications from therapy. This is the rationale routinely used in prophylaxis with subcutaneous heparin to prevent postoperative thrombi.

Uses

Heparin is used to treat DVT, PE, peripheral arterial embolism, and MI and for PCIs. It is used in the treatment of patients with heart valve prostheses. It is also used prophylactically during cardiovascular surgery; in postoperative, immobilized patients; and during hemodialysis to prevent active coagulation and clot formation and to maintain patency of venous access devices. When testing for adequate anticoagulation by heparin, the aPTT is measured. The target range for full anticoagulation is 1.5 to 2.5 times the control time (e.g., if the control time is 25 seconds and the patient's aPTT is 38 to 64 seconds, the patient is considered to be adequately anticoagulated). Another laboratory test that is becoming more frequently used is the measurement of anti–factor Xa levels. Therapeutic ranges of anti–factor Xa for heparin are 0.3 to 0.7 units/mL and for LMWHs are 0.5 to 1 units/mL.

Therapeutic Outcomes

The primary therapeutic outcomes from heparin therapy are as follows:

1. When used in low doses prophylactically, heparin prevents DVT.
2. In full doses, heparin is used to treat a thromboembolism and promote neutralization of activated clotting factors, thus preventing the extension of thrombi and the formation of emboli. If therapy is started shortly after the formation of a thrombus, heparin will minimize tissue damage by preventing it from developing into an insoluble stable thrombus.

❖ **Nursing Implications for Heparin**

◆ *Premedication assessment*

1. Take baseline vital signs.
2. Always check the most recent laboratory data (aPTT) to ensure that the results are within the recommended range for heparin therapy.
3. Inspect the skin and mucous membranes for petechiae, ecchymoses, or hematomas. Also monitor for hematuria, bleeding gums, and melena before administering each dose of medication.

◆ *Availability. Subcutaneous, Intravenous (IV):* 1000, 2000, 5000, 10,000, and 20,000 units/mL in various concentrations and sizes of ampules, vials, prefilled syringes, and IV infusion solutions.

◆ Dosage and administration

Accuracy of dose. Always confirm the dosage calculations with two nurses before subcutaneous or IV administration. Be certain the strength is correct. There is a *drastic difference* in clinical response between 1 mL of 1:1000 units and 1 mL of 1:10,000 units of heparin.

Dosage adjustment. Blood samples for laboratory studies (aPTT, anti–factor Xa) are usually drawn 4 to 6 hours after the initiation of a continuous IV infusion. Do not draw blood samples from the same arm being used for heparin infusion. The effects of heparin only last 4 hours, so a continuous infusion is needed. When the aPTT or anti–factor Xa level is too high, the heparin infusion can be stopped for an hour and then restarted at a lower rate. The use of a nomogram may be employed to maintain a steady state of anticoagulation, which adjusts the heparin infusion according to the aPTT or anti–factor Xa when appropriate.

Heparin dosage is considered to be in the normal therapeutic range if the aPTT is 1.5 to 2.5 times the control aPTT value (e.g., if control is 30 seconds, the patient receiving full-dose heparin should have an aPTT of 45 to 75 seconds for optimal therapy). If anti–factor Xa is used, the normal therapeutic range is 0.3 to 0.7 units/mL.

Subcutaneous: Prophylactic: 5000 units every 8 to 12 hours. *Therapeutic:* Initially, 10,000 to 15,000 units. *Maintenance:* Loading dose: 10,000 to 20,000 units, followed by 8000 to 10,000 units every 8 hours, or 15,000 units every 12 hours.

Subcutaneous injection is usually made into the tissue over the abdomen (Fig. 26.2). Do not inject within 2 inches of the umbilicus. The injection site should not be massaged before or after injection, and sites should be rotated for each dose to prevent the development of a massive hematoma.

Needle length and angle need to be adapted to the patient's size so that the drug will be deposited into the subcutaneous tissue. (Usually, a 26- or 27-gauge, ½-inch needle is used.) The injection is usually made at a 90-degree angle to the skin. *Do not* aspirate. This will increase local tissue damage and create the possibility of hematoma formation. *Do not* inject into a hematoma or an area with any infection present. Follow a planned site rotation schedule.

After injection, apply gentle pressure for 1 or 2 minutes to control local bleeding, but do not massage the area. Ice packs may be used on the site after injection; check the institutional policy. At this time, there is little documented evidence that ice packs prevent hematoma formation or affect drug absorption.

Intramuscular (IM): Not recommended because of the development of hematomas.

IV (intermittent): Initial: 10,000-unit bolus. *Maintenance:* 5000 to 10,000 units every 4 to 6 hours. A heparin lock, consisting of a 22- to 29-gauge scalp vein needle attached to a 3½-inch tubing ending in a resealing rubber diaphragm, may be used to administer intermittent IV doses of heparin. Advantages of a heparin lock are the mobility that it provides the patient and fewer venipunctures.

After injecting a bolus of heparin through the rubber diaphragm, flush the line with saline according to individual institutional policy. The heparin flush solution ensures that the patient will receive the entire heparin bolus, and it prevents the formation of a clot in the scalp vein needle.

IV (continuous infusion): Initial: 70- to 100-unit/kg bolus. *Maintenance:* 15 to 25 units/kg/hr. Continuous infusions of heparin provide the advantage of steady heparin levels in the blood. Periodic dosage adjustment is required based on the response of the patient.

When starting a heparin infusion, always have two nurses confirm calculations and the strength of the heparin to be used. As a safety measure, heparin drips should be a single concentration to avoid medication errors (typically 25,000 units in 250 mg [100 units/mL], but confirm with institutional policy). This protects patients from receiving massive doses of heparin should the infusion "run away." Always use a programmable infusion pump for IV infusions. However, the infusion should be monitored at least every 30 to 60 minutes.

Antidote. Protamine sulfate, 1 mg, will neutralize approximately 100 units of heparin, dalteparin, and 1 mg of enoxaparin. If protamine sulfate is given more than 30 minutes after the heparin or LMWHs were administered, give only half the dose. Because excessive doses of protamine may also cause excessive coagulation, it must be used judiciously.

◆ Common adverse effects.

Patients receiving full-dose heparin therapy should be monitored for hematocrit, platelet counts, aPTT, and signs of bleeding.

Adverse effects of heparin therapy are most commonly caused by inappropriate administration technique or overdosage. Factors that can influence the incidence

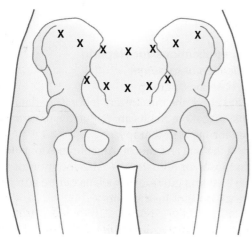

Fig. 26.2 Sites of heparin administration.

of complications include age, weight, gender, and recent trauma. The most common signs of overdosage are petechiae, hematomas, hematuria, bleeding gums, and melena.

Hematologic

Hematoma formation and bleeding at the injection site. Inappropriate administration techniques lead to hematoma formation at the site of injection. **Use proper technique!**

◆ Serious adverse effects
Hematologic

Bleeding. Inspect the skin and mucous membranes for petechiae, ecchymoses, or hematomas; also monitor for bleeding gums. Assess and record vital signs at regular intervals. Always monitor menstrual flow to be certain that it is not excessive or prolonged. Monitor and report signs and symptoms of internal bleeding (e.g., decreasing blood pressure; increasing pulse; cold, clammy skin; feeling faint; disoriented sensorium).

Check urine and stools for blood. Urine may appear red, smoke colored, or brownish. Stools may appear to be dark and tarry. Perform an occult blood test on the stool if necessary. Vomitus may contain bright red blood or may have a coffee-ground appearance.

Assessment of dressings or drainage tubes for any signs of bleeding is necessary for postoperative patients.

Thrombocytopenia. Heparin therapy may cause two types of HIT. Type I HIT results from a direct effect of heparin on platelets, causing sequestration and a fall in the platelet count to as low as $100,000/mm^3$. This reversible form of thrombocytopenia occurs within the first several days of heparin therapy. The patient is asymptomatic, and heparin therapy should be continued if therapeutically indicated. The platelet count should return to normal.

Type II HIT should be suspected when the platelet count falls below $100,000/mm^3$ or falls 50% below the baseline value. This type of thrombocytopenia is an allergic reaction to heparin that causes aggregation of platelets. The onset of falling platelet counts is immediate after heparin therapy is started if the patient has previously received heparin, whereas it occurs after 5 to 22 days in the previously unexposed patient. Type II HIT occurs in about 0.3% to 3% of patients. Patients are at risk for white thrombus formation caused by sudden aggregation of platelets. Heparin therapy should be immediately discontinued if patients develop signs of clot formation, such as pain in an extremity, symptoms of a stroke, or chest pain resembling angina. Warfarin therapy may be initiated or continued when the platelet count is greater than $100,000/mm^3$, and antiplatelet therapy (aspirin) may also be started. Direct thrombin inhibitors such as argatroban or bivalirudin may also be used. Fondaparinux may also be used cautiously. Low-molecular-weight heparins are contraindicated because of the potential for cross-allergenicity. Platelet counts should be monitored daily.

◆ Drug interactions

Drugs that increase therapeutic and toxic effects. Concurrent use of NSAIDs, aspirin, danshen, ginkgo biloba, dipyridamole, clopidogrel, and direct thrombin inhibitors (argatroban, dabigatran, desirudin) may predispose the patient to hemorrhage.

---

warfarin (WĂR-făr-ĭn)
   Coumadin (KŪ-mă-dĭn)
   ⇄ *Do not confuse Coumadin with Cardura, Avandia, or Ambien.*

Actions

Warfarin is a potent anticoagulant that acts by inhibiting the activity of vitamin K, which is required for the activation of clotting factors II, VII, IX, and X and proteins C and S in the blood. Blockade of the activation of these factors prevents clot formation (see Fig. 26.1).

Uses

Warfarin is used for treatment and prophylaxis of venous thrombosis, embolism associated with atrial fibrillation or heart valve replacement, PE, and coronary occlusion. The dosage of warfarin is adjusted based on prolonging the INR. In general, the target range for the INR with warfarin therapy is 2 to 3 when treating atrial fibrillation, embolic stroke, MI, and DVT. When anticoagulating the patient with a mechanical prosthetic heart valve, the target INR range is 2.5 to 3.5.

Therapeutic Outcomes

The primary therapeutic outcomes from warfarin therapy are as follows:

1. Prevention and treatment of venous thrombosis and embolism
2. Prevention and treatment of thromboemboli associated with atrial fibrillation
3. Reduced risk of death, recurrent MI, and thromboembolic events, such as stroke, after MI
4. Prevention and treatment of thromboemboli associated with cardiac valve replacement

❖ Nursing Implications for Warfarin
◆ Premedication assessment

1. Obtain baseline vital signs.
2. Always check the most recent PT or INR results to determine whether they are within the recommended range for warfarin therapy.
3. Inspect the skin and mucous membranes for petechiae, ecchymoses, or hematomas. Also monitor for hematuria, bleeding gums, and melena before administering each dose of medication.
4. Ensure that patients of childbearing age are not pregnant at the time warfarin therapy is initiated. Warfarin therapy should be avoided during pregnancy, particularly in weeks 6 through 12 and at term. Warfarin may be administered during pregnancy

in patients with prosthetic heart valves after discussing the risks and benefits of therapy with the patient.

5. Provide dietary education to include information on those foods high in vitamin K, including green leafy vegetables.

◆ *Availability.* *PO:* Tablets: 1, 2, 2.5, 3, 4, 5, 6, 7.5, and 10 mg.

◆ *Dosage and administration.* **Adult:** *Dosage adjustment:* Dosage during therapy is based on the PT. The PT is expressed as the INR, an internationally accepted standard for adjusting for variability in the PT assay. The optimal dosage is that which prolongs the INR at 2 to 3. Certain medical conditions (e.g., mechanical prosthetic valves, recurrent systemic embolism) require an INR of 2.5 to 3.5 and concurrent antiplatelet therapy.

When warfarin therapy is initiated, the patient should be monitored closely for evidence of hemorrhage because of the drug's cumulative effects.

Stress the need to comply with the prescribed regimen and the need for laboratory data to determine the correct maintenance dose. Instruct the patient to resume a regular schedule if one dose is missed. If two or more doses are missed, the patient should consult the healthcare provider.

PO: Initial: 2 to 5 mg/day, adjusting the dosage every few days until the INR is in the target range. Use of a loading dose is not recommended because it does not anticoagulate the patient any more rapidly than starting with maintenance doses and may result in severe hemorrhagic complications.

Maintenance: 2 to 10 mg daily as determined by the PT (reported as the INR).

Antidote. Vitamin K is a specific antidote for warfarin-induced hemorrhage or reversal of an excessively high INR. Most cases of bleeding induced by warfarin overdose can be controlled by discontinuing warfarin therapy. A prothrombin complex concentrate is available for urgent reversal in patients with acute major bleeding or a need for an urgent surgery/invasive procedure. An alternative in severe hemorrhage is a transfusion with plasma or whole blood.

◆ *Common adverse effects*
Hematologic
Bleeding. Inspect the skin and mucous membranes for petechiae, ecchymoses, or hematomas; also monitor for bleeding gums. Assess and record vital signs at regular intervals. Always monitor menstrual flow to be certain that it is not excessive or prolonged. Monitor and report signs and symptoms of internal bleeding (e.g., decreasing blood pressure; increasing pulse; cold, clammy skin; feelings of faintness; disoriented sensorium).

Check urine and stools for blood. Urine may appear red, smoke colored, or brownish. Stools may appear to be dark and tarry. Perform an occult blood test on the stool if necessary. Vomitus may contain bright red blood or may have a coffee-ground appearance.

Assessment of dressings or drainage tubes for any signs of bleeding is necessary for postoperative patients.

◆ *Drug interactions*
Drugs that enhance therapeutic and toxic effects. The following drugs, foods, and herbal supplements, when used concurrently with warfarin, may enhance its therapeutic and toxic effects:

acetaminophen	fluorouracil	omeprazole
allopurinol	fluoxetine	paclitaxel
amiodarone	flutamide	papaya
anabolic	fluvastatin	phenytoin
steroids	fluvoxamine	piroxicam
aspirin	gemcitabine	propafenone
beta blockers	ginkgo biloba	propranolol
capecitabine	grapefruit	quinidine
cimetidine	ifosfamide	ropinirole
ciprofloxacin	isoniazid	salicylates
cisapride	itraconazole	sertraline
citalopram	ketoconazole	simvastatin
clofibrate	levofloxacin	sulfinpyrazone
cotrimoxazole	lovastatin	sulfonamides
danshen	lyceum	tamoxifen
devil's claw	methyl	tetracyclines
diltiazem	salicylate	thyroid
disulfiram	(oil of	hormones
dong quai	wintergreen)	tolterodine
entacapone	metronidazole	tramadol
erythromycin	miconazole	valproate
ethanol	moricizine	voriconazole
fenofibrate	norfloxacin	zafirlukast
fish oil	NSAIDs	zileuton
fluconazole	ofloxacin	

Drugs that decrease therapeutic effects. The following drugs, foods, and herbal supplements, when used concurrently with warfarin, may decrease its therapeutic activity:

acerola	cholestyramine	ritonavir
aprepitant	coenzyme Q10	rose hip
azathioprine	dicloxacillin	smartweed
black psyllium	etretinate	St. John's wort
blond psyllium	griseofulvin	sucralfate
bosentan	mercaptopurine	terbinafine
cabbage	mesalamine	trazodone
carbamazepine	nafcillin	vitamin C
chlordiazepoxide	phenobarbital	vitamin K
	rifampin	

All prescription and nonprescription medications. Caution the patient not to take any over-the-counter (including herbal supplements) or prescription medications without first consulting a healthcare provider or pharmacist.

DRUG CLASS: THROMBIN INHIBITORS

dabigatran (dă-BĬG-ă-trăn)
Pradaxa (pră-DĂK-să)

Actions

Dabigatran is a direct thrombin inhibitor. Inhibition of thrombin prevents the conversion of fibrinogen to fibrin, which is required for the formation of a thrombus (blood clot). The oral dosage form, dabigatran etexilate, is a prodrug that is rapidly converted to dabigatran, which is further metabolized to four active metabolites. Dabigatran and the four active metabolites also inhibit thrombin-induced platelet aggregation, another essential step in clot formation.

Three other direct thrombin inhibitors—argatroban, bivalirudin, and desirudin—are used in specialized cases (see Uses section).

Uses

Dabigatran is approved and orally administered to:
- Reduce the risk of stroke and systemic embolism in patients with nonvalvular atrial fibrillation
- Treat DVT and PE in patients who have been treated with a parenteral anticoagulant for 5 to 10 days
- Reduce the risk of recurrence of DVT and PE in patients who have been previously treated
- Provide prophylaxis for DVT and PE in patients who have undergone hip replacement surgery

A major advantage of dabigatran is that it does not require monitoring of blood tests with resultant dosage adjustments, as do warfarin and IV heparin.

The other direct thrombin inhibitors are approved for the following uses:
- Argatroban is approved as an anticoagulant for use in patients at risk of HIT undergoing a PCI or in patients being treated for HIT. It is administered intravenously by continuous infusion.
- Bivalirudin is approved as an anticoagulant for patients undergoing PCI, patients with unstable angina undergoing percutaneous transluminal coronary angioplasty, and in patients at risk for or who are being treated for HIT. It is administered intravenously by continuous infusion.
- Desirudin is approved for postoperative prophylaxis for patients undergoing hip replacement surgery. It is administered subcutaneously.

Therapeutic Outcome

The primary therapeutic outcome expected from the direct thrombin inhibitors is prevention and treatment of thrombosis in specialized cases.

❖ Nursing Implications for Dabigatran
◆ Premedication assessment
1. Obtain baseline blood pressure readings in supine and standing positions and apical pulse.
2. Initiate laboratory studies as requested by the healthcare provider (e.g., renal function tests such as serum creatinine, CBC, ECT, TT, and aPTT) to serve as a baseline for future comparison. If the ECT is not available, the aPTT may be used. The PT (INR)

is not a good indicator of dabigatran coagulation activity.
3. Ask whether the patient is pregnant or likely to become pregnant. If so, discuss with the healthcare provider before initiating dabigatran therapy.
4. Obtain a history of bowel elimination patterns and any GI symptoms, frequency of headaches, dizziness, and fatigue.

◆ *Availability.* **PO:** 75-, 110-, and 150-mg capsules.

◆ *Dosage and administration*
Nonvalvular atrial fibrillation. *To reduce the risk of stroke and systemic embolism:* **PO:** 150 mg twice a day. If creatinine clearance is below 30 mL/min, the dose is 75 mg PO twice a day.
DVT and PE. *Treatment and prevention:* **PO:** 150 mg twice daily, after 5 to 10 days of parenteral anticoagulation. *Reduction of recurrence:* **PO:** 150 mg twice daily. *Prophylaxis after hip replacement surgery:* **PO:** 110 mg given 1 to 4 hours after completion of surgery and establishment of hemostasis; if not initiated on the day of surgery, initiate therapy with 220 mg once daily after hemostasis has been achieved. Maintenance: 220 mg once daily (total duration of therapy: 28 to 35 days). *Prophylaxis after knee replacement surgery:* **PO:** 150 or 220 mg once daily for 10 to 35 days with a half-dose 1 to 4 hours after surgery.

> **⚠ Medication Safety Alert**
> - The capsules must be swallowed whole with a full glass of water. Do not crush the capsule or pull it apart and sprinkle the pellets on food. A severe overdose may potentially result.
> - If a dose is not taken at the scheduled time, it should be taken as soon as possible on the same day. If the dose cannot be taken at least 6 hours before the next scheduled dose, it should not be taken. Do not double up on doses at the same time.
> - Dabigatran capsules are sensitive to moisture. Reseal the bottle quickly after taking a capsule out. The container holds 60 capsules that should be taken within 30 days. Once the bottle has been opened, use within 30 days.

Antidote. Idarucizumab (Praxbind) is used as an antidote to reverse bleeding caused by dabigatran.

◆ *Common adverse effects*
Hematologic
Bleeding. A normal physiologic effect of dabigatran is prolongation of bleeding time. Patients should report any incidents of bleeding as soon as possible. Incidents to be reported include nosebleeds; easy bruising; bright red or coffee-ground emesis; hematuria; and dark, tarry stools.

Patients should inform other healthcare practitioners (e.g., another physician, dentist) that they are receiving thrombin inhibitor therapy.

Gastrointestinal

Dyspepsia, reflux, gastritis. These adverse effects may be early indications of GI bleeding. Observe for dark, tarry stools and report to the healthcare provider. Encourage the patient not to discontinue therapy without first consulting the healthcare provider.

◆ *Drug interactions*

Drugs that enhance therapeutic and toxic effects. Heparin, LMWHs, warfarin, aspirin, NSAIDs, fondaparinux, and direct thrombin inhibitors (argatroban, bivalirudin, desirudin) will have an additive bleeding effect in the patient. Monitor very closely for indications of bleeding. Caution should be used when any of these drugs are coadministered with dabigatran.

DRUG CLASS: GLYCOPROTEIN IIB/IIIA INHIBITORS

During PCI procedures, it was found that patients were susceptible to new blood clots forming from the debris often released from atherosclerotic plaque disruption. Antiplatelet and antithrombotic agents such as aspirin and heparin were initially used, but new agents, called glycoprotein IIb/IIIa inhibitors, have been developed. Three of these inhibitors are now available: abciximab (ReoPro), eptifibatide (Integrilin), and tirofiban (Aggrastat).

Actions

The glycoprotein IIb/IIIa inhibitors act by blocking the glycoprotein IIb/IIIa receptor on platelets, preventing platelet aggregation and clot formation. Platelet aggregation inhibition persists during continuous infusion and is reversible on discontinuing the infusion.

Uses

Glycoprotein IIb/IIIa inhibitors are administered intravenously during the PCI procedure and for 12 to 24 hours afterward, significantly reducing the risk of acute MI and death. Other antiplatelet and antithrombotic agents such as aspirin, clopidogrel, and heparin are used in conjunction with the glycoprotein IIb/IIIa inhibitors. Major complications of therapy include bleeding and thrombocytopenia. The hematocrit, platelet counts, and ACT must be monitored closely during and after therapy.

Therapeutic Outcome

The primary therapeutic outcome from glycoprotein IIb/IIIa inhibitor therapy is prevention of clot formation during PCI procedures.

DRUG CLASS: FIBRINOLYTIC AGENTS

There have been significant advances in the treatment of thromboemboli. Enzymes have been discovered that work in the clotting system to dissolve recently formed thrombi. The agents used are called fibrinolytic agents because of their ability to cause the dissolution of fibrin clots.

All fibrinolytic agents increase the risk of bleeding, including intracranial bleeding, and should be used only in eligible patients. In addition, fibrinolytic therapy increases the risk of intracranial hemorrhage in older adult patients.

The goals of fibrinolytic therapy are to lyse the thrombi during the early phase of clot formation, limit the damage to surrounding tissues by restoring circulation to the area distal to the thrombus, and reduce the morbidity and mortality after the formation of a thromboembolism.

Actions

Fibrinolytic agents work by stimulating the body's own clot-dissolving mechanism, converting plasminogen, a naturally occurring substance secreted by endothelial cells in response to injury to the artery, to plasmin (also known as fibrinolysin), which digests fibrin. The clot is then dissolved, restoring blood flow to the area. There are currently four fibrinolytic agents available—streptokinase, alteplase, reteplase, and tenecteplase.

Streptokinase is rarely used; it is being replaced by the newer fibrinolytic agents:

- Alteplase (recombinant tissue plasminogen activator [rtPA]; Activase) is of proven clinical effectiveness, more clot specific (a lower potential for hemorrhage elsewhere in the body), and nonantigenic. Disadvantages are a 10- to 20-fold higher cost, a prolonged administration time, and the need for concurrent heparin therapy.
- Reteplase (rtPA; Retavase) is administered as two boluses to dissolve clots. It is of proven clinical effectiveness, more clot specific (a lower potential for hemorrhage elsewhere in the body), and nonantigenic. Its disadvantage is the need for concurrent heparin therapy.
- Tenecteplase (rtPA; TNKase) is approved for use to treat clots associated with MI. It is the first clot buster that can be administered over 5 seconds in a single dose, offering healthcare providers the fastest administration of a thrombolytic to date in the treatment of heart attack. Tenecteplase is a bioengineered variant of alteplase. The ease of administration may allow this drug to be administered outside the hospital while the patient is being transported to a cardiovascular center, buying potentially lifesaving time.

Uses

The fibrinolytic agents are used to dissolve clots secondary to coronary artery occlusion (MI, also known as acute coronary syndrome), PE, and stroke. Alteplase is used to treat cerebral embolism (stroke). The decisions for use and selection of the agent depend on the location of the thrombus, clinical condition and age of the patient, preference of the patient care team, and availability of alternative therapies, such as angioplasty or bypass graft surgery. A key factor in the successful treatment of these conditions is the early treatment with a fibrinolytic agent. Fibrinolytic agents tend to be much more successful against the soluble fibrin clot in restoring circulation to the obstructed area, rather than older, insoluble clots.

Alteplase and reteplase may also be used to reopen IV catheters, including central venous catheters, obstructed by blood clots.

Therapeutic Outcome

The primary therapeutic outcome from fibrinolytic therapy is reperfusion of the tissues obstructed by the thrombus.

Get Ready for the NCLEX® Examination!

Key Points

- Diseases caused by intravascular clotting are major causes of death and must be treated rapidly to reduce tissue damage associated with thrombosis.
- The major pharmacologic therapeutic agents are platelet inhibitors, factor Xa inhibitors, anticoagulants, thrombin inhibitors, glycoprotein IIb/IIIa inhibitors, and fibrinolytic agents.
- Nurses can play a significant role, especially in the nonpharmacologic prevention and treatment of thromboembolic disease, which includes patient education on how to prevent venous stasis and appropriate use of prescribed medicines.

Additional Learning Resources

SG   Go to your Study Guide for additional Review Questions for the NCLEX® Examination, Critical Thinking Clinical Situations, and other learning activities to help you master this chapter content.

Go to your Evolve website (https://evolve.elsevier.com/Clayton) for additional online resources.

Review Questions for the NCLEX® Examination

1. The nurse knows that patients who are immobile are at risk for developing clots, as well as patients with which of these conditions? *(Select all that apply.)*
   1. Cancer of the lung
   2. Trauma to the lower extremities
   3. Allergic reactions to drugs
   4. Pregnancy
   5. Vasospasms of the lower extremities

2. Which of the following conditions are reasons for having patients receive anticoagulant therapy? *(Select all that apply.)*
   1. Atrial fibrillation
   2. History of pulmonary emboli
   3. Recent hip surgery
   4. Hematuria
   5. Asthma

3. A patient was started on aspirin to prevent a stroke because aspirin has which effect?
   1. Prevents the clotting cascade from being activated
   2. Prevents thrombus formation
   3. Prevents platelet aggregation
   4. Decreases bleeding time

4. The direct thrombin inhibitor dabigatran (Pradaxa) is used for which purpose?
   1. To break up an existing thrombus
   2. To prevent the extension of an existing thrombus
   3. To prevent strokes or thrombus formation in patients with atrial fibrillation
   4. To prevent thrombus formation after hip surgery

5. Fibrinolytic agents such as alteplase are often used for which reason? *(Select all that apply.)*
   1. To prevent the extension of a thrombus
   2. To reopen a central venous catheter
   3. To maintain patency of a stent after PCI
   4. To dissolve a thromboemboli once formed
   5. To prevent a stroke in patients with atrial fibrillation

6. Which laboratory tests are used to monitor the dosage of warfarin?
   1. INR and PT
   2. INR and WBC
   3. INR and ACT
   4. PT and aPTT

7. The nurse initiated discharge teaching for a patient who is to be maintained on warfarin (Coumadin) after hospitalization for thrombophlebitis. Which statement by the patient indicates that further teaching is needed?
   1. "I should change my diet to include more green leafy vegetables."
   2. "I will check with my physician or pharmacist before I begin or stop any medication."
   3. "I should wear a Medic-Alert bracelet to indicate I am on anticoagulant therapy."
   4. "I will need to have my blood drawn routinely to monitor the effects of the Coumadin."

8. The nurse administering enoxaparin (Lovenox) made certain to follow which safety precautions? *(Select all that apply.)*
   1. Rotate the injection site.
   2. Remove the air bubble from the prefilled syringe.
   3. Rub the site after injection to ensure distribution of the drug.
   4. Inject the medication in the subcutaneous tissue in the abdomen.
   5. Dispose of the needle and syringe in the proper sharps container.

Objectives

1. Explain heart failure in terms of the body's compensatory mechanisms.
2. Identify the goals of treatment for heart failure.
3. Identify the primary actions on heart failure of digoxin, angiotensin-converting enzyme inhibitors, angiotensin

receptor blockers, the combination of a neprilysin inhibitor with an angiotensin receptor blocker, and beta blockers.
4. Describe digoxin toxicity and ways to prevent it.
5. Identify essential assessment data and nursing interventions needed for a patient with heart failure.

Key Terms

systolic dysfunction (sĭs-TŎL-ĭk dĭs-FŪNK-shŭn) (p. 420)
diastolic dysfunction (dī-ă-STŎL-ĭk dĭs-FŪNK-shŭn) (p. 420)
inotropic agents (ĭn-ō-TRŌ-pĭk Ā-jĕnts) (p. 422)
digitalis toxicity (dĭ-jĭ-TĂL-ĭs tŏk-SĬS-ĭ-tē) (p. 427)

positive inotropy (PŎZ-ĭ-tĭv ī-nō-TRŌ-pē) (p. 431)
negative chronotropy (NĔG-ĕ-tĭv krō-nō-TRŌ-pē) (p. 431)
digitalization (dĭ-jĭ-tăl-ī-ZĀ-shŭn) (p. 431)

HEART FAILURE

The incidence of heart failure (previously known as *congestive heart failure*)—unlike that of other cardiovascular diseases—continues to increase as a result of population aging and improved survival after acute myocardial infarction (MI). The lifetime risk of developing heart failure is 20% to 45% for Americans at 45 to 95 years of age. An estimated 6.5 million Americans have this disabling condition; more than 960,000 patients develop heart failure annually, and more than 300,000 people die from heart failure each year. The 5-year mortality rate for heart failure is approximately 50%. The economic burden is staggering, with an estimated total cost of $30 billion for managing heart failure in the United States (Benjamin et al, 2017).

Heart failure involves a cluster of signs and symptoms that arise when the left or right ventricle or both ventricles lose the ability to pump enough blood to meet the body's circulatory needs. The most common type of heart failure is **systolic dysfunction** (also known as *contracting dysfunction*). Normally, the heart pumps at a rate that supports the body's need for blood flow and oxygenation of the vital organs and muscles. Systolic heart failure results when the heart lacks sufficient force to pump all the blood (resulting in decreased cardiac output) with which it is presented to meet the body's oxygenation needs (causing decreased tissue perfusion). Early clinical symptoms are decreased exercise tolerance and poor perfusion to the peripheral tissues. As the condition progresses, the left ventricle chamber enlarges

(left ventricular hypertrophy) and an increase in blood volume is required to fill the expanding ventricle to maintain cardiac output. Causes of systolic dysfunction are those that cause damage to the heart muscle itself. The most common is coronary artery disease that leads to MI. Other causes include dysrhythmias, cardiomyopathies, and congenital heart disease. Usually the left ventricle fails first and, as the disease progresses, the right ventricle also enlarges due to increased pulmonary resistance, and it eventually fails.

Diastolic dysfunction (or *filling dysfunction*) causes heart failure because the left ventricle develops a "stiffness" and fails to relax enough between contractions to allow adequate filling before the next contraction. Symptoms of diastolic dysfunction include pulmonary congestion and peripheral edema. There are many reasons why diastolic dysfunction develops, including constrictive pericarditis, ventricular muscle hypertrophy caused by chronic hypertension, valvular heart disease that results in flow resistance, and aortic stenosis.

The general pathogenesis of heart failure is diagrammed in Fig. 27.1. When the vital organs and peripheral tissues are not adequately perfused, compensatory mechanisms begin to overcome the inadequate output of the heart. The natriuretic system is activated primarily by volume expansion. The natriuretic peptides released are beneficial, causing a decrease in blood pressure and diuresis. The sympathetic nervous system releases epinephrine and norepinephrine, which produce tachycardia and increase contractility. The increased

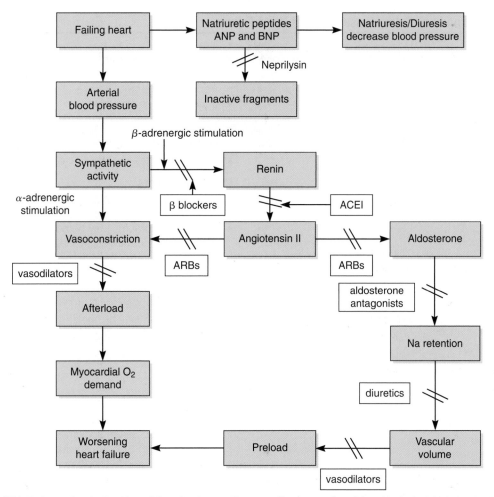

Fig. 27.1 Pathway showing how heart failure develops and how specific classes of medicines block physiologic mechanisms to reduce the worsening of heart failure. Cardiac glycosides and phosphodiesterase inhibitors are also used to increase myocardial contractility. *ACEI,* Angiotensin-converting enzyme inhibitor; *ANP,* atrial natriuretic peptide; *ARBs,* angiotensin II receptor blockers; *BNP,* B-type natriuretic peptide; *β blockers,* beta-adrenergic blocking agents.

sympathetic stimulation also increases peripheral vasoconstriction, which results in an increased afterload against which the heart must pump, causing a further decrease in cardiac output (see Fig. 27.1). The renin-angiotensin-aldosterone system stimulates renal distal tubule sodium and water retention in an effort to increase circulating blood volume, which increases preload to the heart. There is also an increased production of vasopressin (antidiuretic hormone) from the pituitary gland that increases water recovery from the kidneys and increases intravascular volume and preload. With decreased perfusion secondary to low cardiac output, the kidneys also increase sodium reabsorption in the proximal tubules to help expand circulating blood volume. The increased intravascular volume initially improves tissue perfusion; however, over time, excessive amounts of sodium and water are retained, causing increased pressure within the capillaries, resulting in edema formation.

Early symptoms of heart failure vary depending on the underlying cause of the disease. Traditionally, the signs and symptoms of heart failure have been classified on the basis of whether failure is developing in the right ventricle or the left ventricle. However, it has been found that, because of the complexity of the syndrome, the symptoms overlap to such an extent that it is difficult to attribute a particular clinical indicator to a specific ventricle. It is also important to recognize that the clinical indicators vary considerably over time in response to the treatments being applied (Box 27.1).

TREATMENT OF HEART FAILURE

The overall goals for treating heart failure are to reduce the signs and symptoms associated with fluid overload, increase exercise tolerance, improve quality of life, and prolong life. If the heart failure is acute, the patient must be hospitalized for a diagnostic workup to determine the underlying cause. A combination of the American College of Cardiology Foundation and the American Heart Association (ACCF/AHA) and the New York Heart Association (NYHA) Functional Classification System is commonly used to group patients with heart failure according to the degree of impairment

Box 27.1 Clinical and Laboratory Presentation of Heart Failure

GENERAL

Patient presentation may range from asymptomatic to cardiogenic shock.

SYMPTOMS
- Dyspnea, particularly on exertion
- Orthopnea
- Paroxysmal nocturnal dyspnea
- Exercise intolerance
- Tachypnea
- Cough
- Fatigue
- Nocturia
- Hemoptysis
- Abdominal pain
- Anorexia
- Nausea
- Bloating
- Poor appetite; early satiety
- Ascites
- Mental status changes
- Weight gain or loss

SIGNS
- Pulmonary crackles
- Pulmonary edema
- S_3 gallop
- Cool extremities
- Pleural effusion
- Cheyne-Stokes respiration

- Tachycardia
- Narrow pulse pressure
- Cardiomegaly
- Peripheral edema
- Jugular venous distention
- Hepatojugular reflux
- Hepatomegaly
- Venous stasis changes
- Lateral displacement of apical impulse

LABORATORY TESTS
- B-type natriuretic peptide (BNP) level >100 pg/mL
- N-terminal proBNP level >300 pg/mL
- *Electrocardiography:* May be normal or could show numerous abnormalities, including acute ST-T wave changes from myocardial ischemia, atrial fibrillation, bradycardia, and left ventricular hypertrophy
- *Serum creatinine:* May be increased as a result of hypoperfusion; preexisting renal dysfunction can contribute to volume overload
- *Complete blood count:* Useful to determine if heart failure is caused by reduced oxygen-carrying capacity
- *Chest radiography:* Useful for detection of cardiac enlargement, pulmonary edema, and pleural effusions
- *Echocardiography:* Used to assess left ventricular size, valve function, pericardial effusion, wall motion abnormalities, and ejection fraction
- *Hyponatremia:* Serum sodium level <130 mEq/L is associated with reduced survival and may indicate worsening volume overload or disease progression

From Parker RB, Nappi JM, Cavallari LH. Chronic heart failure. In: DiPiro JP, Talbert RL, Yee G, et al, eds. *Pharmacotherapy: A Pathophysiologic Approach.* 9th ed. New York: McGraw-Hill; 2014.

(Table 27.1). The ACCF/AHA stages of heart failure focus on the development and progression of disease and are used to describe individuals and populations, whereas the NYHA classes emphasize clinical aspects such as exercise capacity and symptoms of heart failure. Fig. 27.2 illustrates an updated classification scheme that includes treatment guidelines from the ACCF/AHA. Heart failure is treated by correcting the underlying disease (e.g., coronary artery disease, hypertension, dyslipidemia, thyroid disease), smoking cessation, regular exercise when able, bed rest when necessary, following a sodium-restricted diet, and controlling symptoms with a combination of pharmacologic agents. Healthcare institutions are evaluated according to the core measures that promote quality outcomes for patients with heart failure. These include providing discharge education that is specific to the disease management of heart failure as well as to smoking cessation, measuring left ventricular function during hospitalization, prescribing an angiotensin-converting enzyme (ACE) inhibitor or an angiotensin II receptor blocker (ARB) for patients with left ventricular dysfunction, and reporting the 30-day mortality rate of patients with heart failure.

DRUG THERAPY FOR HEART FAILURE

ACTIONS

Heart failure is treated with a combination of vasodilator, diuretic, and inotropic therapy (see Fig. 27.1). If the failure is acute, most therapy will be administered by the intravenous (IV) route in an intensive care unit. Vasodilators are used to reduce the strain on the left ventricle by reducing the systemic vascular resistance (afterload) against which the left ventricle is working. The reduced vascular resistance will also increase tissue perfusion to vital organs and muscles. The second goal of vasodilator use is to reduce preload so that the high volume of blood returning to the heart is decreased. The reduction in preload decreases pulmonary congestion and allows the patient to breathe more easily (Fig. 27.3). As renal perfusion is improved, potent diuretics are administered to enhance sodium and water excretion. This provides substantial symptomatic relief to the patient in addition to reducing the workload on the heart.

Inotropic agents stimulate the heart to increase the force of contractions, thereby boosting cardiac output. This also helps reduce pulmonary congestion and improve tissue perfusion.

Table 27.1	Comparison of ACCF/AHA Stages of Heart Failure and the NYHA Functional Classification System[a]		
		NYHA FUNCTIONAL CLASSIFICATION SYSTEM	
ACCF/AHA Stages of Heart Failure		**Functional Capacity**	**Objective Assessment**
A	At risk for heart failure but no structural heart disease or symptoms	No classification	
B	Structural heart disease but without signs or symptoms	Class I: Patients who have cardiac disease but without limitation of physical activity. Ordinary physical activity does not cause undue fatigue, palpitation, dyspnea, or anginal pain.	No objective evidence of cardiovascular disease.
C	Structural heart disease with prior or current symptoms of heart failure	Class I: as above Class II: Patients who have cardiac disease resulting in slight limitation of physical activity. Comfortable at rest. Ordinary physical activity results in fatigue, palpitation, dyspnea, or anginal pain.	Objective evidence of minimal cardiovascular disease.
		Class III: Patients who have cardiac disease resulting in marked limitation of physical activity. They are comfortable at rest. Less-than-ordinary activity causes fatigue, palpitation, dyspnea, or anginal pain.	Objective evidence of moderately severe cardiovascular disease.
D	Refractory heart failure requiring specialized interventions	Class IV: Patients who have cardiac disease resulting in inability to carry on any physical activity without discomfort. Symptoms of heart failure or the anginal syndrome may be present even at rest. If any physical activity is undertaken, discomfort is increased.	Objective evidence of severe cardiovascular disease.

[a]Functional Capacity and Objective Assessment are independent categories. Functional Capacity is an estimate of what the patient's heart will allow the patient to do and should not be influenced by the character of the structural lesions or by any opinion regarding the patient's treatment or prognosis. Objective Assessment is based on parameters such as electrocardiograms, stress tests, x-ray studies, echocardiograms, and radiologic images.
ACCF, American College of Cardiology Foundation; *AHA*, American Heart Association; *NYHA*, New York Heart Association.
From The Criteria Committee of the New York Heart Association. *Nomenclature and Criteria for Diagnosis of Diseases of the Heart and Great Vessels.* 9th ed. Boston: Little, Brown; 1994; and Yancy CW, Jessup M, Bozkurt B, et al. ACCF/AHA guideline for the management of heart failure: executive summary: a report of the American Colleges of Cardiology Foundation/American Heart Association Task Force on practice guidelines. *Circulation.* 2013;128(16):1810-1852.

USES

Intravenous nitroglycerin (see Chapter 24), nitroprusside (see Chapter 22), and nesiritide are used as vasodilators to reduce preload and afterload in critically ill patients. Angiotensin-converting enzyme inhibitors or ARBs (see Chapter 22) are the mainstays of oral vasodilator therapy for treating chronic heart failure. Most patients with heart failure require a loop diuretic such as furosemide or bumetanide (see Chapter 28) to help reduce fluid and sodium overload.

Studies have indicated that certain patients will also benefit from the use of beta-adrenergic blocking agents. A major component of the pathophysiologic causes of heart failure is increased sympathetic activity. Carvedilol, a noncardioselective beta blocker and an alpha-1 blocker, blocks adrenergic activity while lowering systemic vascular resistance as a vasodilator (see Chapters 12 and 22). Other vasodilators used include isosorbide (see Chapter 24) and hydralazine (see Chapter 22).

A combination product containing hydralazine and isosorbide dinitrate (BiDil) has been approved by the US Food and Drug Administration. It has been shown to reduce hospitalizations, improve quality of life, and reduce mortality among African Americans with hypertension and heart failure. Guidelines also recommend that ARBs (see candesartan, Chapter 22) and aldosterone antagonists (see eplerenone, Chapter 22; and spironolactone, Chapter 28) may provide additional benefit for patients who are still symptomatic while receiving full therapeutic doses of an ACE inhibitor and a beta blocker, or those who have developed adverse effects from the standard therapies.

Ivabradine and a combination product containing valsartan and sacubitril (Entresto) have been approved for the management of heart failure. Due to the availability of these new pharmacologic therapies, the American College of Cardiology, the AHA, and the Heart Failure Society of America published a focused update of the 2013 ACCF/AHA guideline for the management of heart failure (Yancy et al, 2017).

Inotropic agents used to treat acute failure include IV dobutamine (see Chapter 12) and milrinone. Digoxin, a digitalis glycoside, has been used for decades to treat heart conditions when an oral inotropic agent is needed.

❖ NURSING IMPLICATIONS FOR HEART FAILURE THERAPY

◆ Assessment

History of heart disease. Obtain the patient's history of prior treatment for heart disease, related cardiovascular disease (e.g., hypertension, hyperlipidemia), diabetes mellitus, and lung disease.

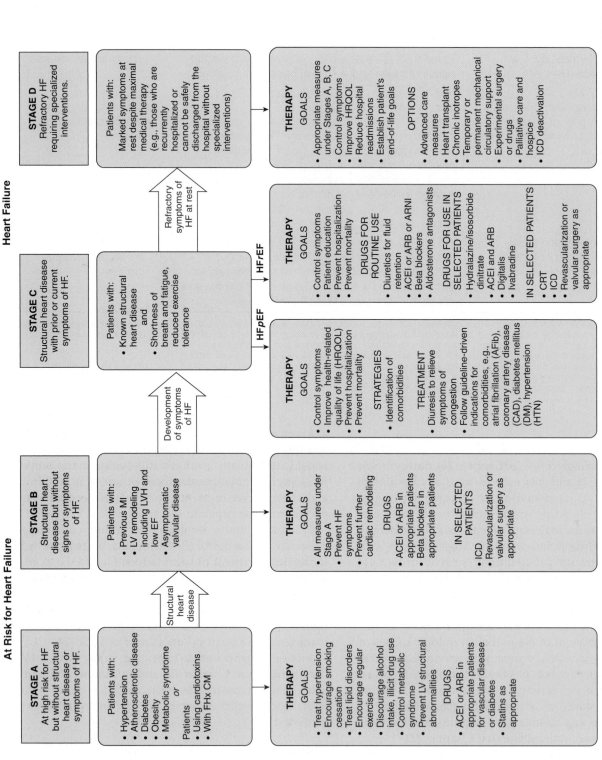

Fig. 27.2 Stages in the development of heart failure (*HF*) and recommended therapy by stage. *ACEI*, Angiotensin-converting enzyme inhibitor; *ARB*, angiotensin II receptor blocker; *ARNI*, angiotensin receptor-neprilysin inhibitor; *CRT*, cardiac resynchronization therapy; *EF*, ejection fraction; *FHx CM*, family history of cardiomyopathy; *CR/XL*, controlled release/extended release; *HFpEF*, heart failure with preserved ejection fraction; *HFrEF*, heart failure with reduced ejection fraction; *ICD*, implantable cardioverter-defibrillator; *LV*, left ventricular; *LVH*, left ventricular hypertrophy; *MI*, myocardial infarction. (Adapted from Hunt SA, Abraham WT, Chin MH, et al. 2009 Focused update incorporated into the ACC/AHA 2005 guidelines for the diagnosis and management of heart failure in adults: a report of the American College of Cardiology Foundation/American Heart Association Task Force on Practice Guidelines Developed in Collaboration With the International Society for Heart and Lung Transplantation. *J Am Coll Cardiol*. 2009;53[15];e1-e90. doi.org/10.1016/j.jacc.2008.11.013.)

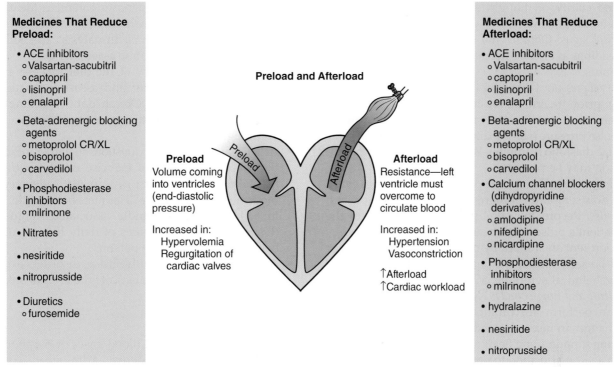

Medicines That Reduce Preload:

- ACE inhibitors
  - Valsartan-sacubitril
  - captopril
  - lisinopril
  - enalapril
- Beta-adrenergic blocking agents
  - metoprolol CR/XL
  - bisoprolol
  - carvedilol
- Phosphodiesterase inhibitors
  - milrinone
- Nitrates
- nesiritide
- nitroprusside
- Diuretics
  - furosemide

Preload and Afterload

Preload
Volume coming into ventricles (end-diastolic pressure)

Increased in:
Hypervolemia
Regurgitation of cardiac valves

Afterload
Resistance—left ventricle must overcome to circulate blood

Increased in:
Hypertension
Vasoconstriction

↑Afterload
↑Cardiac workload

Medicines That Reduce Afterload:

- ACE inhibitors
  - Valsartan-sacubitril
  - captopril
  - lisinopril
  - enalapril
- Beta-adrenergic blocking agents
  - metoprolol CR/XL
  - bisoprolol
  - carvedilol
- Calcium channel blockers (dihydropyridine derivatives)
  - amlodipine
  - nifedipine
  - nicardipine
- Phosphodiesterase inhibitors
  - milrinone
- hydralazine
- nesiritide
- nitroprusside

Fig. 27.3 Medicines that reduce preload and afterload to reduce heart failure.

Medication history. Obtain details of all medications that have been prescribed to the patient. Tactfully determine whether the prescribed medications are being taken regularly. If they are not being taken, ask why not. Ask the patient for a list of all over-the-counter medications and any herbal products being taken. Perform focused assessments to determine the effectiveness and the adverse effects of any pharmacologic interventions.

History of six cardinal signs of heart disease

1. *Dyspnea (difficulty breathing):* Record whether dyspnea occurs while the patient is resting, if it occurs on exertion, or if it occurs while the patient is asleep at night (paroxysmal nocturnal dyspnea). Are symptoms of dyspnea accompanied by a productive or nonproductive cough? Ask the patient to describe his or her sputum. (With heart failure, sputum is frothy and may be tinged with blood.) How has the patient been coping with any orthopneic problems?
2. *Chest pain:* Because heart failure results in decreased cardiac output and lower oxygenation of tissue, the heart may experience inadequate tissue perfusion, which can result in chest pain. Record data regarding the time of onset as well as the frequency, duration, and quality of the chest pain. Note any conditions that the patient has found to aggravate or relieve the chest pain.
3. *Fatigue:* Determine whether fatigue occurs only at specific times of the day, such as toward evening. Ask the patient if fatigue subsides in relation to a decrease in activity level or if it is present at about the same time each day.
4. *Edema:* Record the presence or absence of edema. If edema is present, record its location, any assessment data (e.g., degree of pitting present; ankle, midcalf, or thigh circumference), the appearance of the skin (e.g., shiny, weeping with pressure), and any measures that the patient has used to eliminate it. Chart the time of day that the edema is present (e.g., when rising in the morning, before bedtime) and the specific parts on the body where it is present. When performing the patient's daily weights, use the same scale, weigh the patient at the same time of day, and be sure that the patient is wearing similar clothing each time.
5. *Syncope:* Ask the patient about the conditions surrounding any episodes of syncope. Record the degree of symptoms, such as general muscle weakness, the inability to stand upright, feeling faint, or any loss of consciousness. Record what activities (if any) bring on these syncopal episodes.
6. *Palpitations:* Record the patient's description of palpitations, such as, "My heart skips some beats." Ask if these conditions are preceded by strenuous or mild exercise and how long the palpitations last.

Indications of altered cardiac function

- *Basic mental status:* Identify the individual's level of consciousness (e.g., drowsiness, lethargy, confusion; orientation to date, time, and place). Assess the clarity of thought present. Both the level of consciousness and clarity of thought are indicators of adequate cerebral perfusion.

- *Vital signs:* Obtain vital signs and pulse oximetry readings as often as necessary to monitor the patient's status.
- *Blood pressure:* Obtain baseline readings and a history of prior treatment for hypertension. Monitor the patient at specific intervals and report a narrowing pulse pressure (i.e., the difference between the systolic and diastolic readings). With heart failure, hypotension may be present.
- *Temperature:* Record the patient's temperature every 8 hours; monitor it more frequently if it is elevated.
- *Pulse:* Record the rate, quality, and rhythm of the patient's pulse. With heart failure, tachycardia may represent an attempt by the body to compensate for decreased cardiac output. Tachycardia is often the first clinical symptom of heart failure.
- *Heart and lung sounds:* Nurses with advanced skills can perform auscultation and percussion to note changes in heart size and in the patient's heart and lung sounds. Lung fields are assessed with the patient in a sitting position to detect abnormal lung sounds (e.g., wheezes, crackles). (Refer to a medical-surgical or critical care nursing textbook for details about how to perform these skills.)
- *Skin color:* Note the color of the patient's skin, mucous membranes, tongue, earlobes, and nail beds. Chart the exact location of any pallor or cyanosis that is present.
- *Neck veins:* Record any jugular venous distention.
- *Clubbing:* Inspect the patient's fingernails and toenails for clubbing. Perform the blanching test on the fingernails and toenails.
- *Central venous pressure:* If ordered, obtain baseline and subsequent readings at specified intervals. Report alterations within parameters indicated by the healthcare provider.
- *Abdomen:* Inspect the patient's abdomen, noting size, shape, softness, and any distention. Read the patient's history to obtain any data related to liver enlargement.
- *Fluid volume status:* Continue to assess the patient's intake and output at intervals that are appropriate to the patient's condition (every hour during an acute exacerbation of heart failure). Report intake that exceeds output. Ask the patient about the frequency of nocturia. (Nocturia often occurs with heart failure because renal perfusion is improved when the patient lies down and fluid moves from the interstitial spaces back into the general circulation.)
- *Diagnostic tests:* Review laboratory and diagnostic test results and promptly report any abnormal results to the healthcare provider. Tests include serum electrolytes, especially potassium, calcium, magnesium, and sodium levels; B-type natriuretic peptide, arterial blood gases, and serum lipid levels; electrocardiography; echocardiography, which includes left ventricular function, a diagnostic parameter identified as an indicator in the core measures; nuclear imaging studies; chest x-ray films; urinalysis; and kidney function and hemodynamic assessments.
- *Nutrition:* Take a history of the diet that has been prescribed to the patient and assess the patient's adherence to the diet. Obtain data regarding the patient's appetite and the presence of nausea and vomiting.
- *Activity and exercise:* Ask questions to gather information about the effect of exercise on the patient's functioning. Is the person normally sedentary or moderately or very active? Has there been a reduction in activity level to handle associated fatigue or dyspnea? Are the activities of daily living (ADLs) being performed by the person?
- *Anxiety level:* Patients with cardiac disorders exhibit varying degrees of anxiety. Note the level of anxiety or depression present.

◆ Implementation

- Obtain baseline arterial blood gases or monitor the pulse oximeter, as ordered. Administer oxygen therapy as prescribed and periodically review the patient's results.
- Position the patient in a Fowler's or semi-Fowler's position to maximize lung expansion and oxygenation. Reposition the patient at least every 2 hours, and provide skin care to prevent breakdown.
- Auscultate lung sounds at specified intervals consistent with the patient's condition. Assess the patient for neck vein distention.
- Weigh the patient daily at the same time (usually before breakfast), using the same scale, and with the patient wearing similar clothing. Record and report any significant weight changes. (Weight gains and losses are the single best indicator of fluid gain or loss.) As appropriate to the patient's condition, obtain and record abdominal girth measurements.
- When fluid restrictions are prescribed, half of the fluid is usually given with meals and the other half is divided over the rest of the day. Generally, the nurse should encourage the patient to write down the amount of liquid intake throughout the day to better understand how to follow any fluid restriction.
- Maintain the degree of dietary sodium restriction prescribed.
- Avoid using salt substitutes when potassium-sparing diuretics are being given to the patient.
- Administer prescribed medications (e.g., bronchodilators, ACE inhibitors, nitrates, digoxin, diuretics, antianxiety agents) on a schedule or as needed. Monitor the degree of response achieved and report any ineffectiveness.
- Pace nursing activities to avoid undue patient fatigue; implement exercise gradually while monitoring the patient's vital signs before and after ambulation.

Assess for signs and symptoms of fatigue or poor oxygenation before, during, and after exercise.

- Do not plan exercise or ambulation within 1 hour after eating to avoid excessive oxygen depletion.
- Monitor the patient's vital signs and oximeter readings, and perform a focused assessment of heart and respiratory functions at specified intervals.
- Perform neurologic assessments to determine changes in the patient's mental status.
- Deal calmly with an anxious patient, offer explanations of procedures being performed, and listen to his or her concerns and intervene appropriately.
- Monitor the rate of IV infusions carefully; contact the patient's primary care provider regarding the concentration of admixtures of drugs to IV infusion solution when the limitation of fluids is indicated.
- Give the patient stool softeners to avoid the patient straining while trying to pass a hard stool, which could cause syncope by inducing the Valsalva maneuver.

◆ Patient Education

- Teach the patient and significant others about the functional changes caused by heart failure. Emphasize the need for lifelong treatment and adherence to drug therapy, diet, and exercise regimens to obtain maximum control of the disease process.
- Assess the patient's understanding of symptoms that indicate when to call a healthcare provider: dyspnea; a productive cough; worsening fatigue; edema in the feet, ankles, or legs; weight gain of 2 pounds or more in a 2-day period; and development of angina, chest pain, palpitations, or confusion.
- Provide the patient with instructions for taking vital signs such as blood pressure, pulse, and respirations. Give him or her information about the acceptable parameters for each as prescribed by the healthcare provider.
- Explain any oxygen therapy that has been prescribed. If the patient is being discharged on oxygen, tell him or her where to obtain oxygen equipment and supplies, the rate of administration, and how to care for and maintain the equipment.
- Demonstrate to the patient how to get into a Fowler's position. Discuss the adaptations needed at home to use these positions for relief of dyspnea. Explain that an upright position provides maximum oxygenation.
- Teach the patient about good skin care and the need to change position at least every 2 hours, especially when edema is present. Have the patient inspect his or her ankles, feet, and abdomen daily for edema. If the patient is using a recliner or bed, the sacral area should also be checked regularly for edema.
- Discuss the importance of spacing the ADLs to conserve energy and avoid fatigue. Review the prescribed activity level and stress monitoring pulse, dyspnea, and fatigue levels as a guide to when the patient is overexerting.

- Explore the coping mechanisms that the person uses in response to stress. Discuss how the patient is adapting to the needed changes in his or her lifestyle to manage the disease process. Address depression issues, if present.
- Diet therapy is an integral part of the treatment of heart failure. Schedule meetings with the nutritionist to enable the patient to learn how to manage specific dietary modifications that have been prescribed (these usually include a low-sodium, high-potassium diet with weight reduction parameters for obese patients). If possible, have the patient practice food selection using the daily menus while he or she is still in the hospital. Take cultural food preferences into consideration and offer guidance from the nutrition staff as well as the nurses. Teach the patient about foods that are low in sodium and high in potassium. Potassium restrictions may be indicated if the patient is taking a potassium-sparing diuretic: salt substitutes are high in potassium, so their use must be limited. Alcohol intake should be eliminated from the diet.
- Teach the patient about the importance of maintaining a regular, mild exercise routine as prescribed by the healthcare provider. At one time it was thought that exercise was harmful with this condition; however, mild regular exercise is now prescribed, with limitations defined by the healthcare provider.
- Fluid restrictions may be imposed, usually for patients with moderate to advanced heart failure; discuss specific ways to manage these limitations.
- Teach the patient about the signs and symptoms of potassium deficiency or excess, depending on the medications prescribed.

Medication regimen

- Heart failure requires lifelong treatment, and adherence to prescribed therapy is imperative to control the disease.
- Teach the patient the signs and symptoms of **digitalis toxicity** (e.g., anorexia, nausea, vomiting, bradycardia, visual disturbances, psychiatric disturbances). Explain medication administration parameters: if the pulse is less than 60 or more than 100 beats/min, do not administer digoxin without checking with the prescriber. (An antidote is available for digoxin toxicity.) Tell the patient that it is important to report for blood draws to check serum levels of the drug at the specific times scheduled.
- Diuretics should be taken in the morning to avoid nighttime diuresis. Depending on the type of diuretic prescribed, potassium supplements may be necessary. However, if a potassium-sparing diuretic is ordered, limiting potassium intake may be appropriate. Salt substitutes should be avoided because they are high in potassium.
- Tell the patient to perform daily weights using the same scale, wearing similar clothing, at the same time each day (usually before breakfast). Record and

report significant weight changes, because weight gains and losses are the best indicators of fluid gain or loss. Usually a gain of 2 pounds in 2 days should be reported.

- When ACE inhibitors are ordered, hypotension, hyperkalemia, and a persistent cough are possible. Discuss the management of these adverse effects.

Fostering health maintenance

- Throughout the course of treatment, discuss medication information and how it will benefit the patient.
- Drug therapy is one component of the treatment of heart failure, and it is critical that the medications be taken as prescribed. Provide the patient and his or her significant others with the important information contained in the specific drug monographs for the drugs prescribed. Additional health teaching and nursing interventions for common and serious adverse effects can be found in each drug monograph.
- It is important to control the underlying condition causing the heart failure (e.g., hypertension, hyperlipidemia). The patient and his or her family must understand the importance of complying with diet, exercise, and other prescribed treatments designed to maximize the patient's degree of oxygenation.
- Seek cooperation and understanding of the following points so that medication adherence is increased: the name of the medication; its dosage, route, and times of administration; and common and serious adverse effects.

Patient self-assessment. Enlist the patient's help with developing and maintaining a written record of monitoring parameters (e.g., pulse rate, blood pressure, degree of dyspnea and what precipitates it, chest pain, edema). See the Patient Self-Assessment Form for Cardiovascular Agents on the Evolve website. Complete the Premedication Data column for use as a baseline to track the patient's response to drug therapy. Ensure that the patient understands how to use the form and instruct the patient to bring the completed form to follow-up visits. During the follow-up visits, focus on issues that will foster adherence with the therapeutic interventions prescribed.

DRUG CLASS: ANGIOTENSIN-CONVERTING ENZYME INHIBITORS

Actions

Angiotensin-converting enzyme inhibitors represent a major breakthrough in the treatment of heart failure. Large studies show that ACE inhibitors reduce the morbidity and mortality associated with heart failure. The ACE inhibitors reduce afterload by blocking angiotensin-II–mediated peripheral vasoconstriction, and they help reduce circulating blood volume (preload) by inhibiting the secretion of aldosterone. (See Chapter 22 for a more complete description of the mechanism of action of ACE inhibitors.)

Uses

The ACE inhibitors reduce blood pressure (afterload), preserve cardiac output, and increase renal blood flow. They are now recommended as the drugs of choice over digoxin for the treatment of mild to moderate systolic dysfunction heart failure.

Therapeutic Outcomes

The primary therapeutic outcomes expected from ACE inhibitors are improved cardiac output resulting in improved tissue perfusion and improved tolerance to activity as demonstrated by the ability to perform ADLs without supplemental oxygen therapy or fatigue.

❖ **Nursing Implications for Angiotensin-Converting Enzyme Inhibitors**

See Chapter 22 for a more complete description of the nursing implications related to ACE inhibitors.

DRUG CLASS: NATRIURETIC PEPTIDES

nesiritide (nĕ-SĬR-ĭ-tīd)
Natrecor (NĂT-rĕ-kŏr)

Actions

Nesiritide was the first of a new class of drugs: the human B-type natriuretic peptides. It is a hormone normally secreted by the cardiac ventricles in response to fluid and pressure overload. It helps the heart recover from deteriorating cardiac function by reducing preload and afterload pressures, increasing diuresis and sodium excretion, suppressing the renin-angiotensin-aldosterone system, and reducing secretion of norepinephrine.

Uses

Nesiritide is used as a vasodilator in patients with severe heart failure who have dyspnea at rest or with minimal activity.

Therapeutic Outcomes

The primary therapeutic outcomes of nesiritide are reduction of workload on the heart and improvement in symptoms associated with heart failure.

◆ *Availability.* *IV:* 1.5-mg single-use vials.

◆ *Dosage and Administration.* *Initial dose:* An IV bolus of 2 mcg/kg followed by a continuous infusion at a dosage of 0.01 mcg/kg/min. *Dosage titration:* Up to 0.03 mcg/kg/min. *Duration:* No longer than 96 hours.

DRUG CLASS: ANGIOTENSIN RECEPTOR BLOCKER–NEPRILYSIN INHIBITOR

valsartan-sacubitril (văl-SĂR-tăn; săk-Ū-bĭ-trĭl)
Entresto (ĕn-TRĚS-tō)

Actions

Entresto is a combination product containing an ARB (valsartan) (see Chapter 22) and a neprilysin inhibitor (sacubitril). The ARB treats heart failure by reducing afterload by blocking angiotensin-mediated peripheral vasoconstriction with resultant vasodilation, and decreases preload by reducing circulating blood volume by inhibiting the secretion of aldosterone. Aldosterone inhibition results in a natriuresis (excretion of sodium in the urine) and diuresis (excretion of water in the urine).

Sacubitril inhibits the enzyme neprilysin. Neprilysin normally inactivates natriuretic peptides and bradykinin. Inhibition of neprilysin increases the levels of natriuretic peptides secreted by the atrial and ventricular heart muscles, resulting in blood vessel dilation (reduction in afterload) and reduction in circulating blood volume (reduced preload) by enhanced sodium and water excretion by the kidneys. Thus the ingredients in Entresto work by different mechanisms to reduce preload and afterload, improving cardiac output and reducing heart failure.

Uses

Valsartan-sacubitril is used in the management of heart failure, usually in conjunction with other heart failure medications such as diuretics and beta blockers. It is used in place of an ACE inhibitor or another ARB. The combination reduces the risk of hospitalization and cardiovascular death in patients with chronic heart failure (NYHA Classes II-IV).

Therapeutic Outcomes

The primary therapeutic outcomes are reduced risk of hospitalization and of cardiovascular death from heart failure.

❖ Nursing Implications for Valsartan-Sacubitril

◆ *Premedication assessment*

1. Take the patient's blood pressure in both the supine and standing positions. Record the pulse rate, rhythm, and regularity.
2. Obtain the baseline laboratory studies ordered by the healthcare provider (e.g., complete blood count).
3. Obtain baseline weight.
4. Perform a baseline assessment of the patient's degree of alertness and orientation to name, place, and time before initiating therapy.

◆ *Availability. PO:* tablets: sacubitril/valsartan 24 mg/ 26 mg, 49 mg/51 mg, and 97 mg/103 mg.

◆ *Dosage and administration. Patients **not** currently taking an ACE inhibitor or an ARB: PO:* Initial: sacubitril/ valsartan 24 mg/26 mg twice daily. Double the dose as tolerated every 2 to 4 weeks to the target maintenance dose of sacubitril/valsartan 97 mg/103 mg twice daily.

Patients previously taking more than 10 mg/day of enalapril or more than 160 mg/day of valsartan or equivalent dose of

another ACE inhibitor or ARB: PO: Initial: sacubitril/ valsartan 49 mg/51 mg twice daily. Double the dose as tolerated after 2 to 4 weeks to the target maintenance dose of sacubitril/valsartan 97 mg/103 mg twice daily.

Patients previously taking low doses of an ACE inhibitor (≤10 mg/day of enalapril or an equivalent dose of another ACE inhibitor) or ARB (≤160 mg/day of valsartan or an equivalent dose of another ARB): PO: Initial: sacubitril/ valsartan 24 mg/26 mg twice daily. Double the dose as tolerated every 2 to 4 weeks to the target maintenance dose of sacubitril/valsartan 97 mg/103 mg twice daily.

 Medication Safety Alert

Do not administer Entresto to a patient receiving an ACE inhibitor or ARB. If the patient is currently receiving an ACE inhibitor, wait at least 36 hours before starting Entresto.

◆ *Common adverse effects*

Cardiovascular

Orthostatic hypotension (dizziness, weakness, faintness). Although these adverse effects are infrequent and usually mild, certain patients, particularly those also receiving diuretics, may suffer some degree of orthostatic hypotension, especially when therapy is initiated. Observe the patient closely for at least 2 hours after the initial dose is given and for at least an additional hour until blood pressure has stabilized. Monitor the blood pressure in both the supine and standing positions. Anticipate the development of postural hypotension and take measures to prevent an occurrence. Teach the patient to rise slowly from a supine or sitting position and to sit or lie down if feeling faint.

Inflammatory

Chronic cough. Patients receiving valsartan-sacubitril may develop a chronic, dry, nonproductive, persistent cough. This is thought to be caused by an accumulation of bradykinin by the neprilysin inhibitor. It may appear from 1 week to 6 months after initiation of therapy. Patients should be told to contact the healthcare provider if the cough becomes troublesome. The cough usually resolves after discontinuation of therapy.

◆ *Serious adverse effects*

Pregnancy. Medications that act directly on the renin-angiotensin-aldosterone system can cause fetal and neonatal harm. There is concern about the potential for birth defects in neonates whose mothers receive valsartan-sacubitril, especially during the second and third trimesters of pregnancy. Women who wish to become pregnant or who become pregnant while receiving valsartan-sacubitril should discuss alternative therapies with the healthcare provider as soon as possible.

Cardiovascular

Hypotension. Hypotension may occur upon initiation, particularly in patients with heart failure or post-MI.

It may also occur in patients receiving high-dose diuretics who may be volume depleted. Patients should be warned that this may occur and should sit or lie down immediately if dizziness develops.

Swelling of the face, eyes, lips, and tongue; difficulty breathing. Angioedema has been reported to occur in a small number of patients receiving ARBs, especially after the first dose. The patient should be cautioned to discontinue further therapy and seek medical attention immediately.

Renal

Hyperkalemia. Because valsartan-sacubitril both inhibit aldosterone, patients may develop slight increases in serum potassium levels. Most cases resolve without discontinuation of therapy. Patients most susceptible to the development of hyperkalemia are those with renal impairment or diabetes mellitus and those already receiving a potassium supplement or a potassium-sparing diuretic. Many symptoms associated with altered fluid and electrolyte balance are subtle and interspersed with general symptoms of drug toxicity or the disease process itself.

Gather data relative to changes in the patient's mental status (e.g., alertness, orientation, and confusion), muscle strength, muscle cramps, tremors, nausea, and general appearance (e.g., drowsy, anxious, or lethargic). Always check the electrolyte reports for early indications of electrolyte imbalance. Keep accurate records of intake and output, daily weights, and vital signs.

Nephrotoxicity. Patients who are receiving valsartan-sacubitril, particularly those with preexisting renal impairment and those also taking nonsteroidal antiinflammatory drugs, have developed increased blood urea nitrogen and serum creatinine levels. These elevations have usually been minor and transient, especially when administered concomitantly with a diuretic. Renal function should be monitored during the first few weeks of therapy. Report increasing blood urea nitrogen and creatinine levels. Dosage reduction of valsartan-sacubitril or possible discontinuation of the nonsteroidal antiinflammatory drug or diuretic may be required.

◆ *Drug interactions*

Drugs that enhance therapeutic and toxic effects. These include diuretics, antipsychotics, alcohol, beta-adrenergic blocking agents (e.g., metoprolol, carvedilol), and other antihypertensive agents. ACE inhibitors and ARBs are contraindicated. Monitor the blood pressure response to the cumulative effects of antihypertensive agents. Take the blood pressure in supine and standing positions.

Drugs that reduce therapeutic effects. Nonsteroidal antiinflammatory drugs may reduce the effects of valsartan-sacubitril and may cause a significant decrease in renal function. Monitor serum creatinine closely.

Lithium. Angiotensin II receptor blockers may induce lithium toxicity. Monitor for lithium toxicity manifested by nausea, anorexia, fine tremors, persistent vomiting, profuse diarrhea, hyperreflexia, lethargy, and weakness.

Hyperkalemia. Valsartan-sacubitril may cause small increases in potassium levels by inhibiting aldosterone secretion. Patients should not take dietary supplements of potassium, potassium-containing salt substitutes, or potassium-sparing diuretics (e.g., triamterene, spironolactone, amiloride) without specific approval from the healthcare provider. If a patient has received spironolactone or eplerenone up to several months before valsartan-sacubitril therapy, the serum potassium level should be monitored closely because the potassium-sparing effect of spironolactone or eplerenone may persist. Serum potassium levels should be monitored when the antibiotic trimethoprim is used with valsartan-sacubitril.

DRUG CLASS: BETA-ADRENERGIC BLOCKING AGENTS

Actions

The beta-adrenergic blocking agents (beta blockers; see Table 12.3) inhibit cardiac response to sympathetic nerve stimulation by blocking the beta receptors. As a result, the heart rate, cardiac output, aggravating hypertension—and consequently the blood pressure—are reduced. Beta blockers also reduce blood pressure as they inhibit renin release, diminishing the cascade of the renin-angiotensin-aldosterone system that would induce vasoconstriction and sodium reabsorption.

Uses

The beta-adrenergic blocking agents are agents of another class that have been shown to reduce the morbidity and mortality associated with heart failure. The exact mechanism whereby beta blockers increase survival in patients with heart failure is unknown, but it is thought to include inhibition of renin release, suppression of the effect of elevated circulating catecholamines, and secondary prevention of angina and MI. Because beta-adrenergic blocking agents and ACE inhibitors act through different mechanisms, beta blockers and ACE inhibitors are commonly used together to treat heart failure. There is a question of whether all beta blockers have the same clinical effect. The agents that are the most well studied and shown to be effective in treating heart failure are bisoprolol, long-acting metoprolol (Toprol-XL), and carvedilol.

Therapeutic Outcomes

The primary therapeutic outcomes are reduced risk of hospitalization and of cardiovascular death from heart failure.

❖ **Nursing Implications for Beta-Adrenergic Blocking Agents**

See Chapter 22 for a more complete description of the nursing implications related to the beta-adrenergic blocking agents.

DRUG CLASS: DIGITALIS GLYCOSIDES

digoxin (dĭ-JŎKS-ĭn)
⇄ *Do not confuse digoxin with Doxepin.*
Lanoxin (lă-NŎKS-ĭn)
⇄ *Do not confuse Lanoxin with Inapsine, Lomotil,*
Levoxyl, Levsin, Lovenox, or Xanax.

Actions

The digitalis glycosides are among the oldest therapeutic agents used to treat heart failure. Their use in medicine dates to the 18th century; in 1785, William Withering, an English physician and botanist, published excellent observations regarding the treatment of various ailments with digoxin. Once derived naturally from the dried leaves of *Digoxin purpurea* (purple foxglove), the drug is now prepared synthetically. Digoxin is the only digitalis glycoside currently available in the United States.

Digoxin has two primary actions on the heart: (1) increasing the force of contraction (**positive inotropy**) and (2) slowing the heart rate (**negative chronotropy**), thus reducing the conduction velocity and prolonging the refractory period at the atrioventricular node. The exact mechanisms of these actions are unknown, but the net result is that the heart is able to fill and empty more completely, thereby improving cardiac output and circulation. With improved circulation, there is a reduction in systemic and pulmonary congestion, in heart size (i.e., returning toward normal), and in peripheral edema because of the increased perfusion of blood through the kidneys, which extract water and electrolytes.

Uses

Digoxin is used to treat mild to severe systolic heart failure that does not respond to diuretics, beta blockers, or ACE inhibitors. Digoxin may also be used to treat atrial fibrillation, atrial flutter, and paroxysmal tachycardia. Digoxin is not used to treat diastolic heart failure, and it may actually worsen this condition.

The goal of treatment for heart failure is to give adequate doses of digoxin so that the most optimal cardiac effects are achieved: cardiac output is increased, pulse rate is slowed, and vasoconstriction decreases, resulting in the disappearance of many of the signs and symptoms of heart failure (i.e., dyspnea, orthopnea, edema). The once-standard approach to giving loading doses (**digitalization**) of digoxin over a period of hours or days is no longer thought to be necessary in most cases to produce the desired cardiac effect. A maintenance dosage is now given, usually once a day. Many patients must continue to take digoxin preparations for the remainder of their lives.

Therapeutic Outcomes

The primary therapeutic outcomes expected from digoxin therapy are improved cardiac output resulting in improved tissue perfusion and improved tolerance to activity as demonstrated by the ability to perform ADLs without supplemental oxygen therapy or fatigue.

❖ **Nursing Implications for Digoxin**
◆ *Premedication assessment*

1. Take the patient's apical pulse for 1 full minute and follow institutional guidelines for withholding the drug (e.g., if the pulse is <60 or >100 beats/min). NOTE: In the long-term care setting, a radial pulse may be acceptable.
2. Before initiating therapy, obtain baseline patient data such as vital signs, lung sounds, weight, and laboratory values (e.g., serum electrolytes, liver and kidney function studies).
3. As therapy progresses, monitor the patient for the development of digoxin toxicity, hypokalemia, hypomagnesemia, or a sudden increase in a previously normal or low pulse rate.

◆ *Availability. PO:* 0.0625-, 0.125-, 0.187.5- and 0.25-mg tablets; pediatric elixir, 0.05 mg/mL.
IV: 0.1 mg/mL in 1 mL ampules; 0.25 mg/mL in 2-mL ampules.

◆ *Implementation*
Digitalization. Digitalization is the administration of a larger dose of digoxin for an initial period of 24 hours. After this initial loading period, the patient is switched to a daily maintenance dose. Be sure to monitor the patient carefully for signs of digoxin toxicity.

Pulse variations. Always take the apical pulse for 1 full minute before administering any digoxin preparation. Do not administer the drug when the pulse rate in an adult is less than 60 beats/min until the prescriber is consulted. In a child, report a pulse rate of less than 90 beats/min because the prescriber may decide to withhold the medication.

Accurate identification. Digoxin is often given in minute amounts. Always have the mathematical computations checked by another professional nurse.

Use the correct type of syringe to facilitate the accuracy of the dosage measurement. Always question any order that is unusual before administration. Read the medication label carefully for proper drug and strength.

◆ *Dosage and administration.* Give digoxin after meals to minimize gastric irritation. NOTE: It is recommended that a baseline electrocardiogram be obtained before the initiation of therapy.

Assuming that the patient has not ingested digoxin during the preceding 2 weeks, the following dosages apply:

Adult: *PO: Digitalizing:* 0.5 to 0.75 mg initially followed by 0.125 to 0.375 mg every 6 to 8 hours until adequate digitalization is achieved. *Maintenance:* 0.125 to 0.25 mg daily. Some patients may require 0.375 to 0.5 mg daily.

IV: Digitalizing: Same as for PO administration. The drug may be administered undiluted or diluted with sterile water for injection, normal saline, or dextrose 5% to a volume at least fourfold the volume of digoxin. Administer over at least 5 minutes to avoid complications. *Maintenance:* Same as for PO administration. Adult therapeutic blood levels are 0.5 to 2.0 ng/mL.

 Life Span Considerations
Digoxin Toxicity

Older adults frequently experience digoxin toxicity as a result of digoxin's long half-life. Early symptoms of toxicity are anorexia and mild nausea, but they are frequently overlooked or are not associated with drug toxicity. Any change in pulse rhythm and rate or central nervous system signs (e.g., mental status, orientation, hallucinations, behavioral changes) should be investigated and reported. In children, digoxin toxicity is often first detected by the development of atrial dysrhythmias.

Serum levels. Serum levels of digoxin are measured to determine the amount of digoxin in the bloodstream. Blood should be drawn before the daily dose of medication is given or at least 6 hours after administration. It is important to be consistent with regard to the time of drawing blood and administering the dose.

Treatment of digoxin toxicity. The basic treatment of digoxin-induced dysrhythmias consists of stopping the digoxin and any potassium-depleting diuretics, checking the potassium level (i.e., administering potassium as indicated), and administering antidysrhythmic drugs (e.g., phenytoin). In some cases, atropine may be prescribed for sinus bradycardia. A pacemaker may be necessary to correct continuing bradycardia.

Antidote for severe digoxin intoxication. Digoxin immune fab (ovine) (Digibind).

◆ **Serious adverse effects**
Digoxin toxicity
Cardiac rhythm. Constantly monitor the patient for the development of a pulse deficit, bradycardia (heart rate <60 beats/min), and tachycardia (heart rate >100 beats/min). These may be signs of developing heart block. Whenever the patient is attached to a monitor, the pattern should be closely watched for any type of abnormal cardiac rhythms. In children, digoxin toxicity is often first detected by the development of atrial dysrhythmias.

 Life Span Considerations
Digoxin Dosage

Pediatric dosages for digoxin are extremely small and should be measured in a tuberculin syringe using the metric scale. All dosage calculations should be checked with a second qualified nurse in accordance with the institution's policy.

Noncardiac effects. Noncardiac symptoms of digoxin toxicity are often vague and difficult to separate from symptoms of heart disease. Any patient taking digoxin

products who develops the following symptoms should be evaluated for digoxin toxicity:

- *Gastrointestinal:* loss of appetite, nausea, vomiting
- *Neurologic:* extreme fatigue, weakness of the arms and legs
- *Psychological:* psychiatric disturbances (e.g., nightmares, agitation, listlessness, hallucinations)
- *Sensory:* visual disturbances (e.g., hazy or blurred vision, difficulty reading, difficulty with red-green color perception)

Electrolyte balance. Adverse effects of digoxin may also be induced by electrolyte imbalance (see Drug Interactions section later). Monitor the patient's laboratory reports, and notify the prescriber of deviations from the normal range of 3.6 to 4.5 mEq/L of potassium because hypokalemia potentiates the effects of digoxin and can lead to toxicity. Always monitor the pulse carefully if the potassium level is abnormal. Hypokalemia is especially likely to occur in a patient with nausea, vomiting, diarrhea, or heavy diuresis. Replacing potassium before administering digoxin is an accepted practice.

Other diseases. The patient's other clinical conditions may also induce digoxin toxicity. Patients who suffer from hypothyroidism, acute MI, renal disease, severe respiratory disease, or far-advanced heart failure may require lower-than-normal doses of digoxin; monitor closely.

◆ **Drug interactions**
Drugs that enhance therapeutic and toxic effects. Quinidine, diltiazem, verapamil, ranolazine, macrolide antibiotics (e.g., clarithromycin, erythromycin), propafenone, beta blockers (e.g., atenolol, esmolol, nadolol, propranolol), succinylcholine, thiazide and loop diuretics, calcium gluconate, and calcium chloride enhance the therapeutic and toxic effects of digoxin. Monitor patients taking these drugs for signs and symptoms of digoxin toxicity.

Drugs that reduce therapeutic effects. St. John's wort, aminoglycoside antibiotics (e.g., gentamicin, tobramycin, neomycin), cholestyramine, colestipol, rifampin, and antacids reduce the therapeutic effects of digoxin. Monitor patient symptoms for response to therapy; recurrence or intensification (exacerbation) of the patient's disease should be reported to the healthcare provider.

Drugs that may alter electrolyte balance, thus altering digoxin response. Drugs that may alter digoxin response, and thus the incidence of any of the adverse effects, by altering the electrolyte balance include the following:

MAY CAUSE HYPOKALEMIA

amphotericin B	furosemide (Lasix)
bumetanide	metolazone (Zaroxolyn)
chlorthalidone	thiazide diuretics
corticosteroids	torsemide (Demadex)
ethacrynic acid (Edecrin)	

MAY CAUSE HYPERKALEMIA

amiloride (Midamor)	potassium gluconate
angiotensin-converting enzyme inhibitors	penicillin G potassium potassium supplements (e.g.,
angiotensin receptor blocking agents	K-Lyte, Kaon, K-Lor)
beta-adrenergic blockers	salt substitutes
eplerenone	spironolactone
heparin	succinylcholine
mannitol infusions	triamterene
potassium chloride	trimethoprim

MAY CAUSE HYPOMAGNESEMIA

bumetanide	furosemide (Lasix)
chlorthalidone	metolazone (Zaroxolyn)
ethacrynic acid (Edecrin)	neomycin
ethanol	thiazide diuretics

DRUG CLASS: MISCELLANEOUS AGENT

ivabradine (ī-VĀB-ră-dēn)
Corlanor (cor' la- nor)

Actions
Ivabradine selectively and specifically inhibits the cardiac pacemaker electrical current in the sinoatrial node, resulting in a reduction in heart rate. Ivabradine does not affect the contractility of the heart or vascular system. Ivabradine decreases heart rate, which reduces the risk of hospitalization for worsening heart failure.

Uses
Ivabradine is used to reduce the risk of hospitalization from worsening heart failure in patients with stable, symptomatic chronic heart failure who are in sinus rhythm with a resting heart rate greater or equal to 70 beats per minute. The patient should also be on maximally tolerated doses of beta blockers or have a contraindication to beta blockers. Ivabradine does not significantly reduce the risk of cardiovascular death.

Therapeutic Outcome
The primary therapeutic outcome expected from ivabradine is to decrease frequency of hospitalizations due to heart failure.

❖ **Nursing Implications for Ivabradine**
◆ **Premedication assessment**
1. Take the patient's apical pulse for 1 full minute and follow institutional guidelines for withholding the drug (e.g., if the pulse is <60 or >100 beats/min). NOTE: In the long-term care setting, a radial pulse may be acceptable.
2. Before initiating therapy, obtain baseline patient data such as vital signs, lung sounds, and weight.
3. Obtain laboratory values (e.g., serum electrolytes, liver and kidney function studies).

◆ *Availability.* *PO:* 5- and 7.5-mg tablets.

◆ *Dosage and administration.* **Adult:** *PO: Initial:* 5 mg twice daily or 2.5 mg twice daily in patients who may experience hemodynamic compromise due to bradycardia. After 2 weeks, adjust dose to achieve a resting heart rate between 50 and 60 beats/min. Thereafter adjust dose as needed based on resting heart rate and tolerability. *Maximum dose:* 7.5 mg twice daily.
Ivabradine should be taken with meals, and grapefruit juice should be avoided.
Dosage adjustment based on resting heart rate:
• Heart rate >60 beats/min: Increase dose by 2.5 mg twice daily (maximum dose: 7.5 mg twice daily).
• Heart rate 50 to 60 beats/min: Maintain dose.
• Heart rate <50 beats/min or signs and symptoms of bradycardia: Decrease dose by 2.5 mg twice daily; if current dose is 2.5 mg twice daily, discontinue therapy.

◆ *Common adverse effects*
Cardiovascular
Hypotension and hypertension. Monitor blood pressure regularly and report changes in trend to the healthcare provider.
Visual. Ivabradine has been associated with visual impairment presenting as transiently enhanced brightness, halos, or colored bright lights. This may start within the first 2 months of therapy and may subside spontaneously during treatment.

◆ *Serious adverse effects*
Cardiac
Rhythm disturbances. Regularly monitor the patient for the development of a pulse deficit, bradycardia (heart rate <60 beats/min), and tachycardia (heart rate >100 beats/min). These may be signs of developing heart block. Patients particularly susceptible to rhythm disturbances are those concurrently receiving amiodarone, beta blockers, or digoxin.

◆ *Drug interactions*
Drugs that enhance therapeutic and toxic effects. Diltiazem, verapamil, digoxin, beta blockers, grapefruit juice, amiodarone, macrolide antibiotics (e.g., clarithromycin, erythromycin), and itraconazole enhance the therapeutic and toxic effects of ivabradine.
Drugs that reduce therapeutic effects. St. John's wort, rifampin, phenobarbital, and carbamazepine reduce the therapeutic effects of ivabradine. Monitor patient symptoms for response to therapy.
Drugs that may alter electrolyte balance, thus altering ivabradine response. Drugs that may alter ivabradine response, and thus the incidence of any of the adverse effects, by altering the electrolyte balance include the following: loop diuretics (bumetanide, furosemide, torsemide), hydrochlorothiazide, indapamide, and chlorthalidone.

DRUG CLASS: PHOSPHODIESTERASE INHIBITORS

milrinone (MĬL-rĭ-nōn)

Actions
Milrinone is an inotropic agent that increases the force and velocity of myocardial contractions by inhibiting phosphodiesterase enzymes in the heart muscle. It is also a vascular smooth muscle relaxant that causes vasodilation, thereby reducing preload and afterload.

Uses
Milrinone is used for the short-term management of severe systolic dysfunction heart failure in patients who have not responded adequately to digoxin, diuretics, or vasodilator therapy. The inotropic effects of milrinone are additive to those of digoxin, and milrinone can be used in fully digitalized patients. Milrinone is usually not used to treat diastolic heart failure, and it may indeed worsen this condition.

Therapeutic Outcomes
The primary therapeutic outcomes expected from milrinone therapy are increased cardiac output that results in improved tissue perfusion and reduced dyspnea, orthopnea, and fatigue.

❖ Nursing Implications for Milrinone
◆ *Premedication assessment*
1. Obtain the patient's baseline vital signs, including pain rating.
2. Obtain the baseline laboratory studies ordered by the healthcare provider (e.g., complete blood count).

◆ *Availability. IV:* 1 mg/mL in 10-, 20-, and 50-mL vials. *Premixed infusion:* 200 mcg/mL in 100 and 200 mL of dextrose 5% for injection.

◆ *Dosage and administration. Diluents:* 0.45% or 0.9% sodium chloride or dextrose 5% for injection may be used to prepare dilutions of milrinone for IV infusion.

Adult: *IV:* A loading dose is not necessary. Initiate therapy with a maintenance infusion of 0.5 mcg/kg/min. In general, the total daily dose should not exceed 1.13 mg/kg/24 hr.

◆ *Serious adverse effects*
Cardiovascular
Dysrhythmias, hypotension. The cardiovascular adverse effects of dysrhythmias (12%) and hypotension (1.3%) are the most commonly reported adverse effects. Monitor the patient's blood pressure and heart rate and rhythm closely during therapy. These adverse effects are often related to the dosage size, and they will respond to a reduction in infusion rate. Contact the healthcare provider immediately if dysrhythmias or significant hypotension develops.
Hematologic
Thrombocytopenia. Thrombocytopenia with platelet counts below $100,000/mm^3$ has been reported in 0.4% of patients. This condition appears to be dose dependent, occurring within 48 to 72 hours after initiation of therapy, and is more common in patients receiving higher-than-recommended dosages. Platelet counts should be obtained before and periodically during therapy. If thrombocytopenia does occur, discontinuation of therapy should be considered, especially when platelet counts decrease to less than $50,000/mm^3$. The nadir in platelet count appears to be variable, but it occurs within 1 to 4 weeks.

◆ *Drug interactions*
Furosemide. Milrinone and furosemide are chemically incompatible. When furosemide is mixed with milrinone, a precipitate forms immediately. Do not infuse these two drugs into the same IV line.

Get Ready for the NCLEX® Examination!

Key Points

- Heart failure involves a cluster of signs and symptoms that arise when the left or right ventricle or both ventricles lose the ability to pump enough blood to meet the body's circulatory needs. It is an illness that is growing in frequency as the general population ages.
- The morbidity and mortality associated with heart failure can be reduced through medication, diet, exercise, and health monitoring.
- The major pharmacologic agents used to treat heart failure are valsartan-sacubitril, ivabradine, ACE inhibitors, beta-adrenergic blocking agents, and diuretics. Other agents that may play an active role are calcium channel blockers, ARBs, aldosterone antagonists, and digoxin.

- Nurses can play a significant role in discussing treatment options, planning for lifestyle changes, counseling before discharge, and reinforcing key points during office visits. The best results are attained when the patient, the family, and the nurse work together to develop the care plan.

Additional Learning Resources

SG Go to your Study Guide for additional Review Questions for the NCLEX® Examination, Critical Thinking Clinical Situations, and other learning activities to help you master this chapter content.

Go to your Evolve website (https://evolve.elsevier.com/Clayton) for additional online resources.

Review Questions for the NCLEX® Examination

1. The sympathetic nervous system is activated in a patient with heart failure, causing which effect? *(Select all that apply.)*
   1. Tachycardia
   2. Peripheral vasoconstriction
   3. Increased contractility
   4. Peripheral vasodilation
   5. Bradycardia

2. A 59-year-old male patient with chronic heart failure asks the nurse what else he can do besides drug therapy to control the disease process. Which statement by the nurse would be appropriate? *(Select all that apply.)*
   1. "You need to remain active and continue to participate in the types of exercises you have done in the past, as tolerated."
   2. "The type of diet that is recommended is one low in calories, low in fat, and low in sodium."
   3. "It is important to conserve energy and avoid becoming fatigued."
   4. "If you find that not being able to use salt is hard, you can use salt substitutes on a salt-restricted diet."
   5. "You will need to weigh yourself every day and let your healthcare provider know if you are gaining or losing weight too rapidly."

3. The nurse caring for a patient with heart failure knows that inotropic agents are used for which effect on the heart?
   1. Dilating the left ventricle
   2. Increasing the force of contractions
   3. Slowing the heart rate
   4. Increasing the heart rate

4. The nurse knows that ACE inhibitors are used in heart failure for which result?
   1. To reduce blood pressure (i.e., afterload)
   2. To decrease renal flow
   3. To increase peripheral vascular resistance
   4. To cause vasoconstriction

5. Which of the following conditions place a patient at greater risk for developing digitalis toxicity? *(Select all that apply.)*
   1. Hyperkalemia
   2. Reduced renal function
   3. Liver disease
   4. Hypokalemia
   5. Hypernatremia

6. The nurse knows to watch for which symptoms of heart failure? *(Select all that apply.)*
   1. Decreased exercise tolerance
   2. Poor perfusion to the peripheral tissues
   3. Anorexia and nausea
   4. Edema present around the ankles
   5. Widening pulse pressure

7. One of the body's compensatory mechanisms that occurs in response to decreases in heart function is which symptom?
   1. Increased energy
   2. Increased urination
   3. Increased fatigue
   4. Increased peripheral perfusion

Objectives

1. Identify the nursing assessments used to evaluate a patient's state of hydration and renal function.
2. Describe the actions of diuretics and their effects on blood pressure and electrolytes.
3. Explain the rationale for administering diuretics cautiously to older adults and individuals with impaired renal function, cirrhosis of the liver, or diabetes mellitus.
4. Identify the nursing assessments needed to monitor the therapeutic response or the development of common or serious adverse effects of diuretic therapy.

Key Terms

tubule (TŪ-byŭl) (p. 436)
aldosterone (ăl-DŎS-tĕr-ōn) (p. 436)
edema (ĕ-DĒ-mă) (p. 438)
loop of Henle (HĔN-lē) (p. 440)

orthostatic hypotension (ŏr-thō-STĂT-ĭk hī-pō-TĔN-shŭn) (p. 441)
electrolyte imbalance (ĕ-LĔK-trō-līt ĭm-BĂL-ĕns) (p. 441)
hyperuricemia (hī-pĕr-yŭr-ĭ-SĒ-mē-ă) (p. 441)

DRUG THERAPY WITH DIURETICS

ACTIONS

Diuretics are drugs that act to increase the flow of urine. The purpose of diuretics is to increase the net loss of water from the body. To achieve this, they act on the kidneys in different locations of the nephron to enhance the excretion of sodium (see Fig. 28.1). The osmotic diuretics (glycerol, mannitol) and the carbonic anhydrase inhibitors (acetazolamide) act at the proximal tubule (Fig. 28.1-1). The loop diuretics (e.g., bumetanide, furosemide) act on the ascending limb of the loop of Henle (Fig. 28.1-2) and thiazides act directly on the distal kidney tubules (Fig. 28.1-3) to inhibit the reabsorption of sodium and chloride from the lumen of the tubule. Spironolactone, triamterene, and amiloride inhibit tubular reabsorption of sodium by inhibiting aldosterone, a hormone that induces reabsorption of sodium in the distal tubule and collecting duct (Fig. 28.1-4). Antidiuretic hormone (vasopressin) acts in the collecting duct to reabsorb water, making the urine more concentrated (Fig. 28.1-5). Sodium and chloride that are not reabsorbed are excreted into the collecting ducts and then into the ureters to the bladder, taking large volumes of water to be excreted from the body through urination.

USES

Diuretics are mainstays of treatment in two major diseases affecting the cardiovascular system, heart failure and hypertension. They are routinely used for patients with heart failure to remove excessive sodium and water in order to relieve symptoms associated with pulmonary congestion and edema. The Eighth Report of the Joint National Coordinating Committee on the Detection, Evaluation and Treatment of High Blood Pressure recommends that, after lifestyle modifications, diuretics (often in addition to other antihypertensive agents) should be used as primary agents to treat hypertension because they have been shown to reduce cardiovascular morbidity and mortality associated with hypertension.

Diuretics have a variety of other medical uses as well. Mannitol reduces cerebral edema, acetazolamide is used to reduce intraocular pressure associated with glaucoma, spironolactone can be effective in reducing ascites associated with liver disease, and furosemide may be used to treat hypercalcemia.

❖ NURSING IMPLICATIONS FOR DIURETIC THERAPY

The information the nurse obtains about the patient's general clinical symptoms is important to the healthcare provider when analyzing data for the diagnosis and success of therapy. In addition to assessing overall clinical symptoms, the nurse should include the following data for subsequent evaluation of the patient's response to prescribed therapies that act on the urinary system.

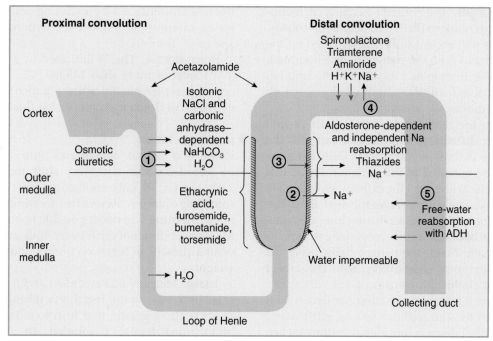

Fig. 28.1 Sites of actions of diuretics within the nephron.

◆ Assessment

History of related causative disorders and factors. Ask the patient questions relating to any history of disorders that contribute to fluid volume excess: heart disorders (e.g., myocardial infarction, heart failure, valvular disease, dysrhythmias); liver disease (e.g., ascites, cirrhosis, cancer of the liver); renal disease (e.g., renal failure); and factors such as immobility, hypertension, pregnancy, and use of corticosteroid agents.

History of current symptoms. Ask the patient questions to ascertain information relating to the onset, duration, and progression of specific symptoms relating to edema, weakness, fatigue, dyspnea, productive cough, and weight gain.

Pattern of urination. Ask the patient to describe his or her current urination pattern and to cite any changes. Details such as frequency, dysuria, incontinence, changes in the urine stream, hesitancy when starting to void, hematuria, nocturia, and urgency are all significant. Provide assistance with voiding for people with impaired mobility, fatigue, or other impairments.

Medication history. Obtain information from the patient about all prescribed and over-the-counter medications being taken. Tactfully ask questions about adherence to the medication regimen.

Hydration status. Obtain the patient's baseline vital signs. Note a pulse that is bounding and full or irregular (i.e., indicating possible dysrhythmias); check the respiratory rate and quality; listen to the lung sounds to detect the presence of crackles; ask the patient about a history of recent weight gain or loss; assess for edema of the extremities; and assess for neck vein distention. Blood pressure may also be elevated.

Dehydration. Assess, report, and record significant signs of dehydration in the patient. Observe for inelastic skin turgor, sticky oral mucous membranes, a shrunken or deeply furrowed tongue, crusted lips, weight loss, deteriorating vital signs, soft or sunken eyeballs, weak pedal pulses, delayed capillary filling, excessive thirst, a high urine specific gravity (or no urine output), and possible mental confusion.

Skin turgor. Check the patient's skin turgor by gently pinching the skin together over the sternum, on the forehead, or on the forearm. Elasticity is present when the skin rapidly returns to a flat position in the well-hydrated patient. In dehydrated patients, the skin will remain in a peaked or pinched position and return very slowly to the flat, normal position. Skin turgor is not a reliable indicator in older adults because of the natural aging changes of the skin.

Oral mucous membranes. With adequate hydration, the membranes of the mouth feel smooth and glisten. With dehydration, they appear dull and are sticky. Assess skin turgor, oral mucosa, and firmness of eyeballs.

Laboratory changes. The patient's hematocrit, hemoglobin, blood urea nitrogen (BUN), creatinine, osmolality, and electrolytes will appear to fluctuate, based on the state of hydration. When the patient is overhydrated, the values appear to drop as a result of hemodilution. A dehydrated patient will show higher values because of hemoconcentration.

Overhydration. Increases in abdominal girth, weight gain, neck vein distention, and circumference of the medial malleolus indicate overhydration. Daily measurements should be obtained of the patient's abdominal girth at the umbilical level and the extremities bilaterally at a level approximately 5 cm above the medial malleolus. The development of crackles during lung auscultation is also a sign of overhydration, especially in patients with heart failure. Weigh the patient daily using the same scale, at the same time of day, with the patient wearing similar clothing.

Edema. *Edema* is a term used to describe excess fluid accumulation in the extracellular spaces, particularly in the lower limbs. Edema is considered "pitting" when an indentation remains in the tissue after pressure is exerted against a bony part, such as the shin, ankle, or sacrum. The degree is usually recorded as +1 (slight) to +4 (deep).

Pale, cool, tight, shiny skin is another sign of edema. Also listen to lung sounds to detect the presence of excess fluid (crackles) in the lungs.

Assess for the presence of edema and record the degree of pitting. Obtain a baseline measurement of abdominal girth when edema is present, and check for the presence of fluid waves in the abdomen.

Electrolyte imbalance. Because the symptoms of most electrolyte imbalances are similar, the nurse should obtain information related to changes in the patient's mental status (i.e., alertness, orientation, confusion), muscle strength, muscle cramps, tremors, nausea, and general appearance.

Susceptible people. Those who are particularly susceptible to the development of electrolyte disturbances frequently have a history of renal or cardiac disease, hormonal disorders, or massive trauma or burns, or are receiving diuretic or steroid therapy. Review the patient's available electrolyte studies.

Hypokalemia. This is indicated by a serum potassium (K^+) level of less than 3.5 mEq/L. Hypokalemia is especially likely to occur when a patient exhibits vomiting, diarrhea, or heavy diuresis. All diuretics, except the potassium-sparing type, are likely to cause hypokalemia.

Hyperkalemia. This is indicated by a serum potassium (K^+) level of more than 5.5 mEq/L. Hyperkalemia occurs most commonly when a patient is given excessive amounts of potassium supplementation, either intravenously or orally. It may also occur as an adverse effect of potassium-sparing diuretics or with renal disease.

Hyponatremia. This is indicated by a serum sodium (Na^+) level of less than 135 mEq/L. Remember the following phrase: "Where sodium goes, water goes."

Because diuretics act by excreting sodium as well as water, monitor the patient for hyponatremia during and after diuresis.

Hypernatremia. This is indicated by a serum sodium (Na^+) level of more than 145 mEq/L. Hypernatremia occurs most frequently when a patient is given intravenous (IV) fluids in excess of the fluid excreted.

◆ **Implementation**

Intake and output. Intake and output (I&O) should be recorded accurately every shift and totaled every 24 hours for all patients having renal evaluations or receiving diuretics. Remember to administer diuretics in the morning whenever possible to prevent nocturia. Measure abdominal girth every shift, record degree of edema present in legs every shift, and obtain a daily weight.

Intake. Measure and record *accurately* all fluids taken (e.g., oral, parenteral, rectal, via tubes). Ice chips and foods such as gelatin that turn to a liquid state must be included. Irrigation solutions should be carefully measured so that the difference between what is instilled and what is returned can be recorded as intake.

Remember to enlist the help of the patient, family, and other visitors in this process. Ask them to keep a record of how many glasses or cups of liquids (e.g., water, juice, soda, tea, coffee) are consumed by the patient. The nurse then converts the household measurements to milliliters.

Nutrition. Patients with edema are routinely placed on a restricted sodium diet to help control edema associated with heart failure. Depending on the type of diuretic prescribed (potassium sparing or non–potassium sparing), the patient may be placed on potassium restrictions or potassium supplements.

Diet therapy for renal disease is directed at keeping a normal equilibrium of the body while decreasing the excretory load on the kidneys. See a nutrition text for modifications specific to acute and chronic renal failure.

Output. Record all output from the mouth, urethra, rectum, wounds, and tubes (e.g., surgical drains, nasogastric tubes, indwelling catheters). Liquid stools should be recorded according to consistency, color, and quantity. Urine output should include information on quantity, color, pH, odor, and specific gravity.

All other secretions should be characterized by color, consistency, volume, and changes from previous collections, if possible.

Daily output is usually 1200 to 1500 mL, or 30 to 50 mL/hr for the adult patient. Always report urine output below this hourly rate. Low hourly output may indicate dehydration, renal failure, or cardiac disease.

Keep the urinal or bedpan readily available. Tell patients and their visitors the importance of not dumping the bedpan or urinal. Instruct them to use the call light and allow the hospital personnel to empty and record all output.

Renal diagnostics. Many laboratory tests are ordered throughout the treatment of renal dysfunction (e.g., BUN, serum creatinine, creatinine clearance, serum osmolalities, urine osmolalities). Plan schedules for appropriate timing of collections of blood and urine samples.

Serum electrolytes. Monitor serum electrolyte reports; notify the healthcare provider of deviations from normal values.

Nutrition. Order a prescribed special diet, depending on the underlying pathologic condition. If fluid restrictions are prescribed, state the amount of fluid to be taken on each tray and the amount that may be taken orally each shift in the patient's computer chart.

◆ **Patient Education**
Purposes of diuresis
- If the disease process is hypertension, stress the importance of following the prescribed methods to deal with emotions and the dietary and medicinal regimens that can control the disease (see discussion of the nursing process for hypertensive therapy in Chapter 22).
- Teach the patient and significant others the functional changes that are caused by hypertension and heart failure. Emphasize the need for lifelong treatment and adherence to drug therapy, diet, and exercise regimens to obtain maximum control of the disease process.
- Diuretics are used in the treatment of several disease processes—for example, hypertension, glaucoma, ascites, hypercalcemia, heart failure, and renal disease. Be certain that the patient understands the medication administration schedule and desired therapeutic outcome for the prescribed therapy.

Medication considerations
- Diuretics should be taken in the morning to avoid nocturia.
- When the diuretic is prescribed on a scheduled pattern other than daily, assist the patient with developing ways to remember when to take the medication (e.g., using a calendar on which to mark dosages or using a medication holder marked with the days of the week that is loaded weekly with the medications to be taken).
- Instruct the patient to perform daily weights using the same scale, in similar clothing, and at the same time daily, usually before breakfast. Record and report significant weight changes because weight gains and losses are the best indicator of fluid loss or gain. Usually a gain of 2 pounds in 2 days should be reported.
- Potassium supplements may be prescribed concurrently with diuretics other than potassium-sparing diuretics.

- Diuretic therapy may produce postural hypotension. Teach the patient to rise slowly from a supine or sitting position, and encourage the patient to sit or lie down if feeling faint.

Nutrition
- The healthcare provider usually prescribes dietary modifications appropriate to the underlying pathologic condition, such as weight reduction or sodium restriction.
- Patients receiving potassium-sparing diuretics should be taught which foods are high in potassium content. These foods should be moderately restricted but not withheld from the diet. Salt substitutes should be avoided because they are high in potassium.
- When taking diuretics other than the potassium-sparing type, the patient is required to eat potassium-rich foods.

Fostering health maintenance
- Throughout the course of treatment, discuss medication information and how it will benefit the patient. Stress the importance of nonpharmacologic interventions and the long-term effects that compliance with the treatment regimen can provide.
- Provide the patient and significant others with important information contained in the specific drug monographs for the medicines prescribed. Additional health teaching and nursing interventions for the common and serious adverse effects are described in the drug monographs that follow.
- Seek cooperation and understanding of the following points so that medication compliance is increased: name of medication; dosage, route, times of administration; and common and serious adverse effects.

Patient self-assessment. Enlist the patient's aid in developing and maintaining a written record of monitoring parameters. See Patient Self-Assessment Form for Diuretics on the Evolve website. Complete the Premedication Data column for use as a baseline to track response to drug therapy. Ensure that the patient understands how to use the form, and instruct the patient to bring the completed form to follow-up visits. During follow-up visits, focus on issues that will foster adherence with the therapeutic interventions prescribed.

DRUG CLASS: CARBONIC ANHYDRASE INHIBITOR

acetazolamide (ă-sē-tă-ZŌL-ă-mīd)
Diamox (DĪ-ă-mŏks)

Actions

Acetazolamide is a weak diuretic that acts by inhibiting the enzyme carbonic anhydrase in the kidneys, brain, and eyes. As a diuretic, it promotes the excretion of sodium, potassium, water, and bicarbonate.

Uses

Acetazolamide is not used frequently as a diuretic because of the availability of more effective medications. However, it is used to reduce intraocular pressure in patients with glaucoma (see Chapter 42).

DRUG CLASS: SULFONAMIDE-TYPE LOOP DIURETICS

Actions

The loop diuretics are potent diuretics that act primarily by inhibiting sodium and chloride reabsorption from the ascending limb of the loop of Henle in the kidneys, enhancing sodium, potassium, chloride, phosphate, magnesium, and bicarbonate excretion into the urine.

Furosemide also acts to increase renal blood flow and glomerular filtration rate and inhibits electrolyte absorption in the proximal and distal tubules. The maximum diuretic effect occurs 1 to 2 hours after oral administration and lasts for 4 to 6 hours. (The brand name "Lasix" is derived from "lasts six hours.") Diuresis occurs 5 to 10 minutes after IV administration, peaks within 30 minutes, and lasts approximately 2 hours.

Bumetanide also acts by increasing renal blood flow into the glomeruli and inhibiting electrolyte absorption in the proximal tubule, but does not act on the distal tubule. Its diuretic activity starts 30 to 60 minutes after oral administration, peaks within 1 to 2 hours, and lasts 4 to 6 hours. Following IV injection, diuresis begins within minutes and reaches maximum levels in 15 to 30 minutes.

Torsemide does not appear to affect glomerular filtration rate or renal blood flow, or block reabsorption of sodium from the proximal or distal tubule. Maximum diuretic effect occurs 1 to 2 hours after oral administration and lasts 6 to 8 hours. Diuresis occurs 5 to 10 minutes after IV administration, peaks within 60 minutes, and lasts up to 6 hours.

Uses

Bumetanide, furosemide, and torsemide are used to treat edema resulting from heart failure, cirrhosis of the liver, and renal disease, including nephrotic syndrome. Furosemide and torsemide may also be used for the treatment of hypertension, alone or in combination with other antihypertensive therapy. Furosemide is also used in combination with 0.9% sodium chloride infusions to enhance the excretion of calcium in patients with hypercalcemia and to treat edema and heart failure.

Therapeutic Outcome

The primary therapeutic outcome associated with sulfonamide loop diuretic therapy is diuresis, with reduction of edema and improvement in symptoms related to excessive fluid accumulation. Reduction of blood pressure is an outcome also expected of furosemide and torsemide.

❖ **Nursing Implications for Sulfonamide-Type Loop Diuretics**

◆ *Premedication assessment*
1. Obtain baseline data such as vital signs, lung sounds, weight, degree of edema present, and laboratory studies (e.g., serum electrolytes, liver and renal function tests) before initiating therapy.
2. Obtain data relating to the patient's mental status (orientation, alertness, confusion), muscle strength, muscle cramps, tremors, nausea, and general appearance.
3. Patients with diabetes require baseline measurement of blood glucose levels.
4. Check for symptoms of acute gout. If present, notify the healthcare provider.
5. Note any reduction in hearing.

◆ *Availability.* See Table 28.1.

◆ *Dosage and administration.* **Adult:** *PO: Do not* exceed the maximum dosages identified in Table 28.1. Administer with food or milk to reduce gastric irritation. *Do not* administer after midafternoon to prevent nocturia.
   Adult: *IM or IV:*
   • *Bumetanide:* The IV and oral doses are equivalent. Administer IV doses over 1 to 2 minutes.

Table 28.1   Sulfonamide-Type Loop Diuretics

GENERIC NAME	BRAND NAME	DOSAGE FORMS AVAILABLE	DOSAGE RANGE
bumetanide	—	Tablets: 0.5, 1, 2 mg Injection: 0.25 mg/mL in 2-, 4-, and 10-mL vials	0.5-10 mg
furosemide ⇄ *Do not confuse furosemide with famotidine, fluoxetine, fosinopril, or minoxidil.*	Lasix ⇄ *Do not confuse Lasix with Lanoxin or Luvox.*	Tablets: 20, 40, 80 mg Oral solution: 8, 10 mg/mL IV: 10 mg/mL in 2-, 4-, and 10-mL vials	20-600 mg
torsemide ⇄ *Do not confuse torsemide with topiramate.*	Demadex ⇄ *Do not confuse Demadex with Demerol.*	Tablets: 5, 10, 20, and 100 mg	5-200 mg

- *Furosemide:* The IV dose is half the oral dose. Administer slowly over 2 to 4 minutes.

◆ Common adverse effects
Gastrointestinal

Oral irritation, dry mouth. Start regular oral hygiene measures when the therapy is initiated. Suggest the use of 1 teaspoon of hydrogen peroxide in 6 to 8 ounces of water as a mouthwash. Commercial mouthwashes contain alcohol, which may cause further drying and oral irritation. Another method to alleviate dryness is sucking on ice chips or hard candy.

Cardiovascular

Orthostatic hypotension. Although orthostatic hypotension (e.g., dizziness, weakness, faintness associated with a drop in blood pressure) is infrequent and generally mild, all diuretics may cause it to some degree, particularly when therapy is being initiated. Monitor the blood pressure daily in both the supine and standing positions. Anticipate the development of postural hypotension and take measures to prevent an occurrence. Teach the patient to rise slowly from a supine or sitting position, and encourage the patient to sit or lie down if feeling faint.

◆ Serious adverse effects
Gastrointestinal

Gastric irritation, abdominal pain. If gastric irritation occurs, administer with food or milk. If symptoms persist or increase in severity, report to the healthcare provider for evaluation.

Metabolic, renal

Electrolyte imbalance, dehydration. The electrolytes most commonly altered are potassium (K^+), sodium (Na^+), and chloride (Cl^-). Hypokalemia and hyponatremia are most likely to occur. Many symptoms associated with fluid and electrolyte imbalance are subtle and interspersed with general symptoms of drug toxicity or the disease process itself. Gather data about changes in the patient's mental status (alertness, orientation, confusion), muscle strength, muscle cramps, tremors, nausea, and general appearance. Always check the electrolyte reports for early indications of electrolyte imbalance. Keep accurate records of I&O, daily weights, and vital signs.

Hyperuricemia. Furosemide may inhibit the excretion of uric acid, resulting in hyperuricemia. Patients who have had previous attacks of gouty arthritis are particularly susceptible to additional attacks as a result of hyperuricemia. Monitor the laboratory reports for early indications of hyperuricemia. Report this to the healthcare provider, who may then add a uricosuric agent or allopurinol to the patient's medication regimen. (See Chapter 44 for more information on gout.)

Hyperglycemia. Diabetic or prediabetic patients must be monitored for the development of hyperglycemia, particularly during the early weeks of therapy. Assess regularly for hyperglycemia with a fingerstick blood sample and home glucometer, and report to the healthcare provider if it occurs with any frequency. Patients receiving oral hypoglycemic agents or insulin may require an adjustment in dosage.

Hypersensitivity

Hives, pruritus, rash. Report symptoms for further evaluation by the healthcare provider. Pruritus may be relieved by adding baking soda to the bathwater.

 Medication Safety Alert

Patients who are allergic to sulfonamides may also be allergic to sulfonamide-type loop diuretics. Use cautiously in these patients.

◆ Drug interactions

Alcohol, sedative-hypnotics, opioids. Orthostatic hypotension associated with sulfonamide-type loop diuretic therapy may be aggravated by these agents.

Digoxin. Sulfonamide-type loop diuretics may cause excessive potassium excretion, leading to hypokalemia. If the patient is also receiving digoxin, monitor closely for digitalis toxicity (anorexia, nausea, fatigue, blurred or colored vision, bradycardia, dysrhythmias).

 Clinical Goldmine

Remember, low potassium levels may cause digitalis toxicity. **Always check potassium levels for patients receiving diuretics prior to administration of digoxin.**

Aminoglycosides. The potential for ototoxicity from the aminoglycosides (e.g., gentamicin, tobramycin, amikacin) is increased. Assess the patient for gradual, often subtle, changes in hearing. Note whether the patient seems to speak more loudly, asks for statements to be repeated, or turns the television or radio progressively louder.

Cisplatin. The potential for ototoxicity from the combination of cisplatin and the sulfonamide-type loop diuretics is increased. Assess the patient for gradual, often subtle, changes in hearing. Note whether the patient seems to speak more loudly, asks for statements to be repeated, or turns the television or radio progressively louder.

Nonsteroidal antiinflammatory drugs. Nonsteroidal antiinflammatory drugs (NSAIDs) (e.g., indomethacin, ibuprofen, naproxen) inhibit the diuretic activity of the sulfonamide-type loop diuretics. The dose of diuretic may have to be increased or the NSAID discontinued. Maintain accurate I&O records and monitor for a decrease in diuretic activity.

Corticosteroids. Corticosteroids (e.g., prednisone) may enhance the loss of potassium. Check potassium levels and monitor more closely for hypokalemia when these two agents are used concurrently.

Metolazone. When used concurrently, there is a considerably greater diuresis than when either agent is used alone. Monitor closely for dehydration and electrolyte imbalance.

ethacrynic acid (ĕth-ă-KRĬN-ĭk)
Edecrin (Ĕ-dĕ-krĭn)

Actions

Ethacrynic acid is another diuretic that acts primarily on the ascending limb of the loop of Henle but also the proximal and distal tubules to prevent sodium and chloride reabsorption. Ethacrynic acid does not appear to affect renal blood flow or the glomerular filtration rate. Its diuretic activity begins within 30 minutes, peaks in approximately 2 hours, and lasts 6 to 8 hours.

Uses

Ethacrynic acid is used to treat edema resulting from heart failure, cirrhosis of the liver, renal disease, and malignancy and for hospitalized pediatric patients with congenital heart disease. It is thought that because ethacrynic acid inhibits the reabsorption of sodium to a much greater extent than other diuretics, it may be more effective for patients with significant renal failure. It is also used in conjunction with 0.9% sodium chloride infusions to enhance excretion of calcium in patients with hypercalcemia.

Therapeutic Outcome

The primary therapeutic outcome associated with ethacrynic acid therapy is diuresis with reduction of edema and improvement in symptoms related to excessive fluid accumulation.

❖ Nursing Implications for Ethacrynic Acid

◆ **Premedication assessment**

1. Obtain baseline data such as vital signs, lung sounds, weight, degree of edema present, and laboratory studies (e.g., serum electrolytes, liver and renal function tests) before initiating therapy.
2. Obtain data relating to the patient's mental status (orientation, alertness, confusion), muscle strength, muscle cramps, tremors, nausea, and general appearance.
3. Patients with diabetes require baseline measurement of blood glucose levels.

◆ *Availability.* *PO:* 25-mg tablets.
   IV: 50 mg/vial.

◆ *Dosage and administration.* **Adult:** *PO:* 50 to 100 mg initially, followed by 50 to 200 mg daily. *Do not* exceed 400 mg/day. Administer with food or milk to reduce gastric irritation. *Do not* administer after midafternoon to prevent nocturia.

Adult: *IV:* 50 mg or 0.5 to 1 mg/kg. Add 50 mL of dextrose 5% or saline solution to 50 mg of ethacrynic acid. This solution is stable for 24 hours. Administer over several minutes through the tubing of a running infusion or by direct IV line. Occasionally, the addition of a diluent may result in a cloudy solution. These solutions should *not* be used. Do not mix with blood derivatives.

Pediatric: *PO:* 1 mg/kg once daily; may increase up to 3 mg/kg/day. Adjust dosage at intervals of 2 to 3 days. Always monitor vital signs and I&O at regular intervals when administering this agent intravenously. Report blood pressure that decreases steadily or a narrowing pulse pressure, which may indicate hypovolemia.

◆ *Common adverse effects*
   Cardiovascular

Orthostatic hypotension. Although this effect is infrequent and generally mild, all diuretics may cause some degree of orthostatic hypotension (dizziness, weakness, faintness associated with a drop in blood pressure), particularly when therapy is initiated or dosages are increased. Monitor the blood pressure daily in both the supine and standing positions. Anticipate the development of postural hypotension and take measures to prevent its occurrence. Teach the patient to rise slowly from a supine or sitting position and encourage the patient to sit or lie down if feeling faint.

◆ *Serious adverse effects*
   Metabolic, renal

Electrolyte imbalance, dehydration. The electrolytes most commonly altered are potassium (K^+), sodium (Na^+), and chloride (Cl^-). Hypokalemia and hyponatremia are most likely to occur. Many symptoms associated with electrolyte imbalance are subtle and interspersed with general symptoms of drug toxicity or the disease process itself. Gather data about changes in the patient's mental status (alertness, orientation, confusion), muscle strength, muscle cramps, tremors, nausea, and general appearance. Always check the electrolyte reports for early indications of electrolyte imbalance. Keep accurate records of I&O, daily weights, and vital signs.

Dizziness, deafness, tinnitus. People with impaired renal function may experience these symptoms. Assess the patient for gradual, often subtle, changes in balance and hearing. Note whether the patient seems more unsteady when standing, speaks loudly, asks for statements to be repeated, or turns the television or radio progressively louder.

Gastrointestinal

Gastrointestinal bleeding. Observe for coffee-ground vomitus or dark, tarry stools, particularly in patients receiving IV therapy.

Diarrhea. Diarrhea may become severe. Report to the healthcare provider and monitor the patient for dehydration and fluid and electrolyte imbalance.

Endocrine

Hyperglycemia. Diabetic or prediabetic patients must be monitored for the development of hyperglycemia, particularly during the early weeks of therapy. Assess regularly for hyperglycemia with a fingerstick blood sample and a glucometer, and report to the healthcare provider if it occurs with any frequency. Patients receiving oral hypoglycemic agents or insulin may require an adjustment in dosage.

◆ *Drug interactions*

Aminoglycosides. The potential for ototoxicity from the aminoglycosides (e.g., gentamicin, tobramycin, amikacin) is increased. Assess the patient for gradual, often subtle, changes in hearing. Note whether the patient seems to speak loudly, asks for statements to be repeated, or turns the television or radio progressively louder.

Nonsteroidal antiinflammatory drugs. Nonsteroidal antiinflammatory drugs (e.g., indomethacin, ibuprofen, naproxen) inhibit the diuretic activity of ethacrynic acid. The dose of ethacrynic acid may have to be increased or the NSAID discontinued. Maintain accurate I&O records and monitor for a decrease in diuretic activity.

Digoxin. Ethacrynic acid may cause excess potassium excretion, leading to hypokalemia. If the patient is also receiving digoxin, monitor closely for digitalis toxicity (anorexia, nausea, fatigue, blurred or colored vision, bradycardia, dysrhythmias).

Corticosteroids. Corticosteroids (e.g., prednisone) may enhance the loss of potassium. Check potassium levels and monitor more closely for hypokalemia when these two agents are used concurrently.

DRUG CLASS: THIAZIDE DIURETICS

Actions

Benzothiadiazides, more commonly called thiazides, have been an important and useful class of diuretic and antihypertensive agents since the 1960s. As diuretics, thiazides act primarily on the distal tubule of the kidney to block the reabsorption of sodium and chloride ions from the tubule. The sodium and chloride ions that are not reabsorbed are passed into the collecting ducts, taking molecules of water with them, resulting in a diuresis.

Uses

Thiazides are used as diuretics in the treatment of edema associated with heart failure, renal disease, hepatic disease, pregnancy, obesity, premenstrual syndrome, and administration of adrenocortical steroids. The antihypertensive properties of thiazides result from a direct vasodilatory action on the peripheral arterioles

(see Chapter 22). Thiazide diuretics tend to lose their diuretic action after about 6 weeks of therapy, but the antihypertensive properties continue. Thiazide diuretics also tend to lose their diuretic effect when creatinine clearance is less than 30 mL/min.

Therapeutic Outcomes

The primary therapeutic outcomes associated with thiazide therapy are diuresis with reduction of edema and improvement in symptoms related to excessive fluid accumulation, and reduction in elevated blood pressure.

❖ Nursing Implications for Thiazide Diuretics

◆ *Premedication assessment*

1. Obtain baseline data such as vital signs, lung sounds, weight, degree of edema present, and laboratory studies (e.g., serum electrolytes, liver and renal function tests) before initiating therapy.
2. Obtain data relating to the patient's mental status (orientation, alertness, confusion), muscle strength, muscle cramps, tremors, nausea, and general appearance.
3. Patients with diabetes require baseline measurement of blood glucose levels.
4. Note any reduction in hearing.
5. Check for any symptoms of acute gout. If present, notify the healthcare provider.

◆ *Availability.* Tables 28.2 and 28.3 list thiazide diuretics and diuretics chemically related to the thiazides. Most of the diuretics listed are administered in divided daily dosages for the treatment of hypertension. However, a single daily dosage may be most effective for mobilization of edema fluid.

◆ *Dosage and administration.* See Tables 28.2 and 28.3. Administer with food or milk to reduce gastric irritation. *Do not* administer after midafternoon to prevent nocturia.

◆ *Common adverse effects*

Cardiovascular

Orthostatic hypotension. Although orthostatic hypotension (dizziness, weakness, faintness associated with a drop in blood pressure) is infrequent and generally mild, all diuretics may cause some degree of orthostatic

Table 28.2 Thiazide Diuretics

GENERIC NAME	BRAND NAME	DOSAGE FORMS AVAILABLE	DOSAGE RANGE
chlorothiazide	Diuril	Tablets: 250, 500 mg Oral suspension: 250 mg/5 mL Injection: 500 mg	500-1000 mg once or twice daily
hydrochlorothiazide ⇄ *Do not confuse hydrochlorothiazide with hydroxychloroquine.*	—	Tablets: 12.5, 25, 50 mg Capsules: 12.5 mg	12.5-200 mg

Table 28.3 **Thiazide-Related Diuretics**

GENERIC NAME	BRAND NAME	DOSAGE FORMS AVAILABLE	DOSAGE RANGE
chlorthalidone ⇄ Do not confuse chlorthalidone with chlorpromazine or chlorothiazide.	—	Tablets: 25, 50 mg	50-200 mg
indapamide	—	Tablets: 1.25, 2.5 mg	1.25-5 mg
metolazone ⇄ Do not confuse metolazone with medroxyprogesterone, metaxalone, methotrexate, metoclopramide, or metoprolol.	Zaroxolyn ⇄ Do not confuse Zaroxolyn with Zyprexa.	Tablets: 2.5, 5, 10 mg	2.5-20 mg

hypotension, particularly when therapy is being initiated. Monitor the blood pressure daily in both the supine and standing positions. Anticipate the development of postural hypotension and take measures to prevent it. Teach the patient to rise slowly from a supine or sitting position, and encourage the patient to sit or lie down if feeling faint.

◆ *Serious adverse effects*
Gastrointestinal
Gastric irritation, nausea, vomiting, constipation. If gastric irritation occurs, administer with food or milk. If symptoms persist or increase in severity, report to the healthcare provider for evaluation.

Metabolic, renal
Electrolyte imbalance, dehydration. Use of thiazides may cause or aggravate electrolyte imbalance; therefore patients should be observed regularly for signs such as dry mouth, drowsiness, confusion, muscular weakness, and nausea. The electrolytes most commonly altered are potassium (K^+), sodium (Na^+), and chloride (Cl^-). Hypokalemia is most likely to occur, and supplementary potassium is often prescribed to prevent or treat it. Many symptoms associated with altered fluid and electrolyte balance are subtle and interspersed with general symptoms of drug toxicity or the disease process itself. Gather data about changes in the patient's mental status (alertness, orientation, confusion), muscle strength, muscle cramps, tremors, nausea, and general appearance. Always check the electrolyte reports for early indications of electrolyte imbalance. Keep accurate records of I&O, daily weights, and vital signs.

Hyperuricemia. The plasma uric acid level is frequently elevated by the thiazides, which inhibit the excretion of uric acid. Patients who have had previous episodes of hyperuricemia or attacks of gouty arthritis are particularly susceptible to additional attacks when receiving thiazide therapy. Monitor the laboratory reports for early indications of hyperuricemia. Report to the healthcare provider, who may then add a uricosuric agent or allopurinol to the patient's medication regimen. (See Chapter 44 for more information on gout.)

Endocrine
Hyperglycemia. The thiazides may induce hyperglycemia and aggravate cases of preexisting diabetes mellitus. Diabetic or prediabetic patients must be monitored for the development of hyperglycemia, particularly during the early weeks of therapy. Assess regularly for hyperglycemia using a fingerstick blood sample and glucometer, and report to the healthcare provider if it occurs with any frequency. Dosages of oral hypoglycemic agents and insulin may need adjustment in patients with diabetes mellitus who also require diuretic therapy.

Hypersensitivity
Hives, pruritus, rash. Report symptoms for further evaluation by the healthcare provider. Pruritus may be relieved by adding baking soda to the bathwater.

◆ *Drug interactions*
Digoxin. Thiazide diuretics may cause excessive excretion of potassium, resulting in hypokalemia. If the patient is also receiving digoxin, monitor closely for signs of digitalis toxicity (e.g., anorexia, nausea, fatigue, blurred or colored vision, bradycardia, dysrhythmias).

Corticosteroids. Corticosteroids (e.g., prednisone) may enhance the loss of potassium. Check potassium levels and monitor more closely for hypokalemia when these two agents are used concurrently.

Lithium. Thiazide diuretics may induce lithium toxicity. Monitor patients for lithium toxicity manifested by nausea, anorexia, fine tremors, persistent vomiting, profuse diarrhea, hyperreflexia, lethargy, and weakness.

Nonsteroidal antiinflammatory drugs. Nonsteroidal antiinflammatory drugs (e.g., indomethacin, ibuprofen, naproxen) inhibit the diuretic activity of this agent. The dose of thiazide may have to be increased or the NSAID discontinued. Maintain accurate I&O records and monitor for a decrease in diuretic activity.

Oral hypoglycemic agents, insulin. Because of the hyperglycemic effects of the thiazide diuretics, dosage adjustments of insulin and oral hypoglycemic agents are often required.

DRUG CLASS: POTASSIUM-SPARING DIURETICS

amiloride (ă-MĬL-ōr-īd)
  Midamor (MĬ-dă-mōr)

Actions

Amiloride is a potassium-sparing diuretic that also has weak antihypertensive activity. Its mechanism of action is unknown, but it acts at the distal renal tubule to retain potassium and excrete sodium, resulting in a mild diuresis.

Uses

Amiloride is usually used in combination with other diuretics in patients with hypertension or heart failure to help prevent hypokalemia that may result from other diuretic therapy.

Therapeutic Outcome

The primary therapeutic outcome associated with amiloride therapy is diuresis with reduction of edema and improvement in symptoms related to excessive fluid accumulation.

❖ Nursing Implications for Amiloride
◆ *Premedication assessment*
1. Obtain baseline data such as vital signs, lung sounds, weight, degree of edema present, and laboratory studies (e.g., serum electrolytes, liver and renal function tests) before initiating therapy.
2. Obtain data relating to the patient's mental status (orientation, alertness, confusion), muscle strength, muscle cramps, tremors, nausea, and general appearance.

◆ *Availability.* *PO:* 5-mg tablets.

◆ *Dosage and administration.* **Adult:** *PO:* Initially, 5 mg daily. Dosage may be increased in 5-mg increments up to 20 mg daily with close monitoring of electrolytes. Administer with food or milk to reduce gastric irritation. *Do not* administer after midafternoon to prevent nocturia.

◆ *Common adverse effects*
Gastrointestinal
Anorexia, nausea, vomiting, flatulence. These adverse effects should be mild, particularly if the dose is administered with food. Persistent nausea and vomiting should be evaluated for other causes, as well as for the development of electrolyte imbalance.
Neurologic
Headache. Monitor the blood pressure at regularly scheduled intervals because amiloride is used for hypertension. Additional readings should be taken during headaches to determine if headaches are caused by the agents or by hypertension. Report persistent headaches to the healthcare provider.

◆ *Serious adverse effects*
Metabolic, cardiovascular
Electrolyte imbalance, dehydration. The electrolytes most commonly altered are potassium (K^+), sodium (Na^+), and chloride (Cl^-). Hyperkalemia is most likely to occur.

Report potassium levels higher than 5 mEq/L to the healthcare provider. Many symptoms associated with altered fluid and electrolyte balance are subtle and interspersed with general symptoms of drug toxicity or the disease process itself. Gather data about changes in the patient's mental status (alertness, orientation, confusion), muscle strength, muscle cramps, tremors, nausea, and general appearance. Always check the electrolyte reports for early indications of electrolyte imbalance. Keep accurate records of I&O, daily weights, and vital signs.

◆ *Drug interactions*
Lithium. Amiloride may induce lithium toxicity. Monitor patients who take lithium for lithium toxicity as manifested by nausea, anorexia, fine tremors, persistent vomiting, profuse diarrhea, hyperreflexia, lethargy, and weakness.

Potassium supplements, salt substitutes. Amiloride inhibits potassium excretion. *Do not* administer with potassium supplements or use salt substitutes high in potassium because of the potentially dangerous effects of hyperkalemia.

Hyperkalemia. Angiotensin-converting enzyme (ACE) inhibitors (e.g., captopril, lisinopril, ramipril), angiotensin II receptor blockers (ARBs; e.g., losartan, candesartan), and aldosterone receptor blocking agents (e.g., eplerenone, spironolactone) inhibit aldosterone. Patients may develop hyperkalemia (K^+ above 5.7 mEq/L). Most cases resolve without discontinuation of therapy. Patients most susceptible to the development of hyperkalemia are those with renal impairment or diabetes mellitus and those already receiving a potassium supplement. In general, potassium-sparing diuretics (e.g., amiloride, triamterene) should not be taken concurrently with these antihypertensive agents.

Nonsteroidal antiinflammatory drugs. Nonsteroidal antiinflammatory drugs (e.g., indomethacin, ibuprofen, naproxen) inhibit the diuretic activity of amiloride. The dose of amiloride may have to be increased or the NSAID discontinued. Maintain accurate I&O records and monitor for a decrease in diuretic activity.

---

spironolactone (spī-rō-nō-LĂK-tōn)
Aldactone (ăl-DĂK-tōn)

Actions

Spironolactone blocks the sodium-retaining and potassium-excreting and magnesium-excreting properties of aldosterone, resulting in a loss of water with the increased sodium excretion.

Uses

Spironolactone is a diuretic that is particularly useful in relieving edema and ascites that do not respond to the usual diuretics. It may be given with thiazide diuretics to increase its effect and reduce the hypokalemia often induced by the thiazides. Spironolactone has also been shown to further reduce morbidity and mortality for patients with heart failure who are also being treated with an ACE inhibitor and a loop diuretic.

Therapeutic Outcome

The primary therapeutic outcome associated with spironolactone therapy is diuresis, with reduction of edema and improvement in symptoms related to excessive fluid accumulation and heart failure.

❖ Nursing Implications for Spironolactone

◆ *Premedication assessment*

1. Obtain baseline data such as vital signs, lung sounds, weight, degree of edema present, and laboratory studies (e.g., serum electrolytes, liver and renal function tests) before initiating therapy.
2. Obtain data relating to the patient's mental status (orientation, alertness, confusion), muscle strength, muscle cramps, tremors, nausea, and general appearance.
3. Tactfully ask about any preexisting problems with libido.

◆ *Availability.* **PO:** 25-, 50-, and 100-mg tablets; oral suspension: 25 mg/5 mL in 118- and 473-mL bottles.

◆ *Dosage and administration.* **Adult: PO:** Initially, 100 mg daily. Maintenance dosage is usually 25 to 200 mg daily, but doses up to 400 mg may be prescribed. Administer with food or milk to reduce gastric irritation. *Do not* administer after midafternoon to prevent nocturia.

◆ *Common and serious adverse effects*

Neurologic

Mental confusion. Perform a baseline assessment of the patient's alertness; drowsiness; lethargy; and orientation to time, date, and place before starting drug therapy. Compare subsequent mental status and assess on a regular basis.

Headache. Monitor blood pressure at regularly scheduled intervals because this agent is used for hypertension. Additional readings should be taken during headaches to determine if headaches are caused by the agent or the hypertension. Report persistent headaches to the healthcare provider.

Gastrointestinal

Diarrhea. The onset of new symptoms occurring after initiating the drug therapy requires evaluation if persistent.

Metabolic

Electrolyte imbalance, dehydration. The electrolytes most commonly altered are potassium (K^+), sodium (Na^+), and chloride (Cl^-). Hyperkalemia is most likely to occur. Report potassium levels higher than 5 mEq/L to the healthcare provider. Many symptoms associated with altered fluid and electrolyte balance are subtle and interspersed with general symptoms of drug toxicity or the disease process itself. Gather data about changes in the patient's mental status (alertness, orientation,

confusion), muscle strength, muscle cramps, tremors, nausea, and general appearance. Always check the electrolyte reports for early indications of electrolyte imbalance. Keep accurate records of I&O, daily weights, and vital signs.

Endocrine

Gynecomastia, reduced libido, breast tenderness. Because the chemical structure of spironolactone is similar to that of estrogen hormones, an occasional male patient will report gynecomastia, reduced libido, and diminished erection. Women may complain of breast soreness and menstrual irregularities. These effects are reversible after therapy is discontinued.

◆ *Drug interactions*

Potassium supplements, salt substitutes. Spironolactone inhibits potassium excretion. *Do not* administer with potassium supplements or use salt substitutes high in potassium because of potentially dangerous effects from hyperkalemia.

Hyperkalemia. Angiotensin-converting enzyme inhibitors (e.g., captopril, lisinopril, ramipril), ARBs (e.g., losartan, candesartan), and aldosterone receptor blocking agents (e.g., eplerenone, spironolactone) inhibit aldosterone. Patients may develop hyperkalemia (K^+ above 5.7 mEq/L). Most cases resolve without discontinuation of therapy. Patients most susceptible to the development of hyperkalemia are those with renal impairment or diabetes mellitus and those already receiving a potassium supplement. In general, potassium-sparing diuretics should not be taken concurrently with these antihypertensive agents.

Nonsteroidal antiinflammatory drugs. Nonsteroidal antiinflammatory drugs (e.g., indomethacin, ibuprofen, naproxen) inhibit the diuretic activity of spironolactone. The dosage of spironolactone may have to be increased or the NSAID discontinued. Maintain accurate I&O records and monitor for a decrease in diuretic activity.

---

triamterene (trī-ĂM-tĕr-ēn)
 Dyrenium (dī-RĒ-nē-ŭm)

Actions

Triamterene is a very mild diuretic that acts by blocking the exchange of potassium for sodium in the distal tubule of the kidney, resulting in retention of potassium with excretion of sodium and water.

Uses

Triamterene is an effective agent to use in conjunction with the potassium-excreting diuretics, such as the thiazides, and the loop diuretics.

Therapeutic Outcome

The primary therapeutic outcome associated with triamterene therapy is diuresis with reduction of edema and improvement in symptoms related to excessive fluid accumulation.

❖ **Nursing Implications for Triamterene**

◆ *Premedication assessment*

1. Obtain baseline data such as vital signs, lung sounds, weight, degree of edema present, and laboratory studies (e.g., serum electrolytes, liver and renal function tests) before initiating therapy.

2. Obtain data relating to the patient's mental status (orientation, alertness, confusion), muscle strength, muscle cramps, tremors, nausea, and general appearance.

◆ *Availability.* **PO:** 50- and 100-mg capsules.

◆ *Dosage and administration.* **Adult: *PO:*** 100 to 300 mg/day given once or twice daily; maximum dose: 300 mg daily.

◆ *Common and serious adverse effects*

Metabolic

Electrolyte imbalance, dehydration, leg cramps, weakness. The electrolytes most commonly altered are potassium (K^+), sodium (Na^+), and chloride (Cl^-). Hyperkalemia is most likely to occur. Report potassium levels higher than 5 mEq/L to the healthcare provider. Many symptoms associated with altered fluid and electrolyte balance are subtle and interspersed with general symptoms of drug toxicity or the disease process itself. Gather data about changes in the patient's mental status (alertness, orientation, confusion), muscle strength, muscle cramps, tremors, nausea, and general appearance (drowsy, anxious, lethargic). Always check the electrolyte reports for early indications of electrolyte imbalance. Keep accurate records of I&O, daily weights, and vital signs.

Gastrointestinal

Nausea, vomiting. These adverse effects should be mild, particularly if the dose is administered with food. Persistent nausea and vomiting should be evaluated for other causes, as well as for the development of electrolyte imbalance.

Hypersensitivity

Hives, pruritus, rash. Report symptoms for further evaluation by the healthcare provider. Pruritus may be relieved by adding baking soda to the bathwater.

◆ *Drug interactions*

Salt substitutes, potassium supplements. Triamterene inhibits potassium excretion. *Do not* administer with potassium supplements or use salt substitutes high in potassium because of the potentially dangerous effects from hyperkalemia.

Hyperkalemia. Angiotensin-converting enzyme inhibitors (e.g., captopril, lisinopril, ramipril), ARBs (e.g., losartan, candesartan), and aldosterone receptor blocking agents (e.g., eplerenone, spironolactone) inhibit aldosterone. Patients may develop hyperkalemia (K^+ above 5.7 mEq/L). Most cases resolve without discontinuation of therapy. Patients most susceptible to the development of hyperkalemia are those with renal impairment or diabetes mellitus and those already receiving a potassium supplement. In general, potassium-sparing diuretics should not be taken concurrently with these antihypertensive agents.

Nonsteroidal antiinflammatory drugs. Nonsteroidal antiinflammatory drugs (e.g., indomethacin, ibuprofen, naproxen) inhibit the diuretic activity of triamterene. The dosage of triamterene may have to be increased or the NSAID discontinued. Maintain accurate I&O records and monitor for a decrease in diuretic activity.

DRUG CLASS: COMBINATION DIURETIC PRODUCTS

A common problem associated with thiazide diuretic therapy is hypokalemia. In an attempt to minimize this adverse effect, several products have been manufactured that contain a potassium-sparing diuretic combined with a thiazide diuretic (Table 28.4). The goal of these combination products is to promote diuresis and antihypertensive effect through different mechanisms of action while maintaining normal serum potassium levels. Patients receiving a combination product are at risk for adverse effects resulting from any of the component drugs. Many cases of hyperkalemia and hyponatremia have been reported after the use of the combination products.

Combination products should not be used as initial therapy for edema or hypertension. Therapy with individual products should be adjusted for each patient. If the fixed combination represents the appropriate dosage for each component, the use of a combination product may be more convenient for patient compliance. Patients must be reevaluated periodically for appropriateness of therapy and to prevent electrolyte imbalance.

Table 28.4   Combination Diuretics

GENERIC NAME	BRAND NAME	DOSAGE RANGE
spironolactone 25 mg, hydrochlorothiazide 25 mg	Aldactazide-25	1-8 tablets daily
spironolactone 50 mg, hydrochlorothiazide 50 mg	Aldactazide-50	1-4 tablets daily
triamterene 37.5 mg, hydrochlorothiazide 25 mg	Dyazide	1 to 2 capsules once daily
triamterene 37.5 mg, hydrochlorothiazide 25 mg	Maxzide-25	1 to 2 tablets once daily
triamterene 50 mg, hydrochlorothiazide 25 mg	—	1 to 2 tablets once daily
triamterene 75 mg, hydrochlorothiazide 50 mg	Maxzide	1 tablet daily
amiloride 5 mg, hydrochlorothiazide 50 mg	—	1 or 2 tablets daily with meals

Get Ready for the NCLEX® Examination!

Key Points

- Diuretics are drugs that act at various locations in the nephron to increase the flow of urine.
- The purpose of diuretics is to increase the net loss of water.
- Diuretics are mainstays in the symptomatic treatment of heart failure, hypertension, and renal disease.
- Diuretics also have a variety of other medical uses, such as reducing cerebral edema, intraocular pressure, ascites, and hypercalcemia.
- The information that the nurse obtains about the patient's general clinical symptoms is important to the healthcare provider when analyzing data for diagnosis and success of therapy.

Additional Learning Resources

SG Go to your Study Guide for additional Review Questions for the NCLEX® Examination, Critical Thinking Clinical Situations, and other learning activities to help you master this chapter content.

Go to your Evolve website (https://evolve.elsevier.com/Clayton) for additional online resources.

Review Questions for the NCLEX® Examination

1. The nurse is assessing a patient taking diuretics for signs of dehydration. What should the nurse assess for? *(Select all that apply.)*
   1. Elastic skin turgor
   2. Lower lab values of hematocrit and hemoglobin from baseline
   3. Dry and sticky oral mucous membranes
   4. Lab values of hematocrit and hemoglobin elevated from baseline

2. Which adverse effect will the nurse watch for in patients with renal impairment while taking amiloride (Midamor)?
   1. Hyperkalemia
   2. Hypokalemia
   3. Hyponatremia
   4. Hypernatremia

3. A nurse is assessing a patient receiving diuretic therapy for signs of electrolyte imbalance. Which of the following are signs or symptoms of electrolyte imbalance? *(Select all that apply.)*
   1. Peripheral edema
   2. Muscle cramps
   3. Nausea with episodes of vomiting
   4. Confusion
   5. Crackles in the lungs

4. The nurse was discussing the possible adverse effects of thiazide diuretic therapy with a patient. The nurse recognized further education was needed when the patient made which statement?
   1. "I understand that, since I am taking this hydrochlorothiazide, I can expect my kidneys to shut down."
   2. "So you are saying that if my ears start to ring continuously then I need to let my doctor know."
   3. "I will need to get my blood work done periodically to determine if this drug is making my potassium level drop."
   4. "I know that I am taking this for my high blood pressure, so I should expect that it will control it better once I get started on this."

5. The nurse reviews which laboratory tests to determine the status of renal function?
   1. Blood sugar and hemoglobin A_{1c}
   2. Serum creatinine and BUN
   3. Uric acid and serum calcium
   4. Serum potassium and chloride

6. The nurse was caring for a patient who asked for a pain pill (ibuprofen) for a recent arm fracture and was currently taking the diuretic furosemide (Lasix). What would be an appropriate response by the nurse?
   1. "Sure, no problem; the two medications do not interact."
   2. "Since these two medications have a known interaction, I will not be allowed to give you any for pain."
   3. "If I give you the pain pill, it will affect the diuretic and you will have an increased effect from the diuretic."
   4. "This pain medication may require an increased dosage of the diuretic."

7. The nurse knows that individuals with impaired renal function, cirrhosis of the liver, or diabetes mellitus need to be given diuretics cautiously because they are known to cause what effect? *(Select all that apply.)*
   1. Diabetic patients may experience hyperglycemia.
   2. Patients with cirrhosis of the liver may develop orthostatic hypotension.
   3. Patients with renal disease tend to develop electrolyte imbalances.
   4. Diabetic patients may experience hypoglycemia.
   5. Patients with renal disease will develop edema secondary to diuretics.

8. The nurse monitoring a patient using diuretics to reduce peripheral edema will watch for which therapeutic response?
   1. A reduction in cerebral edema and headaches
   2. A reduction in edema and an increased urine output
   3. A reduction in ascites associated with liver congestion
   4. An improvement in renal function

9. A nurse assessing a patient for fluid overload will assess for which symptoms? *(Select all that apply.)*
   1. Elastic skin turgor
   2. Moist shiny oral mucous membranes
   3. Pitting edema around the ankle
   4. Neck vein distention
   5. Lab values of hematocrit and hemoglobin elevated from baseline

Drugs Used to Treat Upper Respiratory Disease

https://evolve.elsevier.com/Clayton

Objectives

1. Describe the function of the respiratory system and list the common upper respiratory diseases.
2. Discuss the causes of allergic rhinitis, nasal congestion, and rhinitis medicamentosa.
3. Explain the major actions (effects) of sympathomimetic, antihistaminic, and corticosteroid decongestants and cromolyn.
4. Explain why all decongestant products should be used cautiously by people with hypertension, hyperthyroidism, diabetes mellitus, cardiac disease, increased intraocular pressure, or prostatic disease.
5. Discuss the premedication assessments and nursing assessments needed during therapy to monitor the therapeutic response to and the common and serious adverse effects of decongestant drug therapy.

Key Terms

rhinitis (rī-NĪ-tĭs) (p. 450)
sinusitis (sī-nyū-SĪ-tĭs) (p. 451)
allergic rhinitis (ă-LĔR-jĭk rī-NĪ-tĭs) (p. 451)
antigen-antibody (ĂN-tĭ-jĕn ĂN-tĭ-bŏ-dē) (p. 451)
histamine (HĬS-tă-mēn) (p. 451)
rhinorrhea (rī-nō-RĒ-ă) (p. 451)

decongestants (dē-kŏn-JĔS-tănts) (p. 451)
rhinitis medicamentosa (rī-NĪ-tĭs mĕd-ĭ-kŏ-mĕn-TŌ-să) (p. 451)
antihistamines (ăn-tĭ-HĬS-tă-mēnz) (p. 452)
antiinflammatory agents (ăn-tī-ĭn-FLĂ-mă-tō-rē) (p. 453)

UPPER RESPIRATORY TRACT ANATOMY AND PHYSIOLOGY

The respiratory system is a series of airways that start with the nose and mouth and end at the alveolar sacs within the lungs. The upper respiratory tract is composed of the nose and its turbinates, the sinuses, the nasopharynx, the pharynx, the tonsils, the eustachian tubes, and the larynx (Fig. 29.1). The nose and its structures serve two functions: olfactory (i.e., smell) and respiratory. The olfactory region is located in the upper part of each nostril. It is an area of specialized tissue cells (i.e., olfactory cells) that contain microscopic hairs that react to odors in the air and then stimulate the olfactory cells. The olfactory cells in turn send signals to the brain, which processes the sensation that people perceive as a particular smell.

The respiratory function of the nose is to warm, humidify, and filter the air inhaled to prepare it for the lower respiratory airways. Both nasal passages have folds of skin called *turbinates* that significantly increase the surface area of the passages and contain massive numbers of blood vessels. The blood circulating through the membranes lining the turbinates warms and humidifies inhaled air. The inhaled air is also filtered of particulate matter. The hairs at the entrance to the nostrils remove large particles, and the turbinates and narrowness of the nasal passages cause turbulence of the airflow passing through with each inhalation. All of the surfaces of the nose are coated with a thin layer of mucus, which is secreted by goblet cells. Because of the turbulence of the airflow, particles are thrown against the walls of the nasal passages and become trapped in the mucosal secretions. The epithelial cells lining the posterior two-thirds of the nasal passages contain cilia that sweep the particulate matter back toward the nasopharynx and pharynx. Once in the pharynx, the particulate matter is expectorated or swallowed. The warming, humidification, and filtration processes continue as the air passes into the trachea, bronchi, and bronchioles.

The nasal structures are innervated by the autonomic nervous system. Cholinergic stimulation causes vasodilation of the blood vessels lining the nasal mucosa

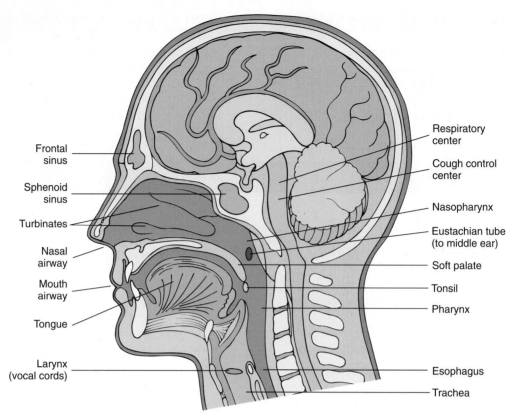

Fig. 29.1 The upper respiratory tract.

and sympathetic (primarily alpha-adrenergic) stimulation causes vasoconstriction. The cholinergic fibers also innervate the secretory glands. When stimulated, they produce serous and mucous secretions within the nostrils.

The paranasal sinuses are hollow, air-filled cavities in the cranial bones on both sides of and behind the nose. There are eight sinuses (four on each side). The purpose of the paranasal sinuses appears to be to act as resonating chambers for the voice and as a means of lightening the bones of the head. The sinuses are lined with the same mucous membranes and ciliated epithelia as those of the upper respiratory tract. The sinuses are connected to the nasal passages by ducts that drain secretions into the nasal cavity from activity of the ciliated cells.

On either side of the oral pharynx is a pharyngeal tonsil, a collection of lymphoid tissue that is called the *adenoids* when enlarged. The tonsils are located in an area where mucus laden with particulate matter (e.g., virus particles, bacteria) accumulates from the ciliary action of cells in the nasopharynx above. The lymphoid tissue is rich in immunoglobulins and is thought to play a role in the immunologic defense mechanisms of the upper airway.

Sneezing is a physiologic reflex used by the body to clear the nasal passages of foreign matter. The sneeze reflex is initiated by irritation of the nasal mucosa by

foreign particulate matter. It is similar to the cough reflex, which clears the lower respiratory airways of secretions and foreign matter.

COMMON UPPER RESPIRATORY DISEASES

Rhinitis is inflammation of the nasal mucous membranes. Signs and symptoms include sneezing, nasal discharge, and nasal congestion. Rhinitis is often subclassified as acute or chronic on the basis of the duration of the signs and symptoms. The most common causes of acute rhinitis are the common cold (viral infection), bacterial infection, presence of a foreign body, and drug-induced congestion (rhinitis medicamentosa). Common causes of chronic rhinitis are allergy, nonallergic perennial rhinitis, chronic sinusitis, and a deviated septum.

The common cold is actually a viral infection of the upper respiratory tissues. When considering the amount of time lost from school and work and the number of healthcare provider office visits that this condition causes annually, it is probably the single most expensive illness in the United States. Seasons in which viral infections reach near-epidemic proportions are midwinter, spring, and early fall (i.e., a few weeks after school starts). Six different virus families, including 120 to 200 subtypes, cause cold-like symptoms; the most common are the rhinoviruses and coronaviruses. Viruses are spread from person to person by direct contact and sneezing. The earliest symptoms of a cold are a clear, watery nasal discharge and sneezing. Nasal congestion from engorgement of the nasal blood vessels and swelling of nasal turbinates quickly follows. Over the next 48 hours the discharge becomes cloudy and much more viscous. Other symptoms include coughing, a "scratchy" or mildly sore throat (pharyngitis), and hoarseness (laryngitis). Other symptoms that occur less frequently are headache, malaise, chills, and fever. A few patients may develop a fever up to 100°F (37.8°C). Symptoms should subside within 5 to 7 days.

Complications occasionally develop as a result of the challenge to the body's immune system initiated by cold viruses. Complications can also arise from thick, tenacious mucus obstructing the sinus ducts or the eustachian tubes to the middle ears. Bacteria are easily trapped behind these obstructions in the sinuses and ears, resulting in bacterial **sinusitis** or otitis media (infection of the middle ear). Viral infections are also a common cause of exacerbations of obstructive lung disease and of acute asthmatic attacks in susceptible individuals. If symptoms of the cold do not begin to resolve after several days or if symptoms become worse or additional symptoms appear (e.g., temperature higher than 100°F [37.8°C], earache), a healthcare provider should be consulted.

Allergic rhinitis is inflammation of the nasal mucosa as a result of an allergic reaction. Patients with allergic rhinitis have had previous exposure to one or more allergens (e.g., pollens, grasses, house dust mites) and have developed antibodies to those allergens. After this exposure, when the person inhales the allergen, an **antigen-antibody** reaction occurs, causing inflammation and swelling of the nasal passages. One of the major causes of symptoms associated with an allergy is the release of histamine during the antigen-antibody reaction.

Histamine is a compound derived from an amino acid called *histidine* that is stored in small granules in most body tissues. Its physiologic functions are not completely known, but it is released in response to allergic reactions and tissue damage caused by trauma or infection.

When histamine is released in the area of tissue damage or at the site of an antigen-antibody reaction (e.g., a pollen inhaled into the nose of a patient who is allergic to that specific pollen), it reacts with the histamine-1 (H_1) receptors in the area and the following reactions take place:

1. The arterioles and capillaries in the region dilate, allowing increased blood flow to the area that results in redness.
2. The capillaries become more permeable, resulting in the outward passage of fluid into the extracellular spaces, causing edema (this is manifested by congestion in the mucous membranes and turbinates of the patient's nose).
3. Nasal, lacrimal, and bronchial secretions are released, resulting in a runny nose (**rhinorrhea**) and watery eyes (conjunctivitis) noted in patients with allergies.

Patients with allergic rhinitis also complain of itching of the palate, ears, and eyes. Most patients with asthma have an allergic component to the disease that triggers acute asthma attacks.

When large amounts of histamine are released (e.g., during a severe allergic reaction), there is extensive arteriolar dilation. Blood pressure drops (hypotension), the skin becomes flushed and edematous, and severe itching (urticaria) develops. Constriction (narrowing) and spasm of the bronchial tubes make respiratory effort more difficult (dyspnea), and copious amounts of pulmonary and gastric secretions are released.

Allergies may be seasonal or perennial. Seasonal allergies occur when a particular allergen is abundant— tree pollen is prevalent from late March to early June; ragweed is abundant from early August until the first hard freeze in October; and grasses pollinate from the middle of May to the middle of July. Weather conditions (e.g., rainfall, humidity, temperature) affect the amount of pollen produced during a particular year but not the actual onset or termination of the specific allergen's season. It is common for a person to be allergic to more than one allergen simultaneously, so seasonal allergies may overlap or may occur more than once per year. People who have allergies to multiple antigens (e.g., smoke, molds, animal dander, feathers, house dust mites, pollens) have varying degrees of symptoms all year round and are said to have *perennial allergies.* Allergy symptoms need to be treated, not only for symptomatic relief but also to prevent irreversible changes within the nose, such as thickening of the mucosal epithelium, loss of cilia, loss of smell, recurrent sinusitis and otitis media, growth of connective tissue, and development of nasal or sinus polyps that aggravate rhinitis and secondary infections.

Overuse of topical **decongestants** may lead to a rebound of nasal secretions known as *rhinitis medicamentosa.* This secondary congestion is thought to be caused by excessive vasoconstriction of the blood vessels and by direct irritation of the nasal membranes by the solution. When the vasoconstrictor effects wear off, the irritation causes excessive blood flow to the passages, causing swelling and engorgement to reappear; the nose feels stuffier and more congested than it did before treatment. Over the following few weeks a vicious cycle develops, involving more frequent use of the topical decongestant to relieve nasal passage swelling and obstruction. Rhinitis medicamentosa may develop as early as 3 to 5 days after use of long-acting topical decongestants such as oxymetazoline and xylometazoline, but it usually does not develop until after 2 to 3 weeks of regular use of short-acting topical decongestants such as phenylephrine.

TREATMENT OF UPPER RESPIRATORY DISEASES

COMMON COLD

Treatment of the common cold is limited to relieving the symptoms associated with rhinitis and, if present, pharyngitis and laryngitis; reducing the risk of complications; and preventing the spread of viral infection to others. Decongestants are the most effective agent for relieving nasal congestion and rhinorrhea.

Life Span Considerations
Decongestants

Sympathomimetic amines, more commonly called *decongestants*, and antihistamines are frequently used in combination with analgesics in cold and flu remedies. People are often not fully aware of the ingredients of over-the-counter (OTC) combination products.

Patients with diabetes mellitus, hypertension, or ischemic heart disease should use products containing decongestants only if advised to do so by a healthcare provider or pharmacist.

A paradoxical effect from antihistamines often seen in young children and older adults is central nervous system stimulation rather than sedation, which may cause insomnia, nervousness, and irritability. Antihistamines may also cause urinary retention and should be used with caution by older men who have an enlarged prostate gland.

The use of **antihistamines** (H$_1$-receptor antagonists) for symptomatic relief of cold symptoms has been controversial. Studies indicate that preschool-age children do not benefit from the use of antihistamines; however, older children, adolescents, and adults do receive some benefit.

Depending on whether fever, pharyngitis, or cough is present, patients may also benefit from the use of analgesics (see Chapter 19), antipyretics, expectorants, and antitussive agents (see Chapter 30). Laryngitis should be treated by resting the vocal cords as much as possible. Inhaling cool mist vapor several times daily to humidify the larynx may be beneficial, but putting medication into the inhaled vapor is of no value. Lozenges and gargles do nothing to relieve hoarseness because they do not reach the larynx.

ALLERGIC RHINITIS

The first steps in treating allergic rhinitis are to (1) identify the allergens—through skin testing—and (2) avoid exposure, if possible. Unfortunately, it often is not possible to eliminate exposure to many allergens without severe lifestyle restrictions. Medicines must then be used to block the allergic reaction or treat the symptoms. The pharmacologic agents typically used include antihistamines, decongestants, and intranasal corticosteroid antiinflammatory agents. Saline nasal sprays can be effective in reducing nasal irritation

between doses of other pharmacologic agents. If the patient is physically able, vigorous exercise for 15 to 30 minutes once or twice daily increases sympathetic output and induces vascular vasoconstriction.

Mild allergic rhinitis can be well treated by an oral second-generation antihistamine (e.g., loratadine, desloratadine, cetirizine, fexofenadine) or a nasal corticosteroid alone. Patients who have moderate to severe symptoms of allergic rhinitis with nasal congestion often require both an oral second-generation antihistamine and a nasal corticosteroid. Immunotherapy may be required if symptoms are only partially controlled, if high doses of intranasal or oral corticosteroids are required, or if the allergic rhinitis is complicated by asthma or sinusitis. Therapy should be started before the anticipated appearance of allergens and continue during the time of exposure.

RHINITIS MEDICAMENTOSA

The best treatment of rhinitis medicamentosa is prevention. Unfortunately, most patients are not aware of the condition until it becomes a problem. Following the directions for a daily dosage and limiting the duration of therapy to that described on the topical decongestant product are the best ways to avoid the condition.

Several strategies have been successful in treating rhinitis medicamentosa. Regardless of the approach used, the patient must understand what caused the rebound congestion and why it is important to eliminate the problem. One method is to withdraw the topical decongestant completely at once. The patient is likely to be congested and uncomfortable for the next week, but use of a saline nasal spray can help moisturize irritated nasal tissues. Nasal steroid solutions can also be used, but they still take several days to reduce inflammation and congestion. Probably the most successful approach, although the longest to complete, is to have the patient work to clear one nostril at a time. Start by reducing the strength and frequency of the decongestant used in the left nostril while continuing with the normal dosage in the right nostril. Saline or corticosteroid nasal spray can be used every other dose in the left nostril. Eventually, the saline can be used more frequently and the decongestant can be discontinued in the left nostril. Once the patient can breathe normally through the left nostril, the same approach can be started in the right nostril. Frequent follow-up with the patient and reinforcement of progress made are important to the success of this treatment.

DRUG THERAPY FOR UPPER RESPIRATORY DISEASES

ACTIONS AND USES

Antihistamines, or H$_1$-receptor antagonists, are the drugs of choice for treating allergic rhinitis. Because they are administered orally and thus distributed systemically, they also reduce the symptoms of nasal itching, sneezing, rhinorrhea, lacrimation, and conjunctival itching. However, antihistamines do not reduce nasal congestion.

Decongestants are alpha-adrenergic stimulants that cause vasoconstriction of the nasal mucosa, which significantly reduces nasal congestion. When treating allergic rhinitis, decongestants are often administered in conjunction with antihistamines to reduce nasal congestion and counteract the sedation caused by many antihistamines.

Antiinflammatory agents administered intranasally are used to treat nasal symptoms resulting from mild to moderate allergic rhinitis. In general, antiinflammatory agents are not used to treat symptoms associated with a cold because the symptoms start to resolve before the antiinflammatory agents can become effective. The antiinflammatory agents used to treat allergic rhinitis are corticosteroids and cromolyn sodium.

❖ NURSING IMPLICATIONS FOR UPPER RESPIRATORY DISEASES

Nasal congestion, allergic rhinitis, and sinusitis are treated with prescription or OTC medicines. The roles of the nurse in the healthcare provider's office are to perform the initial assessment of symptoms and then focus on teaching the proper techniques for self-administering and monitoring of the medication therapy. Always review the patient's history for other diseases currently being treated (e.g., hypertension, glaucoma, asthma, prostatic hyperplasia) that may contraindicate the concurrent use of some upper respiratory medications used as OTC or prescribed treatments.

◆ Assessment
Description of symptoms
- Which symptoms are present (e.g., frequency of sneezing or coughing, hoarseness, nasal congestion, presence of nasal secretions and type [watery, viscous, color])?
- When did the symptoms start?
- Does the patient have a history of allergies? If yes, what are the known allergens? Are the symptoms associated with a particular time of year or the release of pollen from plants? Are the symptoms triggered by exposure to household environmental factors (e.g., animal dander, dust, molds, certain foods)?
- Has the individual recently been exposed to someone with a common cold or upper respiratory tract infection?
- Is the individual having pain or discomfort? What are the specific areas affected and the degree of pain?

History of treatment
- What prescribed or OTC medicines have been used? Have any been effective?
- When allergies are suspected, has skin or blood testing been completed to determine what specific allergens are initiating the attacks?

- If pain is present, how has pain relief been obtained? Is the degree of pain relief satisfactory?

History of concurrent medical problems. Ask specific questions to determine whether the patient has concurrent medical problems (e.g., glaucoma, prostatic hyperplasia, asthma, hypertension, diabetes mellitus) as described in the drug monograph preassessments.

◆ Patient Education
- Make sure that the patient understands the importance of adequate rest, hydration, and personal hygiene (i.e., handwashing) to prevent the spread of infection, when present.
- Discuss the specific medications prescribed, the therapeutic effects that can be expected, and when to contact a healthcare provider if therapy does not yield the expected benefit. Explain which symptoms should be reported to the healthcare provider that would indicate a poor response to therapy (e.g., escalation of symptoms, pain, or fever with sinusitis).
- Make sure that the patient understands when to take the medicine (e.g., if treating symptoms of allergy, antihistamines should be taken 45 to 60 minutes before exposure to the allergen).
- Proper technique is important to therapy success. Explain the procedures for proper instillation of nose drops or nasal sprays associated with the prescribed treatment regimen. Document and verify that the patient can self-administer the medication as recommended.
- Teach the patient to monitor temperature, pulse, respirations, and blood pressure as appropriate to the underlying diagnosis and the medicines used to treat the diagnosed condition.

Fostering health maintenance
- Throughout the course of treatment, discuss medication information and how it will benefit the patient. Recognize that nonadherence may occur, especially when treatment response is not immediate.
- Seek cooperation and understanding regarding the following points so that medication adherence is increased: the name of the medication; its dosage, route, and times of administration; and its common and serious adverse effects. Numerous OTC preparations may be contraindicated when other medications or coexisting diseases are present. For example, patients taking antihypertensive medicines should not take decongestants. (See the individual drug monographs for details.)

DRUG CLASS: SYMPATHOMIMETIC DECONGESTANTS

Actions
Sympathomimetic nasal decongestants (Table 29.1) stimulate the alpha-adrenergic receptors of the nasal

Table 29.1 Nasal Decongestants

GENERIC NAME	BRAND NAME	AVAILABILITY	ADULT DOSAGE RANGE
oxymetazoline	Afrin, Dristan Spray	Solution: 0.05%	Nasal: 2-3 drops or sprays twice daily; use less than 3 days
phenylephrine ⇄ Do not confuse phenylephrine with epinephrine, phenytoin, or norepinephrine.	Neo-Synephrine Cold & Sinus ⇄ Do not confuse Neo-Synephrine with epinephrine.	Solution: 0.25%, 0.5%, 1%	Nasal: 2-3 drops or sprays in each nostril q4h; use less than 3 days
pseudoephedrine ⇄ Do not confuse pseudoephedrine with prednisone.	Sudafed Sudafed 12 hr Sudafed 24 hr	Tablets: 30, 60 mg Liquid: 15, 30 mg/5 mL Syrup: 30 mg/5 mL 120 mg 240 mg	PO: 30-60 mg q4-6h; do not exceed 240 mg/24 hr
	Sudafed PE Congestion	Tablets: 10 mg; Oral solution 2.5 mg/5 mL; Oral liquid 2.5 mg/mL	Oral: 10 to 20 mg every 4 hr

mucous membranes, causing vasoconstriction. This constriction reduces blood flow in the engorged nasal area, resulting in shrinkage of the engorged turbinates and mucous membranes and promoting sinus drainage, improving nasal air passage, and relieving the feelings of stuffiness and obstruction.

Uses

Decongestants are the drugs of choice for relieving congestion associated with rhinitis caused by the common cold. They are also often used in conjunction with antihistamines when treating allergic rhinitis to reduce nasal congestion and to counteract the sedation caused by many antihistamines.

Decongestants can be administered orally or applied directly to the nose (topically) in the form of nasal sprays or drops to treat rhinitis. An advantage of topical administration is that it has essentially no systemic effects. Disadvantages of nasal sprays and drops are their lack of effect on conjunctival symptoms, their inconvenience, and their potential to cause rhinitis medicamentosa.

Nasal decongestants provide temporary relief of symptoms, but it is important for the patient to follow the directions on the label carefully. Initially, the stuffiness or blocked sensation will be relieved. However, misuse—including excessive use or frequency of administration—may cause a rebound swelling (i.e., rhinitis medicamentosa) of the nasal passages.

Alpha-adrenergic agents used as nasal decongestants can stimulate alpha receptors at other sites in the body as well. Therefore they should be used with caution when taken orally by patients with hypertension, hyperthyroidism, diabetes mellitus, cardiac disease, increased intraocular pressure, or prostatic hyperplasia.

Many states have enacted laws regulating and tracking the amount of pseudoephedrine-containing decongestants that can be purchased by an individual. Pseudoephedrine is one of the ingredients used in the manufacturing of methamphetamine, an illicit drug with significant potential for abuse.

Therapeutic Outcome

The primary therapeutic outcome associated with sympathomimetic decongestant therapy is reduced nasal congestion with easier breathing.

❖ Nursing Implications for Sympathomimetic Decongestants

◆ *Premedication assessment*

1. Check the patient's history for evidence of hypertension, hyperthyroidism, diabetes mellitus, cardiac dysrhythmias, glaucoma, or prostatic hyperplasia. If any one of these conditions is present, consult the healthcare provider before initiating therapy.
2. Inquire about urinary pattern, particularly in male patients over the age of 55 who may be developing prostatic hyperplasia.
3. Obtain the patient's baseline vital signs.
4. Assess nasal and sinus congestion prior to therapy.

◆ *Availability, dosage, and administration.* See Table 29.1; see Chapter 7 for techniques for administering nose drops and nasal spray.

◆ *Common adverse effects*

Respiratory

Mild nasal irritation. Burning or stinging may be felt when sympathomimetic decongestants are administered to the nasal membranes. This may be avoided by using a weaker solution.

◆ *Serious adverse effects*

Genitourinary

Urinary retention. Some patients, particularly males with prostatic hyperplasia, may develop urinary partial obstruction—difficulty with starting a stream of urine—when taking oral decongestants. The obstruction is dose related and will resolve with metabolism of the drug. This adverse effect can be eliminated by using only topical decongestants rather than oral decongestants.

Cardiovascular

Hypertension. Excessive use of decongestants may result in significant hypertension. Patients already receiving antihypertensive therapy should avoid using decongestants. When sympathomimetic decongestants are used, blood pressure monitoring should be initiated; the healthcare provider should be contacted if the patient's blood pressure becomes elevated.

Metabolic

Hyperglycemia. Patients with prediabetes or diabetes must be monitored for the development of hyperglycemia.

◆ Drug interactions

Drugs that enhance toxic effects. Monoamine oxidase inhibitors (e.g., tranylcypromine, phenelzine, isocarboxazid) may enhance the toxic effects of sympathomimetic decongestants and result in significant hypertension.

Methyldopa and reserpine. Frequent decongestant use inhibits the antihypertensive activity of methyldopa and reserpine. Concurrent therapy is not recommended.

DRUG CLASS: ANTIHISTAMINES

Actions

Antihistamines, or H$_1$-receptor antagonists, are chemical agents that compete with the allergy-liberated histamine for H$_1$-receptor sites in the patient's arterioles, capillaries, and secretory glands in the mucous membranes. Antihistamines do not prevent histamine release, but they reduce the symptoms of an allergic reaction if the concentration of the antihistamine exceeds the concentration of histamine at the receptor site. Antihistamines are therefore more effective if they are taken before histamine is released or when symptoms first appear.

Uses

Antihistamines are the drugs of choice for the systemic treatment of allergic rhinitis and conjunctivitis. These agents reduce rhinorrhea, lacrimation, nasal and conjunctival pruritus, and sneezing. However, antihistamines do not stop nasal congestion. The antihistamines shown in Table 29.2 have similar histamine-blocking effects when they are taken in recommended dosages, but they vary in duration of action, sedative effects, and anticholinergic effects. Occasionally, a patient may develop a tolerance to the antihistaminic effects; changing to another antihistamine is usually effective when this occurs.

Antihistamines work best if taken on a scheduled basis rather than as needed during the allergy season. These agents are much more effective if they are taken before exposure to the allergen (e.g., 45 to 60 minutes before going outdoors during pollen season).

There is no evidence that one agent is particularly better than another at treating symptoms of allergic rhinitis, although there are differences among products regarding their frequency and type of associated adverse effects. The most common adverse effect of many antihistaminic agents is sedation. Most patients acquire a tolerance to this effect with continued therapy. Reducing the dosage or changing to another antihistamine may occasionally be necessary. The most sedating antihistamines are diphenhydramine, cyproheptadine, clemastine, and doxylamine (doxylamine and diphenhydramine are the active ingredients in OTC sleep aids). The least sedating antihistamines are fexofenadine, loratadine, cetirizine, levocetirizine, and desloratadine. Although some patients do not feel a sense of sedation after taking an antihistamine, their cognitive functions (e.g., attention, memory, coordination, psychomotor performance) can be significantly impaired. A disturbing observation by these patients is that they often are not aware that their cognitive abilities are impaired. This is particularly important when patients who are taking antihistamines perform potentially dangerous activities (e.g., driving).

All antihistamines display anticholinergic adverse effects, particularly when higher dosages are used. Symptoms include dry mouth, stuffy nose, blurred vision, constipation, and urinary retention. Patients with asthma, prostatic enlargement, or glaucoma should take antihistamines only with a healthcare provider's supervision. The drying effects may also make respiratory mucus more viscous and tenacious. Antihistamines should be used with caution in patients who have a productive cough. If the cough continues but becomes nonproductive, consider additional hydration and discontinue the antihistamine.

Therapeutic Outcome

The primary therapeutic outcome associated with antihistamine therapy is reduced symptoms of allergic rhinitis (e.g., rhinorrhea, lacrimation, itching, conjunctivitis).

❖ Nursing Implications for Antihistamines
◆ Premedication assessment

1. Review the patient's history for evidence of glaucoma, prostatic hyperplasia, or asthma. If any one of these is present, consult the healthcare provider before initiating therapy.
2. Inquire about urinary pattern, particularly in male patients over the age of 55 who may be developing prostatic hyperplasia.
3. Assess the patient's work environment and consider whether drowsiness will affect safety and work performance.
4. Because antihistamines are prescribed for a variety of symptoms (e.g., hay fever, dermatologic reactions, drug hypersensitivity, rhinitis, transfusion reactions), it is necessary to individualize the patient assessments with regard to the underlying pathologic condition.

◆ Availability, dosage, and administration. See Table 29.2.

◆ Common adverse effects
Neurologic

Sedative effects. The types of antihistamines ordered can produce varying degrees of sedation. Tolerance may be produced over time, thus diminishing the effect.

Table 29.2	Antihistamines[a]				
GENERIC NAME	**BRAND NAME**	**AVAILABILITY**	**SEDATION[b]**	**ADULT DOSAGE RANGE**	**MAXIMUM DAILY DOSAGE**
azelastine	Astepro	Nasal spray: 0.1, 0.15 %; 137 mcg/spray	−	2 sprays per nostril twice daily	—
cetirizine ⇅ *Do not confuse cetirizine with cyclobenzaprine.*	Zyrtec Allergy ⇅ *Do not confuse Zyrtec with Zantac, Zestril, or Zyprexa.*	Tablets: 5, 10 mg Oral solution: 5 mg/5 mL Tablets, chewable: 5, 10 mg Orally disintegrating tablet: 10 mg	±	5-10 mg once daily	10 mg
chlorpheniramine maleate	Chlor-Trimeton	Tablets: 4 mg Tablets, extended release (12 hr): 12 mg Liquid: 2 mg/mL in 60 mL bottle Syrup: 2 mg/5 mL in 118, 473 mL bottles	+	4 mg q4-6h	24 mg
clemastine fumarate	Tavist Allergy	Tablets: 1.34, 2.68 mg	+++	1.34-2.68 mg two or three times daily	8 mg
cyproheptadine hydrochloride ⇅ *Do not confuse cyproheptadine with cyclobenzaprine.*	—	Tablets: 4 mg Syrup: 2 mg/5 mL in 473 mL bottle	+	4 mg three times daily	32 mg
desloratadine	Clarinex	Tablets: 5 mg Syrup: 0.5 mg/mL in 473 mL bottle Orally disintegrating tablets: 2.5, 5 mg	±	5 mg once daily	5 mg
diphenhydramine hydrochloride ⇅ *Do not confuse diphenhydramine with dicyclomine or dipyridamole.*	Benadryl Allergy	Injection: 50 mg/mL in 1 mL vials Capsules: 25, 50 mg Tablets: 25, 50 mg Syrup: 12.5 mg/5 mL Elixir: 12.5 mg/5 mL	+++	25-50 mg q4-8h	300 mg
fexofenadine	Allegra ⇅ *Do not confuse Allegra with Adalat CC, Asacol, or Viagra.*	Tablets: 60, 180 mg Oral suspension: 30 mg/5 mL in 120 and 240 mL bottle Orally disintegrating tablets: 30 mg	±	60 mg twice daily; 180 mg extended-release formulation daily	180 mg
levocetirizine	Xyzal Allergy 24	Tablets: 5 mg Oral solution: 2.5 mg/5 mL	±	2.5-5 mg once daily in the evening	5 mg
loratadine ⇅ *Do not confuse loratadine with losartan.*	Claritin	Tablets: 10 mg Tablets, chewable: 5 mg Tablets, disintegrating: 5 mg, 10 mg Capsules: 10 mg Syrup: 5 mg/mL Oral solution: 5 mg/mL	±	10 mg daily	10 mg
olopatadine	Patanase	Nasal spray: 0.6%	−	2 sprays per nostril two times daily	No established dosage
promethazine hydrochloride[c] ⇅ *Do not confuse promethazine with phenazopyridine or prochlorperazine.*	Phenergan	Injection: 25, 50 mg/mL Tablets: 12.5, 25, 50 mg Syrup: 6.25 mg/5 mL Oral solution: 6.25 mg/5 mL Suppository: 12.5, 25, 50 mg	+++	6.25-12.5 mg three times daily	100 mg

[a]Many of these antihistamines are also available in combination with decongestants.
[b]Sedation index: +++, high; ++, moderate; +, low; ±, low to none; −, none.
[c]Promethazine is a phenothiazine with antihistaminic properties.

Operating machinery or motor vehicles may be hazardous. Warn the patient to be cautious.

Cognitive impairment. Although newer antihistamines are less sedating, patients should still be cautioned about the possibility of impaired memory, coordination, and psychomotor performance. In many states it is a crime to operate a motor vehicle while under the influence of medicines (in addition to alcohol). Operating machinery or motor vehicles may be hazardous. Caution patients to watch closely for signs of impairment (e.g., forgetfulness, poor coordination) in these situations.

Respiratory

Drying effects. Monitor the patient's cough and degree of sputum production when antihistamines are used. Because of their drying effects, antihistamines may impair expectoration. Give adequate fluids concurrently with the use of antihistamines. Maintain fluid intake at 8 to 10 eight-ounce glasses daily.

Anticholinergic

Blurred vision; constipation; urinary retention; dryness of mouth, throat, and nose mucosa. These symptoms are the anticholinergic effects produced by antihistamines. Patients taking these medications should be monitored for these effects.

Mucosa dryness may be alleviated by sucking hard candy or ice chips or by chewing gum. Caution the patient that blurred vision may occur, and make appropriate suggestions for the personal safety of the individual.

◆ *Serious adverse effects*

Genitourinary

Urinary retention. Some patients, particularly males with prostatic hyperplasia, may develop urinary partial obstruction—difficulty with starting a stream of urine—when taking oral antihistamines, particularly with first-generation antihistamines (e.g., diphenhydramine). The obstruction is dose related and will resolve with metabolism of the drug. This adverse effect can be eliminated by using only topical antihistamines (e.g., azelastine) or second-generation antihistamines (e.g., loratadine, desloratadine, fexofenadine) rather than first-generation antihistamines.

◆ *Drug interactions*

Central nervous system depressants. Central nervous system depressants—including sleep aids, analgesics, tranquilizers, and alcohol—will potentiate the sedative effects of antihistamines. People who work around machinery, operate motor vehicles, or perform other duties that require constant mental alertness should be particularly cautious until they know how the medication affects them and should not take these medications while working.

DRUG CLASS: RESPIRATORY ANTIINFLAMMATORY AGENTS

intranasal corticosteroids (ĭn-tră-NĀ-zăl cŏr-tĭ-cō-STĔR-ŏydz)

Actions

The exact mechanism by which corticosteroids reduce inflammation is unknown.

Uses

Patients with allergic seasonal rhinitis who do not respond to antihistamines and sympathomimetic agents may be given corticosteroids to relieve the symptoms of their allergies. Corticosteroids—whether they are applied topically or administered systemically—have been shown to be highly effective for the treatment of allergic rhinitis. Intranasal corticosteroids are successful in controlling nasal symptoms associated with mild to moderate allergic rhinitis, but systemic steroids are required for severe cases.

Topically active aerosol steroids (e.g., beclomethasone, budesonide, fluticasone, flunisolide) are highly effective with few adverse effects. Their therapeutic effect (i.e., the reduction of sneezing, nasal itching, stuffiness, and rhinorrhea) is usually observed by the third day, although maximal effects may not be evident for 2 weeks. If symptoms do not improve within 3 weeks, therapy is discontinued. To minimize the development of adrenal suppression, these corticosteroids should be used only for short courses of therapy for acute seasonal allergies.

Therapeutic Outcomes

The primary therapeutic outcomes associated with intranasal corticosteroid therapy are reduced rhinorrhea, rhinitis, itching, and sneezing.

❖ **Nursing Implications for Intranasal Corticosteroid Therapy**

◆ *Premedication assessment*

1. Blocked nasal passages should be treated with a topical decongestant just before beginning intranasal corticosteroids.
2. Ask the patient to blow the nose thoroughly before administering intranasal therapy.

◆ *Availability, dosage, and administration.* See Table 29.3; see Chapter 7 for techniques for administering intranasal spray.

Counseling. The therapeutic effects—unlike those of sympathomimetic decongestants—are not immediate. This should be explained to the patient in advance to ensure cooperation and the continuation of treatment with the prescribed dosage regimen. The full therapeutic benefit requires regular use, and it is usually evident within a few days, although a few patients may require up to 3 weeks for maximum benefit.

Preparation before administration. Patients with blocked nasal passages should be encouraged to use a decongestant just before intranasal corticosteroid administration to ensure adequate penetration. Patients should also be advised to clear their nasal passages of secretions before use.

Table 29.3   Intranasal Corticosteroids

GENERIC NAME	BRAND NAME	AVAILABILITY	ADULT DOSAGE RANGE
beclomethasone dipropionate, monohydrate	Beconase AQ, Qnasl Children ⇌ *Do not confuse Beconase with Beclovent.* Qnasl	Nasal spray: 40, 42, mcg/actuation	1 or 2 sprays (42-84 mcg) in each nostril twice daily
		Nasal spray: 80 mcg/actuation	2 sprays in each nostril once daily
budesonide	Rhinocort Allergy	Nasal aerosol: 120 doses/canister; (32 mcg/ actuation)	1-4 sprays in each nostril once daily
ciclesonide	Omnaris Zetonna	Nasal spray: 50 mcg/actuation Nasal spray: 37 mcg/actuation	2 sprays in each nostril daily 1 spray in each nostril daily
flunisolide	—	Nasal spray: 200 doses/bottle; 25 mcg/actuation	2 sprays in each nostril two or three times daily; maximum daily dosage is 8 sprays (400 mcg) in 24 hr
fluticasone	Flonase Sensimist	Nasal spray: 27.5 mcg/actuation; 60, 120 metered-dose bottles	Up to 2 sprays (55 mcg) per nostril daily
	Flonase Allergy Relief ⇌ *Do not confuse Flonase with Flovent.*	Nasal spray: 50 mcg/actuation, 120 actuations/bottle	Up to 2 sprays (100 mcg each) in each nostril once daily
mometasone	Nasonex	Nasal spray: 120 actuations/bottle; 50 mcg/actuation	2 sprays (100 mcg) in each nostril once daily
triamcinolone	Nasacort Allergy 24 Hr ⇌.	Nasal spray: 55 mcg/actuation	2 sprays (110 mcg each) in each nostril once daily; maximum daily dosage is 2 sprays in each nostril in 24 hr

Maintenance therapy. After the desired clinical effect is obtained, the maintenance dosage should be reduced to the smallest amount necessary to control the symptoms.

◆ *Common adverse effects*
Respiratory
Nasal irritation. Nasal burning is usually mild and tends to resolve with continued therapy. Encourage the patient not to discontinue therapy without first consulting the healthcare provider.

◆ *Drug interactions.* No significant drug interactions have been reported.

cromolyn sodium (KRŌ-mō-lĭn)
  NasalCrom (NĀ-zăl-krŏm)
  ⇌

Actions
Cromolyn sodium is a mast cell stabilizer that inhibits the release of histamine and other mediators of inflammation, making it an indirect antiinflammatory agent. It must be administered before the body receives a stimulus to release histamine, such as an antigen that initiates an antigen-antibody allergic reaction.

Uses
Cromolyn is recommended for use in conjunction with other medications in treating patients with severe allergic rhinitis to prevent the release of histamine, which results in symptoms of allergic rhinitis. It is also used as part of the prophylactic management of bronchospasm and asthma.

Cromolyn has no direct bronchodilatory, antihistaminic, or anticholinergic activity, and it does not relieve nasal congestion. The concomitant use of antihistamines or nasal decongestants may be necessary during initial treatment with cromolyn. A 2- to 4-week course of therapy is usually required to determine the patient's clinical response. Therapy should be continued only if there is a decrease in the severity of allergic symptoms during treatment.

Therapeutic Outcomes
The primary therapeutic outcomes associated with cromolyn therapy are reduced rhinorrhea, itching, and sneezing and fewer incidents of bronchospasm and asthmatic exacerbations.

❖ **Nursing Implications for Cromolyn Sodium**
◆ *Premedication assessment*
1. Cromolyn must be taken before exposure to the stimulus that initiates an allergic response.
2. Check to see if the concurrent use of antihistamines or nasal decongestants has been ordered by the healthcare provider, especially during the initiation of cromolyn therapy.
3. Have the patient blow his or her nose before the nasal instillation of this drug.

◆ *Availability.* *Nasal spray:* 5.2 mg/actuation in 13-mL (100 sprays) and 26-mL (200 sprays) metered-spray devices.

Inhalation with nebulizer: 20 mg/2 mL in 2-mL plastic containers.

Oral concentrate: 100 mg/5 mL in 5-mL ampules.

◆ *Dosage and administration.* See Chapter 7 for techniques to use to administer nasal spray.

Counseling. The therapeutic effects of these drugs—unlike those of sympathomimetic amines—are not immediate. This should be explained to the patient in advance to ensure cooperation and continuation of treatment with the prescribed dosage regimen. The full therapeutic benefit requires regular use, and it is usually evident within 2 to 4 weeks. Therapy must be continued even when the patient is free of symptoms.

Nasal spray. Adult patients with blocked nasal passages should be encouraged to use a decongestant just before intranasal cromolyn administration to ensure adequate penetration. Patients should also be advised to clear their nasal passages of secretions and then inhale through the nose during administration. One spray is placed in each nostril three or four times daily at regular intervals. The maximum dosage is six sprays in each nostril daily.

◆ *Common adverse effects*
Respiratory

Nasal irritation. The most common adverse effect is irritation manifested by sneezing, nasal itching, burning, and stuffiness. Patients usually develop a tolerance to the irritation, but this is rarely a cause for discontinuing intranasal therapy.

◆ *Serious adverse effects*
Respiratory

Bronchospasm and coughing. Notify the healthcare provider if inhalation causes bronchospasm or coughing.

◆ *Drug interactions.* No significant drug interactions have been reported.

Get Ready for the NCLEX® Examination!

Key Points

- Rhinitis is defined as the inflammation of the nasal mucous membranes that causes sneezing, nasal discharge, and nasal congestion.
- The most common causes of acute rhinitis are the common cold, allergies, bacterial infection, the presence of a foreign body, and drug-induced congestion (i.e., rhinitis medicamentosa).
- The roles of the nurse when working with patients with rhinitis are to perform the initial assessment of symptoms and then to focus on teaching the proper techniques for self-administering and monitoring medication therapy. Frequent follow-up with the patient and the reinforcement of gains made are important to the success of these treatments.

Additional Learning Resources

SG Go to your Study Guide for additional Review Questions for the NCLEX® Examination, Critical Thinking Clinical Situations, and other learning activities to help you master this chapter content.

Go to your Evolve website (https://evolve.elsevier.com/Clayton) for additional online resources.

Review Questions for the NCLEX® Examination

1. A patient asks the nurse about the frequent upper respiratory illnesses that he has been experiencing. The nurse responds with which appropriate statement?
   1. "When you have an infection, the normal functioning of your upper respiratory system can be impaired. Avoid irritants such as smoke, chemicals, or allergens that might make your nasal passages more susceptible to infections."
   2. "Sometimes when this happens your respiratory system will stop working properly and you will need to get a flu shot to get it back on track."
   3. "Studies show that once you get an infection, it never really leaves your system, so you will be having this problem regularly."
   4. "Your respiratory system can become overwhelmed with too many infections and then it doesn't work anymore."

2. After explaining allergic rhinitis to the patient, the nurse realized further teaching was needed when the patient made which statement?
   1. "I have to be careful with nasal decongestants so I don't get that rebound effect, where after I take them, once the drug wears off, my nose gets stuffy again and then I wind up taking it again."
   2. "So this antihistamine will stop my running nose and itchy eyes as well as my nasal congestion."
   3. "As I understand it, I need to take my antihistamine before I am exposed to the pollen outside."
   4. "So my nasal congestion is caused from reacting to the pollen in the air, which I will get every season."

3. The nurse is teaching a patient about an antihistamine recently prescribed. Which statement by the patient indicates that further teaching is needed?
   1. "I should drink 8 to 10 glasses of water every day."
   2. "If my vision starts to blur, I will need to call my doctor."
   3. "I can suck on candy or chew gum when my mouth gets dry from this drug."
   4. "I will be able to drive without any problem because I will know when I am impaired."

4. The nurse knows that intranasal corticosteroids are used for short periods to treat seasonal allergies, and explains to the patient that which of the following needs to be done before application?
   1. Rinse mouth prior to application
   2. Blow nose prior to application
   3. Suck on hard candy or ice chips before application
   4. Drink 8 ounces of water before application

5. Before initiating antihistamine medications, the nurse knows that the patient's history should be checked for which of the following? *(Select all that apply.)*
   1. Hypertension
   2. Hypothyroidism
   3. Glaucoma
   4. Urinary retention
   5. Asthma

6. When cromolyn sodium is prescribed for patients with severe allergic rhinitis, the nurse knows this drug will have which of the following effects?
   1. Bronchodilator
   2. Antihistamine
   3. Antiinflammatory
   4. Decongestant

7. The nurse administered levocetirizine (Xyzal) to a patient who asks what the drug is for. The nurse makes which appropriate response?
   1. "This drug is for your cold symptoms and will help with your nasal congestion."
   2. "This drug is for your seasonal allergy to ragweed and is an antihistamine."
   3. "This drug will help reduce the effects the nasal congestion you have from rhinitis medicamentosa."
   4. "This drug will help prevent the release of histamine to relieve your allergy symptoms."

Drugs Used to Treat Lower Respiratory Disease

https://evolve.elsevier.com/Clayton

Objectives

1. Compare the physiologic responses of the respiratory system to emphysema, chronic bronchitis, and asthma.
2. Cite nursing assessments used to evaluate the respiratory status of a patient.
3. Distinguish the mechanisms of action of expectorants, antitussives, and mucolytic agents.
4. Describe the nursing assessments needed to monitor therapeutic response and the development of adverse effects from beta-adrenergic bronchodilator therapy.

5. Discuss the nursing assessments needed to monitor therapeutic response and the development of adverse effects from anticholinergic bronchodilator therapy.
6. List the lower respiratory conditions that use anticholinergic bronchodilators and corticosteroid inhalant therapy.

Key Terms

ventilation (věn-tǐ-LĀ-shŭn) (p. 461)
diffusion (dǐ-FYŪ-zhŭn) (p. 462)
goblet cells (GŎB-lĕt SĔLZ) (p. 462)
obstructive airway diseases (ŏb-STRŬK-tǐv ĀR-wā dǐ-ZĒ-zĕz) (p. 462)
bronchospasm (BRŎN-kō-spăz-ĕm) (p. 463)
restrictive airway diseases (rē-STRĬK-tǐv ĀR-wā) (p. 463)
chronic obstructive pulmonary disease (COPD) (KRŎN-ĭk ŏb-STRŬK-tǐv PŬL-mō-nār-ē) (p. 463)
chronic airflow limitation disease (CALD) (KRŎN-ĭk ĀR-flō lǐ-mǐ-TĀ-shŭn) (p. 463)
arterial blood gases (ABGs) (ăr-TĒR-ē-ăl BLŬD GĂS-ĕz) (p. 463)

oxygen saturation (ŎKS-ĕ-jĕn să-chŭr-Ā-shŭn) (p. 463)
spirometry (spǐ-RŎM-ĕ-trē) (p. 464)
cough (KŎF) (p. 464)
asthma (ĂZ-mă) (p. 464)
bronchitis (brŏn-KĪ-tǐs) (p. 466)
emphysema (ĕm-fǐ-SĒ-mă) (p. 466)
expectorants (ĕk-SPĔK-tōr-ănts) (p. 468)
antitussives (ăn-tǐ-TŬS-ǐvz) (p. 468)
mucolytic agents (myū-kō-LĬ-tǐk) (p. 468)
bronchodilators (brŏn-kō-DĪ-lā-tǒrz) (p. 468)
antiinflammatory agents (ăn-tī-ǐn-FLĂ-mă-tō-rē) (p. 468)
immunomodulators (ǐm-yū-nō-MŎD-yū-lā-tǒrz) (p. 468)

LOWER RESPIRATORY TRACT ANATOMY AND PHYSIOLOGY

The respiratory system is a series of airways that start with the nose and mouth and end at the alveolar sacs. The nose and mouth airways connect at the pharynx. Passing out of the pharynx, the airways divide into the esophagus of the gastrointestinal (GI) tract and the larynx (voice box) and trachea of the respiratory tract. The trachea divides into the right and left mainstem bronchi, which enter the lungs. The bronchi subdivide in each lung into many smaller bronchioles, which further subdivide into many smaller airways called alveolar ducts that terminate in alveolar sacs. The alveolar sacs are surrounded by capillaries of the blood circulatory system. Human lungs contain 300 to 500 million sacs for gaseous exchange and have a surface area approximately equal to that of a tennis court. The anatomic parts of the body associated with the lower respiratory system are the larynx, trachea, bronchi, bronchioles, and alveolar sacs (Fig. 30.1).

The primary function of the lower respiratory tract is the ventilatory cycle. **Ventilation** is the movement of air into and out of the lungs. Inhalation is the process of transport of air containing oxygen to the alveolar sacs, exchange of oxygen for carbon dioxide across the alveolar membranes containing blood capillaries, and exhalation of "stale air," including carbon dioxide. Ventilation of the lungs is accomplished by contraction and relaxation of the diaphragmatic and intercostal muscles (muscles between the ribs). During inspiration, the diaphragmatic and intercostal muscles contract, creating a vacuum in the lungs and pulling air in through the mouth and nose. During exhalation, relaxation of the muscles allows the chest to return to its unexpanded position, forcing air out of the lungs.

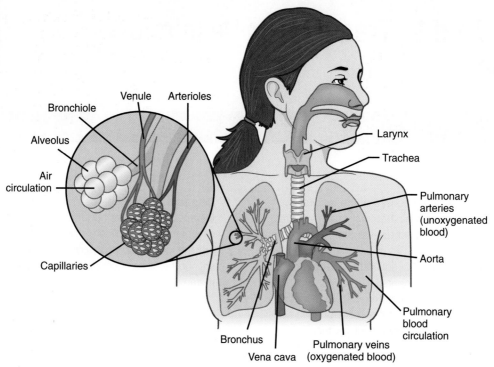

Fig. 30.1 The respiratory tract and the alveoli.

Blood flow through the pulmonary arteries to the capillaries surrounding the alveoli and then to the pulmonary veins is called *perfusion*. **Diffusion** is the process by which oxygen (O_2) passes across the alveolar membrane to the blood in the capillaries and carbon dioxide (CO_2) passes from the blood to the alveolar sacs for exhalation. Oxygen is transported by combining with hemoglobin in red blood cells or by dissolving in the blood plasma. Blood circulation provides distribution of oxygen to the body's cells for the sustenance of life. Ventilation and perfusion must be equal to maintain homeostasis.

The fluids of the respiratory tract originate from specialized mucous glands (**goblet cells**) and serous glands that line the respiratory tract. The goblet cells produce gelatinous mucus that forms a thin layer over the interior surfaces of the trachea, bronchi, and bronchioles. Secretion of mucus is increased by exposure to irritants, such as smoke, airborne particulate matter, and bacteria. The serous glands are controlled by the cholinergic nervous system. When stimulated, the serous glands secrete a watery fluid to the interior surface of the bronchial tree. There the mucous secretions of the goblet cells and the watery secretions of the serous glands combine to form respiratory tract fluid.

Normally, respiratory tract fluid forms a protective layer over the trachea, bronchi, and bronchioles. Foreign bodies, such as smoke particles and bacteria, are caught in the respiratory tract fluid and are swept upward by ciliary hairs that line the bronchi and trachea to the larynx, where they are removed by the cough reflex. The expectorated (coughed up) material contains pulmonary mucus secretions, foreign particulate matter such as smoke and bacteria, and epithelial cells sloughed from the lining of the airways. Common names given to the expectorated mass are *sputum* and *phlegm*. If too much mucus is secreted as a result of chronic irritation, cilia are destroyed by chronic inhalation of smoke, dehydration dries the mucus, or anticholinergic agents inhibit watery secretions from the serous glands, the mucus becomes viscous, forming thick plugs in the bronchiolar airways (Fig. 30.2). These thick plugs are difficult to eliminate. The resultant colonization of pathogenic microorganisms in the lower respiratory tract causes inflammation and additional mucus secretions and the possible development of pneumonia from trapped bacteria.

The smooth muscle of the tracheobronchial tree is innervated by the parasympathetic and sympathetic branches of the autonomic nervous system. Stimulation of the cholinergic nerves causes bronchial constriction and increased mucus secretion. Sympathetic stimulation of adrenergic nerves causes dilation of bronchial and bronchiolar airways and inhibition of respiratory tract fluids. Both beta-1 and beta-2 adrenergic receptors are present, but the beta-2 receptors predominate.

COMMON LOWER RESPIRATORY DISEASES

Respiratory diseases are often divided into two types: obstructive and restrictive. **Obstructive airway diseases** are those that narrow air passages, create turbulence, and increase resistance to airflow. Diseases cause

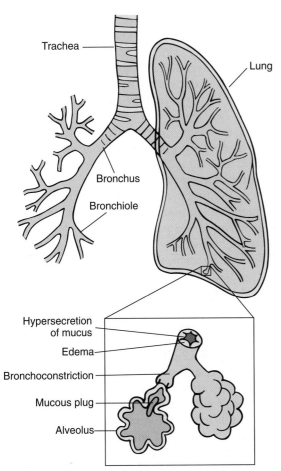

Fig. 30.2 Factors restricting the airway. Major factors include hypersecretion of mucus, mucosal edema, and bronchoconstriction. Mucous plugs may form in the alveoli. (From Clark JB, Queener SF, Karb VB. *Pharmacological Basis of Nursing Practice.* 3rd ed. St. Louis: Mosby–Year Book; 1982.)

Table **30.1**	Arterial Blood Gases Used to Assess Respiratory Function	
TEST	**NORMAL VALUE**	**RESULTS**
pH	7.35-7.45 (arterial)	>7.45 = Alkalosis <7.35 = Acidosis
$PaCO_2$	35-45 mm Hg	Abnormalities indicate respiratory acid-base imbalance. ↑ = Hypercapnia = respiratory acidosis ↓ = Hypocapnia = respiratory alkalosis
HCO_3	24-28 mEq/L	Abnormalities indicate metabolic acid-base imbalance. ↑ = Metabolic alkalosis ↓ = Metabolic acidosis
PaO_2	80-100 mm Hg	Measures the amount of oxygen moving through pulmonary alveoli into blood for transport to other tissues; depends on the amount of inspired oxygen. ↓ = Hypoxemia, hypoventilation ↑ = Hyperventilation
SaO_2	95%	Measures the ratio of actual oxygen content of hemoglobin compared with the hemoglobin's oxygen-carrying capacity. When decreased, either there is an impairment of oxygen binding to hemoglobin (e.g., metabolic acidosis) or inadequate amounts of oxygen are being inspired.

narrowing of the airways through smooth muscle constriction (**bronchospasm**), edema, inflammation of the bronchial walls, or excess mucus secretion. Examples of obstructive lung disease are asthma and acute bronchitis. **Restrictive airway diseases** are those in which lung expansion is limited from loss of elasticity (e.g., pulmonary fibrosis) or physical deformity of the chest (e.g., kyphoscoliosis). Chronic bronchitis and emphysema are examples of both restrictive and obstructive lung diseases. Patients who have persistent airflow limitation associated with chronic inflammation in the airways and lung tissue due to noxious particles and gases are referred to as having **chronic obstructive pulmonary disease (COPD)** or **chronic airflow limitation disease (CALD)**; the terms are used interchangeably. Chronic obstructive pulmonary disease is a leading cause of disability and death among individuals over age 40 in the United States.

Pulmonary function tests have been developed to assess the ventilation and diffusion capacity of the lungs to assist in diagnosis and to give an objective assessment of improvement or deterioration of the patient's clinical condition. The best indicators of overall pulmonary

function (ventilation and diffusion) are the partial pressure of **arterial blood gases (ABGs)** (e.g., arterial partial pressure of oxygen [PaO_2] and arterial partial pressure of carbon dioxide [$PaCO_2$]) and pH (Table 30.1). To determine ABGs, a sample of arterial blood must be drawn and immediately analyzed to measure the pH and partial pressures of oxygen and carbon dioxide in the blood. Another measure that is more readily available and noninvasive is the oxygen saturation of hemoglobin. **Oxygen saturation** (SaO_2) is the ratio, expressed as a percentage, of the oxygen actually bound to hemoglobin compared with the maximum amount of oxygen that could be bound to hemoglobin (see Table 30.1). Oxygen saturation is routinely used because a transcutaneous monitor or pulse oximeter is easily attached to the skin to measure and report oxygen saturation continuously. Oxygen saturations should generally be greater than

Table 30.2 **Terminology Used With Spirometry**

TERM	DEFINITION
Tidal volume (TV)	Volume of air inspired or expired during normal breathing
Vital capacity (VC)	Volume of air exhaled after maximal inspiration to full expiration
Residual volume (RV)	Volume of air left in lungs after maximal exhalation
Functional residual capacity (FRC)	Volume of air left in lungs after normal exhalation
Total lung capacity (TLC)	Vital capacity plus residual volume (VC + RV = TLC)
Forced expiratory volume (FEV)	Volume of air forced out of the lungs by maximal exhalation
Forced expiratory volume in 1 second (FEV_1)	Volume of air forced out in 1 sec to give the rate of flow
Forced vital capacity (FVC)	Maximal volume of air exhaled with maximal forced effort after maximal inhalation
Peak expiratory flow rate (PEFR)	Maximal rate of airflow produced during forced expiration

90%; in patients with normal lung function, SaO_2 values should be 95% to 99%.

Spirometry studies are routinely used to assess the capability of the patient's lungs, thorax, and respiratory muscles for moving volumes of air during inhalation and exhalation. It is recommended that spirometry be used to diagnose airway obstruction in symptomatic patients, but it should not be used as a screening tool for asymptomatic patients. A spirometer measures volumes of air. Terms used with spirometry are listed in Table 30.2. Patients with obstructive disease usually have a normal total lung capacity (TLC), difficulty with expiration, decreased vital capacity (VC), and increased residual volume (RV). Patients with restrictive disease have a decrease in all measured lung volumes. The forced expiratory volume in 1 second (FEV_1) and the forced vital capacity (FVC) are the most commonly used pulmonary function tests. The FEV_1 is used to determine the reversibility of airway disease and the effectiveness of bronchodilator therapy. The peak expiratory flow rate (PEFR) meter is not as accurate but is much less costly and more readily available than other pulmonary function test equipment. This meter is routinely used by patients at home and by healthcare providers to assess the benefits of therapy for treating acute and chronic asthmatic symptoms. A patient is considered to have significant reversibility of airway obstruction if there is a 15% to 20% improvement in the FEV_1 or PEFR after bronchodilator therapy.

One of the first symptoms of a respiratory disease is the presence of a **cough**, a reflex initiated by irritation of the airway. It is a protective beneficial mechanism for clearing excess secretions from the tracheobronchial tree. The same irritants responsible for asthma or allergy may stimulate the cough receptors, or congestion of the nasal mucosa from a cold may cause a postnasal drip into the back of the throat that stimulates the cough.

A cough is productive if it helps remove accumulated secretions and phlegm from the tracheobronchial tree. A nonproductive cough results when irritants repeatedly stimulate the cough receptors but are not removed by the coughing reflex. Excessive coughing, particularly if it is dry and nonproductive, is not only uncomfortable but also tends to be self-perpetuating because the rapid air expulsion further irritates the tracheobronchial mucosa.

Asthma is a common chronic airway disease and major health concern that affects children and adults (Box 30.1). It is responsible for an excessive number of hospitalizations, emergency department visits, healthcare provider office visits, and deaths. Asthma is an inflammatory disease of the bronchi and bronchioles. There are intermittent periods of acute, reversible airflow obstruction (bronchoconstriction) caused by bronchiolar inflammation and hyperresponsiveness to a variety of stimuli. Examples of stimuli that trigger bronchospasm and inflammation are respiratory viral infections, inhaled allergens, cold air, dry air, emotional stress, and smoke. Symptoms of asthma include cough, wheezing, shortness of breath, tightness of the chest, and increased mucus production. The exact causes of asthma are unknown. Asthmatic patients are often subdivided into categories based on severity of disease: intermittent, mild persistent, moderate persistent, and severe persistent (Fig. 30.3).

Fig. 30.3 Stepwise management of chronic asthma in adults. Therapy is stepped up to the next level of therapy if control is not achieved at the current step with proper use of medication. Step-down, or reduction of dosages, should be considered when the desired outcomes have been achieved and sustained for several weeks at the current step. Step-down therapy is desired to identify the minimum dosages of therapy required to maintain the desired outcomes. FEV_1, Forced expiratory volume in 1 second; *FVC*, forced vital capacity; *PEF*, peak expiratory flow; *PRN*, as needed. (Modified from National Asthma Education and Prevention Program, National Heart, Lung and Blood Institute. *Expert Panel Report: Guidelines for the Diagnosis and Management of Asthma: Update on Selected Topics, 2002.* Washington, DC: National Institutes of Health; 2003. NIH publication 02-5074; and Third Expert Panel on the Management of Asthma, National Asthma Education and Prevention Program, National Heart, Lung and Blood Institute. *Expert Panel Report 3: Guidelines for the Diagnosis and Management of Asthma.* Washington, DC: National Institutes of Health; 2007. NIH publication 07-4051; and Global Initiative for Asthma. *Global strategy for asthma management and prevention, 2018.* Retrieved from https://ginasthma.org.)

Clinical characteristics	Therapy (must include patient education)		Outcome

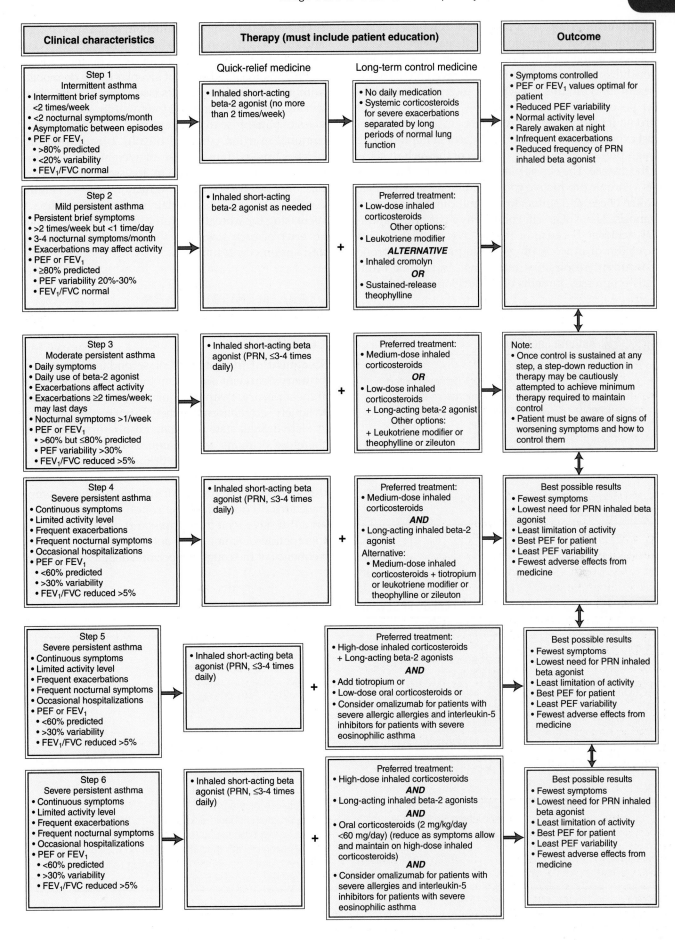

Therapy (must include patient education)

Quick-relief medicine   **Long-term control medicine**

Step 1
Intermittent asthma
- Intermittent brief symptoms <2 times/week
- <2 nocturnal symptoms/month
- Asymptomatic between episodes
- PEF or FEV$_1$
  - >80% predicted
  - <20% variability
- FEV$_1$/FVC normal

- Inhaled short-acting beta-2 agonist (no more than 2 times/week)

- No daily medication
- Systemic corticosteroids for severe exacerbations separated by long periods of normal lung function

- Symptoms controlled
- PEF or FEV$_1$ values optimal for patient
- Reduced PEF variability
- Normal activity level
- Rarely awaken at night
- Infrequent exacerbations
- Reduced frequency of PRN inhaled beta agonist

Step 2
Mild persistent asthma
- Persistent brief symptoms
- >2 times/week but <1 time/day
- 3-4 nocturnal symptoms/month
- Exacerbations may affect activity
- PEF or FEV$_1$
  - ≥80% predicted
  - PEF variability 20%-30%
- FEV$_1$/FVC normal

- Inhaled short-acting beta-2 agonist as needed

Preferred treatment:
- Low-dose inhaled corticosteroids
  Other options:
- Leukotriene modifier
  ALTERNATIVE
- Inhaled cromolyn
  OR
- Sustained-release theophylline

Step 3
Moderate persistent asthma
- Daily symptoms
- Daily use of beta-2 agonist
- Exacerbations affect activity
- Exacerbations ≥2 times/week; may last days
- Nocturnal symptoms >1/week
- PEF or FEV$_1$
  - >60% but ≤80% predicted
  - PEF variability >30%
- FEV$_1$/FVC reduced >5%

- Inhaled short-acting beta agonist (PRN, ≤3-4 times daily)

Preferred treatment:
- Medium-dose inhaled corticosteroids
  OR
- Low-dose inhaled corticosteroids + Long-acting beta-2 agonist
  Other options:
  + Leukotriene modifier or theophylline or zileuton

Note:
- Once control is sustained at any step, a step-down reduction in therapy may be cautiously attempted to achieve minimum therapy required to maintain control
- Patient must be aware of signs of worsening symptoms and how to control them

Step 4
Severe persistent asthma
- Continuous symptoms
- Limited activity level
- Frequent exacerbations
- Frequent nocturnal symptoms
- Occasional hospitalizations
- PEF or FEV$_1$
  - <60% predicted
  - >30% variability
- FEV$_1$/FVC reduced >5%

- Inhaled short-acting beta agonist (PRN, ≤3-4 times daily)

Preferred treatment:
- Medium-dose inhaled corticosteroids
  AND
- Long-acting inhaled beta-2 agonist
  Alternative:
  - Medium-dose inhaled corticosteroids + tiotropium or leukotriene modifier or theophylline or zileuton

Best possible results
- Fewest symptoms
- Lowest need for PRN inhaled beta agonist
- Least limitation of activity
- Best PEF for patient
- Least PEF variability
- Fewest adverse effects from medicine

Step 5
Severe persistent asthma
- Continuous symptoms
- Limited activity level
- Frequent exacerbations
- Frequent nocturnal symptoms
- Occasional hospitalizations
- PEF or FEV$_1$
  - <60% predicted
  - >30% variability
- FEV$_1$/FVC reduced >5%

- Inhaled short-acting beta agonist (PRN, ≤3-4 times daily)

Preferred treatment:
- High-dose inhaled corticosteroids + Long-acting beta-2 agonists
  AND
- Add tiotropium or
- Low-dose oral corticosteroids or
- Consider omalizumab for patients with severe allergic allergies and interleukin-5 inhibitors for patients with severe eosinophilic asthma

Best possible results
- Fewest symptoms
- Lowest need for PRN inhaled beta agonist
- Least limitation of activity
- Best PEF for patient
- Least PEF variability
- Fewest adverse effects from medicine

Step 6
Severe persistent asthma
- Continuous symptoms
- Limited activity level
- Frequent exacerbations
- Frequent nocturnal symptoms
- Occasional hospitalizations
- PEF or FEV$_1$
  - <60% predicted
  - >30% variability
- FEV$_1$/FVC reduced >5%

- Inhaled short-acting beta agonist (PRN, ≤3-4 times daily)

Preferred treatment:
- High-dose inhaled corticosteroids
  AND
- Long-acting inhaled beta-2 agonists
  AND
- Oral corticosteroids (2 mg/kg/day <60 mg/day) (reduce as symptoms allow and maintain on high-dose inhaled corticosteroids)
  AND
- Consider omalizumab for patients with severe allergies and interleukin-5 inhibitors for patients with severe eosinophilic asthma

Best possible results
- Fewest symptoms
- Lowest need for PRN inhaled beta agonist
- Least limitation of activity
- Best PEF for patient
- Least PEF variability
- Fewest adverse effects from medicine

Chronic **bronchitis** is a condition in which chronic irritation causes inflammation and edema, with excessive mucus secretion leading to airflow obstruction. Chronic bronchitis refers to a chronic productive cough that is present for 3 months in each of 2 successive years and has no other identifiable cause. Common causes of chronic irritation are cigarette smoke, grain and coal dust exposure, and air pollution. A persistent productive cough present on most days is one of the earliest signs of the disease. The classic patient with chronic bronchitis has a chronic productive cough and moderate dyspnea, is often obese, and suffers from significant hypoxia with cyanosis. The ABGs will confirm hypoxia and respiratory acidosis. Because of mucus overproduction and formation of mucous plugs, these patients are prone to recurrent respiratory infections. As chronic bronchitis progresses, patients often develop polycythemia (increased red blood cell production) to transport oxygen and right-sided heart failure (cor pulmonale) secondary to the lung disease and pulmonary hypertension.

Emphysema is a disease of alveolar tissue destruction without fibrosis. Alveolar sacs lose elasticity and collapse during exhalation, trapping air within the lung. The classic patient with emphysema is dyspneic with minimal exertion (short of breath), breathes through pursed lips, is thin because of weight loss, is barrel chested from increased use of accessory muscles, and has only scanty sputum production with a minimal cough. These patients maintain normal oxygenation by increasing their breathing rate. Table 30.3 classifies the severity of each stage of COPD based on symptoms and spirometry test results.

TREATMENT OF LOWER RESPIRATORY DISEASES

COUGH

Treatment of the cough is of secondary importance; primary treatment is aimed at the underlying disorder. If the air is dry, a vaporizer or humidifier may be used to liquefy secretions so that they do not become irritating. A dehydrated state thickens respiratory secretions; therefore drinking large amounts of fluids will help reduce secretion viscosity (thickness). Patients can also suck on hard candies to increase saliva flow to coat the throat, thereby reducing irritation. If these simple measures do not reduce the cough, an expectorant or an antitussive (cough suppressant) may be used. The therapeutic outcome is to decrease the intensity and frequency of the cough yet permit adequate elimination

---

Box **30.1**   Asthma Fact Sheet

In 2015:
- 6.2% of physician office visits were asthma related.
- There were 1.7 million visits to emergency departments.

In 2015:
- There were 3615 deaths due to asthma.

In 2016:
- 20.4 million, or 8.3%, of adults 18 years and older had asthma.
- 6.1 million, or 8.3%, of children under 18 years of age had asthma.

From Centers for Disease Control and Prevention, National Center for Health Statistics. FastStats: Asthma; 2017. Retrieved from https://www.cdc.gov/nchs/fastats/asthma.htm.

Table **30.3** Classification of Airway Limitation Severity, Classification of Group, and Therapy		
AIRFLOW LIMITATION[a]	**GROUP CLASSIFICATION**[b]	**THERAPY**[b]
GOLD 1: mild $FEV_1 \geq 80\%$ predicted	Group A: Mild symptoms and 0-1 exacerbations not leading to hospitalization	Add a bronchodilator (short acting). Continue if symptom benefit is documented.
GOLD 2: Moderate $50\% \leq FEV_1 < 80\%$ predicted	Group B: Moderate to severe symptoms and 0-1 exacerbations not leading to hospitalization	Start with a LABA or long-acting anticholinergic agent. Patients with persistent symptoms should use two bronchodilators.
GOLD 3: Severe $30\% \leq FEV_1 < 50\%$ predicted	Group C: Mild symptoms and greater than 2 exacerbations or 1 that led to hospitalization	Start with a long-acting anticholinergic agent. Patients with further exacerbations should use two bronchodilators or a LABA plus an ICS.
GOLD 4: Very Severe $FEV_1 < 30\%$ predicted	Group D: Moderate to severe symptoms and greater than 2 exacerbations or 1 that led to hospitalization	Start with a long-acting anticholinergic agent and a LABA or a LABA plus an ICS. Patients with further exacerbations should add an ICS to the combination of long-acting bronchodilators or add a long-acting anticholinergic agent to the LABA and ICS. If further exacerbations occur, consider adding roflumilast if patient has chronic bronchitis.

[a]Based on forced expiratory volume in 1 second (FEV_1).
[b]Based on symptoms and risk of exacerbations.
GOLD, Global Initiative for Chronic Obstructive Lung Disease; *ICS,* inhaled corticosteroid; *LABA,* long-acting beta-2 agonist.
Data from Vogelmeier CF, Criner GJ, Martinez FJ, et al. Global strategy for the diagnosis, management, and prevention of chronic obstructive lung disease 2017 report. GOLD executive summary. *Am J Respir Crit Care Med.* 2017;195(5):557-582.

of tracheobronchial phlegm. In severe cases of pulmonary congestion, a mucolytic agent may be required.

ASTHMA

The National Asthma Education and Prevention Program (NAEPP) of the National Heart, Lung and Blood Institute has published *Expert Panel Report 3: Guidelines for the Diagnosis and Management of Asthma* (2007; updated 2012). The Global Initiative for Asthma also published the Global Strategy for Asthma Management and Prevention (2017; available at https://ginasthma.org/). Both publications recommend the following goals of therapy for asthma: maintain normal activity levels; maintain near-normal pulmonary function rates; prevent chronic and troublesome symptoms (e.g., coughing or breathlessness in the night, in the early morning, or after exertion); prevent recurrent exacerbations; minimal use of short-acting inhaled beta-2 agonist (<2 days/wk); and avoid adverse effects from asthma medications. The guidelines describe four components to asthma therapy—patient education, environmental control, comprehensive pharmacologic therapy, and objective monitoring measures (e.g., regular use of a peak flowmeter). The guidelines also recommend a stepwise approach to asthma therapy for three different age groups: 0 to 4 years, 5 to 11 years, and 12 years and older. Fig. 30.3 provides an algorithm for the recommended therapy for asthma patients age 12 years and older. Medicines used to treat asthma can be divided into two groups: long-term control medications to achieve and maintain control of persistent asthma and quick-relief medications to treat symptoms and exacerbations. Long-term control medications are the inhaled corticosteroids, cromolyn sodium, long-acting beta-2 agonists (LABAs), leukotriene modifiers, long-acting anticholinergic agents, and immunomodulators. The quick-relief medications are short-acting inhaled beta-2 agonists, short-acting inhaled anticholinergic agents, and systemic corticosteroids.

Even with maximal efforts at following the NAEPP guidelines, there are some patients who remain poorly controlled despite high-dose inhaled corticosteroids and long-acting beta agonists. Subtypes of asthma are being discovered and classified based on pathogenic pathway (e.g., eosinophilic asthma, airborne allergy asthma). Identification of these pathways creates more targeted therapy, such as the immunomodulators, to achieve asthma control in patients who are failing treatment standard protocols.

CHRONIC OBSTRUCTIVE PULMONARY DISEASE

It is common for patients with obstructive lung disease to have symptoms of both bronchitis and emphysema, but one usually predominates and overall treatment is similar. According to the *Global Strategy for the Diagnosis, Management, and Prevention of Chronic Obstructive Pulmonary Disease, 2017 Report* (also known as the GOLD

Guidelines—2017) the goals of effective COPD management are the following:

- Reduce symptoms
  - Relieve symptoms
  - Improve exercise tolerance
  - Improve health status
- Reduce risk
  - Prevent disease progression
  - Prevent and treat exacerbations
  - Reduce mortality

Management principles include ensuring that the patient understands the disease process, the rationale for various procedures used to treat the disease, and the goals of therapy. Spirometry tests should be completed periodically to assess treatment success. Patients must also be taught appropriate nutrition; exercise; proper coughing techniques; chest percussion and postural drainage to mobilize mucus secretions and plugs; and elimination of risk factors such as smoking, occupational dusts, fumes and gases, and indoor or outdoor pollutants. All these efforts must be balanced with the patient's perceptions of quality of life.

None of the existing medications for COPD have been shown to modify the long-term decline in lung function associated with obstructive disease. Medicines are used for symptomatic relief and to minimize frequency of complications. Bronchodilators are the cornerstone of COPD, but the extent to which they are effective depends on how much reversibility there is to the patient's airway narrowing. Regularly scheduled treatment with long-acting inhaled bronchodilators is more effective and convenient than treatment with short-acting bronchodilators. The anticholinergic agents and the beta-adrenergic agonists are equally effective to start therapy. Pharmacotherapy recommendations are based on the patient's symptoms and history of exacerbations. According to the GOLD guidelines, patients are classified in Group A, B, C, or D (see Table 30.3). Patients in all groups should be taught to avoid risk factors that cause their COPD to flare up and should receive vaccinations for influenza yearly and pneumococcal disease when appropriate. Patients in Group A may start therapy with a short- or long-acting bronchodilator. Patients in Group B initiate therapy with either a long-acting beta or anticholinergic bronchodilator. Adding regular treatment with inhaled corticosteroids to bronchodilator treatment is appropriate for symptomatic COPD patients who are in Group C or Group D. In some patients, such as those with both asthma and COPD, a corticosteroid (e.g., prednisone) may be added for short courses of therapy during an acute exacerbation of asthma or COPD. The phosphodiesterase-4 (PDE-4) inhibitor roflumilast may be useful in reducing exacerbations in patients in Group D. Long-term treatment with systemic corticosteroids should be avoided. Each of these agents should be used sequentially and the patient reevaluated at each step before a new drug is added. If spirometry tests or symptoms do not show improvement with a particular agent, another agent with a different mechanism of action may be added. Pulmonary rehabilitation may also be helpful in assisting the patient with COPD by reducing the frequency of exacerbations. The use of antibiotics is not indicated in COPD, other than for treating infectious exacerbations and other bacterial infections.

Oxygen therapy may also be used if the patient is chronically hypoxemic, has nocturnal or exercise-induced hypoxemia, or has an acute exacerbation of obstructive disease and the O_2 drops below 55 mm Hg. Normal doses for oxygen therapy are 2 to 3 L/min.

DRUG THERAPY FOR LOWER RESPIRATORY DISEASES

ACTIONS AND USES

Expectorants liquefy mucus by stimulating the secretion of natural lubricant fluids from the serous glands. The flow of serous fluids helps liquefy thick mucus masses that may plug the narrow bronchioles. A combination of ciliary action and coughing will then expel the phlegm from the pulmonary system. Expectorants are used to treat nonproductive cough, bronchitis, and pneumonia, in which mucous plugs inhibit the expulsion of irritants and bacteria that cause bronchitis or pneumonia.

Antitussives act by suppressing the cough center in the brain. They are used when the patient has a dry, hacking, nonproductive cough. These agents will not stop the cough completely but should decrease the frequency and suppress the severe spasms that prevent adequate rest at night. Under normal circumstances, it is not appropriate to suppress a productive cough, so antitussives should not be used in patients with a productive cough.

Mucolytic agents reduce the stickiness and viscosity of pulmonary secretions by acting directly on the mucous plugs to cause dissolution. This eases the removal of the secretions by suction, postural drainage, and coughing. Mucolytic agents are most effective in removing mucous plugs obstructing the tracheobronchial airway. They are used in treating patients with acute and chronic pulmonary disorders, before and after bronchoscopy, after chest surgery, and as part of the treatment of tracheostomy care.

Bronchodilators relax the smooth muscle of the tracheobronchial tree. This allows an increase in the opening of the bronchioles and alveolar ducts, which decreases the resistance to airflow into the alveolar sacs. Asthma and bronchitis cause reversible obstruction of the airways. The airway constriction associated with emphysema is somewhat reversible, depending on the severity and duration of the disease. The primary bronchodilators used in the treatment of airway obstructive diseases include beta-adrenergic agonists and anticholinergic aerosols. Combining bronchodilators that have different mechanisms of action (e.g., combining a long-acting anticholinergic agent with a long-acting

beta agonist) and duration of action may increase the degree of bronchodilation and lung function for equivalent or fewer side effects.

Antiinflammatory agents play an important role in the treatment of asthma to reduce inflammation. Corticosteroids are the most effective agents and the mainstay of all asthma therapy. Most commonly used are those administered by inhalation, often in combination with beta-adrenergic agonists (see Table 30.6 later in this chapter). Inhalation places the medicine at the site of inflammation with minimal systemic adverse effects. Depending on the frequency and severity of acute attacks, some asthmatic patients will require short "bursts" of systemic steroids, usually prednisone, for 1 to 2 weeks of therapy. An occasional patient with asthma may require alternate-day or daily steroid administration to control symptoms. All efforts must be made to optimize other forms of treatment before resorting to regular systemic steroid administration because of the potential serious adverse effects that accompany this.

Other antiinflammatory agents used are the leukotriene modifiers cromolyn sodium and roflumilast. Leukotriene modifiers are a class of antiinflammatory agents that block leukotriene formation, which is part of the inflammatory pathway that causes bronchoconstriction. Cromolyn acts as a mast cell stabilizer, preventing the release of histamines and other chemicals that activate the inflammation cascade. Roflumilast is the first of a new class of agents, the selective PDE-4 inhibitors. This agent inhibits the release of inflammatory mediators and inhibits immune cell activation. None of these antiinflammatory agents has bronchodilating properties.

Immunomodulators—omalizumab, reslizumab, or mepolizumab—may be prescribed for patients who have been diagnosed with subtypes of asthma. Reslizumab and mepolizumab are used to treat eosinophilic asthma, and omalizumab is used to treat airborne allergenic asthma. The immunomodulators are used in addition to other maintenance treatment (corticosteroids, bronchodilators) to reduce the frequency of asthma exacerbations.

❖ NURSING IMPLICATIONS FOR LOWER RESPIRATORY DISEASES

The nurse must first understand normal respiratory function before proceeding to the assessment of pathophysiologic conditions of the respiratory tract, such as asthma, chronic bronchitis, and emphysema. *COPD* and *CALD* are terms that are used interchangeably. Both emphysema and chronic bronchitis are progressive diseases with little reversibility, whereas asthma is an inflammatory process with reversible airflow obstruction.

◆ Assessment
History of respiratory symptoms
- What pulmonary symptoms has the individual experienced (e.g., childhood or adult allergies,

pulmonary infections, pneumonia, tuberculosis, chest trauma, surgeries)? Has the individual had any respiratory problems that have required recent healthcare provider treatment or emergency department treatment? If yes, get details. When coughing, wheezing, or difficulty breathing occurs, what measures have helped to relieve the symptoms?

- What is the work environment of the individual? Ask about exposure to allergens, dust, and chemicals.
- Ask specifically for details of smoking or exposure to secondhand smoke. History of smoking is usually recorded in pack-years. (Multiply the number of packs of cigarettes smoked per day times the number of years of smoking. For example, if a person smoked 1½ packs of cigarettes per day for 20 years, the patient is said to have a 30 pack-year [1½ × 20 = 30] history of smoking.)
- Is there a family history of respiratory disease or disorders? If so, obtain details (e.g., diagnosis of disease, people affected).

History of respiratory medication
- What prescribed medications, over-the-counter medications, or herbal products are being used or have been used for the treatment of the same or similar respiratory problems? Do any medications, such as aspirin or nonsteroidal antiinflammatory drugs (e.g., ibuprofen [Advil]), precipitate an asthma attack?
- How effective have the medications been in treating prior or current symptoms?

Description of current symptoms
- What is the patient's chief complaint?
- When did the symptoms start? Does the patient have any idea what triggered them?
- Ask the patient to describe the symptoms. What effect do the symptoms have on the patient's ability to carry on activities of daily living?

Respiratory assessment. NOTE: The extent of the pulmonary examination (inspection, palpation, percussion, auscultation) must be adapted to the nurse's education level and assessment skills.

- Observe the patient's general appearance and degree of respiratory impairment. Adapt the assessment and prioritization of the examination to the degree of respiratory impairment present.
- Take and record baseline vital signs and pulse oximetry level.
- *Respiratory pattern:* Assess the rate, depth, and regularity of the patient's breathing. The normal respiratory rate is approximately 14 to 22 breaths/min in adults and up to 44 breaths/min in infants.
  - Rapid shallow breathing may be caused by an elevated diaphragm, restrictive lung disease, or pleuritic chest pain. Rapid deep breathing may be

caused by exercise, anxiety, or metabolic acidosis. Kussmaul's respiration is deep breathing associated with metabolic acidosis. It may be fast, normal, or slow. It is most often found in patients with diabetic ketoacidosis.
  - Breathing associated with obstructive lung disease has a prolonged expiratory phase because of increased airway resistance. If the respiratory rate increases, the patient lacks time for full expiration. The chest overexpands with trapped air and breathing becomes shallow.
  - Cheyne-Stokes respiration is a cyclic breathing pattern in which periods of deep breathing alternate with periods of apnea. Children and older people normally show this pattern while asleep. Other causes include heart failure, drug-induced respiratory depression, uremia, and stroke.
- *Cough:* Note whether a cough is productive or nonproductive. Record sputum color, consistency, amount, and any appearance of frothiness or blood (hemoptysis). Has the patient experienced any sudden episodes of severe coughing, wheezing, or shortness of breath? Does the patient have coughing or wheezing during certain seasons of the year or when exposed to certain places or conditions (e.g., cats, dogs, smoke, medications, foods)? Does exercise induce coughing?
- *Mental status:* As the oxygen level in the body diminishes and carbon dioxide accumulates, the mental status will deteriorate from alertness to progressively lower levels of functioning (alert → restless → drowsy → unconscious → death).

Inspection
- *Skin color:* Is the skin color normal, or is the patient cyanotic? Where is the cyanosis visible? Peripheral cyanosis is defined as a bluish coloring of an isolated area of the body (e.g., earlobes, toes, feet, fingers). Central cyanosis indicates a general lack of oxygen in the hemoglobin. The entire body has a slight bluish tinge. It is most readily observed on the lips and mucous membranes of the mouth (circumoral cyanosis).
- *Dyspnea:* Note whether dyspnea occurs at rest or with exertion. Observe the breathing pattern (e.g., pursed lip, exertion required to exhale).
- *Muscle involvement:* Elevating the shoulders, retracting the spaces between the ribs, and using the abdominal muscles are associated with advanced respiratory disease.
- *Posture:* Dyspneic patients usually sit upright or lean forward from the waist, resting the elbows on the knees. This helps give the chest maximal expansion.
- *Chest contour:* Note changes in chest contour, such as barrel chest (increased anteroposterior diameter), kyphosis, or scoliosis. Measure and record the chest circumference.
- *Fingernail clubbing:* Assess for flattening or an increase in the angle between the fingernail and the nail base

of the fingers. Clubbing has many causes, including hypoxia and lung cancer.

Palpation. Perform palpation of the chest, noting any tender or painful areas, masses, and increased or decreased tactile fremitus. Note diminished expansion of the chest wall on inspiration.

Auscultation. Perform auscultation of the chest; note the intensity, pitch, and relative duration of inspiratory and expiratory phases. Identify additional sounds (e.g., crackles, rhonchi, wheezes). Are the abnormal sounds inspiratory, expiratory, or both? Where are they located? Do they clear with deep breathing or coughing?

Cardiovascular assessment. As appropriate to the symptoms and the diagnosis, perform a cardiovascular assessment (see Chapters 22 through 27). Whenever dyspnea is severe, do not overlook the possibility of cardiovascular involvement—perform a cardiac assessment.

Sleep pattern. Ask whether the individual has had difficulty sleeping; determine the number of pillows he or she requires. Obtain details.

Psychosocial assessment. Ask specifically about the presence and degree of depression, anxiety, and social isolation experienced as a result of the disease process, as well as adaptive or maladaptive responses. Identify support systems in place to assist in providing for the individual's care.

Laboratory and diagnostic data. Review pulmonary function tests, ABGs, hematology, sputum tests, and x-ray reports as available and appropriate to the diagnosis. Allergy testing may be appropriate for some individuals. If alpha-1 antitrypsin deficiency is suspected, an alpha-1 antitrypsin test and proteinase inhibitor typing may be ordered to determine which type of alpha-1 antitrypsin deficiency is present.

◆ **Implementation**
- Perform physical assessments of the patient in accordance with clinical site policies (e.g., every 4 or 8 hours, depending on the patient's status).
- Assist the patient, as needed, to perform self-care activities. Note the degree of impairment or dyspnea seen with and without oxygen.
- During an acute asthma attack, continual respiratory assessments are performed. Monitor oxygen saturation. Compare pulmonary function tests with normal levels and report findings outside the parameters specified by the healthcare provider.
- Administer oxygen as ordered and as needed. Record spirometer readings when ordered.
- Administer prescribed medications and treatments that can best alleviate the patient's symptoms and provide the maximum level of comfort.

- Encourage physical activity as prescribed. Do not allow the patient to overexert or become fatigued.
- Maintain patient hydration consistent with any coexisting diagnoses (e.g., heart failure). Provide humidification as prescribed.
- Institute measures to reduce anxiety. Support the patient in a calm manner.

◆ **Patient Education**

Peak flowmeter. People with asthma are routinely taught how to use a peak flowmeter to measure the peak expiratory flow (PEF) to assess the severity of their symptoms. The following can be determined using the PEF as a guide:
- The green zone is where the PEF is at 80% to 100% of the patient's personal best PEF. When in the green zone, the patient is breathing well and having no coughing, wheezing, or chest tightness and should continue therapy as prescribed.
- The yellow zone is where the PEF is at 50% to 80% of the personal best PEF. In the yellow zone, the patient is starting to become symptomatic, having symptoms such as coughing, wheezing, or chest tightness. It is time to use quick-relief medicine (inhaled beta-2 agonist).
- The red zone is where the PEF is less than 50% of the patient's personal best PEF. When in the red zone, the patient should contact the healthcare provider immediately. Quick-relief medicine is continued, and corticosteroids are often started at this point.

Avoiding irritants. Smoking, pollen, and environmental pollutants commonly aggravate respiratory disorders. Check the home and work environment for allergens that may be precipitating or worsening an asthmatic attack. Medicines alone will not alleviate the problem. The control of triggers for the attacks is of paramount importance.

Activity and exercise
- Fatigue and resulting dyspnea may require adjustments in physical activity and employment.
- Support the patient's concerns.
- Plan for rest periods to alternate with activity.
- Provide oxygenation before or during activities as appropriate to the patient's needs.
- Initiate the use of an inhaled beta-2 agonist 30 minutes before undertaking exercise known to induce an asthma attack.

Nutritional status
- A well-balanced diet that prevents excessive weight loss or gain is important.
- Encourage patients with dyspnea to eat several small servings throughout the day and to take small bites. A nutritional supplement for patients with respiratory disease (e.g., Pulmocare) may be prescribed as an

adjunct to limited daily food intake. Avoid foods known to increase production of mucus (e.g., milk, chocolate).

- For COPD patients requiring oxygen, administer oxygen via nasal cannula during mealtime.
- Patients who experience asthma attacks during or following the ingestion of processed potatoes, shrimp, or dried fruits or when drinking beer or wine should avoid these items.

Preventing infections
- Encourage patients to avoid exposure to people with infection, practice good hygiene such as handwashing, get adequate rest, and dispose of secretions properly.
- Patients should seek medical attention at the earliest sign of suspected infection (e.g., increased cough, increased fatigue, dyspnea, temperature elevation, change in characteristics of secretions).
- Annual influenza vaccinations are recommended for patients having persistent asthma attacks; consider pneumonia vaccine.

Increased fluid intake. Unless contraindicated, encourage patients to increase fluid intake. This will aid in decreasing secretion viscosity. Patients should drink 8 to 10 (or more) 8-ounce glasses of water daily as directed by the healthcare provider.

Environmental elements. People experiencing difficulty in breathing can benefit from proper temperature, humidification of the air, or ventilation of the immediate surroundings. Moist air from a humidifier can readily relieve nose or throat dryness.

Breathing techniques. If ordered by the healthcare provider, teach postural drainage and pursed-lip breathing or abdominal breathing and coughing; referrals to pulmonary rehabilitation may be indicated. Record peak flow readings and institute prescribed treatments as indicated by the healthcare provider.

Sleep patterns. Discuss adaptations that the individual can make in daily routines to ensure adequate rest. As the disease progresses, sleeping in a recliner or in an upright position may be necessary.

Psychosocial behavior
- Encourage open discussion of the person's fears and expectations regarding therapy.
- Discuss the expectations of therapy (e.g., level of exercise, degree of pain relief if pain is present, tolerance, frequency of therapy, relief of dyspnea, ability to maintain activities of daily living and work, other issues as indicated by the underlying pathologic condition).
- Identify support people who can assist the individual during periods of breathlessness and make them, as well as the patient, aware of community resources

available, such as the Visiting Nurse Association and home healthcare agencies.

Medications
- Explain the purpose and method of administration of each prescribed medication. Be certain that the individual understands the delivery method for administration of the medication (e.g., aerosol therapy, metered-dose inhalers, nebulizer, peak expiratory flowmeter). The care and cleaning of equipment used for delivery of drugs to the respiratory tract should be explained to prevent bacterial growth.
- When administering medicines by aerosol therapy to a child or an older adult, make sure that the patient has the strength and dexterity to operate the equipment before discharge. When muscle coordination is not fully developed, as in a younger child, or when dexterity has diminished, as in an older patient, it may be beneficial to use a spacer device for medicines administered by inhalation (see Fig. 7.12). Have the patient demonstrate use of the inhaler at each office or emergency department visit. Confirm that the patient exhales completely before initiating the first inhalation of a medication and that the breath is held for approximately 10 seconds during inhalation of the medication. Whenever both a bronchodilator and a steroid are prescribed, administer the bronchodilator as the first puff of medication and then wait a few minutes before administering the steroid as the second medication. This will allow bronchodilation so that when the steroid, or any second drug, is given, the drug is more likely to reach the lower portions of the airway. Advise the patient to rinse the mouth (rinse and spit) following inhalation of steroid medications.
- Oxygen therapy must be explained in detail. The patient who is in a continual hypoxic state must understand that it is not beneficial and may be harmful to increase the oxygen flow above the prescribed rate.
- Be certain that the individual understands the proper use of bronchodilators and antiinflammatory agents prescribed. Drugs prescribed for PRN use or use during an acute attack of asthma must be thoroughly explained. Teach the patient to check whether an inhaler is full or empty.

Fostering health maintenance
- Throughout the course of treatment, discuss medication information, the importance of adequate airway clearance, dietary and hydration needs, breathing exercises, physical exercise, pulmonary hygiene, environmental control, the need to balance activities with abilities, and stress reduction and how each of these measures can benefit the patient.
- *Filtration systems:* The use of specialized filtration systems on furnaces and air conditioners can significantly reduce exposure to pollen and fungal spores when used with the windows and outside doors

closed. Filters must be changed regularly for full effect. Water-based air-conditioning units must be cleaned regularly to prevent fungal growth, which could exacerbate allergy symptoms.

- *Dust mites:* The most common cause of allergy from indoor sources, the dust mite, is found in carpeting and mattresses and is not removed by air cleaners. To kill dust mites, wash bedding frequently in hot water and wash or steam porous surfaces; stuffed animals and pillows can be placed inside a plastic bag and put in the freezer overnight. Encase mattresses, pillows, and box springs in nonallergenic covers. When cleaning, use a damp cloth to remove rather than spread the dust.
- *Pets:* Cats, dogs, and birds are frequently a source of asthma triggers. Pets should be removed from the home or kept outside if at all possible.
- *Smoking:* All smoking must cease; provide smoking cessation education and counseling.
- *Mold:* Molds are often asthma triggers. Remove house plants. Do not allow wet clothing to lie around without prompt drying.
- Seek cooperation and understanding of the following points to increase medication adherence: name of medication; dosage, route, and times of administration; and common and serious adverse effects.
- It is critical to teach the individual using an inhaler the proper technique of use. Evaluate whether a spacer is needed.
- Teach breathing techniques such as diaphragmatic or abdominal breathing and the pursed-lip technique that will facilitate breathing.
- Humidified air may be required, but when used, it is essential that the humidifier be cleaned thoroughly daily to prevent mold growth.
- Teach the patient to schedule daily activities, including rest, to conserve energy. Eating smaller meals more frequently spaced throughout the day will help provide energy, and less energy will be consumed metabolizing larger meals.
- Teach the patient relaxation therapy to avoid anxiety and stress, known triggers of bronchospasm and asthma attacks.
- Pulmocare, a specifically designed nutritional supplement for patients with respiratory diseases, may be ordered. Avoid caffeine-containing beverages because caffeine is a weak diuretic. Diuresis promotes thickening of lung secretions, making it more difficult to expectorate them. Milk and chocolate are also known to increase the thickness of secretions and may need to be eliminated from the diet.
- Make the patient and family aware of the community resources available.

Patient self-assessment. Enlist the patient's aid in developing and maintaining a written record of monitoring parameters (e.g., respirations, pulse, daily weights, degree of dyspnea relief, exercise tolerance, secretions

being expectorated). See Patient Self-Assessment Form for Respiratory Agents on the Evolve website. Complete the Premedication Data column for use as a baseline to track response to drug therapy. Ensure that the patient understands how to use the form, and instruct the patient to bring the completed form to follow-up visits. During follow-up visits, focus on issues that will foster adherence with the therapeutic interventions prescribed. Teach the patient to contact the healthcare provider if the PEF is deteriorating or if shortness of breath or wheezing persists despite taking prescribed medications.

DRUG CLASS: EXPECTORANTS

guaifenesin (gwĭ-FĔN-ĕ-sĭn)
Robitussin (rō-bĭ-TŬS-sĭn)

Actions
Guaifenesin is an expectorant that acts by enhancing the output of respiratory tract fluid. The increased flow of secretions decreases mucus viscosity and promotes ciliary action. A combination of ciliary action and coughing then expels the phlegm from the pulmonary system.

Uses
Guaifenesin is used for the symptomatic relief of conditions characterized by mucus in the respiratory tract with a dry, nonproductive cough. Such conditions include the common cold, bronchitis, laryngitis, pharyngitis, and sinusitis. Guaifenesin is often combined with bronchodilators, decongestants, antihistamines, or antitussive agents to aid in making a nonproductive cough more productive. Guaifenesin is more effective if the patient is well hydrated at the time of therapy.

Guaifenesin should not be given to a patient if there is a dry persistent cough that lasts more than 1 week; if there is a chronic, persistent cough, such as that which accompanies asthma, bronchitis, and emphysema; or if the cough is accompanied by excessive production of phlegm. These may be indications of more serious conditions for which the patient should seek medical attention.

Therapeutic Outcome
The primary therapeutic outcome expected from guaifenesin therapy is thinning of bronchial secretions for expectoration of mucus in the respiratory tract and reduced frequency of nonproductive cough.

❖ **Nursing Implications for Guaifenesin**
◆ *Premedication assessment.* Record characteristics of the cough before initiating therapy.

◆ *Availability. PO:* tablets: 200 and 400 mg; extended-release tablets: 600, 1200 mg; oral granules: 100 mg/packet; liquid: 100 mg/5 mL; syrup: 100 mg/5 mL. It is also available in individual products in combination with pseudoephedrine, dextromethorphan, codeine phosphate, and phenylephrine.

◆ *Dosage and administration.* **Adult:** *PO:* 100 to 400 mg every 4 to 6 hours; do not exceed 2400 mg/day.

Pediatric: *PO:* For children 6 to 11 years old, give 100 to 200 mg every 4 hours; do not exceed 1200 mg/day. For children 2 to 5 years old, give 50 to 100 mg every 4 hours; do not exceed 600 mg/day.

Fluid intake. Maintain fluid intake of 8 to 12 eight-ounce glasses of water daily.

Humidification. Suggest the concurrent use of a humidifier.

◆ *Common adverse effects*
Gastrointestinal
Gastrointestinal upset, nausea, vomiting. Development of these adverse effects is rare.

◆ *Drug interactions.* No significant drug interactions have been reported.

DRUG CLASS: SALINE SOLUTIONS

Actions
Saline solutions act by hydrating mucus, reducing its viscosity.

Uses
Saline solutions of varying concentrations can be effective expectorants when administered by nebulization. When administered by inhalation, hypotonic solutions (0.4% or 0.65% sodium chloride) are thought to provide deeper penetration into the more distant airways; a hypertonic solution (1.8% sodium chloride) hydrates and stimulates a productive cough by irritating the respiratory passages. Isotonic saline solutions (0.9% sodium chloride) administered by nebulization are used to hydrate respiratory secretions.

Saline nose drops are sometimes ordered for patients experiencing nasal congestion secondary to low humidity to clear the nasal passages and aid in breathing.

Therapeutic Outcomes
The primary therapeutic outcomes expected from nasal and respiratory saline therapy are moisturized mucous membranes for less irritation from dryness and a more productive cough because of less viscous mucus.

❖ **Nursing Implications for Saline Therapy**
◆ *Premedication assessment.* Record characteristics of cough and mucus production before initiating therapy.

DRUG CLASS: ANTITUSSIVE AGENTS

Actions
Antitussive agents (cough suppressants) act by suppressing the cough center in the brain.

Uses
Antitussive agents are used when the patient has a bothersome, dry, hacking, nonproductive cough. These agents will not stop the cough completely but should decrease its frequency and suppress the severe spasms that prevent adequate rest at night. Under normal circumstances, it is not appropriate to suppress a productive cough.

Codeine is an effective cough suppressant and the standard against which other antitussive agents are compared. In the relatively low doses and short duration used to suppress cough, addiction is not a problem; dependence may develop, however, after long-term continuous use. Codeine should not be used for patients with chronic pulmonary disease who may have respiratory depression or patients who have a documented allergy to codeine (rash, pruritus).

> **! Medication Safety Alert**
>
> The US Food and Drug Administration and Health Canada issued a warning that codeine should not be used in children under 12 years and in some adolescents between 12 and 18 years of age who are obese, following tonsillectomy and/or adenoidectomy, have genetic factors (e.g., ultra rapid metabolism leading to respiratory depression), or have conditions that increase the risk of serious breathing problems (e.g., obstructive sleep apnea, severe lung disease).

Dextromethorphan is a cough suppressant. It does not cause respiratory depression or addiction. The American Academy of Pediatrics warns against the use of dextromethorphan for respiratory illnesses in children younger than 4 years of age. Serious adverse effects including death have been reported.

Diphenhydramine is an anticholinergic agent with both antihistaminic and antitussive properties. As with most other antihistamines, diphenhydramine has significant sedative properties. This is often detrimental during the day, especially if the person must be mentally alert, but it is an excellent agent to suppress cough during sleep. Like other anticholinergic agents, diphenhydramine should not be taken by patients with closed-angle glaucoma or those with prostatic hyperplasia. It also may cause mucus to dry, making it thickened and more viscous, especially if the patient is not well hydrated. In addition, it should be used cautiously with other central nervous system depressants, such as sedatives, hypnotics, alcohol, or antidepressants.

Therapeutic Outcome
The primary therapeutic outcome expected from antitussive therapy is reduced frequency of nonproductive cough.

❖ **Nursing Implications for Antitussive Therapy**
◆ *Premedication assessment.* Record characteristics of cough and mucus before initiating therapy.

Table 30.4   Antitussive Agents

GENERIC NAME	BRAND NAME	AVAILABILITY	ADULT ORAL DOSAGE RANGE
benzonatate ⇄ *Do not confuse benzonatate with benazepril or benztropine.*	Tessalon Perles	Capsules: 100, 150, 200 mg	100-200 mg three times daily
codeine[a]	—	Tablets: 15, 30, 60 mg	10-20 mg q4-6h
dextromethorphan	Robitussin 12 Hour Cough ⇄ *Do not confuse Robitussin with Reglan.* Delsym	Lozenges: 5, 7.5 mg Capsules: 15 mg Syrup: 5, 7.5, 10 mg/5 mL Liquid: 7.5, 10, 12.5, 15 mg/5 mL Gel: 7.5 mg/5 mL Suspension, extended release: 30 mg/5 mL	10-20 mg q4h or 30 mg q6-8h; 60 mg q12h (sustained release); do not exceed 120 mg/24 hr
diphenhydramine ⇄ *Do not confuse diphenhydramine with dicyclomine or dipyridamole.*	Diphen Allergy Relief	Syrup, liquid: 12.5 mg/5 mL Capsules and tablets: 25, 50 mg	25 to 50 mg every 4 to 6 hr; maximum dose: 300 mg/day

[a]An ingredient in combination antitussive products.

◆ *Availability, dosage, and administration.* See Table 30.4.

◆ *Common adverse effects*

Neurologic

Drowsiness. All the antitussive agents cause some sedation, but diphenhydramine has the most sedative effect. Caution patients about being alert when driving and operating machinery.

Gastrointestinal

Constipation. Codeine is the most constipating of the antitussive agents. This effect can be minimized by keeping the patient well hydrated and by the use of bulk stool softeners if the patient requires more than 1 or 2 days of codeine therapy.

◆ *Drug interactions*

Central nervous system depressants. The following agents may enhance the depressant effects of antitussive agents: phenothiazines, antidepressants, sedative-hypnotics, antihistamines, and alcohol.

DRUG CLASS: MUCOLYTIC AGENTS

acetylcysteine (ăs-ĕ-tēl-SĬS-tēn)

Actions

Acetylcysteine acts by dissolving chemical bonds within the mucus itself, causing it to separate and liquefy, reducing viscosity.

Uses

Acetylcysteine is used to dissolve abnormally viscous mucus that may occur in chronic emphysema, emphysema with bronchitis, asthmatic bronchitis, and pneumonia. The reduced viscosity allows easier removal of secretions by coughing, percussion, and postural drainage. Acetylcysteine is also used to treat acetaminophen toxicity and to prevent renal failure secondary to contrast media used to visualize organs or locations of blood clots.

Therapeutic Outcome

The primary therapeutic outcome expected from acetylcysteine therapy is improved airway flow, with more comfortable breathing.

❖ **Nursing Implications for Acetylcysteine Therapy**

◆ *Premedication assessment*

1. Record the characteristics of cough and bronchial secretions before starting therapy.
2. Obtain and record baseline vital signs and pulse oximetry.
3. Observe for and record any GI symptoms before starting therapy.
4. Perform a baseline assessment of the patient's mental status (e.g., degree of anxiety, nervousness, alertness).

◆ *Availability.* **Inhalation:** 10% and 20% solutions in 4-, 10-, and 30-mL vials.

◆ *Dosage and administration.* **Adult:** *Nebulization:* The recommended dosage for most patients is 3 to 5 mL of the 20% solution three or four times daily.

Direct application into an intratracheal catheter or tracheostomy: 1 to 2 mL of a 20% solution every 1 to 4 hours. After administration, the volume of bronchial secretions may increase. Some patients with inadequate cough reflex may require mechanical suctioning to maintain an open airway.

Nebulizer. This solution tends to concentrate as it is used. When three-fourths of the original amount in the nebulizer is used, dilute the remaining solution with sterile water.

After therapy, wash the patient's face and hands because the drug is sticky and irritating. Thoroughly cleanse equipment used.

Storage. Store the opened solution of the drug in a refrigerator for up to 96 hours. Discard the unused portion.

Discoloration. Use medication stored only in plastic or glass containers. Contact with metals other than stainless steel can cause the solution to discolor.

◆ *Common adverse effects*
Gastrointestinal

Nausea, vomiting. Acetylcysteine has a pungent odor (similar to rotten eggs) that may cause nausea and vomiting; have an emesis basin available. Do not, however, suggest it by having the basin in clear view.

◆ *Serious adverse effects*
Respiratory

Bronchospasm. Acetylcysteine may occasionally cause bronchoconstriction and bronchospasm. Concurrent use of a bronchodilator may be necessary.

◆ *Drug interactions*
Antibiotics. Acetylcysteine inactivates most antibiotics. Do not mix together for aerosol administration. Schedule administration of inhalation antibiotics 1 hour after administration of acetylcysteine.

DRUG CLASS: BETA-ADRENERGIC BRONCHODILATING AGENTS

Actions

Beta-adrenergic agonists stimulate the beta receptors in the smooth muscle of the tracheobronchial tree to relax, opening the airway passages to greater volumes of air.

Uses

Beta-adrenergic bronchodilators reverse airway constriction caused by acute and chronic bronchial asthma, bronchitis, and emphysema. Agents with more selective beta-2 receptor activity (e.g., albuterol, terbutaline, formoterol, salmeterol, arformoterol, indacaterol, olodaterol, vilanterol) have more direct bronchodilating activity and fewer systemic adverse effects. (See Chapter 12 for a discussion of selective beta receptor activity.)

Unfortunately, the receptors stimulated by sympathomimetic agents, causing relaxation of the smooth muscle in the tracheobronchial tree, are not found only in the pulmonary system. These receptors are also found in the muscles of the heart; in blood vessels; in the uterus; and in the GI, urinary, and central nervous systems. They also help regulate fat and carbohydrate metabolism. Therefore there are many adverse effects from these agents, particularly if used too frequently or in higher-than-recommended doses. Those administered by inhalation generally have fewer systemic effects because inhalation places the drug at the site of action so that smaller dosages may be used.

The short-acting beta agonists (e.g., albuterol, levalbuterol, terbutaline, metaproterenol) have a rapid onset (a few minutes) and are used to treat acute bronchospasm. During acute exacerbations, these agents can be used every 3 to 4 hours. If a patient is using an increased amount of these inhaled bronchodilators on a daily basis, it is an indication of worsening asthma. Patients then must be reassessed for adherence, inhalation technique, improved environmental control, and the possible addition of corticosteroids to the therapeutic regimen.

Salmeterol, arformoterol, formoterol, indacaterol, and olodaterol are long-acting inhaled bronchodilators, sometimes known as *long-acting beta-2 agonists (LABAs)*. Salmeterol and arformoterol have an onset of action in 10 to 15 minutes with a duration of action up to 12 hours. Therefore they are administered twice daily. Salmeterol is approved for both asthma and COPD. Arformoterol is approved for use in COPD only.

Formoterol, indacaterol, and olodaterol have an onset of action in 5 to 15 minutes with a duration of action of 24 hours, and are therefore administered only 1 time daily. Formoterol is approved for use in asthma and COPD, whereas indacaterol and olodaterol are approved only for COPD. The LABAs are not used to treat acute episodes of asthma or COPD, but are used for long-term control of respiratory effort to prevent acute exacerbations of asthma and COPD.

There is concern that although LABAs decrease the frequency of asthmatic attacks, they may actually make the attacks that do occur more severe. In February 2010, the US Food and Drug Administration issued an advisory on LABA use in asthma (but not COPD), stating that:

- Use of LABAs is contraindicated without the use of an asthma controller medicine such as an inhaled corticosteroid.
- LABAs should only be used long-term in patients whose asthma cannot be adequately controlled on asthma controller medicines.
- LABAs should be used for the shortest duration of time required to achieve control of asthma symptoms and discontinued, if possible, once asthma control is achieved. Patients should then be maintained on asthma controller medicines.

Patients known to have hypertension, hyperthyroidism, diabetes mellitus, or cardiac disease with dysrhythmias may be particularly sensitive to adverse reactions and must be observed closely.

Therapeutic Outcome

The primary therapeutic outcome associated with beta-adrenergic bronchodilator therapy is bronchodilation resulting in reduced wheezing and easier breathing.

❖ **Nursing Implications for Beta-Adrenergic Bronchodilators**

◆ *Premedication assessment*

1. Obtain and record baseline vital signs and pulse oximetry.

2. Assess the patient for the presence of palpitations and dysrhythmias before administration of beta-adrenergic agents. If suspected, notify the healthcare provider and ask whether therapy should be started.
3. Perform an assessment of the patient's baseline mental status (e.g., degree of anxiety, nervousness, alertness).

◆ *Availability, dosage, and administration.* See Table 30.5. Patients using inhaled bronchodilators should wait approximately 10 minutes between inhalations. This allows the medicine to dilate the bronchioles so that the second dose can be inhaled more deeply into the lungs for a more therapeutic effect. Assure that patients understand how to use the inhaler as described in the manufacturer's leaflet that accompanies the inhaler.

◆ *Serious adverse effects*
Cardiovascular
Tachycardia, palpitations. Because most symptoms are dose related, alterations should be reported to the healthcare provider. Monitor the patient's heart rate and rhythm at regular intervals throughout therapy with bronchodilators. An increase of 20 beats/min or more after treatment should be reported to the prescriber. Always report palpitations and suspected dysrhythmias to the healthcare provider.
Neurologic
Tremors. Tell the patient to notify the healthcare provider if tremors develop after starting any of these medications. A dosage adjustment may be necessary.
Nervousness, anxiety, restlessness, headache. Perform a baseline assessment of the patient's mental status (e.g., degree of anxiety, nervousness, alertness); compare subsequent, regular assessments with the baseline.
Dizziness. Provide for patient safety during episodes of dizziness. Report episodes of dizziness to the healthcare provider for further evaluation.
Gastrointestinal
Nausea, vomiting. Monitor all aspects of the development of these symptoms. Question the patient concerning other medications being taken and any other symptoms that have also developed. Administer the medication with food and a full glass of water or milk. Report if the symptoms are not relieved.

◆ *Drug interactions*
Drugs that enhance toxic effects. Tricyclic antidepressants (e.g., imipramine, amitriptyline, nortriptyline, doxepin), monoamine oxidase inhibitors (e.g., tranylcypromine, phenelzine), and other sympathomimetic agents (e.g., metaproterenol, isoproterenol) enhance the toxic effects of beta-adrenergic bronchodilators. Monitor for increases in severity of drug effects, such as nervousness, tachycardia, tremors, and dysrhythmias.
Drugs that reduce therapeutic effects. Beta-adrenergic blocking agents (e.g., propranolol, nadolol, pindolol)

reduce the therapeutic effects of beta-adrenergic bronchodilators. Higher dosages or use of another class of bronchodilator may be required.
Antihypertensive agents. Sympathomimetic agents may reduce the therapeutic effects of antihypertensive agents. Monitor blood pressure for an indication of loss of antihypertensive control.

DRUG CLASS: ANTICHOLINERGIC BRONCHODILATING AGENTS

Anticholinergic agents have been used as bronchodilators for treating obstructive pulmonary disease for more than 200 years, but the potent anticholinergic adverse effects (e.g., throat irritation, dry mouth, reduced mucous secretions, increased secretion viscosity, mydriasis, cycloplegia, urinary retention, tachycardia) and the availability of selective sympathomimetic agents have limited their use for pulmonary disorders. When administered by inhalation, anticholinergic agents (aclidinium, glycopyrrolate, ipratropium, tiotropium, umeclidinium) have substantially fewer systemic side effects and are well tolerated.

Actions

Anticholinergic agents produce bronchodilation by competitive inhibition of cholinergic receptors on bronchial smooth muscle, blocking the bronchoconstriction action of vagal efferent impulses. There is minimal effect on ciliary activity, mucus secretion, sputum volume, and viscosity with these agents.

Uses

Ipratropium is a short-acting bronchodilating agent, whereas aclidinium, glycopyrrolate, tiotropium, and umeclidinium are long-acting bronchodilators. Ipratropium is administered every 6 hours, aclidinium and glycopyrrolate every 12 hours, and tiotropium and umeclidinium every 24 hours. All of the anticholinergic bronchodilating agents are used in long-term treatment of reversible bronchospasm associated with COPD, including bronchitis and emphysema. Ipratropium, in combination with a short-acting beta-agonist such as albuterol, is also used in the management of patients with asthma exacerbations. Tiotropium is also used in the long-term management of asthma. Anticholinergic bronchodilating agents should not be used as a rescue medicine in acute episodes of bronchospasm.

Therapeutic Outcome

The primary therapeutic outcome associated with anticholinergic bronchodilating agents is bronchodilation resulting in reduced wheezing and easier breathing.

❖ **Nursing Implications for Anticholinergic Bronchodilators**
◆ *Premedication assessment*
1. Record baseline vital signs and pulse oximetry.

Table 30.5   Bronchodilators

GENERIC NAME	BRAND NAME	AVAILABILITY	ADULT DOSAGE RANGE
Beta-Adrenergic Agonists			
albuterol ⇄ *Do not confuse albuterol with acebutolol.*	Proventil-HFA Ventolin HFA	Tablets: 2, 4 mg Syrup: 2 mg/5 mL Tablets, extended release (12 hr): 4, 8 mg Aerosol: 90 mcg/actuation Solution for inhalation: 0.083%, 0.5%, 0.63, 1.25 mg/3 mL	PO: 2-4 mg three or four times daily; maximum dose 32 mg daily PO: Extended release: 8 mg q12h; maximum dose 32 mg/24 hr Inhale: 2 inhalations q4-6h; maximum dose 12 inhalations/24 hr See manufacturer's recommendations
arformoterol	Brovana	Solution for inhalation: 15 mcg/2 mL	Inhale: 15 mcg twice daily
formoterol	Perforomist	Solution for inhalation: 20 mcg/2 mL	Nebulizer: 20 mcg q12h
indacaterol	Arcapta Neohaler	Inhalation powder: 75 mcg	Inhale: 1 capsule q24h using Neohaler inhaler at same time daily
levalbuterol	Xopenex Xopenex HFA	Solution for inhalation: 0.31, 0.63, 1.25 mg/3 mL; 1.25 mcg/0.5 mL Aerosol: 45 mcg/actuation	0.31-1.25 mg q8h Inhale: 1-2 inhalations q4-6h
metaproterenol	—	Tablets: 10, 20 mg Syrup: 10 mg/5 mL	PO: 10-20 mg three or four times daily
olodaterol	Striverdi Respimat	Aerosol: 2.5 mcg/actuation	Two actuations once daily at the same time of the day
salmeterol	Serevent Diskus ⇄ *Do not confuse Serevent with Atrovent.*	Powder for inhalation: 50 mcg/ inhalation	Inhale: 1 inhalation q12h
terbutaline ❶		Tablets: 2.5, 5 mg Injection: 1 mg/mL	PO: 5 mg q6h Subcutaneous: 0.25 mg; repeat, if needed, in 30 min
Combination Anticholinergic and Beta-Adrenergic Bronchodilators			
glycopyrrolate/ formoterol	Bevespi Aerosphere	Aerosol: glycopyrrolate 9 mcg and formoterol 4.8 mcg/ inhalation	Inhale: 2 inhalations twice a day
glycopyrrolate/ indacaterol	Utibron Neohaler	Powder for inhalation: glycopyrrolate 15.6 mcg and indacaterol 27.5/inhalation	Inhale: 1 capsule twice daily using Neohaler
ipratropium/albuterol	Combivent Respimat	Aerosol: ipratropium 20 mcg and albuterol 100 mcg/inhalation Inhalation Solution: Ipratropium bromide 0.5 mg and albuterol 2.5 mg/3 mL	Inhale: 1 inhalation four times a day Nebulize: 1 vial (3 mL) via nebulization every 6 hours
umeclidinium/vilanterol	Anoro Ellipta	Aerosol powder: umeclidinium 62.5 mcg and vilanterol 25 mcg/inhalation	Inhale: 1 inhalation per 24 hr
tiotropium/olodaterol	Stiolto Respimat	Aerosol powder: tiotropium 2.5 mcg and olodaterol 2.5 mcg/actuation	Inhale: 2 inhalations at the same time per 24 hr

❶ High-alert medication.

Table 30.6   Inhaled Anticholinergic Bronchodilators

GENERIC NAME	BRAND NAME	AVAILABILITY	ADULT DOSAGE RANGE
aclidinium	Tudorza Pressair	Powder for inhalation: 400 mcg/actuation	Inhale: 1 inhalation twice daily
glycopyrrolate	Seebri Neohaler	Powder for inhalation: 15.6 mg/inhalation	Inhale: 1 capsule twice daily using Neohaler
	Lonhala Magnair	Inhalation Solution: 25 mcg/mL in 1 mL vial	Nebulize: 1 vial (25 mcg) inhaled twice daily; using only Magnair
ipratropium	Atrovent HFA	Aerosol: 17 mcg/actuation Inhalation Solution: 0.2%/2.5 mL vial	Inhale: 2 inhalations 4 times daily; maximum dose: 12 inhalations per 24 hr Nebulize: 1 unit-dose vial q6-8h
tiotropium	Spiriva HandiHaler Spiriva Respimat	18-mcg capsule: 1.25 mcg and 2.5 mcg per actuation	Handihaler–Inhaler: 1 capsule once daily (to ensure drug delivery, the contents of each capsule should be inhaled twice) COPD: 2 inhalations (5 mcg) once daily Asthma: 2 inhalations (2.5 mcg) once daily
umeclidinium	Incruse Ellipta	Powder for inhalation: 62.5 mcg/actuation	Inhale: 1 inhalation once daily

2. Check the medical record to determine whether the patient has a history of closed-angle glaucoma. If so, reconfirm the administration order with the healthcare provider before administration of anticholinergic bronchodilators.

◆ *Availability and dosage.* See Table 30.6.

◆ *Administration.* Ensure that the patient understands how to use the inhaler that accompanies the medication. Read the manufacturer's instructions for administration for the various types of inhalers available.

> **! Medication Safety Alert**
>
> Use anticholinergic bronchodilators with caution in patients with the potential for closed-angle glaucoma, prostatic hyperplasia, or bladder neck obstruction.

◆ *Common adverse effects*
   Gastrointestinal
   Mouth dryness, throat irritation. These adverse effects are usually mild and tend to resolve with continued therapy. Encourage the patient not to discontinue therapy without first consulting the healthcare provider. Other measures to alleviate dryness include sucking on ice chips or hard candy.

◆ *Serious adverse effects*
   Anticholinergic
   Tachycardia, urinary retention, exacerbation of pulmonary symptoms. Instruct the patient to consult the prescriber before continuing with further therapy.

◆ *Drug interactions.* No significant interactions have been reported.

DRUG CLASS: RESPIRATORY ANTIINFLAMMATORY AGENTS—CORTICOSTEROIDS USED FOR OBSTRUCTIVE AIRWAY DISEASE

Actions
Corticosteroids (see Chapter 37), whether applied by aerosol or administered systemically, have been shown to be highly effective for treating obstructive airway disease. The mechanisms of action are not completely known, but corticosteroids have a direct effect on smooth muscle relaxation; they enhance the effect of beta-adrenergic bronchodilators and inhibit inflammatory responses that may result in bronchoconstriction.

Uses
Because inflammation is a key component of asthma, daily use of inhaled corticosteroids has become the preferred long-term control medicine for mild, moderate, and severe persistent asthma. Patients with severe COPD who are unresponsive to bronchodilators may have corticosteroids added to the medication regimen to provide enhanced airway flow.

For patients with COPD, the first course of therapy is often a short course (5 to 7 days) of systemic corticosteroids (e.g., prednisone), with intervals of several weeks or months without steroid treatment. Alternate-day therapy (a single dose every other morning) is the next preferable program. Aerosolized corticosteroids may be used daily by certain patients instead of alternate-day therapy.

If the patient has not previously been receiving corticosteroid therapy, several weeks may pass before the full benefits from the aerosolized medication are achieved, but a single aerosol "burst" does produce noticeable benefits in reducing bronchoconstriction. It is important to remember that corticosteroid aerosols should not be regarded as true bronchodilators and should not be used for rapid relief of bronchospasm. (See Chapter 29 for the use of intranasal corticosteroids.)

Therapeutic Outcome

The primary therapeutic outcome associated with corticosteroid therapy is decreased pulmonary inflammation, resulting in easier breathing with less effort.

❖ **Nursing Implications for Corticosteroid Therapy**

◆ *Premedication assessment.* Inspect the oral cavity for the presence of any type of infection.

◆ *Availability and dosage.* See Table 30.7.

◆ *Administration*

Counseling, adherence. The therapeutic effects, unlike those of sympathomimetic bronchodilators, are not immediate. This should be explained to the patient before therapy begins to ensure cooperation and continuation of treatment with the prescribed dosage regimen, even when the patient is asymptomatic. Full therapeutic benefit requires regular use and may require up to 4 weeks of therapy for maximum benefit.

Preparation before administration. Patients receiving bronchodilators by inhalation should be advised to use the bronchodilator before the corticosteroid inhalant to enhance penetration of the corticosteroid into the bronchial tree. After using the bronchodilator, the patient should wait several minutes before the corticosteroid is inhaled to allow time for the bronchodilator to relax the smooth muscle.

Maintenance therapy. After the desired clinical effect has been obtained, the maintenance dose should be reduced to the smallest amount necessary to control symptoms.

Severe stress or asthma attack. During periods of stress or a severe asthma attack, patients may require treatment with systemic steroids. Exacerbation of asthma that occurs during the course of corticosteroid inhalant therapy should be treated with a short course of a systemic steroid. Instruct patients not to use the corticosteroid inhaler when taking systemic steroids because the aerosol not only may cause irritation and exacerbate symptoms, but also may not penetrate deep enough into the bronchial tree because of inflammation and swelling from the asthmatic attack.

◆ *Common adverse effects*

Gastrointestinal

Hoarseness, dry mouth. Hoarseness and dry mouth are usually mild and tend to resolve with continued therapy. Encourage the patient not to discontinue therapy without first consulting the healthcare provider.

◆ *Serious adverse effects*

Gastrointestinal

Fungal infections (thrush). Increased risk factors for the development of oral thrush include concomitant antibiotic use, diabetes, improper aerosol administration, large oral doses of corticosteroids, and poor dental hygiene. Patients should be instructed on good oral hygiene technique and told to gargle and rinse the mouth with a mouthwash after each aerosol treatment. Commercial mouthwashes contain alcohol, which may cause further drying and oral irritation. If thrush develops, it is usually not sufficiently troublesome to require discontinuing steroid aerosol therapy. An antifungal mouthwash such as nystatin will generally eradicate the oral candidiasis (thrush).

◆ *Drug interactions.* No significant drug interactions have been reported.

DRUG CLASS: ANTILEUKOTRIENE AGENTS

When inflammatory cells are triggered by irritants such as smoke, allergens, or viruses, the phospholipid membrane of the epithelial lining of the airways is disrupted, causing a series of chemical reactions from arachidonic acid that releases leukotrienes, prostaglandins, thromboxanes, and eicosanoids. The leukotrienes produced cause many of the signs and symptoms of asthma, such as bronchoconstriction, vascular permeability leading to edema, and mucus hypersecretion.

montelukast (mŏn-tĕ-LŪ-kăst)
Singulair (SĬN-gyū-lār)

Actions

Montelukast is a selective and competitive receptor antagonist of the cysteinyl leukotriene receptor. This is the receptor that leukotriene D_4 stimulates to trigger symptoms of asthma.

Uses

Montelukast is approved for use in conjunction with other medications for the prophylactic and chronic treatment of asthma. It has been shown to reduce early and late-phase bronchoconstriction, bronchial hyperresponsiveness, daytime asthma symptoms, and nighttime awakening; reduce beta-adrenergic agonist use; and improve pulmonary function tests. The NAEPP recommends antileukotriene agents as alternatives to low-dose inhaled corticosteroids for mild persistent asthma and with low to medium doses of inhaled corticosteroids for moderate persistent asthma.

Montelukast is not a bronchodilator and should not be used to treat acute episodes of asthma. However, treatment with montelukast can be continued during acute exacerbations of asthma. Montelukast use should be continuous, even during acute asthma exacerbations and symptom-free periods.

Table 30.7 Oral Inhalant Corticosteroids

GENERIC NAME	BRAND NAME	AVAILABILITY	ADULT DOSAGE RANGE
Inhalant Corticosteroids			
beclomethasone dipropionate	Qvar Redihaler	Aerosol: 40, 80 mcg/actuation; 100 doses/inhaler	Inhale: 1 or 2 inhalations (80 mcg) twice daily; maximum 640 mcg daily
budesonide phosphate	Pulmicort ⇄ Do not confuse Pulmicort with Pulmozyme. Pulmicort Flexhaler	Suspension via inhaler: 0.25, 0.5, 1 mg/2 mL Aerosol powder: 90, 180 mcg/actuation	Inhale: 2 inhalations twice daily; maximum 4 inhalations twice daily
ciclesonide	Alvesco	Aerosol solution: 80, 160 mcg/actuation	80-160 mcg twice daily
flunisolide	Aerospan	80 mcg/actuation	320 mcg twice daily
fluticasone propionate	Flovent HFA ⇄ Do not confuse Flovent with Flonase.	Aerosol: 44, 110, 220 mcg/actuation	88-440 mcg twice daily
	Flovent Diskus ⇄ Do not confuse Flovent with Flonase.	Powder for inhalation: 50, 100, 250 mcg/dose	100-500 mcg twice daily
fluticasone furoate	Arnuity Ellipta	Powder for inhalation: 50, 100, 200 mcg/inhalation	50-200 mcg daily
mometasone furoate	Asmanex HFA Asmanex Metered doses	Powder for inhalation: 100, 200 mcg/inhalation Powder, breath activated: 110, 220 mcg/inhalation	200-400 mcg twice daily
Inhalant Corticosteroid–Beta-Adrenergic Bronchodilator			
budesonide/formoterol	Symbicort	Aerosol: 80 mcg budesonide and 4.5 mcg formoterol/actuation; 160 mcg budesonide and 4.5 mcg formoterol/actuation	Inhale: 2 inhalations twice daily for maintenance on a regularly scheduled basis; not for acute bronchospasm
fluticasone/salmeterol	Advair Diskus ⇄ Do not confuse Advair with Advicor.	Powder for inhalation: 100 mcg fluticasone and 50 mcg salmeterol; 250 mcg fluticasone and 50 mcg salmeterol; 500 mcg fluticasone and 50 mcg salmeterol	Inhale: 1-2 inhalations twice daily for maintenance therapy on regularly scheduled basis; not for acute bronchospasm
	Advair HFA	Aerosol inhalation: 45 mcg fluticasone and 21 mcg salmeterol; 115 mcg fluticasone and 21 mcg salmeterol; 230 mcg fluticasone and 21 mcg salmeterol	Inhale: 2 inhalations twice daily for maintenance therapy on regularly scheduled basis; not for acute bronchospasm
fluticasone/vilanterol	Breo Ellipta	Aerosol inhalation: 100 mcg fluticasone and 25 mcg vilanterol; 200 mcg fluticasone and 25 mcg vilanterol	Inhale: 1 inhalation once daily
mometasone/formoterol	Dulera	Aerosol inhalation: 100 mcg mometasone and 5 mcg formoterol/actuation; 200 mcg mometasone and 5 mcg formoterol/actuation	Inhale: 2 inhalations twice daily for maintenance on regularly scheduled basis; not for acute bronchospasm
Inhalant Corticosteroid-Beta Adrenergic-Anticholinergic Bronchodilator			
fluticasone/vilanterol/umeclidinium	Trelegy Ellipta	Fluticasone 100 mcg/ Vilanterol 25 mcg/ umeclidinium 62.5 mcg per actuation	Inhale: 1 inhalation once daily

Therapeutic Outcome

The primary therapeutic outcome associated with montelukast therapy is fewer episodes of acute asthmatic symptoms.

❖ Nursing Implications for Montelukast

◆ *Premedication assessment.* Obtain and record baseline vital signs, pulse oximetry, and pulmonary function tests.

◆ *Availability. PO:* 10-mg tablets; 4- and 5-mg chewable tablets; 4-mg granules.

◆ *Dosage and administration.* **Adult: *PO:*** 10 mg taken once daily in the evening. Doses greater than 10 mg appear to be of no value. Continue other therapy for asthma as prescribed.

Pediatric age 2 to 5 years: *PO;* 4 mg once daily.

◆ *Common adverse effects*
Gastrointestinal
Nausea, dyspepsia. These symptoms are usually mild and disappear with continued therapy. Encourage the patient not to discontinue therapy without first consulting the healthcare provider. Administration with food or milk may help minimize discomfort.
Neurologic
Headache. This adverse effect is usually mild and tends to resolve with continued therapy. Encourage the patient not to discontinue therapy without first consulting the healthcare provider.

◆ *Drug interactions.* No clinically significant drug interactions have been reported.

DRUG CLASS: PHOSPHODIESTERASE-4 INHIBITOR

roflumilast (rō-FLŪ-mĭ-lăst)
Daliresp (dă-lĭ-RĔSP)

Actions

Intracellular cyclic adenosine monophosphate (cAMP) plays a key role in blocking inflammation in many tissues of the body. It is normally metabolized by PDE-4, a key enzyme in lung tissue. Roflumilast is a PDE-4 inhibitor that blocks PDE-4 from metabolizing cAMP, allowing it to accumulate and reduce inflammation.

Uses

Roflumilast is used to reduce the frequency of exacerbations (flare-ups) of inflammation (with consequent constriction of airways) in patients with chronic bronchitis and severe COPD. Roflumilast is not a bronchodilator and has no value in the acute treatment of bronchospasms. It may be used in conjunction with bronchodilators and corticosteroids in the overall management of COPD. Roflumilast is contraindicated in patients with severe liver impairment (Child-Pugh classification B or C). These patients are unable to metabolize roflumilast and toxic levels may result.

Therapeutic Outcome

The primary therapeutic outcome expected from roflumilast is fewer exacerbations of COPD.

❖ Nursing Implications for Roflumilast

◆ *Premedication assessment*
1. Obtain and record baseline vital signs, pulse oximetry, and pulmonary function tests.
2. Obtain a history of bowel elimination patterns and any GI symptoms, frequency of headaches, dizziness, and fatigue that may be present before therapy is started.
3. Record baseline data on the level of insomnia and anxiety present.
4. Obtain baseline weight; schedule weekly weight measurement.

◆ *Availability. PO:* 250-, 500-mcg tablets.

◆ *Dosage and administration. PO:* Initially, 250 mcg once daily for 4 weeks to improve tolerability. The actual therapeutic maintenance dose is 500 mcg once daily with or without food.

◆ *Common adverse effects*
Gastrointestinal
Dyspepsia, cramps, nausea, diarrhea. These adverse effects are usually mild and tend to resolve with continued therapy. Encourage the patient not to discontinue therapy without first consulting the healthcare provider.
Metabolic
Weight loss. Some patients lose weight (5% to 10% of body weight) with roflumilast therapy. Monitor patients for unexplained or clinically significant weight loss.
Neurologic
Headache. This adverse effect is usually mild and tends to resolve with continued therapy. Encourage the patient not to discontinue therapy without first consulting the healthcare provider.

◆ *Serious adverse effects*
Psychiatric/neurologic
Insomnia, anxiety, depression. Patients and caregivers should watch for the emergence or worsening of insomnia, anxiety, depression, suicidal thoughts, or other mood changes. In clinical trials, an increase in these symptoms was reported more frequently in those patients receiving the drug compared to those patients receiving a placebo. Suicidal ideation and behavior have been reported.

◆ *Drug interactions*
Drugs that enhance therapeutic and toxic effects. Ketoconazole, enoxacin, fluvoxamine, and cimetidine increase

serum concentrations of roflumilast. Monitor the patient closely for adverse effects.

Drugs that reduce therapeutic effects. Rifampin, phenobarbital, carbamazepine, and phenytoin enhance the metabolism of roflumilast. Monitor the frequency of COPD exacerbations as an indication of therapeutic effect or loss of effect.

DRUG CLASS: IMMUNOMODULATOR AGENTS

benralizumab (ben-rah-LIZ-u-mab)
  Fasenra (fa-SEN-rah)
mepolizumab (me-pol-LIZ-u-mab)
  Nucala (new-CAL-ah)
omalizumab (ō-mă-LĪZ-ū-măb)
  Xolair (ZŌ- lār)
reslizumab (res-LIZ-u-mab)
  Cinqair (sink-air)

Actions

Four immunomodulators are used in the management of severe asthma to achieve control in patients who have failed standard treatment: benralizumab, mepolizumab, reslizumab, and omalizumab. Benralizumab, mepolizumab, and reslizumab are humanized monoclonal antibodies that bind to interleukin-5. Interleukin-5 is responsible for the differentiation, maturation, recruitment, and activation of human eosinophils. By binding to interleukin-5, benralizumab, mepolizumab, and reslizumab block its biologic function, reducing eosinophilic production and action. The exact mechanism by which these immune modulators reduce acute episodes of asthma is not known.

Omalizumab, a DNA-derived humanized immunoglobulin G monoclonal antibody, binds to the circulating immunoglobulin E (IgE) antibodies in the blood, decreasing the number of IgE antibodies available to bind to mast cells, thereby inhibiting the mast cell's release of those inflammatory chemicals that can lead to the symptoms of asthma.

Uses

Benralizumab, mepolizumab, and reslizumab are used with other asthma medicines for the maintenance treatment of severe eosinophilic asthma. When added to other medicines for asthma, these immunomodulators help prevent severe asthma attacks (exacerbations) and can improve breathing in patients whose asthma is not controlled with the current asthma medicines. Benralizumab and mepolizumab are used in patients aged 12 years and older, and reslizumab in patients 18 years and older. Omalizumab is used in patients who are at least 12 years old, have moderate to severe persistent asthma, have a positive skin reaction to a perennial airborne allergen, and have symptoms that are not adequately controlled with inhaled corticosteroids. Omalizumab decreases the incidence of asthma exacerbations in these patients.

Immunomodulators do not stop acute exacerbations of asthma and should not be used to treat acute bronchospasm or status asthmaticus. Patients should be counseled that it may take a few weeks before the immunomodulator has a noticeable effect on their asthma, so it is important that they continue taking all other asthma medicines unless otherwise instructed by their healthcare provider. Systemic or inhaled corticosteroids should not be abruptly discontinued when an immunomodulator is initiated. Reductions in corticosteroid dosage should be very gradual and done only under the supervision of a healthcare provider.

Therapeutic Outcome

The primary therapeutic outcome associated with immunomodulator agents is reduced frequency of acute asthmatic exacerbations.

❖ Nursing Implications for Immunomodulator Agents
◆ *Premedication assessment*
1. Review the patient's medication history to ensure that the patient does not have an allergy to any immunomodulator agents. If the patient does, inform the charge nurse and the healthcare provider immediately. Do not administer the medication without specific approval.
2. Review the patient's medical history to ensure that the patient has positive skin reactions to at least one airborne allergen or has been diagnosed with eosinophilic asthma.
3. Before administering the first dose of omalizumab, ensure that serum IgE levels have been measured; this helps determine the dose of the omalizumab to be administered. Following administration of omalizumab, serum total IgE levels become elevated because of the formation of omalizumab-IgE complexes. Further measurement of serum IgE levels is not necessary.
4. Obtain and record baseline vital signs and pulmonary function test results.

◆ *Availability and dosage.* See Table 30.8.

◆ *Preparation and administration.* Preparation and administration of benralizumab is as follows:
1. Prior to administration, remove prefilled syringe from refrigerator and allow to warm at room temperature for about 30 minutes. **Do Not Shake!**
2. The solution is clear to opalescent, colorless to slight yellow liquid. Particles may be present in the solution that appear translucent or white to off-white; do not use if cloudy or discolored.
3. Syringe may contain a small air bubble; do not expel the air bubble prior to administration.
Preparation and administration of mepolizumab is as follows:
1. Draw 1.2 mL of sterile water for injection USP into a 3-mL syringe equipped with a 1-inch, 21-gauge needle.

Table 30.8   Immunomodulator Agents

GENERIC NAME	BRAND NAME	AVAILABILITY	DOSAGE
benralizumab	Fasenra	Subcutaneous: 30 mg/mL in 1 mL prefilled syringe	Twelve years old and older: Subcutaneous: 30 mg every 4 weeks for 3 doses, then once every 8 weeks.
mepolizumab	Nucala	Subcutaneous: 100-mg single-use vials in powder form	Twelve years old and older: *Subcutaneous:* 100 mg once every 4 wk into the upper arm, thigh, or abdomen.
omalizumab	Xolair	Subcutaneous: 150-mg single-use vials in powder form	Twelve years old and older: *Subcutaneous:* 150-375 mg every 2-4 wk, based on patient weight and immunoglobulin E serum level. Doses of more than 150 mg (1.2 mL) should be divided and administered at more than one site.
reslizumab	Cinqair	Intravenous: 100 mg/10 mL solution in single-use vials	Twelve years old and older: *Intravenous infusion:* 3-mg/kg infusion over 20-50 min once every 4 wk

2. Place the vial upright on a flat surface; using standard aseptic technique, insert the needle and inject the sterile water directly onto the center of the powder cake.

3. Gently swirl the vial for 10 seconds with a circular motion at 15 second intervals until the powder is dissolved. **Do Not Shake!** Reconstitution is typically complete within 5 minutes. Final concentration is 100 mg/mL.

4. The solution is clear to opalescent, colorless to pale yellow or pale brown. The solution should be essentially particle free; if particulate matter remains in the solution or if the solution appears cloudy or milky, discard the solution. Do not mix with other medicines for administration.

5. Replace the 21-gauge needle with a 21- to 27-gauge, 0.5-inch needle for subcutaneous injection. For the 300-mg dose, administer in 3 separate 100-mg injections into the upper arm, thigh, or abdomen. **Do Not Shake** the vial to prevent foaming or precipitation.

6. The reconstituted solution may be stored for up to 8 hours below 86° F but do not freeze. Discard if not used within 8 hours of reconstitution.

Preparation and administration of omalizumab is as follows:

1. Draw 1.4 mL of sterile water for injection USP into a 3-mL syringe equipped with a 1-inch, 18-gauge needle.

2. Place the vial upright on a flat surface; using standard aseptic technique, insert the needle and inject the sterile water directly onto the powder.

3. Keeping the vial upright, gently swirl the upright vial for approximately 1 minute to wet the powder evenly. **Do Not Shake!**

4. Gently swirl the vial for 5 to 10 seconds approximately every 5 minutes to dissolve any remaining solids. There should be no visible gelatinous particles in the solution. NOTE: Some powders in vials may take longer than 20 minutes to dissolve completely. Repeat this step until there are no visible gelatinous particles in the solution. It is acceptable to have small bubbles or foam around the edge of the vial. Do not use if the contents of the vial do not dissolve completely within 40 minutes.

5. Invert the vial for 15 seconds to allow the solution to drain toward the stopper. Note that it is a rather viscous solution. Using a new 3-mL syringe equipped with a 1-inch, 18-gauge needle, insert the needle into the inverted vial. Position the needle tip at the very bottom of the solution in the vial when drawing the solution into the syringe. Before removing the needle from the vial, be sure to remove all the solution from the inverted vial.

6. Replace the 18-gauge needle with a 25-gauge needle for subcutaneous injection.

7. Expel air, large bubbles, and any excess solution to obtain the required 1.2-mL dose. A thin layer of small bubbles may remain at the top of the solution in the syringe. Because the solution is slightly viscous, the injection may take 5 to 10 seconds to administer.

Preparation and administration of reslizumab is as follows:

1. Remove the vial from the refrigerator. **Do Not Shake** to prevent foaming.

2. The solution should be clear to slightly hazy or opalescent, colorless to slightly yellow in color. Translucent to white protein particles may be visible in the solution. Do not administer if discolored.

3. Withdraw the calculated dose and slowly inject (to prevent foaming) into a 50-mL normal saline infusion bag. Gently invert the bag, **Do Not Shake!** Allow the infusion bag to come to room temperature.

4. Administer intravenously using an infusion set with an inline, low protein-binding filter (pore size, 0.2 micron). Infuse over 20 to 50 minutes and then flush the IV administration set with normal saline after the infusion is complete. Do not administer as an IV push or bolus, and do not administer concurrently in the same IV line with other medicines.

5. Observe the patient during and after the infusion to the development of signs of an allergic reaction.

> ⚠ **Medication Safety Alert**
>
> Allergic reactions and anaphylaxis have occurred within hours of administration of benralizumab, mepolizumab, omalizumab, and reslizumab. Symptoms include urticaria and throat and/or tongue edema. Patients should be observed after administration of benralizumab, mepolizumab, omalizumab, or reslizumab and medications for the treatment of allergic reactions (e.g., oxygen, epinephrine, diphenhydramine) should be readily available.

◆ *Common and serious adverse effects*
Hypersensitivity

Injection site reactions. The most commonly reported adverse effect for benralizumab, mepolizumab, and omalizumab is injection site reaction, including bruising, redness, warmth, burning, stinging, itching, hive formation, pain, indurations, mass, and inflammation. Most injection site reactions occur within 1 hour after injection, last less than 8 days, and generally decrease in frequency with subsequent dosing. Immediately report a rash or pruritus, with or without fever, and withhold additional injections until approved by the healthcare provider.

Musculoskeletal. Infusion of reslizumab was associated with oropharyngeal pain, chest pain, neck pain, muscle spasms, extremity pain, muscle fatigue, and musculoskeletal pain.

◆ *Drug interactions.* No drug interactions have been reported.

DRUG CLASS: MISCELLANEOUS ANTIINFLAMMATORY AGENTS

cromolyn sodium (KRŌ-mō-lĭn)

Actions

Cromolyn sodium is a mast cell stabilizer that inhibits the release of histamine and other mediators of inflammation, making it an indirect antiinflammatory agent. It must be administered before the body is given a stimulus to release histamine, such as an antigen that initiates an antigen-antibody allergic reaction.

Uses

Cromolyn is recommended for use in conjunction with other medications for treating patients with severe bronchial asthma or allergic rhinitis to prevent the release of histamine that results in asthmatic attacks or symptoms of allergic rhinitis. It is also used for the prophylactic management of exercise-induced bronchospasm and asthma.

Cromolyn has no direct bronchodilating, antihistaminic, or anticholinergic activity. Concomitant use of antihistamines or nasal decongestants may be necessary during initial treatment with cromolyn. A 2- to 4-week course of therapy is usually required to determine clinical

response. Therapy should be continued only if there is a decrease in the severity of asthmatic symptoms.

Therapeutic Outcome

The primary therapeutic outcome associated with cromolyn therapy is reduced frequency of episodes of allergic rhinitis, bronchospasm, and asthmatic attacks.

❖ **Nursing Implications for Cromolyn Sodium**
◆ *Premedication assessment*

1. This medication must be taken before exposure to the stimulus that initiates an attack of allergic rhinitis or bronchial asthma. Inhalation during an attack of bronchospasm or asthma may exacerbate symptoms.
2. Check to see whether the concurrent use of antihistamines or nasal decongestants has been ordered by the healthcare provider, especially during initiation of cromolyn therapy.

◆ *Availability. Inhalation:* Solution for inhalation: 20 mg/2 mL.

◆ *Dosage and administration.* **Adult:** *Inhalation: For chronic control:* 20 mg via nebulizer, four times daily. Inhalation during an acute asthma attack may aggravate symptoms because the powder form of the drug can increase the irritation in the respiratory passage and result in more bronchospasm.

For prevention of exercise-induced bronchospasm or bronchospasm associated with cold air or environmental substances: 20 mg (single dose) via nebulizer; administer 10 to 15 minutes prior to exercise or allergen exposure.

Counseling. The therapeutic effects of cromolyn, unlike those of beta-adrenergic decongestants, are not immediate. This should be explained to the patient in advance to ensure cooperation and continuation of treatment with the prescribed dosage regimen. Full therapeutic benefit requires regular use and is usually evident within 2 to 4 weeks. Therapy must be continued, even if the patient is symptom free.

◆ *Common adverse effects*
Gastrointestinal

Oral irritation, dry mouth. The most common adverse effect is irritation of the throat and trachea caused by inhaling the dry powder. This may be manifested by nasal itching and burning, nasal stuffiness, sneezing, coughing, and bronchospasm. Start regular oral hygiene measures when the therapy is initiated. Commercial mouthwashes contain alcohol, which may cause further drying and oral irritation. Other measures to alleviate dryness include sucking on ice chips or hard candy.

◆ *Serious adverse effects*
Respiratory

Bronchospasm, coughing. Notify the prescriber if inhalation causes bronchospasm or coughing.

◆ *Drug interactions.* No significant drug interactions have been reported.

Get Ready for the NCLEX® Examination!

Key Points

- Chronic obstructive pulmonary diseases, also known as chronic airflow limitation diseases, include chronic bronchitis and emphysema, both of which are progressive, irreversible diseases that usually cause death after a long debilitating illness.
- Asthma is an inflammatory disease that has airflow limitations; however, the episodes are intermittent and the limitations are reversible.
- Regular use of preventive medicine and removal of triggers such as allergens are key to the long-term treatment of asthma.
- Emphasize taking medications *before* exposure to a suspected trigger of an attack; treat all respiratory infections early.
- Regular use of a peak flowmeter and appropriate use of an inhaler are integral to treating asthma successfully.
- Nurses can teach patients with irreversible chronic airflow disorders techniques to manage their symptoms (e.g., adequate fluid intake to decrease secretion viscosity, breathing techniques, exercise conditioning to strengthen respiratory muscles, controlled coughing, positioning).
- Nurses can play a significant role in public education efforts, monitoring for nonadherence and encouraging patients to make changes in lifestyle to reduce the severity of chronic obstructive pulmonary diseases.
- Nurses can help the patient and/or family identify community resources available in the immediate vicinity.

Additional Learning Resources

SG Go to your Study Guide for additional Review Questions for the NCLEX® Examination, Critical Thinking Clinical Situations, and other learning activities to help you master this chapter content.

Go to your Evolve website (https://evolve.elsevier.com/Clayton) for additional online resources.

Review Questions for the NCLEX® Examination

1. During a respiratory assessment of a patient, the nurse noted the patient was coughing frequently and the oxygen saturation was less than 90%. Which of the following lower respiratory diseases/conditions could be the cause of these findings? *(Select all that apply.)*
   1. Asthma
   2. Pulmonary embolism
   3. Smoking
   4. Pneumonia
   5. Chronic obstructive pulmonary disease

2. During an evaluation of a patient who came into the clinic complaining of shortness of breath and increased sputum production, the nurse asks the patient for further information by which of the following statements? *(Select all that apply.)*
   1. "Tell me about your cough. Does it wake you at night?"
   2. "What activities would you say make you short of breath?"
   3. "When you cough up sputum, what color is it?"
   4. "Is there anyone at home to help you?"
   5. "Have you had any constipation or diarrhea recently?"

3. The nurse is preparing the antitussive agent benzonatate (Tessalon Perles) for a patient with a dry cough and knows the action of this drug will have which effect?
   1. It will dissolve thick, sticky mucus.
   2. It will suppress the cough reflex response in the brain.
   3. It will stimulate an increase in bronchial gland secretions.
   4. It will reduce the release of leukotrienes.

4. The expectorant guaifenesin (Robitussin), used for relief of conditions such as the common cold and bronchitis, works by which actions? *(Select all that apply.)*
   1. Suppressing the cough reflex response in the brain
   2. Decreasing mucus viscosity
   3. Stimulating an increase in bronchial secretions
   4. Promoting ciliary action
   5. Reducing the release of leukotrienes

5. The nurse is preparing to administer the beta-adrenergic bronchodilator albuterol but first performs which of the following preassessments on the patient? *(Select all that apply.)*
   1. Checks liver function test results
   2. Checks for a history of glaucoma, diabetes mellitus, or peptic ulcer disease
   3. Performs an assessment of the baseline mental status
   4. Asks about concurrent use of antihistamines or nasal decongestants
   5. Assesses for the presence of palpitations and dysrhythmias

6. The nurse instructing the patient on the drug tiotropium bromide (Spiriva), which was being started instead of continuing ipratropium bromide (Atrovent), realized further teaching was needed after the patient made which statement?
   1. "As I understand it, the effects of Spiriva last much longer than Atrovent so I only have to take it once a day."
   2. "This drug is used to treat an acute attack, like a rescue drug."
   3. "I can follow the instructions on the package for how to use this drug."
   4. "When I take this drug, I should notice a reduced amount of wheezing and easier breathing."

7. The nurse is preparing to administer both a bronchodilator and a steroid by inhalation and knows which medication should be administered first?
   1. Administer the steroid first.
   2. Administer the bronchodilator first.
   3. It does not make a difference.
   4. Bronchodilators and steroids should not be taken together.

8. After the administration of inhaled steroid medications, the nurse instructs the patient to do the which of the following? *(Select all that apply.)*
   1. Hold the breath for 30 seconds.
   2. Rinse the mouth and swallow.
   3. Rinse the mouth with water and spit out the water.
   4. Nothing is required.
   5. Use the bronchodilator first before the inhaled steroid when both are ordered.

Drugs Used to Treat Oral Disorders

31

https://evolve.elsevier.com/Clayton

Objectives

1. Explain common oral disorders and their treatments.
2. Describe therapy used for oral health.
3. Identify nursing assessments and interventions associated with treatment of mucositis.

Key Terms

cold sores (fever blisters) (KŌLD SŌRZ) (p. 487)
canker sores (KĂN-kĕr SŌRZ) (p. 488)
candidiasis (kăn-dĭ-DĪ-ă-sĭs) (p. 488)
mucositis (myū-kō-SĪ-tĭs) (p. 488)
plaque (PLĂK) (p. 488)
dental caries (DĔN-tŭl KĂR-ēz) (p. 488)

tartar (TĂR-tĕr) (p. 489)
gingivitis (jĭn-jĭ-VĪ-tĭs) (p. 489)
halitosis (hăl-ĭ-TŌ-sĭs) (p. 489)
xerostomia (zĕr-ŏ-STŌ-mē-ă) (p. 489)
dentifrices (DĔN-tĭ-frĭs-ĕz) (p. 492)

ORAL ANATOMY

The mouth, or oral cavity, is the beginning of the digestive tract and contains all the essential structures needed to consume food and drink to feed the body. The mouth consists of the upper and lower lips, which are outside of the oral cavity, as well as the jaw bone, the tongue, the pharynx, the teeth (including the surrounding gums), the cheeks (mucous membranes inside of the mouth), the hard and soft palate (the roof of the mouth), the uvula, and the tonsils. Salivary glands are also part of the oral cavity that produce saliva to lubricate the oral cavity and to provide enzymes secreted during eating to help aid digesting of food (Fig. 31.1).

MOUTH DISORDERS

Common disorders affecting the mouth are cold sores on the lip; canker sores and candidal infections of soft tissues of the tongue, cheeks, and gums; and plaque and calculus affecting the gums and teeth. Xerostomia, or lack of saliva, originates from nonoral causes. Halitosis can arise from oral or nonoral diseases. A much less common problem, but one that causes significant discomfort, is oral mucositis.

Cold sores (fever blisters) are caused by the herpes simplex type 1 virus (herpes simplex labialis) and are most commonly found at the junction of the mucous membrane and the skin of the lips or nostrils, although they can occur inside the mouth, especially affecting the gums and hard and soft palate. It is estimated that at least half of all Americans ages 20 to 40 years have had cold sores. Most victims were infected before 5 years of age. About half of patients will develop recurrent outbreaks of the lesions, often in the same location, separated by latent periods. The recurrence rate and extent of lesions are highly variable. Patients often predict when an outbreak may occur because of predisposing factors, such as systemic illnesses accompanied by fever or cold (hence the names fever blisters and cold sores) or by flu, menstruation, extreme physical stress and fatigue, or sun and wind exposure. Chemotherapy or radiation therapy that depresses the immune system also triggers cold sores.

Patients often report that a flare-up of the sores is preceded by a prodrome of burning, itching, and/or numbness in the area where the lesion develops. The lesions first become visible as small, red papules that develop into fluid-filled vesicles (blisters) 1 to 3 mm in diameter. Smaller lesions often coalesce into larger lesions. Pain is intense, fever may be present, and increased salivation and mouth odor occur. Often, the lymph nodes in the neck are swollen because of the body's response to infection. Over the next 10 to 14 days, a crust develops over the top of many coalesced, burst vesicles; the base is erythematous. The liquid from the vesicles contains live virus that is contagious if transferred to other people by direct contact (e.g.,

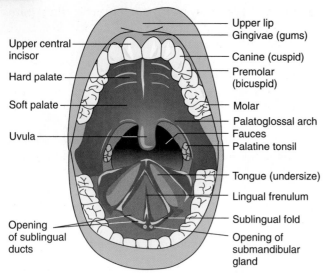

Fig. 31.1 The oral cavity. (From VanMeter KC, Hubert RJ. *Gould's Pathophysiology for the Health Professions.* 5th ed. St. Louis: Saunders; 2015.)

Table 31.1	World Health Organization Oral Mucositis Scale	
GRADE	**CLINICAL FEATURES**	
0	No mucositis present	
1	Oral soreness with erythema	
2	Oral erythema, ulcers, solid diet tolerated	
3	Oral ulcers, liquid diet tolerated	
4	Oral feeding not possible	

From Sonis ST, Elting LS, Keefe D, et al. Perspectives on cancer therapy-induced mucosal injury: pathogenesis, measurement, epidemiology, and consequences for patients. *Cancer.* 2004;100(9 suppl):1995-2025.

kissing). If pus develops in the vesicles or under the crust of a cold sore, a secondary bacterial infection may be present and should be evaluated for antibiotic therapy.

Canker sores, also known as *recurrent aphthous stomatitis,* affect 20% to 50% of people in the United States. The exact cause is unknown, but precipitating factors appear to be stress and local trauma (e.g., chemical irritation, toothbrush abrasion, irritation from orthodontic braces, biting the inside of the cheeks or lips). The lesions are not viral infections, as was once thought, and they are not contagious. There appears to be a familial factor as well as nutritional, emotional, and physiologic factors. They can develop at any age and affect both genders in equal numbers. Canker sores can appear as ulcers 0.5 to 2 cm in diameter on surfaces that are not attached to bone, such as the tongue, gums, or inner lining of the cheeks and lips. The lesion is usually gray to whitish yellow, with an erythematous halo of inflamed tissue surrounding the ulcer crater. Lesions do not form blisters and usually do not grow together. Patients may experience a single lesion or as many as 30 or more at one time. The lesions can be painful and can inhibit normal eating, drinking, talking, and swallowing as well as oral hygiene. There are usually no swollen lymph glands or fever unless the sore becomes secondarily infected. Most canker sores last 10 to 14 days and heal without scarring.

Candidiasis is a fungal infection caused by *Candida albicans,* the most common organism associated with oral infections. It is often called "the disease of the diseased" because it appears in debilitated patients and patients taking a variety of medicines. The most common predisposing factors are physiologic (e.g., early infancy, pregnancy, old age), diabetes mellitus, malnutrition, malignancies, and radiation therapy. Medicines that predispose a patient to candidiasis are those that depress defense mechanisms (e.g., immunosuppressants,

corticosteroids, cytotoxics, broad-spectrum antibiotics) and those that cause xerostomia (e.g., anticholinergics, antidepressants, antipsychotics, antihypertensives, antihistamines).

There are several forms of candidiasis, but the most common is the acute pseudomembranous form that is often referred to as *thrush.* It is characterized by white, milk curd–appearing plaques attached to the oral mucosa. These plaques usually can be easily detached, and erythematous, bleeding, sore areas appear beneath them. Thrush is most common in infants, pregnant women, and debilitated patients. Treatment requires local or systemic therapy with antifungal agents, such as nystatin (Mycostatin) suspension or clotrimazole lozenges (see discussion of antifungal agents in Chapter 45).

Mucositis (once called *stomatitis*) is a general term used to describe a painful inflammation of the mucous membranes of the mouth. It is commonly associated with chemotherapy and radiation therapy. Mucositis develops 5 to 7 days after antineoplastic therapy or radiation therapy has been administered. The sores are erythematous ulcerations intermixed with white, patchy mucous membranes. Candidal infections are often present.

Several scales and criteria are commonly used to standardize the evaluation of mucositis and its therapy. These include the World Health Organization Oral Mucositis Scale (Table 31.1), the Oral Assessment Guide, the Oral Mucositis Index, the Oral Mucositis Assessment Scale, and various visual analog scales. Of the many oral assessment tools available, there is no standard scale—all the scales are used to try to determine the degree of pain and ulceration. Mucositis is often a primary complaint associated with cancer therapy because it can diminish a patient's perception of quality of life. It can be severely debilitating, with pain and difficulty in swallowing, eating, drinking, and talking.

Plaque is the primary cause of most tooth, gum (gingiva), and periodontal disease. Plaque, the whitish yellow substance that builds up on teeth and gum lines around the teeth, is thought to originate from saliva. Plaque forms a sticky meshwork that traps bacteria and food particles. If not removed regularly, it thickens and bacteria proliferate. The bacteria secrete acids that eat into the enamel of teeth, causing **dental caries** (cavities).

If the plaque is not removed within 24 hours, it begins to calcify, forming calculus or **tartar**. The calculus forms a foundation for additional plaque to form, eventually eroding under the gum line and causing inflammation (**gingivitis**) and periodontal disease.

Halitosis is the term used to describe a very foul mouth odor. A temporary foul odor at certain times is normal in healthy individuals, such as "morning breath" or after eating certain foods (e.g., garlic, onions). Halitosis can also signify an underlying pathologic condition. Halitosis comes from oral and nonoral sources. Nonoral causes of halitosis include sinusitis, tonsillitis, and rhinitis; pulmonary diseases such as tuberculosis or bronchiectasis; and elimination of chemicals from the blood, such as acetone exhaled by patients with diabetic ketoacidosis. Paraldehyde and dimethyl sulfoxide are two medicinal agents excreted primarily through the lungs that leave a characteristic foul odor to the breath. "Smoker's breath" caused by cigarette smoking is a fairly common cause of halitosis. Oral causes of halitosis include decaying food particles, plaque-coated tongue and teeth, dental caries, poor oral or denture hygiene, periodontal disease, and xerostomia.

Xerostomia is a condition in which the flow of saliva is either partially or completely stopped. About 20% of those older than 65 years report a change in consistency, a decrease in production, or a discontinuation of salivary flow. Xerostomia causes loss of taste, difficulty in chewing and swallowing food, and difficulty in talking, and it increases tooth decay. Xerostomia can also cause a burning sensation of the tongue, cause mucositis, and reduce how long dentures can be worn each day. The most common causes of xerostomia are medicines (e.g., anticholinergic agents, diuretics, antidepressants, certain antihypertensive agents), diseases (e.g., diabetes mellitus, depression), and functional conditions (e.g., smoking, mouth breathing).

☀ Life Span Considerations

Salivary Flow

About 20% of people older than 65 years report a change in consistency, decrease in production, or discontinuation of salivary flow. The most common causes of xerostomia are medicines such as anticholinergic agents, diuretics, and antidepressants and certain antihypertensive medicines.

DRUG THERAPY FOR MOUTH DISORDERS

COLD SORES

The goals of treatment are to control discomfort, allow healing, prevent spread to others, and prevent complications. The cold sore should be kept moist to prevent drying and cracking that may make it more susceptible to secondary bacterial infection. Docosanol (Abreva) is the only US Food and Drug Administration–approved product clinically proven to shorten healing time as well as the duration of symptoms such as tingling, pain, burning, and itching. It must be applied five times daily starting at the first sign of outbreak (e.g., tingling, redness, itching). Local anesthetics (e.g., benzocaine, dibucaine, lidocaine) in emollient creams, petrolatum, or protectants (e.g., Zilactin-B [benzocaine 10%]) can temporarily relieve the pain and itching and prevent drying of the lesion.

Topical analgesics (e.g., Blistex [allantoin, menthol, camphor, phenol]) are safe and effective for temporarily reducing pain. Oral analgesics (e.g., aspirin, acetaminophen, ibuprofen, naproxen) may also provide significant pain relief. Broad-brimmed hats and ultraviolet blockers (e.g., ChapStick Moisturizer, Natural Ice) with a sun protection factor of at least 15 can be used for patients whose cold sores occur with sun exposure. Secondary infections can be treated with a topical antibiotic ointment such as Neosporin.

CANKER SORES

The goals of treatment are similar to those for cold sores: to control discomfort and promote healing. Topical anesthetics to control discomfort, such as benzocaine (Kank-A Mouth Pain [benzocaine 20% in oral mucosal protectant]), are particularly effective if applied just before eating or performing oral hygiene. Oral analgesics (e.g., aspirin, acetaminophen, ibuprofen, naproxen) may also provide significant pain relief. Aspirin should not be placed on the lesions because of the high risk of severe chemical burns with necrosis.

Oxygen-releasing agents (carbamide peroxide [Gly-Oxide], hydrogen peroxide [Peroxyl Spot Treatment]) can be used as debriding and cleansing agents up to four times daily for 7 days. Long-term safety has not been established, and tissue irritation and black hairy tongue have been reported. Saline rinses (1 to 3 teaspoons of table salt in 4 to 8 ounces of warm tap water) may be soothing and can be used before topical application of medication. Sustained use of products containing menthol, phenol, camphor, and eugenol should be discouraged because they cause tissue irritation and damage or systemic toxicity if overused. Silver nitrate should not be used to cauterize lesions because it may damage healthy tissue surrounding the lesion and predispose the area to later infection.

MUCOSITIS

Basic oral hygiene is an important component of care for any patient with cancer. The purpose is to decrease the complications associated with pain, oral microorganisms, and bleeding. Prior to cancer therapy, a baseline pretreatment oral mucosal assessment should be completed to rule out preexisting conditions or infections that might aggravate impending mucositis. Although it takes 5 to 7 days for mucositis to develop after a patient begins chemotherapy or radiation therapy, oral hygiene regimens should be started when chemotherapy or radiation therapy is initiated. Oral hygiene, oral irrigations, and methods to relieve dry mouth and lips can be very effective in providing comfort.

Pain associated with oral mucositis can be a major complication that contributes to poor nutrition and hydration. To be effective, topical applications of medications for pain must come into contact with the tissue. Therefore it is advisable to schedule these routines before cleaning the oral cavity. In addition to the previously described protectants, local anesthetics, and analgesics, the following are routine approaches to treating pain in the oral area:

- Viscous lidocaine 2% can be used before meals to relieve pain. Frequent applications are required, and the sense of taste is diminished. Care must be taken to make sure the patient is not burned by the food because the entire mouth and throat are anesthetized. The gag reflex may also be anesthetized, allowing for the potential to choke on food. Proper positioning while eating is important to prevent choking.
- Milk of magnesia can be used to rinse the mouth and coat the mucous membranes.
- Nystatin liquid suspension can be swished in the mouth for 1 minute and then swallowed ("swish and swallow" routine), or clotrimazole lozenges may be dissolved slowly in the mouth and then swallowed to reduce candidal oral infections.
- Sucralfate suspensions applied topically have been reported to provide effective pain relief.
- Oral or parenteral analgesics (e.g., morphine) should be administered for severe pain.
- Palifermin (Kepivance)—recombinant human keratinocyte growth factor—has been approved specifically for stimulating epithelial cell proliferation to prevent or treat the mucositis that develops in hematologic malignancies in patients undergoing chemotherapy before bone marrow transplantation.

PLAQUE

Plaque is controlled by brushing teeth, flossing between teeth, and using mouthwashes. If plaque is removed regularly, calculus will not form. Using a dentifrice (toothpaste) and flossing between teeth help remove dental plaque and stain, resulting in less halitosis and periodontal disease and fewer dental caries. Other devices, such as oral irrigators (Waterpik), sponge-tipped applicators, or electric toothbrushes, can be used for patients who wear orthodontic appliances, are physically or mentally handicapped, or lack manual dexterity and require someone else to clean their teeth. Therapeutic mouthwashes also help reduce plaque accumulated above the gum line.

HALITOSIS

Halitosis is treated most easily by eliminating the causes, such as smoking and certain foods. Regularly brushing the teeth or dentures and using dental floss between teeth can remove particles of decaying food. Mouthwashes and breath mints can mask halitosis but usually last less than 1 hour. If halitosis is persistent and has no readily identifiable cause such as smoking or diet, a dentist should be consulted for a thorough examination to ensure that no other pathologic condition is the underlying cause.

XEROSTOMIA

Xerostomia is treated by changing the medicines that cause dry mouth or with artificial saliva. Artificial saliva products do not stimulate natural saliva production, but mimic the viscosity, mineral content, and taste. Patients with xerostomia should be seen by a dentist regularly to help avoid additional dental caries and ensure proper denture fit to prevent gum irritation. Commercially available saliva substitutes include Mouth Kote, Biotène, Aquoral, and Caphosol. All are available as sprays for easy administration.

❖ NURSING IMPLICATIONS FOR ORAL HEALTH THERAPY

◆ Assessment

Drug history. Obtain a history of recent drug therapy. Some drugs, such as phenytoin (Dilantin), may cause alterations in the gums, and oral mucositis is common after chemotherapy and radiation therapy.

Dental history
- Obtain a dental history that includes frequency of visits to the dentist and a brief summary of dental procedures that have been performed within the past 1 to 3 years.
- Ask about usual hygiene practices, such as number of times per day brushing or flossing is done, type of toothbrush used, and oral products used (e.g., toothpaste, mouthwashes).
- Ask about tobacco and alcohol use, frequency, and amounts.
- Ask about any difficulty chewing, swallowing, or speaking.
- Ask about any recent changes in the taste of foods or alterations within the mouth, such as burning or tingling.

Oral cavity
- Put on gloves and inspect the oral cavity with the aid of a flashlight and tongue blade. Visually inspect the mucous membranes covering the lips, hard and soft palates, gums, tongue, pharynx, and teeth.
- Note the color of the mucous membranes and the moisture present.
- Inspect the mucous membranes for inflamed or receding gums, ulcerations, crusts, changes in color (e.g., white patches), and sores from poorly fitting dentures. Inquire how well the dentures fit and how long each day they are worn. Assess for the presence of teeth, dental caries, and plaque.

- Observe the amount and consistency of the saliva present.
- Note the presence or absence of halitosis. Its presence may indicate poor dental hygiene practices or an oral infection. Some odors occur from a variety of causes (e.g., garlic, smoking, ingestion of alcohol) and some from systemic diseases (e.g., acetone from diabetes, ammonia from liver disease).
- Biopsy of the soft tissues of the oral cavity may be completed to confirm diagnosis of the oral lesion.

◆ **Implementation**
- Develop a schedule for oral hygiene measures to be performed consistent with type and severity of mouth disorder.
- Make necessary referrals to the dentist, especially before starting chemotherapy.
- Order prescribed oral hygiene supplies and medications; list medications used as rinses or "swish and swallows" in the medication administration record.
- Develop a teaching plan to promote maintaining a healthy oral cavity and promote daily hygienic practices.

Cold sores
- Patients who develop cold sores should be taught that the lesions are common and may occur at any time from childhood into adulthood. The cold sores are also contagious when an active lesion is present. Teach the patient to avoid contaminating other individuals.
- Cold sores should be kept clean by gentle washing with mild soap solutions. Cold sores should be kept moist to prevent drying and cracking. Cracking may render the cold sore more susceptible to secondary bacterial infection, delay healing, and increase discomfort. Therefore highly astringent products (e.g., tannic acid, zinc sulfate) should be avoided.
- Apply docosanol (Abreva), local anesthetics, and ultraviolet blockers or oral analgesics as prescribed.
- When secondary infections are present, apply topical antibiotic ointment to the cold sore.

Canker sores
- Apply topical anesthetics before the patient eats or performs oral hygiene.
- Apply amlexanox (Aphthasol) after meals and oral hygiene, four times daily.
- Administer oral analgesics; apply oxygen-releasing agents for debridement and cleansing agents at appropriate intervals.
- Saline rinses using 1 to 3 teaspoons of table salt dissolved in 4 to 8 ounces of warm tap water may be soothing and can be used before topical medications are applied.
- Changes in diet can also reduce irritation to the sores. Avoid sharp-edged foods, such as potato chips and crackers, and spicy foods, pineapple, citrus

fruits, and chocolate. Drinking acidic juices and soft drinks through a straw can minimize contact and irritation.

Mucositis. Oral hygiene regimens should be started at the time of chemotherapy or radiation therapy. Oral hygiene should include a soft-bristled brush, a Waterpik on low setting, or a sponge-tipped applicator (in the case of severe lesions). With advanced lesions, pain and discomfort may be severe and other devices, such as a gravity flow irrigating system or an oral syringe, may be helpful.

Commercially prepared mouthwashes containing alcohol are usually not recommended because they dry and irritate the mouth rather than relieve symptoms of mucositis. Alternative preparations for oral hygiene solutions are 1 tablespoon of salt or ½ teaspoon of baking soda in 8 ounces of water or 1.5% to 6% solutions of hydrogen peroxide as a mouthwash. Although each of these solutions has disadvantages, they remain the standard for irrigating solutions.

The frequency of oral irrigations is important. Irrigations should be performed immediately before and after meals and at bedtime if symptoms are mild. With moderate lesions, increase the frequency to every 2 hours. In patients with severe symptoms, the mouth may be rinsed hourly. When fungal infections are present, the cleansing regimen should be performed immediately before administering the topical agents (e.g., nystatin liquids as a "swish and swallow" or clotrimazole lozenges). Performing the cleansing routine immediately before the medication is given will improve the contact of the medicine with the denuded surface of the oral mucosa. Caution the patient not to take food or drink for approximately 15 minutes after the medication has been given.

Mouth dryness can be relieved by chewing gum and sucking on ice chips or ice pops. Dry lips can be coated with cocoa butter, K-Y jelly, petroleum jelly, or lip balm. Artificial saliva is available.

Administer pain preparations according to prescribed routines using viscous lidocaine 2% or milk of magnesia rinses, nystatin liquid as a "swish and swallow," or sucralfate suspension topically. Use oral or parenteral analgesics for severe pain.

Plaque. Perform toothbrushing and dental flossing and use mouthwashes on a scheduled basis daily to prevent plaque.

Halitosis. Brushing dentures and teeth regularly and using dental floss can remove particles of decaying food. Mouthwashes and breath mints can mask halitosis but usually last less than 1 hour.

Xerostomia. Monitor the medication routine, report xerostomia to the healthcare provider, and use artificial saliva if prescribed.

Dentures. Dentures should be cleaned each time oral hygiene is performed. For neutropenic patients, dentures should be worn only for eating. Poorly fitting dentures must be repaired to prevent further tissue breakdown.

◆ Patient Education
- Teach the patient proper cleansing techniques for oral hygiene consistent with the conditions present (e.g., normal healthy tissue, mucositis, jaw wiring).
- Instruct patients who are to receive radiation or chemotherapy to start oral hygiene on a scheduled regimen immediately rather than waiting until mucositis develops.
- Teach the patient with pain the proper use of prescribed analgesics and comfort measures.
- Discuss dietary practices that may relieve symptoms, such as bland foods. For dry mouth, instruct the person to use gravies or sauces to moisten foods. When mucous membranes are irritated, suggest avoiding hot and spicy foods, alcohol, and tobacco.
- Persistent halitosis that is not relieved by brushing and flossing may have a medical basis. The individual should be told to discuss the matter with the healthcare provider or dentist to ensure appropriate therapy.
- Fluoride supplements may be recommended in areas of the United States in which the water supply is not fluoridated or the fluoride level is low.

Fostering health maintenance
- Discuss hygiene practices and medications prescribed for discomfort, infections, or mucosal breakdown.
- Seek cooperation and understanding of the following points to ensure that medication compliance is increased: name of medication; dosage, route, and times of administration; and common and serious adverse effects.
- Discuss a specific schedule for performing oral hygiene measures and include details of products to be used to relieve oral dryness or pain. Discuss basic dietary modifications needed while oral lesions are present (e.g., avoid citrus juices and spicy foods). With severe oral lesions, discuss supplemental nutrition formulas (e.g., Ensure, Boost). Cold drinks generally are more soothing to the oral tissue than hot foods.
- Report to the healthcare provider conditions that are not relieved by the prescribed therapies.

DRUG CLASS: DENTIFRICES

Actions
Dentifrices contain one or more abrasive agents, a foaming agent, and flavoring materials. They are available in powder, paste, or gel and are best used with a soft nylon toothbrush. Although dentifrices vary, degree of abrasiveness is an essential property for removing plaque. Some toothpastes contain higher concentrations of abrasive agents (e.g., silicates, dicalcium phosphate,

calcium pyrophosphate, calcium carbonate) and are advertised as "smokers' toothpastes" to remove tobacco stains.

The most common therapeutic agent added to dentifrices is fluoride for its anticaries activity. Chemicals such as sanguinarine, zinc citrate, triclosan, thymol, and eucalyptol have antibacterial properties that may reduce plaque. Dentifrices advertised as tooth whiteners contain oxidizing ingredients, such as hydrogen peroxide, carbamide peroxide, and perhydrol urea. Zinc chloride, zinc citrate, and soluble pyrophosphates prevent or retard the formation of new calculus from plaque but will not remove calculus already formed. Potassium nitrate is used for relieving sensitivity to hot and cold liquids and foods in otherwise normal teeth.

Uses
If possible, everyone should brush at least twice daily with a fluoride toothpaste. If the teeth and gums are normal, select a fluoride-containing dentifrice that has an acceptable taste. Those of all ages should use toothpastes that are the least abrasive to the teeth while controlling tooth decay and gum disease. This is especially important to patients with receding gums. People who have a sensitivity to hot or cold liquids and foods may want to try a sensitivity toothpaste containing potassium nitrate. About 2 weeks of regular use is necessary to eliminate sensitivity to hot or cold beverages and food.

Therapeutic Outcomes
The primary therapeutic outcomes expected from dentifrices are as follows:
1. Reduction in plaque formation and cavities
2. Pleasant, refreshing taste

DRUG CLASS: MOUTHWASHES

Toothbrushing and flossing are optimal for good oral hygiene; however, they may not be possible for the patient who has undergone oral surgery or who has experienced facial trauma. Mouthwashes may be temporarily effective in removing disagreeable tastes and reducing halitosis. Therapeutic mouthwashes are also available to reduce plaque.

Actions
Mouthwashes are solutions of flavoring, coloring, water, surfactants, and sometimes therapeutic ingredients. Flavoring agents are used to give a pleasant taste and freshen the breath. Coloring suggests a certain type of mouthwash: green or blue for minty, red for spicy, white for whitening, and brown for medicinal. Surfactants are foaming agents that aid in removing debris. Alcohol is often present, adding a bite and enhancing flavor (especially in the medicinal type of product) and solubilizing other ingredients. Therapeutic ingredients include fluoride for anticaries protection

and antimicrobial agents (e.g., benzoic acid, thymol, eucalyptol, menthol, cetylpyridinium chloride, domiphen bromide, chlorhexidine) to kill bacteria to reduce plaque formation and decaying food odor. Phenol is a local anesthetic, antiseptic, and antibacterial agent that penetrates and reduces plaque formation. Zinc citrate and zinc chloride are astringents that neutralize sulfur-smelling compounds from decaying debris in the mouth.

Uses

Mouthwashes can be subdivided into cosmetic and therapeutic products based on ingredients. Cosmetic mouthwashes freshen the breath and rinse out some debris, although the odor-reducing effect lasts only 10 to 30 minutes.

Certain mouthwashes are for specific purposes. The most common are the fluoride-containing mouthwashes used to prevent dental caries. Medicinal mouthwashes (e.g., Listerine) reduce plaque accumulation and gingivitis. Chlorhexidine (Peridex) is an antibacterial agent used to treat oral mucositis. Products containing zinc chloride are used as astringents for temporarily decreasing bleeding or irritation. A 0.9% solution of sodium chloride (normal saline) is an effective gargle. It can provide temporary, soothing relief of pharyngeal irritation from nasogastric tubes, endotracheal tubes, sore throat, or oral surgery. Solutions containing hydrogen peroxide cleanse and debride minor lesions; however, use should be limited to 7 to 10 days to prevent further tissue irritation. Lidocaine, a local anesthetic, is available as an oral viscous solution (Lidocaine Viscous 2%). The viscous solution is a longer-lasting local anesthetic and can be used as a gargle for patients with sore throats or mouth ulcers. This product is frequently used for immunosuppressed patients with painful candidal infections of the mouth and throat. Caution the patient not to eat or drink anything for at least 30 minutes following use of viscous lidocaine because of the absence of the gag reflex and potential risk for aspiration.

Unless a mouthwash is being used to treat a specific medical condition (e.g., oral mucositis), it should *not* become a substitute for normal oral hygiene. Primary oral hygiene includes proper toothbrushing and flossing.

All mouthwashes have specific dosage recommendations. It is important not to exceed these recommendations without a healthcare provider's order because many of the therapeutic ingredients (e.g., lidocaine, fluoride) can be systemically absorbed, resulting in potentially toxic levels. Most mouthwashes are designed to be used as a rinse (mouthwash is held in the mouth, swished around, and expectorated). Again, prolonged swallowing of mouthwashes may lead to systemic toxicities. Patients should be advised to refrain from smoking, eating, or drinking for at least 30 minutes after use.

Therapeutic Outcomes

The primary therapeutic outcomes expected from mouthwashes are as follows:

1. Temporary reduction in bleeding or irritation
2. Relief of discomfort
3. A refreshing taste
4. Improvement in halitosis

Get Ready for the NCLEX® Examination!

Key Points

- Common disorders affecting the mouth are cold sores on the lip; canker sores and candidal infections of soft tissues of the tongue, cheeks, and gums; and plaque and calculus affecting the gums and teeth. Xerostomia (lack of saliva) originates from nonoral causes.
- Halitosis can arise from oral or nonoral causes. A much less common problem but one that causes significant discomfort is oral mucositis.
- Health teaching should start with teaching children to carry out regular brushing, flossing, and dental care. Stress regular dental checkups, have problems treated promptly when they occur, and if wearing dentures, be certain that they fit properly.

Additional Learning Resources

SG Go to your Study Guide for additional Review Questions for the NCLEX® Examination, Critical Thinking Clinical Situations, and other learning activities to help you master this chapter content.

Go to your Evolve website (https://evolve.elsevier.com/Clayton) for additional online resources.

Review Questions for the NCLEX® Examination

1. The nurse discussing halitosis with a patient should include which of these causes? *(Select all that apply.)*
   1. Smoking
   2. Canker sores
   3. Sinusitis
   4. Dimethyl sulfoxide
   5. *Candida albicans*

2. The nurse educating a patient with painful oral lesions discusses the best approach to oral hygiene that includes which instruction?
    1. "You should wait until the oral lesions are all healed before going back to routine oral care."
    2. "You should start using commercial mouthwashes for rinsing after meals and at bedtime."
    3. "You could think about using normal saline, baking soda, or half-strength hydrogen peroxide rinses for these lesions."
    4. "You need to get a prescription for pain medication."

3. A patient was asking the nurse to explain canker sores. What is the appropriate response by the nurse? *(Select all that apply.)*
    1. "The causes of canker sores are not known."
    2. "Sometimes canker sores are brought on by stress and trauma to the mouth."
    3. "Canker sores are lesions that are really viral infections."
    4. "Canker sores are not contagious."
    5. "If you take aspirin, it will promote healing of the canker sores."

4. The nurse knows that thrush can occur in which of these patient populations? *(Select all that apply.)*
    1. Infants
    2. Pregnant women
    3. Debilitated patients
    4. Teens
    5. Older adults

5. The nurse can expect that a patient who recently underwent chemotherapy will develop mucositis during which time frame?
    1. Within 2 to 3 days of starting chemotherapy
    2. Within 5 to 7 days of starting chemotherapy
    3. Within 10 to 12 days of starting chemotherapy
    4. Within 2 weeks of starting chemotherapy

6. Which drug has been approved specifically for use in preventing and treating the mucositis that develops in leukemia or lymphoma patients undergoing chemotherapy before bone marrow transplantation?
    1. Nystatin
    2. Sucralfate
    3. Viscous lidocaine
    4. Palifermin

Drugs Used to Treat Gastroesophageal Reflux and Peptic Ulcer Disease

32

Objectives

1. Describe the physiology of the stomach.
2. Cite common stomach disorders that require drug therapy.
3. Identify factors that prevent breakdown of the body's normal defense barriers resulting in ulcer formation.
4. Discuss the drug classifications and actions used to treat stomach disorders.
5. Identify interventions that incorporate pharmacologic and nonpharmacologic treatments for an individual with stomach disorders.

Key Terms

chief cells (CHĒF) (p. 495)
parietal cells (pă-RĪ-ĕ-tŭl) (p. 495)
hydrochloric acid (hī-drō-KLŎR-ĭk) (p. 495)
mucous cells (MŪ-kŭs SĔLZ) (p. 495)
gastroesophageal reflux disease (GERD) (găs-trō-ĕs-ŏf-ĕ-JĒ-ŭl RĒ-flŭks) (p. 495)

heartburn (HĂRT-bŭrn) (p. 495)
peptic ulcer disease (PUD) (PĔP-tĭk ŬL-sŭr) (p. 496)
Helicobacter pylori (hĕl-ĭ-kō-BĂK-tŭr pī-LŎR-ē) (p. 496)

PHYSIOLOGY OF THE STOMACH

As a major part of the gastrointestinal (GI) tract, the stomach has three primary functions: (1) storing food until it can be processed in the lower GI tract; (2) mixing food with gastric secretions until it is a partially digested, semisolid mixture known as chyme; and (3) slowly emptying the stomach at a rate that allows proper digestion and absorption of nutrients and medicine from the small intestine.

Three types of secretory cells line portions of the stomach—chief, parietal, and mucous cells. The **chief cells** secrete pepsinogen, an inactive enzyme. **Parietal cells** secrete **hydrochloric acid** by way of a hydrogen ion pump, which activates pepsinogen to pepsin, providing the optimal pH for pepsin to start protein digestion. Stimulation of histamine-2 (H_2) receptors on the stomach's parietal cells also causes secretion of hydrochloric acid. Cholinergic nerve fibers that innervate the stomach will also increase parietal cell secretion of hydrochloric acid when stimulated by acetylcholine. Normal pH in the stomach ranges from 1 to 5, depending on the presence of food and medications. Hydrochloric acid also breaks down muscle fibers and connective tissue ingested as food and kills bacteria that enter the digestive tract through the mouth. The parietal cells also secrete intrinsic factor needed for absorption of vitamin B_{12}. The **mucous cells** secrete mucus, which coats the stomach wall. The 1-mm-thick coat is alkaline and protects the stomach wall from damage by hydrochloric acid and the digestive enzyme pepsin. It also contributes lubrication for food transport. Small amounts of other enzymes are also secreted in the stomach: lipases digest fats and gastric amylase digests carbohydrates. Other digestive enzymes are also carried into the stomach from swallowed saliva.

Prostaglandins play a major role in protecting the stomach walls from injury by stomach acids and enzymes. Prostaglandins are produced by cells lining the stomach and prevent injury by inhibiting gastric acid secretion, maintaining blood flow, and stimulating mucus and bicarbonate production.

COMMON STOMACH DISORDERS

Gastroesophageal reflux disease (GERD), more commonly referred to as *heartburn*, *acid indigestion*, or *sour stomach*, is a common stomach disorder (Fig. 32.1). Approximately one-third of the US population experiences heartburn once each month, and 5% to 7% have heartburn daily. Common symptoms are a burning sensation, bloating, belching, and regurgitation. Other symptoms that are reported less frequently are nausea, a "lump in the throat," hiccups, and chest pain.

Gastroesophageal reflux disease is the reflux of gastric secretions, primarily pepsin and hydrochloric acid, up into the esophagus. Causes of GERD are a weakened lower esophageal sphincter, delayed gastric emptying,

495

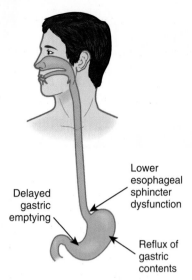

Delayed gastric emptying

Lower esophageal sphincter dysfunction

Reflux of gastric contents

Fig. 32.1 Causes of gastroesophageal reflux disease. (From Lewis SL, Bucher L, Heitkemper MM. *Medical-Surgical Nursing: Assessment and Management of Clinical Problems.* 10th ed. St. Louis: Elsevier; 2017.)

hiatal hernia, obesity, overeating, tight-fitting clothing, and increased acid secretion. Acid secretions are increased by smoking, alcohol, carbonated beverages, coffee, and spicy foods.

Most cases of GERD pass quickly with only mild discomfort, but frequent or prolonged bouts of acid reflux cause inflammation, tissue erosion, and ulcerations in the lower esophagus. Anyone who has recurrent or continuous symptoms of reflux, especially if the symptoms interfere with activities, should be referred to a healthcare provider. These symptoms may also accompany more serious conditions, such as ischemic heart disease, scleroderma, and gastric malignancy.

> **Clinical Pitfall**
>
> Nurses need to be aware that the symptoms of GERD may also accompany more serious conditions, such as ischemic heart disease, scleroderma, and gastric malignancy. It is important to do a thorough physical assessment whenever a patient presents with heartburn or acid indigestion and not simply dismiss the symptoms as GI in origin.

Peptic ulcer disease (PUD) refers to several stomach disorders that result from an imbalance between acidic stomach contents and the body's normal defense barriers, causing ulcerations in the GI tract. The most common illnesses are gastric and duodenal ulcers. It is estimated that approximately 10% of all Americans will develop an ulcer at some time in their lives. The incidence in men and women is approximately the same. Race, economic status, and psychological stress do not correlate with the frequency of ulcer disease. Often the only symptom reported is epigastric pain, described as burning, gnawing, or aching. Patients often report that varying degrees of pain are present for a few weeks and are then gone, only to recur a few weeks later. The

pain is most often noted when the stomach is empty, such as at night or between meals, and is relieved by food or antacids. Other symptoms that cause patients to seek medical attention are bloating, nausea, vomiting, and anorexia.

Ulcers appear to be caused by a combination of acid and a breakdown in the body's defense mechanisms that protect the stomach wall. Proposed mechanisms are oversecretion of hydrochloric acid by excessive numbers of parietal cells; injury to the mucosal barrier, such as that resulting from prostaglandin inhibitors (nonsteroidal antiinflammatory drugs [NSAIDs], including aspirin); and infection of the mucosal wall by *Helicobacter pylori*. It had been thought that no bacterium could survive in the highly acidic environment of the stomach; however, *H. pylori* was first isolated from patients with gastritis in 1983. The bacterium seems able to live below the mucous barrier, where it is protected from stomach acid and pepsin. *Helicobacter pylori* is now thought to be associated with as many as 90% of duodenal and 70% of gastric ulcers. The exact mechanism whereby *H. pylori* contributes to ulcer formation is not known, but several hypotheses are being tested.

Several risk factors increase the likelihood of PUD:
1. There seems to be a genetic predisposition to PUD. Some families have a much greater history of PUD than others.
2. It is a commonly held belief that stress causes ulcers, but no well-controlled studies have supported this.
3. Cigarette smoking increases acid secretion, alters blood flow in the stomach wall, and retards prostaglandin synthesis needed for defense mechanisms.
4. Nonsteroidal antiinflammatory drugs have a twofold effect: they inhibit prostaglandins that protect the mucosa and directly irritate the stomach wall. Once ulcerations have formed, NSAIDs also slow healing.
5. It is commonly thought that certain foods (e.g., spicy foods) and alcohol contribute to ulcer formation. It is true that certain foods increase acid secretion and that alcohol irritates the stomach lining, but results from studies have not corroborated this concept.

GOALS OF TREATMENT

The goals of treatment of GERD are to relieve symptoms, decrease the frequency and duration of reflux, heal tissue injury, and prevent recurrence. The most important treatment is a change in lifestyle, which includes losing weight (if significantly over the ideal body weight), reducing or avoiding foods and beverages that increase acid production, reducing or stopping smoking, avoiding alcohol, and consuming smaller meals. Additional therapy includes remaining upright for 2 hours after meals, not eating before bedtime, and avoiding tight clothing over the abdominal area. Lozenges may be used to increase saliva production, and antacid therapy may provide relief for patients who experience infrequent heartburn. If the patient's symptoms do not improve within 2 to 3 weeks, or if the condition is severe, additional pharmacologic measures should be tried to reduce irritation. About 5% to 10% of patients with GERD require surgery.

The treatment of PUD and GERD is somewhat similar: relieve symptoms, promote healing, and prevent recurrence. Lifestyle changes that eliminate risk factors for PUD, such as cigarette smoking and foods (and alcohol) that increase acid secretion, should be initiated. Patients rarely need to be restricted to a bland diet. If NSAIDs are being taken, consideration should be given to switching to acetaminophen if feasible. For decades, ulcer treatment focused on reducing acid secretions (anticholinergic agents, H_2 antagonists, gastric acid pump inhibitors), neutralizing acid (antacids), or coating ulcer craters to hasten healing (sucralfate). Major changes in therapy have come about because of the approval of antibiotics to eradicate *H. pylori*. Several large studies are underway to refine the healing and reduce ulcer recurrence rates. Various combinations of antimicrobial agents (e.g., amoxicillin, tetracycline, metronidazole, clarithromycin), bismuth, and antisecretory agents (e.g., H_2 antagonists, proton pump inhibitors [PPIs]) are used to eradicate *H. pylori*. Antibiotics are not recommended for individuals who are asymptomatic with *H. pylori* because there is concern that resistant strains of bacteria may develop.

DRUG THERAPY

ACTIONS

- Antacids neutralize gastric acid, thereby causing the gastric contents to be less acidic.
- Coating agents provide a protective covering over the ulcer crater.
- Histamine-2 antagonists decrease the volume of hydrochloric acid produced, which increases the gastric pH and thereby results in decreased irritation to the gastric mucosa.
- Proton pump inhibitors block the formation of hydrochloric acid, reducing irritation of the gastric mucosa.
- Prokinetic agents increase the lower esophageal sphincter muscle pressure and peristalsis, hastening emptying of the stomach to reduce reflux.

USES

- Antacids decrease hyperacidity associated with PUD, GERD, gastritis, and hiatal hernia.
- Coating agents provide a protective barrier for the mucosal lining where hydrochloric acid may come into contact with inflamed eroded areas. They are used to treat existing ulcer craters on the gastric mucosa.
- Histamine-2 antagonists are used to treat acute gastric and duodenal ulcers and gastroesophageal

disease, as well as for maintenance to prevent ulcer recurrence.
- Proton pump inhibitors are used to treat hyperacidity conditions (e.g., GERD, Zollinger-Ellison syndrome) and peptic and gastric ulcer disease.
- Prokinetic agents are used to treat GERD.

❖ NURSING IMPLICATIONS FOR AGENTS USED FOR STOMACH DISORDERS

◆ Assessment

Nutritional assessment. Obtain patient data about current height, weight, and any recent weight gain or loss. Identify the normal pattern of eating, including snacking habits. Use a food guide such as the Healthy Eating Plate (see Fig. 46.3) as a guide when asking questions to identify the usual foods eaten by the individual. Ask about any nutritional or cultural restrictions associated with dietary practices. Are there any food allergies (obtain details) or foods that particularly cause gastric distress when eaten? Does the individual take any nutritional supplements? How often and how much fast food is eaten?

Esophagus, stomach. Ask patients to describe symptoms. Question in detail what is meant by the terms *indigestion, heartburn, upset stomach, nausea,* and *belching.*

Pain, discomfort
- Ask the patient to describe the onset, duration, location, and characteristics of pain or discomfort. Determine whether there is a relationship between the ingestion of certain types of food or drinks and the onset of pain. Ask specifically about coffee, tea, cola, chocolate, and alcohol intake.
- What has the patient done to relieve the pain or discomfort? Have there been any changes in taste (e.g., bitterness, sourness)? Record pain levels using a rating scale before and after medications are administered.

Activity, exercise. Ask specifically what type of work or activities the individual performs that may increase intraabdominal pressure (e.g., lifting heavy objects, bending over frequently).

History of diseases or disorders
- What other diagnoses have been made for diseases or disorders (e.g., ulcer, gallbladder, liver, jaundice, irritable bowel syndrome)?
- Have there been any changes in bowel elimination or stool color, consistency, or frequency?

Medication history
- What self-medications have been tried?
- What prescribed medications are being taken?
- What is the schedule of medication administration (e.g., how frequently and when are antacids taken)?

Anxiety or stress level. Ask the patient to describe his or her lifestyle. What does the patient think are stressors and how often do they occur?

Smoking. What is the frequency of smoking?

◆ Implementation

- *Routine orders:* Most healthcare providers order antacids 1 hour before meals, 2 to 3 hours after meals, and at bedtime. As-needed (PRN) medication dosages must be discussed.
- Each type of medication used to treat GERD or PUD may require somewhat different scheduling to avoid drug interactions. When developing the time frames for administration of medications on the medication administration record, schedule the other prescribed drugs 1 hour before or 2 hours after antacids.
- Changes in diet require careful planning with the patient and the person responsible for purchasing and cooking the meals. Schedule teaching sessions appropriately. Not only may some foods need to be altered, but also the number of meals per day may need to be increased with a smaller serving at each meal.

◆ Patient Education

Nutrition

- Implement prescribed dietary changes: eat small, more frequent meals to support optimal energy requirements and healing; avoid overdistention of the stomach; avoid any seasonings that are intolerable or that aggravate the condition; and avoid coffee, teas, colas, alcoholic beverages (including beer), carbonated beverages, peppermint, spearmint, and citric juices, which may produce discomfort in those with GERD.
- Avoid late-night snacks or meals that could result in increased gastric secretions.
- Observe for foods that aggravate the condition and eliminate these from the diet. Drink only small amounts of fluid with the meal and drink mostly between meals. Increase protein foods and decrease fats to about 45 g/day or less; use nonfat milk.

Pain, discomfort. Keep a written record (see Patient Self-Assessment later) of the onset, duration, location, and precipitating factors for any pain. Sit upright at the table when eating and do not lie down for at least 2 hours after eating. When a hiatal hernia is present, elevate the head of the bed by 6 to 8 inches using bed blocks to prevent reflux during sleep. Have the patient keep a log of the pain, including time of day, any factors that might have precipitated the pain, and degree of pain relief from medications used.

Medications

- Take prescribed medications at recommended times to promote optimal healing. See individual drug monographs for suggested scheduling.

- Avoid NSAIDs and aspirin-containing medicines that irritate the gastric mucosa. Consult the prescriber or pharmacist regarding scheduling of or discontinuation of these medications.

Lifestyle changes

- Discuss stress and its effects on the person, and implement needed lifestyle changes.
- Encourage a significant reduction or cessation of smoking.
- Implement plans to gain sufficient rest.

Fostering health maintenance

- Discuss medication information and how it will benefit the course of treatment to produce an optimal response. Medications used in the treatment of hyperacidity are important measures to alleviate the irritating effects on the mucosal tissue; stress the importance of not discontinuing treatment and the need for continued medical follow-up.
- Seek cooperation and understanding of the following points so that medication adherence is increased: name of medication; dosage, route, and times of administration; and common and serious adverse effects. Stress the need to complete a full course of treatment for *H. pylori* so that the organisms are indeed killed and not only suppressed; *H. pylori* can regrow if medications are discontinued too early.

Patient self-assessment. Enlist the patient's aid in developing and maintaining a written record of monitoring parameters (e.g., a list of foods causing problems, degree of pain relief). See Patient Self-Assessment form for Agents Affecting the Digestive System on the Evolve website. Complete the Premedication Data column for use as a baseline to track response to drug therapy. Ensure that the patient understands how to use the form and instruct the patient to bring the completed form to follow-up visits. During follow-up visits, focus on issues that will foster adherence with the therapeutic interventions prescribed.

DRUG CLASS: ANTACIDS

Actions

Antacids lower the acidity of gastric secretions by buffering the hydrochloric acid (normal pH is 1 to 2) to a lower hydrogen ion concentration. Buffering hydrochloric acid to a pH of 3 to 4 is highly desired because the proteolytic action of pepsin is reduced and the gastric juice loses its corrosive effect.

Uses

Antacids are commonly used for heartburn, excessive eating and drinking, and PUD. They are no longer first-line agents in the treatment of stomach disorders but are often the first agents used by consumers to self-treat these conditions. However, nurses and patients must be aware that not all antacids are alike. They should be used judiciously, particularly by certain types of patients (e.g., those with heart failure, hypertension, or renal failure). Long-term self-treatment with antacids may also mask symptoms of serious underlying diseases, such as a bleeding ulcer.

The most effective antacids available are combinations of aluminum hydroxide, magnesium oxide or hydroxide, and calcium carbonate. All act by neutralizing gastric acid. Combinations of these ingredients must be used because any compound used alone in therapeutic quantities may produce severe systemic adverse effects. Other ingredients found in antacid combination products include simethicone and bismuth. Simethicone is a defoaming agent that breaks up gas bubbles in the stomach, reducing stomach distention and heartburn. It is effective in patients who have overeaten or who have heartburn, but it is not effective in treating PUD. Bismuth compounds have little acid-neutralizing capacity and are therefore poor antacids.

The following principles should be considered when antacid therapy is planned:

- For indigestion, antacids should not be administered for more than 2 weeks. If after this time the patient is still experiencing discomfort, the healthcare provider should be contacted.
- Patients with edema, heart failure, hypertension, renal failure, pregnancy, or salt-restricted diets should use low-sodium antacids, such as Maalox. Therapy should continue only on the recommendation of the healthcare provider.
- Antacid tablets should be used only for the patient with occasional indigestion or heartburn. Tablets *do not* contain enough antacid to be effective in treating PUD.
- A common complaint of patients consuming large quantities of calcium carbonate or aluminum hydroxide is constipation. Excess magnesium results in diarrhea. If a patient experiences these symptoms and still has stomach discomfort, the healthcare provider should be consulted.
- Effective management of acute ulcer disease requires large volumes of antacids. The selection of an antacid and the quantity to be taken depend on its neutralizing capacity. Any patient with coffee-ground emesis, bloody stools, or recurrent abdominal pain should seek medical attention immediately and not attempt to self-treat the disorder.
- Calcium carbonate and sodium bicarbonate may cause rebound hyperacidity.
- Patients with renal failure should not use large quantities of antacids containing magnesium. The magnesium ions cannot be excreted and may produce hypermagnesemia and toxicity.
- Most antacids have similar ingredients. Selection of an antacid for occasional use should be determined by quantity of each ingredient, cost, taste,

and frequency of adverse effects. Patients may need to try more than one product and weigh the advantages and disadvantages of each.

Therapeutic Outcomes

The primary therapeutic outcomes expected from antacid therapy are relief of discomfort, reduced frequency of heartburn, and healing of irritated tissues.

❖ **Nursing Implications for Antacids**
◆ *Premedication assessment*

1. Check renal function test results to ensure that renal function is normal. When renal failure is present, patients should not take large quantities of antacids containing magnesium. Monitor the patient's renal function tests, including blood urea nitrogen, creatinine, and serum electrolyte levels (including magnesium and potassium). Magnesium and potassium ions cannot be excreted when patients have renal failure and may produce hypermagnesemia, hyperkalemia, and toxicity.
2. Check the pattern of bowel elimination for diarrhea or constipation.
3. Record the pattern of gastric pain being experienced; report coffee-ground emesis, bloody stools, or recurrent abdominal pain to the healthcare provider for prompt attention.
4. If the patient is pregnant or has edema, heart failure, hypertension, or salt restrictions, ensure that a low-sodium antacid has been prescribed.
5. Schedule other prescribed medications to be taken 1 hour before or 2 hours after antacids are to be administered.

Life Span Considerations
Antacids

Those older than 65 years are the most common purchasers of antacid products. Gastrointestinal disorders such as PUD, NSAID-induced ulcers, and GERD occur more often in this age group. Magnesium-containing antacids are often used as laxatives. Although the primary symptom of ulcer disease in a younger person is usually burning epigastric pain, the symptoms in an older person, if present at all, usually include complaints of vague abdominal discomfort, anorexia, and weight loss.

◆ *Availability.* See Table 32.1.

- Liquid forms of antacid preparations should be used for treatment of PUD because tablets do not contain enough of the active ingredients to be effective.
- Antacid tablets may be used for occasional episodes of heartburn. They should be well chewed before swallowing for a more rapid onset of action.

Table 32.1   **Ingredients of Commonly Used Antacids**

PRODUCT	FORM	CALCIUM CARBONATE	ALUMINUM HYDROXIDE	MAGNESIUM OXIDE, HYDROXIDE, OR CARBONATE	SODIUM BICARBONATE	SIMETHICONE	OTHER INGREDIENTS
Baking soda	Powder	—	—	—	×	—	—
Gelusil	Tablet	—	×	×	—	×	—
Maalox Advanced Maximum Strength	Suspension	—	×	×	—	×	—
Phillips' Milk of Magnesia	Tablet, suspension	—	—	×	—	—	—
Riopan Plus	Tablet, suspension	—	—	—	—	×	magaldrate
Rolaids	Tablet	×	—	×	—	—	—
Tums	Tablet	×	—	—	—	—	—

◆ *Common adverse effects*

Chalky taste. A chalky taste is a common problem with antacids. Suggest a change in brands or flavors. Suggest using a liquid instead of tablets.

◆ *Serious adverse effects*

Gastrointestinal

Diarrhea, constipation. Diarrhea or constipation is a common problem when antacids are used in therapeutic dosages to treat ulcers. Alternating between calcium- or aluminum-containing compounds and magnesium-containing compounds should help alleviate the problem.

◆ *Drug interactions*

Tetracycline antibiotics, fluoroquinolone antibiotics, phenytoin, phenothiazines, captopril, ketoconazole, corticosteroids, digoxin, iron supplements. The absorption of these medicines is inhibited by antacids. These medications should be administered 1 hour before or 2 to 3 hours after antacids.

Levodopa, valproic acid. The absorption of levodopa is increased by magnesium-aluminum antacids. When antacid therapy is added, toxicity may result in the patient with Parkinson's disease whose condition is well controlled on a certain dosage of levodopa. If the patient's parkinsonism symptoms are well controlled on levodopa and antacid therapy, withdrawal of antacids may result in a recurrence of parkinsonian symptoms.

Quinidine, amphetamines. Frequent use of sodium bicarbonate–containing antacid therapy may result in increased urinary pH. Renal excretion of quinidine and amphetamines may be inhibited and toxicity may occur.

DRUG CLASS: HISTAMINE-2 RECEPTOR ANTAGONISTS

Actions

One of the primary mechanisms of hydrochloric acid secretion has to do with histamine stimulation of H_2 receptors on the stomach's parietal cells. The H_2 antagonists act by blocking the H_2 receptors, resulting in a decrease in the volume of acid secreted. The pH of the stomach contents rises as a consequence of a reduction in acid.

Uses

The H_2 antagonists (cimetidine, ranitidine, nizatidine, famotidine) are used to treat GERD, duodenal ulcers, and pathologic hypersecretory conditions, such as Zollinger-Ellison syndrome, and for preventing and treating stress ulcers in critically ill patients. Unapproved uses include prevention of aspiration pneumonitis, stress ulcer prophylaxis, acute upper GI bleeding, hives, and hyperparathyroidism. All of the H_2 antagonists have products that are available for over-the-counter purchase for symptomatic relief of overeating and heartburn.

Cimetidine was the first approved H_2 antagonist but differs from the other agents by its extensive liver metabolism and antiandrogenic effect that may result in gynecomastia. It also has many drug-drug interactions that are not seen with the others. Consequently, cimetidine is used less frequently than the other H_2 antagonists.

Famotidine is similar in action and use to cimetidine but has the advantages of once-daily dosing, fewer drug interactions, and no antiandrogenic effect. A parenteral dosage form is available.

Ranitidine is similar in action and use to cimetidine but has the advantages of twice-daily dosing, fewer drug interactions, and no antiandrogenic effect. A parenteral dosage form is also available.

Nizatidine is similar to ranitidine and famotidine but, in contrast to the other agents, is not available in a parenteral dosage form.

Therapeutic Outcomes

The primary therapeutic outcomes expected from H_2 antagonist therapy are relief of discomfort, reduced frequency of heartburn, and healing of irritated tissues.

❖ Nursing Implications for H₂ Antagonists

◆ *Premedication assessment.* Perform a baseline assessment of the patient's mental status for comparison with subsequent mental status evaluations to detect central nervous system alterations that may occur, particularly with cimetidine therapy.

◆ *Availability, dosage, and administration.* See Table 32.2.
- All H₂ antagonists may be administered with or without food.
- Because antacid therapy is often continued during early therapy of PUD, administer 1 hour before or 2 hours after the H₂ antagonist dose.

◆ *Common adverse effects.* Approximately 1% to 3% of patients develop these adverse effects. They are usually mild and resolve with continued therapy. Encourage patients not to discontinue therapy without first consulting the healthcare provider.

Neurologic
Dizziness, headache, somnolence. Provide for patient safety during episodes of dizziness. If the patient develops somnolence and lethargy, encourage the use of caution when working around machinery, driving a car, or performing other duties that require mental alertness.

Gastrointestinal
Diarrhea, constipation. Maintain the patient's state of hydration and obtain an order for stool softeners or bulk-forming laxatives if necessary. Encourage the inclusion of sufficient roughage (fresh fruits, vegetables, whole-grain products) in the diet.

◆ *Serious adverse effects*
Neurologic
Confusion, disorientation, hallucinations. If high dosages (particularly of cimetidine) are used in patients with liver or renal disease or in patients older than 50 years, mental confusion, slurred speech, disorientation, and hallucinations may occur. These adverse effects dissipate over 3 or 4 days after therapy has been discontinued. Perform a baseline assessment of the patient's degree of alertness and orientation to name, place, and time before starting therapy. Make regularly scheduled subsequent mental status evaluations, and compare findings. Report alterations in mental status.

Endocrine
Gynecomastia. Mild bilateral gynecomastia and breast soreness may occur with long-term use (longer than 1 month) of cimetidine but will resolve after discontinuing therapy. Report findings of gynecomastia for further observation and possible laboratory tests.

Gastrointestinal
Hepatotoxicity. Although rare, hepatotoxicity in patients taking H₂ antagonists has been reported. The symptoms

Table 32.2   Histamine-2 (H₂) Receptor Antagonists

GENERIC NAME	BRAND NAME	AVAILABILITY	DOSAGE RANGE
cimetidine	Tagamet HB Apo-Cimetidine ✿	Tablets: 200, 300, 400, 800 mg Suspension: 300 mg/5 mL	*Duodenal and gastric ulcers:* PO: 800-1600 mg at bedtime, 400 mg twice daily, or 300 mg four times daily *GERD:* PO: 800 mg twice daily or 400 mg four times daily
famotidine ⇄ Do not confuse famotidine with fluoxetine.	Pepcid ⇄ Do not confuse Pepcid with Prevacid. Teva-Famotidine ✿	Tablets: 10, 20, 40 mg Suspension: 40 mg/5 mL Injection: 10 mg/mL	*Duodenal and gastric ulcers:* PO: 40 mg once daily at bedtime or 20 mg twice daily *GERD:* PO: 20 mg twice daily
nizatidine ⇄ Do not confuse nizatidine with tizanidine.	– Apo-Nizatidine ✿	Capsules: 150, 300 mg Oral solution: 15 mg/mL	*Duodenal and gastric ulcers:* PO: 300 mg at bedtime or 150 mg twice daily *GERD:* PO: 150 mg twice daily
ranitidine ⇄ Do not confuse ranitidine with amantadine or rimantadine.	Zantac; Zantac 75, Zantac 150 ⇄ Do not confuse Zantac with Xanax or Zyrtec. pms-Ranitidine ✿	Tablets: 75, 150, 300 mg Capsules: 150, 300 mg Syrup: 15 mg/mL Suspension: 22.4 mg/mL in 250 mL bottle Injection: 25 mg/mL	*Duodenal and gastric ulcers:* PO: 300 mg at bedtime or 150 mg twice daily *GERD:* PO: 150 mg twice daily

✿ Available in Canada.
GERD, Gastroesophageal reflux disease.

of hepatotoxicity are anorexia, nausea, vomiting, jaundice, hepatomegaly, splenomegaly, and abnormal liver function test results (elevated bilirubin, aspartate aminotransferase, alanine aminotransferase, gamma-glutamyl transferase, and alkaline phosphatase levels; increased prothrombin time).

◆ *Drug interactions*

Benzodiazepines. Cimetidine inhibits the metabolism or excretion of the following benzodiazepines: alprazolam, chlordiazepoxide, diazepam, clorazepate, flurazepam, and triazolam. Patients taking cimetidine and a benzodiazepine concurrently should be observed for increased sedation; a reduction in dosage of the benzodiazepine may be required. The metabolism of oxazepam, temazepam, and lorazepam does not appear to be affected.

Beta-adrenergic blocking agents. Beta-adrenergic blocking agents (e.g., propranolol, labetalol, metoprolol) may accumulate as a result of inhibited metabolism. Monitor for signs of toxicity, such as hypotension and bradycardia.

Phenytoin. Cimetidine inhibits the metabolism of phenytoin. Monitor patients with concurrent therapy for signs of phenytoin toxicity: nystagmus, sedation, and lethargy. Serum levels may be ordered, and a reduced dosage of phenytoin may be required.

Antacids. Administer 1 hour before or 2 hours after administration of cimetidine.

Warfarin. Cimetidine may enhance the anticoagulant effects of warfarin. Observe for the development of petechiae; ecchymoses; nosebleeds; bleeding gums; dark, tarry stools; and bright red or coffee-ground hematemesis. Monitor the prothrombin time (international normalized ratio [INR]), and reduce the dosage of warfarin if necessary.

Calcium antagonists. Cimetidine may inhibit the metabolism of diltiazem, nifedipine, and verapamil. Patients should be monitored for increased effects from the calcium antagonists (e.g., bradycardia, hypotension, dysrhythmias, fatigue).

Tricyclic antidepressants. Cimetidine may inhibit the excretion of imipramine, desipramine, and nortriptyline, usually within 3 to 5 days after the start of cimetidine therapy. If anticholinergic effects or toxicity becomes apparent, a decreased dosage of the antidepressant may be required. If cimetidine is discontinued, the patient should be monitored for a decreased response to the antidepressant.

Famotidine, nizatidine, ranitidine. In general, there appear to be only minor interactions with these H₂ antagonists. There are conflicting data, however. Studies indicate that patients receiving higher doses of ranitidine may be more susceptible to drug interactions between ranitidine and other drugs. When used concurrently, monitor for toxic effects of warfarin, theophylline, procainamide, and glipizide.

DRUG CLASS: GASTROINTESTINAL PROSTAGLANDIN

misoprostol (mǐs-ō-PRŎS-tŏl)
Cytotec (SĪ-tō-tĕk)

Actions

Misoprostol is a synthetic prostaglandin E series drug. Prostaglandins are normally present in the GI tract to inhibit gastric acid and pepsin secretion to protect the stomach and duodenal lining against ulceration. The prostaglandin E analogues may also induce uterine contractions.

Uses

Misoprostol is used to prevent and treat gastric ulcers caused by prostaglandin inhibitors (e.g., NSAIDs, including aspirin). Whereas prostaglandin inhibition is effective in reducing pain and inflammation, especially in arthritis, prostaglandin inhibition in the stomach by NSAIDs makes the patient more predisposed to peptic ulcers.

Therapeutic Outcomes

The primary therapeutic outcomes expected from misoprostol therapy are relief of discomfort and healing of irritated tissues.

❖ **Nursing Implications for Misoprostol Therapy**
◆ *Premedication assessment*
1. Determine if the patient is pregnant. This drug is a uterine stimulant and may induce miscarriage.
2. Check the pattern of bowel elimination; misoprostol may induce diarrhea.

◆ *Availability. PO:* 100- and 200-mcg tablets.

 Medication Safety Alert

Misoprostol is contraindicated during pregnancy and in women at risk of becoming pregnant. As a uterine stimulant, it may induce miscarriage.

◆ *Dosage and administration.* **Adult:** *PO:* 100- to 200-mcg tablets four times daily with food during NSAID therapy.

◆ *Common adverse effects*
Gastrointestinal
Diarrhea. Diarrhea associated with misoprostol therapy is dose related and usually develops after approximately 2 weeks of therapy. It often resolves after about 8 days, but a few patients require discontinuation of misoprostol therapy. Diarrhea can be minimized by taking misoprostol with meals and at bedtime and avoiding magnesium-containing antacids (e.g., Maalox liquid, Mylanta). Encourage the patient not to discontinue

therapy without first consulting the healthcare provider. Encourage the patient to include sufficient roughage or fiber (fresh fruits, vegetables, whole-grain products) in the diet.

Contraindication

Pregnancy. It is crucial that therapy be discontinued if the patient is pregnant because misoprostol may cause spontaneous abortion. The patient must receive attention from the healthcare provider who prescribed the misoprostol, as well as an obstetrician. The question of alternative therapies to NSAIDs must also be considered.

◆ *Drug interactions.* No significant drug interactions have been reported.

DRUG CLASS: PROTON PUMP INHIBITORS

Actions

Proton pump inhibitors inhibit gastric secretion of hydrochloric acid by inhibiting the gastric acid (hydrogen ion pump) of the stomach's parietal cells. These inhibitors have no anticholinergic or H_2 receptor antagonist actions, so some hydrochloric acid continues to be secreted unless anticholinergics or H_2 antagonists are also administered.

Uses

Proton pump inhibitors are used to treat severe esophagitis, GERD, gastric and duodenal ulcers, and hypersecretory disorders, such as Zollinger-Ellison syndrome. They may also be used in combination with antibiotics (e.g., amoxicillin, clarithromycin) to eradicate *H. pylori,* a common cause of PUD. Proton pump inhibitors (e.g., Nexium) are also available over the counter to treat intermittent heartburn.

Therapeutic Outcomes

The primary therapeutic outcomes expected from PPIs are relief of discomfort, reduced frequency of heartburn, and healing of irritated tissues.

❖ **Nursing Implications for Proton Pump Inhibitor Therapy**

◆ *Premedication assessment.* Check pattern of bowel elimination; the PPIs may induce diarrhea.

◆ *Availability, dosage, and administration.* See Table 32.3. Omeprazole, lansoprazole, and esomeprazole need to be taken before a meal. Capsules and tablets should be swallowed whole; instruct the patient not to open, chew, or crush.

◆ *Common adverse effects.* The following symptoms are relatively mild and rarely result in the discontinuation of therapy. Encourage the patient not to discontinue therapy without first consulting the healthcare provider.

Gastrointestinal

Diarrhea. Maintain the patient's state of hydration. Encourage the inclusion of sufficient roughage or

fiber (fresh fruits, vegetables, whole-grain products) in the diet.

Neurologic. Headache, fatigue.
Musculoskeletal. Muscle pain.

◆ *Serious adverse effects*

Skeletal

Risk of fractures. Patients who are over the age of 50 years who received high doses of PPIs or used them for more than 1 year are at greater risk for fractures of the hip, wrist, and spine. Patients who continue to receive PPIs and who are at risk for osteoporosis should receive vitamin D and calcium supplementation and have their bone status monitored. Patients should not stop taking their PPI unless told to do so by their healthcare provider. Short-term, low-dose use of over-the-counter products is not likely to cause an increased risk of fractures.

Electrolytes

Hypomagnesemia. Hypomagnesemia has been reported with as little as 3 months of PPI therapy, but it more commonly occurs in patients receiving PPIs for more than 1 year. Hypomagnesemia can cause serious adverse events, including tetany, tremors, seizures, Q–T interval prolongation, and cardiac arrhythmias. Healthcare providers should consider obtaining serum magnesium levels prior to beginning long-term PPI therapy, especially in patients receiving digoxin or patients receiving diuretics or other medicines known to cause hypomagnesemia. Magnesium supplementation may resolve the hypomagnesemia, but discontinuation of the PPI may be necessary. Magnesium levels return to normal within about a week of discontinuing PPI therapy. Patients should not stop PPI therapy without first discussing it with their healthcare provider. Use of over-the-counter PPIs taken according to directions and for a limited duration has not been associated with hypomagnesemia.

Vitamin B_{12} deficiency. Treatment with PPIs for more than 2 years may lead to vitamin B_{12} malabsorption and subsequent vitamin B_{12} deficiency. However, patients should not be routinely screened for vitamin B_{12} deficiency. There is no evidence for or against testing for B_{12} deficiency for patients taking PPIs for longer than 2 years.

Integumentary

Rash. Persistent vesicular rash from omeprazole may be cause for discontinuing therapy. Report rashes to the healthcare provider for further observation and possible laboratory tests.

◆ *Drug interactions*

Diazepam, triazolam, flurazepam. Omeprazole and esomeprazole significantly increase the half-life of diazepam, triazolam, and flurazepam by inhibiting their metabolism. Observe patients for increased sedative effects from these medicines. Caution against hazardous tasks, such as driving and operating machinery. The

Table 32.3 Proton Pump Inhibitors

GENERIC NAME	BRAND NAME	AVAILABILITY	DOSAGE RANGE
dexlansoprazole	Dexilant	Capsules: 30, 60 mg	PO: Initial: 60 mg once daily for 4-8 wk Maintenance: 30 mg once daily
esomeprazole ⇄ *Do not confuse esomeprazole with omeprazole.*	Nexium Apo-Esomeprazole ❦	Tablets, delayed release (24 hr): 20 mg Capsules, sustained release (24 hr): 20, 40, 49.3 mg Powder for suspension: 2.5-, 5-, 10-, 20-, 40-mg unit dose IV: 20, 40 mg	IV, PO: Initial: 20-40 mg once daily for 4-8 wk Maintenance: 20 mg daily
lansoprazole	Prevacid ⇄ *Do not confuse Prevacid with Prinivil, Pepcid, Pravachol, Premarin, or Prilosec.* Teva-Lansoprazole ❦	Capsules, sustained release (24 hr): 15, 30 mg Tablets, dispersible: 15, 30 mg Suspension: 3 mg/mL in 90, 150, 300 mL bottles	PO: Initial: 15-30 mg once daily 30 min before a meal for 4 wk Maintenance: 15 mg once daily Maximum: 30 mg once daily before a meal
omeprazole ⇄ *Do not confuse omeprazole with esomeprazole.*	Prilosec ⇄ *Do not confuse Prilosec with Prinivil, prednisone, Prevacid, Prinivil, or Prozac.* Losec ❦	Capsules, sustained release: 10, 20, 40 mg Tablets, sustained release: 20 mg Powder: 2.5, 10 mg Suspension: 2 mg/mL in 90-, 150- and 300-mL bottles	PO: Initial: 20 mg once daily for 4 wk Maintenance: 20 mg daily *Zollinger-Ellison syndrome:* Maximum: 120 mg three times daily
pantoprazole	Protonix ⇄ *Do not confuse Protonix with Lotronex.* Pantoloc ❦	Tablets, delayed release: 20, 40 mg Powder for oral suspension: 40 mg IV: 40 mg/vial	PO: Initial: 40 mg once daily for 8 wk Maintenance: 40 mg daily IV: Initial: 40 mg once daily for up to 7-10 days; switch to oral dosages
rabeprazole	Aciphex, Aciphex Sprinkle ⇄ *Do not confuse Aciphex with Accupril, Adipex-P, or Aricept.* Pariet ❦	Tablets, delayed release: 20 mg Capsules, sprinkle: 5, 10 mg	PO: Initial: 20 mg daily after morning meal for up to 4 wk Maintenance: 20 mg once daily Maximum: 60 mg twice daily

❦ Available in Canada.

dosages of diazepam, triazolam, and flurazepam may have to be reduced.

Phenytoin. Omeprazole slows the metabolism of phenytoin. Observe for nystagmus, sedation, and lethargy. The dosage of phenytoin may have to be reduced.

Clopidogrel. There has been a controversy in the literature as to whether PPIs prevent conversion of clopidogrel to its active therapeutic metabolite. A consensus statement by the American College of Cardiology Foundation, the American Heart Association, and the American College of Gastroenterology reports that clopidogrel alone and aspirin alone and their combination are associated with an increased risk of GI bleeding; that the risk of GI bleeding increases as the number of risk factors increases (such as prior GI bleeding, advanced age, concurrent use of anticoagulants); that PPIs are appropriate in patients with multiple risk factors for GI bleeding who are also receiving antiplatelet therapy

such as clopidogrel; that a clinically significant interaction cannot be excluded in subgroups who are poor metabolizers of clopidogrel; and that until solid evidence exists to support staggering PPIs with clopidogrel, the dosing of PPIs should not be altered.

Warfarin. Omeprazole may reduce the rate of metabolism of warfarin. Monitor the patient closely for signs of bleeding tendencies and monitor the prothrombin time (INR) closely. Reduction of warfarin dosage may be required.

Sucralfate. Sucralfate inhibits the absorption of PPIs. Administer PPIs at least 30 minutes before sucralfate.

Altered absorption. The reduction in gastric acid secretion may alter absorption of food and drugs as follows:

- *Ketoconazole, itraconazole capsules, iron:* These medicines require an acid medium for absorption. They should be administered at least 30 to 45 minutes before PPI therapy.

- *Insulin:* The absorption of food may be altered and an adjustment in timing or dosage of insulin in patients with diabetes may be required.

DRUG CLASS: COATING AGENTS

sucralfate (sū-KRĂL-fāt)
   Carafate (KĂR-ă-fāt)

Actions

When swallowed, sucralfate forms a complex that adheres to the crater of an ulcer, thereby protecting it from aggravators such as acid, pepsin, and bile salts. However, sucralfate does not inhibit gastric secretions (as do the H_2 antagonists) or alter gastric pH (as do antacids).

Uses

Sucralfate is used to treat duodenal ulcers, particularly in those patients who do not tolerate other forms of therapy.

Therapeutic Outcomes

The primary therapeutic outcomes expected from sucralfate therapy are relief of discomfort and healing of irritated tissues.

❖ **Nursing Implications for Sucralfate Therapy**
◆ *Premedication assessment.* Check pattern of bowel elimination; sucralfate may induce constipation.

◆ *Availability. PO:* 1-g tablets; 1-g/10-mL suspension.

◆ *Dosage and administration.* **Adult:** *PO:* 1 tablet four times a day 1 hour before each meal and at bedtime, all on an empty stomach. Because antacid therapy is often continued during early therapy of ulcer disease, administer antacids at least 30 minutes before or after sucralfate.

◆ *Common adverse effects.* The following adverse effects are usually mild and tend to resolve with continued therapy. Encourage the patient not to discontinue therapy without first consulting the healthcare provider.
   Gastrointestinal
   Constipation, dry mouth. Measures to alleviate dry mouth include sucking on ice chips or hard candy. Avoid mouthwashes that contain alcohol because they cause further drying and irritation. Maintain the patient's state of hydration, and obtain an order for stool softeners or bulk-forming laxatives if necessary. Encourage the inclusion of sufficient roughage (e.g., fresh fruits, vegetables, whole-grain products) in the diet.
   Neurologic
   Dizziness. Provide for patient safety during episodes of dizziness.

◆ *Drug interactions*
   Tetracyclines. Sucralfate may interfere with the absorption of tetracycline. Administer tetracyclines 1 hour before or 2 hours after sucralfate.

DRUG CLASS: PROKINETIC AGENTS

metoclopramide (mět-ō-KLŌ-pră-mīd)
   Reglan (RĚG-lăn)

Actions

Metoclopramide is a gastric stimulant whose mechanisms of action are not fully known. It increases lower esophageal sphincter pressure, thereby reducing reflux; increases stomach contractions; relaxes the pyloric valve; and increases peristalsis in the GI tract, resulting in an increased rate of gastric emptying and intestinal transit. Metoclopramide is an antiemetic that blocks dopamine in the chemoreceptor trigger zone. It inhibits serotonin (5-hydroxytryptamine) when administered in higher dosages.

Uses

Metoclopramide is used to relieve the symptoms of gastric reflux esophagitis and diabetic gastroparesis, as an aid in small bowel intubation, and to stimulate gastric emptying and intestinal transit of barium after radiologic examination of the upper GI tract. It is also given as an antiemetic to patients undergoing cancer chemotherapy. Treatment should be limited to less than 12 weeks.

Therapeutic Outcomes

The primary therapeutic outcomes expected from metoclopramide therapy are relief of discomfort, reduced frequency of heartburn, and healing of irritated tissues.

❖ **Nursing Implications for Metoclopramide Therapy**
◆ *Premedication assessment*
   1. Determine if other drugs being taken may induce extrapyramidal symptoms; do not administer metoclopramide concurrently.
   2. Check for a history of epilepsy. If present, check with the healthcare provider before starting drug therapy.
   3. Do not administer to an individual with symptoms of GI perforation, mechanical obstruction, or hemorrhage.
   4. For diabetic patients, food absorption may be altered and more frequent monitoring for hypoglycemia may be required.

◆ *Availability. PO:* 5- and 10-mg tablets; 5-, 10-mg disintegrating tablets; 5-mg/5-mL solution.
   Injection: 5 mg/mL in 2 mL.

◆ *Caution.* Approximately 1 in 500 patients may develop extrapyramidal symptoms manifested by restlessness, involuntary movements, facial grimacing, and possibly oculogyric crisis, torticollis, or rhythmic tongue protrusion. Children and young adults are most susceptible, as are patients receiving higher doses of metoclopramide as an antiemetic. Metoclopramide should not be used in patients with epilepsy or those receiving drugs likely to cause extrapyramidal reactions (e.g., phenothiazines) because the frequency and severity of seizures or extrapyramidal reactions may be increased. Metoclopramide must not be used in patients when increased gastric motility may be dangerous, such as with GI perforation, mechanical obstruction, or hemorrhage.

◆ *Dosage and administration.* **Adult:** *PO: Diabetic gastroparesis:* 10 mg four times a day 30 minutes before each meal and at bedtime. Duration of therapy depends on response and continued well-being after discontinuation of therapy. It is not recommended to use for more than 12 weeks.

Adult: *PO: Gastroesophageal reflux:* 10 to 15 mg up to 4 times daily 30 minutes before meals and at bedtime. It is not recommended to use for more than 12 weeks.

Adult: *IV: Chemotherapy antiemesis:* Initially two doses, 1 to 2 mg/kg, or 2 mg/kg if highly emetogenic chemotherapy is being used. If vomiting is suppressed, follow with 1 mg/kg. Dilute the dose in 50 mL of parenteral solution (dextrose 5% in water, normal saline [0.9%], dextrose 5%/0.45% saline, Ringer's solution, or lactated Ringer's solution). Infuse over at least 15 minutes, 30 minutes before beginning chemotherapy. Repeat every 2 hours for two doses, followed by one dose every 3 hours for three doses.

> **! Medication Safety Alert**
>
> Rapid IV infusion of metoclopramide (Reglan) may cause sudden, intense anxiety and restlessness, followed by drowsiness. If extrapyramidal symptoms should develop, treat with diphenhydramine.

◆ *Common adverse effects.* The following adverse effects are usually mild and tend to resolve with continued therapy. Encourage the patient not to discontinue therapy without first consulting the healthcare provider.

Neurologic

Drowsiness, fatigue, lethargy, dizziness. People who work around machinery, drive a car, or perform other duties that require mental alertness should be particularly cautious. Provide patient safety during episodes of dizziness.

Gastrointestinal. Nausea.

◆ *Serious adverse effects*

Extrapyramidal symptoms. Provide for patient safety and then report extrapyramidal symptoms to the healthcare provider immediately.

◆ *Drug interactions*

Drugs that increase sedative effects. Antihistamine, alcohol, analgesics, phenothiazines, and sedative-hypnotics increase the sedative effects of metoclopramide. Monitor the patient for excessive sedation and reduce dosage if necessary.

Drugs that decrease therapeutic effects. Anticholinergic agents (e.g., atropine, benztropine, antihistamines, dicyclomine) and opiate agonists (e.g., meperidine, morphine, oxycodone) decrease the therapeutic effects of metoclopramide. Instruct the patient to avoid taking these agents while using metoclopramide.

Altered absorption. The GI stimulatory effects of metoclopramide may alter absorption of food and drugs as follows:

- *Digoxin:* Monitor for decreased activity (e.g., return of edema, weight gain, heart failure).
- *Levodopa:* Metoclopramide may decrease the effects of levodopa. Monitor for increased parkinsonian activity (e.g., restlessness, nightmares, hallucinations, additional involuntary movements such as bobbing of head and neck, facial grimacing, active tongue movements).
- *Alcohol:* Monitor for signs of sedation and intoxication with smaller amounts of alcohol.
- *Insulin:* The absorption of food may be altered, and an adjustment in timing or dosage of insulin in patients with diabetes mellitus may be required.

Get Ready for the NCLEX® Examination!

Key Points

- Gastroesophageal reflux disease and PUD continue to be common illnesses that are often self-treated initially. Once medication therapy has been instituted, it is important to explain thoroughly the medications prescribed and adverse effects that should be expected or reported. Some medications taken for GERD and ulcer disease can have significant adverse effects that will need healthcare provider management.

- Solicit information about whether symptoms have decreased and whether the patient is experiencing adverse effects from therapy. Have the patient maintain a record of the pain using a standard pain rating scale. Also, have the patient record the degree of relief obtained at a specified interval after medications have been taken.
- Assess and make recommendations regarding lifestyle changes that are necessary to prevent symptom recurrence. If symptoms have not begun to diminish over 2 weeks, the nurse should encourage the person to seek medical attention.

Additional Learning Resources

SG Go to your Study Guide for additional Review Questions for the NCLEX® Examination, Critical Thinking Clinical Situations, and other learning activities to help you master this chapter content.

Go to your Evolve website (https://evolve.elsevier.com/Clayton) for additional online resources.

Review Questions for the NCLEX® Examination

1. The stomach functions to digest food by secreting pepsinogen from the secretory cells known as what?
   1. Parietal cells
   2. Chief cells
   3. Mucous cells
   4. Salivary cells

2. Proton pump inhibitors and antibiotics are often used in combination to eradicate which common cause of PUD?
   1. *Giardia lamblia*
   2. *Clostridium difficile*
   3. *Helicobacter pylori*
   4. *Listeria monocytogenes*

3. A nurse caring for a patient with diabetes who was diagnosed with gastroparesis would expect which drug to work as a gastric stimulant?
   1. Pantoprazole (Protonix)
   2. Metoclopramide (Reglan)
   3. Sucralfate (Carafate)
   4. Misoprostol (Cytotec)

4. Which statement by the patient would indicate to the nurse that further teaching is needed about how the defense mechanisms of the stomach can be compromised to cause PUD?
   1. "I should be careful about taking aspirin because it may cause damage to my stomach lining."
   2. "My doctor tells me that my stomach has an infection called *H. pylori* that caused this ulcer."
   3. "As I understand it, I have an overproduction of stomach acid that caused my ulcer."
   4. "I need to be careful about drinking too much orange juice because it is acidic and can damage my stomach lining."

5. The nurse was discussing the mechanism of action for pantoprazole with a patient diagnosed with GERD and realized further education was needed after the patient made which statement?
   1. "I understand that pantoprazole will inhibit my stomach from producing acid."
   2. "So this drug will coat the lining of my stomach so I do not get GERD symptoms."
   3. "When I take this, it will not affect how fast my food is digested."
   4. "I can expect that pantoprazole will relieve my symptoms of heartburn."

6. The nurse instructing a patient on how to reduce acid production in the stomach to prevent GERD indicated that which measures should be taken? *(Select all that apply.)*
   1. Decrease or stop smoking.
   2. Decrease the amount of coffee consumed.
   3. Increase the amount of spicy foods consumed.
   4. Decrease the amount of alcohol intake.
   5. Increase the amount of carbonated beverages.

7. Which common stomach disorders are treated with proton pump inhibitors? *(Select all that apply.)*
   1. Duodenal ulcers
   2. GERD
   3. Esophagitis
   4. Gastroparesis
   5. Hypersecretory disorders

Drugs Used to Treat Nausea and Vomiting

Objectives

1. Describe the six common causes of nausea and vomiting.
2. Discuss the three types of nausea associated with chemotherapy and the nursing considerations for these.
3. Identify the therapeutic classes of antiemetics.
4. Discuss the scheduling of antiemetics for maximum benefit.

Key Terms

nausea (NŎ-zē-ă) (p. 508)
vomiting (VŎ-mĭt-ĭng) (p. 508)
emesis (ĔM-ĕ-sĭs) (p. 508)
retching (RĔCH-ĭng) (p. 508)
regurgitation (rē-gŭr-jĭ-TĀ-shŭn) (p. 508)
postoperative nausea and vomiting (PONV) (pōst-ŎP-ĕr-ă-tĭv) (p. 509)
hyperemesis gravidarum (hī-pĕr-ĔM-ĕ-sĭs gră-vĭ-DĂR-ŭm) (p. 510)

psychogenic vomiting (sī-kō-JĔN-ĭk) (p. 510)
chemotherapy-induced nausea and vomiting (CINV) (kē-mō-THĔR-ă-pē) (p. 510)
anticipatory nausea and vomiting (ăn-TĬ-sĕ-pĕ-tō-rē) (p. 510)
emetogenicity (ĕ-MĔ-tō-gĕ-NĬ-sĭ-tē) (p. 510)
delayed emesis (p. 511)
radiation-induced nausea and vomiting (RINV) (p. 511)

NAUSEA AND VOMITING

Nausea is the sensation of abdominal discomfort that is intermittently accompanied by a desire to vomit. **Vomiting** is the forceful expulsion of gastric contents (**emesis**) up the esophagus and out the mouth. Nausea may occur without vomiting and sudden vomiting may occur without prior nausea, but the two symptoms often occur together. **Retching** is the involuntary labored, spasmodic contractions of the abdominal and respiratory muscles without emesis (also known as *dry heaves*). Nausea and vomiting accompany almost any illness, are experienced by virtually everyone at one time or another, and have a wide variety of causes (Box 33.1).

The primary anatomic areas involved in vomiting are shown in Fig. 33.1. The vomiting center (VC; more recently referred to as the *central pattern generator*), located in the medulla of the brain, coordinates the vomiting reflex. Nerves from sensory receptors in the pharynx, stomach, intestines, and other tissues connect directly with the VC through the vagus and splanchnic nerves and produce vomiting when stimulated. The VC also responds to stimuli originating in other tissues, such as the cerebral cortex, the vestibular apparatus of the inner ear, and blood. These stimuli travel first to the chemoreceptor trigger zone (CTZ), which then activates the VC to induce vomiting. The CTZ is also located in the medulla. An important function of the CTZ is to sample blood and spinal fluid for potentially toxic

substances and, when detected, to initiate the vomiting reflex. The CTZ cannot initiate vomiting independently, but only by stimulating the VC. Both the VC and the CTZ are much smaller than shown in Fig. 33.1.

The cerebral cortex of the brain can be a source of stimulus or suppression of the VC (see Fig. 33.1). Vomiting can occur as a conditioned response (e.g., see Anticipatory Nausea and Vomiting later in this chapter) or as a reaction to unpleasant sights and smells. Suppression of motion sickness by the person's concentration on some mental activity is an example of cortical control of the vomiting reflex. Psychological factors can play an important role (see Psychogenic Vomiting later in this chapter).

When the VC is stimulated, nerve impulses are sent to the salivary, vasomotor, and respiratory centers. The vomiting reflex begins with a sudden deep inspiration that increases abdominal pressure, which is further increased by contraction of the abdominal muscles. The soft palate rises and the epiglottis closes, thus preventing aspiration of vomitus into the lungs. The pyloric sphincter contracts and the cardiac sphincter and esophagus relax, allowing stomach contents to be expelled. The flow of saliva increases to aid the expulsion. Autonomic symptoms of pallor, sweating, and tachycardia cause additional discomfort associated with vomiting. **Regurgitation** occurs when the gastric or esophageal contents rise to the pharynx because of greater pressure (gas bubbles, tight clothing, body

Box 33.1 Causes of Nausea and Vomiting

- Infection
- Gastrointestinal disorders (e.g., gastritis; liver, gallbladder, or pancreatic disease)
- Overeating or irritation of the stomach by certain foods or liquids
- Motion sickness
- Drug therapy (nausea and vomiting are the most common adverse effects of drug therapy)
- Surgical procedures (e.g., abdominal surgery, extraocular and middle ear manipulations, testicular traction)
- Emotional disturbances and mental illness
- Pregnancy
- Pain and unpleasant sights and odors

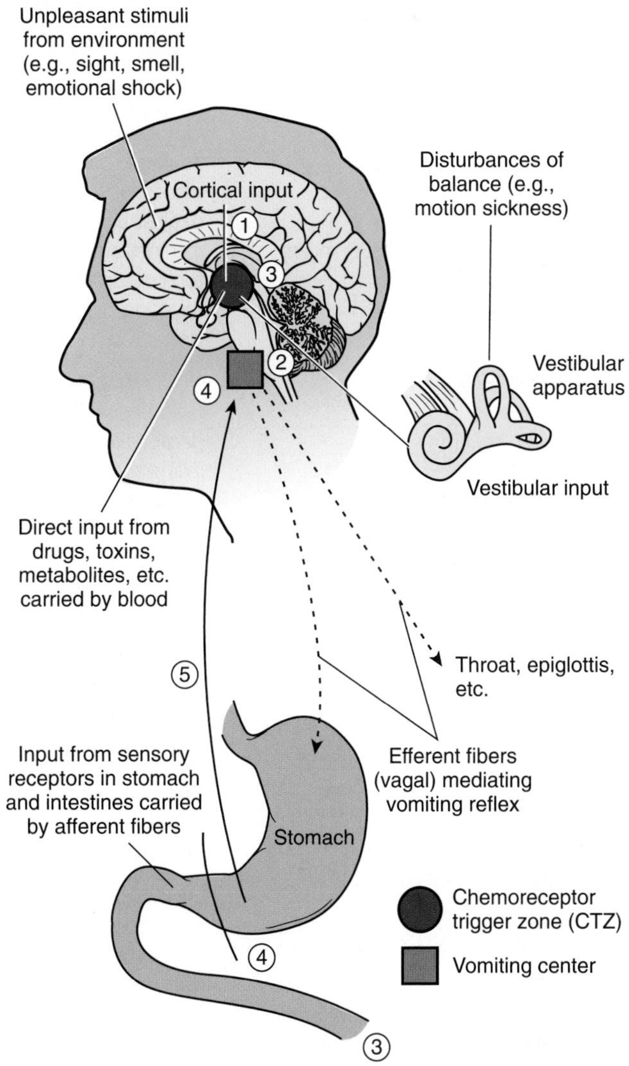

Fig. 33.1 Sites of action of antiemetic medicines. *1,* Cerebral cortex: anxiolytic agents; *2,* vestibular apparatus: antihistamine and anticholinergic agents; *3,* chemoreceptor trigger zone and gastrointestinal (GI) tract: dopamine antagonists; *4,* serotonin receptors in GI tract and vomiting center (VC): serotonin antagonists; *5,* neurokinin receptors in VC: neurokinin-1 receptor antagonists. (Adapted from Clayton BD, Brown BK. Nausea and vomiting. In: Helms RA, Quan DJ, Herfindel ET, Gourley DR, eds. *Textbook of Therapeutics: Drug and Disease Management.* 8th ed. Philadelphia: Lippincott Williams & Wilkins; 2006.)

position) in the stomach and should not be confused with vomiting.

COMMON CAUSES OF NAUSEA AND VOMITING

POSTOPERATIVE NAUSEA AND VOMITING

Postoperative nausea and vomiting (PONV) constitute a relatively common complication after surgery. The incidence of nausea and vomiting varies with the surgical procedure, gender, age, obesity, anesthetic procedure, and analgesia used. A previous history of motion sickness and PONV also is an indicator of the likelihood of developing this postoperative complication. Factors associated with obesity that may contribute to a higher incidence of nausea and vomiting are a larger residual gastric volume, increased esophageal reflux, and increased risk for gallbladder and gastrointestinal (GI) disease. Fat-soluble anesthetics may also accumulate in adipose tissue and continue to be released long after anesthesia is discontinued. Pain not treated with appropriate analgesia may also induce nausea and vomiting. Surgical procedures that have a higher incidence of PONV are extraocular muscle and middle ear manipulations, testicular traction, and abdominal surgery. Women have a higher incidence of PONV, possibly because of hormonal differences. Children ages 11 to 14 years have the highest incidence based on age group. Patients who have had general anesthesia have a higher incidence of PONV than those who have had regional anesthesia; spinal anesthesia is generally associated with less PONV than general anesthesia, and peripheral regional anesthesia is the least emetogenic. Analgesics (e.g., morphine, fentanyl, alfentanil) used as premedication or with regional anesthetics frequently induce nausea and vomiting. Patients under nitrous oxide anesthesia have a higher incidence of nausea and vomiting than do those under enflurane or isoflurane. Swallowed blood and gas accumulation in the stomach may also induce nausea and vomiting.

MOTION SICKNESS

Nausea and vomiting associated with motion are thought to result from stimulation of the labyrinth system of the ear, with subsequent transmission of this stimulus to the vestibular network located near the VC. When there is strong or frequent stimulation, such as from a rocking ship or airplane, the vestibular network is bombarded with an abnormally high number of stimuli that radiate by cholinergic nerve impulses to the adjacent VC. Thus drugs that inhibit the cholinergic nerve impulses from the vestibular network to the VC should be effective in treating motion sickness.

NAUSEA AND VOMITING IN PREGNANCY

The percentage of women reporting vomiting during the first 16 weeks of gestation is relatively constant at about 40%, decreasing to 20% from 17 to 20 weeks;

only 9% of women report vomiting after 20 weeks of pregnancy. Vomiting is much more common among primigravidas, younger women, nonsmokers, African Americans, and obese women. Contrary to commonly held beliefs, vomiting is not more common in women who have experienced prior fetal losses or women with hypertension, proteinuria, or diabetes. There is also no association between vomiting and cohabitation; unplanned pregnancy; or gallbladder, liver, or thyroid disease.

Although traditionally described as "morning sickness," most women report that symptoms of nausea and vomiting tend to persist to varying degrees throughout the day. The cause of morning sickness is unknown, but its occurrence and severity appear to be related to the levels of free and bound estradiol and sex hormone–globulin-binding capacity.

A woman with severe persistent vomiting that interferes with nutritional, fluid, and electrolyte balance may be experiencing hyperemesis gravidarum, a condition in which starvation, dehydration, and acidosis are superimposed on the vomiting syndrome. Hospitalization for fluid, electrolyte, and nutritional therapy may be required.

PSYCHOGENIC VOMITING

Psychogenic vomiting can be self-induced, or it can occur involuntarily in response to situations that the person considers threatening or distasteful (e.g., eating food whose origin is considered repulsive).

CHEMOTHERAPY-INDUCED NAUSEA AND VOMITING

Chemotherapy-induced nausea and vomiting (CINV) is the most unpleasant adverse effect associated with the use of cancer chemotherapy. Many patients regard it as the most stressful aspect of their disease, more so even than the prospect of dying. Because the object of cancer therapy is at least to prolong life, the effect of CINV on the quality of life must be considered.

Three types of emesis have been identified in patients receiving antineoplastic therapy: anticipatory nausea and vomiting, acute CINV, and delayed emesis.

Anticipatory nausea and vomiting is a conditioned response triggered by the sight or smell of the clinic or hospital or by the knowledge that treatment is imminent. The onset of anticipatory nausea and vomiting is usually 2 to 4 hours before treatment and is most severe at the time of chemotherapy administration. Patients who experience anticipatory nausea and vomiting are more likely to be younger and to have received about twice as many courses of chemotherapy, with more drugs, for about three times as long as patients who do not experience this complication.

Acute CINV may be stimulated directly by chemotherapeutic agents. These agents have emetogenicity, which refers to having the ability to cause emesis. This type of emesis may begin 1 to 6 hours after chemotherapy

has been administered and may last for up to 24 hours. The emetogenicity of antineoplastic drugs is highly variable, ranging from an incidence of almost 100% with high-dose cisplatin to less than 10% with chlorambucil. Table 33.1 summarizes chemotherapeutic agents in terms of emetogenicity. Emetogenicity also is influenced by dosage, duration, and frequency of administration.

Table **33.1**	Potential of Emesis With Intravenous Antineoplastic Agents[a]	
High (>90%)		
anthracycline/cyclophosphamide combination	cyclophosphamide ≥1500 mg/m^2	
carmustine	dacarbazine	
cisplatin	mechlorethamine	
	streptozotocin	
Moderate (30%-90%)		
alemtuzumab	epirubicin	
azacitidine	idarubicin	
bendamustine	ifosfamide	
carboplatin	irinotecan	
clofarabine	oxaliplatin	
cyclophosphamide <1500 mg/m^2	romidepsin	
cytarabine >1 g/m^2	temozolomide	
daunorubicin	thiotepa	
doxorubicin	trabectedin	
Low (10%-30%)		
aflibercept	5-fluorouracil	
atezolizumab	gemcitabine	
belinostat	ipilimumab	
blinatumomab	ixabepilone	
bortezomib	methotrexate	
brentuximab vedotin	mitomycin	
cabazitaxel	mitoxantrone	
carfilzomib	paclitaxel	
catumaxomab	panitumumab	
cetuximab	pemetrexed	
cytarabine ≤1000 mg/m^2	pertuzumab	
docetaxel	temsirolimus	
eribulin	topotecan	
etoposide	trastuzumab-emtansine	
elotuzumab	vinflunine	
Minimal		
bevacizumab	pixantrone	
bleomycin	pralatrexate	
busulfan	ramucirumab	
cladribine (2-chlorodeoxyadenosine)	rituximab	
fludarabine	trastuzumab	
nivolumab	vinblastine	
ofatumumab	vincristine	
pembrolizumab	vinorelbine	

[a]Estimated incidence without prophylaxis.
Data from Roila F, Moassiotis A, Aapro M, et al. 2016 MASCC and ESMO guideline update for the prevention of chemotherapy- and radiotherapy-induced nausea and vomiting and of nausea and vomiting in advanced cancer patients. *Ann Oncol.* 2016;27:19-33; and Hesketh PJ, Kris MG, Basch E, et al. Antiemetics: American Society of Clinical Oncology Clinical Practice Guideline Update. *J Clin Oncol.* 2017;35:3240-3261.

Patient factors also affect acute CINV. The incidence and severity are generally higher in younger people, women, those in poor general health, and those with metabolic disorders (e.g., uremia, dehydration, infection, GI obstruction). Patients with a history of motion sickness seem to be more sensitive to the emetic effects of cytotoxic agents. The patient's outlook and attitude about cancer and therapy can significantly influence the frequency and severity of nausea and vomiting.

Delayed emesis occurs 24 to 120 hours after the administration of chemotherapy. The mechanisms are not known, but delayed emesis in patients receiving chemotherapy may be induced by metabolic by-products of the chemotherapeutic agent or by destruction of malignant cells. The emesis experienced is usually less severe than that which occurs acutely, but it still can be significant in reducing activity, nutrition, and hydration. Patients who have incomplete control of acute emesis often experience delayed emesis. Events that often trigger delayed nausea and vomiting are brushing teeth, using mouthwash, manipulating dentures, seeing food, and quickly standing up while getting out of bed after awakening in the morning.

RADIATION-INDUCED NAUSEA AND VOMITING

Another common cause of emesis associated with the treatment of cancer is **radiation-induced nausea and vomiting (RINV)**. The use of high-energy radiation (also known as *radiotherapy*) from x-rays, gamma rays, neutrons, and other sources to kill cancer cells and shrink tumors also induces nausea and vomiting, especially when concurrent chemotherapy is used. Radiation may come from a machine outside the body (external beam radiation therapy), or it may come from radioactive material placed in the body near cancer cells (internal radiation therapy, implant radiation). The frequency of RINV depends on the treatment site, field exposure, dose of radiation delivered per fraction, and total dose delivered.

DRUG THERAPY FOR SELECTED CAUSES OF NAUSEA AND VOMITING

Control of vomiting is important for relieving the obvious distress associated with it and preventing aspiration of gastric contents into the lungs, dehydration, and electrolyte imbalance. Primary treatment of nausea and vomiting should be directed at the underlying cause. Because this is not always possible, treatment with nondrug and drug measures is appropriate. Most medicines (antiemetics) used to treat nausea and vomiting act either by suppressing the action of the VC or by inhibiting the impulses going to or coming from the center. These agents are generally more effective if administered before the onset of nausea, rather than after it has started. The seven classes of agents used as antiemetics are dopamine antagonists, serotonin antagonists, anticholinergic agents, corticosteroids, benzodiazepines, cannabinoids, and neurokinin-1 (NK1) receptor antagonists.

POSTOPERATIVE NAUSEA AND VOMITING

As noted, there is no single cause of PONV, and therefore successful treatment with a single pharmacologic agent for all cases is unlikely. Measures such as limiting patient movement and preventing gastric distention can reduce PONV. Adequate analgesia can also forestall this complication. Nonsteroidal antiinflammatory analgesics are not emetogenic (opioids are emetogenic) and should be given consideration if appropriate to the type of surgical procedure. Antiemetics used include dopamine antagonists, anticholinergic agents, and serotonin antagonists. The histamine-2 antagonists (e.g., cimetidine, ranitidine) are also used to reduce gastric secretions to minimize nausea and vomiting.

Postoperative nausea and vomiting is usually managed with an as-needed (PRN) order, but patients who are considered to be at moderate to high risk should be considered for prophylactic antiemetic therapy. In addition to minimizing the risk factors listed, a multimodal treatment approach is recommended because of the variety of receptor types associated with PONV. Therapy may include hydration, supplemental oxygen, a benzodiazepine for anxiolysis, a combination of antiemetics that work by different mechanisms (e.g., droperidol, dexamethasone, serotonin antagonist), intravenous (IV) anesthesia induction agents (e.g., propofol and remifentanil), and analgesia with a nonsteroidal antiinflammatory drug (e.g., ketorolac) rather than an opioid. Nonpharmacologic techniques prior to surgery using acupuncture, transcutaneous electrical nerve stimulation, and acupressure stimulation have also been shown to reduce PONV.

The first step in treating PONV is to identify the cause. If a nasogastric (NG) tube is in place, check its patency and placement in preventing abdominal distention. Do not move an NG tube that was inserted during surgery (e.g., gastric resection); in this case, there is a danger of penetrating the suture line. Irrigation of a blocked NG tube may alleviate the nausea and vomiting. (A healthcare provider's order to irrigate the NG tube is required.) Administration of PRN antiemetics when the patient first reports nausea will often prevent vomiting.

MOTION SICKNESS

Most agents used to reduce nausea and vomiting from motion sickness are chemically related to antihistamines. The effectiveness of antihistamines in motion sickness probably results from their anticholinergic properties, not from their ability to block histamine.

NAUSEA AND VOMITING IN PREGNANCY

In most cases, morning sickness can be controlled by dietary measures alone. The woman should be advised to eat small, frequent, dry meals and to avoid fatty foods and other foods found to cause problems. Sometimes it may be difficult or impossible to work in the kitchen around food, and assistance may be required.

In about 10% to 15% of cases, dietary measures alone will be insufficient and drug therapy should be considered. Drugs that have been widely used for treating morning sickness are vitamin B_6, antihistamines (doxylamine, diphenhydramine, dimenhydrinate, meclizine), and phenothiazines such as promethazine and prochlorperazine. Ginger, an herb (see Chapter 47), is used in many cultures to treat pregnancy-induced nausea and vomiting. From a safety standpoint, vitamin B_6 and doxylamine are generally recommended first. If persistent vomiting threatens maternal nutrition, promethazine may be considered. If antidopaminergic antiemetic therapy is required, prochlorperazine is the safest time-tested medicine. Ondansetron and metoclopramide have been shown to be effective antiemetics in treating hyperemesis gravidarum, and no teratogenic effects have been reported to date.

PSYCHOGENIC VOMITING

When a person has chronic or recurrent vomiting, a diagnosis of psychogenic vomiting is made after eliminating all other possible causes. The person with psychogenic vomiting usually does not lose weight and can control vomiting in certain situations (e.g., in public). Identification of the causes of psychogenic vomiting and successful resolution of the problem may not be possible. After an extensive workup eliminates other potential causes, a short course of an antiemetic drug (e.g., metoclopramide) or an antianxiety drug may be prescribed, along with counseling.

ANTICIPATORY NAUSEA AND VOMITING

People with a negative attitude toward therapy, such as the belief that it will be of no benefit, are more likely to develop anticipatory nausea and vomiting. It tends to become more severe as treatments progress unless behavior therapy modifies the conditioned response. Such treatments include progressive muscle relaxation, guided imagery, hypnosis, self-hypnosis, systematic desensitization, music therapy, acupressure, and benzodiazepines (alprazolam, lorazepam). Nurses can play a significant role by maintaining a positive supportive attitude with the patient and making sure that the patient receives antiemetic therapy before each course of chemotherapy.

CHEMOTHERAPY-INDUCED NAUSEA AND VOMITING

Antiemetic therapy to minimize acute CINV is based on the emetogenic potential of the antineoplastic agents used. Combinations of antiemetics are often used, based on the assumption that antineoplastic agents produce emesis by more than one mechanism. In general, all patients being treated with chemotherapeutic agents of moderate to high emetogenic potential should receive prophylactic antiemetic therapy before chemotherapy is started. Combinations of a serotonin antagonist (ondansetron, dolasetron, granisetron, or palonosetron) with dexamethasone, aprepitant, rolapitant, and possibly lorazepam are often used. There is also an oral fixed-dose combination of an NK1 receptor antagonist (netupitant) and palonosetron available for chemotherapy-induced nausea and vomiting. Antiemetic therapy should be continued for 2 to 4 days to prevent delayed vomiting. Emesis induced by moderately emetogenic agents may be treated prophylactically with a similar regimen, and therapy should be continued for 24 hours. Dexamethasone with or without a phenothiazine (prochlorperazine) or metoclopramide is recommended if the chemotherapy has low emetic potential. Lorazepam may be added to the antiemetic regimen if necessary. Antiemetic therapy is not recommended with medications with minimum emetic risk, although dexamethasone, metoclopramide, or prochlorperazine may be used to prevent delayed emesis. All antiemetics should be given an adequate amount of time before chemotherapy is initiated and should be continued for an appropriate time after the antineoplastic agent has been discontinued.

DELAYED EMESIS

In general, patients who have complete control of acute emesis have a much lower incidence of delayed-onset emesis. A combination of prochlorperazine and lorazepam given orally has successfully controlled delayed emesis. Recent studies have indicated that providing optimal antiemetic therapy with the chemotherapy will significantly reduce the frequency of delayed emesis. Adding aprepitant, fosaprepitant, or rolapitant, the NK1 antagonists, in combination with a serotonin antagonist plus dexamethasone, and the fixed-dose combination of netupitant and palonosetron plus dexamethasone significantly reduces the incidence of delayed emesis.

RADIATION-INDUCED NAUSEA AND VOMITING

Clinical guidelines recommend that patients who will be receiving total body irradiation or those receiving single-exposure, high-dose radiation therapy to the upper abdomen should receive preventive antiemetic therapy. The serotonin antagonists (e.g., granisetron, ondansetron), with or without dexamethasone, are approved and recommended to treat RINV. Patients at low to intermediate risk for RINV should receive serotonin antagonists or prochlorperazine before each dose of radiation. Rescue medicines used to treat RINV include prochlorperazine and metoclopramide. Patients who require rescue antiemetic therapy should be pretreated with a serotonin antagonist before the next dose of radiation therapy.

❖ NURSING IMPLICATIONS FOR NAUSEA AND VOMITING

Nausea and vomiting are associated with illnesses of the GI tract and other body systems and with adverse effects of medications and food intolerance. Nursing care must be individualized to the patient's diagnosis and needs at all times.

◆ Assessment

History

- Obtain a history of the patient's symptoms—onset, duration, frequency, volume, and description of the vomitus (e.g., color: dark brown or black [coffee-ground emesis], greenish yellow, red-tinged; consistency; presence of undigested food particles).
- Ask the patient's perception of precipitating factors, such as foods, odors, medications, stress, or treatment (e.g., chemotherapy, radiation therapy, surgery). Is there actual emesis, or is it primarily retching?
- Is there a history of obstruction, asthma, and/or narrow-angle glaucoma?

Medications

- Ask the patient to list all current over-the-counter medications being taken (including herbal supplements) or those prescribed by a healthcare provider. Are any used to treat nausea and vomiting?
- Schedule prescribed medications on the medication profile, and requisition the medicines from the pharmacy.
- Ensure that antiemetics to be given before chemotherapy or irradiation therapy are marked precisely as ordered on the medication profile, along with around-the-clock or PRN orders.

Basic assessment. Individualize the assessment procedure to the underlying cause of the symptoms if known.

- *Vital signs:* Obtain baseline vital signs, height, and weight.
- *Abdomen:* Assess bowel sounds in all four quadrants of the abdomen. Observe the size and shape of the abdomen. Note any signs of distention, ascites, or masses.
- *Hydration:* Assess and record signs of dehydration, such as nonelastic skin turgor, sticky oral mucous membranes, excessive thirst, shrunken and deeply furrowed tongue, crusted lips, weight loss, deteriorating vital signs, soft or sunken eyeballs, delayed capillary filling, high urine specific gravity or no urine output, and possible mental confusion.

Laboratory studies. Review laboratory reports for indications that include malabsorption, protein depletion, or dehydration (fluid, electrolytes, blood urea nitrogen, creatinine, and acid-base imbalances), and for other values (e.g., K^+, Cl^-, pH, partial pressure of CO_2, bicarbonate, hemoglobin, hematocrit, urinalysis [specific gravity], serum albumin, total protein). The scope of laboratory data gathered will depend on the underlying cause of the nausea and vomiting and severity of the symptoms.

Nursing considerations

- Record intake and output, vital signs every shift or more frequently depending on patient's status, and daily weights.
- Schedule oral hygiene measures.

◆ Implementation

Nutrition

- Obtain specific orders relating to nutrition. Diet orders will depend on the underlying cause and severity of the nausea and vomiting.
- Obtain specific orders for diet, such as nothing by mouth (NPO) with NG suction, IV fluids, or enteral or parenteral nutrition.
- As the patient's condition improves, obtain orders for a gradual progression of diet.
- Maintain hydration via oral or parenteral forms as prescribed by the prescriber.
  - *Adults:* The usual treatment includes discontinuation of solid foods and ingestion of oral rehydration solutions or clear juices. Depending on the severity of the condition or underlying cause, the patient may be NPO with an NG tube in place for decompression of the stomach to reduce the risk of vomiting. As the patient's condition improves, the diet is advanced from clear liquids to small, frequent, low-fat feedings to bland or normal diet. Generally, high-fat foods, milk products, whole grains, and raw fruits and vegetables are initially avoided.
  - *Infants:* Formula, milk products, and solid foods usually are discontinued. Fluids are offered every 30 to 60 minutes in small amounts (30 to 60 mL). The volume is gradually increased as tolerance improves. Oral rehydration solutions (e.g., Pedialyte, diluted gelatin, water, decarbonated colas, ginger ale) may be offered. Monitor for lactose intolerance when formula is reintroduced. Formula is generally given in a diluted form when reinitiated and gradually increased to full strength.
- Monitor hydration status using vital signs, skin turgor, daily weights, and moisture of mucous membranes, as well as intake and output.
- Perform a physical assessment every shift and a focused assessment at intervals consistent with the patient's status and underlying pathologic condition.
- Initiate hygiene measures to provide patient comfort during and after emesis. Oral hygiene should be scheduled at regular intervals, every 2 hours during waking hours, whenever an NG tube is in place, when the patient has stomatitis, or if the condition warrants it.
- Patients with significant central nervous system (CNS) depression may have lost the gag reflex; therefore institute aspiration precautions as appropriate.
- Initiate measures to eliminate factors that contribute to nausea and vomiting (e.g., irritating foods, odors, or medications).

- Give antiemetics as prescribed or recommended. With postsurgical patients, administer when symptoms of nausea first occur. Administer before chemotherapy or radiation therapy; depending on treatment, schedule on an around-the-clock basis following chemotherapy or radiation therapy. Administer 30 to 60 minutes before undertaking an activity known to precipitate motion sickness. If a transdermal patch is to be worn during travel, it can be applied behind the ear 4 hours before departure.
- If young children experience motion sickness while riding in a car, position them so they face forward and can see the horizon; try covering the side windows with screens so they do not have to turn their heads suddenly to watch rapidly passing objects.
- Provide diversional activities.
- Monitor nutritional needs and status on a continuum.

◆ Patient Education
Nutritional status
- Ensure the patients', parents', or significant others' understanding of all aspects of the diet, fluid, and nutritional regimen during hospitalization, as well as at discharge for home management.
- Stress the importance of maintaining hydration and following the parameters that must be reported to the healthcare provider (e.g., weight loss of 2 pounds in a specified period, recurrence of nausea and vomiting).
- For patients receiving cancer treatments, the American Cancer Society has pamphlets with suggestions for supplementing dietary needs. These include, but are not limited to, giving small, frequent, low-fat meals; food temperature; and increasing protein content of meals with the use of powdered milk added to puddings, shakes made with nutritional supplements, and frozen yogurt.
- If constipation is present, help patients with cardiac disease prevent straining and the Valsalva (vasovagal) reflex by giving stool softeners or bulk-forming laxatives as needed. Ensure that bulk-forming laxatives are rehydrated with juice, water, or milk before ingestion. Maintain overall body hydration. (See Chapter 34 for more information.) For patients with degenerative neurologic disorders, a bowel program may be necessary, usually performed every other day. Glycerin or bisacodyl suppositories or digital stimulation may be required as part of the regimen.
- Discuss ways to decrease environmental stimuli to vomit, such as removing the emesis basin from sight.
- Antiemetics cause some degree of sedation, and patients are often fatigued after receiving chemotherapy or radiation therapy; therefore caution patients not to drive or operate power equipment until these effects have subsided.

Medications. Verify the patient's and significant others' understanding of all prescribed medications to be given on a scheduled or PRN basis.

Fostering health maintenance
- Provide the patient and significant others with important information described in the monographs for drugs prescribed. Additional health teaching and nursing interventions, as well as common and serious adverse effects, are described in each monograph.
- Seek cooperation and understanding of the following points so that medication adherence is increased: name of medication; dosage, route, and times of administration; and adverse effects.

Patient self-assessment. Enlist the patient's aid in developing and maintaining a written record of monitoring parameters (e.g., weight, details of when nausea occurs and amount and appearance of vomitus, food diary of what is being eaten, which foods initiate or aggravate the symptoms) (see Appendix B: Template for Developing a Written Record for Patients to Monitor Their Own Therapy). Complete the Premedication Data column for use as a baseline to track response to drug therapy. Ensure that the patient understands how to use the form, and instruct the patient to bring the completed form to follow-up visits. During follow-up visits, focus on issues that will foster adherence with the therapeutic interventions prescribed.

DRUG CLASS: DOPAMINE ANTAGONISTS

Actions
The dopamine antagonists are the phenothiazines, butyrophenones (e.g., haloperidol, droperidol, trimethobenzamide), and metoclopramide. These medications inhibit dopamine receptors that are part of the pathway to the VC. Unfortunately, dopamine receptors in other parts of the brain are also blocked, potentially producing extrapyramidal symptoms of dystonia, parkinsonism, and tardive dyskinesia (see Chapters 14, 17, and 32) in some patients, especially when higher dosages are required.

Uses
The phenothiazines are primarily used as antiemetics for the treatment of mild to moderate nausea and vomiting associated with anesthesia and surgery, radiation therapy, and cancer chemotherapy. Prochlorperazine and promethazine are the phenothiazines most widely used as antiemetics.

The butyrophenones are seldom used as antiemetics in surgery and cancer chemotherapy. These agents tend to cause less hypotension than the phenothiazines, but they produce more sedation. The more widely used butyrophenones are haloperidol and trimethobenzamide. Droperidol must be administered parenterally and requires an electrocardiogram prior to and after administration because of increased risk of Q–T interval prolongation. Due to the additional monitoring required, droperidol is used much less frequently.

Metoclopramide is an antagonist of both dopamine and serotonin receptors. In addition to acting on receptors in the brain, it acts on similar receptors in the GI tract, thus making it particularly useful for treating nausea and vomiting associated with GI cancers, gastritis, peptic ulcer, radiation sickness, gastroparesis, and migraine. High-dose metoclopramide was routinely used to treat nausea and vomiting associated with certain cancer chemotherapies until the serotonin antagonists (e.g., ondansetron) became available. In higher doses, extrapyramidal symptoms are more common with metoclopramide; therefore many cancer chemotherapy protocols now include both high-dose metoclopramide and routine doses of diphenhydramine when highly emetogenic anticancer agents are used. Metoclopramide appears to be of little value in treating motion sickness.

Therapeutic Outcomes
The primary therapeutic outcome expected from the dopamine antagonist antiemetics is relief of nausea and vomiting.

❖ **Nursing Implications for Dopamine Antagonists**
◆ *Premedication assessment*
1. Collect data regarding emesis (type, amount, and frequency, on a continuum).
2. Assess data relative to the underlying cause of nausea and vomiting (e.g., pregnancy, postsurgical state, chemotherapy, radiation, bowel obstruction).
3. Obtain baseline data about the patient's degree of alertness before starting therapy because these medications tend to produce some degree of sedation.

◆ *Availability, dosage, administration, and adverse effects.* See Table 33.2. For additional information on phenothiazines and haloperidol, see Chapter 17. For additional information on metoclopramide, see Chapter 32.

DRUG CLASS: SEROTONIN ANTAGONISTS

Actions
The serotonin (5-hydroxytryptamine) type 3 receptor (5-HT$_3$) antagonists have made major inroads in the treatment of emesis associated with CINV, RINV, and PONV over the past few years. Serotonin receptors of the 5-HT$_3$ type are located centrally in the CTZ of the medulla and specialized cells of the GI tract and play a significant role in inducing nausea and vomiting. The serotonin antagonists block these receptors and have been shown to control nausea and vomiting associated with cisplatin and several other emetogenic chemotherapeutic agents.

Uses
Studies of ondansetron and metoclopramide demonstrate that ondansetron is more effective than metoclopramide in the control of high-dose cisplatin-induced nausea and vomiting. Studies comparing the efficacy and safety of ondansetron, dolasetron, granisetron, and palonosetron in the control of cisplatin-induced acute emesis and PONV conclude that there are no significant differences among the treatment groups with respect to emetic control, nausea, or adverse reactions. Granisetron and ondansetron are approved to treat nausea and vomiting associated with RINV. Palonosetron has been approved to treat acute and delayed nausea and vomiting associated with CINV and PONV. A particular advantage to this group of compounds is that there is minimal to no dopaminergic blockade, so extrapyramidal adverse effects are rare.

Therapeutic Outcomes
The primary therapeutic outcome expected from the serotonin antagonist antiemetics is relief of nausea and vomiting.

❖ **Nursing Implications for Serotonin Antagonists**
◆ *Premedication assessment*
1. Collect data regarding emesis (type, amount, and frequency, on a continuum).
2. Assess data relative to the underlying cause of nausea and vomiting (e.g., pregnancy, postsurgical state, chemotherapy, radiation, bowel obstruction).
3. Obtain baseline data about the patient's degree of alertness before initiation of therapy because these medications tend to produce some degree of sedation.

◆ *Availability, dosage, and administration.* See Table 33.2.
◆ *Common adverse effects.* These adverse effects are fairly mild, especially in relation to the prevention of nausea and vomiting. Because only a few doses are administered, the frequency and duration of adverse effects are minimal.
   Neurologic. Headache, sedation.
   Gastrointestinal. Diarrhea, constipation.
   Cardiovascular. Prolongation of the Q–Tc interval, inducing potentially fatal dysrhythmias, has been reported for all drugs in the class, but is more frequently reported with ondansetron. Thus the maximum dose for ondansetron IV is 16 mg as a single dose.

◆ *Drug interactions*
   Apomorphine. The use of serotonin antagonists with apomorphine is contraindicated. Profound hypotension and loss of consciousness have been reported.

DRUG CLASS: ANTICHOLINERGIC AGENTS

Actions
Motion sickness is thought to be caused by an excess of acetylcholine at the CTZ and the VC by cholinergic nerves receiving impulses from the vestibular network of the inner ear. Anticholinergic agents are used to counterbalance the excessive amounts of acetylcholine present.

Table 33.2 Antiemetic Agents

GENERIC NAME	BRAND NAME	AVAILABILITY	ANTIEMETIC DOSAGE RANGE		COMMENTS
			ADULTS	CHILDREN	
Dopamine Antagonists					
Phenothiazines					**Comments for All Phenothiazines**
prochlorperazine	–Compro pms-Prochlorperazine ✦	Tablets: 5, 10 mg Rectal suppositories: 25 mg Injection: 5 mg/mL	PO: 5-10 mg q6-8h Rectal: 25 mg twice daily IM: 5-10 mg q3-4h; do not exceed 40 mg/24 hr	PO or Rectal: 20-29 lb: 2.5 mg once or twice daily (maximum of 7.5 mg daily) 30-39 lb: 2.5 mg two or three times daily (maximum of 10 mg daily) 40-85 lb: 2.5 mg three times daily or 5 mg twice daily (maximum of 15 mg daily) IM: 0.132 mg/kg three to four times per day; same oral maximum limits apply to IM dosing	Phenothiazines may suppress the cough reflex. Ensure that the patient does not aspirate vomitus. Use with caution in patients, especially children, with undiagnosed vomiting. Phenothiazines can mask signs of toxicity of other drugs or mask symptoms of other diseases, such as brain tumor, Reye's syndrome, or intestinal obstruction. Use with extreme caution in patients with seizure disorders. Discontinue if rashes develop. May cause orthostatic hypotension.
promethazine	Phenergan, Promethegan pms-Promethazine ✦	Tablets: 12.5, 25, 50 mg Syrup: 6.25 mg/5 mL Oral solution: 6.25 mg/5 mL Suppositories: 12.5, 25, 50 mg Injection: 25, 50 mg/ mL in 1-mL ampules	PO/PR: 12.5-25 mg q4-6h IM/IV: Adults: 12.5-25 mg deep IM or IV; may repeat q4-6h	PO/PR: Children >2 yr: 0.25-1 mg/kg up to 25 mg q4-6h IM/IV: Children ≥2 years and adolescents: 0.25-1 mg/kg IM or IV (maximum: 25 mg/dose) q4-6h as needed; IVPB is preferred method of delivery	
Butyrophenones					
haloperidol[a]					See earlier comments for phenothiazines.
metoclopramide[b]					
trimethobenzamide	Tigan ⇅ *Do not confuse Tigan with Tiazac.*	Capsules: 300 mg Injection: 100 mg/mL	PO: 300 mg three or four times daily IM: 200 mg three or four times daily	Trimethobenzamide is generally not recommended for use in children	Injectable form contains benzocaine. Do not use in patients allergic to benzocaine or local anesthetics. Inject in upper, outer quadrant of gluteal region. Avoid escape of solution along the route. May cause burning, stinging, pain on injection.

Serotonin Antagonists

Generic Name	Brand Name	Availability	Dosage	Notes
dolasetron	Anzemet ⇅ Do not confuse Anzemet with Aricept.	Tablets: 50, 100 mg	PO: 100 mg within 1 hr before chemotherapy; PO: 1.8 mg/kg 60 min before chemotherapy	NOTE: PO medication is approved for chemotherapy-induced nausea and vomiting.
granisetron	—	Tablets: 1 mg; Injection: 0.1, 1 mg/mL	PO: 1 mg up to 1 hr before chemotherapy, followed by a second dose 12 hr later; or 2 mg once daily. Radiation therapy: 2-mg tablet once daily or 10 mL of oral solution within 1 hr of radiation therapy. IV: 10 mcg/kg infused over 5 min beginning 30 min before chemotherapy. IV: Children 2-16 yr: 10 mcg/kg infused over 5 min beginning 30 min before chemotherapy	Recommended for prevention of nausea and vomiting associated with cancer chemotherapy and radiation therapy.
	Sancuso (transdermal patch)	Transdermal patch: 3.1 mg/24 hr	Transdermal patch: Apply one patch to the upper outer arm 24-48 hr before chemotherapy. Patch may be worn for 7 days; do not remove for at least 24 hr after chemotherapy.	
	Sustol (subcutaneous injection)	Subcutaneous: 10 mg/0.4 mL	Subcutaneous for moderately emetogenic chemotherapy: 10 mg at least 30 min prior to chemotherapy on day 1	

Continued

Table 33.2   Antiemetic Agents—cont'd

			ANTIEMETIC DOSAGE RANGE		
GENERIC NAME	**BRAND NAME**	**AVAILABILITY**	**ADULTS**	**CHILDREN**	**COMMENTS**
ondansetron	Zofran, Zofran ODT ⬆⬇ *Do not confuse Zofran with Reglan, Zantac, or Zosyn.* Zuplenz ◆Dom-Ondansetron	Tablets: 4, 8, 24 mg Tablets, orally disintegrating: 4, 8 mg Injection: 2 mg/mL; 40 mg/20 mL Liquid: 4 mg/5 mL Oral film: 4, 8 mg	*Chemotherapy:* PO: Moderately emetogenic chemotherapy: 8 mg 30 min before chemotherapy, followed by 8 mg 8 hr later; then give 8 mg q12h for 1-2 days after completion of chemotherapy Highly emetogenic chemotherapy: 24 mg 30 min before chemotherapy Radiation therapy: 8 mg three times daily IV: 0.15 mg/kg/dose (maximum: 16 mg/dose) administered over 15 min for 3 doses, beginning 30 min prior to chemotherapy, followed by subsequent doses 4 and 8 hr after the first dose *PONV:* PO: 16 mg 1 hr before induction of anesthesia IV: 4 mg just before induction of anesthesia	*Chemotherapy:* 6 mo to 18 yr: IV: 0.15 mg/ kg 30 min before chemotherapy and 0.15 mg/kg 4 and 8 hr after the first dose of ondansetron 4-11 yr: PO: 4 mg 30 min before chemotherapy and repeated 4 and 8 hr after initial dose of ondansetron, then continue q8h for 1-2 days posttreatment 12 yr: PO: 8 mg 30 min before chemotherapy and 4 and 8 hr after initial dose of ondansetron, then continue q8h for 1-2 days posttreatment *PONV:* IV: 1 mo to 12 yr: <40 kg: 0.1 mg/kg; >40 kg: 4 mg	Recommended for prevention of nausea and vomiting associated with cancer chemotherapy, PONV, and radiation therapy.
palonosetron	Aloxi	Injection: 0.25 mg/5 mL in 5-mL vials	*Chemotherapy:* IV: 0.25 mg 30 min before start of chemotherapy; *do not* repeat within 2 days *PONV:* 0.075 mg over 10 sec immediately before anesthesia induction	*Chemotherapy:* IV: 20 mcg/kg infused over 15 min beginning 30 min prior to the start of chemotherapy Not approved for PONV in children	Recommended for prevention of nausea and vomiting associated with cancer chemotherapy, prevention of delayed nausea and vomiting from chemotherapy, and PONV.

Anticholinergic Agents Used for Motion Sickness

		Availability	Adult Dosage	Pediatric Dosage	Remarks
dimenhydrinate	Dramamine Apo-Dimenhydrinate	Tablets: 50 mg; Chewable tablet: 50 mg; Injection: 50 mg/mL	PO: 50-100 mg q4-6h; do not exceed 400 mg/24 hr; IM: 50 mg as needed	PO: 6-12 yr: 25-50 mg q6-8h; do not exceed 150 mg/24 hr; 2-5 yr: up to 25 mg q6-8h; do not exceed 75 mg/24 hr	May cause sedation. Caution patient against operating machinery.
diphenhydramine ⇅ *Do not confuse diphenhydramine with dicyclomine or dipyridamole.*	—	Tablets: 12.5, 25, 50 mg; Orally disintegrating strips: 12.5, 25 mg; Capsules: 25, 50 mg; Elixir: 12.5 mg/5 mL; Injection: 50 mg/mL; Liquid: 12.5, 25 mg/5 mL	PO: 25-50 mg three or four times daily; IM: 10-50 mg; do not exceed 400 mg/24 hr	PO: 12.5-25 mg 3 or 4 times a day; do not exceed 300 mg/24 hr; IM: 5 mg/kg/24 hr, in four divided doses; do not exceed 300 mg/24 hr	
meclizine	—	Tablets: 12.5, 25 mg; Chewable tablet: 25 mg	PO: 25-50 mg; may be repeated every 24 hr	Not approved for use in children under 12 yr of age	
scopolamine, transdermal	Transderm-Scop	Transdermal patch: 1.5 mg delivered over 72 hr	Patch: Apply to skin behind ear at least 4 hr before antiemetic effect is required; replace in 72 hr if continued therapy required. *Do not cut patches!*	Not approved for use in children	

Corticosteroids

		Availability	Adult Dosage	Pediatric Dosage	Remarks
dexamethasone		Tablets: 0.5, 0.75, 1, 1.5, 2, 4, 6 mg; Elixir: 0.5 mg/5 mL; Injection: 4, 10 mg/mL; Liquid: 1 mg/mL, 0.5 mg/5 mL	PO: 4-16 mg on day 1; IV: 8-20 mg before administration of chemotherapy	As for adults	Recommended for prevention of nausea and vomiting associated with chemotherapy. Used in combination with other antiemetics

Benzodiazepines

		Availability	Adult Dosage	Pediatric Dosage	Remarks
lorazepam ⇅ *Do not confuse lorazepam with loperamide.*	Ativan ⇅ *Do not confuse Ativan with Ambien.*	Tablets: 0.5, 1, 2 mg; Injection: 2, 4 mg/mL; Liquid: 2 mg/mL	PO: 0.5-2 mg q6h; IV: 0.5-2 mg q6h	Not recommended	Recommended for prevention and treatment of nausea and vomiting associated with chemotherapy.

Continued

Table 33.2 Antiemetic Agents—cont'd

GENERIC NAME	BRAND NAME	AVAILABILITY	ANTIEMETIC DOSAGE RANGE		COMMENTS
			ADULTS	CHILDREN	
Cannabinoids					
dronabinol (THC)	Marinol	Capsules: 2.5, 5, 10 mg	PO: Initial 5 mg/m^2 1-3 hr before chemotherapy, then q2-4h for a total of 4-6 doses/day Maximum: 15 mg/m^2/dose	Not recommended	Schedule III controlled substance. Common adverse effects include drowsiness, dizziness, muddled thinking, and possible impairment of coordination, sensory, and perceptual functions. Use with caution in patients with hypertension or heart disease. Syndros is a Schedule II controlled substance requiring a new prescription.
	Syndros	Oral solution: 5 mg/mL (30 mL)	PO: 4.2 mg/m^2 1-3 hours prior to chemotherapy and then q2-4h after chemotherapy for a total of 4 to 6 doses/day Maximum: 12.6 mg/m^2/dose and 4 to 6 doses/day.		
nabilone	Cesamet	Capsules: 1 mg	PO: 1-2 mg two or three times daily Maximum: 6 mg daily in 3 doses	Not recommended	Schedule II controlled substance. Because of its potential for dysphoria, it should be used only when the patient can be supervised by a responsible individual.
Neurokinin-1 Receptor Inhibitor Antagonists					
aprepitant	Emend	Capsules: 40, 80, 125 mg Oral suspension: 125 mg Intravenous Emulsion: 130 mg/18 mL	*Chemotherapy:* PO: 125 mg 1 hr before chemotherapy on day 1; 80 mg daily in the morning of days 2 and 3 IV: 100-130 mg 30 minutes prior to chemotherapy on day 1 *PONV:* PO: 40 mg within 3 hr before induction of anesthesia	*Chemotherapy:* Children at least 12 yr old and at least 30 kg: As for adults	In combination with other antiemetics (dexamethasone, serotonin antagonist), recommended for prevention of acute and delayed nausea and vomiting associated with initial and repeat courses of highly emetogenic cancer chemotherapy, including high-dose cisplatin. Also approved for prevention of PONV in adults.
	Cinvanti				

			Chemotherapy	PONV	Uses
fosaprepitant	Emend	Injection: 150 mg	*Chemotherapy:* IV: 150 mg administered over 15-20 min 30 min before chemotherapy on day 1 only	Not recommended	Same as aprepitant but not approved for PONV.
rolapitant	Varubi	Tablets: 90 mg; Intravenous emulsion: 166.5 mg/92.5 mL	*Chemotherapy:* PO: 180 mg 1-2 hr before chemotherapy in combination with dexamethasone and a serotonin antagonist; IV: 166.5 mg within 2 hours prior to initiation of chemotherapy on day 1	Not recommended	Use in combination with other antiemetics for the prevention of delayed nausea and vomiting in adults receiving highly emetogenic cancer chemotherapy.
Fixed-dose combination: netupitant and palonosetron	Akynzeo	Capsule: netupitant 300 mg and palonosetron 0.5 mg; Intravenous: fosnetupitant 235 mg and palonosetron 0.25 mg	*Chemotherapy:* PO: 1 capsule ~1 hr prior to initiation of chemotherapy on day 1 in combination with dexamethasone; IV: 235/0.25 mg 30 minutes before chemotherapy on day 1 in combination with dexamethasone	Not recommended	Prevention of acute and delayed nausea and vomiting associated with initial and repeat courses of cancer chemotherapy, including, but not limited to, highly emetogenic chemotherapy.

[a]For information on haloperidol, see the Drug Class: Antipsychotic Agents section in Chapter 17 and Table 17.1.
[b]For a drug monograph for metoclopramide, see the Drug Class: Prokinetic Agents section in Chapter 32.
♦ Available in Canada.
CINV, Chemotherapy-induced nausea and vomiting; *IVPB*, intravenous piggyback; *PONV*, postoperative nausea and vomiting; *THC*, tetrahydrocannabinol.

Uses

Anticholinergic agents, such as scopolamine, and antihistamines (e.g., diphenhydramine, dimenhydrinate, meclizine, promethazine) are used to treat motion sickness and, in the case of the antihistamines, nausea and vomiting associated with pregnancy. The choice of drug depends on both the period for which antinausea protection is required and the adverse effects. Scopolamine is the drug of choice for short periods of motion, and an antihistamine is preferred for longer periods. Of the antihistamines, promethazine is the drug of choice. Higher doses act longer, but sedation is usually a problem. Meclizine has fewer adverse effects than promethazine but has a shorter duration of action and is less effective for severe conditions. Diphenhydramine has a long duration, but excessive sedation is often a problem, especially after the boat, plane, or car ride is over. For very severe conditions, sympathomimetic drugs such as ephedrine are used in combination with scopolamine or an antihistamine. Anticholinergic agents are usually not effective in CINV.

Therapeutic Outcome

The primary therapeutic outcome expected from the anticholinergic antiemetics is relief of nausea and vomiting.

❖ Nursing Implications for Anticholinergic Agents
◆ Premedication assessment
1. Collect data regarding emesis (type, amount, and frequency, on a continuum).
2. Assess data relative to the underlying cause of nausea and vomiting (e.g., pregnancy, postsurgical state, chemotherapy, radiation, bowel obstruction).
3. Obtain baseline data about the patient's degree of alertness before initiation of therapy because these medications tend to produce some degree of sedation.
4. Check the patient's history to screen for presence of closed-angle glaucoma; use of an anticholinergic agent would be contraindicated.

◆ *Availability, dosage, and administration.* See Table 33.2.

◆ *Common adverse effects*
Neurologic
Sedative effects. Tolerance may develop over time, thus diminishing the effect. Caution patients to avoid operating power equipment or motor vehicles.
Anticholinergic effects
Blurred vision; constipation; urinary retention; dry mucosa of the mouth, throat, and nose. These symptoms are the anticholinergic effects produced by these agents. Patients should be monitored for these adverse effects. Maintain fluid intake at 8 to 10 eight-ounce glasses daily. Dryness of the mucosa may be relieved by sucking hard candy or ice chips, or by chewing gum. Stool softeners, such as docusate, or the occasional use of a stimulant laxative, such as Bisacodyl, may be required for constipation. Caution the patient that blurred vision may occur, and make appropriate suggestions for his or her personal

safety. Patients who develop urinary hesitancy should discontinue the medication and contact their healthcare provider for further evaluation.

◆ *Drug interactions*
Enhanced sedation. Central nervous system depressants, including sleeping aids, analgesics, benzodiazepines, phenothiazines, and alcohol, will enhance the sedative effects of antihistamines. People who work around machinery, drive a car, or perform other duties in which they must remain mentally alert should not take these medications while working.

DRUG CLASS: CORTICOSTEROIDS

Actions
Several studies have shown that dexamethasone and methylprednisolone can be effective antiemetics, either as single agents or in combination with other antiemetics. The mechanism of action is unknown. Other actions of the corticosteroids, such as mood elevation, increased appetite, and a sense of well-being, may also help in patient acceptance and control of emesis.

Uses
A particular advantage of the steroids, apart from their efficacy, is their relative lack of adverse effects. Because only a few doses are administered, the usual complications associated with long-term therapy do not arise.

Therapeutic Outcome
The primary therapeutic outcome expected from the corticosteroids as antiemetics is relief of nausea and vomiting.

❖ Nursing Implications for Corticosteroids
◆ Premedication assessment
1. Collect data regarding emesis (type, amount, and frequency, on a continuum).
2. Assess data relative to the underlying cause of nausea and vomiting (e.g., pregnancy, postsurgical state, chemotherapy, radiation, bowel obstruction).
3. Obtain baseline data about the patient's degree of alertness before initiation of therapy because these medications tend to produce some degree of sedation.

◆ *Availability, dosage, and administration.* See Table 33.2.

◆ *Common and serious adverse effects.* Adverse effects are infrequent because few doses are administered for nausea and vomiting. See also Chapter 37.
◆ *Drug interactions.* See Chapter 37.

DRUG CLASS: BENZODIAZEPINES

Actions
Benzodiazepines act as antiemetics through a combination of effects, including sedation, reduction in anxiety,

possible depression of the VC, and an amnesic effect. Of these, the amnesic effect appears to be most important in treating cancer patients and, in this respect, lorazepam and midazolam are superior to diazepam.

Uses

Benzodiazepines (e.g., lorazepam, midazolam, diazepam) are effective in reducing not only the frequency of nausea and vomiting but also the anxiety often associated with chemotherapy. Clinically, benzodiazepines are most useful in combination with other antiemetics, such as metoclopramide, dexamethasone, and serotonin antagonists.

Therapeutic Outcome

The primary therapeutic outcome expected from benzodiazepine antiemetics is relief of nausea and vomiting.

❖ Nursing Implications for Benzodiazepines
◆ *Premedication assessment*
1. Collect data regarding emesis (type, amount, and frequency, on a continuum).
2. Assess data relative to the underlying cause of the nausea and vomiting (e.g., pregnancy, postsurgical state, chemotherapy, radiation therapy, bowel obstruction).
3. Obtain baseline data about the patient's degree of alertness before initiation of therapy because these medications tend to produce some degree of sedation.

◆ *Availability, dosage, and administration.* See Table 33.2.

◆ *Common adverse effects, serious adverse effects, and drug interactions.* See Chapter 15.

DRUG CLASS: CANNABINOIDS

Actions

After numerous reports that smoking marijuana reduces the frequency of nausea, the antiemetic properties of the active ingredient tetrahydrocannabinol (THC) and its synthetic analogues, such as dronabinol and nabilone, have been studied. The cannabinoids act through several mechanisms to inhibit pathways to the VC; however, there is no dopamine antagonist activity.

Uses

Cannabinoids have been shown to be more effective than placebo and equally as effective as prochlorperazine in patients receiving moderately emetogenic chemotherapy. They are less effective than metoclopramide. Because of the mind-altering effects and potential for abuse, the cannabinoids serve as antiemetics only in patients receiving chemotherapy. The cannabinoids are of more use in those younger patients who are refractory to other antiemetic regimens and in whom combination therapy may be more effective.

Therapeutic Outcome

The primary therapeutic outcome expected from the cannabinoids is relief of nausea and vomiting.

❖ Nursing Implications for Cannabinoids
◆ *Premedication assessment*
1. Collect data regarding emesis (type, amount, and frequency, on a continuum).
2. Assess data relative to the underlying cause of nausea and vomiting (e.g., pregnancy, postsurgical state, chemotherapy, radiation, bowel obstruction).
3. Obtain baseline data about the patient's degree of alertness before initiation of therapy because these medications tend to produce some degree of sedation.

◆ *Availability, dosage, and administration.* See Table 33.2.

◆ *Common and serious adverse effects*
   Psychological
   Dysphonic effects. Depressed mood, hallucinations, dreaming or fantasizing, distortion of perception, paranoid reactions, and elation are more frequent with moderate to high doses. Younger patients appear to tolerate these adverse effects better than older patients or patients who have not previously used marijuana. Patients should be specifically warned not to drive, operate machinery, or engage in any hazardous activity until it is determined that they are able to tolerate the drug and to perform such tasks safely. Patients should remain under the supervision of a responsible adult during initial use of dronabinol and after dosage adjustments.

◆ *Drug interactions*
   Drugs that increase toxic effects. Antihistamines, alcohol, analgesics, benzodiazepines, phenobarbital, antidepressants, muscle relaxants, and sedative-hypnotics increase toxic effects. Monitor the patient for excessive sedation and reduce the dosage of the other sedative agents, if necessary.

DRUG CLASS: NEUROKININ-1 RECEPTOR ANTAGONISTS

Actions

Another neurotransmitter thought to play a role in the vomiting process is substance P. Substance P is a neuropeptide found in high concentrations in the area of the CNS responsible for vomiting, and it coexists with serotonin in the enterochromaffin cells and vagal afferent nerves of the GI tract. The actions of substance P are mediated through the NK1 receptor. NK1 antagonists block the effects of substance P in the CNS and have no affinity for serotonin, dopamine, or corticosteroid receptors. The NK1 receptor antagonists are aprepitant, fosaprepitant, and rolapitant. There is also a fixed-dose combination of netupitant, an NK1 receptor antagonist, and palonosetron, a 5-HT$_3$ antagonist.

Uses

Neurokinin-1 antagonists are used for the prevention of acute and delayed CINV caused by highly emetogenic antineoplastic agents. They are used in combination with a corticosteroid and a 5-HT$_3$ receptor antagonist. Their greatest effect appears to be in reducing the frequency of delayed emesis; they do not treat CINV once it has started. Aprepitant is also used to treat pain.

Therapeutic Outcome

The primary therapeutic outcome expected from NK1 antagonists is prevention of nausea and vomiting.

❖ Nursing Implications for Neurokinin-1 Receptor Antagonists

◆ *Premedication assessment*

1. Collect data regarding emesis (type, amount, and frequency, on a continuum).
2. Assess data relative to the underlying cause of nausea and vomiting (e.g., pregnancy, postsurgical state, chemotherapy, radiation therapy, bowel obstruction).
3. Assess premedication bowel pattern since diarrhea or constipation may occur posttherapy.

◆ *Availability.* See Table 33.2.

◆ *Dosage and administration*

Postoperative nausea and vomiting. See Table 33.2.

◆ *Common and serious adverse effects.* The most common adverse effects with NK1 antagonists are tiredness, nausea, hiccups, constipation, diarrhea, loss of appetite, headache, neutropenia, and hair loss. Because NK1 antagonists are taken only for up to 3 days at a time, adverse effects are short-lived and rarely troublesome.

◆ *Drug interactions*

Drugs that increase toxic effects of NK1 antagonists. Ketoconazole, itraconazole, nefazodone, clarithromycin, ritonavir, nelfinavir, and diltiazem may inhibit the metabolism of aprepitant, rolapitant, and netupitant. Monitor the patient for signs of toxicity.

Drugs that reduce therapeutic effects of NK1 antagonists. Rifampin, carbamazepine, paroxetine, and phenytoin induce the metabolism of aprepitant, rolapitant, and netupitant, reducing their therapeutic effect.

Oral contraceptives. Female patients receiving aprepitant who take oral contraceptives should be advised to use an alternative or additional method of birth control for the next month because aprepitant may enhance the metabolism of estrogens.

Dexamethasone and methylprednisolone. Aprepitant inhibits the metabolism of these corticosteroids. Oral doses of dexamethasone and methylprednisolone should be reduced by approximately 50% when prescribed concurrently with aprepitant. Intravenous methylprednisolone dosages should be reduced by 25%.

Netupitant also inhibits the metabolism of dexamethasone. The oral dose of dexamethasone should be reduced.

Warfarin. Patients receiving warfarin therapy should be instructed to have an international normalized ratio (INR) checked approximately 7 to 10 days after aprepitant therapy because coadministration with aprepitant may result in increased metabolism of warfarin and a reduced INR.

Thioridazine. Concurrent use with rolapitant is contraindicated.

Get Ready for the NCLEX® Examination!

Key Points

- Nausea and vomiting vary from a minor inconvenience to severe debilitation.
- The six common causes of nausea and vomiting are PONV, motion sickness, nausea and vomiting in pregnancy, psychogenic vomiting, CINV, and RINV.
- Nonpharmacologic treatments, such as eliminating noxious substances, avoiding fatty or spicy foods, and restricting activity to bed and chair rest to avoid vestibular irritation, are equally important in reducing the frequency of nausea and vomiting.
- The causes of nausea and vomiting should be assessed before treatment is begun, and specific therapy should be selected for each of the causes.
- Drug therapy for treatment of nausea and vomiting includes dopamine antagonists, serotonin antagonists, anticholinergic agents, corticosteroids, benzodiazepines, cannabinoids, and neurokinin-1 receptor antagonists.

Additional Learning Resources

SG Go to your Study Guide for additional Review Questions for the NCLEX® Examination, Critical Thinking Clinical Situations, and other learning activities to help you master this chapter content.

Go to your Evolve website (https://evolve.elsevier.com/Clayton) for additional online resources.

vary, a careful history must be obtained to determine the change in a particular patient's bowel elimination pattern. An important fact to remember about diarrhea is that diarrhea is a symptom rather than a disease.

CAUSES OF DIARRHEA

Intestinal Infections

Intestinal infections are most frequently associated with ingestion of food contaminated with bacteria or protozoa (food poisoning) or eating or drinking water that contains bacteria foreign to the patient's gastrointestinal (GI) tract. People traveling, especially to other countries, develop what is known as *traveler's diarrhea* from ingestion of microorganisms that are pathogenic to their GI tracts but not to those of the local residents.

Spicy or Fatty Foods

Spicy or fatty foods may produce diarrhea by irritating the lining of the GI tract. Diarrhea occurs particularly when the patient does not routinely eat these types of foods. This type of diarrhea may occur while an individual is traveling or on vacation (e.g., eating fresh oysters daily while visiting coastal regions).

Enzyme Deficiencies

Patients with deficiencies of digestive enzymes, such as lactase or amylase, have difficulty digesting certain foods. Diarrhea usually develops because of irritation from undigested food.

Excessive Use of Laxatives

People who use laxatives on a routine, chronic basis but are not under the care of a healthcare provider for a specific GI problem are laxative abusers. Some do it for weight control, and others use laxatives under the misconception that a person is not normal if the bowels do not move daily.

Drug Therapy

Diarrhea is a common adverse effect caused by irritation of the GI lining by ingested medication. Diarrhea may also result from the use of antibiotics that may kill certain bacteria that live in the GI tract and help digest food.

Emotional Stress

Diarrhea is a common symptom of emotional stress and anxiety.

Hyperthyroidism

Hyperthyroidism induces increased GI motility, resulting in diarrhea.

Inflammatory Bowel Disease

Inflammatory bowel diseases such as diverticulitis, ulcerative colitis, gastroenteritis, and Crohn's disease cause inflammation of the GI lining, resulting in muscle spasm and diarrhea.

Surgical Bypass

Surgical bypass procedures of the intestine often result in chronic diarrhea because of the decreased absorptive area remaining after surgery. Incompletely digested food and water rapidly pass through the GI tract.

TREATMENT OF ALTERED ELIMINATION

CONSTIPATION

Constipation that does not have a specific cause can often be treated without the use of laxatives. A high-fiber diet (e.g., fruits, grains, nuts, vegetables), adequate hydration (e.g., 8 to 10 eight-ounce glasses of water daily), and daily exercise (e.g., for physical activity, stress relief) can eliminate most cases of constipation. Laxatives, other than when treating acute constipation from a specific cause (e.g., a change in routine such as traveling for long hours in a car or plane), should be avoided. The ingredients of laxative products frequently cause adverse effects and may be contraindicated in certain patients. The following patients should not take over-the-counter (OTC) laxatives and should be referred to a healthcare provider: those with severe abdominal discomfort or pain; those who have nausea, vomiting, or fever; those with a preexisting condition (e.g., diabetes mellitus, abdominal surgery); those taking medicines that cause constipation (e.g., iron, aluminum antacids, antispasmodics, muscle relaxants, opioids); those who have used other laxatives without success; and laxative abusers.

DIARRHEA

Diarrhea may be acute or chronic, mild or severe. Because it may be a defense mechanism to rid the body of infecting organisms or irritants, it is usually self-limiting. Chronic diarrhea may indicate a disease of the stomach or small or large intestine, may be psychogenic, or may be one of the first symptoms of cancer of the colon or rectum. If diarrhea is severe or prolonged, it may cause dehydration, electrolyte depletion, and physical exhaustion. Specific antidiarrheal therapy depends on the cause of the diarrhea.

❖ NURSING IMPLICATIONS FOR CONSTIPATION AND DIARRHEA

◆ Assessment
History
- Obtain a history of the patient's usual bowel pattern and changes that have occurred in the frequency, consistency, odor, color, and number of stools per day. Ask whether the patient has a usual time of defecation (e.g., mornings or afternoon or after meals). Does the individual respond immediately to the urge to defecate or delay toileting until a more convenient time?
- Ask whether the onset of diarrhea or constipation is recent and if it can be associated with travel or stress. Has there been a change in water source

or foods lately? Ask what measures (whether prescribed by a healthcare provider or by self-treatment) the patient has already initiated to correct the problem, and ask about the degree of success achieved.

- Obtain a detailed history of the individual's health. Are any acute or chronic conditions being treated—for example, cancer, GI disorders, neurologic conditions, or intestinal obstruction?
- Plan to perform a focused assessment consistent with the symptoms and the underlying pathology.

Medications, treatments, and diagnostics

- Ask the patient to provide a list of all current medications prescribed by a healthcare provider, as well as all OTC medications that are being taken. Are any used to treat diarrhea or constipation? Are any of these medications known to slow intestinal transit time (e.g., opioids, aluminum-containing antacids, anticholinergic agents)? Are any known to cause diarrhea (e.g., magnesium-containing antacids)?
- Order baseline laboratory studies requested by the healthcare provider. Schedule prescribed treatments (e.g., enema administration) and diagnostic procedures (e.g., abdominal radiographs, colonoscopy, anorectal manometry).

Activity and exercise

- Ask the patient about daily activity level and exercise. Does the patient play vigorous sports, take walks or jog, or have a sedentary job and hobby?

Elimination pattern. What is the individual's usual pattern of stool elimination (i.e., frequency of the urge to defecate, usual stool consistency, presence of bloating or flatus, fecal incontinence)? Does the individual have a history of, or currently have, anal fissures, hemorrhoids, or abscesses? Assess intake and output, and any presence of blood.

Nutrition

- Ask questions to determine the patient's usual dietary practices. How much coffee, tea, soft drinks (caffeinated or decaffeinated), water, fruit juice, and alcoholic beverages are consumed each day?
- Ask for a description of what the patient has eaten over the past 24 hours. Evaluate the data to identify whether foods from all levels of the food pyramid (see Fig. 46.4) are being eaten. Are there good sources of dietary fiber? Has the patient introduced foods not usually eaten into the diet?
- Obtain specific orders relating to nutrition. Diet orders depend on the cause of constipation or diarrhea. A dietary consult may be indicated. Schedule fluid intake of at least 3000 mL/day, unless contraindicated by coexisting conditions (e.g., heart failure, renal disease). Rehydration solutions may be required with

severe diarrhea. Does the patient have any food intolerances or foods known to produce diarrhea or constipation?

Basic assessment

- Obtain and record baseline vital signs, height, and weight.
- Assess bowel sounds in all four quadrants. Observe the size and shape of the abdomen. Note any signs of distention, ascites, or masses.
- Assess and record signs of dehydration. Examine the patient for inelastic skin turgor, sticky oral mucous membranes, excessive thirst, a shrunken and deeply furrowed tongue, crusted lips, weight loss, deteriorating vital signs, soft or sunken eyeballs, delayed capillary filling, high urine specific gravity or no urine output, and possible mental confusion.

Laboratory studies

- Review laboratory reports for indications of problems such as malabsorption, dehydration, and fluid, electrolyte, and acid-base imbalances (e.g., K^+, Cl^-, pH, partial pressure of carbon dioxide, bicarbonate, hemoglobin, hematocrit, urinalysis [specific gravity], serum albumin, total protein).
- Check reports of stool specimen sent for laboratory examination.

◆ Implementation

- Maintain hydration with oral or parenteral solutions as prescribed by the healthcare provider. Monitor the hydration status with volume of intake, urine output, skin turgor, moisturization of mucous membranes, and daily weights.
- Assess for bowel sounds in all four quadrants. Report absence of bowel sounds immediately to the healthcare provider. Assess abdomen for distention; measure abdominal girth if necessary.
- Give enemas prescribed according to hospital procedures. (These are not used for long-term treatment of constipation.) Oil retention enemas may be required to soften the fecal material.
- Initiate nutritional interventions such as high-fiber foods and adequate fluid intake.
- Give prescribed laxatives or stool softeners. Monitor for effectiveness and adverse effects.
- Administer prescribed antidiarrheal agents, antiperistaltic agents (except to patients known to have infectious diarrhea), and antibiotics for infection-based diarrhea.
- Initiate hygiene measures to prevent perianal skin breakdown. Cleanse the perianal area thoroughly after each stool. Apply protective ointment (e.g., zinc oxide) as prescribed; with severe diarrhea, a fecal collection apparatus may be helpful.
- Monitor vital signs, daily weights, and stool cultures and perform a focused assessment appropriate to the underlying cause of the constipation or diarrhea.

◆ **Patient Education**

Nutritional status

- Be certain that the individual, parent, or significant other understands all aspects of the diet and fluid orders prescribed. Ask specifically what should and should not be avoided and how much he or she should be drinking.
- Stress the inclusion of high-fiber foods and adequate fluids to maintain hydration and alleviate constipation.
- Depending on the underlying cause of the symptoms, health teaching is appropriate regarding proper food preparation, storage, and prevention of contamination.
- During travel, advise using bottled water when appropriate.

Activity and exercise

- Encourage regular exercise.

Medications

- Explain the consequences of regular use of laxatives and the benefits of handling constipation with diet, exercise, and adequate fluid intake.
- When opioids are used regularly for pain control in cancer patients, it is imperative that the patients know that stool softeners should be initiated and continued as long as constipating medications are being taken.
- If laxatives or enemas are prescribed to cleanse the intestines before diagnostic examination, be certain that the individual has written instructions for use, the time and amount to be administered, and where the laxative or enema can be purchased. Review the correct procedure for self-administering an enema with the patient, or instruct a family member.
- Emphasize the need to be in proximity to a bathroom when taking laxatives such as GoLYTELY (a poly- ethylene glycol–electrolyte solution).

Fostering health maintenance

- Fecal-oral contamination may cause diarrhea. Teach proper handwashing and cleansing or disinfection of the toilet, bedpan, or commode.
- For diarrhea associated with chronic GI diseases, it is imperative to reinforce all aspects of health teaching relating to the specific disease underlying the symptomatology.
- Provide the patient and significant others with impor- tant information contained in the individual drug monographs to identify drugs that cause constipation or diarrhea. Additional health teaching and nursing interventions for common and serious adverse effects are described in each drug monograph.
- Seek cooperation and understanding of the following points for judicious use of laxatives or antidiarrheals: name of medication; dosage, route, and times of administration; and common and serious adverse effects. For infectious diarrhea, teach the patient precautions to prevent its spread to others. For all patients with diarrhea, teach the need for adequate fluid intake and any dietary restrictions.

DRUG CLASS: LAXATIVES

Actions

Laxatives are chemicals that act to promote the evacu- ation of the bowel. They are usually subclassified based on the mechanism of action (Table 34.1).

Stimulant laxatives. Stimulant laxatives (bisacodyl, sennosides A and B) act directly on the intestine, causing an irritation that promotes peristalsis and evacuation. If given orally, these agents act within 6 to 10 hours. If administered rectally, they act within 60 to 90 minutes.

Osmotic laxatives. Osmotic laxatives (e.g., lactulose, polyethylene glycol, glycerin) are hypertonic compounds that draw water into the intestine from surrounding tissues. Lactulose has an onset of action within 24 to 48 hours. Polyethylene glycol usually acts within 24 to 96 hours, and glycerin suppositories usually act within 15 to 30 minutes.

Polyethylene glycol–electrolyte solution is a relatively new approach to osmotic laxative therapy. It is a mixture of a nonabsorbable ion exchange solution and electrolytes that acts as an osmotic agent. When taken orally, it pulls electrolytes and water into the solution in the lumen of the bowel and exchanges sodium ions to replace those removed from the body. The result is a diarrhea that cleanses the bowel for colonoscopy and barium enema x-ray examination with no significant dehydration or loss of electrolytes.

Saline laxatives. Saline laxatives (e.g., magnesium hydroxide, magnesium citrate, sodium phosphates) are hypertonic compounds that work in the small and large intestine, drawing water into the lumen of the intestine from surrounding tissues. The accumulated water affects stool consistency and distends the bowel, causing peristalsis. The magnesium-containing products also stimulate muscle peristalsis, helping evacuate the bowel. These agents usually act within 1 to 3 hours and up to 6 hours for sodium phosphates. Continued use of these products significantly alters electrolyte balance and may cause dehydration.

Chloride channel activator. Lubiprostone (Amitiza) induces secretion of chloride-rich intestinal fluid without altering sodium or potassium concentrations in the serum. Increasing intestinal fluid secretion increases intestinal motility with passage of feces.

Guanylate cyclase C agonists. Linaclotide (Linzess) and plecanatide (Trulance) are guanylate cyclase-C agonists, the newest class of drugs approved for chronic idiopathic constipation. They both activate guanylate cyclase-C, which stimulates secretion of chloride and bicarbonate

Table 34.1 Laxatives

GENERIC NAME	BRAND NAME	LAXATIVE TYPE
bisacodyl	Dulcolax tablets	Stimulant
docusate sodium	Colace	Stool softener
glycerin	Glycerin suppositories	Osmotic
lactulose	Constulose	Osmotic
linaclotide	Linzess	Guanylate cyclase-C agonist
lubiprostone	Amitiza	Chloride channel activator
magnesium citrate	Citrate of Magnesia	Saline
magnesium hydroxide	Phillips' Milk of Magnesia	Saline
methylcellulose	Citrucel	Bulk-forming
methylnaltrexone	Relistor	Peripheral opioid antagonist
mineral oil	Mineral Oil	Lubricant
naldemedine	Symproic	Peripheral opioid antagonist
naloxegol	Movantik	Peripheral opioid antagonist
plecanatide	Trulance	Guanylate cyclase-C agonist
polycarbophil	FiberCon	Bulk-forming
polyethylene glycol 3350	MiraLAX	Osmotic
polyethylene glycol–electrolyte solution	CoLyte / GoLYTELY / MoviPrep	Osmotic / Osmotic / Osmotic
psyllium hydrophilic mucilloid	Metamucil	Bulk-forming
sennosides	Ex-Lax / Black Draught / Senokot	Stimulant / Stimulant / Stimulant
sennosides and docusate sodium	Peri-Colace	Stool softener plus stimulant
sodium phosphates	Osmo-Prep	Saline

because the action is highly dependent on the individual patient's normal GI transit time. Peristaltic activity does not appear to be increased. If used frequently, these oils may inhibit the absorption of fat-soluble vitamins.

Bulk-forming laxatives. Psyllium, calcium polycarbophil, and methylcellulose are approved bulk-forming laxatives. Psyllium increases stool frequency in patients with chronic constipation, but evidence is lacking for the efficacy of the other approved bulk-forming laxatives. Bulk-forming laxatives must be administered with a full glass of water. The laxative causes water to be retained within the stool. This increases bulk, which stimulates peristalsis. Onset of action is usually 12 to 24 hours but may be as long as 72 hours, depending on the patient's GI transit time. Bulk-forming agents are usually considered the safest laxatives, even when taken routinely. Fresh fruits, vegetables, and cereals such as wheat bran are natural bulk-forming products.

Stool softeners. Stool softeners, also known as *wetting agents,* draw water into the stool, causing it to soften. Docusate calcium and docusate sodium are US Food and Drug Administration approved, but there is little evidence that they are effective in treating chronic constipation. Psyllium is more effective in improving stool frequency than stool softeners. Stool softeners do not stimulate peristalsis and may require up to 72 hours to aid in a soft bowel movement. Action from these agents depends on the patient's state of hydration and the GI transit time.

Peripheral opioid antagonists. Methylnaltrexone (Relistor), naloxegol (Movantik), and naldemedine (Symproic) are mu-opioid receptor antagonists that bind to opioid receptors in the GI tract, inhibiting the constipation-producing effects of opioid drugs. Methylnaltrexone, naloxegol, and naldemedine do not cross the blood-brain barrier and do not interfere with the analgesic effects of the opioids.

Uses
Stimulant, osmotic, chloride channel activator, guanylate cyclase-C agonist, and saline laxatives. Stimulant, osmotic, and saline laxatives may be used individually to relieve acute constipation. They are also effective when used in higher doses and in combination for cleaning out the gut prior to bowel surgery or colonoscopy. Polyethylene glycol, lactulose, and lubiprostone are effective in treating chronic constipation. Lubiprostone is approved to treat chronic idiopathic constipation, opioid-induced constipation in adults with chronic noncancer pain, and irritable bowel syndrome with constipation. Smaller doses of lactulose or polyethylene glycol can be taken to regulate stool consistency and frequency. Larger doses of polyethylene glycol are routinely used as bowel preparations to remove gas and feces before radiologic examination of the kidneys, colon, intestine,

into the intestinal lumen, increasing intestinal fluid secretion, which can soften stools and increase motility with passage of feces.

Lubricant laxatives. Lubricant laxatives (e.g., mineral oil) lubricate the intestinal wall and soften the stool, allowing a smooth passage of fecal contents. Onset of action is often 6 to 8 hours but may be up to 48 hours or gallbladder. These products should be used only intermittently because chronic use may cause loss of normal bowel function and dependency on the agent for bowel evacuation. The guanylate cyclase-C agonists linaclotide and plecanatide are used in the treatment of chronic idiopathic constipation and in the treatment of irritable bowel syndrome with constipation. The most common adverse effect is diarrhea.

Lubricant laxatives. Lubricant laxatives are helpful for producing a soft stool without causing significant bowel spasm. Lubricants are also used prophylactically in patients who should not strain during defecation. Lubricants should not be administered to debilitated patients who are constantly in a recumbent position. The oil can be aspirated into the lungs, where it may cause lipid pneumonia. Lubricant laxatives may be used in geriatric and pregnant patients because there is little cramping accompanying their use.

Bulk-forming laxatives. Bulk-forming laxatives are generally considered the drug of choice for someone who is incapacitated and needs a laxative regularly. These agents may also be used in patients with irritable bowel syndrome to provide a softer consistency to the stools if a high-fiber diet is not adequate. Bulk-forming laxatives are also used to control certain types of diarrhea by absorbance of the irritating substance, thus allowing its removal from the bowel during defecation. Bulk-forming laxatives may be used in geriatric and pregnant patients because there is little cramping accompanying their use. Pediatric patients should also be treated with a change in diet to include cereals, fruits, and grains. Constipation in infants can be treated with malt soup extract, a bulk-forming laxative. It is important that bulk-forming laxatives be dispersed in a glass of water or juice before administration. If adequate volumes of water are not taken, obstruction within the GI tract may result from a bulk laxative that forms a sticky mass.

Stool softeners. Stool softeners are routinely used for prophylactic purposes to prevent constipation or straining at stool (e.g., in patients recovering from myocardial infarction or abdominal surgery).

Peripheral opioid antagonists. Methylnaltrexone, naloxegol, and naldemedine are used for the treatment of opioid-induced constipation in patients with advanced illness who are receiving palliative care when their response to laxative therapy has not been adequate.

Therapeutic Outcomes

The primary therapeutic outcomes expected from laxative therapy are as follows:

1. Relief from abdominal discomfort.
2. Passage of bowel contents within a few hours of administration.

❖ **Nursing Implications for Laxative Therapy**

◆ *Premedication assessment*

1. Determine the usual pattern of elimination.
2. Ask specifically about symptoms that may indicate undiagnosed abdominal pain, such as symptoms associated with intestinal obstruction or appendicitis.

> [!] **Medication Safety Alert**
>
> Do not administer laxatives to patients with undiagnosed abdominal pain or inflammation of the GI tract, such as gastritis, appendicitis, or colitis.

◆ *Availability.* For drugs not listed here, see drug monographs for individual products for information on available formulations.

- Lubiprostone: 8- and 24-mcg capsules
- Methylnaltrexone: 8 mg in a 0.4-mL syringe; 12 mg in a 0.6-mL vial and syringe; 150-mg tablets
- Naldemedine: 0.2-mg tablets
- Naloxegol: 12.5- and 25-mg tablets

◆ *Dosage and administration.* For drugs not listed here, see drug monographs for individual products for information on dosage and administration.

Bulk-forming laxatives: PO: Be sure to administer with adequate water to prevent esophageal, gastric, intestinal, or rectal obstruction.

Lubiprostone. *Chronic idiopathic constipation and opioid-induced constipation: PO:* 24 mcg taken twice daily with food and water.

Irritable bowel syndrome with constipation: PO: 8 mcg twice daily with food and water.

Methylnaltrexone. *Opioid-induced constipation with chronic noncancer pain: Subcut:* 12 mg once daily. *PO:* 450 mg once daily with water on an empty stomach at least 30 minutes before the first meal of the day.

Opioid-induced constipation with advanced illness (receiving palliative care): Treatment of opioid-induced constipation in adult patients with advanced illness who are receiving palliative care and have an inadequate response to conventional laxative regimens is based on patient weight:

PATIENT WEIGHT	METHYLNALTREXONE DOSAGE
<38 kg	0.15 mg/kg
38-62 kg	8 mg
62-114 kg	12 mg
>114 kg	0.15 mg/kg

- In patients with a creatinine clearance lower than 30 mL/min, reduce the dosage by one-half.
- Administer by subcutaneous injection every other day, as needed, but no more than once every 24 hours.

Naldemedine. *Opioid-induced constipation with chronic noncancer pain: PO:* 0.2 mg daily.

Naloxegol. *Opioid-induced constipation with noncancer pain: PO:* 25 mg once daily in the morning on an empty stomach. If not tolerated, reduce dose to 12.5 mg once daily.

◆ *Common adverse effects*

Gastrointestinal

Abdominal spasms, abdominal discomfort with flatulence, nausea. The most common adverse effect is excessive bowel stimulation that results in abdominal spasms and diarrhea. Patients who are severely constipated may develop abdominal cramps. The patient should first experience the urge to defecate, then defecate and feel a sense of relief.

◆ *Serious adverse effects*

Gastrointestinal

Abdominal tenderness, pain, bleeding, vomiting, diarrhea, increasing abdominal girth. Failure to defecate or defecation of only a small amount may indicate the presence of an impaction. These also are symptoms of an acute abdominal condition.

◆ *Drug interactions*

Bisacodyl. Do not administer with milk, antacids, cimetidine, famotidine, nizatidine, or ranitidine. These products may allow the enteric coating to dissolve prematurely, resulting in nausea, vomiting, and cramping.

Psyllium. Do not administer products containing psyllium (e.g., Metamucil) at the same time as salicylates, nitrofurantoin, or digoxin, because the psyllium may inhibit absorption. Administer salicylates, nitrofurantoin, or digoxin at least 1 hour before or 2 hours after psyllium.

Mineral oil. Daily administration of mineral oil for more than 1 to 2 weeks may cause a deficiency of the fat-soluble vitamins.

Docusate. Docusate enhances the absorption of mineral oil. Concurrent use is not recommended.

Methylnaltrexone, lubiprostone, linaclotide, and plecanatide. There are no reported drug interactions for these medications.

Naldemedine and naloxegol

Drugs that increase toxic effects of naldemedine and naloxegol. Fluconazole, aprepitant, diltiazem, verapamil, erythromycin, itraconazole, ketoconazole, clarithromycin, and ritonavir may inhibit the metabolism of naldemedine and naloxegol. Monitor for signs of toxicity.

Drugs that reduce therapeutic effects of naldemedine and naloxegol. Rifampin, carbamazepine, phenytoin, and St. John's wort can induce the metabolism of naldemedine and naloxegol, reducing their therapeutic effect.

DRUG CLASS: ANTIDIARRHEAL AGENTS

Actions

Antidiarrheal agents include a wide variety of drugs that can be divided into two broad categories—locally acting agents and systemic agents. Locally acting agents such as activated charcoal, pectin, and psyllium absorb excess water to cause a formed stool and adsorb irritants or bacteria that are causing the diarrhea. Bismuth subsalicylate acts locally to stop secretion of fluids into the GI tract that promote diarrhea; it may also have local antimicrobial effects, killing bacteria and viruses that may be inducing diarrhea. *Lactobacillus acidophilus* is used to promote normal bacterial growth in the intestinal tract with chronic (not acute) diarrhea.

The systemic agents act through the autonomic nervous system to reduce peristalsis and motility of the GI tract, allowing the mucosal lining to absorb nutrients, water, and electrolytes, leaving a formed stool in the colon. Representatives of the systemically acting agents are loperamide (without atropine) and diphenoxylate and difenoxin with atropine to prevent abuse (see Table 34.2).

The systemically acting agents are associated with more adverse effects (see Table 34.2) and should not be used to treat diarrhea caused by substances toxic to the GI tract, such as bacterial contaminants or other irritants. Because these agents act by reducing GI motility, the systemically acting antidiarrheals tend to allow the toxin to remain in the GI tract longer, causing further irritation.

Uses

Although the ingredients of the antidiarrheal products are, in general, benign and the majority are available OTC, the decision to recommend treatment or to refer the patient to a healthcare provider is not to be taken lightly.

Antidiarrheal products are usually indicated under the following conditions:

- The diarrhea is of sudden onset, has lasted more than 2 or 3 days, and is causing significant fluid and water loss. Young children and elderly patients are more susceptible to rapid dehydration and electrolyte imbalance and therefore should start antidiarrheal therapy earlier.
- Patients with inflammatory bowel disease develop diarrhea. Rapid treatment shortens the course of the incapacitating diarrhea and allows the patient to live a more normal lifestyle. Other agents, such as adrenocorticosteroids or sulfonamides, may also be used to control the underlying bowel disease.
- Post–GI surgery patients develop diarrhea. These patients may require chronic antidiarrheal therapy to allow adequate absorption of fluids and electrolytes.
- The cause of the diarrhea has been diagnosed, and the healthcare provider determines that an antidiarrheal product is appropriate for therapy. Because many cases of diarrhea are self-limiting, therapy may not be necessary.

Therapeutic Outcome

The primary therapeutic outcome expected from antidiarrheal therapy is relief from the incapacitation and discomfort of diarrhea.

Table 34.2	**Antidiarrheal Agents**			
GENERIC NAME	BRAND NAME	AVAILABILITY	ADULT DOSAGE RANGE	COMMENTS
Systemic Action				
difenoxin with atropine	Motofen	Tablets: 1 mg difenoxin with 0.025 mg atropine	PO: 2 tablets, then 1 tablet after each loose stool or every 3-4 hr as needed; do not exceed 8 tablets in 24 hr	Inhibits peristalsis Atropine added to minimize potential overdose or abuse May cause drowsiness or dizziness; use caution in performing tasks requiring alertness Do not use in children younger than 2 yr
diphenoxylate with atropine	Lomotil	Tablets: 2.5 mg diphenoxylate with 0.025 mg atropine Liquid: 2.5 mg diphenoxylate with 0.025 mg atropine/5 mL	PO: 5 mg three or four times daily; do not exceed 20 mg per 24 hr	Inhibits peristalsis Atropine added to minimize potential overdose or abuse May cause drowsiness or dizziness; use caution in performing tasks requiring alertness Do not use in children younger than 2 yr
loperamide	Imodium A-D	Tablets: 2 mg Capsules: 2 mg Liquid: 1 mg/5 mL; 1 mg/7.5 mL	PO: 4 mg initially, followed by 2 mg after each unformed movement; do not exceed 16 mg/day	Inhibits peristalsis Used in acute, nonspecific diarrhea and to reduce volume of discharge from ileostomy
Local Action				
Lactobacillus acidophilus	Lactinex	Capsules, granules	PO: 2-4 capsules, two to four times daily, with milk Granules: 1 packet added to cereal, fruit juice, or milk three or four times daily	Bacteria used to recolonize GI tract in an attempt to treat chronic diarrhea Do not use in acute diarrhea
bismuth subsalicylate	Pepto-Bismol	Tablets, chewable; 262 mg suspension; 262 mg/15 mL, 525 mg/15 mL	PO: 524 mg every 30 to 60 min or 1050 mg every 60 min as needed; Maximum dosage: Approximately 4200 mg (8 doses of 262 mg; 4 doses of 525 mg) per 24 hr	In the GI tract, bismuth subsalicylate dissociates; the salicylate stops secretions of fluids into the GI tract, and the bismuth has antimicrobial action against bacterial and viral enteropathogens

❖ **Nursing Implications for Antidiarrheal Agents**
◆ *Premedication assessment*
1. Confer with patient regarding medications that may be contributing to diarrhea, including antacids containing magnesium or laxative products, antibiotics, or products containing large quantities of sorbitol.
2. Review history of onset of diarrhea and precipitating factors. Refer to a healthcare provider if in doubt about administering antidiarrheal agents.

◆ *Availability, dosage, and administration.* See Table 34.2.
   PO: Follow directions on the container. Be sure to give adequate water with bulk-forming agents to prevent esophageal, gastric, intestinal, or rectal obstruction.

◆ *Common adverse effects*
   Gastrointestinal
   Abdominal distention, nausea, constipation. Locally acting agents have essentially no adverse effects, but if used excessively, they may cause abdominal distention, nausea, and constipation.

◆ *Serious adverse effects*
   Gastrointestinal
   Prolonged or worsened diarrhea. This may be an indication that toxins are present in the gut and that the systemically acting antidiarrheal is causing retention of these toxins. Refer the patient to a healthcare provider for medical attention.

◆ *Drug interactions*

Diphenoxylate, difenoxin. The chemical structure of these two antidiarrheal agents is similar to meperidine. These agents should not be used in a patient receiving monoamine oxidase inhibitors (e.g., phenelzine, isocarboxazid, tranylcypromine) because of the potential for a hypertensive crisis.

Sedatives, alcohol, phenothiazines. Sedation caused by diphenoxylate and difenoxin is potentiated by other medications with central nervous system depressant properties.

Get Ready for the NCLEX® Examination!

Key Points

- Constipation and diarrhea are common disorders of the GI tract that most people experience occasionally throughout their lives. Most cases are self-limiting and do not require pharmacologic treatment.
- Constipation is most frequently treated by adding bulk and water to the diet and by exercising regularly. If drug treatment is required, laxatives that act by a variety of mechanisms are available: bulk-forming agents, stimulants, osmotics, lubricants, stool softeners, and opioid antagonists.
- Acute diarrhea is usually a symptom of an underlying problem, such as a GI infection. A detailed history of recent events must be taken to assess whether to recommend treatment with antidiarrheal agents.

Additional Learning Resources

SG Go to your Study Guide for additional Review Questions for the NCLEX® Examination, Critical Thinking Clinical Situations, and other learning activities to help you master this chapter content.

Go to your Evolve website (https://evolve.elsevier.com/Clayton) for additional online resources.

Review Questions for the NCLEX® Examination

1. A nurse is providing education to a patient who has complained about frequent bouts of constipation. Which statement by the patient indicates further teaching is needed?
   1. "If I exercise for at least 30 minutes every day, my bowels will move more regularly."
   2. "Drinking adequate amounts of water can keep constipation from occurring."
   3. "Taking pain medications regularly will not affect my bowel habits."
   4. "Eating a diet rich in fiber should help alleviate any irregular bowel movements."
2. A nurse preparing the drug Metamucil explains to the patient that oral, bulk-forming laxatives usually relieve constipation by which time frame?
   1. "You should have relief from constipation in about half an hour."
   2. "This drug takes about 1 to 3 hours to work."
   3. "Since this drug takes a while to work, do not expect results for at least 6 to 10 hours."
   4. "This drug works by absorbing water into the stool, causing a softer stool, and takes about 12 to 24 hours."

3. The patient with an ileostomy is receiving loperamide (Imodium A-D) for treatment of diarrhea because of which effects? *(Select all that apply.)*
   1. This drug will soften the stool.
   2. This drug will inhibit peristalsis.
   3. This drug uses an antimicrobial action.
   4. This drug stops the secretion of fluids into the GI tract.
   5. This drug allows more time for the intestines to absorb excess water to cause a formed stool.
4. The nurse teaching a patient about the antidiarrheal agent *Lactobacillus acidophilus* (Lactinex) knows that which statement by the patient indicates further teaching is needed?
   1. "When I take Lactinex, I can add it to my cereal or juice in the morning."
   2. "This drug Lactinex has a stimulating effect on my bowels."
   3. "As I understand it, I take Lactinex so that bacteria can recolonize my gut."
   4. "This drug will not have any systemic effect, so side effects are not a worry."
5. Which type of laxative should not be administered to debilitated patients who are in a recumbent position most of the time?
   1. Osmotic
   2. Stimulant
   3. Lubricant
   4. Bulk forming
6. Stimulant laxatives have an onset of action of how many hours?
   1. 1 to 4
   2. 2 to 5
   3. 6 to 10
   4. 12 to 18
7. Which antidiarrheal agent is contraindicated for use in children younger than the age of 2 years?
   1. Diphenoxylate (Lomotil)
   2. Loperamide (Imodium A-D)
   3. Bismuth subsalicylate (Pepto-Bismol)
   4. *Lactobacillus acidophilus* (Lactinex)
8. Which type of laxative may cause electrolyte imbalance and dehydration?
   1. Osmotic
   2. Stimulant
   3. Lubricant
   4. Bulk forming

Drugs Used to Treat Diabetes Mellitus

35

https://evolve.elsevier.com/Clayton

Objectives

1. Identify normal fasting blood glucose levels and differentiate between the symptoms of type 1 and type 2 diabetes mellitus.
2. Identify the major nursing considerations associated with the management of the patient with diabetes (e.g., nutritional evaluation, dietary prescription, activity and exercise, and psychological considerations).
3. Compare the signs, symptoms, and management of hypoglycemia and hyperglycemia.
4. Describe the action and use of insulin to control diabetes mellitus.
5. Discuss the action and use of oral hypoglycemic agents to control diabetes mellitus.
6. Discuss the educational needs for patients with complications from diabetes.

Key Terms

diabetes mellitus (dī-ă-BĒ-tēz měl-Ī-tĭs) (p. 535)
hyperglycemia (hī-pěr-glī-SĒ-mē-ă) (p. 535)
type 1 diabetes mellitus (p. 536)
type 2 diabetes mellitus (p. 536)
gestational diabetes mellitus (GDM) (jĕs-TĀ-shŭn-ăl) (p. 537)
impaired glucose tolerance (IGT) (GLŪ-kōs) (p. 537)
impaired fasting glucose (IFG) (p. 537)
prediabetes (prē-dī-ă-BĒ-tēz) (p. 537)

microvascular complications (mīk-rō-VĂS-kyū-lăr) (p. 537)
macrovascular complications (măk-rō-VĂS-kyū-lăr) (p. 537)
neuropathies (nŷr-ŎP-ě-thēz) (p. 538)
paresthesia (păr-ĕs-THĒ-zē-ă) (p. 538)
medical nutrition therapy (MNT) (mĕd-ĭ-KŬL nū-TRĬSH-ĕn THĒR-ě-pē) (p. 538)
hypoglycemia (hī-pō-glī-SĒ-mē-ă) (p. 538)
intensive therapy (p. 539)

DIABETES MELLITUS

Diabetes mellitus is a group of diseases characterized by hyperglycemia (fasting plasma glucose level >100 mg/dL) and abnormalities in fat, carbohydrate, and protein metabolism that lead to microvascular, macrovascular, and neuropathic complications. Several pathologic processes are associated with the development of diabetes, and patients often have impairment of insulin secretion, as well as defects in insulin action, resulting in hyperglycemia. It is now recognized that different pathologic mechanisms are involved that affect the development of the different types of diabetes. "Diabetes is a complex, chronic illness requiring continuous medical care with multifactorial risk-reduction strategies beyond control of blood glucose" (American Diabetes Association [ADA], 2015, p. S1).

Diabetes mellitus is occurring with increasing frequency in the United States as the population increases in weight and age. In the United States, the Centers for Disease Control and Prevention's National Diabetes Statistics Report (CDC, 2017) estimates that the prevalence of diabetes in the general population is approximately 9.4% (23.1 million people, 7.2 million of whom are undiagnosed). Direct expenditures of medical care totaled $327 billion in 2017. An additional $90 billion was attributed to lost productivity at work, disability, and premature death. Diabetes is listed as the sixth leading cause of death in the United States. Most diabetes-related deaths are the result of cardiovascular disease because the risk of heart disease and stroke is two to four times greater in patients with diabetes compared with those without the disease.

Undiagnosed diabetic adults, with few or no symptoms, present a major challenge to the health profession. Because early symptoms of diabetes are minimal, many of these people do not seek medical advice. Indications of the disease are discovered only at the time of routine physical examination. Those with a predisposition to developing diabetes include people who have relatives with diabetes (they have a 2.5 times greater incidence of developing the disease), obese people (85% of all diabetic patients are overweight), and older people (four out of five diabetic patients are older than 45 years).

The incidence of diabetes is higher in African Americans, Hispanics, American Indians, Alaskan Natives, and women. There also appears to be a significant increase in diabetes among those younger than 20 years.

The National Diabetes Data Group of the National Institutes of Health and the World Health Organization Expert Committee on Diabetes have classified diabetes by the underlying pathology causing hyperglycemia (Box 35.1).

Type 1 diabetes mellitus, formerly known as *insulin-dependent diabetes mellitus (IDDM),* is present in 5% to 10% of the diabetic population. It is caused by an autoimmune destruction of the beta cells in the pancreas. It occurs more frequently in juveniles, but patients can become symptomatic for the first time at any age. The onset of this form of diabetes usually has a rapid progression of symptoms (a few days to a few weeks) characterized by polydipsia (increased thirst), polyphagia (increased appetite), polyuria (increased urination), increased frequency of infections, loss of weight and strength, irritability, and often ketoacidosis. Because there is no insulin secretion from the pancreas, patients require administration of exogenous insulin. Insulin dosage adjustment is easily affected by inconsistent patterns of physical activity and dietary irregularities. It is common for patients with type 1 diabetes mellitus to go into remission in the early stages of the disease, requiring little or no exogenous insulin. This condition may last for a few months and is referred to as the *honeymoon period.*

Type 2 diabetes mellitus, formerly known as *non–insulin-dependent diabetes mellitus (NIDDM),* is present in 90% to 95% of the diabetic population. In contrast to type 1 diabetes mellitus, type 2 diabetes is characterized by a decrease in beta cell activity (insulin deficiency), insulin resistance (reduced uptake of insulin by peripheral muscle cells), or an increase in glucose production by the liver. Over time, the beta cells of the pancreas fail, and exogenous insulin injections may be required. Most people with type 2 diabetes mellitus also have metabolic syndrome, also known as *insulin resistance syndrome* (see Chapter 20). Type 2 diabetes onset is usually more insidious than that of type 1 diabetes. The pancreas still maintains some capacity to produce and secrete insulin. Consequently, symptoms (polyphagia, polydipsia, polyuria) are minimal or absent for a prolonged period. The patient may seek medical attention several years later only after symptoms of the disease are apparent (see next section on Complications of Diabetes Mellitus). Fasting hyperglycemia can be controlled by diet in some patients, but most patients require the use of supplemental insulin or oral antidiabetic agents, such as metformin or glyburide. Although the onset is usually after the fourth decade of life, type 2 diabetes can occur in younger patients who do not require insulin for control. See Table 35.1 for a comparison of the characteristics of type 1 and type 2 diabetes mellitus.

Box 35.1 Classification of Diabetes Mellitus by Pathologic Cause

I.   Type 1 diabetes (beta cell destruction, usually leading to absolute insulin deficiency)[a]
   • Immune mediated
   • Idiopathic
II. Type 2 diabetes (due to a progressive insulin secretory defect aggravated by insulin resistance)[a]
III. Other specific types
   • Genetic defects of beta cell function
   • Genetic defects in insulin action
   • Disease of the exocrine pancreas (such as cystic fibrosis)
   • Endocrinopathies
   • Drug or chemical induced (such as after organ transplantation)
   • Infections
   • Uncommon forms of immune-mediated diabetes
   • Other genetic syndromes sometimes associated with diabetes
IV. Gestational diabetes mellitus

Modified from American Diabetes Association. Classification and diagnosis of diabetes. *Diabetes Care.* 2017;40(suppl 1):S11.
[a]Patients with any form of diabetes may require insulin treatment at some stage of their disease. Such use of insulin does not, in itself, classify the patient.

Table 35.1 Features of Type 1 and Type 2 Diabetes Mellitus[a]

FEATURE	TYPE 1 DIABETES	TYPE 2 DIABETES
Age (yr)	<20[b]	>40[b]
Onset	Over a few days to weeks	Gradual
Insulin secretion	Falling to none	Oversecretion for years
Body image	Lean	Obese
Early symptoms	Polyuria, polydipsia, polyphagia	Often absent until complications arise
Ketones at diagnosis	Yes	No
Insulin required for treatment	Yes	No[c]
Acute complications	Diabetic ketoacidosis	Hyperosmolar hyperglycemia
Microvascular complications at diagnosis	No	Common
Macrovascular complications at diagnosis	Uncommon	Common

[a]Clinical presentation is highly variable.
[b]Age of onset is most commonly younger than 20 years, but onset may occur at any age. As the rates of obesity increase, type 2 diabetes is becoming much more prevalent in children, adolescents, and young adults in all ethnic groups.
[c]May eventually require insulin therapy over time.

A third subclass of diabetes mellitus (see Box 35.1) includes additional types that have causes other than those that cause type 1 and type 2 diabetes mellitus. They are part of other diseases having features not generally associated with the diabetic state. Diseases that may have a diabetic component include pheochromocytoma, cystic fibrosis, acromegaly, and Cushing's syndrome. Other disorders included in this category are malnutrition, infection, drugs and chemicals that induce hyperglycemia, defects in insulin receptors, and certain genetic syndromes.

The fourth category of classification, known as *gestational diabetes mellitus (GDM)*, is reserved for women who show abnormal glucose tolerance during pregnancy. Gestational diabetes is diagnosed in about 7% of all pregnancies in the United States, resulting in about 200,000 cases per year. (The range is 1% to 14%, depending on the population studied and the diagnostic criteria used.) It does not include diabetic women who become pregnant. Women with diabetes in the first trimester are classified as having type 2 diabetes. Gestational diabetes mellitus is diabetes diagnosed in the second or third trimester of pregnancy that is not clearly overt diabetes. Most gestational diabetic women have a normal glucose tolerance postpartum. Gestational diabetic patients must be reclassified 6 weeks after delivery into one of the following categories: diabetes mellitus, impaired fasting glucose, impaired glucose tolerance, or normoglycemia. Gestational diabetic patients have been put into a separate category because of the special clinical features of diabetes that develop during pregnancy and the complications associated with fetal involvement, such as neonatal macrosomia, large-for-gestational-age births, and shoulder dystocia. These women are also at a greater risk of developing diabetes 5 to 10 years after pregnancy.

There is a group of patients found to have an **impaired glucose tolerance (IGT)** or **impaired fasting glucose (IFG)**. These patients are often normally euglycemic, but develop hyperglycemia when challenged with an oral glucose tolerance test. In many of these patients, the glucose tolerance returns to normal or persists in the intermediate range for years. This intermediate stage between normal glucose homeostasis and diabetes is now known as *prediabetes*. It is now thought that patients with IGT or IFG are at a higher risk for developing type 1 or type 2 diabetes and cardiovascular disease in the future. The CDC has estimated that 84 million American adults over the age of 18 had prediabetes in 2015. Without lifestyle changes to improve their health, 15% to 30% of people with prediabetes will develop type 2 diabetes within 5 years. Categories of fasting plasma glucose (FPG) levels are the following:

- FPG less than 100 mg/dL = normal fasting glucose
- FPG at 100 mg/dL or greater but less than 126 mg/dL = IFG
- 2-hour plasma glucose level at 140 or greater but less than 199 mg/dL = IGT

Table 35.2 Criteria for Diagnosis of Diabetes Mellitus[a]

DIABETES MELLITUS	PREDIABETES
Hemoglobin A_{1c} ≥6.5% in certified laboratory using DCCT assay *Or*	5.7%-6.4%
Symptoms of diabetes and a casual[b] plasma glucose level ≥200 mg/dL *Or*	N/A
FPG level ≥126 mg/dL[c] *Or*	100-125 mg/dL (IFG)
2-hr plasma glucose level ≥200 mg/dL during an OGTT	140-199 mg/dL (IGT)

[a]In the absence of unequivocal hyperglycemia, these criteria should be confirmed by repeat testing on a different day. The OGTT is not recommended for routine clinical use but may be required in the evaluation of patients with IFG or when diabetes is still suspected despite a normal FPG, as with the postpartum evaluation of women with gestational diabetes mellitus.
[b]*Casual* is defined as any time of day without regard to time since last meal. The classic symptoms of diabetes include polyuria, polydipsia, and unexplained weight loss.
[c]*Fasting* is defined as no caloric intake for at least 8 hours.
DCCT, Diabetes Control and Complications Trial; *FPG*, fasting plasma glucose; *IFG*, impaired fasting glucose; *IGT*, impaired glucose tolerance; *OGTT*, oral glucose tolerance test.
Adapted from American Diabetes Association. Standards of medical care in diabetes—2018. *Diabetes Care.* 2018;41(suppl 1):S13-S27.

See Table 35.2 for criteria for the diagnosis of types 1 and 2 diabetes mellitus.

COMPLICATIONS OF DIABETES MELLITUS

Long-standing hyperglycemia and abnormalities in fat, carbohydrate, and protein metabolism lead to microvascular, macrovascular, and neuropathic complications. **Microvascular complications** are those that arise from destruction of capillaries in the eyes, kidneys, and peripheral tissues. Diabetes has become the leading cause of end-stage renal disease and adult blindness. **Macrovascular complications** are those associated with atherosclerosis of middle to large arteries, such as those in the heart and brain. Macrovascular complications, stroke, myocardial infarction, and peripheral vascular disease account for 75% to 80% of mortality in patients with diabetes. Complications of diabetes mellitus that often arise include the following (Fig. 35.1):

- Hypertension
- Cardiovascular disease (atherosclerosis) leading to myocardial infarction and stroke
- Retinopathy leading to blindness
- Renal disease leading to end-stage renal disease and the need for dialysis
- Peripheral arterial disease leading to nonhealing ulcers, infections, and lower extremity amputations
- Neuropathies with sexual dysfunction, bladder incontinence, paresthesias, and gastroparesis
- Periodontal disease with loss of teeth

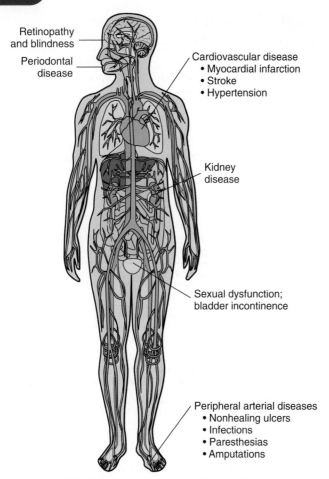

Fig. 35.1 Complications of diabetes mellitus.

Symptoms associated with complications of diabetes may be the first indication of the disease's presence. Patients may complain of weight gain or loss. Blurred vision may indicate hyperglycemia or diabetic retinopathy. Neuropathies may first be observed as numbness or tingling of the extremities (paresthesia), loss of sensation, orthostatic hypotension, impotence, vaginal yeast (candidiasis) infections, and difficulty in controlling urination (neurogenic bladder). Nonhealing ulcers of the lower extremities may indicate chronic vascular disease. Diabetic complications can be delayed or prevented with continuous normoglycemia, accomplished by monitoring blood glucose levels, drug therapy, and treatment of comorbid conditions as they arise.

TREATMENT OF DIABETES MELLITUS

Although the classification system of the National Diabetes Data Group and the World Health Organization Expert Committee on Diabetes was developed to facilitate clinical and epidemiologic investigation, the categorization of patients can also be helpful in determining general principles for therapy. Because a cure for diabetes mellitus is unknown at present, the minimal purpose of treatment is to prevent ketoacidosis and symptoms resulting from hyperglycemia. The long-term objective of control of the disease must involve mechanisms to stop the progression of the complications. Major determinants of success are a balanced diet, insulin or oral antidiabetic therapy, routine exercise, and good hygiene.

Patients with diabetes can lead full and satisfying lives. However, unrestricted diets and activities are not possible. Dietary treatment of diabetes using medical nutrition therapy (MNT) and exercise constitutes the basis for management of most patients, especially those with the type 2 form of the disease. With adequate weight reduction, exercise, and dietary control, patients may not require the use of exogenous insulin or oral antidiabetic drug therapy. People with type 1 diabetes will always require exogenous insulin injections and dietary control because the pancreas has lost the capacity to produce and secrete insulin. The aims of dietary control are the prevention of excessive postprandial hyperglycemia, the prevention of hypoglycemia (blood glucose level less than 60 mg/dL) in those patients being treated with antidiabetic agents or insulin, the achievement and maintenance of an ideal body weight, and a reduction of lipids and cholesterol. A return to normal weight is often accompanied by a reduction in hyperglycemia. The diet should also be adjusted to reduce elevated cholesterol and triglyceride levels in an attempt to retard the progression of atherosclerosis.

To help maintain adherence to dietary restrictions, the diet should be planned using the MNT recommendations of the ADA in relation to the patient's food preferences, economic status, occupation, and physical activity. Emphasis should be placed on what food the patient may have and what exchanges are acceptable. Food should be measured for balanced portions, and the patient should be cautioned not to omit meals or between-meal and bedtime snacks.

Patient education and reinforcement are extremely important to successful therapy. The intelligence and motivation of the diabetic patient and his or her awareness of potential complications contribute significantly to the ultimate outcome of the disease and the quality of life that the patient may lead.

All diabetic patients must receive adequate instruction on personal hygiene, especially regarding care of the feet, skin, and teeth. Infection is a common precipitating cause of ketosis and acidosis and must be treated promptly.

Patients with diabetes must also be aggressively treated for comorbid diseases (smoking cessation [including e-cigarettes], treatment of dyslipidemia, blood pressure control, antiplatelet therapy, influenza and pneumococcal vaccinations) to help prevent microvascular and macrovascular complications. The ADA and the American Association of Clinical Endocrinologists (AACE) have developed programs of intensive diabetes self-management that applies to type 1 and type 2 diabetes mellitus. These programs include the concepts of care, the responsibilities of the patient and the healthcare provider, and the appropriate intervals for

Table **35.3**	Treatment Goals for Diabetes and Comorbid Diseases[a]		
DISEASE	**MONITORING PARAMETER**	**ADA THERAPEUTIC GOALS**[b]	**AACE THERAPEUTIC GOALS**[c]
Diabetes	Hemoglobin A_{1c}	<7%[d]	≤6.5%
	Preprandial plasma glucose	80-130 mg/dL	<110 mg/dL
	Postprandial plasma glucose	<180 mg/dL	<140 mg/dL
Hypertension	Blood pressure	<140/90 mm Hg	<130/80 mm Hg
Dyslipidemia	LDL cholesterol	See Chapter 21, Table 21.1	<55 mg/dL for extreme risk patient
			<70 mg/dL for very high risk patient
			<100 mg/dL for high risk patient
	Non-HDL cholesterol		<80 mg/dL for extreme risk patient
			<100 mg/dL for very high risk patient
			<130 mg/dL for high risk patient
	HDL cholesterol	>40 mg/dL in males	
		>50 mg/dL in females	
	Triglycerides	<150 mg/dL	<150 mg/dL
Weight	Weight loss	BMI <25 kg/m² (see Chapter 20, Table 20.2)	BMI <25 kg/m² (see Chapter 20, Table 20.2)
		Asian Americans: BMI <23 kg/m²	Reduce weight at least 5%-10%; avoid weight gain

[a]Recommended by the American Diabetes Association (ADA) and the American Association of Clinical Endocrinologists (AACE).
[b]See American Diabetes Association. Standards of medical care in diabetes—2017. Diabetes Care. 2017;40(suppl 1):S75-S87.
[c]See Garber AJ, Abrahamson MJ, Barzilay, JI, et al. Consensus statement by the American Association of Clinical Endocrinologists and American College of Endocrinology on the Comprehensive Type 2 Diabetes Management Algorithm—2017 Executive Summary. *Endocr Pract.* 2017;23:207-238.
[d]The goal hemoglobin A_{1c} level for patients in general is less than 6.5% to 7%, but more or less stringent goals may be appropriate for individual patients (<6.5%-<8%). The ideal goal for individual patients is as close to normal (<6%) as possible without significant hypoglycemia.
BMI, Body mass index; *HDL,* high-density lipoprotein; *LDL,* low-density lipoprotein.

laboratory testing and follow-up. Patient education, understanding, and direct participation by the patient in his or her treatment are key components of long-term success in disease management. **Intensive therapy** describes a comprehensive program of diabetes care that includes patient-centered communication, a team approach to care, self-monitoring of blood glucose four or more times daily, MNT, exercise, and, for those patients with type 1 diabetes, three or more insulin injections daily or use of an insulin pump for continuous insulin infusion. See Table 35.3 for the treatment goals recommended by the ADA and the AACE.

DRUG THERAPY FOR DIABETES MELLITUS

"Hyperglycemia defines diabetes, and glycemic control is fundamental to diabetes management" (ADA, 2018, p. S59). The primary treatment goal of type 1 and type 2 diabetes is normalization of blood glucose levels. Insulin is required to control type 1 diabetes and other types of diabetes in patients whose blood glucose cannot be controlled by an MNT diet, exercise, weight reduction, or other antidiabetic agents. Patients normally controlled with other antidiabetic agents require insulin during situations of increased physiologic and psychological stress, such as pregnancy, surgery, and infections. The dosage of insulin is usually adjusted according to the blood glucose levels. The patient should test the blood

glucose level before each meal and at bedtime while the insulin and food intake are being regulated.

The ADA now recommends that patients with prediabetes be treated to prevent or delay the onset of type 2 diabetes. Patients should be referred to an effective ongoing support program targeting weight loss of 7% of body weight and increasing physical activity to at least 150 minutes per week of moderate activity such as walking. The 2018 ADA standards of care also recommend that people should be encouraged to limit the amount of time they spend being sedentary by breaking up extended amounts of time (>90 min) spent sitting. Metformin therapy should be considered for treatment of prediabetes, especially in those patients whose body mass index (BMI) is greater than 35 kg/m², in those who are older than 60 years, and in women with prior GDM. Patients should be monitored at least annually for the development of diabetes mellitus.

Other antidiabetic agents are used in the therapy of type 2 diabetes. They are recommended only for those patients whose diabetes cannot be controlled by an MNT diet and exercise alone and who are not prone to develop ketosis, acidosis, or infections. Patients most likely to benefit from treatment are those who have developed diabetes after age 40 and who require less than 40 units of insulin daily.

A combination of antidiabetic agents working by different mechanisms is often required to control hyperglycemia successfully (Fig. 35.2):

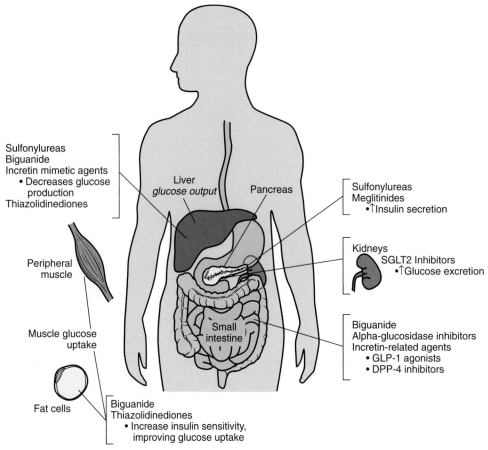

Fig. 35.2 Sites and mechanisms of action of antidiabetic agents.

- *Biguanide:* The only biguanide available in the United States is metformin. Unless contraindicated, it is the initial drug of choice for treatment of type 2 diabetes. Metformin decreases hepatic glucose production by inhibiting glycogenolysis and gluconeogenesis, reducing absorption of glucose from the small intestine, and increasing insulin sensitivity, which improves glucose uptake in peripheral muscle and adipose cells. The net result is a significant decrease in fasting and postprandial blood glucose and hemoglobin A_{1c} (A_{1c}) concentrations.
- *Secretagogues:* The sulfonylureas (e.g., glyburide, glipizide, glimepiride) and the meglitinides (repaglinide, nateglinide) stimulate the pancreas to secrete more insulin. The sulfonylureas also diminish hepatic glucose production and metabolism of insulin by the liver. The net effect is a normalization of insulin and glucose levels.
- *Thiazolidinediones (TZDs):* The TZDs (e.g., pioglitazone, rosiglitazone) increase tissue sensitivity to insulin, causing greater glucose uptake in muscle, adipose, and liver tissue. They also diminish glucose production by the liver.
- *Alpha-glucosidase inhibitors:* Acarbose and miglitol inhibit enzymes in the small intestine that metabolize complex carbohydrates. This slows the absorption of carbohydrates, reducing postprandial hyperglycemia.

- *Sodium-glucose cotransporter 2 (SGLT2) inhibitors*: These agents block the reabsorption of glucose by the kidneys, causing the sugar to be excreted in the urine, lowering blood glucose. The SGLT2 inhibitors are canagliflozin, dapagliflozin, empagliflozin, and ertugliflozin.
- *Incretin-related therapy:* It is thought that patients with type 2 diabetes have a suppressed incretin hormone system. The incretin hormones act in the gastrointestinal tract to control blood glucose levels by enhancing insulin secretion, suppressing glucagon secretion from the liver, suppressing glucose output from the liver, delaying gastric emptying (thus slowing carbohydrate and lipid absorption), reducing postprandial hyperglycemia, reducing appetite, and maintaining beta cell function. There are currently two classes of agents that increase incretin activity: (1) incretin mimetics (the glucagon-like peptide-1 [GLP-1] agonists dulaglutide, exenatide, exenatide ER, liraglutide, lixisenatide, and semaglutide) and (2) the dipeptidyl peptidase-4 (DPP-4) inhibitors (alogliptin, sitagliptin, saxagliptin, and linagliptin).

Initial antidiabetic therapy for type 2 diabetes is highly dependent on the patient's success with lifestyle modification and diet control. A consensus statement endorsed by the ADA recommends metformin in combination with MNT and exercise as initial treatment

Table 35.4 Summary of Physiologic Effects of Antidiabetic Agents

DRUG	INSULIN SECRETION	DECREASE IN FASTING BLOOD GLUCOSE LEVEL	REDUCTION IN HEMOGLOBIN A$_{1c}$ LEVEL	WEIGHT GAIN
Insulin	Decrease	Significant	Significant	Yes
Sulfonylureas	Increase	40-60 mg/dL	1%-2%	Yes
Meglitinides	Increase	30 mg/dL	1.1%	Yes
Biguanide (metformin)	No change	53 mg/dL	1%-2%	No; mild
Thiazolidinediones	No change	25-55 mg/dL	0.5%-1.4%	Yes
Alpha-glucosidase inhibitors	No change	20-30 mg/dL	0.5%-0.8%	No
Glucagon-like peptide-1 agonists	Increase	—	1.0%-1.5%	No
Dipeptidyl peptidase-4 inhibitors	Increase	—	0.5%-0.8%	No
Sodium-glucose cotransporter 2 inhibitors	Decrease	—	0.7%-1%	No

Data from Feld S. The American Association of Clinical Endocrinologists medical guidelines for the management of diabetes mellitus: the ACCE system of intensive diabetes self-management—2002 update. *Endocr Pract.* 2002;8(suppl 1):S52; Nathan DM, Buse JB, Davidson MB, et al. Medical management of hyperglycemia in type 2 diabetes mellitus: a consensus algorithm for the initiation and adjustment of therapy. *Diabetolgia.* 2009;52:17-30; Clinical Resource, Comparison of GLP-1 Agonists. *Pharmacist's Letter/Prescriber's Letter.* January 2017; Clinical Resource, Drugs for Type 2 DM. *Pharmacist's Letter/Prescriber's Letter.* July 2017; U.S. Department of Health and Human Services and U.S. Department of Agriculture. *2015-2020 Dietary Guidelines for Americans.* 8th ed. December 2015 Available at: https://health.gov/dietaryguidelines/2015/guidelines/.

of type 2 diabetes mellitus. If the goal A$_{1c}$ level less than 7% has not been achieved with this monotherapy within 3 to 6 months and the patient does not have atherosclerotic cardiovascular disease, add another agent such as a sulfonylurea, a TZD, an incretin-related DPP-4 inhibitor, or GLP-1 agonist, or basal insulin should be added based on the individual patient. If the patient has atherosclerotic cardiovascular disease, add an agent proven to reduce cardiovascular events and/or cardiovascular mortality, such as canagliflozin, empagliflozin, liraglutide, and semaglutide. If the A$_{1c}$ level is not at goal, another member of a drug class not already being used in the initial therapy should be added. An alpha-glucosidase inhibitor may be added if postprandial hyperglycemia is a problem. See Table 35.4 for a comparison of antidiabetic agents and their effects on lowering blood glucose levels and A$_{1c}$ concentrations.

❖ NURSING IMPLICATIONS FOR PATIENTS WITH DIABETES MELLITUS

A major challenge in nursing is to teach the recently diagnosed diabetic patient all the necessary information to manage self-care and the disease process and to prevent complications. The patient must be taught the entire therapeutic regimen—diet, activity level, blood or urine testing, medication, self-injection techniques, prevention of complications, illness management, and effective management of hypoglycemia or hyperglycemia. Patient education may begin in the hospital and continue for several weeks in the outpatient setting. Dietitians, nurses, diabetic nurse educators, and pharmacists are all actively involved in educating the patient and family. A referral to the ADA serves as an excellent resource in the community for the patient and family. Many diabetic patients have difficulty understanding the critical balance that must be maintained among

the dietary prescription, prescribed medication, and maintenance of general health. All are important to the control and effective management of the disease process.

◆ Assessment and Implementation
Description of current symptoms
- Ask the reasons for seeking the current appointment or admission.

Patient's understanding of diabetes mellitus
- Assess the individual's current knowledge of the treatment of diabetes mellitus. Gather additional data about the person's current educational needs with regard to self-management of the disease process. Answer questions that the patient has, including rationale for actions being recommended.
- Will other family members or significant others be providing part of the care or participating in the health education portion of the individual's care?
- Patients who are readmitted must be assessed for the understanding of the treatment regimen and for adherence with the prescribed diet, medications, and exercise.
- For pregnant women, risk assessment for GDM should be performed at the first prenatal visit. High-risk women who have an initial negative testing for diabetes should be retested between 24 and 28 weeks of gestation.

Psychosocial assessment
- *Mental status:* Ask specific information to evaluate the patient's current level of consciousness, alertness, comprehension, and appropriateness of responses. Evaluate the person's judgment capabilities and ability to solve problems about the management of the diabetes.

- *Adaptation to disease:* Ask specifically about the person's adjustment to the diagnosis of diabetes mellitus; in a recently diagnosed individual, identify prior coping mechanisms used successfully to deal with life events.
- *Feelings:* Assess for fears and the person's perspective of the impact of the disease on his or her life. Encourage expression of the patient's feelings and concerns; address the patient's concerns first. Involve support personnel, as appropriate, in the delivery of care or planning for home management of the diabetes.
- *Support system:* Obtain information regarding who can provide support for the patient. Does the individual live alone? What effect does the disease have on other members of the family structure (e.g., children who are diabetic, people with renal or visual complications)? Does the patient participate in a support group for patients with diabetes?

Nutrition

- Is the patient on a prescribed MNT diet? The recently diagnosed diabetic patient requires a thorough nutritional assessment. Information collected by the nurse or dietitian should include identification of the patient's average daily diet, the ability and willingness to prepare foods, food budget, and level of daily activity and exercise.
- Ask about diet prescription—total daily calories and distribution pattern of carbohydrates, fats, and proteins.
- Have there been any problems encountered in purchasing or preparing the foods? Has it been difficult to comply with the diet? If so, what are the problems encountered?
- How much alcohol is consumed and how often?
- Has the individual experienced any weight loss or gain recently?
- If the patient is a child, obtain data relating to the individual's growth and development patterns.

Activity and exercise

- Does the individual experience weakness or fatigue with daily activities? Does the patient get regular exercise? What type, intensity, and duration is the exercise? Has there been any significant variation in the degree of exercise recently?
- Has the patient made any adjustments in the insulin, oral antidiabetic agents, or diet to offset an increase or decrease in exercise?
- Has there been a change in occupation that has affected the level of exercise?

Medications

- What medications have been prescribed, and what is the degree of adherence with the regimen? Monitor for common and serious adverse effects and document associated monitoring parameters in the medical records (e.g., blood glucose, ketone testing). If the patient is taking insulin, ask specifically about the type and dose being taken and the times of administration. Assess the ability and accuracy to self-administer injections. If a family member gives the insulin, assess his or her ability and accuracy in giving injections.
- What over-the-counter medications (including herbal medicines) does the patient take and how often?

Monitoring. Ask the patient to bring a record of self-monitoring of insulin or antidiabetic agents taken, as well as any blood glucose testing or A_{1c} testing that was done. Has the patient done any testing for ketones? If so, what were the results? Other tests to be performed periodically include the fasting lipid profile, which includes measurement of lipid levels (high-density lipoprotein [HDL], low-density lipoprotein [LDL] cholesterol, triglycerides), as well as serum creatinine and microalbuminuria. When hypertension is present, perform a urinalysis and check for albuminuria. If protein is negative, microalbumin testing should be performed to determine the presence of protein in the urine. Annual monitoring of LDL, triglyceride, and A_{1c} levels is recommended.

◆ Physical Assessment

Generally, data are collected about all body systems to serve as a baseline for subsequent evaluations throughout the course of treatment. Periodic focused assessments are completed to detect signs and symptoms of complications commonly associated with diabetes mellitus.

- *Hypoglycemia:* Have there been any episodes of hypoglycemia? If so, obtain details of the occurrences (e.g., has the patient eaten the prescribed diet, taken the prescribed medications, or altered the exercise level?). If a hypoglycemic reaction occurs, notify the team leader or primary nurse, who will then contact the healthcare provider. The underlying cause of the hypoglycemia must be identified to prevent further occurrences. If in doubt about whether a hypoglycemic reaction is taking place, treat as though a hypoglycemic reaction is occurring to prevent neurologic damage from prolonged reduction in glucose to the nerve cells (e.g., brain cells). Record all prescription and over-the-counter medications being taken to assess whether any drug interactions may be causing the hypoglycemia.
- *Hyperglycemia:* With any hyperglycemic reaction, notify the team leader or primary nurse, who will then contact the healthcare provider. The goals of treatment include maintaining normal fluid and electrolyte balance and restoring a normal serum glucose level.
- *Illnesses, stress:* Have there been any recent illnesses, infections, or stressful events? If so, what treatments have been initiated? Ask specifically about any sores on the skin and feet, periodontal disease, and occurrence of urinary tract or vaginal (candidiasis) infections.

- *Vascular changes:* Obtain baseline vital signs. Does the person have any symptoms of, or is the patient being treated for, cerebrovascular, peripheral vascular, or cardiovascular disease (including hypertension) or diabetic retinopathy or nephropathy? Obtain a current history of the patient's blood pressure and details of any medications being taken to treat hypertension.
- *Neuropathy:* Ask about specific symptoms of paresthesias (numbness or tingling sensations), foot injuries and ulcerations, diarrhea, postural hypotension, impotence, or neurogenic bladder.
- *Smoking:* Obtain a history of smoking and tobacco use from all patients with diabetes mellitus.

◆ **Patient Education**

The ADA has developed areas of diabetic education. Not all aspects of the care outlined in these recommendations are presented in the sample teaching plan for a patient with diabetes mellitus taking one type of insulin (see Chapter 5, Box 5.2: "Sample Teaching Plan for a Patient With Diabetes Mellitus Taking One Type of Insulin"). The recommendations must be adapted to the individual's needs. It may not be possible to teach the entire program during the hospitalization period. Teach the individual specifics regarding the type of diabetes that has been diagnosed.

- Type 1 diabetes mellitus results from damage to the beta cells of the pancreas, where insulin is normally produced. Insulin is needed to transport the glucose required by the body cells from the bloodstream to the individual cells to be used as an energy source. Without beta cells, no insulin is produced and the glucose accumulates in the blood (hyperglycemia).
- Type 1 diabetes mellitus requires the administration of insulin injections to replace the insulin that the body is no longer able to make. The patient must follow a prescribed diet and exercise program, perform glucose testing, and, when hyperglycemia is present, test for ketones in the urine.
- Type 2 diabetes mellitus is an illness characterized by abnormal beta cell function, resistance to insulin action, and increased hepatic glucose production. Type 2 diabetes mellitus requires a prescribed diet and exercise program, weight loss to a near-ideal body level, glucose testing, and an oral antidiabetic agent or antihyperglycemic agent if the diabetes cannot be managed with diet and exercise alone. During times of illness, or if the oral treatment stops being effective, insulin may be required. Special adjustments may be required for patients who are pregnant or nursing.

Psychological adjustment

- When first diagnosed, the patient may experience varying degrees of grief, anger, denial, or acceptance. Let the patient express these concerns, and address those items that are considered to be of greatest importance first.

- Encourage the idea that the patient can control most aspects of diabetes by careful management of diet, medications, and activities. Having a sense of control is important to everyone. Stress that learning to manage the disease process is the best long-term approach.
- Discuss the individual's lifestyle, travel, work or school schedules, and activities and individualize the care needs.
- Discuss the need for continued regular monitoring of the diabetes to minimize the effect that the disease may have on the patient and family.

Smoking. Healthcare providers should emphasize the need for smoking (including e-cigarettes) cessation as a priority of care for all patients with diabetes.

Nutrition

- Diet is used alone or in combination with insulin or oral antidiabetic agents to control diabetes mellitus. The patient with diabetes, whether type 1 or 2, must follow a prescribed diet to achieve optimal control of the disease.
- The dietary prescription is based on the nutritional and energy requirements necessary to maintain an appropriate weight and lifestyle and normal growth and development. Diabetic patients are encouraged to maintain a reasonable body weight based on height, gender, and frame size.
- Medical nutrition therapy is now being recommended for patients with diabetes. Standardized calorie-level meal patterns based on exchange lists have traditionally been used to plan meals for hospitalized patients. Other meal planning systems include menus based on the *2015–2020 Dietary Guidelines for Americans* (US Department of Health and Human Services and US Department of Agriculture, 2015), regular hospital menus, individualized meal plans, or menus using carbohydrate counting. A new system, called the *consistent-carbohydrate diabetes meal plan,* is being developed that uses meal plans without a specific calorie level; instead, it incorporates a consistent carbohydrate content for each meal and snack. The meal plan also includes appropriate fat and protein modifications and emphasizes consistent timing of meals and snacks. A typical day's meals and snacks provide 1500 to 2000 calories with 45% to 65% of the calories from carbohydrate, 10% to 35% from protein, and 20% to 35% from fat. If a patient's nutritional needs are more or less than provided by these meal plans, individualized adjustments may be required. Patients who often require adjustments include children, adolescents, metabolically stressed patients, pregnant women, and older adult patients.
- Weight loss is recommended for all adults who are overweight (BMI = 25 to 29.9 kg/m^2) or obese (BMI ≥30 kg/m^2) or who have or are at risk for developing

type 2 diabetes. The primary approach for achieving weight loss is therapeutic lifestyle change, which includes a reduction in energy (food) intake and/or an increase in physical activity. A moderate decrease in caloric balance (500 to 1000 kcal/day) will result in slow but progressive weight loss (1 to 2 lb/wk). For most patients, weight loss diets should supply at least 1000 to 1200 kcal/day for women and 1200 to 1600 kcal/day for men.

- Additional goals for MNT include maintaining a blood glucose level in the normal range to reduce the risk of complications of diabetes, a normal lipid profile to reduce the risk for microvascular disease, and normal blood pressure levels to reduce the risk for vascular disease.

- The ADA no longer endorses any single meal plan or specified percentages of macronutrients as it has in the past. The Institute of Medicine and the ADA recommend, in general, that the diet be composed of 45% to 65% carbohydrates, 15% to 20% protein (0.8 to 1 g protein/kg of body weight), and no more than 30% fat. Monounsaturated and polyunsaturated fats should be the primary fat sources; saturated fats should be limited to no more than 10% of the diet and cholesterol intake to 300 mg or less daily. *Trans*-fatty acids should be avoided when possible. Including high-fiber foods in the diet (e.g., legumes, oats, barley) assists in lowering both blood glucose and blood cholesterol levels. Reduced sodium, alcohol, and caffeine consumption is also advisable (see also Chapter 46). The ADA has several cookbooks and pamphlets on nutrition available for the diabetic person.

- Patients with diabetes, as well as all individuals, need to be encouraged to consume an adequate intake of vitamins and minerals from natural food sources.

- Inclusion of sucrose is now permitted in limited amounts in the diabetic diet; however, the amount eaten must be calculated as part of the carbohydrate intake for the day. Meal plans such as "no concentrated sweets," "no added sugar," "low sugar," and "liberal diabetic diets" are no longer appropriate. These diets do not reflect the diabetes nutrition recommendations and unnecessarily restrict sucrose. Such meal plans may perpetuate the false notion that simply restricting sucrose-sweetened foods will improve blood glucose control.

- The US Food and Drug Administration has approved the use of four artificial sweeteners as sugar substitutes: saccharin, aspartame (NutraSweet), sucralose (Splenda), and acesulfame potassium.

- Patients with diabetes should adhere to the same guidelines for ingestion of alcohol as for all Americans—no more than two drinks daily for men and one drink daily for women. People with good control of their diabetes may ingest alcohol in moderation. However, drinking can result in hypoglycemia or hyperglycemia in diabetics. The effects of alcohol are influenced by the amount ingested, if ingested on an empty stomach, or if used chronically or excessively. Many alcoholic beverages are high in sugar and should be used with caution; light beer or dry wines are alternatives. One drink is defined as 12 ounces of beer, 5 ounces of wine, or 1.5 ounces of distilled spirits, each of which contains 15 grams of alcohol. Because alcohol affects the blood sugar, it may be prudent to test the blood glucose level before and after drinking to identify how the alcohol reacts in a particular patient. Abstinence is recommended for pregnant patients, those with known medical problems aggravated by its use, and those with a history of alcohol abuse.

- Dietary considerations for children and adolescents with type 1 or 2 diabetes are similar to the needs for all other children. They need to maintain a steady intake of a balanced diet aimed at maintaining normal growth and development. It is important to obtain height and weight values and to compare these to the normal growth curve found on charts to ascertain whether the dietary intake is adequate, deficient, or excessive. The individual's meal planning must be done in such a way as to accommodate irregular meal times and schedules and the varying activity levels of the child or adolescent.

- All women have similar nutritional needs during pregnancy and lactation whether they have diabetes or not. A woman with GDM is given education on food choices that are appropriate for normal weight gain, normoglycemia, and absence of ketones. Some patients with GDM may require a modest restriction in carbohydrates.

- In older adults, a change in body weight of more than 10 pounds or 10% of the body weight in less than 6 months is considered sufficient reason to investigate for nutrition-related causes. In general, older people with diabetes in long-term care settings tend to be underweight rather than overweight. Administering a daily vitamin supplement to older adults, especially those with decreased energy intake, may be advisable. Specialized diets do not appear to be beneficial to the older adult in a long-term care setting, where food choices are decidedly limited. It is preferable to make medication adjustments to control blood glucose rather than implement food restrictions in the long-term care setting. Physical activity should be encouraged.

Activity and exercise

- Maintenance of a normal lifestyle is to be encouraged. This includes exercise and activities enjoyed by the individual. The normal daily energy level is used in determining the dietary and medication requirements for the patient. The ADA recommends that initial therapy be modest and based on the patient's willingness and ability, gradually increasing the duration and frequency to 30 to 45 minutes of moderate aerobic activity 3 to 5 days per week (150 minutes per week) when possible. Greater activity levels of at least 1 hour daily of moderate (walking) or 30 minutes daily of vigorous (jogging) activity may be needed to achieve successful long-term weight loss.

- As with all individuals who are about to undertake exercise, a proper period of warm-up and cool-down consisting of 5 to 10 minutes of aerobic activity at a low intensity should be done. It is very important to maintain proper foot care in a diabetic patient who is to start exercising. Use silica gel or air insoles, as well as polyester-cotton blend socks to prevent blisters, and keep the feet as dry as possible. Visible inspection of the feet surfaces before and after exercise is an important component of an exercise regimen and is especially important for diabetic patients who already have peripheral neuropathy. Persons with loss of protective sensation should not use step exercises, jogging, prolonged walking, or treadmills as an exercise regimen. Rather, they should substitute swimming, bicycling, rowing, chair exercises, arm exercises, or other non–weight-bearing exercises.
- Just as it is important for the patient to maintain a certain diet, it is equally important to maintain a certain activity level. Patients who suddenly increase or decrease their activity level are susceptible to developing episodes of hyperglycemia or hypoglycemia. Both dietary and medication prescriptions may require adjustment if patients do not plan to resume the previous exercise level. Patients should consult with the prescriber before initiating an exercise program.
- Additional self-monitoring of the blood glucose level may be advisable before, during, and approximately 30 minutes after exercise to provide the prescriber with data to analyze regarding the effects of exercise on the individual's blood glucose level. The ADA recommends that the diabetic patient not exercise if his or her glucose level is above 250 mg/dL. Conversely, exercising with hypoglycemia is not advisable. A snack high in carbohydrates (10 to 20 g) should be taken before exercising if the blood glucose level is less than 100 mg/dL.
- Exercise helps the cells use glucose; therefore exercise lowers the glucose level.
- Drink sufficient fluids without caffeine when exercising to prevent dehydration.
- Stop exercising if feeling weak, sick, or dizzy or if experiencing any type of pain.

Medication

- Insulin or oral antidiabetic agent therapy may be required to control diabetes mellitus. No changes in therapy should be made without medical supervision.
- A variety of combinations of insulin or insulin and oral antidiabetic agents may be used to provide control of the blood glucose level. The goal of therapy is to consistently maintain the blood glucose level within normal range. Administration schedules have

evolved over the years to accomplish this goal. The schedules commonly used are as follows:

1. Divided doses of intermediate-acting insulin (two-thirds in the morning, one-third in the evening before dinner)
2. A combination of rapid- or short-acting and intermediate-acting insulin in the morning, followed by rapid- or short-acting insulin at dinner and intermediate-acting insulin before bedtime
3. Rapid- or short-acting insulin before each meal and intermediate-acting or long-acting insulin at bedtime
4. Rapid-acting or short-acting and long-acting insulin before breakfast, rapid-acting or short-acting insulin before lunch, and rapid-acting or short-acting and long-acting insulin again before dinner
5. Continuous infusion of rapid- or short-acting insulin using a small, portable insulin infusion pump

- The regimen chosen depends on each person's response to medications, schedule of daily activities, and compliance with blood glucose monitoring, insulin injections, and diet.
- Medication preparation, dosage, frequency, storage, and refilling should be discussed and taught in detail. See Fig. 10.3 for administration of subcutaneous injections and Fig. 9.26 for mixing of insulins. Also, discuss proper disposal of used syringes and needles in the home setting.
- Be certain that the patient understands how to refill prescriptions for insulin or oral antidiabetic agents. When purchasing insulin, ask the patient to double-check the type, concentration (usually U-100), and expiration date. Insulin types should not be changed without the approval of the prescribing healthcare provider. The insulin should be stored in the refrigerator (not the freezer) before use. Once it is opened and being used, it can be stored at room temperature for up to 1 month. The patient or nurse should mark the date on the bottle when first opened and used. The patient should always have a spare bottle of each type of prescribed insulin available for use.
- When a patient is experiencing an acute illness, injury, or surgery, hyperglycemia may result. When ill, the patient should continue with the regular diet plan and increase noncaloric fluids such as broth, water, and other decaffeinated drinks. The patient should continue to take the oral agents and/or insulin as prescribed and monitor the blood glucose level at least every 4 hours. If the glucose level is higher than 240 mg/dL, urine should be tested for ketones (see Urine Testing for Ketones later in this section). If the patient is unable to eat the normal caloric intake, he or she should continue to take the same dose of oral agents and/or insulin prescribed, but supplement food intake with carbohydrate-containing fluids such as soups, regular juices, and decaffeinated soft drinks.

The healthcare provider should be notified immediately if the patient is unable to "keep anything down." Patients should understand that medication for diabetes, including insulin, should not be withheld during times of illness because counterregulatory mechanisms in the body often increase the blood glucose level dramatically. Food intake is also necessary because the body requires extra energy to deal with the stress of illness. Extra insulin may also be necessary to meet the demand of illness.

- If pregnancy is suspected, the patient should consult an obstetrician as soon as possible about continuing and adjusting medication therapy during pregnancy.
- Patients with diabetes should receive an annual influenza vaccination and at least one pneumococcal vaccination before the age of 65. The pneumococcal vaccination should be repeated at least 5 years later and after the patient turns 65 years of age.

Hypoglycemia. Hypoglycemia, or low blood sugar, can occur from too much insulin, a sulfonylurea, insufficient food intake to cover the insulin given, imbalances caused by vomiting and diarrhea, and excessive exercise without additional carbohydrate intake.

Symptoms. Recognize and assess early symptoms of hypoglycemia; these include nervousness, tremors, headache, apprehension, sweating, cold and clammy skin, and hunger. If uncorrected, hypoglycemia progresses to blurring of vision, lack of coordination, incoherence, coma, and death. Children younger than 6 to 7 years may not have the cognitive abilities to recognize and initiate self-treatment of hypoglycemia.

Treatment. If the patient is conscious and able to swallow, give 2 to 4 ounces of fruit juice, 1 cup of skim milk, or 4 ounces of a nondiet soft drink, or give a piece of candy such as a gumdrop. An alternative is to carry a glucose-containing product (e.g., Glutose gel, Dex4 glucose tablets) and take as recommended when hypoglycemic. Repeat in 10 to 15 minutes if relief of symptoms is not evident. Do not use hard candy if there is a danger of aspiration. If the patient is unconscious, having a seizure, or unable to swallow, administer glucagon or 20 to 50 mL of glucose 50% intravenously. (People taking insulin should have a family member, significant other, or coworker who is able to administer glucagon.) Obtain a blood glucose level at the time of hypoglycemia, if possible.

Hyperglycemia. Hyperglycemia (elevated blood sugar) occurs when the glucose available in the body cannot be transported into the cells for use because of a lack of insulin necessary for the transport mechanism. Hyperglycemia can be caused by nonadherence, overeating, acute illness, or acute infection.

Symptoms. Symptoms of hyperglycemia are headache, nausea and vomiting, abdominal pain, dizziness, rapid pulse, rapid shallow respirations, and a fruity odor to the breath from acetone. If untreated, hyperglycemia may also cause coma and death. Glucose levels higher than 240 mg/dL and ketones present in the urine are early indications of diabetic ketoacidosis.

Treatment. Treatment of hyperglycemia often requires hospitalization with close monitoring of hydration status; administration of intravenous (IV) fluids and insulin; and blood glucose, urine ketone, and potassium levels. Hyperglycemia usually occurs because of another cause; therefore the problem, often an infection, must also be identified and treated.

Prevention. The risk of hyperglycemia can be minimized by taking the prescribed dose of insulin or oral antidiabetic agent; adhering to the prescribed diet and exercise; reporting fevers, infection, or prolonged vomiting or diarrhea to the healthcare provider; and maintaining an accurate written record for the healthcare provider to analyze to determine the individual patient's needs. Self-monitoring of blood glucose results and evaluation of urine ketones can provide the prescriber with valuable information to manage the treatment of the individual effectively.

Self-monitoring of blood glucose

- Home blood glucose monitoring (self-monitoring) is an accepted practice for managing diabetes mellitus. It is used to evaluate the degree of control of the blood glucose. It can also be used to evaluate when additional insulin must be taken or to determine the effect of exercise on insulin needs.
- Educate the individual using the equipment for self-monitoring that will be used at home. Teach the person all details of the operation, including calibration, care, handling, and cleansing of the glucose monitor.
- The best time to check blood glucose levels is just before meals, 1 to 2 hours after meals, before bed, and between 2 and 3 AM. The prescriber will give specific instructions regarding how often and when glucose testing should be done. When the person is ill, it is important to increase the frequency of glucose monitoring.
- A small sample of capillary blood is obtained, generally using an automatic finger-sticking lancet. The blood sample is applied to a reagent strip, which is then placed into an electronic device that reads the amount of color change and converts this into a numerical value representing the blood glucose level. There also are meters and sensors that do not use reagent strips for delivering the glucose results. "Talking" glucometers are on the market for those who are visually impaired. Written records of the blood glucose results should be maintained and taken to all follow-up visits with the healthcare provider for analysis.

Urine testing for ketones

- Teach the patient to perform urine testing for ketones at least four times daily during times of stress, with an infection, or when signs or symptoms of hyperglycemia are suspected or present. (Ketone testing should be done when the blood glucose level is consistently higher than 300 mg/dL, during pregnancy, or when symptoms of ketoacidosis, such as nausea, vomiting, or abdominal pain, are present.) The healthcare provider may suggest additional times when ketones should be monitored, depending on the type of regimen prescribed for controlling blood glucose. An accurate written record of the results should be maintained. Guidelines for reporting abnormal results to the prescriber should be discussed at the time of discharge. First morning urine tests from pregnant women and up to 30% of first morning specimens in individuals who are fasting may have positive readings. Several drugs also may interfere with the results of ketone urine testing, giving false-positive values. Blood ketone testing methods that quantify beta-hydroxybutyric acid are available for home testing and are preferred over urine ketone testing for monitoring and diagnosing ketoacidosis.

- Suggest that ketone testing be initiated when an illness occurs and the serum glucose is elevated above the individual's usual range. Explain when to call the healthcare provider. Suggest increasing fluid intake whenever ketones are positive.

Other laboratory glucose testing

- The A_{1c} test measures the percentage of hemoglobin that has been irreversibly glycosylated because of high blood glucose levels. This provides a reflection of the average blood glucose level attained over the past 2 to 3 months. This test is used in conjunction with home glucose self-monitoring to assess overall glycemic control.
- The fructosamine test measures the amount of glucose bonded to the protein fructosamine. This reflects the average blood level attained over the past 1 to 3 weeks.

Complications associated with diabetes mellitus

Cardiovascular disease. Men and women with diabetes are at an increased risk of dying from complications of cardiovascular disease. Aspirin therapy is a primary prevention strategy for both diabetic men and women with type 1 or type 2 diabetes who have a 10-year cardiovascular risk greater than 10%. This includes most men over 50 years of age or women over 60 years of age who have at least one additional major risk factor (family history of cardiovascular disease, hypertension, smoking, dyslipidemia, or albuminuria). Enteric-coated aspirin in doses of 75 to 162 mg daily is taken by individuals who do *not* have an aspirin sensitivity. Aspirin therapy is no longer recommended for those who do not meet the criteria.

Peripheral vascular disease. The person with diabetes mellitus is more likely to suffer from peripheral vascular disease than the general population. Reduced blood supply to the extremities may result in intermittent claudication, numbness and tingling, and a greater likelihood of foot infection. The following are

symptoms the patient should look for in caring for the extremities:

- *Color:* Observe the color of each hand, finger, leg, and foot; report cyanosis or reddish-blue discolorations. Inspect the skin of the extremities for any signs of ulceration.
- *Temperature:* Feel the temperature in each hand, finger, leg, and foot. Report paleness and coldness. Note that these symptoms will be increased if the limbs are elevated above the level of the heart.
- *Edema:* Report edema, its extent, and whether relieved or unchanged when in a dependent position.
- *Limb pain:* Pain with exercise that is relieved by rest may be from claudication and should be reported to the healthcare provider.
- *Care of the extremities:* Prevent ulcers, injury, and infection in the lower extremities with meticulous regular care. Use lotion to prevent dryness. Inspect the feet daily for any signs of skin breakdown or loss of sensation; report to the healthcare provider and do not attempt to self-treat. The presence of redness, warmth, or calluses may signal an impending breakdown. Always cut toenails straight across and seek foot care from a podiatrist if problems are noted.

Visual alterations. Visual changes are common in the patient with diabetes mellitus. These patients frequently suffer from blurred vision associated with an elevated blood glucose level. Any diabetic person with intermittently blurred vision should contact the healthcare provider for a check of the blood glucose level. Once the hyperglycemia is controlled, the blurred vision usually resolves.

Blindness. In advanced stages of diabetes mellitus, the patient may suffer from changes (microangiopathies) in the small blood vessels of the eyes. Retinal hemorrhages, degeneration of retinal vascular tissue, cataracts, and eventual blindness may occur. The patient with diabetes should have regular eye examinations to allow early treatment of any apparent alterations.

Renal disease. People with diabetes mellitus are more susceptible to urinary tract infections; therefore symptoms such as burning on urination or low back pain should be evaluated promptly. Patients are also more susceptible to renal disease. Routine periodic monitoring of protein in the urine determines the presence of renal disease. In patients with type 1 or 2 diabetes who have microalbuminuria, even a small reduction in protein intake has been shown to improve the glomerular filtration rate and reduce urinary albumin excretion rates.

Infection. Any type of infection can cause a significant loss of control of diabetes mellitus. Patients should check themselves carefully for any signs of redness, tenderness, swelling, or drainage that may occur when there is any break in the skin. Patients should be taught to report immediately early signs of infection, such as fever or sore throat. During an infection the dosage of insulin may require an adjustment to compensate for a change in metabolic rate, diet, and exercise. Contact the health-care provider for specific directions.

Neuropathies. Explain to appropriate individuals the complication of degeneration of nerves when it exists. Ask the patient to describe sensations (e.g., numbness, tingling) in the extremities. Inspect the feet for blisters, ulcerations, ingrown toenails, or sores. Occasionally, the patient will not be aware of these lesions because of the degeneration of nerves in the area. When numbness and lack of sensation are present, always test the water temperature before immersing a limb. Because of impaired sensation, it is easy to burn the skin, and the patient may be unaware of the burn until later.

Impotence. Impotence may occur from a number of causes and should be discussed on an individual basis with the healthcare provider.

Hypertension. All patients with diabetes should have a blood pressure measurement, including orthostatic measurements, completed on every routine office visit. The ADA (2018) recommends that most patients with diabetes and hypertension should be treated to a blood pressure goal of less than 140/90 mm Hg. A lower blood pressure goal of less than 130/80 mm Hg may be appropriate in individuals at high risk of cardiovascular disease if it can be achieved without adverse effects.

Fostering health maintenance

- Throughout the course of treatment, discuss medication, diet, exercise, and the need to achieve and maintain good glucose control to prevent the complications associated with diabetes mellitus. The patient must achieve a high degree of understanding of diabetes mellitus and its management. The patient and family members must be included in the entire educational program.
- With shorter hospitalizations, it may be necessary to incorporate follow-up care by a health professional from a visiting nurse association or a home health agency in the discharge planning.
- Seek cooperation and understanding of the following points so that medication compliance is increased: name of medication; dosage, route, and time of administration; and common and serious adverse effects.

At discharge. Develop a list of specific equipment and supplies that the patient will need when discharged. Keep in mind the cost of these supplies. Consider the following:

1. *Syringes:* Disposable syringes are convenient and presterilized but are more expensive. Be sure to tell the patient that disposable syringes are designed to be used once and then discarded. However, recent literature refers to the repeated use of the same syringe by an individual patient as long as the needle remains sharp and is kept clean and covered. *Check with the individual prescriber before instituting this practice.* Diabetics are susceptible to infection and healing may be a problem. The newer, smaller 30- and 31-gauge needles can become bent with even one use, forming a hook at the end of the needle. If the needle is reused, the hook may result in a laceration to the tissue and lead to adverse effects. Syringes being reused should be stored at room temperature. The potential benefits of storing a syringe and needle for reuse in the refrigerator or of wiping the needle with alcohol are unknown. Cleansing the needle with alcohol may disrupt the silicone coating on the needle, resulting in increased pain at the injection site. Syringes are available in 0.3-, 0.5-, 1-, and 2-mL capacities. In some cases, the insulin pen may also be prescribed for use by appropriate individuals. Several medical devices have been developed to reduce the incidence of needlesticks and other sharps injuries. When performing patient education on the self-administration of insulin, it is important to use the type of syringe and needle device that will be used at home to ensure that the patient knows how to manipulate the device correctly. Insulin can also be administered using a jet injector for those with a phobia of needles or unable to use a syringe. They are not a routine option for use in all patients with diabetes.

2. *Insulin pumps:* An insulin pump uses regular insulin or the rapid-acting insulin analogues such as lispro, aspart, or glulisine. The use of mixtures of insulins in insulin pumps is not recommended because this approach has not been evaluated.

3. *Needles:* Disposable needles are more convenient but also more expensive. Patients usually use a 27-, 28-, 29-, 30-, or 31-gauge ½- or ⅝-inch needle, but needles should be adjusted to the individual. An obese patient may require a 1- to 1½-inch-long needle to inject the insulin properly. Several lengths of needles are available, and blood glucose should be monitored when changing from one needle length to another. Always dispose of insulin syringes, needles, and lancets in sharps containers. (See Chapter 9 for further discussion of syringes, needles, and safety during use.)

4. *Specialized equipment:* BD Magni-Guides (Becton, Dickinson and Company, Franklin Lakes, NJ) are available for the visually impaired patient. This device holds the vial of insulin, acts as a guide in withdrawing insulin, and has a magnifying glass to make reading the syringe scale easier. Insulin pens are available for blind or neurologically impaired patients. A talking glucose-measuring device is also available for the visually impaired individual to perform self-monitoring of capillary blood glucose levels. Persons with diabetes desiring more information on insulin delivery aids can contact the ADA.

5. *Self-monitoring equipment for blood glucose:* Be certain that the individual has or understands where to purchase the supplies used with the specific brand of self-monitoring glucose machine to be used at home. Because a number of models of self-monitoring equipment are available, it is important that the individual be trained on the specific equipment that will be used at home.

Patient self-assessment. Enlist the patient's aid in developing and maintaining a written record of monitoring parameters (e.g., blood glucose, insulin dosage, pertinent stress factors, exercise level, illnesses, major changes in diet or other routine). See the Patient Self-Assessment Form for Antidiabetic Agents on the Evolve website. Complete the Premedication Data column for use as a baseline to track response to drug therapy. Ensure that the patient understands how to use the form, and instruct the patient to bring the completed form to follow-up visits. During follow-up visits, focus on issues that will foster adherence with the therapeutic interventions prescribed.

Life Span Considerations
Children With Diabetes Mellitus

For children who have diabetes, it is essential that the appropriate faculty of the school, whether a day care, preschool, or regular school environment, be familiar with the child's health needs. Fig. 35.3 is a diabetes healthcare plan for use in school and day care.

DRUG CLASS: INSULINS

Actions

Insulin, a hormone produced in the beta cells of the pancreas, is a key regulator of metabolism. Insulin is required for the entry of glucose into skeletal and heart muscle and fat. It also plays a significant role in protein and lipid metabolism. It is not required for glucose transport into the brain, kidney, gastrointestinal, or liver tissue.

The pancreas secretes insulin at a steady rate of 0.5 to 1 unit/hr. It is released in greater quantities when the blood glucose level rises above 100 mg/dL such as after a meal. The average rate of insulin secretion in an adult is 30 to 50 units daily.

Insulin deficiency reduces the rate of transport of glucose into cells, producing hyperglycemia. Other metabolic reactions also are inhibited by the lack of insulin and intracellular glucose, resulting in the conversion of protein to glucose (gluconeogenesis), hyperlipidemia, ketosis, and acidosis.

Insulins from the pancreases of different animals have similar activity and were used in human beings for many years. Biosynthetic human insulin is now used by most patients, especially people newly diagnosed with diabetes. It has fewer allergic reactions associated with it than do animal-origin insulins.

Uses

Three factors—onset, peak, and duration—are important in the use of insulin therapy. *Onset* is the time required for the medication to have an initial effect or action, *peak* is when the insulin will have the maximum effect, and *duration* is how long the agent remains active in the body. When monitoring insulin therapy, it is important to understand these terms and to associate them with the type of insulin being administered to ascertain when a patient is most susceptible to hyperglycemia or hypoglycemia.

Four types of insulin, based on onset, peak, and duration, are in use today: rapid-acting, short-acting, intermediate-acting, and long-acting insulins (Table 35.5). The most rapid-acting insulins are the insulin analogues, newer synthetic forms called lispro, aspart, and glulisine. They are clear solutions that may be injected separately or mixed in the same syringe with an intermediate-acting insulin. Aspart and lispro are as potent as human regular insulin but have a more rapid onset and shorter duration of activity. Aspart appears to have a slightly more rapid onset than lispro. Glulisine has an onset of action similar to lispro and aspart but has a slightly shorter duration of action. Their rapid onset of action is related to a more rapid absorption rate from subcutaneous tissue than is the case with regular insulin. Aspart, lispro, and glulisine are usually administered within 10 to 15 minutes of a meal. The rationale for the development and use of these newer insulins is that when a meal is ingested, the blood glucose rises for about 2 to 3 hours. After injection, regular insulin takes 30 minutes to start acting, peaks at $2\frac{1}{2}$ to 5 hours, and may have a duration of 5 to 10 hours. Lispro and aspart start to act within 10 minutes of injection, peak within 1 to 2 hours, and are gone by 3 to 5 hours. Glulisine has a similar onset of action but peaks in 30 to 90 minutes with a duration of action up to 4 hours. Consequently, the newer rapid-acting, shorter-duration insulins are used to control hyperglycemia associated with meals without having longer-lasting effects with the potential for hypoglycemia. These insulins may also be used without any other insulin in patients with type 2 diabetes who only have hyperglycemia associated with ingestion of meals (postprandial hyperglycemia). Aspart and glulisine may also be injected intravenously.

Regular insulin has long been used for its short onset of activity and relatively short duration of action. But, as noted in Table 35.5, regular insulin is slower in its onset and longer in duration than the rapid-acting insulins. Regular insulin is approved to be injected by both IV and subcutaneous routes of administration. Human regular insulin is usually administered 30 to 60 minutes before meals.

Diabetes Care Plan for _____(name of student)_____ School _____ Effective Dates: _____

To be completed by parents/health care team and reviewed with necessary school staff. Copies should be kept in student's classrooms and school records.

Date of Birth: _____ **Grade:** _____ **Homeroom Teacher:** _____

Contact information:
Parent/guardian #1: _____ Address: _____
   Telephone - Home: _____ Work: _____ Cell Phone: _____
Parent/guardian #2: _____ Address: _____
   Telephone - Home: _____ Work: _____ Cell Phone: _____
Student's Doctor/Health Care Provider: _____ Telephone: _____
   Nurse Educator: _____ Telephone: _____
Other emergency contact: _____ Relationship: _____
   Telephone - Home: _____ Work: _____ Cell Phone: _____
Notify parent/guardian in the following situations: _____

Blood Glucose Monitoring
Target range for blood glucose: _____ mg/dL to _____ mg/dL   Type of blood glucose meter student uses: _____
Usual times to test blood glucose: _____
Times to do extra tests (check all that apply):   _____ Before exercise   _____ When student exhibits symptoms of hyperglycemia
                                    _____ After exercise   _____ When student exhibits symptoms of hypoglycemia
                                      _____ Other (explain): _____

Can student perform own blood glucose tests?   Yes   No   Exceptions: _____
School personnel trained to monitor blood glucose level and dates of training: _____

Insulin
Times, types, and dosages of insulin injections to be given during school:
Time   Type(s)   Dosage
_____   _____   _____
_____   _____   _____

School personnel trained to assist with insulin injection and dates of training: _____

Can student give own injections?   Yes   No
Can student determine correct amount of insulin?   Yes   No
Can student draw correct dose of insulin?   Yes   No

For Students with Insulin Pumps:
Type of pump: _____
Insulin/carbohydrate ratio: _____
Correction factor: _____

Is student competent regarding pump?   Yes   No
Can student effectively troubleshoot problems   Yes   No
(e.g., ketosis, pump malfunction)?
Comments: _____

Meals and Snacks Eaten at School (The carbohydrate content of the food is important in maintaining a stable blood glucose level.)

	Time	Food content/amount
Breakfast	_____	_____
AM snack	_____	_____
Lunch	_____	_____
PM snack	_____	_____
Dinner	_____	_____

Snack before exercise?
    Yes   No
Snack after exercise?
    Yes   No

Other times to give snacks (content/amount): _____

A source of glucose such as _____ should be readily available at all times.
Preferred snack foods: _____
Foods to avoid, if any: _____
Instructions for when food is provided to the class, (e.g., as part of a class party or food sampling): _____

Hypoglycemia (Low Blood Sugar)
Usual symptoms of hypoglycemia: _____

Treatment of hypoglycemia: _____

School personnel trained to administer glucagon and dates of training: _____

Glucagon should be given if the student is unconscious, having a seizure (convulsion), or unable to swallow. If required, glucagon should be administered promptly and then 911 (or other emergency assistance) and parents should be called.

Hyperglycemia (High Blood Sugar)
Usual symptoms of hyperglycemia: _____

Treatment of hyperglycemia: _____

Circumstances when urine or blood ketones should be tested: _____

Treatment for ketones: _____

Exercise and Sports
A snack such as _____ should be readily available at the site of exercise or sports.
Restrictions on activity, if any: _____
Student should not exercise if blood glucose is below _____ mg/dL.

Supplies and Personnel
Location of supplies: Blood glucose monitoring equipment: _____   Insulin administration supplies: _____
                         Glucagon emergency kit: _____   Ketone testing supplies: _____
                         Snack foods: _____
Personnel trained in the symptoms and treatment of low and high blood sugar and dates of training: _____

Signatures
Reviewed by: _[student's health provider/date]_   Acknowledged/received by: _[guardian/date]_   Acknowledged/received by: _[school representative/date]_

Fig. 35.3 Diabetes healthcare plan. (From American Diabetes Association. Care of children with diabetes in the school and day care setting. _Diabetes Care._ 2003;26[suppl 1]:S131-S135.)

Table 35.5   Commercially Available Forms of Insulin[a]

TYPE OF INSULIN	MANUFACTURER	STRENGTH (UNITS/ML)	ONSET (HR)	PEAK (HR)	DURATION[b] (HR)	HYPERGLYCEMIA[c]	HYPOGLYCEMIA[c]
Rapid-Acting Insulin							
Insulin Analogue Injection							
NovoLog (aspart)	Novo Nordisk	100	0.2–0.33	1–3	3–5	After lunch (3)	Within 1–3 hr
Humalog (lispro)	Lilly	100	0.2–0.33	0.5–2.5	3–5	After lunch (3)	Within 1–3 hr
Apidra (glulisine)	Sanofi-Aventis	100	0.2–0.33	0.5–1.5	3–4	After lunch (3)	Within 1–3 hr
Short-Acting Insulin							
Insulin Injection							
Humulin R (human)	Lilly	100, 500	0.5–1	2.5–5	5–10	Early AM (1)	Before lunch (3)
Novolin R (human)	Novo Nordisk	100	0.5–1	2.5–5	8	Early AM	Before lunch
Intermediate-Acting Insulin							
Isophane Insulin Suspension (NPH)							
Humulin N (human)	Lilly	100	1–2	4–12	16–28	Before lunch (2)	3 PM to supper (3)
Novolin N (human)	Novo Nordisk	100	1–2	4–12	24	Before lunch	3 PM to supper
Isophane Insulin Suspension (NPH) and Insulin Injection (Regular)							
Humulin 70/30 (human) (70% NPH/30% regular)	Lilly	100	0.5–1	4–12	24	Before lunch	3 PM to supper
Novolin 70/30 (human) (70% NPH/30% regular)	Novo Nordisk	100	0.5–1	2–12	24	Before lunch	3 PM to supper
Insulin Analogue Protamine Suspension and Insulin Analogue Injection							
Humalog Mix 75/25 (75% lispro protamine/25% lispro)	Lilly	100	0.25–0.5	0.5–1.5	14–24	—	3 PM to supper
NovoLog Mix 70/30 (70% aspart protamine/30% aspart)	Novo Nordisk	100	0.2–0.33	2.4	18–24	—	3 PM to supper
Long-Acting Insulin							
Lantus (glargine)	Sanofi-Aventis	100	1.1	—[d]	24	Mid-AM to mid-PM (1)	—[d]
Toujeo (glargine)	Sanofi-Aventis	300	1.1	—[d]	24	Mid-AM to mid-PM	—[d]
Basaglar (glargine)	Lilly	100	1	—[d]	Up to 24	mid-PM	—[d]
Levemir (detemir)	Novo Nordisk	100	1	—[d]	Up to 24	Mid-AM to mid-PM (1)	—[d]
Tresiba (degludec)	Novo Nordisk	100, 200	1	—[d]	Up to 42	Mid-AM to mid-PM (1)	—[d]
Long-Acting Insulin Plus Rapid-Acting Insulin							
Ryzodeg 70/30 (70% degludec/30% aspart)	Novo Nordisk	100	0.2–0.33	1.15	Greater than 24	—	Mid-AM to mid-PM

[a]All forms of insulin listed are from a semisynthetic source.
[b]The times listed are averages based on a newly diagnosed diabetic patient. Factors modifying these times include patient variation, site and route of administration, and dosage.
[c]Most often occurs when insulin is administered (1) at bedtime the previous night, (2) before breakfast the previous day, or (3) before breakfast the same day.
[d]No pronounced peak activity.
NPH, Neutral protamine Hagedorn.

Neutral protamine Hagedorn (NPH) insulin is an intermediate-acting insulin containing specific amounts of regular insulin and protamine. The protamine binds to the insulin. When administered subcutaneously, the insulin is slowly released from the protamine and becomes active, giving it the intermediate-acting classification.

Lispro and aspart insulin may also be mixed with protamine to prolong their duration of action. Two products are available: 75% lispro protamine suspension and 25% lispro solution (Humalog Mix 75/25) and 70% aspart protamine suspension and 30% aspart solution (NovoLog Mix 70/30). The combined effect is a rapid-acting onset with an intermediate duration of action of 14 to 24 hours (Novolog 70/30 is 18 to 24 hours, while Humalog 75/25 is 14 to 24 hours).

Insulin glargine, insulin detemir, and insulin degludec are biosynthetic long-acting insulins. They are absorbed from the subcutaneous tissue in a uniform manner without large fluctuations in insulin levels, reducing the possibility of hypoglycemic reactions. Most commonly injected in the evening, these products provide a 24-hour basal source of insulin for the body. Rapid-acting insulin is then injected just before meals to control hyperglycemia secondary to the meal, or intermediate-acting NPH can be injected in the morning and late afternoon to treat hyperglycemia from meals. Neither insulin glargine, detemir, nor degludec should be mixed with other insulins.

Storage of Insulin

Insulin should not be allowed to freeze and should not be heated above a temperature of 98°F. A general rule of thumb is that the bottle of insulin should be stored in the refrigerator (not the freezer) until opened. Because patients find it uncomfortable to inject cold insulin, the bottle (and insulin cartridges for insulin pens) may then be kept at room temperature (68° to 75°F) until gone. For all insulins other than regular, lispro, aspart, or glulisine, the vial should be gently rolled in the palms of the hands (not shaken) to warm and resuspend the insulin. Once an insulin vial is opened, it should be discarded within 30 days. Even though the insulin has not deteriorated, there is concern that the contents are no longer sterile and the vial may become a reservoir for infection, especially with patients who reuse needles.

At sustained temperatures above room temperature, insulins lose potency rapidly. Do not leave in a hot car throughout the day.

Excess agitation should be avoided to prevent loss of potency, clumping, or precipitation. When insulins are prefilled in syringes, the syringes should be stored in a refrigerator for up to 30 days in a vertical position with the needle facing upward. Prior to use, the syringe should be taken out of the refrigerator, allowed to warm to room temperature, and then gently rolled between the hands to remix the insulin before administration.

Therapeutic Outcomes

The primary therapeutic outcomes expected from insulin therapy are as follows:

1. A decrease in both fasting blood glucose levels and A_{1c} concentrations in the range defined as acceptable for the individual patient
2. Fewer long-term complications associated with poorly controlled diabetes mellitus

❖ Nursing Implications for Insulin

◆ Premedication assessment

1. Confirm that a blood glucose level was recently measured and was acceptable for the individual patient.
2. Confirm that the patient has had a level of activity reasonable for that patient and that the anticipated level of activity planned for the next several hours is balanced with the insulin dose.
3. Confirm that the prescribed diet is being consumed as planned and that no changes in diet are anticipated in relation to insulin dosage over the next several hours (e.g., with patients on nothing by mouth [NPO] status, consider holding medication).

◆ Availability, dosage, and administration. See Table 35.5, Fig. 9.26, and Chapter 10 for information regarding availability and administration. Maintenance therapy for newly diagnosed diabetic patients should incorporate the following information:

• Effective control of diabetes mellitus requires a balanced food intake, exercise, blood glucose levels measured several times daily, and insulin dosage adjustments based on the blood glucose levels.

• Several methods have been developed to initiate insulin therapy. The method chosen depends on such issues as fluctuation of the patient's blood glucose; ability of the patient to measure, mix, and administer the insulin; and adherence to planned exercise and diet.

• Before starting a standardized regimen, the diet and physical exercise level must be stabilized. A standard approach is to calculate the initial total daily dose of insulin based on 0.5 to 0.8 unit/kg of whole-body (not lean-body) weight. NPH (human) insulin is often used to initiate therapy. This total daily dosage is then split into two doses so that two-thirds are administered in the morning before breakfast and one-third is administered 30 minutes before the evening meal. The insulin dosage is then adjusted over the next several weeks based on blood glucose measurements taken (usually) four times daily and on A_{1c} levels. Diet and exercise may also require adjustment.

Mixing insulins. Many patients with diabetes mix rapid-acting insulin with intermediate-acting or long-acting insulin to manage the hyperglycemia that follows a meal or snack. See Table 35.6 and Chapter 9 for the technique to follow when mixing insulins. When regular

Table 35.6 Compatibility of Insulin Combinations

COMBINATION	RATIO	MIX BEFORE ADMINISTRATION
regular + NPH	Any combination	2-3 mo
aspart + NPH	Any combination	Immediately
lispro + NPH	Any combination	Immediately
glulisine + NPH	Any combination	Immediately
glargine	Do not mix with other insulin	
detemir	Do not mix with other insulin	
degludec	Do not mix with other insulin	

NPH, Neutral protamine Hagedorn.

insulin, insulin lispro, or insulin aspart is combined with another insulin in the same syringe, the rapid-acting insulin should be drawn into the syringe first to avoid contaminating the rapid-acting insulin vial with the longer-acting insulin, which may happen if the longer-acting insulin was drawn into the syringe first and then the needle was inserted into the rapid-acting insulin to draw it into the syringe.

Life Span Considerations
Insulin

Almost all patients receiving insulin will experience a hypoglycemic reaction at some point. Symptoms of a hypoglycemic reaction vary from patient to patient. Be aware that confusion and lethargy are signs of hypoglycemia but may sometimes be overlooked in older adult patients because slowness and confusion can be interpreted as signs of aging.

◆ Common and serious adverse effects
Metabolic

Hyperglycemia. Diabetic or prediabetic patients must be monitored for the development of hyperglycemia, particularly during the early weeks of therapy. Assess regularly for abnormal blood glucose levels and, in certain patients as requested by the healthcare provider, for glycosuria and ketones. If symptoms occur frequently, the healthcare provider should be notified and the patient's written records of the results of self-testing should be supplied to the healthcare provider for analysis. Patients receiving insulin may require an adjustment in dosage.

Hypoglycemia. Insulin overdose or decreased carbohydrate intake may result in hypoglycemia. If untreated, irreversible brain damage may occur. Hypoglycemia occurs most frequently when the administered insulin reaches its peak action (see Table 35.5). Hypoglycemia must be treated immediately.

The following conditions may predispose a patient with diabetes to a hypoglycemic (insulin) reaction: improper measurement of insulin dosage, excessive exercise, insufficient food intake, concurrent ingestion of hypoglycemic drugs, and discontinuation of drugs that cause hyperglycemia (see Drug Interactions later in this section). Monitor the patient for the following signs

of hypoglycemia: headache, nausea, weakness, hunger, lethargy, decreased coordination, general apprehension, sweating, or blurred or double vision.

Hypersensitivity, immune system

Allergic reactions. Allergic reactions, manifested by itching, redness, and swelling at the site of injection, are common in patients receiving insulin therapy. These reactions may be caused by modifying proteins in NPH insulin, the insulin itself, the alcohol used to cleanse the injection site, the patient's injection technique, or the intermittent use of insulin.

Spontaneous desensitization frequently occurs within a few weeks. Local irritation may be reduced by changing to insulins derived from biosynthetic sources (e.g., "human" insulin), by using unscented alcohol swabs and disposable syringes and needles, and by checking the patient's injection technique. Acute rashes covering the whole body and anaphylactic symptoms are rare, but if they occur, they must be treated with antihistamines, epinephrine, and steroids.

Lipodystrophies. Rotation of injection sites is important to avoid atrophy or hypertrophy of subcutaneous fat tissue. This dermatologic condition may occur at the site of frequent insulin injections. The hypertrophic areas tend to be used more frequently by diabetic patients because the fat pad becomes anesthetized. In addition to the adverse cosmetic effects, the absorption rate of insulin from these sites becomes significantly prolonged and erratic. Loss of diabetic control may result, particularly in patients with unstable type 1 diabetes.

◆ Drug interactions

Hyperglycemia. The following medications may produce hyperglycemia, especially in prediabetic and diabetic patients (insulin dosages may require adjustment): albuterol, asparaginase, calcitonin, clozapine, olanzapine, corticosteroids, cyclophosphamide, diltiazem, diuretics (e.g., thiazides, furosemide, bumetanide), dobutamine, epinephrine, glucagon, isoniazid, lithium, morphine, niacin, nicotine, oral contraceptives, pentamidine, phenothiazines, phenytoin, protease inhibitors, terbutaline, somatropin, and thyroid hormones.

Diabetic or prediabetic patients must be monitored for the development of hyperglycemia, particularly during the early weeks of therapy. Assess the patient regularly for elevated blood glucose level or glycosuria and notify the healthcare provider if either occurs with any frequency.

Hypoglycemia. The following drugs may cause hypoglycemia, thereby decreasing insulin requirements, in diabetic patients: anabolic steroids, angiotensin-converting enzyme (ACE) inhibitors, alcohol, nonselective beta-adrenergic blocking agents, calcium, clonidine, fluoxetine, ethanol, fibrates, lithium, insulin, monoamine oxidase inhibitors (MAOIs), pentamidine, pentoxifylline, pyridoxine, salicylates, sulfonamides, and sulfonylureas.

Monitor for the following signs of hypoglycemia: headache, nausea, weakness, hunger, lethargy, decreased coordination, general apprehension, sweating, or blurred or double vision. Notify the healthcare provider if any of these symptoms appear.

Beta-adrenergic blocking agents. Beta blockers (e.g., propranolol, nadolol, metoprolol) may mask many of the symptoms of hypoglycemia. Notify the healthcare provider if you suspect that any of these symptoms appear intermittently.

DRUG CLASS: BIGUANIDE ORAL ANTIDIABETIC AGENT

metformin (mĕt-FŎR-mĭn)
Glucophage (GLŪ-kō-fāj)
⇄ *Do not confuse metformin with metronidazole.*

Actions
Metformin represents a class of oral antihyperglycemic agents known as the biguanides. It decreases hepatic glucose production by inhibiting glycogenolysis and gluconeogenesis, reduces absorption of glucose from the small intestine, and increases insulin sensitivity, improving glucose uptake in peripheral muscle and adipose cells. Metformin may also stimulate glucose metabolism by anaerobic glycolysis. The net result is a significant decrease in fasting and postprandial blood glucose and A_{1c} concentrations. Insulin must be present for metformin to be active, and therefore metformin is not effective in type 1 diabetes.

Uses
Metformin is used as an adjunct to the diet to lower blood glucose levels in patients with type 2 diabetes mellitus whose hyperglycemia cannot be controlled by diet and exercise alone. It has the particular advantage that it will not cause hypoglycemia, as can occur with insulin and the sulfonylureas. It may also be used in combination with other oral antidiabetic agents to lower blood glucose because the agents act by different mechanisms.

Metformin has two other beneficial effects: it does not cause weight gain and actually may cause weight loss, contrary to the actions of the sulfonylureas, meglitinides, and insulin; and it also has a favorable effect on triglycerides. It produces a modest decrease in concentrations of serum triglycerides and total and LDL cholesterol, with modest increases in concentrations of HDL cholesterol. See the Medication Safety Alert in the Dosage and Administration section later regarding patients with renal function problems, heart failure, and liver impairment.

Therapeutic Outcomes
The primary therapeutic outcomes expected from biguanide oral antidiabetic agent therapy are as follows:

1. A decrease in fasting blood glucose and A_{1c} concentrations in the range defined as "acceptable" for the individual patient

2. Fewer long-term complications associated with poorly controlled type 2 diabetes mellitus

❖ **Nursing Implications for Metformin**
◆ *Premedication assessment*
1. Confirm that blood glucose and A_{1c} levels were recently measured and were acceptable for the individual patient.
2. Confirm that the prescribed diet is being consumed as planned and that no changes in diet are anticipated in relation to oral hypoglycemic agent dosage over the next several hours (e.g., in patients on NPO status, consider holding medication).

◆ *Availability. PO:* 500-, 850-, and 1000-mg tablets; 500-, 750-, and 1000-mg tablets, extended release (24 hr); 500 mg/5 mL oral solution.

◆ *Dosage and administration.* **Adult:** *PO: Immediate-release tablet or solution:* Initial: 500 mg twice daily *or* 850 mg once daily; titrate in increments of 500 mg weekly or 850 mg every other week; may also titrate from 500 mg twice a day to 850 mg twice a day after 2 weeks. If a dose greater than 2000 mg/day is required, it may be better tolerated in three divided doses. Maximum recommended dose: 2550 mg/day.

PO: Extended-release tablet: Initial: 500 to 1000 mg once daily; dosage may be increased by 500 mg weekly up to a maximum of 2500 mg/day. Doses can be administered twice a day at maximum dose.

If a patient's blood glucose level is not controlled with the maximum dosage, a sulfonylurea, a TZD, a DPP-4 inhibitor, a GLP-1 agonist, SGLT2 inhibitor, or basal insulin may be added to the regimen.

⚠ **Medication Safety Alert**

Lactic acidosis is a rare but potentially life-threatening complication that can occur during treatment with metformin. It is recommended that metformin therapy *not* be initiated in the following patients:

- Patients with an estimated glomerular filtration rate of 30 to 45 mL/min/1.73 m²
- Patients with tissue hypoperfusion, such as in heart failure, shock, or septicemia, and patients at risk for developing metabolic acidosis
- Patients with clinical or laboratory evidence (hyperbilirubinemia; elevated aspartate aminotransferase [AST] and/or alanine aminotransferase [ALT] levels) of liver disease
- Patients scheduled to receive IV radiopaque dyes. Radiopaque dyes often induce temporary renal insufficiency, so in patients with an eGFR 30 to 60 mL/min/1.73 m² or lower, metformin should be discontinued 24 to 48 hours before procedures in which radiopaque dye will be administered (e.g., kidney studies). Metformin should not be reinitiated for 2 to 3 days, until normal renal function has been proven.

◆ *Common adverse effects*
Gastrointestinal

Nausea, vomiting, anorexia, abdominal cramps, flatulence. These adverse effects are most common and are the reason for slow dose titration. They are usually mild and tend to resolve with continued therapy. Taking the medication with meals will help reduce these adverse effects. Encourage the patient not to discontinue therapy without first consulting the healthcare provider.

◆ *Serious adverse effects*
Metabolic

Malaise, myalgias, respiratory distress, hypotension. A rare adverse effect of metformin is lactic acidosis. A gradual onset of these symptoms may be an early indication of the development of lactic acidosis. Patients with reduced renal function, poor circulation, and/or excessive alcohol intake are most susceptible to developing lactic acidosis.

◆ *Drug interactions*

Drugs that may enhance toxic effects. Amiloride, cimetidine, digoxin, furosemide, morphine, quinidine, ranitidine, triamterene, trimethoprim, and vancomycin are excreted by the same route through the kidneys that metformin depends on for excretion. There is a possibility that these drugs may block the excretion of metformin, potentially causing lactic acidosis. Monitor for signs of lactic acidosis (refer to earlier discussion).

Ethanol. Patients should be cautioned against excessive alcohol intake, acute or chronic, when taking metformin, because alcohol potentiates the effects of metformin on lactate metabolism.

Hyperglycemia. The following drugs, when used concurrently with metformin, may decrease its therapeutic effects: corticosteroids, phenothiazines, diuretics, oral contraceptives, thyroid replacement hormones, phenytoin, and lithium carbonate.

Diabetic and prediabetic patients must be monitored for the development of hyperglycemia, particularly during the early weeks of therapy. Assess regularly for elevated blood glucose level or glycosuria and notify the healthcare provider if either occurs with any frequency.

Nifedipine. Nifedipine appears to increase the absorption of metformin. Reducing the dosage of metformin may minimize adverse effects.

DRUG CLASS: SULFONYLUREA ORAL HYPOGLYCEMIC AGENTS

Actions
The sulfonylureas lower blood glucose levels by stimulating the release of insulin from the beta cells of the pancreas. The sulfonylureas also diminish glucose production and metabolism of insulin by the liver.

Uses
The sulfonylureas are effective in type 2 diabetes patients in whom the pancreas still has the capacity to secrete insulin, but they are of no value in the patient with type 1 diabetes who has no beta cell function. Sulfonylureas may be effective in the treatment of type 2 diabetes mellitus that cannot be controlled by diet and exercise if the patient is not susceptible to developing ketosis, acidosis, or infections. Patients most likely to benefit from oral hypoglycemic treatment are those who develop signs of diabetes after age 40 years and who require less than 40 units of insulin per day (indicating that some insulin is still being secreted by the beta cells). Sulfonylureas may induce hypoglycemia due to overproduction of insulin.

Therapeutic Outcomes
The primary therapeutic outcomes expected from sulfonylurea oral hypoglycemic therapy are as follows:
1. A decrease in fasting blood glucose and A_{1c} concentrations in the range defined as acceptable for the individual patient
2. Fewer long-term complications associated with poorly controlled diabetes mellitus

❖ **Nursing Implications for Sulfonylurea Oral Hypoglycemic Agents**
◆ *Premedication assessment*
1. Confirm that blood glucose and A_{1c} levels were recently measured and were hyperglycemic for the individual patient.
2. Confirm that the patient has had a level of activity "reasonable" for that patient and that the anticipated level of activity planned for the next several hours is balanced with the oral hypoglycemic agent dosage.
3. Confirm that the prescribed diet is being consumed as planned and that no changes in diet are anticipated in relation to the oral hypoglycemic agent dosage over the next several hours (e.g., in patients on NPO status, consider holding medication).

◆ *Availability, dosage, and administration.* See Table 35.7. Individual dosage adjustment is essential for the successful use of oral hypoglycemic agents. A patient should receive a 1-month trial on maximum dosage of the sulfonylurea being used before the medication can be considered a primary failure. If a patient represents a secondary failure (a patient initially controlled on oral agents), changing to an alternative sulfonylurea is occasionally successful in controlling blood glucose levels.

 Medication Safety Alert

In general, sulfonylureas should not be administered to patients who are allergic to sulfonamides. These patients may also be allergic to sulfonylureas.

◆ *Common adverse effects*
Gastrointestinal

Nausea, vomiting, anorexia, abdominal cramps. These adverse effects are usually mild and tend to resolve

Table 35.7   Sulfonylurea Oral Hypoglycemic Agents

GENERIC NAME	BRAND NAME	AVAILABILITY	INITIAL DOSAGE	DOSAGE RANGE	DURATION[a] (HR)
First Generation					
chlorpropamide ⇄ *Do not confuse chlorpropamide with chlorpromazine.*	—	Tablets: 100, 250 mg	100 mg daily	100-750 mg daily	24-60
tolazamide	—	Tablets: 250, 500 mg	100 mg daily	0.1-1 g daily	12-24
tolbutamide	—	Tablets: 500 mg	1 g twice daily	0.25-3 g daily	6-12
Second Generation					
glimepiride	Amaryl ⇄ *Do not confuse Amaryl with Altace, Avandia, Reminyl*	Tablets: 1, 2, 4 mg	1-2 mg daily	1-8 mg daily	24
glipizide	Glucotrol Glucotrol XL	Tablets: 5, 10 mg Tablets, extended release (24 hr): 2.5, 5, 10 mg	5 mg daily 2.5-10 mg	15-40 mg daily 20 mg daily	10-24 24
glyburide		Tablets: 1.25, 1.5, 2.5, 3, 5, 6 mg	2.5-5 mg daily	1.25-20 mg daily	24
	Glynase	Tablets: 1.25, 2.5, 5 mg	2.5-5 mg daily	1.25-20 mg daily	24
		Tablets micronized 1.5, 3, 6 mg	1.5-3 mg daily	0.75-12 mg daily	24

[a]The times listed are averages based on a newly diagnosed diabetic patient. Factors modifying these times include patient variation and dosage.

with continued therapy. Encourage the patient not to discontinue therapy without first consulting the healthcare provider.

◆ *Serious adverse effects*

Metabolic

Hypoglycemia. Patients receiving oral hypoglycemic therapy are as susceptible to hypoglycemia as diabetic patients on insulin therapy. Consequently, blood glucose levels must be monitored closely, especially in the early stages of therapy. Monitor for the following signs of hypoglycemia: headache, nausea, weakness, hunger, lethargy, decreased coordination, general apprehension, sweating, or blurred or double vision. Notify the healthcare provider immediately if any of these symptoms appear.

Hypoglycemia must be treated immediately. Mild symptoms may be controlled by the oral administration of a glucose source (e.g., a lump of sugar, orange juice, carbonated cola beverage [not diet], candy [not chocolate]) or ingestion of a commercially prepared product such as Glutose. Severe symptoms may be relieved by the administration of IV glucose, and parenteral glucagon may be prescribed in some cases. If in doubt about whether the patient is hypoglycemic or hyperglycemic, always treat the individual for hypoglycemia to prevent the possible neurologic complications that can occur from untreated hypoglycemia. The dosage of oral hypoglycemic agents may also have to be reduced.

Gastrointestinal

Hepatotoxicity. The symptoms of hepatotoxicity are anorexia, nausea, vomiting, jaundice, hepatomegaly, splenomegaly, and abnormal liver function (e.g., elevated bilirubin, AST, ALT, gamma-glutamyltransferase [GGT], and alkaline phosphatase levels; increased prothrombin time).

Hematologic

Blood dyscrasias. Routine laboratory studies (e.g., red blood cell and white blood cell counts, differential counts) should be scheduled. Stress the need for the patient to return for this laboratory work.

Immune system. Monitor for the development of a sore throat, fever, purpura, jaundice, or excessive and progressively increasing weakness.

Dermatologic reactions. Report a rash or pruritus immediately. Withhold additional doses pending approval by the healthcare provider.

◆ *Drug interactions*

Hypoglycemia. The following drugs may enhance the hypoglycemic effects of the sulfonylureas: azole antifungal agents (e.g., fluconazole), fluoroquinolone antibiotics, ethanol, androgens (e.g., methandrostenolone), warfarin, beta-adrenergic blocking agents, salicylates, sulfonamides (e.g., sulfamethoxazole-trimethoprim), and MAOIs.

Monitor the patient for the following signs of hypoglycemia: headache, nausea, weakness, hunger, lethargy, decreased coordination, general apprehension, sweating, or blurred or double vision. Notify the healthcare provider if any of these symptoms appear.

Hyperglycemia. The following drugs, when used concurrently with the sulfonylureas, may decrease the therapeutic effects of the sulfonylureas: corticosteroids, fluoroquinolone antibiotics, thiazide diuretics, phenothiazines, oral contraceptives, thyroid replacement hormones, phenytoin, and lithium carbonate.

Diabetic or prediabetic patients must be monitored for the development of hyperglycemia, particularly during the early weeks of therapy. Assess regularly for elevated blood glucose level or glycosuria and notify the healthcare provider if either occurs with any frequency.

Patients receiving insulin may require an adjustment in dosage.

Beta-adrenergic blocking agents. Beta blockers (e.g., propranolol, nadolol, metoprolol, carvedilol) may induce hypoglycemia but may also mask many of the symptoms of hypoglycemia. Notify the healthcare provider if any of these symptoms appear intermittently.

Alcohol. Ingestion of alcoholic beverages during sulfonylurea therapy may infrequently result in an Antabuse-like reaction, manifested by facial flushing, pounding headache, feeling of breathlessness, and nausea.

In patients who develop an Antabuse-like reaction to alcohol, the use of alcohol and preparations containing alcohol (e.g., over-the-counter cough medications, mouthwashes) should be avoided during therapy and for up to 5 days after discontinuation of sulfonylurea therapy.

DRUG CLASS: MEGLITINIDE ORAL HYPOGLYCEMIC AGENTS

meglitinides (mĕ-GLĬ-tĭ-nīdz)

Actions
The meglitinides are nonsulfonylurea oral hypoglycemic agents. They lower blood glucose levels by stimulating the release of insulin from the beta cells of the pancreas.

Uses
The meglitinides are effective in patients with type 2 diabetes mellitus in whom the pancreas still has the capacity to secrete insulin, but they are of no value in patients with type 1 diabetes mellitus who have no beta cell function. The meglitinides may be effective in the treatment of type 2 diabetes mellitus that cannot be controlled by diet and exercise if the patient is not susceptible to developing ketosis, acidosis, or infections. Patients most likely to benefit from oral hypoglycemic treatment are those who develop signs of diabetes after age 40 and who require less than 40 units of insulin daily (indicating that some insulin is still being secreted by the beta cells). The meglitinides may be used alone

or in combination with metformin to control hyperglycemia. The meglitinides have the advantage of having a short duration of action, thus reducing the potential for hypoglycemic reactions. On the other hand, having to take doses up to four times daily may reduce compliance. The meglitinides may be of particular use for patients normally well controlled on diet but who may have periods of transient loss of control, such as during an infection.

Therapeutic Outcomes
The primary therapeutic outcomes expected from meglitinide oral hypoglycemic therapy are as follows:
1. A decrease in fasting blood glucose and the A_{1c} concentrations in the range defined as "acceptable" for the individual patient
2. Fewer long-term complications associated with poorly controlled diabetes mellitus

❖ **Nursing Implications for Meglitinide Therapy**
◆ *Premedication assessment*
1. Confirm that blood glucose and A_{1c} levels were recently measured and were hyperglycemic for the individual patient.
2. Confirm that the patient has had a level of activity "reasonable" for that patient and that the anticipated level of activity planned for the next several hours is balanced with the oral hypoglycemic agent dosage.
3. Confirm that the prescribed diet is being consumed as planned and that no changes in diet are anticipated in relation to the oral hypoglycemic agent dosage over the next several hours (e.g., in patients on NPO status, consider holding medication).

◆ *Availability, dosage, and administration.* See Table 35.8. Doses may be administered within 1 to 30 minutes of the meal.
- Individual dosage adjustment is essential for the successful use of the meglitinides. Dosages may be adjusted weekly, based on fasting blood glucose.
- Doses may be taken preprandially two, three, or four times daily in response to changes in the patient's meal pattern.

> **! Medication Safety Alert**
> Patients should skip a scheduled dose if they skip a meal so that the risk of hypoglycemia is reduced.

◆ *Common and serious adverse effects*
Metabolic
Hypoglycemia. Patients receiving oral hypoglycemic therapy are as susceptible to hypoglycemia as diabetic patients on insulin therapy. Consequently, blood glucose levels must be monitored closely, especially in the early stages of therapy. Monitor for the following signs of hypoglycemia: headache, nausea, weakness, hunger, lethargy, decreased coordination, general apprehension,

Table 35.8 Meglitinide Oral Hypoglycemic Agents

GENERIC NAME	BRAND NAME	AVAILABILITY	DAILY DOSAGE RANGE	MAXIMUM DAILY DOSAGE
nateglinide	Starlix	Tablets: 60, 120 mg	Initially, 60-120 mg before each meal	360 mg
repaglinide	Prandin ⇄ Do not confuse Prandin with Avandia.	Tablets: 0.5, 1, 2 mg	Initially, 0.5 mg before each meal	16 mg

sweating, or blurred or double vision. Notify the healthcare provider immediately if any of these symptoms appear.

Hypoglycemia must be treated immediately. Mild symptoms may be controlled by the oral administration of a glucose source (e.g., a lump of sugar, orange juice, carbonated cola beverage [not diet], candy [not chocolate]) or ingestion of a commercially prepared product such as Glutose. Severe symptoms may be relieved by administering IV glucose, and parenteral glucagon may be prescribed in some cases. If in doubt about whether the patient is hypoglycemic or hyperglycemic, always treat the individual for hypoglycemia to prevent the possible neurologic complications that can occur from untreated hypoglycemia. The dosage of oral hypoglycemic agents also may have to be reduced.

◆ Drug interactions

Hypoglycemia. The following drugs may enhance the hypoglycemic effects of repaglinide and nateglinide: ethanol, erythromycin, clarithromycin, nonsteroidal antiinflammatory drugs, sulfonylureas, gemfibrozil, itraconazole, ketoconazole, androgens (e.g., methandrostenolone), warfarin, salicylates, sulfonamides (e.g., sulfamethoxazole-trimethoprim), fluoroquinolones (e.g., ciprofloxacin, levofloxacin, moxifloxacin), probenecid, and MAOIs.

Monitor for the following signs of hypoglycemia: headache, nausea, weakness, hunger, lethargy, decreased coordination, general apprehension, sweating, or blurred or double vision. Notify the healthcare provider if any of these symptoms appear.

Hyperglycemia. The following drugs, when used concurrently with the meglitinides, may decrease the therapeutic effects of the meglitinides: corticosteroids, phenothiazines, diuretics, estrogens, oral contraceptives, thyroid replacement hormones, niacin, sympathomimetics, calcium channel blockers, phenytoin, and lithium carbonate.

Beta-adrenergic blocking agents. Beta blockers (e.g., propranolol, nadolol, metoprolol, carvedilol) may induce hypoglycemia but may also mask many of the symptoms of hypoglycemia. Notify the healthcare provider if you suspect that any of these symptoms appear intermittently.

Carbamazepine, barbiturates, rifampin. These agents may increase repaglinide metabolism. Monitor blood glucose levels closely when any of these agents are started or discontinued.

Erythromycin, clarithromycin, ketoconazole. These agents may inhibit repaglinide metabolism. Monitor closely for hypoglycemia if any of these agents are started in a patient receiving repaglinide.

DRUG CLASS: THIAZOLIDINEDIONE ORAL ANTIDIABETIC AGENTS

thiazolidinediones (thī-ă-zŏl-ĭ-dēn-DĪ-ōnz)

Actions

The TZDs lower blood glucose levels by increasing the sensitivity of muscle and fat tissue to insulin, allowing more glucose to enter the cells in the presence of insulin for metabolism. Thiazolidinediones also may inhibit hepatic gluconeogenesis and decrease hepatic glucose output. Unlike sulfonylureas or meglitinides, TZDs do not stimulate the release of insulin from the beta cells of the pancreas, but insulin must be present for these agents to work.

Uses

Thiazolidinediones are effective in patients with type 2 diabetes mellitus in whom the pancreas still has the capacity to secrete insulin but are of no value in the person with type 1 diabetes who has no beta cell function. Thiazolidinediones may be effective in the treatment of type 2 diabetes mellitus that cannot be controlled by diet and exercise if the patient is not susceptible to developing ketosis, acidosis, or infections. They are not indicated as initial therapy for patients with type 2 diabetes mellitus. Rosiglitazone and pioglitazone may be used as monotherapy (with diet and exercise) or in combination with insulin, sulfonylureas, or metformin to control blood glucose levels. Therapy often takes 4 to 6 weeks for notable effect and several months for full therapeutic effect. Thiazolidinediones should not be used in patients with New York Heart Association class III or IV heart failure (see Chapter 27).

Therapeutic Outcomes

The primary therapeutic outcomes expected from TZD oral antidiabetic therapy are as follows:

1. A decrease in fasting blood glucose and A_{1c} concentrations in the range defined as "acceptable" for the individual patient
2. Fewer long-term complications associated with poorly controlled diabetes mellitus

❖ Nursing Implications for Thiazolidinedione Therapy

◆ Premedication assessment

1. Confirm that blood glucose and A_{1c} levels were recently measured and were hyperglycemic for the individual patient.
2. Perform scheduled baseline laboratory tests. Liver function, including bilirubin, AST, ALT, GGT, and alkaline phosphatase tests, should be determined before initiation of therapy, once a month for the first year, and quarterly after the first year. A baseline test should also be completed for body weight; hemoglobin and hematocrit; white blood cell count; and total cholesterol, HDL cholesterol, LDL cholesterol, and triglyceride levels.
3. Confirm that the prescribed diet is being consumed as planned and that no changes in diet are anticipated in relation to the oral hypoglycemic agent dosage over the next several hours (e.g., in patients on NPO status, consider holding medication).
4. Premenopausal, anovulatory women should be informed that TZDs might induce the resumption of ovulation. These women may be at risk for pregnancy if adequate contraception is not used (see Oral Contraceptives in the Drug Interactions section later).

◆ Availability, dosage, and administration.
See Table 35.9. Individual dosage adjustment is essential for the successful use of hypoglycemic agents. A patient should be given a multiweek trial (12 weeks for rosiglitazone and pioglitazone therapy) before adjusting the dosage or adding other hypoglycemic agents.

◆ Common adverse effects

Gastrointestinal

Nausea, vomiting, anorexia, abdominal cramps. These adverse effects are usually mild and tend to resolve with continued therapy. Encourage the patient not to discontinue therapy without first consulting the healthcare provider.

◆ Serious adverse effects

Metabolic

Hypoglycemia. Patients receiving TZDs are not susceptible to hypoglycemia unless they are also receiving other hypoglycemic therapy, such as insulin or sulfonylureas. If patients are receiving multiple hypoglycemic therapies, blood glucose levels must be monitored closely, especially in the early stages of therapy. Monitor for the following signs of hypoglycemia: headache, nausea, weakness, hunger, lethargy, decreased coordination, general apprehension, sweating, or blurred or double vision. Notify the healthcare provider immediately if any of the previously mentioned symptoms appear.

Hypoglycemia must be treated immediately. Mild symptoms may be controlled by the oral administration of a glucose source (e.g., a lump of sugar, orange juice, carbonated cola beverage [not diet], candy [not chocolate]) or ingestion of a commercially prepared product such as Glutose. Severe symptoms may be relieved by IV administration of glucose, and parenteral glucagon may be prescribed in some cases. If in doubt about whether the patient is hypoglycemic or hyperglycemic, always treat the individual for hypoglycemia to prevent the possible neurologic complications that can occur from untreated hypoglycemia. The dosage of oral hypoglycemic agents also may have to be reduced.

Weight gain. Weight gain of a few pounds is a common adverse effect of TZD therapy. It also may be a sign of fluid accumulation and increased plasma volume. Monitor patients for signs of edema and heart failure and report to the healthcare provider if present.

Gastrointestinal

Hepatotoxicity. The symptoms of hepatotoxicity are anorexia, nausea, vomiting, jaundice, hepatomegaly, splenomegaly, and abnormal liver function (elevated bilirubin, AST, ALT, GGT, and alkaline phosphatase levels; increased prothrombin time).

◆ Drug interactions

Hypoglycemia. The following drugs may enhance the hypoglycemic effects of TZDs: sulfonylureas, ethanol, androgens (e.g., methandrostenolone), warfarin, salicylates, sulfonamides (e.g., sulfamethoxazole-trimethoprim), fluoroquinolones (ciprofloxacin, levofloxacin, norfloxacin), and MAOIs.

Monitor for the following signs of hypoglycemia: headache, nausea, weakness, hunger, lethargy, decreased coordination, general apprehension, sweating, or blurred or double vision. Notify the healthcare provider if any of these symptoms appear.

Table 35.9 Thiazolidinedione Oral Hypoglycemic Agents

GENERIC NAME	BRAND NAME	AVAILABILITY	DAILY DOSAGE RANGE	MAXIMUM DAILY DOSAGE
pioglitazone	Actos ⇄ Do not confuse Actos with Actonel.	Tablets: 15, 30, 45 mg	PO: Initially, 15-30 mg once daily	45 mg
rosiglitazone	Avandia ⇄ Do not confuse Avandia with Amaryl, Atacand, or Avelox.	Tablets: 2, 4 mg	PO: Initially, 2 mg twice daily or 4 mg once daily	8 mg

Hyperglycemia. The following drugs, when used concurrently with TZDs, may decrease the therapeutic effects of TZDs: corticosteroids, phenothiazines, diuretics, oral contraceptives, thyroid replacement hormones, phenytoin, and lithium carbonate.

Diabetic or prediabetic patients need to be monitored for the development of hyperglycemia, particularly during the early weeks of therapy. Assess regularly for elevated blood glucose level or glycosuria and notify the healthcare provider if it occurs with any frequency. Patients receiving insulin may require an adjustment in dosage.

Beta-adrenergic blocking agents. Beta blockers (e.g., propranolol, nadolol, metoprolol, carvedilol) may induce hypoglycemia but may also mask many of the symptoms of hypoglycemia. Notify the healthcare provider if you suspect that any of these symptoms appear intermittently.

Oral contraceptives. Pioglitazone may enhance the metabolism of ethinyl estradiol and norethindrone, which may cause a resumption of ovulation in patients taking oral contraceptives. Counseling regarding alternative methods of birth control (e.g., contraceptive foam, condoms) should be planned. This interaction has not been reported with rosiglitazone.

Drugs that inhibit metabolism. Erythromycin, ketoconazole, itraconazole, calcium channel blockers, corticosteroids, cyclosporine, triazolam, and 3-hydroxy-3-methylglutaryl coenzyme A (HMG-CoA) reductase inhibitors (statins) may inhibit the metabolism of pioglitazone. If a TZD hypoglycemic agent is indicated for a patient already receiving one of these agents, rosiglitazone should be considered over pioglitazone because these agents do not inhibit its metabolism.

DRUG CLASS: ALPHA-GLUCOSIDASE INHIBITOR AGENTS

acarbose (Ă-kăr-bōs)
  Precose (PRĒ-kōs)
miglitol (MĬG-lĭ-tŏl)
  Glyset (GLĪ-sĕt)

Actions

Acarbose and miglitol are classified as an antihyperglycemic agents. They are enzyme inhibitors that inhibit pancreatic alpha-amylase and gastrointestinal alpha-glucoside hydrolase enzymes used in the digestion of sugars. In patients with diabetes, this enzyme inhibition results in delayed glucose absorption and a lowering of postprandial hyperglycemia.

Uses

Acarbose and miglitol are used as an adjunct to the diet to lower blood glucose levels in patients with type 2 diabetes mellitus whose hyperglycemia cannot be controlled by diet and exercise alone. The particular advantage of the alpha-glucosidase inhibitors is that they will not cause hypoglycemia, as can occur with insulin and the sulfonylureas. They also may be used in combination with the sulfonylureas or metformin to lower the blood glucose level because the agents act by different mechanisms.

Therapeutic Outcomes

The primary therapeutic outcomes expected from acarbose and miglitol therapy are as follows:
1. A decrease in postprandial blood glucose and A_{1c} concentrations in the range defined as "acceptable" for the individual patient
2. Fewer long-term complications associated with poorly controlled type 2 diabetes mellitus

❖ Nursing Implications for Acarbose and Miglitol
◆ Premedication assessment
1. If the patient is also receiving an oral hypoglycemic agent or insulin therapy, ensure that the dosages of these medications are well adjusted before starting acarbose or miglitol therapy.
2. Review the patient's history to ensure that there is no gastrointestinal malabsorption syndrome or obstruction present.
3. Review the patient's medical history to ensure that no liver abnormalities are present before starting acarbose.

◆ Availability, dosage, and administration
See Table 35.10.

◆ Common adverse effects
Gastrointestinal
Abdominal cramps, diarrhea, flatulence. These adverse effects are caused by the metabolism of carbohydrates in the large intestine that were blocked from metabolism in the small intestine by acarbose and miglitol. These adverse effects are usually mild and tend to resolve with continued therapy. Encourage the patient not to discontinue therapy without first consulting the healthcare provider.

◆ Serious adverse effects
Metabolic
Hypoglycemia. Although acarbose and miglitol do not cause hypoglycemia, they can enhance the hypoglycemia caused by a sulfonylurea or insulin. Consequently, blood glucose levels must be monitored closely, especially in the early stages of therapy. Monitor for the following signs of hypoglycemia: headache, nausea, weakness, hunger, lethargy, decreased coordination, general apprehension, sweating, or blurred or double vision. Notify the healthcare provider immediately if any of these symptoms appear.

Hypoglycemia must be treated immediately. Treatment should be initiated with oral dextrose (Glutose)

Table 35.10 Alpha-Glucosidase Inhibitor Agents

GENERIC NAME	BRAND NAME	AVAILABILITY	DAILY DOSAGE RANGE	MAXIMUM DAILY DOSE
acarbose	Precose	Tablets: 25, 50, 100 mg	PO: 25-100 mg three times a day	≤132 lb (60 kg): 50 mg three times a day >132 lb (60 kg): 100 mg three times a day
miglitol	Glyset	Tablets: 25, 50, 100 mg	PO: 25-100 mg three times a day	100 mg three times a day

because its metabolism is not blocked by acarbose or miglitol. Do not use sucrose (table sugar) because its metabolism is blocked by acarbose and miglitol. Severe symptoms may be relieved by IV administration of glucose, and parenteral glucagon may be prescribed in some cases. If in doubt about whether the patient is hypoglycemic or hyperglycemic, always treat the individual for hypoglycemia to prevent the possible neurologic complications that can occur from untreated hypoglycemia. The dosage of oral hypoglycemic agents may also have to be reduced.

Gastrointestinal

Hepatotoxicity. Acarbose has been reported to cause elevations of serum aminotransferase levels (AST and ALT). In rare cases, it causes hyperbilirubinemia. It is recommended that serum aminotransferase concentrations be checked every 3 months during the first year of treatment and periodically thereafter.

◆ *Drug interactions*

Hyperglycemia. The following drugs, when used concurrently with acarbose and miglitol, may decrease the therapeutic effects of acarbose and miglitol: corticosteroids, phenothiazines, diuretics, oral contraceptives, thyroid replacement hormones, phenytoin, diazoxide, and lithium carbonate.

Digestive enzymes, intestinal adsorbents. Digestive enzymes (e.g., amylase, pancreatin) and intestinal adsorbents (e.g., charcoal) may reduce the effect of acarbose and miglitol. Concurrent therapy is not recommended.

Digoxin. Acarbose may inhibit the absorption of digoxin. Monitor serum digoxin levels and therapeutic effects to assess whether the dosage of digoxin needs to be adjusted. Monitor closely when the dosage of acarbose is increased or discontinued.

DRUG CLASS: SODIUM-GLUCOSE COTRANSPORTER 2 INHIBITORS

Actions

In normal physiology, SGLT2 proteins located in the epithelial cells of the proximal tubules of the nephron (kidneys) reabsorb about 80% to 90% of the glucose filtered across the glomerulus, transporting it back into the circulating blood. In type 2 diabetes, SGLT2 is oversecreted, reabsorbing even more glucose back into the blood that may aggravate hyperglycemia.

Sodium-glucose cotransporter 2 inhibitors block the secretion of the SGLT2 protein, dropping glucose reabsorption from 90% to less than 10%, causing the glucose to be excreted in the urine.

Uses

Sodium-glucose cotransporter 2 inhibitors are a new class of antidiabetic agents used to treat hyperglycemia in type 2 diabetes by reducing renal glucose reabsorption in the proximal convoluted tubule, enhancing increased urinary glucose excretion. They are used as adjuncts to diet and exercise to improve blood glucose control in adults with type 2 diabetes. They may be used as monotherapy or in combination with metformin, sulfonylureas, TZDs, DPP-4 inhibitors, and insulin. With continuous use, the A_{1c} is lowered about 0.7%, similar to the reduction with other adjunctive antidiabetic agents. Patients who have type 1 diabetes or who are susceptible to ketoacidosis are not candidates for SGLT2 inhibitor therapy.

Therapeutic Outcomes

The primary therapeutic outcomes expected from SGLT2 inhibitor therapy are as follows:

1. A decrease in postprandial blood glucose and A_{1c} concentrations in the range defined as "acceptable" for the individual patient
2. Fewer long-term complications associated with poorly controlled type 2 diabetes mellitus

❖ **Nursing Implications for SGLT2 Inhibitors**
◆ *Premedication assessment*

1. Ensure that the dosages of concurrent antidiabetic therapy are well adjusted before starting SGLT2 inhibitor therapy.
2. Confirm that blood glucose and A_{1c} levels were recently measured and were hyperglycemic for the individual patient.
3. Review the estimated glomerular filtration rate (eGFR) as a renal function test to assure that the SGLT2 inhibitor being prescribed is acceptable based on the patient's glomerular filtration rate. Monitor the eGFR periodically during therapy because SGLT2 inhibitors may reduce renal function.
4. In patients starting canagliflozin therapy, ensure that the patient's serum potassium level is normal before starting therapy. Patients predisposed to hyperkalemia (including those with renal impairment or

taking potassium-sparing diuretics, ACE inhibitors, and angiotensin II receptor blockers) are more likely to develop hyperkalemia; monitor serum potassium levels after initiation in those who are predisposed.

5. Discuss with patients their compliance with current antidiabetic therapy and ability to do self-monitoring of blood glucose levels.

6. Ensure that the patient and family understand the signs and symptoms of hypoglycemia and its causes and treatment.

7. Ensure that the patient and family understand the signs and symptoms of ketoacidosis. Risk factors that may predispose to ketoacidosis include reduction in insulin therapy, caloric restriction, alcohol abuse, extensive exercise, myocardial infarction, stroke, severe infection, or other extreme stress event.

8. Patients receiving SGLT2 inhibitor therapy are at twice the risk of requiring a lower limb amputation such as toe, midfoot, or above or below knee amputations. Risk factors include prior amputation, peripheral vascular disease, neuropathy, and diabetic foot ulcers. Counsel patients on the importance of preventive foot care. SGLT2 inhibitor therapy should be discontinued if symptoms of a new infection, new pain or tenderness, or sores/ulcers involving the lower limbs are reported.

9. Discuss with both male and female patients their histories of urinary tract and genital fungal infections. Assure that the patients know the signs and symptoms of these infections and the need to report to their healthcare provider.

10. Identify whether the patient is pregnant or breastfeeding.

11. Monitor the patient's weight prior to beginning therapy and on a regular basis thereafter. This class of medicine is not associated with weight gain as are some of the other antidiabetic medicines. Weight losses of 4 to 7 pounds were reported in clinical trials.

◆ *Availability, dosage, and administration*
See Table 35.11.

◆ *Common and serious adverse effects*
Cardiovascular
Hypotension. Sodium-glucose cotransporter 2 inhibitors may induce vascular dehydration due to excretion of water along with hypertonic concentrations of glucose in the urine. Patients may develop hypotension with low systolic blood pressure, particularly in elderly patients and those concurrently taking antihypertensive medications and diuretics for other conditions. Maintain adequate hydration, especially when initiating therapy.

Increases in low-density lipoprotein cholesterol. It was noted in clinical trials that LDL cholesterol increased 5% to 7% in patients participating in the trials. The clinical significance of this mild elevation is unknown. The healthcare provider will decide whether or not to treat the LDL cholesterol.

Metabolic
Hypoglycemia. Hypoglycemia is quite rare in patients using the SGLT2 inhibitors as monotherapy but is more common in concurrent therapy with insulin and those agents that secrete insulin (secretagogues) (e.g., insulin, sulfonylureas, meglitinides). When using lower doses of insulin, the secretagogues or the SGLT2 inhibitors may be necessary to reduce the incidence of hypoglycemia.

Glycosuria. Based on the mechanism of action of SGLT2 inhibitors, patients will commonly spill glucose in the urine. Patients who test urine to monitor their diabetes should stop doing so because the results will be meaningless for monitoring.

Genitourinary
Genitourinary tract infections. All patients prescribed an SGLT2 inhibitor are at slightly greater risk of developing bacterial and fungal infections of the genitourinary tract due to glucosuria. Those patients with chronic or recurrent genitourinary infections are more likely to develop infections. Report symptoms to the healthcare provider for appropriate treatment.

Increased urination. Excretion of additional urine glucose may result in polyuria and nocturia in 2% to 5% of patients.

Table 35.11   Sodium-Glucose Cotransporter 2 Inhibitors

GENERIC NAME	BRAND NAME	AVAILABILITY	DAILY DOSAGE RANGE	MAXIMUM DAILY DOSAGE
canagliflozin	Invokana	Tablets: 100, 300 mg	PO: 100 mg once daily	300 mg; adjust dose in renal impairment; not recommended in patients with eGFR <45 mL/min/1.73 m^2; do not use in patients with eGFR of <30 mL/min/1.73 m^2
dapagliflozin	Farxiga	Tablets: 5, 10 mg	PO: 5 mg once daily	10 mg; do not use in patients with eGFR <60 mL/min/1.73 m^2
empagliflozin	Jardiance	Tablets: 10, 25 mg	PO: 10 mg once daily	25 mg; do not use in patients with eGFR <45 mL/min/1.73 m^2
ertugliflozin	Steglatro	Tablets: 5, 15 mg	PO: 5 mg once daily	15 mg; do not use in patients with eGFR <60 mL/min/1.73 m^2

eGFR, Estimated glomerular filtration rate; *GFR*, glomerular filtration rate.

◆ *Drug interactions*

Antihypertensive agents. Patients taking antihypertensive agents (ACE inhibitors, beta blockers, alpha blockers, calcium channel blockers, diuretics) may be more susceptible to orthostatic hypotension and hypotensive episodes induced by hypovolemic dehydration caused by SGLT2 inhibitors.

INCRETIN-RELATED ANTIDIABETIC THERAPY

In normal physiology there are two proteins known as incretin peptides: glucagon-like peptide-1 (GLP-1) and glucose-dependent insulinotropic polypeptide (GIP). (The term *glucose-dependent* means that they are secreted only when glucose levels start to rise.) These hormones are released from L cells in the distal ileum and colon in response to ingestion of carbohydrates and fats. The incretins help control blood glucose levels by the following mechanisms:

- Enhancing insulin secretion
- Suppressing glucagon secretion from the liver, thereby suppressing glucose output from the liver
- Delaying gastric emptying, thus slowing carbohydrate and lipid absorption and reducing postprandial hyperglycemia
- Reducing appetite
- Maintaining beta cell function

These actions result in reduction in basal glucose concentration and elevation of postprandial glucose concentration. There is also a reduced appetite, with subsequent weight reduction.

One of the pathophysiologies associated with type 2 diabetes mellitus is low incretin levels. A new approach to the treatment of this form of diabetes is to enhance the activity of incretin hormones. There are currently two classes of agents that support the incretins: the incretin mimetic agents (dulaglutide, exenatide, exenatide ER, liraglutide, lixisenatide, and semaglutide), which are GLP-1 agonists that improve GLP-1 levels, and the DPP-4 inhibitors (alogliptin, linagliptin, saxagliptin, and sitagliptin).

DRUG CLASS: INCRETIN MIMETIC AGENTS (GLUCAGON-LIKE PEPTIDE-1 AGONISTS)

Actions

Glucagon-like peptide-1 agonists mimic the actions of this incretin for self-regulating glycemic control, resulting in an increase in serum insulin and a reduction in glucose concentrations.

Uses

Glucagon-like peptide-1 agonists are used as additional therapy to reduce elevated fasting and postprandial hyperglycemia in patients with type 2 diabetes mellitus who are taking metformin, a sulfonylurea, or a combination of metformin and a sulfonylurea, but who have not achieved adequate glycemic control. Particular

benefits of GLP-1 agonists are that they enhance insulin secretion only in the presence of hyperglycemia, and insulin secretion decreases as the blood glucose level approaches normal levels.

Exenatide ER, semaglutide and dulaglutide are administered once weekly, whereas liraglutide and lixisenatide are administered once daily and exenatide must be administered twice daily. All are available in prefilled syringes for injection.

Dulaglutide, exenatide ER, liraglutide, and semaglutide are contraindicated for use in patients with a personal or family history of medullary thyroid cancer (MTC) and in patients with multiple endocrine neoplasia syndrome type 2 (MEN2). All patients should be monitored for symptoms of thyroid tumors (e.g., mass in the neck, dysphagia, dyspnea, persistent hoarseness).

Therapeutic Outcomes

The primary therapeutic outcomes expected from GLP-1 agonist therapy are as follows:

1. A decrease in fasting and postprandial blood glucose levels and A_{1c} concentrations in the range defined as "acceptable" for the individual patient
2. Fewer long-term complications associated with poorly controlled type 2 diabetes mellitus

❖ **Nursing Implications for GLP-1 Agonists**
◆ *Premedication assessment*

1. Ensure that the dosages of concurrent oral antidiabetic agents are well adjusted before starting GLP-1 therapy.
2. Assess the patient's or family member's ability to self-administer injections.

◆ *Availability, dosage, and administration.* See Table 35.12. Administer GLP-1 agonists as a subcutaneous injection in the thigh, abdomen, or upper arm. Exenatide is a twice-daily administration, whereas liraglutide is a once-daily administration independent of meals. Do *not* administer exenatide after a meal. Based on clinical response, the dose of the agonist may be increased.

The GLP-1 agonists are used in conjunction with metformin and/or a sulfonylurea. Dosage adjustment of the metformin is not necessary, but a dosage reduction of the sulfonylurea might be necessary to reduce the risk of hypoglycemia.

Glucagon-like peptide-1 pens should be stored refrigerated at 36°F to 46°F (2.2°C to 7.8°C). Do not freeze or use the pen if it has been frozen. Warm to room temperature before use. After first use, the pens may be stored at room temperature (59°F to 86°F [15°C to 30°C]). The pens should be discarded 30 days after first use, even if some of the drug remains in the pen.

◆ *Common adverse effects*
Gastrointestinal

Nausea, vomiting, diarrhea, constipation. These adverse effects are usually mild to moderate and tend to resolve with continued therapy. Encourage the patient not to

Table 35.12   Glucagon-like Peptide-1 Agonists

GENERIC NAME	BRAND NAME	AVAILABILITY	DOSAGE RANGE	MAXIMUM DOSAGE
dulaglutide	Trulicity	Prefilled pen for one-time use: 0.75, 1.5 mg	Subcutaneous: 0.75 mg or 1.5 mg one time weekly	1.5 mg; 1 injection weekly
exenatide	Byetta	Prefilled pen cartridges: 1.2 mL of solution to deliver 5 mcg per injection; 2.4 mL of solution to deliver 10 mcg per injection (each prefilled pen will deliver 60 doses to provide a 30-day supply of the twice-daily medication)	Subcutaneous: 5 mcg twice daily within 60 min of morning and evening meals; 6 or more hr apart	10 mcg twice daily
exenatide ER	Bydureon	Subcutaneous suspension: 2 mg/vial	2 mg once weekly at any time of day, with or without meals	2 mg; 1 injection weekly
liraglutide	Victoza	Prefilled pen cartridge: 18 mg/3 mL	Subcutaneous: 0.6 mg once daily at any time for 1 wk May increase dose to 1.2 mg once daily May increase to 1.8 mg for glycemic control	Use with caution in patients with renal or hepatic impairment No dosage adjustment is required for these conditions.
lixisenatide	Adlyxin	Adlyxin Starter Pack: Prefilled pen: 10 mcg/0.2 mL in 3 mL prefilled pen and 20 mcg/0.2 mL in 3 mL prefilled pen; Prefilled Pen injector 20 mcg/0.2 mL in 3 mL	Subcutaneous: 10 mcg once daily for 14 days; on day 15 increase to 20 mcg once daily. Maintenance dose: 20 mcg once daily	20 mcg once daily
semaglutide	Ozempic	Prefilled pen 0.25 mg or 0.5 mg per dose (2 mg/1.5 mL); 1 mg per dose (2 mg/1.5 mL)	Subcutaneously: 0.25 mg once weekly for 4 weeks; after 4 weeks on the initial dose, increase to 0.5 mg subcutaneously once weekly for at least 4 weeks	1 mg once weekly
Combination Insulin and Glucagon-like Peptide-1 Agonists				
degludec and liraglutide	Xultophy	Prefilled pen: degludec 100 units/mL and liraglutide 3.6 mg/mL in 3 mL	Subcutaneous: 16 units of degludec and 0.58 mg of liraglutide once daily	Maximum daily dosage: 50 units of degludec and 1.8 mg of liraglutide
glargine and lixisenatide	Soliqua	Prefilled pen: glargine 100 units/mL and lixisenatide 33 mcg/mL in 3 mL	In patients inadequately controlled on <30 units of basal insulin or on lixisenatide: Subcutaneous: 15 units glargine/5 mcg lixisenatide given once daily In patients inadequately controlled on 30-60 units of basal insulin: Subcutaneous: 30 units glargine/10 mcg lixisenatide once daily	Maximum dosage: 60 units glargine/20 mcg lixisenatide

discontinue therapy without first consulting the healthcare provider.

Neurologic

Headache. This adverse effect is usually mild to moderate and tends to resolve with continued therapy.

Encourage the patient not to discontinue therapy without first consulting the healthcare provider.

Immune system, respiratory

Upper respiratory infection. In clinical trials with GLP-1 agonists there was a higher rate of upper respiratory infection in the GLP-1 agonist–treated group than in the placebo-treated group. Notify the healthcare provider if symptoms of nasal congestion and sore throat develop during GLP-1 therapy.

◆ *Serious adverse effects*
Metabolic
Hypoglycemia. Although GLP-1 agonists do not cause hypoglycemia by themselves, they can enhance the hypoglycemia that may be caused by a sulfonylurea or other secretagogues. Consequently, blood glucose levels must be monitored closely, especially in the early stages of therapy. Monitor for the following signs of hypoglycemia: headache, nausea, weakness, hunger, lethargy, decreased coordination, general apprehension, sweating, or blurred or double vision. Notify the healthcare provider immediately if any of these symptoms appear.

Hypoglycemia must be treated immediately. Mild symptoms may be controlled by the oral administration of a glucose source (e.g., a lump of sugar, orange juice, carbonated cola beverage [not diet], candy [not chocolate]) or ingestion of a commercially prepared product such as Glutose. Severe symptoms may be relieved by IV administration of glucose, and parenteral glucagon may be prescribed in some cases. If in doubt about whether the patient is hypoglycemic or hyperglycemic, always treat the individual for hypoglycemia to prevent the possible neurologic complications that can occur from untreated hypoglycemia. The dosage of oral antidiabetic agents may also have to be reduced.

Pancreatitis. Glucagon-like peptide-1 agonists may rarely cause pancreatitis, particularly when treatment is started and following increases in dosage. Observe for signs and symptoms of pancreatitis, including persistent, severe abdominal pain that may radiate around to the back and may be accompanied by vomiting. If symptoms develop, hold the dose of medication and contact the healthcare provider.

◆ *Drug interactions*
Hypoglycemia. The following drugs may enhance the hypoglycemic effects of the sulfonylureas and GLP-1 agonists: ethanol, androgens (e.g., methandrostenolone), warfarin, beta-adrenergic blocking agents (e.g., propranolol, metoprolol, carvedilol), salicylates, sulfonamides (e.g., sulfamethoxazole-trimethoprim), fluoroquinolones (e.g., ciprofloxacin, levofloxacin, moxifloxacin), and MAOIs.

Monitor for the following signs of hypoglycemia: headache, nausea, weakness, hunger, lethargy, decreased coordination, general apprehension, sweating, and blurred or double vision. Notify the healthcare provider if any of these symptoms appear.

Hyperglycemia. The following medications, when used concurrently with GLP-1 agonists, may decrease the therapeutic effects of GLP-1 agonists: corticosteroids, phenothiazines, diuretics, oral contraceptives, thyroid replacement hormones, phenytoin, diazoxide, and lithium carbonate.

DRUG CLASS: DIPEPTIDYL PEPTIDASE-4 INHIBITORS

Actions
The incretin hormones GIP and GLP-1 are quickly metabolized by DPP-4, which results in hyperglycemia. Dipeptidyl peptidase-4 inhibitors prolong the life of active GLP-1 and GIP, prolonging the beneficial effects of the incretin hormones in reducing hyperglycemia.

Uses
Dipeptidyl peptidase-4 inhibitors may be used as monotherapy or as additional therapy as an adjunct to diet and exercise to reduce elevated fasting and postprandial hyperglycemia in patients with type 2 diabetes mellitus who are taking metformin, a sulfonylurea, or a combination of metformin and a sulfonylurea, but who have not achieved adequate glycemic control. Particular benefits of DPP-4 inhibitors are that they enhance insulin secretion only in the presence of hyperglycemia, and insulin secretion decreases as blood glucose approaches normal levels. Saxagliptin has been associated with heart failure that may require hospitalization. Monitor for signs and symptoms of heart failure during therapy and consider discontinuation if condition develops

Therapeutic Outcomes
The primary therapeutic outcomes expected from DPP-4 inhibitor therapy are as follows:
1. A decrease in fasting and postprandial blood glucose levels and A_{1c} concentrations in the range defined as "acceptable" for the individual patient
2. Fewer long-term complications associated with poorly controlled type 2 diabetes mellitus

❖ **Nursing Implications for DPP-4 Inhibitors**
◆ *Premedication assessment.* Ensure that the dosages of concurrent oral antidiabetic therapy are well adjusted before starting DPP-4 inhibitor therapy.

◆ *Availability, dosage, and administration.* See Table 35.13. *Adult:* Administer with or without food. Adjust DPP-4 inhibitor dosage for patients with renal impairment.

 Medication Safety Alert

Dipeptidyl peptidase-4 inhibitors do not cause hypoglycemia by themselves, but their concurrent use with an agent known to cause hypoglycemia (e.g., sulfonylureas) should be closely monitored. Use with caution when given with other agents that may also cause hypoglycemia. A lower dose of the sulfonylurea may be required.

◆ *Common adverse effects*
Gastrointestinal
Nausea, abdominal pain, diarrhea. These adverse effects are usually mild to moderate and tend to resolve with continued therapy. Encourage the patient not to

Table 35.13   Dipeptidyl Peptidase-4 Inhibitors

GENERIC NAME	BRAND NAME	AVAILABILITY	DAILY DOSAGE RANGE	MAXIMUM DAILY DOSAGE
alogliptin	Nesina	Tablets: 6.25, 12.5, 25 mg	PO: 25 mg daily	25 mg; adjust dose in renal impairment
linagliptin	Tradjenta	Tablets: 5 mg	PO: 5 mg once daily	5 mg
saxagliptin	Onglyza	Tablets: 2.5, 5 mg	PO: 2.5-5 mg once daily	5 mg; adjust dose in renal impairment
sitagliptin	Januvia	Tablets: 25, 50, 100 mg	PO: 100 mg once daily	100 mg; adjust dose in renal impairment

discontinue therapy without first consulting the healthcare provider.

Neurologic

Headache. This adverse effect is usually mild to moderate and tends to resolve with continued therapy. Encourage the patient not to discontinue therapy without first consulting the healthcare provider.

Immunologic, respiratory

Upper respiratory infection, nasopharyngitis. In clinical trials with DPP-4 inhibitors, there was a higher rate of upper respiratory infection and nasopharyngitis in the DPP-4 inhibitor–treated group than in the placebo-treated group. Notify the prescriber if symptoms of nasal congestion and sore throat develop during DPP-4 inhibitor therapy.

◆ *Serious adverse effects*

Metabolic

Hypoglycemia. Patients may develop hypoglycemia when DPP-4 inhibitors are used in combination with other agents that may induce hypoglycemia (e.g., sulfonylureas). Consequently, blood glucose levels must be monitored closely, especially in the early stages of therapy. Monitor for the following signs of hypoglycemia: headache, nausea, weakness, hunger, lethargy, decreased coordination, general apprehension, sweating, or blurred or double vision. Notify the healthcare provider immediately if any of these symptoms appear.

Hypoglycemia must be treated immediately. Mild symptoms may be controlled by the oral administration of a glucose source (e.g., a lump of sugar, orange juice, carbonated cola beverage [not diet], candy [not chocolate]) or ingestion of a commercially prepared product such as Glutose. Severe symptoms may be relieved by IV administration of glucose, and parenteral glucagon may be prescribed in some cases. If in doubt about whether the patient is hypoglycemic or hyperglycemic, always treat the individual for hypoglycemia to prevent the possible neurologic complications that can occur from untreated hypoglycemia. The dosage of oral antidiabetic agents may also have to be reduced.

Pancreatitis. Dipeptidyl peptidase-4 inhibitors infrequently cause pancreatitis, particularly when treatment is started and following increases in dosage. Observe for signs and symptoms of pancreatitis, including persistent, severe abdominal pain that may radiate around to the back and may be accompanied with vomiting. If symptoms develop, hold the dose of medication and contact the healthcare provider.

Immunologic

Hypersensitivity. With use of DPP-4 inhibitors there have been infrequent reports of hypersensitivity reactions manifested by skin rashes, angioedema, and anaphylaxis. If symptoms develop, hold the dose of medication and contact the healthcare provider.

Arthralgia. Severe and disabling arthralgia has been reported with DPP-IV inhibitor use; onset may occur within one day to years after treatment initiation and may resolve with discontinuation of therapy. Some patients may experience a recurrence of symptoms if DPP-IV inhibitor therapy is resumed.

◆ *Drug interactions*

Digoxin. Patients taking sitagliptin and digoxin concurrently may experience a 20% increase in digoxin serum levels. In most patients, this is not a particular problem, but monitor for bradycardia. Hold the digoxin dose and contact the prescriber if the heart rate is below 60 beats/min.

Hypoglycemia. The following drugs may enhance the hypoglycemic effects of DPP-4 inhibitors: ethanol, androgens (e.g., methandrostenolone), warfarin, beta-adrenergic blocking agents (e.g., propranolol, metoprolol, carvedilol), salicylates, sulfonamides (e.g., sulfamethoxazole-trimethoprim), fluoroquinolones (ciprofloxacin, moxifloxacin, norfloxacin), and MAOIs.

The following drugs may inhibit the metabolism of saxagliptin, enhancing hypoglycemic effects: ketoconazole, itraconazole, clarithromycin, indinavir, nelfinavir, and ritonavir.

Monitor for the following signs of hypoglycemia: headache, nausea, weakness, hunger, lethargy, decreased coordination, general apprehension, sweating, or blurred or double vision. Notify the healthcare provider if any of these symptoms appear.

Hyperglycemia. The following drugs, when used concurrently with DPP-4 inhibitors, may decrease the therapeutic effects of sitagliptin: corticosteroids, phenothiazines, diuretics, oral contraceptives, thyroid replacement hormones, phenytoin, and lithium carbonate.

The following drugs may enhance the metabolism of linagliptin, reducing the therapeutic effects: rifampin, phenobarbital, phenytoin, and carbamazepine. Change therapy to another DPP-4 inhibitor.

DRUG CLASS: ANTIHYPOGLYCEMIC AGENTS

glucagon (GLŬ-kă-gŏn)

Actions

Glucagon is a hormone secreted by the alpha cells of the pancreas that breaks down stored glycogen to glucose, resulting in elevated blood glucose levels. Glucagon also aids in converting amino acids to glucose (gluconeogenesis). Glucagon is dependent on the presence of glycogen for its action. It has essentially no action in cases of starvation, adrenal insufficiency, or chronic hypoglycemia.

Uses

Glucagon is used to treat hypoglycemic reactions in patients with diabetes mellitus.

Therapeutic Outcome

The primary therapeutic outcome expected from glucagon therapy is elimination of symptoms associated with hypoglycemia.

❖ **Nursing Implications for Glucagon**

◆ *Premedication assessment*

1. Confirm patient unresponsiveness before administration. If patient is conscious, oral antihypoglycemic therapy is usually more appropriate.
2. Hypoglycemia is a medical emergency. If suspected, it should be treated by authorized personnel as soon as possible.

◆ *Availability.* *Subcutaneous, IM, IV*: 1-mg vial.

◆ *Dosage and administration.* **Adult:** *Subcutaneous, IM, IV*: Administer 1 mg. Repeat in 15 minutes as needed. Administer fast-acting and long-acting carbohydrates to patient as soon as possible after response to treatment. If the patient is slow to arouse, consider administering glucose by the IV route.

◆ *Common and serious adverse effects*
   Gastrointestinal
   Nausea, vomiting. These adverse effects may also occur with hypoglycemia. Take precautions to prevent aspiration of vomitus.

◆ *Drug interactions*
   Warfarin. Glucagon may potentiate the anticoagulant effects of warfarin if used for several days. Monitor the patient's international normalized ratio and reduce the dosage of warfarin accordingly.

Get Ready for the NCLEX® Examination!

Key Points

- Diabetes mellitus is a complex group of chronic diseases that is associated with both short- and long-term complications. The long-term objective of control of the disease must involve mechanisms to stop the progression of the complications of the disease.
- Patient education and reinforcement are extremely important to successful therapy. Major determinants to success are the patient's taking responsibility for a balanced diet, insulin or oral hypoglycemic therapy, routine exercise, and good hygiene.
- The nurse plays a critical role as a health educator by discussing treatment options, planning lifestyle changes, counseling before discharge, and reinforcing key points during office visits. Best results are attained when the patient, family, and nurse work together in developing the care plan.

Additional Learning Resources

SG Go to your Study Guide for additional Review Questions for the NCLEX® Examination, Critical Thinking Clinical Situations, and other learning activities to help you master this chapter content.

Go to your Evolve website (https://evolve.elsevier.com/Clayton) for additional online resources.

Review Questions for the NCLEX® Examination

1. The nurse is educating a new diabetic patient on how to manage dietary requirements and prevent hypoglycemia. The nurse realizes the patient needs further teaching after he makes which statement?
   1. "If I increase my carbohydrate intake, I will need to adjust my daily insulin dose."
   2. "So as I understand it, when I increase my protein intake, I can decrease my physical activity without affecting my blood sugar."
   3. "When I take a beta blocker with insulin, it can cause my blood sugar to drop."
   4. "If I take insulin and do not eat enough carbohydrates, I could become hypoglycemic."

2. After learning the symptoms of hypoglycemia, a patient performing teach-back to the nurse included which of the following in the discussion? *(Select all that apply.)*
   1. Hunger
   2. Sweating
   3. Rapid, shallow respirations
   4. Nausea, vomiting, and abdominal pain
   5. Weakness and blurred vision

3. Which types of insulin are considered the rapid-acting types? *(Select all that apply.)*
   1. Lispro
   2. Humulin R
   3. Glargine
   4. Glulisine
   5. Aspart

4. A patient who received insulin at breakfast started to complain around noon about feeling shaky, off balance, sweaty, and unable to focus. The nurse suspected that the patient was experiencing which effect?
   1. Lactic acidosis
   2. Kidney failure
   3. Hyperglycemia
   4. Hypoglycemia

5. During a clinic visit 3 months following a diagnosis of type 2 diabetes, a patient reports following the reduced-calorie diet without any weight loss. The patient has also neglected to bring a record of glucose monitoring results. The best indicator of this patient's control of diabetes since the initial diagnosis and instruction is apparent using which laboratory value?
   1. Fasting glucose level
   2. Potassium level
   3. Hemoglobin A$_{1c}$ level
   4. Urine ketones

6. A nurse is administering insulin subcutaneously to a patient. List in order the actions the nurse will take.
   1. Draw up insulin
   2. Document the medication
   3. Inject insulin
   4. Check the order
   5. Verify the correct patient

7. A newly diagnosed diabetic patient asks the nurse how long it takes for insulin to "kick in." Which response by the nurse would be appropriate?
   1. "Depending on the type of insulin you receive, it can take as long as 2 hours and as short as 15 minutes."
   2. "Insulin lasts as long as there is glucose circulating in your system."
   3. "The half-life of insulin is rather short, which is why you need to take it so frequently."
   4. "Insulin is only effective when it is given before a meal and only lasts as long as it takes to digest the meal."

8. A patient asked the nurse how the antidiabetic drug pioglitazone works to lower blood glucose. Which response by the nurse would be appropriate?
   1. "This medication works by stimulating the release of insulin from beta cells in the pancreas."
   2. "Unfortunately, this medications works by an unknown mechanism of action."
   3. "This is one of the antidiabetic agents that work by increasing muscle and fat tissue sensitivity to allow more glucose to enter the cell in the presence of insulin."
   4. "This medication works by affecting certain enzymes used in the digestion of sugars, which results in delayed glucose absorption."

9. The nurse is educating a patient who was admitted with peripheral edema and acute kidney injury. After discussing the complications of diabetes, the patient was able to correctly identify which examples of neuropathies? *(Select all that apply.)*
   1. Retinopathy
   2. Loss of sensation
   3. Numbness of the extremities
   4. Tingling of the extremities
   5. Myocardial infarction

10. The nurse caring for a type 1 diabetic patient knows this type of diabetes is caused by which pathology?
    1. Genetic defects of beta cell function
    2. Drug or chemically induced
    3. Immune mediated or idiopathic
    4. Progressive insulin resistance

Drugs Used to Treat Thyroid Disease

Objectives

1. Describe the function of the thyroid gland.
2. Identify the two classes of drugs used to treat thyroid disease.
3. Describe the signs, symptoms, treatment, and nursing interventions associated with hypothyroidism and identify the drug of choice for hypothyroidism.
4. Describe the signs, symptoms, treatments, and nursing interventions associated with hyperthyroidism.
5. Discuss the drug interactions associated with thyroid hormones and antithyroid medicines.

Key Terms

thyroid-stimulating hormone (TSH) (THĪ-royd STĬM-yū-lā-tĭng HŌR-mōn) (p. 569)
triiodothyronine (T₃) (trī-ī-ō-dō-THĪ-rō-nēn) (p. 569)
thyroxine (T₄) (thī-RŎKS-ēn) (p. 569)
hypothyroidism (hī-pō-THĪ-royd-ĭzm) (p. 569)

myxedema (mĭk-sĕ-DĒ-mă) (p. 569)
cretinism (KRĒ-tĭn-ĭzm) (p. 570)
hyperthyroidism (hī-pĕr-THĪ-royd-ĭzm) (p. 570)
thyrotoxicosis (thī-rō-tŏk-sĭ-KŌ-sĭs) (p. 570)

THYROID GLAND

The thyroid gland is a large, reddish, ductless gland in front of and on either side of the trachea. It consists of two lateral lobes and a connecting isthmus and is roughly butterfly shaped (Fig. 36.1). It is enclosed in a covering of areolar connective tissue. The thyroid is made up of numerous closed follicles containing colloid matter and is surrounded by a vascular network. This gland is one of the most richly vascularized tissues in the body. It can be palpated by placing fingers on either side of the trachea and asking the patient to swallow (Fig. 36.2).

As with other endocrine glands, thyroid gland function is regulated by the hypothalamus and the anterior pituitary gland. The hypothalamus secretes thyrotropin-releasing hormone (TRH), which stimulates the anterior pituitary gland to release thyroid-stimulating hormone (TSH). Thyroid-stimulating hormone stimulates the thyroid gland to release its hormones, triiodothyronine (T₃) and thyroxine (T₄).

The thyroid hormones regulate general body metabolism. Imbalance in thyroid hormone production may also interfere with the following body functions: growth and maturation; carbohydrate, protein, and lipid metabolism; thermal regulation; cardiovascular function; lactation; and reproduction.

THYROID DISEASES

Hypothyroidism is the result of inadequate thyroid hormone production. Myxedema is hypothyroidism that occurs during adult life. The onset of symptoms is usually mild and vague. Patients develop slowness in motion, speech, and mental processes. They often develop more lethargic, sedentary habits, and they have decreased appetites, gain weight, are constipated, cannot tolerate cold, become weak, and fatigue easily. The body temperature may be subnormal; the skin becomes dry, coarse, and thickened; and the face appears puffy. Patients often have decreased blood pressure and heart rate, have elevated cholesterol levels, and develop anemia. These patients have an increased susceptibility to infection and are sensitive to small doses of sedative-hypnotics, anesthetics, and narcotics. Myxedema may be caused by excessive use of antithyroid drugs to treat hyperthyroidism, radiation exposure, thyroid surgery, acute viral thyroiditis, or chronic thyroiditis.

A rare presentation of hypothyroidism is myxedema coma. Myxedema coma is a severe form of hypothyroidism that can occur as the culmination of severe, long-standing hypothyroidism or be precipitated by an acute event in a poorly controlled hypothyroid patient, such as infection, myocardial infarction, cold exposure,

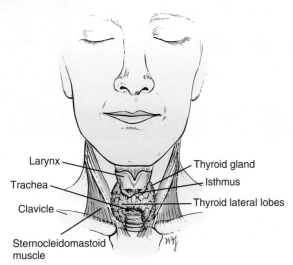

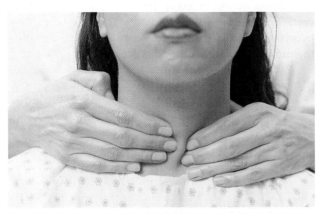

Fig. 36.1 Location of the thyroid gland. (From Swartz MH. *Textbook of Physical Diagnosis: History and Examination.* 7th ed. Philadelphia: Elsevier Inc; 2014.)

Fig. 36.2 Palpation of the thyroid gland. (From Thompson JM, Wilson SF. *Health Assessment for Nursing Practice.* St. Louis: Mosby; 1996.)

or the administration of sedative drugs, especially opioids. It is a medical emergency with a high mortality rate. Fortunately, it is now a rare presentation of hypothyroidism.

Congenital hypothyroidism occurs when a child is born without a thyroid gland or with a gland that is hypoactive. The historic name of the resulting disorder is **cretinism**. Fortunately, this disorder is becoming rare because most states require diagnostic testing of the newborn for hypothyroidism.

Although the symptoms of hypothyroidism in both infants and adults are for the most part classical, the final diagnosis is usually not made until diagnostic tests have been completed. These tests include determining serum levels of circulating T_3 and T_4 hormones. If the levels are low, the patient is considered to be hypothyroid. Further diagnostic testing is required to determine the cause of thyroid hypofunction.

Hyperthyroidism is caused by excess production of thyroid hormones. Disorders that may cause hyperactivity of the thyroid gland are Graves' disease, nodular

goiter, thyroiditis, thyroid carcinoma, overdoses of thyroid hormones, and tumors of the pituitary gland.

The clinical manifestations of hyperthyroidism are a rapid, bounding pulse (even during sleep) as well as cardiac enlargement, palpitations, and dysrhythmias. Patients are nervous and easily agitated. They develop tremors, a low-grade fever, and weight loss, despite an increased appetite. Hyperactive reflexes and insomnia are also usually present. Patients are intolerant of heat; the skin is warm, flushed, and moist, with increased sweating; and edema of the tissues around the eyeballs produces characteristic eye changes, including exophthalmos. Patients develop amenorrhea; dyspnea with minor exertion; hoarse, rapid speech; and an increased susceptibility to infection. Elevated circulating thyroid hormone levels easily diagnose hyperthyroidism. Further diagnostic studies are required to determine the cause.

Excessive formation of thyroid hormones and their secretion into the circulatory system causes hyperthyroidism, potentially leading to *thyrotoxicosis*. Symptoms include increased metabolic rate, increased pulse rate (to perhaps 140 beats/min), increased body temperature, restlessness, nervousness, anxiety, sweating, muscle weakness and tremors, and a sensation of feeling too warm. This condition is treated with antithyroid drugs or surgical removal of the thyroid gland.

TREATMENT OF THYROID DISEASES

The primary goal of therapy for hyperthyroidism and hypothyroidism is to return the patient to a normal thyroid (euthyroid) state. Hypothyroidism can be treated successfully by replacement of thyroid hormones (see drug monographs on individual agents). After therapy is initiated, the dosage of thyroid hormone is adjusted until serum levels of the thyroid hormones are within the normal range.

Three types of treatment can be used to reduce the hyperthyroid state—subtotal thyroidectomy, radioactive iodine, and antithyroid medications. Until treatment is underway, the patient requires nutritional and psychological support.

Life Span Considerations
Treatment of Hypothyroid State

During initial treatment of the hypothyroid state in the older adult patient, be alert for and report increased frequency of angina or symptoms of heart failure.

DRUG THERAPY FOR THYROID DISEASES

Two general classes of drugs are used to treat thyroid disorders: (1) those used to replace thyroid hormones in patients whose thyroid glandular function is inadequate to meet metabolic requirements (hypothyroidism); and (2) antithyroid agents used to suppress synthesis of thyroid hormones (hyperthyroidism). Thyroid hormone replacements available are levothyroxine (T_4), liothyronine (T_3), liotrix, and thyroid USP. Antithyroid drugs interfere with the formation or release of the hormones produced by the thyroid gland. Antithyroid agents include radioactive iodine, propylthiouracil, and methimazole.

❖ NURSING IMPLICATIONS FOR PATIENTS WITH THYROID DISORDERS

Hypothyroidism and hyperthyroidism are treated primarily on an outpatient basis unless surgery is indicated or complications occur. Nurses must be able to offer guidance to the patients requiring treatment on an inpatient or ambulatory basis. In general, body processes are slowed with hypothyroidism and accelerated with hyperthyroidism.

◆ Assessment

Take a history of treatment prescribed for hypothyroidism or hyperthyroidism (e.g., surgery, iodine-131, or hormone replacement). Ask for specific information regarding treatment for any cardiac disease or adrenal insufficiency.

Medications. Request a list of all prescribed and over-the-counter medications being taken. Ask if any of the prescribed medications are taken on a regular basis. If not taken regularly, what factors have caused the patient to decrease administration?

Description of current symptoms. Ask the patient to explain symptoms experienced and what changes in functioning have occurred over the past 2 to 3 months.

Focused assessment. Perform a focused assessment of the body systems generally affected by hypothyroid or hyperthyroid states:

- Implement monitoring parameters for vital signs, intake and output, daily weights, and mental status checks. Schedule regular assessment of intake and output, vital signs, mental status, and daily weights.
- *Cardiovascular:* Take current vital signs, including an apical pulse. Note bradycardia or tachycardia and any alterations in rhythm and pulsations (e.g., bounding or thready), subnormal or elevated temperature, and hypertension. Monitor for cardiac symptoms (e.g., heart failure). Ask whether the pulse rate is decreased or elevated on awakening, before any stimulus. Does the patient experience any palpitations or a feeling that the pulse is rapid and bounding? Record heart sounds and any abnormal characteristics heard (or have a qualified nurse perform this).
- *Respiratory:* Does the patient experience dyspnea? Is it made worse by mild exertion?
- *Gastrointestinal:* Measure the person's height and weight. Monitor the pattern of bowel elimination

and give as-needed (PRN) medications prescribed for diarrhea or constipation. Ask for a history of increase or decrease in weight over the past 3 months. Has there been a change in appetite? Does the individual experience nausea and vomiting? What have the characteristics of the stools been over the past several months—constipation, diarrhea, or normal? Check and record bowel sounds.

- *Integumentary:* Note the temperature, texture, and condition of the skin and the characteristics of the hair and nails. Does the patient complain of intolerance to heat or cold?
- *Musculoskeletal:* What activity level is maintained? Does the person feel or act sluggish or hyperactive? Is the pattern of activity a change from the recent past? If so, when did this become apparent? Is there muscle weakness, wasting, or discomfort? Is dependent edema present?
- *Neurologic:* What is the patient's mental status—is the patient oriented to time, date, and place? What is the degree of alertness and pace of responsiveness (e.g., sluggish and slow in contrast with being quick or fast paced)? Is the individual depressed, stuporous, or hyperactive? Has the individual or family and significant others noticed any change in personality in the recent past? Has the individual had tremors of the hands, eyelids, or tongue? Has the individual experienced insomnia?
- *Sensory:* What is the condition of the eyes? Do the eyelids retract or is exophthalmos present?
- *Reproductive:* Obtain a history of changes in the pattern of menses and libido.
- *Immunologic:* Has the individual had any recent infections? What types of infections and at what frequency has the patient had infections over the last year?

Laboratory and diagnostic studies and surgery. Review laboratory and diagnostic studies available on the patient's record associated with thyroid disorders such as total thyroxine (TT_4) and total triiodothyronine (TT_3) tests, free thyroxine (FT_4) and free triiodothyronine (FT_3) tests, TSH levels, TRH stimulation test, thyroid autoantibodies, thyroglobulin, calcitonin assay, ultrasound, fine-needle biopsy, radioactive iodine uptake, electrocardiography, and thyroid scan. If surgery is scheduled for hyperthyroidism, schedule routine postoperation vital signs and order a tracheostomy set for the bedside. Indicate on the written and/or computer care plan to check dressings for bleeding, perform respiratory assessments, perform voice checks for hoarseness, and monitor for development of tetany for the first 24 to 48 hours, as ordered by the healthcare provider. Gather calcium gluconate and supplies needed for intravenous (IV) administration and have them ready for use.

◆ Implementation
Environment
- For the hyperthyroid individual, plan to provide a cool, quiet, structured environment because the patient lacks the ability to respond to change and anxiety-producing situations and has intolerance to heat.
- For the hypothyroid individual, plan to provide a warm, quiet, structured environment that supports the patient's needs. Provide support and give directions slowly and with patience because the individual may have difficulty processing the information. Incorporate the family into the provision of care, as appropriate.

Nutrition
- *Hyperthyroid*: Order the prescribed diet, usually a high-calorie diet of 4000 to 5000 calories per day with balanced nutrients, and note no caffeine products (e.g., coffee, tea, colas). If diarrhea is present, note any foods with a laxative or stimulating effect such as bran products, fruits, and fresh vegetables.
- *Hypothyroid*: Order the prescribed diet, usually a low-calorie diet with increased bulk to alleviate constipation. Encourage adequate fluid intake, unless comorbidities prohibit it. Encourage the patient to comply with dietary orders.

Psychosocial care
- Monitor the mental status at least every shift.
- Plan to incorporate the family into the health teaching plan because the patient may be unable to understand or implement all facets of the therapeutic regimen.

Activity and exercise. Note the prescribed level of activity ordered by the healthcare provider. Institute safety precautions for individuals with muscle weakness, wasting, or pain that would place them at risk for injury.

Medications. Give prescribed medications and monitor for response to therapy. Thyroid medications usually are scheduled early in the day to prevent insomnia.

◆ Patient Education
Medications
- Stress the need for lifelong administration of medications for the treatment of hypothyroidism and the need for periodic laboratory studies and evaluation by the healthcare provider.
- Stress that several medications interact with thyroid drugs so it is important to inform any prescribing healthcare provider of the thyroid disease and the medications being taken.
- Patients scheduled for outpatient diagnostics must receive detailed written instructions regarding the prescribed medications to be taken in preparation for testing.

- The patient and, as appropriate, family or significant others must understand the anticipated therapeutic response sought from prescribed medications. Teach specific indications of a satisfactory response to pharmacologic therapy. Stress the need to contact the healthcare provider if signs of an excess or deficit in dosage occur. Ensure that the individual can monitor the resting pulse.

Environment. Explain the need for a cool environment for a patient with hyperthyroidism or a warm environment for the person with hypothyroidism.

Nutrition
- In patients with diarrhea secondary to hyperthyroidism, explain the need for a high-calorie diet with reduced roughage.
- Explain the need for a low-calorie diet with increased roughage to the individual with hypothyroidism. Encourage patients with constipation to drink 8 to 10 eight-ounce glasses of water and add roughage to the diet each day.
- As the patient returns to a more normal thyroid function through medication, the caloric requirements of the diet will also change.

Psychosocial. The patient may have had a major personality change, may be depressed, or (at the other end of the spectrum) may be hyperactive. Explain these symptoms to the family and involve them in examining potential interventions that can be used in the home environment.

Activity and exercise
- Provide for patient safety during ambulation if muscle weakness, wasting, or discomfort is present. Discuss measures needed to provide for patient safety with the family and significant others.
- As the patient returns to a more normal thyroid function through medication, the activity level should change. Encourage moderate exercise.

Fostering health maintenance
- Throughout the course of treatment, discuss information about the medication and how it will benefit the patient. Recognize that nonadherence with lifelong treatment, when prescribed, may occur, and stress positive outcomes that result from regular medication adherence.
- Provide the patient and significant others with important information contained in the specific drug monographs for the medications prescribed. Additional health teaching and nursing interventions for the common and serious adverse effects are described in the drug monographs.
- Seek cooperation and understanding of the following points so that medication adherence is increased: name of medication; dosage, route, and times of

administration; and common and serious adverse effects.

- When laboratory studies for thyroid function are scheduled, thyroid preparations may be discontinued for one or more days in advance of the tests. Always consult the prescriber for detailed instructions.

Patient self-assessment. Enlist the patient's aid in developing and maintaining a written record; see Patient Self-Assessment Forms for Thyroid Medications and Antithyroid Medications on the Evolve website. Complete the Premedication Data column for use as a baseline to track response to drug therapy. Ensure that the patient understands how to use the form and instruct the patient to bring the completed form to follow-up visits. During follow-up visits, focus on issues that will foster adherence with the therapeutic interventions prescribed.

DRUG CLASS: THYROID REPLACEMENT HORMONES

Actions

Thyroid hormones either are hormones extracted from animal thyroid glands or are synthetically manufactured to be equivalent to natural thyroid hormones. Triiodothyronine and thyroxine are normally secreted from the properly functioning thyroid gland. Thyroxine is partially metabolized to triiodothyronine, so therapy with thyroxine provides physiologic replacement of both hormones.

Uses

The primary goal of thyroid hormone replacement therapy is to return the patient to a normal thyroid (euthyroid) state. Several forms of thyroid hormone replacement are available from natural and synthetic sources.

Synthetic levothyroxine (T_4) is now considered the drug of choice for hormone replacement in hypothyroidism. All the US Food and Drug Administration (FDA)–approved brands of T_4 are not bioequivalent; there are subtle differences in their composition. The bioavailability of a given brand at a given time after ingestion might be different. That's why endocrinologists recommend that once a brand is started, the patient should stick with the same brand. Changing brands may change the dose slightly, which in turn may change how the patient feels.

Liothyronine is a synthetic form of the natural thyroid hormone T_3. Its onset of action is more rapid than that of levothyroxine, and it is used occasionally as a thyroid hormone replacement when prompt action is necessary. It is not recommended for patients with cardiovascular disease unless a rapid onset of activity is deemed essential.

Liotrix is a synthetic mixture of levothyroxine and liothyronine in a ratio of 4:1, respectively. A few endocrinologists prefer this combination because the

standardized content of the two hormones produces consistent laboratory test results that are more in agreement with the patient's clinical response.

Thyroid USP (desiccated thyroid) is derived from pig, beef, and sheep thyroid glands. Thyroid USP is the oldest thyroid hormone replacement available and the least expensive. Because of its lack of purity, uniformity, and stability, however, it is generally not the drug of choice for the initiation of thyroid replacement therapy.

Therapeutic Outcome

The primary therapeutic outcome expected from thyroid hormone replacement therapy is return of the patient to a euthyroid metabolic state.

❖ Nursing Implications for Thyroid Hormone Replacement Therapy

◆ *Premedication assessment*

1. Record baseline vital signs, including apical pulse, weight, and bowel elimination patterns, before initiating therapy. Establish a once-daily schedule in which these assessments are repeated. Assess for patterns that may indicate early signs of hyperthyroidism (e.g., weight loss, nervousness, diaphoresis, muscle cramps, palpitations, angina pectoris).
2. Ensure that laboratory studies (e.g., thyroid hormone levels) have been completed before administration of the medication.

◆ *Availability and dosage*
See Table 36.1.

◆ *Administration.* **Adult:** *PO:* Therapy may be initiated with low dosages of levothyroxine, such as 50 to 100 mcg daily. Dosages are gradually increased over the next few weeks to an average daily maintenance dosage of 100 to 200 mcg daily. The dose should be taken on an empty stomach at least 45 minutes before ingestion of food. Most patients take it immediately upon arising, 45 minutes before breakfast.

> **⚠ Medication Safety Alert**
>
> The age of the patient, severity of hypothyroidism, and other concurrent medical conditions determine the initial dosage and the interval of time necessary before increasing the dosage. Hypothyroid patients are sensitive to replacement of thyroid hormones. Monitor patients closely for adverse effects.

◆ *Common and serious adverse effects*
  Endocrine

  Signs of hyperthyroidism. Adverse effects of thyroid replacement preparations are dose related and may occur 1 to 3 weeks after changes in therapy have been initiated. Symptoms of adverse effects are tachycardia, anxiety, weight loss, abdominal cramping and diarrhea, cardiac palpitations, dysrhythmias, angina pectoris,

Table 36.1 Thyroid Hormones

GENERIC NAME	BRAND NAME	AVAILABILITY	COMPOSITION	DOSAGE RANGE
levothyroxine ⇄ *Do not confuse levothyroxine with Lanoxin or leucovorin.*	Synthroid Levoxyl ⇄ *Do not confuse Levoxyl with Lanoxin or Luvox.*	Tablets/capsules: 13, 25, 50, 75, 88, 100, 112, 125, 137, 150, 175, 200, 300 mcg Injection: 100, 200, 500 mcg/10-mL vial	L-thyroxine (T_4)	PO: Initial: 12.5-50 mcg daily Maintenance: 100-200 mcg daily
liothyronine	Cytomel –	Tablets: 5, 25, 50 mcg Injection: 10 mcg/mL in 1-mL vials	liothyronine (T_3)	PO: Initial: 5-25 mcg daily Maintenance: 25-75 mcg daily IV: 25-50 mcg Patients with known or suspected cardiovascular disease: 10-20 mcg
liotrix	Thyrolar	Thyrolar-1/4: levothyroxine sodium 12.5 mcg/ liothyronine sodium 3.1 mcg Thyrolar-1/2: levothyroxine sodium 25 mcg/liothyronine sodium 6.3 mcg Thyrolar-1: levothyroxine sodium 50 mcg/liothyronine sodium 12.5 mcg Thyrolar-2: levothyroxine sodium 100 mcg/liothyronine sodium 25 mcg Thyrolar-3: levothyroxine sodium 150 mcg/liothyronine sodium 37.5 mcg	T_4:T_3 = 4:1	PO: Initial: levothyroxine 25 mcg/liothyronine 6.25 mcg once daily Usual maintenance dose: levothyroxine 50-100 mcg/liothyronine 12.5 mcg
thyroid USP	Armour Thyroid	Tablets: 15, 16.25, 30, 32.5, 48.75, 60, 65, 81.25, 90, 97.5, 113.75, 120, 130, 146.25, 162.5, 180, 195, 240, 260, 300, 325 mg	Unpredictable T_4:T_3 ratio	PO: Maintenance: 30-130 mg daily

fever, and intolerance to heat. Symptoms may require a reduction or discontinuation of therapy. Patients may require up to a month without medication for toxic effects to fully dissipate. Therapy must be restarted at lower dosages after symptoms have stopped.

◆ Drug interactions

Warfarin. Patients with hypothyroidism require increased dosage of anticoagulants. If thyroid replacement therapy is initiated while the patient is receiving warfarin therapy, the patient should have frequent prothrombin time (international normalized ratio [INR]) determinations and should be counseled to observe closely for the development of petechiae; ecchymoses; nosebleeds; bleeding gums; dark, tarry stools; and bright red or coffee-ground emesis. The dosage of warfarin may have to be reduced by one-third to one-half over the next 1 to 4 weeks.

Digoxin. Patients with hypothyroidism require a decreased dosage of digoxin. If thyroid replacement therapy is started while the patient is receiving digoxin, a gradual increase in the digoxin will also be necessary to maintain adequate therapeutic activity.

Estrogens. Patients who have no thyroid function and who start estrogen therapy may require an increase in dosage of the thyroid hormone. Estrogens increase thyroid-binding globulin levels, which reduce the level of circulating free T_4. The total level of T_4 is normal or increased. Do not adjust the thyroid hormone dosage until the patient shows clinical signs of hypothyroidism.

Cholestyramine. To prevent binding of thyroid hormones by cholestyramine, administer doses at least 4 hours apart.

Hyperglycemia. Patients with diabetes should be monitored for the development of hyperglycemia, particularly during the early weeks of therapy. Assess regularly for hyperglycemia or glycosuria and report if it occurs with any frequency. Patients receiving oral hypoglycemic agents or insulin may require an adjustment in dosage.

DRUG CLASS: ANTITHYROID MEDICATIONS

iodine-131 (^{131}I) (Ī-ō-dīn WŬN THŬR-tē WŬN)

Actions

The synthesis of thyroid hormones and their maintenance in the bloodstream in adequate amounts depend on sufficient iodine intake through food and water. Iodine is converted to iodide and stored in the thyroid gland before reaching the circulation.

Iodine-131 (^{131}I) is a radioactive isotope of iodine. When administered, it is absorbed into the thyroid gland in high concentrations. The liberated radioactive isotope destroys the hyperactive thyroid tissue, with essentially no damage to other tissues in the body.

Uses

Radioactive iodine is used most commonly for treating hyperthyroidism in the following individuals: older patients who are beyond the childbearing years, those with severe complicating diseases (e.g., heart disease), those with recurrent hyperthyroidism after previous thyroid surgery, those who are poor surgical risks, and those who have unusually small thyroid glands.

It often takes 3 to 6 months after a dose of radioactive iodine to fully assess the benefits gained. Normal thyroid function occurs in about 60% of patients after one dose; the remaining patients require two or more doses. If more than one dose is required, an interval of at least 3 months between doses is necessary.

Therapeutic Outcome

The primary therapeutic outcome expected from radioactive iodine is a return to a normal thyroid state.

❖ Nursing Implications for Radioactive Iodine
◆ *Premedication assessment*

1. Review policy for both institutional personnel and patients regarding precautions, storage, handling, administration, and disposal of radioactive substances.
2. Have all necessary supplies immediately available in case of a spill.
3. Have all supplies needed according to institutional procedure to dispose of patient's waste, such as urine and feces, because it will be a radioactive biohazard.

◆ *Availability*

Each dose is prepared for an individual patient by a nuclear pharmacy.

◆ *Administration*

Administration of a radioactive iodine preparation seems simple—it is added to water and swallowed. It has no color or taste. The radiation, however, is extremely dangerous.

- Minimize exposure as much as possible. Maintain hazardous medication precautions according to the institution's policy. Wear latex gloves whenever administering radioactive iodine or disposing of the patient's urine and feces.
- If the radioactive iodine or the patient's urine or feces spills, follow institutional policy. In general, collect the clothing, bedding, bedpan, urinal, and any other contaminated materials and place them in special containers for radioactive waste disposal.
- *Avoid spills! Report any accidental contamination at once to the supervisor and follow directions for the institution's contamination cleanup technique, and then complete an incident report.*

◆ *Common and serious adverse effects*
Endocrine

Tenderness in the thyroid gland. Adverse effects include radioactive thyroiditis, which causes tenderness over the thyroid area and occurs during the first few days or few weeks after radioactive iodine therapy.

Hyperthyroidism. A return of symptoms of hyperthyroidism occurs in about 40% of patients who have received one dose of radioactive iodine. Additional doses may be required.

Hypothyroidism. Some patients who receive radioactive iodine develop hypothyroidism, which requires thyroid hormone replacement therapy.

◆ *Drug interactions*

Lithium carbonate. Lithium and iodine may cause synergistic hypothyroid activity. Concurrent use may result in hypothyroidism. Monitor patients for both hypothyroidism and bipolar disorder.

---

propylthiouracil (PRŌ-pĭl-thī-ō-YŪ-ră-sĭl)
  ⇄ *Do not confuse propylthiouracil with Purinethol.*
methimazole (mĕ-THĬM-ă-zōl)
  ⇄ *Do not confuse methimazole with methazolamide.*
Tapazole (TĂP-ă-zōl)

Actions

Propylthiouracil and methimazole are antithyroid agents that act by blocking synthesis of T_3 and T_4 in the thyroid gland. They do not destroy any T_3 or T_4 already produced, so there is usually a latent period of a few days to 3 weeks before symptoms improve once therapy has been started.

Uses

Propylthiouracil and methimazole may be used for long-term treatment of hyperthyroidism or for short-term treatment before subtotal thyroidectomy. Therapy for long-term use is often continued for 1 to 2 years to control symptoms. After discontinuation, some patients gradually return to the hyperthyroid state, and antithyroid therapy must be reinitiated.

The US Food and Drug Administration suggests that because of potential hepatotoxicity, it may be appropriate to reserve the use of propylthiouracil for those who cannot tolerate other treatments such as methimazole, radioactive iodine, or surgery. In addition, because of the potential for birth defects that have been observed with the use of methimazole in pregnant women during the first trimester, propylthiouracil may be the treatment of choice during and just before the first trimester of pregnancy.

Therapeutic Outcome

The primary therapeutic outcome expected from propylthiouracil or methimazole is a gradual return to normal thyroid metabolic function.

❖ **Nursing Implications for Propylthiouracil and Methimazole**

◆ *Premedication assessment*

1. Record baseline vital signs, weight, and bowel elimination patterns before initiating therapy. Establish an alternate-day schedule in which these assessments are repeated. Assess for patterns that may indicate early signs of hypothyroidism.

2. Ensure that laboratory studies (e.g., complete blood count with differential; thyroid hormone, TSH, blood urea nitrogen, serum creatinine, and liver enzyme levels) have been completed before administering the medication.

◆ *Availability*

Propylthiouracil. *PO:* 50-mg tablets.
Methimazole. *PO:* 5- and 10-mg tablets.

◆ *Dosage and administration*

Propylthiouracil. Adult: *PO:* Initially, 100 to 150 mg every 8 hours. Dosage ranges up to 900 mg daily. The maintenance dosage is 50 mg two or three times daily.

Methimazole. Adult: *PO:* Initially, 5 to 20 mg every 8 hours. Daily maintenance dosage is 5 to 15 mg.

◆ *Common and serious adverse effects*

Integumentary

Purpuric maculopapular rash. The most common reaction (in 5% of all patients) that occurs with propylthiouracil therapy is a purpuric maculopapular skin eruption. This skin eruption often occurs during the first 2 weeks of therapy and usually resolves spontaneously without

treatment. If pruritus becomes severe, a change to methimazole and the use of short-term oral steroids may be necessary. Cross-sensitivity is uncommon.

This adverse effect is usually mild and tends to resolve with continued therapy. Encourage the patient not to discontinue therapy without first consulting the healthcare provider.

Immunologic

Bone marrow suppression, lymph node enlargement. Routine laboratory studies (e.g., red blood cell, white blood cell, and differential counts) should be scheduled. Stress the importance of the patient's returning for this laboratory work. Monitor the patient for the development of a sore throat, fever, purpura, jaundice, or excessive progressive weakness.

Gastrointestinal

Hepatotoxicity. The symptoms of hepatotoxicity are anorexia, nausea, vomiting, jaundice, hepatomegaly, splenomegaly, and abnormal liver function (e.g., elevated bilirubin, aspartate aminotransferase, alanine aminotransferase, gamma-glutamyl transferase, and alkaline phosphatase levels; increased prothrombin time [INR]).

Salivary gland enlargement, loss of taste.

Renal

Nephrotoxicity. Monitor urinalyses and kidney function tests for abnormal results. Report increased blood urea nitrogen and creatinine levels, decreased urine output or decreased specific gravity (despite amount of fluid intake), casts or protein in the urine, frank blood or smoke-colored urine, or red blood cells in excess of 0 to 3 per high-power field on the urinalysis report.

◆ *Drug interactions*

Warfarin. Patients with hyperthyroidism require reduced dosage of anticoagulants. If antithyroid therapy is initiated while the patient is receiving warfarin therapy, the patient should have frequent prothrombin time (INR) determinations and be counseled to observe closely for the development of petechiae; ecchymoses; nosebleeds; bleeding gums; dark, tarry stools; and bright red or coffee-ground emesis. The dosage of warfarin may have to be increased over the next 1 to 4 weeks.

Digoxin. Patients with hyperthyroidism require an increased dosage of digoxin. If antithyroid replacement therapy is started while the patient is receiving digoxin, a gradual reduction in the digoxin will be necessary to prevent signs of toxicity. Monitor for the development of digoxin toxicity.

Get Ready for the NCLEX® Examination!

Key Points

- Thyroid disease can be manifested as hyperthyroidism or hypothyroidism, depending on the amount of circulating thyroid hormone. These are relatively common disorders that are easily treated.
- Most therapies for hypothyroidism require lifelong treatment to maintain normal thyroid function.
- Nurses can play a significant role in education and reinforcement of the treatment plan. Best results are attained when the patient, family, significant other(s), and nurse work together in reinforcing the care plan.

Additional Learning Resources

[SG] Go to your Study Guide for additional Review Questions for the NCLEX® Examination, Critical Thinking Clinical Situations, and other learning activities to help you master this chapter content.

Go to your Evolve website (https://evolve.elsevier.com/Clayton) for additional online resources.

Review Questions for the NCLEX® Examination

1. The nurse knows the thyroid gland provides which function for the body?
   1. Release of T_3 and T_4
   2. Regulation of body temperature
   3. Release of TSH
   4. Regulation of the metabolism of carbohydrates and proteins

2. A patient receiving levothyroxine (Synthroid) is monitored for which signs and symptoms of overdose?
   1. Bradycardia, weight gain
   2. Cold intolerance, bradycardia
   3. Palpitations, tachycardia, heat intolerance
   4. Sluggish, slow speech; increasing confusion

3. A patient comes in to the clinic complaining of weight gain even though his appetite is poor; he is feeling fatigued, and he has intolerance to cold. The nurse anticipates that the patient may be diagnosed with which condition?
   1. Cretinism
   2. Hyperthyroidism
   3. Hypothyroidism
   4. Thyrotoxicosis

4. The thyroid hormones regulate which general body metabolism? *(Select all that apply.)*
   1. Reproduction
   2. Temperature regulation
   3. Growth and maturation
   4. Stimulating the release of TSH
   5. Maintaining sleep cycles

5. Patients with hyperthyroidism present with which of the following symptoms? *(Select all that apply.)*
   1. Palpitations
   2. Bradycardia
   3. Heat intolerance
   4. Tachycardia
   5. Weight gain

6. A patient with hyperthyroidism has been prescribed propylthiouracil, which works by which action?
   1. Destroying T_3 and T_4
   2. Converting iodine to active iodine
   3. Blocking synthesis of T_3 and T_4 in the thyroid gland
   4. Synthesizing the hormone thyroxine

7. Patients treated for hypothyroidism with levothyroxine require careful management of warfarin to prevent bleeding. What does this management include? *(Select all that apply.)*
   1. Frequent INR checks
   2. Increasing the dose of warfarin slowly over 1 to 4 weeks
   3. Observing for nosebleeds and petechiae
   4. Frequent assessment of TSH levels
   5. Reducing the dose of warfarin slowly over 1 to 4 weeks

8. The nurse assesses a patient for thyroid enlargement by which method?
   1. Palpate the throat and ask the patient to swallow.
   2. Auscultate the throat and ask the patient to cough.
   3. Palpate the throat and ask the patient to cough.
   4. Auscultate the throat and ask the patient to swallow.

Corticosteroids

Objectives

1. Discuss the normal actions of mineralocorticoids and glucocorticoids in the body.
2. Cite the disease states caused by hyposecretion of the adrenal gland.
3. Identify the baseline assessments needed for a patient receiving corticosteroids.
4. Discuss the clinical uses and potential adverse effects associated with corticosteroids.

Key Terms

corticosteroids (kōr-tǐ-kō-STĚR-ōydz) (p. 578)
mineralocorticoids (mǐn-ěr-ăl-ō-KŌR-tǐ-kōydz) (p. 578)

glucocorticoids (glū-kō-kŌR-tǐ-kōydz) (p. 578)
cortisol (KŌR-tǐ-sōl) (p. 582)

CORTICOSTEROIDS

Corticosteroids are hormones secreted by the adrenal cortex of the adrenal gland. Corticosteroids are divided into two categories based on structure and biologic activity. The **mineralocorticoids** (fludrocortisone and aldosterone) maintain fluid and electrolyte balance and are used to treat adrenal insufficiency caused by hypopituitarism or Addison's disease. The **glucocorticoids** (e.g., cortisone, hydrocortisone, prednisone) regulate carbohydrate, protein, and fat metabolism. Glucocorticoids have antiinflammatory, antiallergenic, and immunosuppressant activity.

❖ NURSING IMPLICATIONS FOR CORTICOSTEROID THERAPY

◆ Assessment

The minimum assessment data for a patient receiving corticosteroids include baseline weight, blood pressure, and results of electrolyte and glucose studies. Monitoring all aspects of intake, output, diet, electrolyte balance, and state of hydration is important to the long-term success of corticosteroid therapy. Although many of the parameters used for assessment may initially be normal, it is important that baseline values for these parameters be established so that they may be used to monitor steroid therapy.

- Ask the patient to describe the current problems that initiated this visit or admission.
- How long have the symptoms been present?
- Is this a recurrent problem? If so, how has it been treated?
- If an infectious process is suspected, determine when the patient was last tested for tuberculosis.

History of pain experience. See equivalent subsection under Assessment in the Nursing Implications for Pain Management section of Chapter 19 (Drugs Used for Pain Management).

Medication use. Obtain a detailed history of all prescribed and over-the-counter medications (including herbal medicines). Ask if the patient understands why each is being taken. Ask specifically whether corticosteroids have been taken within the past year and for what purpose. Tactfully determine if the prescribed medications are being taken regularly and if not, why not.

Physical assessment

- *Blood pressure:* Take a baseline blood pressure reading in the sitting, lying, and standing positions. Because patients receiving corticosteroids accumulate fluid and gain weight, hypertension may develop.
- *Temperature:* Record temperature daily and monitor more frequently if elevated. Patients receiving corticosteroids are more susceptible to infection, and fever is often an early indicator of infection. Glucocorticoids, however, sometimes suppress a febrile response to infection.
- *Weight and fat distribution:* Obtain the patient's weight on admission and use as a baseline in assessing therapy. Because patients receiving corticosteroids have a tendency to accumulate fluid and gain weight, the daily weight is an important tool in assessing ongoing therapy. Observe any changes in the distribution of fat and any muscle weakness or muscle wasting.
- *Pulse:* Record rate, quality, and rhythm of pulse.

- *Heart and lung sounds:* Nurses with advanced skills can perform auscultation and percussion to note changes in heart size and heart and lung sounds. (Consult a medical-surgical nursing textbook for details in performing these assessments.) Lung fields are assessed in a sitting position to detect abnormal lung sounds (e.g., wheezes, crackles, and accumulation of fluid).
- *Skin color:* Note the color of the skin, mucous membranes, tongue, earlobes, and nail beds. Note in particular the development of a rash or the development of ecchymoses (bruises).
- *Neck veins:* Record any jugular vein distention. This may be an indication of fluid overload.

Neurologic

- *Mental status:* A patient receiving a higher dosage of corticosteroids is susceptible to psychotic behavioral changes. The most susceptible patient is one with a previous history of mental dysfunction. Perform a baseline assessment of the patient's ability to respond rationally to the environment and the diagnosis of the underlying disease. Check for orientation to date, time, and place and assess for level of confusion, restlessness, or irritability. Make regularly scheduled mental status evaluations and compare the findings.
- *Anxiety:* What degree of apprehension is present? Did stressful events precipitate the anxiety?

Status of hydration

- *Dehydration:* Assess and record significant signs of dehydration in the patient. Observe for the following signs: poor skin turgor, sticky oral mucous membranes, a shrunken or deeply furrowed tongue, crusted lips, weight loss, deteriorating vital signs, soft or sunken eyeballs, weak pedal pulses, delayed capillary filling, excessive thirst, high urine specific gravity (or no urine output), and possible mental confusion.
- *Skin turgor:* Check skin turgor by gently pinching the skin together over the sternum, over the forehead, or on the forearm. In the well-hydrated patient, elasticity is present and the skin rapidly returns to a flat position. With dehydrated patients, the skin remains pinched or peaked and returns very slowly to the flat, normal position.
- *Oral mucous membranes:* When adequately hydrated, the membranes of the mouth feel smooth and glisten. When dehydrated, they are sticky and appear dull.
- *Laboratory changes:* The values of the hematocrit, hemoglobin, blood urea nitrogen, and electrolytes will appear to fluctuate based on the state of hydration. A dehydrated patient will show higher values as a result of hemoconcentration. When a patient is overhydrated, the values appear to drop because of hemodilution.
- *Overhydration:* Increased abdominal girth and increased circumference of the medial malleolus,

weight gain, and neck vein engorgement indicate overhydration. Measure the patient's abdominal girth daily at the umbilical level. Measure the extremities bilaterally every day, approximately 5 cm above the medial malleolus.
- *Edema:* Is edema present? Where is it located? Is it pitting or nonpitting? It may be an indicator of fluid and electrolyte imbalance.

Presence of ulcer disease. Patients receiving corticosteroid therapy have higher incidences of peptic ulcer disease. Ask the patient about any previous treatment for an ulcer, heartburn, or stomach pain. Periodic testing of stools for occult blood may be ordered.

Laboratory tests

- Patients taking corticosteroids are particularly susceptible to the development of electrolyte imbalance. Physiologically, corticosteroids cause sodium retention (hypernatremia) and potassium excretion (hypokalemia); hyperglycemia may be observed with high-dose glucocorticoids.
- Patients most likely to develop electrolyte disturbances are those who, in addition to receiving corticosteroids, have histories of renal or cardiac disease, hormonal disorders, or massive trauma or burns, or are on diuretic therapy.
- Review laboratory tests and report abnormal results to the healthcare provider promptly. Tests may include serum electrolytes, especially sodium, potassium, calcium, and magnesium; arterial blood gases; glucose; electrocardiography; chest x-ray; urinalysis and kidney function; and hemodynamic assessment.
- Because the symptoms of most electrolyte imbalances are similar, the nurse should assess changes in the patient's mental status (alertness, orientation, and confusion), muscle strength, muscle cramps, tremors, nausea, and general appearance.

Nutrition. Obtain a history of the patient's diet. Ask questions regarding appetite and the presence of nausea and vomiting. Anorexia, nausea, and vomiting are early indications of corticosteroid insufficiency.

Hyperglycemia. Corticosteroid therapy may induce hyperglycemia, particularly in prediabetic or diabetic patients. All patients must be monitored for the development of hyperglycemia, especially during the early weeks of therapy. Assess regularly for hyperglycemia and report abnormalities.

Activity and exercise. Ask questions to obtain information about the effect of exercise on the patient's functioning:
- Is the person normally sedentary, moderately active, or very active?
- Has there been a reduction in activity level to cope with associated fatigue or dyspnea?

- Is the person performing the activities of daily living?

◆ **Implementation**

Presence of illness. If an infectious disease process is suspected and tuberculosis testing is planned, it should be performed before initiating corticosteroid therapy.

Medication use. Review prescription medications as well as over-the-counter medications (including herbal medicines) being taken and establish whether they are being taken correctly. Analyze nonadherence issues and plan interventions with the patient. Plan to review drug administration as needed.

Medication administration

- Glucocorticoids may cause hyperglycemia, necessitating the monitoring of blood glucose levels at appropriate intervals. If elevated, insulin therapy may be required. Initiate a diabetic flow sheet, and mark the medication profile or computer care plan to clearly identify the insulin orders.
- During steroid replacement therapy, the administration schedule for the replacement drugs should mimic the body's normal circadian rhythm. Therefore glucocorticoids ordered twice daily are usually scheduled with two-thirds of the dose administered before 9 AM (usually with breakfast) and one-third of the dose in the late afternoon (usually with dinner). Alternate-day therapy is also used in some cases to maintain a more normal body rhythm. Mineralocorticoids are usually given once daily in the evening.
- Steroid replacement therapy is gradually discontinued in small increments (tapered) to ensure that the patient's adrenal glands are able to start secreting steroids appropriately as the drug dosage is reduced.
- Order medications prescribed and schedule these on the medication profile. Corticosteroids should be scheduled to be taken with food. Perform focused assessments to determine effectiveness and adverse effects of pharmacologic interventions. Monitor for hyperglycemia.

Neurologic. Plan for stress reduction education and discussion of effective means of coping with stressful events. Note patient's mental status every shift.

- Perform neurologic assessment to determine changes in mental status.
- Deal calmly with an anxious patient, offer explanations of procedures being performed, and listen to concerns and intervene appropriately.

Fluid volume status. Plan to monitor intake and output at intervals appropriate to the patient's condition. Report intake that exceeds output.

Nutrition. Examine the dietary history to determine if referral to a nutritionist would help the patient understand the diet regimen. Plan interventions needed to deal with dietary nonadherence.

Schedule meetings with the nutritionist to learn how to manage specific dietary modifications prescribed (e.g., a low-sodium, high-potassium diet with weight reduction parameters for obese patients). If possible, instruct the patient to practice food selections from the daily menus while still in the hospital. Teach the patient which foods are low in sodium and high in potassium. Potassium restrictions may be indicated if the patient is taking a potassium-sparing diuretic. Salt substitutes are high in potassium; therefore use must be limited.

Pain management. When pain is present, comfort measures must be implemented to allow the patient to decrease the pain. Fatigue may increase pain perception; spacing activities so that fatigue does not occur is recommended. Maintain a flow sheet of pain ratings and evaluate for the effectiveness of medications in the management of pain.

Vital signs and status of hydration

- Monitor vital signs and perform focused assessment of heart, respiratory, and hydration status at specified intervals.
- Perform daily weights using the same scale, in clothing of approximately the same weight, and at the same time, usually before breakfast. Record and report significant weight changes. (Weight gains and losses are the best indicators of fluid gain or loss.) As appropriate to the patient's condition, obtain and record abdominal girth measurements.
- When fluid restrictions are prescribed, half of the fluids are generally given with meals. The other half is given on a per-shift basis.
- Monitor the rate of intravenous (IV) infusions carefully; contact the healthcare provider regarding the concentration of admixtures of drugs to the IV infusion solution when limited fluids are indicated.

Laboratory tests. Check for and report abnormal laboratory values (e.g., hypokalemia, hyperkalemia, hypoglycemia, hyperglycemia, hyponatremia, hypernatremia), depending on the underlying disease pathology.

◆ **Patient Education**

Contact with healthcare provider's office

- Assess the patient's understanding of symptoms that should be reported to the healthcare provider: dyspnea; productive cough; worsening fatigue; edema in the feet, ankles, or legs; weight gain; or development of angina (chest pain), palpitations, or confusion.
- Instruct the patient to perform daily weights using the same scale, in clothing approximately the same weight, and at the same time of day, usually before breakfast. Record and report significant weight changes; weight gains and losses are the best indicators of fluid gain

or loss. Usually, a gain of 2 pounds in 2 days should be reported.

Skin care. Teach appropriate skin care and the need to change position at least every 2 hours, especially when edema is present. Have the patient inspect the ankles, feet, and abdomen for edema daily. If the patient is using a recliner or bed, the sacral area should also be checked regularly for edema.

Coping with stress

- Patients receiving high doses of corticosteroids do not tolerate stress well. Patients should be instructed to notify the healthcare provider before exposure to additional stress, such as dental procedures. If a patient sustains an accidental injury or sudden emotional stress, the attending healthcare provider should be told that the patient is receiving steroid therapy. An additional steroid dose may be needed to support the patient through a stressful situation.
- Explore the mechanisms that the person uses to cope with stress. Discuss how the patient is adapting to the needed lifestyle changes to manage the disease process. Address depression issues, if present.

Avoidance of infections. Advise the patient to avoid crowds or people known to have infections. Report even minor signs of an infection (e.g., general malaise, sore throat, low-grade fever) to the healthcare provider.

Nutritional status

- Assist the patient in developing a specific schedule for spacing daily fluid intake and planning sodium restrictions, as prescribed by the healthcare provider.
- If weight gain is a specific problem (not related to fluid accumulation), plan for calorie restrictions and spacing of daily intake.
- If a high-potassium diet is prescribed, help the patient become familiar with foods that should be consumed. Teach the signs and symptoms of potassium deficiency or excess, depending on medications prescribed.
- Further dietary needs may include increases in vitamin D and calcium.
- Fluid restrictions may be imposed; discuss specific ways to manage these limitations.

Activity and exercise

- Participation in regular exercise is essential. The patient may resume activities of daily living within the boundaries set by the healthcare provider. Encourage activities such as regular and moderate exercise, meal preparation, resumption of usual sexual activity, and social interactions. Help the patient plan for appropriate alterations, depending on the disease process and degree of impairment.
- Encourage weight-bearing measures to prevent calcium loss. Active and passive range-of-motion exercises maintain mobility and joint and muscle integrity.
- Individuals unable to attain the degree of activity anticipated as a result of drug therapy may become frustrated. Allow for verbalization of feelings and then implement actions appropriate to the circumstances.

Fostering health maintenance

- Throughout the course of treatment, discuss medication information and how the medication will benefit the patient.
- Drug therapy is one component of the treatment of illnesses for which steroids are prescribed; it is critical that the medications be taken as prescribed. Ensure that the patient understands the entire medication regimen, including the importance of not adjusting the dosage without healthcare provider approval. If corticosteroid therapy is to be discontinued, a tapering schedule is used. Stress the importance of not withdrawing the prescribed medication suddenly.
- Patients on steroid therapy should carry identification cards or a bracelet with the name of the healthcare provider to contact in an emergency, as well as the drug name, dosage, and frequency of use. Emphasize situations requiring healthcare provider consultation for drug dosage adjustments (e.g., stress, dental procedures, infection).
- Provide the patient and significant others with the important information contained in the specific drug monographs for the drugs prescribed. Additional health teaching and nursing interventions for common and serious adverse effects are in each drug monograph.
- Seek the patient's cooperation and understanding of the following points to increase medication adherence: name of medication; dosage, route, and times of administration; and common and serious adverse effects.

Patient self-assessment. Enlist the patient's help in developing and maintaining a written record of monitoring parameters (e.g., pulse rate, blood pressure, body weight, edema, exercise tolerance, pain relief). See the Patient Self-Assessment Form for Corticosteroids on the Evolve website. Complete the Premedication Data column for use as a baseline to track response to drug therapy. Ensure that the patient understands how to use the form and instruct the patient to take this written record to follow-up visits. During follow-up visits, focus on issues that will foster adherence with the therapeutic interventions prescribed.

DRUG CLASS: MINERALOCORTICOIDS

fludrocortisone (flū-drō-KOR-tĭ-sōn)

Actions

Fludrocortisone is an adrenal corticosteroid with potent mineralocorticoid and glucocorticoid effects. It affects fluid and electrolyte balance by acting on the distal renal tubules, causing sodium and water retention and potassium and hydrogen excretion.

Uses

Fludrocortisone is used in combination with glucocorticoids to replace mineralocorticoid activity in patients who suffer from adrenocortical insufficiency (Addison's disease) and to treat salt-losing adrenogenital syndrome.

Therapeutic Outcomes

The primary therapeutic outcomes expected from fludrocortisone therapy are as follows.
1. Control of blood pressure
2. Restoration of fluid and electrolyte balance

❖ Nursing Implications for Fludrocortisone
◆ Premedication assessment
1. Check the electrolyte reports for early indications of electrolyte imbalance.
2. Keep accurate records of intake and output, daily weights, and vital signs.
3. Ask the patient about any signs of infection (e.g., sore throat, fever, malaise, nausea, vomiting). Corticosteroid therapy can mask symptoms of infection.
4. Perform a baseline assessment of the patient's degree of alertness; orientation to name, place, and time; and rationality of responses.
5. Ask the patient about previous treatment for an ulcer, heartburn, or stomach pain. Testing stools for occult blood should be done periodically.

◆ Availability. *PO:* 0.1-mg tablets.

◆ Dosage and administration. **Adult:** *PO:* 0.1 mg daily. Dosage may be adjusted as needed. Cortisone or hydrocortisone also is usually administered to provide additional glucocorticoid effect. Because fludrocortisone is a natural hormone, adverse effects such as sodium accumulation and potassium depletion reflect fludrocortisone excess.

◆ Common and serious adverse effects and drug interactions. See equivalent sections under Drug Class: Glucocorticoids.

DRUG CLASS: GLUCOCORTICOIDS

Actions

The major glucocorticoid of the adrenal cortex is cortisol. The hypothalamic-pituitary axis regulates the secretion of cortisol by increasing or decreasing the output of corticotropin-releasing factor (CRF) from the hypothalamus. Corticotropin-releasing factor stimulates the release of adrenocorticotropic hormone (ACTH) from the pituitary gland; ACTH then stimulates the adrenal cortex

to secrete cortisol. As serum levels of cortisol increase, the amount of CRF secreted by the hypothalamus is decreased, resulting in diminished secretion of cortisol from the adrenal cortex.

Uses

Glucocorticoids are usually given because of their antiinflammatory and antiallergenic properties. They do not cure disease, but they relieve the symptoms of tissue inflammation. When glucocorticoids are used to control rheumatoid arthritis, symptom relief is noted within a few days. Joint and muscle stiffness, muscle tenderness and weakness, joint swelling, and soreness are significantly reduced. However, it is important to assess the patient's predrug activity level because pain relief may lead to overuse of the diseased joints. Appetite, weight, and energy levels are increased; fever is reduced; and sedimentation rates are reduced or return to normal. Anatomic changes and joint deformities already present remain unchanged. Symptoms usually return shortly after glucocorticoid withdrawal.

Glucocorticoids are also effective for immunosuppression in the treatment of certain cancers, organ transplantation, autoimmune diseases (e.g., lupus erythematosus, dermatomyositis, rheumatoid arthritis), relief of allergic manifestations (e.g., serum sickness, severe hay fever, status asthmaticus), and treatment of shock. They also may be used to treat nausea and vomiting secondary to chemotherapy (see Chapter 33).

Therapeutic Outcomes

The primary therapeutic outcomes expected from glucocorticoid therapy are as follows:
1. Reduced pain and inflammation
2. Minimized shock syndrome and faster recovery
3. Reduced nausea and vomiting associated with chemotherapy

❖ Nursing Implications for Glucocorticoids
◆ Premedication assessment
1. Check the electrolyte and glucose reports for early indications of electrolyte imbalance or hyperglycemia.
2. Keep accurate records of intake and output, daily weights, and vital signs.
3. Ask the patient about any signs of infection (e.g., sore throat, fever, malaise, nausea, vomiting). Corticosteroid therapy can mask symptoms of infection.
4. Perform a baseline assessment of the patient's degree of alertness; orientation to name, place, and time; and rationality of responses.
5. Ask the patient about previous treatment for an ulcer, heartburn, or stomach pain. Testing stools for occult blood should be done periodically.

◆ Availability, dosage, and administration
See Table 37.1.

When a therapeutic dosage is administered for 3 weeks or longer, it must be assumed that the internal production of corticosteroids is suppressed. General

Table **37.1** **Topical and Systemic Corticosteroid Preparations**[a]

GENERIC NAME	BRAND NAME	DOSAGE FORMS
alclometasone		Cream, ointment
amcinonide		Cream, ointment, lotion
betamethasone	Celestone Soluspan, Luxiq, Sernivo	Injection, cream, ointment, lotion, emulsion, gel, foam, spray
budesonide	Entocort EC, Uceris	Oral extended-release capsule and tablet, rectal foam
clobetasol	Temovate, Clobex, Olux	Cream, ointment, solution, scalp shampoo, lotion, gel, foam
clocortolone	Cloderm	Cream
cortisone		Tablets
desonide	DesOwen, Verdeso	Cream, ointment, lotion, foam, gel
desoximetasone	Topicort	Cream, ointment, gel, liquid
dexamethasone	Decadron	Injection, tablets, elixir, solution
diflorasone	ApexiCon E	Cream, ointment
fludrocortisone		Tablets
fluocinolone	Capex, Derma-Smoothe/FS, Synalar	Cream, ointment, solution, shampoo, oil
fluocinonide ⇄ *Do not confuse fluocinonide with fluorouracil.*	Vanos	Cream, ointment, gel, solution
flurandrenolide	Cordran	Cream, ointment, tape, lotion
fluticasone	Cutivate	Cream, ointment, lotion
halcinonide	Halog	Cream, ointment
halobetasol	Ultravate	Cream, ointment, lotion
hydrocortisone ⇄ *Do not confuse hydrocortisone with hydralazine or hydrocodone.*	Cortef ⇄ *Do not confuse Cortef with Lortab.* Solu-Cortef, Hydrocortone	Cream, ointment, tablets, enema, gel, lotion, solution, suppositories, foam, injection
methylprednisolone ⇄ *Do not confuse methylprednisolone with medroxyprogesterone.*	Solu-Medrol, Depo-Medrol, Medrol	Tablets, injection
mometasone	Elocon	Cream, ointment, lotion, solution
prednicarbate	Dermatop	Cream, ointment
prednisolone	Veripred 20, Pediapred	Tablets, syrup, suspension, solution
prednisone ⇄ *Do not confuse prednisone with potassium, Prilosec, primidone, or pseudoephedrine.*	Deltasone Rayos	Tablets, solution, liquid concentrate Delayed-release tablets
triamcinolone	Kenalog, Triderm	Cream, ointment, lotion, injection, tablets, aerosol, paste

[a]For information on ophthalmic corticosteroid products, see Chapter 42; for information on nasal inhalation corticosteroid products, see Chapter 29; for information on lower respiratory system inhalation corticosteroid products, see Chapter 30.

guidelines are that if a patient has received prednisone 2 mg/kg/day or less, or 20 mg/day for 21 days or less, the patient does not need to be tapered off the corticosteroid. Abrupt discontinuation of glucocorticoids may result in adrenal insufficiency if higher dosages are being received. Therapy should be withdrawn gradually (often called a *steroid taper*). The time required to decrease glucocorticoids depends on the duration of treatment, dosage amount, mode of administration, and glucocorticoid being used.

- *Abrupt discontinuation:* Patients who have received corticosteroids for at least 3 weeks must not abruptly discontinue therapy. Symptoms of abrupt discontinuation include fever, malaise, fatigue, weakness, anorexia, nausea, orthostatic dizziness, hypotension, fainting, dyspnea, hypoglycemia, muscle and joint pain, and possible exacerbation of the disease process.
- *Application:* Topical corticosteroids are applied as directed by the manufacturer. Specific instructions

regarding use of an occlusive dressing should be clarified before application.

- *Alternate-day therapy:* Alternate-day therapy may be used to treat chronic conditions. Corticosteroids are usually given between 6 and 9 AM on alternate days to minimize suppression of normal adrenal function. Administer with meals to minimize gastric irritation.
- *Pediatric patients:* The correct dosage for a child is usually based on the disease being treated rather than the patient's weight. Monitoring of skeletal growth may be required in children if prolonged therapy is required.

> **⚠ Medication Safety Alert**
>
> Glucocorticoids are potent agents that produce many undesirable adverse effects as well as therapeutic benefits. Unless immediate life-threatening conditions exist, other therapeutic methods should be exhausted before corticosteroid therapy is initiated. Many of the adverse effects of the steroids are related to dosage and duration of therapy. These drugs must be used with caution in patients with diabetes mellitus, heart failure, hypertension, peptic ulcer disease, mental disturbance, immunocompromise, and suspected infections.

◆ *Common and serious adverse effects*

Fluid and electrolyte disturbances

Electrolyte imbalance, fluid accumulation. The electrolytes most commonly altered are potassium (K^+), sodium (Na^+), and chloride (Cl^-). Hypokalemia is most likely to occur. Many symptoms associated with altered fluid and electrolyte balance are subtle and interspersed with general symptoms of drug toxicity or the disease process itself. Obtain data about changes in the patient's mental status (alertness, orientation, and confusion), muscle strength, muscle cramps, tremors, nausea, and general appearance (drowsy, anxious, or lethargic). Always check the electrolyte reports for early indications of electrolyte imbalance. Keep accurate records of intake and output, daily weights, blood glucose, and vital signs.

Immune system

Susceptibility to infection. Always question the patient before initiation of therapy about any signs and symptoms of possible infection. Corticosteroid therapy often masks symptoms of infection. Monitor the patient for signs of infection, such as sore throat, fever, malaise, nausea, and vomiting. Encourage the patient to avoid exposure to infections.

Psychological

Behavioral changes. Psychotic behaviors are more likely to occur in patients with previous histories of mental instability. Perform a baseline assessment of the patient's degree of alertness; orientation to name, place, and time; and rationality of responses *before* initiating therapy. Make regularly scheduled mental status evaluations, and compare the findings. Report the development of alterations.

Metabolic

Hyperglycemia. Patients with prediabetes or diabetes must be monitored for the development of hyperglycemia, particularly during early weeks of therapy. Assess regularly for hyperglycemia and report any abnormal findings. Patients receiving oral hypoglycemic agents or insulin may require an adjustment in dosage.

Gastrointestinal

Peptic ulcer formation. Before initiating therapy, ask the patient about any previous treatment for an ulcer, heartburn, or stomach pain. Periodic testing of stools for occult blood may be ordered. Antacids may also be recommended by the prescribing healthcare provider to minimize gastric symptoms.

Integumentary

Delayed wound healing. Patients who have recently had surgery must have their surgical sites monitored closely for signs of dehiscence (the edges of a surgical incision that start to open, pull apart, or separate). Teach surgical patients to splint the wounds while coughing and breathing deeply. Inspect surgical sites and report statements such as, "When I coughed, I felt something pop."

Sensory

Visual disturbances. Visual disturbances noted by patients on long-term therapy must be reported. Glucocorticoid therapy may produce cataracts.

Musculoskeletal

Osteoporosis. Long-term glucocorticoid therapy may produce osteoporosis.

◆ *Drug interactions*

Diuretics (e.g., furosemide, bumetanide, thiazides). Corticosteroids may enhance the loss of potassium. Check potassium levels and monitor the patient more closely for hypokalemia when these agents are used concurrently. Many symptoms of altered fluid and electrolyte balance are subtle and interspersed with general symptoms of drug toxicity or the disease process itself.

Gather data about changes in the patient's mental status (alertness, orientation, and confusion), muscle strength, muscle cramps, tremors, nausea, and general appearance (drowsy, anxious, and lethargic). Always check the electrolyte reports for early indications of electrolyte imbalance. Keep accurate records of intake and output, daily weights, and vital signs.

Warfarin. Steroids may enhance or decrease the anticoagulant effects of warfarin. Observe for the development of petechiae; ecchymoses; nosebleeds; bleeding gums; dark, tarry stools; and bright red or coffee-ground emesis. Monitor the prothrombin time (international normalized ratio) and adjust the dosage of warfarin if necessary. Because of the ulcerogenic potential of steroids, close observation of patients taking anticoagulants is necessary to reduce the possibility of hemorrhage.

Hyperglycemia. Patients with prediabetes or diabetes must be monitored for the development of hyperglycemia, particularly during the early weeks of therapy. Assess regularly for hyperglycemia and report any frequent occurrences. Patients receiving oral hypoglycemic agents or insulin may require an adjustment in dosage.

Rifampin. Rifampin may enhance the metabolism of corticosteroids, thus reducing therapeutic effect. Monitor for diminished therapeutic effect and increase the corticosteroid dose if necessary.

Get Ready for the NCLEX® Examination!

Key Points

- Corticosteroids are potent agents that produce many therapeutic benefits as well as undesirable adverse effects.
- Many of the adverse effects of the steroids are related to dosage and duration of therapy. These drugs must be used with caution in patients with diabetes mellitus, heart failure, hypertension, peptic ulcer disease, mental disturbance, and suspected infections.
- Nurses can play a significant role in helping patients monitor therapy and can assist them in seeking medical attention at the earliest signs of impending trouble.

Additional Learning Resources

SG Go to your Study Guide for additional Review Questions for the NCLEX® Examination, Critical Thinking Clinical Situations, and other learning activities to help you master this chapter content.

Go to your Evolve website (https://evolve.elsevier.com/Clayton) for additional online resources.

Review Questions for the NCLEX® Examination

1. Mineralocorticoids have which of the following actions in the body?
   1. They regulate serum glucose levels.
   2. They help maintain fluid and electrolyte balance.
   3. They are used to treat hyperpituitarism.
   4. They help regulate body temperature.

2. Glucocorticoids regulate carbohydrate, protein, and fat metabolism and have which of the following properties? *(Select all that apply.)*
   1. Antiinflammatory
   2. Antiallergenic
   3. Immunosuppressant
   4. Antihypertensive
   5. Antipyretic

3. The nurse is explaining to the patient the reason for corticosteroids to be prescribed for rheumatoid arthritis. During the teach-back session, which response by the patient indicates that further teaching is needed?
   1. "I know that I can't overdo activity, even though I may be feeling less pain with the prednisone."
   2. "When I take this drug, I can gain water weight, so I need to weigh myself every day."
   3. "I should let my doctor know if I get a sore throat, fever, and start to feel crummy."
   4. "I know that this drug will cure my arthritis."

4. Patients receiving a corticosteroid should be questioned regarding any history of which disorder?
   1. Gastric ulcers
   2. Blood dyscrasias
   3. Heart disease
   4. Respiratory disease

5. Which two types of electrolyte imbalances are most likely to be caused by corticosteroids?
   1. Hyperkalemia and hyponatremia
   2. Hypokalemia and hypernatremia
   3. Hypercalcemia and hypermagnesemia
   4. Hypocalcemia and hypomagnesemia

6. A 35-year-old prediabetic patient was prescribed prednisone 20 mg daily. The nurse knows that this may induce which condition?
   1. Hypoglycemia
   2. Hyperglycemia
   3. Insulin resistance
   4. Hypomagnesemia

7. Steroid replacement therapy needs to be gradually discontinued in small increments because of which effect?
   1. The steroid taper will maintain a more normal body rhythm.
   2. The steroid taper will lessen the risk of adverse effects.
   3. The steroid taper will ensure that the patient's adrenal glands are able to start secreting steroids appropriately.
   4. The steroid taper will decrease the risk of electrolyte imbalance.

8. The nurse administering prednisone to a patient with rheumatoid arthritis knows to watch for which adverse effects? *(Select all that apply.)*
   1. Electrolyte imbalance
   2. Hyperglycemia
   3. Hyperthyroidism
   4. Presence of edema
   5. Bradycardia

Objectives

1. Describe gonads and their function.
2. Discuss the body changes that can be anticipated with the administration of androgens, estrogens, or progesterone.
3. Identify the uses of estrogens and progestins.
4. Compare the adverse effects seen with the use of estrogen hormones with those seen with androgens.

Key Terms

gonads (GŌ-nădz) (p. 586)
testosterone (těs-TŎS-těr-ōn) (p. 586)
androgens (ĂN-drō-jěnz) (p. 586)

ovaries (Ō-văr-ēz) (p. 586)
estrogen (ĔS-trō-jěn) (p. 586)
progesterone (prō-JĔS-těr-ōn) (p. 586)

THE GONADS AND GONADAL HORMONES

The **gonads** are the reproductive glands—the testes of the male and the ovaries of the female. In addition to producing sperm, the testes produce **testosterone**, the male sex hormone. Testosterone controls the development of the male sex organs and influences characteristics such as voice, hair distribution, and male body form. **Androgens** are other steroid hormones that produce masculinizing effects.

The **ovaries** produce estrogen and progesterone. These are hormones that stimulate maturation of the female sex organs. They influence breast development, voice quality, and the broader pelvis of the female body form. Menstruation is established because of the hormone production of the ovaries. **Estrogen** is responsible for most of these changes. **Progesterone** is thought to be associated mainly with body changes that favor the implantation of the fertilized ovum, continuation of pregnancy, and preparation of the breasts for lactation.

❖ NURSING IMPLICATIONS FOR GONADAL HORMONES

◆ Assessment

History. Ask the patient to describe the current problem that initiated this visit. How long have the symptoms been present? Is this a recurrent problem? If so, how was it treated?

Reproductive. Ask female patients to describe the following, as appropriate: age of menarche; usual pattern of menses (i.e., duration, number of pads used, last menstrual period); number of pregnancies, live births, miscarriages, and abortions; vaginal discharges, itching, infections, and how treated; and breast self-examination routine (if not being performed regularly, explain the correct procedure).

Male patients should be asked whether testicular self-examinations are performed (if not being performed regularly, explain the correct procedure). As appropriate, obtain information regarding impotence, sterility, or alterations in libido.

Prior illnesses. Any indication of hypertension, heart or liver disease, thromboembolic disorders, or cancer of the reproductive organs is of particular concern.

Medication. Obtain a detailed history of all prescribed medications, including oral contraceptives; over-the-counter medications, including herbal medicines (e.g., dong quai, black cohosh); and any street drugs (e.g., "muscle-building" steroids). Ask if the patient understands why each is being taken. Tactfully determine if the prescribed medications are being taken regularly and, if not, why not?

Smoking. Does the person smoke?

Physical examination

- A complete physical examination is usually done as part of the preliminary workup before treatment of any disorders using gonadal hormones. With children and adolescent patients, include questions to collect data regarding growth and development (note in particular the development of long bones), changes in hair growth and distribution, and size of the genitalia.
- Record basic patient data: height, weight, and vital signs. Baseline blood pressure readings are of

particular concern so that recordings on future visits can be evaluated for any change.

- Collect urine for urinalysis and blood samples for hemoglobin, hematocrit, measurement of gonadotropic hormones, and other laboratory studies deemed appropriate by the healthcare provider. Usually, patients with family histories of diabetes mellitus should be tested for hyperglycemia before starting gonadal hormone therapy.
- The physical examination for a female patient should include a breast examination and a pelvic examination, including a Papanicolaou (Pap) test. Observe the distribution of body hair and the presence of scars. Stress the need for periodic physical examinations while receiving gonadal hormones.

Psychosocial. Patients requiring androgen therapy may need to be encouraged to discuss feelings relating to sexuality, sterility, or altered libido.

 Life Span Considerations

Diabetes Mellitus

Patients with diabetes mellitus who receive gonadal hormones may experience alterations in the blood glucose levels. Parameters should be established and a written record for glucose monitoring maintained for reporting to the healthcare provider.

Most gonadal hormones are prescribed to patients for prolonged self-administration. Therefore planning should stress patient education specific to the type of gonadal hormone prescribed and its intended actions, including monitoring of common and serious adverse effects. Ensure that the patient understands the dosage and specific time schedule for administration of the prescribed medication.

◆ **Implementation**
Obtain baseline data for subsequent evaluation of therapeutic response to therapy (e.g., weight, vital signs, and blood pressure in sitting, lying, and standing positions). Assist with the physical examination.

◆ **Patient Education**
Expectations of therapy. Discuss the expectations of therapy with the patient (e.g., degree of pain relief, frequency of use of therapy, relief of menopausal symptoms, sexual maturation, regulation of menstrual cycle, sexual activity, maintenance of mobility, activities of daily living and/or work).

Smoking. Explain the risks of continuing to smoke, especially when the patient is receiving estrogen or progestin therapy. The incidence of fatal heart attacks, thromboembolic disorders, and stroke is increased for women older than 35 years who smoke. Provide smoking cessation education.

Physical examination. Stress the need for regular periodic medical examinations and laboratory studies.

Fostering health maintenance. Discuss medication information and how it will benefit the course of treatment to produce an optimal response. Seek cooperation and understanding of the following points so that medication adherence is increased: name of medication; dosage, route, and times of administration; and common and serious adverse effects. If estrogen has been prescribed for the purpose of delaying the advancement of osteoporosis, stress the importance of adhering to the regimen to achieve the maximum effect.

Patient self-assessment. Plan to teach the individual to monitor vital signs and weight daily. Enlist the patient's help in developing and maintaining a written record of monitoring parameters (e.g., blood pressure, pulse, daily weight, degree of pain relief, menstrual cycle information, breakthrough bleeding, nausea, vomiting, cramps, breast tenderness, hirsutism, gynecomastia, masculinization, hoarseness, headaches, sexual stimulation). See Appendix B: Template for Developing a Written Record for Patients to Monitor Their Own Therapy. Complete the Premedication Data column for use as a baseline to track response to drug therapy. Ensure that the patient understands how to use the form, and instruct the patient to take the completed form to follow-up visits. During follow-up visits, focus on issues that will foster adherence to the therapeutic interventions prescribed.

DRUG THERAPY WITH GONADAL HORMONES

DRUG CLASS: ESTROGENS

Actions
The natural estrogenic hormone released from the ovaries is composed of several closely related chemical compounds—estradiol, estrone, and estriol. The most potent is estradiol. It is metabolized to estrone, which is half as potent. Estrone is further metabolized to estriol, which is considerably less potent. Estrogens are responsible for development of the sex organs during growth in utero and for maturation at puberty. They are also responsible for characteristics such as growth of hair, texture of skin, and distribution of body fat. Estrogens affect the release of pituitary gonadotropins; cause capillary dilation, fluid retention, and protein metabolism; and inhibit ovulation and postpartum breast engorgement.

Uses
Estrogen products are used for relief of hot flash symptoms of menopause; for contraception; for hormone replacement therapy after an oophorectomy, in conjunction with appropriate diet, calcium, and physical therapy;

for the prevention of osteoporosis; for treatment of severe acne in females (contained in oral contraceptives); and to slow the disease progress (and minimize discomfort) in patients with advanced prostatic cancer and certain types of breast cancer.

Postmenopausal women with an intact uterus are at an increased risk of developing endometrial cancer with the use of estrogens alone. If estrogen therapy is indicated, it should be accompanied by progestin therapy to reduce the risk of endometrial cancer. There is no evidence that "natural" estrogens are more or less hazardous than "synthetic" estrogens at equiestrogenic dosages.

Results of a controlled study, the Women's Health Initiative (WHI), have indicated that hormone replacement therapy is associated with a small increase in the risk of coronary heart disease (CHD) (Rossouw et al, 2002). Follow-up studies reaffirm that hormone therapy is effective for relief of vasomotor symptoms associated with menopause, and that the risk of CHD tended to be reduced in women close to menopause compared with increased risk in women more distant from menopause. Based on WHI data, use of hormone replacement therapy for fewer than 5 years is a reasonable option for relief of moderate to severe vasomotor symptoms. However, prior to initiation of therapy the patient should have a baseline risk assessment (family history of CHD, age, body weight, diabetes, smoking) and then should be monitored annually. Long-term use of hormone replacement therapy is not recommended due to the risk of stroke, venous thromboembolism, and breast cancer that has been documented in studies completed since 2002 (Rossouw et al, 2013).

Therapeutic Outcomes
The primary therapeutic outcomes expected from estrogen therapy are as follows:
1. Contraception (see Chapter 40)
2. Hormonal balance
3. Prevention of osteoporosis
4. Palliative treatment of prostate and breast cancer
5. Treatment of severe acne in females

❖ Nursing Implications for Estrogen Therapy
◆ Premedication assessment
1. Determine whether the patient is pregnant before starting estrogen therapy; hold the medication and consult the prescriber if there is a possibility of pregnancy.
2. Obtain baseline weight and vital signs, especially accurate blood pressure readings.
3. Ask whether the individual has a history of thromboembolic disorders or cancer of the reproductive organs; if so, hold medication and contact the healthcare provider.

◆ Availability, dosage, and administration
See Table 38.1.

> **! Medication Safety Alert**
>
> The use of estrogens during early pregnancy is contraindicated. Serious birth defects have been reported, and it has been found that the female offspring have an increased risk of developing vaginal or cervical cancer later in life.

◆ Common adverse effects
Neurologic

Headache, migraine, dizziness, insomnia, anxiety, nervousness, emotional lability. These symptoms tend to be mild and resolve with continued therapy. If they do not resolve or become particularly bothersome, the patient should consult the healthcare provider.

Endocrine

Weight gain, edema, breast tenderness, nausea. These symptoms tend to be mild and resolve with continued therapy. If they do not resolve or become particularly bothersome, the patient should consult the healthcare provider.

◆ Serious adverse effects.
The following are all complications associated with estrogen therapy. It is extremely important that the patient be evaluated by her healthcare provider for any of the following symptoms or other symptoms that the patient recognizes to be of concern.

Cardiovascular. Hypertension, thrombophlebitis, and thromboembolism.

Metabolic. Hyperglycemia.

Gynecologic. Breakthrough bleeding may occur. Long-term exposure to estrogens can increase the risks of breast, endometrial, and vaginal cancers in women. Too much estrogen aggravates endometriosis, a painful growth of the uterine lining outside the uterus, whereas too little estrogen weakens bones (osteoporosis).

◆ Drug interactions
Warfarin. This medication may diminish the anticoagulant effects of warfarin. Monitor the prothrombin time (international normalized ratio [INR]) and increase the dosage of warfarin if necessary.

Phenytoin. Estrogens may inhibit the metabolism of phenytoin, resulting in phenytoin toxicity. Monitor patients with concurrent therapy for signs of phenytoin toxicity (e.g., nystagmus, sedation, lethargy). Serum levels may be ordered, and a reduced dosage of phenytoin may be required.

Thyroid hormones. Patients who have no thyroid function and who start estrogen therapy may require an increase in thyroid hormone dosage. Estrogens increase thyroid-binding globulin levels, which reduce the level of circulating free thyroxine (T_4). The total level of T_4 is normal or increased. Do not adjust the thyroid hormone dosage until the patient shows clinical signs of hypothyroidism.

Table 38.1 Estrogens

GENERIC NAME	BRAND NAME	AVAILABILITY	USES	DOSAGE RANGE
conjugated estrogens	Premarin ⇄ *Do not confuse Premarin with Prevacid.* C.E.S. 🍁	Tablets: 0.3, 0.45, 0.625, 0.9, 1.25 mg IV: 25 mg in 5-mL vial Cream: 0.625 mg/g	Menopause, atopic vaginitis Female hypogonadism Ovarian failure or postoophorectomy Osteoporosis (prevention) Breast carcinoma Prostatic carcinoma	PO: 0.3-1.25 mg daily cyclically[a] Intravaginal cream: 0.5-2 g intravaginally daily cyclically[a] PO: 0.3-0.625 mg daily cyclically[a] PO: 1.25 mg daily cyclically[a] PO: 0.3 mg initially daily cyclically[a]; dose may be titrated; use lowest effective dose PO: 10 mg three times daily for at least 3 mo PO: 1.25-2.5 mg three times daily
conjugated estrogens and bazedoxifene	Duavee	Tablet: conjugated estrogens 0.45 mg, bazedoxifene 20 mg	Menopause (moderate to severe vasomotor symptoms); prevention of postmenopausal osteoporosis	PO: 1 tablet daily
esterified estrogen	Menest	Tablets: 0.3, 0.625, 1.25, 2.5 mg	Menopause, atropic vaginitis Female hypogonadism, postoophorectomy, ovarian failure Breast carcinoma Prostatic carcinoma	PO: 0.3-1.25 mg daily cyclically[a] PO: 1.25-7.5 mg daily cyclically[a] PO: 10 mg three times daily PO: 1.25-2.5 mg three times daily
estradiol ⇄ *Do not confuse estradiol with Risperdal.*	Estrace ⇄ *Do not confuse Estrace with Evista.*	Tablets: 0.5, 1, 2 mg Injections: valerate in oil: 10, 20, 40 mg/mL Cream, vaginal: 0.1 mg/g	Menopause, atropic vaginitis, hypogonadism, postoophorectomy, ovarian failure Prostatic carcinoma Breast carcinoma	PO: 1-2 mg daily or cyclically[a] IM: valerate 10-20 mg q4 wk PO: 1-2 mg three times daily IM: valerate 30 mg q1-2 wk PO: 10 mg three times daily for at least 3 mo
	Alora, Vivelle-Dot, Minivelle	Transdermal patch applied twice weekly: 0.025, 0.0375, 0.05, 0.075, 0.1 mg/24 hr	Menopause, female hypogonadism, primary ovarian failure, atropic vaginitis, postoophorectomy, osteoporosis prevention	Transdermal system: patch should be placed on clean, dry area of skin on trunk (usually abdomen or buttock) on cyclic schedule; rotate application site; interval of 1 wk between uses of same site
	Climara	Transdermal patch applied once weekly: 0.025, 0.037, 0.05, 0.06, 0.075, 0.1 mg/24 hr	Menopause, female hypogonadism, primary ovarian failure, atropic vaginitis, postoophorectomy, osteoporosis prevention	Transdermal system: patch should be placed on clean, dry area of skin on trunk (usually abdomen or buttock) on cyclic schedule; rotate application site; interval of 1 wk between uses of same site
	Menostar	Transdermal patch applied once weekly: 0.014 mg/24 hr	Prevention of postmenopausal osteoporosis	Apply one patch weekly to clean, dry area of the lower abdomen; rotate site weekly; remove old patch and discard appropriately
	Divigel	Transdermal gel: 0.25 mg/0.25 g; 0.5 mg/0.5 g; 1 mg/g	Menopause	0.25 g applied once daily; may apply 0.25 to 1 g daily based on symptoms
	Elestrin	Transdermal gel: 0.06%	Menopause	0.87 g applied once daily; may apply 0.87 to 1.7 g daily based on symptoms

Continued

Table 38.1 Estrogens—cont'd

GENERIC NAME	BRAND NAME	AVAILABILITY	USES	DOSAGE RANGE
	EstroGel	Topical gel: 0.06% in pump	Menopause, vaginal atrophy	Topical: apply contents of one pump daily to one arm, spreading from wrist to upper arm on all sides; allow to dry; wash hands with soap and water; if uterus is intact, progestin should also be taken to prevent endometrial cancer; alcohol gel is flammable until dry, so avoid fire, flame, or smoking until dry
	Evamist	Transdermal spray: 1.53 mg/spray	Menopause	Topical: 1 spray once every morning May apply 1-3 sprays daily based on symptoms
	Femring	Vaginal ring: 0.05/24 hours, 0.1 mg/24 hours	Menopause Vaginal atrophy	0.05 mg intravaginally; adjust dose based on clinical response; ring should remain in place for 3 months
estropipate		Tablets: 0.75 mg	Menopause, atropic vaginitis	PO: 0.75-6 mg daily cyclically[a]
			Female hypogonadism, postoophorectomy, ovarian failure	PO: 1.25-9 mg daily cyclically[a]
			Osteoporosis prevention	PO: 0.75 mg daily cyclically[a]

♣ Available in Canada.
[a]Cyclically = 3 weeks of daily estrogen followed by 1 week off; 25 days daily and 5 days off.

DRUG CLASS: PROGESTINS

Actions
Progesterone and its derivatives (the progestins) inhibit the secretion of pituitary gonadotropins, preventing maturation of ovarian follicles and thus inhibiting ovulation.

Uses
Progestins are used primarily to treat secondary amenorrhea, breakthrough uterine bleeding, and endometriosis, but they may also be used in combination with estrogens as contraceptives (see Chapter 40).

Therapeutic Outcomes
The primary therapeutic outcomes expected from progestin therapy are as follows:
1. Contraception
2. Relief of symptoms of endometriosis
3. Hormonal balance to relieve amenorrhea or abnormal uterine bleeding

❖ **Nursing Implications for Progestins**
◆ *Premedication assessment*
1. Determine whether the patient is pregnant before starting progestin therapy; hold the medication and consult the healthcare provider if there is a possibility of pregnancy.

2. Obtain baseline weight and vital signs, especially accurate blood pressure readings.
3. Ask whether the individual has a history of thromboembolic disorders or cancer of the reproductive organs; if so, withhold medication and contact the healthcare provider.

◆ *Availability, dosage, and administration*
See Table 38.2.

 Medication Safety Alert

The use of progestins in early pregnancy has been associated with birth defects. If pregnancy is suspected, the healthcare provider should be consulted immediately.

◆ *Common adverse effects.* These symptoms tend to be mild and resolve with continued therapy. If they do not resolve or become particularly bothersome, instruct the patient to consult the healthcare provider.
  Endocrine. Weight gain, edema, tiredness, oily scalp, acne.
  Gastrointestinal. Nausea, vomiting, diarrhea.

◆ *Serious adverse effects.* The following are complications associated with progestin therapy. If these complications occur, it is extremely important that the patient be

minimize the possibility of renal calculi. Encourage the patient to drink 8 to 12 eight-ounce glasses of water daily. The patient should perform weight-bearing and active and passive exercises to the degree tolerated to minimize loss of calcium from bones.

Endocrine

Masculinization. Women receiving high doses of androgens may develop signs of masculinization. Women should be monitored for signs of masculinization (e.g., deepening of the voice, hoarseness, growth of facial hair, clitoral enlargement, and menstrual irregularities) during androgen therapy. The drug should usually be discontinued when mild masculinization is evident because some adverse androgenic effects (e.g., voice changes) may not reverse with discontinuation of therapy. In consultation with the healthcare provider, the woman may decide that some masculinization is acceptable during treatment for breast cancer. Help patients adjust to a possible change in self-image or self-esteem caused by the effects of masculinization.

Males should be carefully monitored for the development of gynecomastia, priapism, or excessive sexual stimulation. These are indications of androgen overdose.

Gastrointestinal

Hepatotoxicity. The symptoms of hepatotoxicity include anorexia, nausea, vomiting, jaundice, hepatomegaly, splenomegaly, and abnormal liver function test results (e.g., elevated bilirubin, aspartate aminotransferase, alanine aminotransferase, gamma-glutamyltransferase, and alkaline phosphatase levels; increased prothrombin time [INR]).

> **Life Span Considerations**
> **Androgens**
>
> Male children receiving androgens must have the effects of the drug on long bones monitored by periodic radiographs of long bones. Usually, radiographs of long bones are obtained every 3 to 6 months to check the status of the epiphyseal line. Androgens may prematurely close the epiphyseal line, preventing bone elongation.

◆ *Drug interactions*

Warfarin. Androgens may enhance the anticoagulant effects of warfarin. Observe for the development of petechiae; ecchymoses; nosebleeds; bleeding gums; dark, tarry stools; and bright red or coffee-ground emesis. Monitor the prothrombin time (INR), and reduce the dosage of warfarin if necessary.

Oral antidiabetic agents, insulin. Monitor for hypoglycemia; symptoms include headache, weakness, decreased coordination, general apprehension, diaphoresis, hunger, and blurred or double vision. The dosage of the hypoglycemic agent or insulin may need to be reduced. Notify the healthcare provider if any of these symptoms appear.

Corticosteroids. Concurrent use may increase the possibility of electrolyte imbalance and fluid retention.

Get Ready for the NCLEX® Examination!

Key Points

- The gonadal hormones are necessary for the body to grow and mature into the adult form and for reproduction.
- Male and female gonads secrete hormones. The male testes secrete predominantly androgens, and the female ovaries secrete primarily estrogens and progesterone.
- These hormones are responsible for the shape and secondary sex characteristics associated with the male and female body forms.

Additional Learning Resources

SG Go to your Study Guide for additional Review Questions for the NCLEX® Examination, Critical Thinking Clinical Situations, and other learning activities to help you master this chapter content.

Go to your Evolve website (https://evolve.elsevier.com/Clayton) for additional online resources.

Review Questions for the NCLEX® Examination

1. The reproductive glands of both sexes produce hormones that control the development and maturation of the sex organs. Which of the following are gonadal hormones? *(Select all that apply.)*
   1. Testosterone
   2. Cortisol
   3. Progesterone
   4. Luteinizing hormone
   5. Estrogen
2. Androgens, when given to a patient with breast cancer, may result in the development of which adverse effect? *(Select all that apply.)*
   1. Hypertension
   2. Weight gain and edema
   3. Masculinization
   4. Hypercalcemia
   5. Hyperglycemia
3. Estrogens are given to women for which of the following therapeutic outcomes? *(Select all that apply.)*
   1. Hormonal balance
   2. Prevention of osteoporosis
   3. Relief of headaches and insomnia
   4. Treatment of severe acne
   5. Prevention of coronary artery disease

4. Women taking androgens for treatment of discomfort associated with breast cancer may develop which symptoms of masculinization? *(Select all that apply.)*
   1. Growth of long bones
   2. Deeper voice quality
   3. Growth of facial hair
   4. Irregular menses
   5. Shrinking breast tissue

5. Progestin is used to treat which of the following conditions in women? *(Select all that apply.)*
   1. Prevention of ovulation for contraceptive use
   2. Treatment of breakthrough uterine bleeding
   3. Relief of symptoms of endometriosis
   4. Treatment of breast cancer symptoms
   5. Treatment of hypogonadism

6. The patient who is starting on testosterone pellets subcutaneously for treatment of hypogonadism asks the nurse what effects to expect. What is the appropriate response of the nurse?
   1. "You should be able to feel your hormonal balance being restored in one week."
   2. "Your voice may get deeper, and you may grow a fuller beard, as well as have improved libido."
   3. "You can expect to have improved muscle strength and to grow chest hairs."
   4. "You should be able to continue to feel just like you always do; it only affects the blood levels."

Drugs Used in Obstetrics

39

https://evolve.elsevier.com/Clayton

Objectives

1. Identify appropriate nursing assessments during normal labor and delivery.
2. Discuss potential complications of preterm labor and when uterine relaxants and magnesium sulfate are used.
3. Describe when uterine stimulants are administered for induction of labor, augmentation of labor, and postpartum atony and hemorrhage.
4. State the actions and the primary use of clomiphene citrate.
5. Identify the action and proper timing of the administration of $Rh_o(D)$ immune globulin.
6. Cite education needed for care of the neonate, including erythromycin ophthalmic ointment and phytonadione administration.

Key Terms

pregnancy hypertension disorders (PRĔG-nĕn-sē hī-pĕr-TĔN-shŭn) (p. 597)
lochia (LŌ-kē-ă) (p. 598)
precipitous labor and delivery (prē-SĬP-ĭ-tŭs LĀ-bŭr) (p. 605)

augmentation (ŏg-mĕn-TĀ-shŭn) (p. 605)
dysfunctional labor (dĭs-FŬNK-shŭn-ăl LĀ-bŭr) (p. 605)

OBSTETRICS

Obstetrics is the field of healthcare practice associated with pregnancy, the health of the mother and the child, and the process of birth. The current culture is for mothers who are expecting to deliver a child to be admitted to a hospital or birthing center and have the baby under controlled conditions. The labor and delivery process is unpredictable to some extent, and having trained clinicians present during the birth provides a sense of control. Nurses working in obstetrics are trained in assessment of the mother during the trimesters of fetal growth and the baby upon delivery.

❖ NURSING IMPLICATIONS FOR OBSTETRICS

◆ Assessment

Prenatal assessment. Obtain basic historical information about the woman and family concerning acute or chronic conditions, surgeries, and deaths.

- Has the patient been treated for kidney or bladder problems; high blood pressure; heart disease; rheumatic fever; hypothyroidism or hyperthyroidism; diabetes mellitus; allergies to any foods, drugs,

or environmental substances; or sexually transmitted infections (STIs)?
- Has the patient been exposed to any communicable diseases since becoming pregnant?
- Has the patient received blood or blood products?

If the woman answers yes to any of these questions, find out which healthcare provider made the diagnosis, when the condition occurred, and how the condition was treated. Request the approximate date of the last Papanicolaou (Pap) test and results.

Gather data about menstrual pattern (e.g., age of initial onset, duration and frequency of monthly periods, date of last full menstrual cycle, any bleeding since the last full menstrual period) and contraceptive use (e.g., condoms, foam, diaphragm, sponge, oral contraceptives, intrauterine devices).

Take an obstetric history. Ask the woman if she has had any previous live births, stillbirths, or spontaneous or therapeutic abortions. If any of the deliveries were premature, obtain additional information about the infant's gestational age, survival of the child, suspected causes of prematurity, and infections. Ask whether any of the births required a cesarean delivery. If yes, ask

595

why. Ask if $Rh_o(D)$ immune globulin (RhoGAM) has been given for Rh factor incompatibility.

Nutritional history

- What is the patient's usual or prepregnant weight? How much weight has she gained or lost in the past 3 months?
- What are the woman's favorite foods? Are there any foods that she avoids? How often does she eat? What has she eaten in the past 3 days? Does she normally take daily vitamins, minerals, or herbal products?
- Are there any cultural food practices to be maintained during the pregnancy?

Elimination pattern

- What is the patient's elimination pattern?
- How often does she have bowel movements?
- What is the stool consistency and color?
- Is there any bleeding?
- Are laxatives ever needed? If so, how often?

Psychosocial cultural history

- Determine how the woman feels about this pregnancy (e.g., excited, nervous, or if the baby is not intended).
- Determine cultural patterns regarding prenatal care (e.g., language spoken, activities that she cannot do while pregnant, whether she prefers a female caregiver). Ask the pregnant woman what specific cultural practices she would like to follow during the pregnancy.
- Who makes up her support group: husband, boyfriend, friends, partner, family, tribal healer?
- Ask about her employment status and what type of work she performs.
- Determine the woman's level of education, economic status, and general interest in learning more about effective management of the pregnancy. Will referral to social services agencies be necessary?

Medication history. Ask the woman if she takes any prescribed medications, over-the-counter medications, or herbal remedies. If she is not currently taking any medications, ask whether she has taken any over the past 6 months. Determine which have been prescribed and for what purpose.

Determine the use of alcohol and street or recreational drugs of any type, including what, how much, and how frequently.

Physical examination. Assist the woman to undress and prepare for examination, including a pelvic examination and Pap smear.

- *Height and weight:* Record height and weight. (See an obstetrics textbook for a detailed guide to all aspects of a prenatal visit and the initial assessments performed.)
- *Hypertension:* Take the blood pressure. Ask if any treatment has been given for high blood pressure. If so, inquire about the onset, treatment, and degree of control achieved.
- *Heart rate:* At prenatal visits, count the pulse for 1 full minute. Report irregularities in rate, rhythm, or volume. On subsequent visits, anticipate an increase

in rate of approximately 10 beats/min during the course of the pregnancy.

- *Respirations:* Record the rate of respirations. As the pregnancy progresses, observe for hyperventilation and thoracic breathing.
- *Temperature:* If the temperature is elevated, ask about any signs of infection or exposure to people with known communicable diseases.
- *Laboratory and diagnostic studies:* Obtain a urine specimen using the clean-catch method.
- *Blood tests:* Testing for complete blood count (CBC), hemoglobin, hematocrit, hemoglobin electrophoresis, rubella titer, Rh factor, and STIs (e.g., syphilis, gonorrhea, chlamydia) may be ordered at this initial visit. These may include antibody, sickle cell, and thalassemia screens; folic acid level; and, as appropriate, purified protein derivative, human immunodeficiency virus (HIV), hepatitis B, and toxicology screens. With a history of diabetes, hypertension, or renal disease, additional laboratory testing may be ordered (e.g., 1-hour glucose tolerance, creatinine clearance, total protein excretion).

Assessment during first, second, and third trimesters. Assessment done at routine visits during the pregnancy includes weight; measurement of blood pressure, pulse, and respirations; and examination of the abdomen, with measurement of fundal height and fetal heart sounds. Any problems or concerns should be discussed. Hemoglobin and hematocrit may be periodically rechecked.

The pregnant woman who is not experiencing complications is usually examined monthly for the first 6 months, every 2 weeks in the seventh and eighth months, and weekly during the last month. Vaginal examinations are usually performed on the initial visit and are not repeated until 2 to 3 weeks before the estimated date of delivery or estimated date of birth (due date), at which time the cervical status, degree of engagement, and fetal presentation are evaluated. A sonogram may be obtained in early pregnancy.

Assessment of the pregnant patient at risk. Assess for signs and symptoms of potential obstetric complications (see an obstetrics textbook for further details of each complication): infection, hyperemesis gravidarum, spontaneous abortion, preterm labor, premature rupture of membranes (PROM), gestational diabetes, preeclampsia, HELLP (hemolysis, elevated liver enzymes, and low platelet count) syndrome, and intrauterine fetal death.

- *Infection:* Record the patient's temperature. Report any elevations to the healthcare provider immediately for further evaluation. As appropriate, obtain urine for urinalysis.
- *Hyperemesis gravidarum:* Obtain details of persistent, severe vomiting.
- *Early pregnancy loss, placental separation, abortion:* Assess for signs of bleeding. Gather specific information

about the onset, duration, volume (number of pads used), and color, and report any clots or tissue.

- Ask the patient to describe any pain experienced using a scale of 0 to 10. Has she had any backache or pelvic cramping, sharp abdominal pain, faintness, or pain in the shoulder area?
- Vital signs should be taken and compared with baseline data whenever bleeding is suspected. Assess for development of shock—restlessness, perspiration, pallor, clammy skin, dyspnea, tachycardia, and blood pressure changes. Record fetal heart tones at regular intervals.
- *Preterm labor:* Preterm labor is defined as:
  - Labor occurring after 20 and before 37 completed weeks of gestation *plus*
  - Clinically documented uterine contractions (4/20 minutes or 6/60 minutes) *plus*
  - Ruptured membranes *or*
  - Intact membranes and cervical dilation greater than 2 cm *or*
  - Intact membranes and cervical effacement greater than 80% *or*
  - Intact membranes and cervical change during observation.

These can be measured by changes in dilation or effacement, or by changes in cervical length measured clinically, or by ultrasound.

A fetal fibronectin (FFN) test may be ordered to assess the presence of preterm labor in patients whose presenting symptoms are questionable so that early intervention (e.g., tocolytic therapy, corticosteroids, transport to a tertiary care center) can be initiated when indicated or, if negative, unnecessary interventions can be avoided. The FFN test is for women with intact membranes and cervical dilation of less than 3 cm. This test may detect the probability of preterm labor from 24 to 34 weeks' gestation. If the test is negative, the patient is unlikely to experience preterm delivery in the next 7 to 14 days (Fig. 39.1). Home uterine activity monitoring using a tocodynamometer may be used to detect excessive uterine contractions.

- *Premature rupture of membranes:* Assess for and obtain specifics of any signs of leakage of amniotic fluid from the vagina.
- *Gestational diabetes:* Review urinalysis reports for glycosuria. Review history of symptoms, especially during previous pregnancies. Review 1- and 3-hour glucose tolerance blood test results.
- *Pregnancy hypertension disorders:* Assess for and report sudden hypertension (an elevation of systolic pressure 30 mm Hg or more above prior readings, systolic blood pressure of 140 mm Hg or more, or diastolic pressure of 90 mm Hg or more). **Pregnancy hypertension disorders** include preeclampsia (elevated blood pressure; proteinuria due to hypoperfusion secondary to a vasospastic process that affects the fetus, the placenta, and maternal organs and vasculature) and eclampsia (convulsions accompanying preeclampsia).

- Assess for edema of any body parts (e.g., fingers, hands, face, legs, ankles). Assess hydration status, and, in particular, obtain daily weights.
- Review laboratory reports for indications of abnormal electrolytes, elevated uric acid or hematocrit levels, and thrombocytopenia in the blood and for the presence of red blood cells (RBCs) and protein in the urine.
- Assess for signs and symptoms of seizure activity.
- Monitor fetal heart rate and movements.
- Assess for start of labor or signs of other complications, such as pulmonary edema, disseminated intravascular coagulation, heart failure, abruptio placentae, or cerebral hemorrhage.
- When giving magnesium sulfate for preeclampsia, assess deep tendon reflexes, respiratory status (report depression), sedation level, intake and output, seizure precautions, and cardiac status. (Always have calcium gluconate, the antidote for magnesium sulfate, available.)

 Life Span Considerations

The status of the fetus may be assessed by fetal movement counts, contraction stress testing, biophysical profile, and ultrasonography for placental placement and measurement of maturity indicators. Amniocentesis may be performed to assess fetal lung maturity and detect fetal disorders.

Assessment during normal labor and delivery

History of pregnancy. On admission of the pregnant woman to the hospital, obtain the following information:
- Name and age
- Obstetric history (gravida, para, abortions, fetal deaths, birth weight of previous children, and complications during previous deliveries)
- Estimated due date, estimated gestational age, and day of last menstrual period
- Prenatal care (type and amount, any significant problems)
- Prenatal education (type and extent of childbirth preparation)
- Plan for infant feeding
- Status of membranes (intact, ruptured, time ruptured, amount, and color of fluid that escaped)
- Status of labor (time of onset of contractions; frequency, duration, and intensity; how patient is coping with contractions)
- Time of last meal

Physical examination. The physical examination should include the following:
- Height, weight, vital signs (temperature, blood pressure, pulse, and respirations)
- State of hydration, including presence of edema
- Size and contour of abdomen and fundus
- Frequency of contractions
- Fetal heart rate

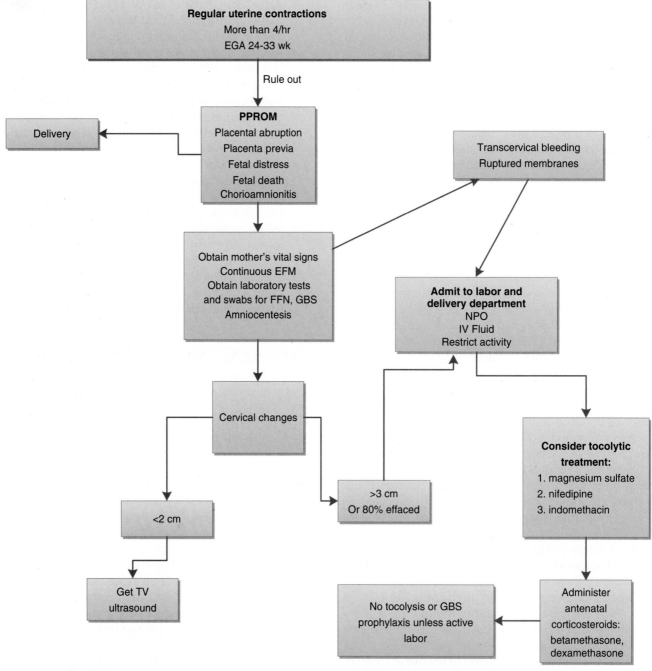

Fig. 39.1 Alternatives to the treatment of preterm labor. *EFM*, External fetal monitor; *EGA*, estimated gestational age; *FFN*, fetal fibronectin (indicates probability of preterm labor); *GBS*, group B streptococcus (if positive, treat with penicillin during labor); *NPO*, nothing by mouth; *PPROM*, preterm premature rupture of membranes; *TV*, transvaginal. NOTE: Tocolysis indicates use of medications to stop preterm labor.

- Vaginal examination: cervical dilation and efface-ment, status of membranes, and presentation and position of fetus

Assessment after delivery and during postpartum care

- The vital signs should be checked every 15 minutes during the first hour after delivery or until the woman is stable, then every 30 minutes for the next 2 hours.
- Inspect the perineum and note any abnormal swelling or bruising.

- Assess fundal height and firmness every 15 minutes for 1 hour, then every 30 minutes for the next 4 hours. Continue to assess fundal height and position until the woman is discharged.
- Describe the amount of lochia (vaginal discharge after delivery) and the color and the presence of clots every 15 minutes for 1 hour, every 30 minutes for 4 hours, and at least every 4 hours for the next 12 hours or as needed (PRN).
- Assess breasts for redness, softness, and nipple condition. Encourage early feedings with normal

newborns as allowed. Check for breast engorgement and discomfort.

Assessment of the neonate
- Ensure a patent airway.
- Observe umbilical cord until pulsations cease, then clamp or ligate it.
- Assess neonate's health status at 1 minute and 5 minutes after delivery using the Apgar scoring system (Table 39.1).
- Perform rapid estimation of gestational age (Fig. 39.2).

◆ Implementation
Prenatal
- Collect information relating to the mother's health status and the pregnancy. Observe for signs of potential complications of pregnancy.
- Assist with routine prenatal examinations and diagnostic procedures.

Table 39.1 Apgar Scoring System

	SCORE		
SIGN	**0**	**1**	**2**
Heart rate (beats/min)	Absent	Slow (below 100)	Over 100
Respiratory effort	Absent	Slow, irregular	Good, crying
Muscle tone	Flaccid	Some flexion of extremities	Active motion
Reflex irritability	No response	Grimace	Cry
Color	Blue, pale	Body pink, extremities blue	Completely pink

NEUROMUSCULAR MATURITY

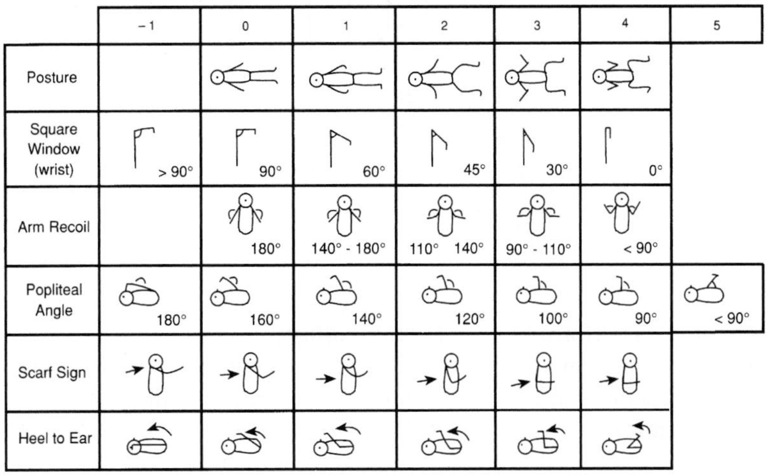

PHYSICAL MATURITY

Skin	sticky friable transparent	gelatinous red, translucent	smooth pink, visible veins	superficial peeling or rash, few veins	cracking pale areas rare veins	parchment deep cracking no vessels	leathery cracked wrinkled
Lanugo	none	sparse	abundant	thinning	bald areas	mostly bald	
Plantar Surface	heel-toe 40-50 mm: -1 <40 mm: -2	>50 mm no crease	faint red marks	anterior transverse crease only	creases ant. 2/3	creases over entire sole	
Breast	imperceptible	barely perceptible	flat areola no bud	stippled areola 1-2 mm bud	raised areola 3-4 mm bud	full areola 5-10 mm bud	
Eye/Ear	lids fused loosely: -1 tightly: -2	lids open pinna flat stays folded	sl. curved pinna; soft; slow recoil	well-curved pinna; soft but ready recoil	formed & firm instant recoil	thick cartilage ear stiff	
Genitals (male)	scrotum flat, smooth	scrotum empty faint rugae	testes in upper canal rare rugae	testes descending few rugae	testes down good rugae	testes pendulous deep rugae	
Genitals (female)	clitoris prominent labia flat	prominent clitoris small labia minora	prominent clitoris enlarging minora	majora & minora equally prominent	majora large minora small	majora cover clitoris & minora	

A

MATURITY RATING

score	weeks
-10	20
-5	22
0	24
5	26
10	28
15	30
20	32
25	34
30	36
35	38
40	40
45	42
50	44

Fig. 39.2 Estimation of gestational age. (A) New Ballard Score for newborn maturity rating. Expanded scale includes extremely premature infants and has been refined to improve accuracy in more mature infants. *Continued*

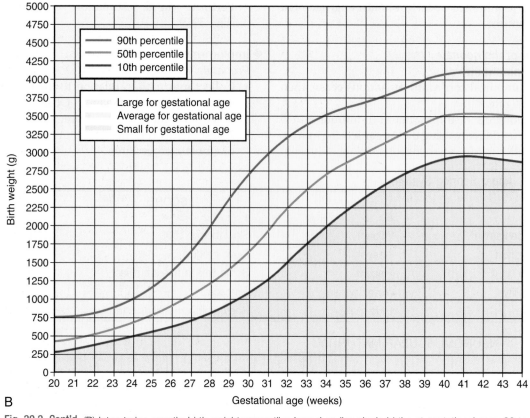

B

Fig. 39.2, Cont'd (B) Intrauterine growth: birth weight percentiles based on live single births at gestational ages 20 to 44 weeks. (A, From Ballard JL, Khoury JC, Wedig K, et al. New Ballard score expanded to include extremely premature infants. *J Pediatr.* 1991;119[3]:417. B, Data from Alexander GR, Himes JH, Kaufman RB, et al. A United States national reference for fetal growth. *Obstet Gynecol.* 1996;87[2]:163-168.)

- Review laboratory and diagnostic studies performed; report abnormal findings to the healthcare provider.
- During the first trimester, initiate discussion of infant feeding options available; provide information needed for parents to make a decision.

Complications of pregnancy
- *Infection:* Monitor for infections and intervene according to the healthcare provider's orders when an infection is confirmed.
- *Hyperemesis gravidarum* (see Chapter 33): Monitor hydration status, daily weight, and vital signs. Provide for dietary needs through intravenous (IV) therapy, nutritional supplements, and gradual progression of diet as tolerated.
- *Bleeding, spontaneous abortion:* Ensure that the patient adheres to bed rest and give sedatives as prescribed. Monitor maternal vital signs, fetal heart rate and activity, and the volume (frequency of change and number of pads used) of bleeding present. When bleeding is present, blood studies for hemoglobin, hematocrit, white blood cells, human chorionic gonadotropin titer, and blood type and crossmatch may be ordered. Other diagnostic procedures, such as culdoscopy, sonography, laparoscopy, fetoscopy, and pregnancy tests, may be performed.

Preterm labor
- Monitor uterine contractions and continue external fetal and uterine monitoring.
- Position the mother on her side, increase fluid intake, and start an IV infusion as ordered. Monitor hydration, maintain accurate intake and output records, and take daily weights.
- Assist with obtaining cervical and vaginal cultures, as ordered.
- Perform cervical examination to determine dilation and effacement. Assess for leakage of amniotic fluid.
- Take maternal vital signs. Record fetal heart rate and frequency and intensity of uterine contractions.
- Administer prescribed uterine relaxants, for example, nifedipine, indomethacin, or magnesium sulfate. (See the magnesium sulfate drug monograph later in this chapter for administration information and monitoring parameters.) Glucocorticoids, usually betamethasone or dexamethasone, may be administered by the intramuscular (IM) route to accelerate lung maturation to minimize fetal respiratory distress syndrome. Either glucocorticoid may be used in cases in which it is anticipated that premature labor should be stopped for only 36 to 48 hours, such as with PROM. There is no evidence to support one glucocorticoid over

another. Review available laboratory studies (e.g., FFN, electrolyte studies, CBC with differential, thrombocytopenia, uric acid level, hematocrit, serum estriol, lecithin-to-sphingomyelin ratio) and report findings to the healthcare provider.

- All patients in preterm labor are considered to be at high risk for neonatal group B streptococcal infection and therefore often receive prophylactic antibiotics. Antibiotics frequently used are penicillin G, ampicillin, or clindamycin for patients allergic to penicillins.
- Provide appropriate psychological support. Involve supportive pastoral care as appropriate.

Premature rupture of membranes
- Check fetal heart tones and fetal activity.
- Describe the color, characteristics, and amount of amniotic fluid leakage.
- Check maternal vital signs; report elevated temperature, chills, or malaise to the healthcare provider immediately.
- Continue to monitor for any leakage of fluid.
- Limit number of cervical exams to prevent infection.

Gestational diabetes mellitus
- Assist with the performance of glucose tolerance testing.
- Perform blood glucose testing four times daily, and assist the patient in administering prescribed insulin. While reviewing the self-monitoring blood glucose levels, ensure that the patient understands her individualized insulin dosage adjustment.
- Encourage adherence to diet and exercise prescribed to achieve tight glucose control to maintain desired weight gain during the pregnancy and to prevent complications (e.g., neonatal hypoglycemia or stillbirth).
- Women with gestational diabetes mellitus (GDM) have twice the risk of developing hypertension as other pregnant women, so the blood pressure should be monitored regularly.
- Monitor for development of hypoglycemia and hyperglycemia. Consult current American Diabetes Association guidelines for monitoring GDM.
- During labor, monitor glucose level every 2 hours; maintain adequate hydration.
- During the postpartum period, continue to monitor glucose levels. (Usually with GDM, the mother's glucose reverts to normal during the postpartum period. Therefore careful monitoring of glucose and adjustment of insulin dosages are required.)

The patient with diabetes should have multiple laboratory tests, including glycosylated hemoglobin (hemoglobin A_{1c}), serum creatinine, urine microalbumin, and other tests consistent with the history. The woman with diabetes must understand the importance of having a sustained record of preconception glycemic control to prevent maternal and fetal complications.

Pregnancy hypertension disorders (preeclampsia, eclampsia)
- Monitor maternal vital signs, fetal heart tones, and fetal movement at appropriate intervals consistent with presenting symptoms. Maintain the patient on bed rest in a lateral position to promote uteroplacental circulation and to reduce compression of the vena cava.
- Maintain hydration by the oral or IV route (usually 1000 mL plus the amount of urine output over the past 24 hours). Maintain accurate intake and output, and obtain daily weights. Salt intake is generally maintained at a normal level, although heavy use should be discouraged.
- Test the urine for protein and specific gravity every hour. Report a steady decrease in hourly output or output of less than 30 mL/hr to the healthcare provider.
- Review available laboratory studies and report findings to the healthcare provider (e.g., electrolyte levels, CBC with differential, thrombocytopenia, liver enzyme levels, uric acid level, hematocrit, serum estriol, lecithin-to-sphingomyelin ratio).
- Monitor deep tendon reflexes and for signs of seizure activity (e.g., increased drowsiness, hyperreflexia, visual disturbances, and development of severe pain). If symptoms are present, report to the healthcare provider immediately.
- If seizures occur, give supportive care, provide a nonstimulating environment, and have oxygen and suction available. Institute seizure precautions.
- Be alert for complications (e.g., start of labor, pulmonary edema, disseminated intravascular coagulation, heart failure, abruptio placentae, cerebral edema).
- Administer prescribed drugs (e.g., diazepam or phenobarbital, antihypertensives). The vasodilator hydralazine is usually administered to control blood pressure. It may be administered orally or intravenously, depending on the severity of the condition. If given intravenously, monitor the maternal and fetal heart rates and the mother's blood pressure every 2 to 3 minutes after the initial dose and every 10 to 15 minutes thereafter. The diastolic pressure is usually maintained at 90 to 100 mm Hg. Anticonvulsants such as magnesium sulfate or phenytoin may be given for seizure activity (see drug monograph for hydralazine for administration and monitoring of the patient during drug therapy).

Termination of pregnancy
- If bleeding occurs near the estimated date of delivery, the infant may be delivered by cesarean birth. If it appears that a spontaneous abortion (i.e., miscarriage) is occurring, the woman may be hospitalized for observation and bed rest, diagnosis for possible causes (e.g., infection), and fluid replacement.
- If a pregnancy is to be terminated (i.e., induced abortion), the following methods may be used:

- *Before 12 weeks' gestation:* Suction curettage or dilation and evacuation
- *From 12 to 20 weeks' gestation:* Intraamniotic instillation of hypertonic saline (20% solution) or prostaglandin administered intraamniotically, intramuscularly, or by vaginal suppository
- *Intrauterine fetal death after 20 weeks' gestation:* Prostaglandin suppositories with or without oxytocin augmentation (see the section on uterine stimulants later in this chapter)
- Encourage the persons involved in the loss of an infant to talk about their feelings of grief, sadness, or anger. Create memories of the experience through photographs and mementos as appropriate. Have chaplains involved in supportive processes as appropriate. Listen and allow feelings to be vented. Give answers (if known) regarding future pregnancies. Refer for other counseling as appropriate. Anticipate that depression may develop over the next few weeks and that the patient may need treatment for depression.
- Administer Rh$_o$(D) immune globulin to an Rh-negative mother within 72 hours of the termination of pregnancy (see drug monograph on Rh$_o$(D) immune globulin later in this chapter). Also check the patient's rubella titer; if low, obtain an order for inoculation immediately after pregnancy.

Normal labor and delivery

- Perform routine admission procedures (e.g., vital signs, fetal heart rate monitoring, birth plan). Determine if there will be someone present during the delivery process who will provide emotional support.
- Follow institutional guidelines regarding activity level of the mother; some permit ambulation during early stages of labor.
- During labor, provide pain relief, alternate side-to-side positioning (avoid lying flat on back), and intervene with comfort measures (e.g., back rub, pelvic rocking, effleurage, warm shower, music). Encourage leg extension and dorsiflexion of the foot to relieve spasms and cramping.
- Provide privacy, and support the woman and coach when necessary.
- Check for bladder distention. Have patient void every 2 hours.
- Maintain adequate hydration by giving ice chips or clear liquids. Check hydration status throughout labor by observing mucous membranes, dryness of lips, and skin turgor. Give oral hygiene frequently. Do not give solid foods unless specifically approved by the healthcare provider.
- As labor progresses, continue to monitor the maternal and fetal vital signs and the frequency, duration, and intensity of uterine contractions.
- Report contractions of 90 seconds or more and those not followed by complete uterine relaxation. Report abnormal patterns on the fetal monitor, such as decreased variability, late decelerations, and variable decelerations of the fetal heart rate.
- Continue to coach when necessary.
- As vaginal discharge increases, wash the perineum with warm water, then dry the area. Change the bed sheets, pad, and gown when necessary.
- Monitor the temperature every 4 hours while membranes are intact and temperature remains within normal range. Monitor every 2 hours if the temperature is elevated or if the membranes have ruptured.
- After delivery, record the time of delivery and position of the infant; the type of tear or episiotomy and type of suture used in repair, if appropriate; any anesthetic or analgesic used during repair; the time of placental delivery; and any complications (e.g., additional bleeding, postpartum hemorrhage, or neonatal distress).
- Administer and record oxytocic agent, as ordered.

Immediate neonatal care. Before delivery, the maternal history through the current stage of labor should be reviewed to identify potential complications that may arise for the neonate. Although a complete physical examination of the neonate will be performed later, a preliminary assessment and recording of data must be completed at the time of birth. The following procedures must be completed by the healthcare provider or nurse immediately after delivery.

Airway. Ensure that the airway remains open. As soon as the head is delivered, suction the oropharynx and nasal passages with a small bulb syringe. Immediately after delivery, hold the newborn with the head lowered at a 10- to 15-degree angle to help drain amniotic fluid, mucus, and blood. Resuction with the bulb syringe as necessary.

Clamping the umbilical cord. Consult with the mother before delivery if she is participating in cord blood banking. If so, special containers must be used for blood storage and registration. When the airway is opened and the respirations have stabilized, the neonate should be held at the same level as the uterus until cord pulsations cease. The cord is then clamped or ligated.

Health status. The health status of the neonate is estimated at 1 minute and 5 minutes after delivery using the Apgar scoring system (see Table 39.1). Rapid estimation of gestational age is also performed (see Fig. 39.2).

Temperature maintenance. The neonate should be dried immediately and body temperature maintained with the use of prewarmed blankets, a heated bassinet, or a radiant warmer. If the neonate is term and in stable condition as assessed by the Apgar score, temperature may be maintained by skin-to-skin contact with the mother.

Eye prophylaxis. It is a legal requirement that every newborn baby's eyes be treated prophylactically for *Neisseria gonorrhoeae.* Another rapidly emerging neonatal conjunctival infection is chlamydial ophthalmia neonatorum, which is caused by *Chlamydia trachomatis*. The neonate may have become infected during birth if the mother is infected. Ophthalmic erythromycin is used for prophylactic treatment of neonatal conjunctivitis caused by *N. gonorrhoeae* or *C. trachomatis* (see drug monograph on erythromycin ophthalmic ointment later in this chapter). Instillation of the ophthalmic agent may be delayed up to 1 hour to facilitate parent-child bonding.

Other procedures. While the parents are bonding with the newborn infant, the nurse should prepare an infant identification bracelet and place it on the baby, as well as a duplicate one on the mother. Examine the placenta and cord for anomalies and verify the presence of one vein and two arteries. Samples of cord blood may be collected for analysis of the Rh factor, blood grouping, and hematocrit. The baby may be held by the parents as long as the infant's condition is stable. Breastfeeding should be initiated. The newborn is cared for in the presence of the family in most institutions while the weight, measurements, and physical examinations are completed. Some healthcare providers also order an IM injection of vitamin K as prophylaxis against hemorrhage along with an IM injection of hepatitis B vaccine. Evaluation of the infant's vital signs and color is performed on a continuum. Alterations from baseline are evaluated and reported.

Postpartum care. Postpartum is defined as the time between delivery and return of the reproductive organs to prepregnancy status.

- An Rh-negative mother may receive $Rh_o(D)$ immune globulin within 72 hours of the completion of the pregnancy.
- If the mother's rubella titer is low, an appropriate time for inoculation is immediately after delivery.
- Continue to assess the fundal height, position, and lochia until the woman is discharged. The lochia normally progresses from blood red (bright) to darker red with some small clots (1 to 3 days postpartum), to pinkish, thin, watery consistency (4 to 10 days), to a yellowish or creamy color (11 to 21 days). The odor should be similar to that of a normal menstrual flow; a foul-smelling odor should be reported to the healthcare provider. Pads should be changed at frequent regular intervals or with each voiding rather than waiting for them to become heavily soiled.
- On delivery, the breasts secrete a thin yellow fluid called *colostrum*. Within the first few days, breast milk becomes available. This may produce some discomfort for the mother as the breasts become full. Engorgement in the breastfeeding mother can be minimized by having the infant nurse more frequently (every 60 to 90 minutes) or massaging and hand-expressing or pumping milk to empty the breasts completely. A warm shower or application of warm, moist heat may also provide relief.

- The quantity of breast milk varies among mothers. Diet, fluid intake, and level of anxiety all affect lactation.
- Monitor and record the number of infant voidings (one wet diaper per day of age until 5 days old and then six to eight wet diapers per day is average) and stools (usually one in 24 hours).
- Weigh the infant daily. It is normal for an infant to lose up to 7% of his or her body weight over the first 3 days. A weight gain of 0.75 to 1 ounce daily indicates that the infant is receiving adequate nutritional intake.
- Help the mother hold the baby correctly and provide instruction and guidance on the correct technique of breastfeeding, bottle feeding, and burping the baby.
- Suppression of lactation in the nonnursing mother includes having the woman wear a supportive, well-fitting bra within 6 hours of delivery. The bra is removed only during bathing. Ice packs may be applied to the axillary area of the breast for 15 to 20 minutes four times daily. Teach the mother to avoid any stimulation of her breasts until the feeling of fullness has subsided (usually 5 to 7 days). The mother should not use a breast pump and when showering should allow the warm water to run down her back to avoid stimulating lactation.
- Encourage the mother who is breastfeeding or formula feeding to eat a well-balanced diet with adequate protein, vitamins, and fluids to help restore the body to the optimal level.
- Continue to provide emotional support to the new mother.
- Afterpains often require a mild analgesic. For the breastfeeding mother who is experiencing afterpains, administering a mild analgesic approximately 40 minutes before nursing may relieve discomfort.
- Check on voiding and return of normal bowel elimination during the postpartum period.
- Check vital signs every shift or more frequently when indicated.
- Monitor laboratory reports during the postpartum period. The hematocrit may rise during the initial period after childbirth; white blood cells, mainly neutrophils, may be elevated as well, making it difficult to diagnose an infection.
- Monitor for thromboembolisms during the postpartum period. Clotting factors and fibrinogen are increased during pregnancy and the immediate postpartum period.

◆ **Patient Education**
- Prenatal pregnancy education starts with open communication with the expectant family. They must be guided to understand the need for prenatal care. Keep emphasizing what the family can do to optimize the chances for a healthy baby, including maintaining general health, nutritional needs, adequate rest, and appropriate exercise and continuing prescribed medication therapy.

- The amount of information provided to the expectant mother or parents is individualized. The following health teaching is an overview of information that may be given (refer to a maternity textbook to cover the areas not addressed).

Adequate rest and relaxation. Assist the individual to plan for adequate rest periods throughout the day to prevent fatigue, irritability, and exhaustion. Talk with the new mother about planning rest periods during lunch breaks at work, when preschoolers are napping, or when another caregiver is home to care for children. A short period of relaxation in a reclining chair or elevation of the feet may be beneficial when there is no time during the day for sleep. Advise the mother to avoid long periods of standing in one place and to perform some daily activities while sitting.

Activity and exercise. Usually, the woman can continue to perform common activities of daily living and her usual exercise regimen. As pregnancy continues, she will need to consult with her healthcare provider regarding exercise limits. New attempts at strenuous exercise (such as jogging or aerobics) should not be started during pregnancy. Daily walks in fresh air are encouraged.

Any changes in activity level should be discussed with the healthcare provider ahead of time.

Encourage good posture and participation in prenatal classes in which exercises are taught to strengthen the abdominal muscles and relax the pelvic floor muscles.

The woman should avoid lifting heavy objects and anything that might cause physical harm, especially as the pregnancy progresses, because pregnancy may affect balance.

Employment. Advice about continued employment should be based on the type of job; working conditions; amount of lifting, standing, or exposure to toxic substances; and the individual's state of health.

General personal hygiene. Encourage maintenance of general hygiene through daily tub baths or showers. The pregnant woman should avoid soaking in a hot tub or whirlpool. Tub baths near the end of pregnancy may be discouraged because of the danger of slipping and falling while getting in and out of the tub. Tub baths should not be taken once the membranes have ruptured.

Encourage the use of plain soap and water to cleanse the perineum and prevent odors. Deodorant sprays should *not* be used because of possible irritation. Tell the pregnant woman that an increase in vaginal discharge is common. Discharge that is yellowish or greenish, is foul smelling, or causes irritation and itching should be reported for further evaluation.

Clothing. Encourage the mother to dress in nonconstricting clothing. As the pregnancy progresses, the mother may be more comfortable with a maternity girdle to support the abdomen. Encourage the mother to wear a well-fitting bra to provide proper breast support. The pregnant woman should avoid any restrictive clothing that would limit lower leg circulation. Encourage low-heeled, well-fitting shoes that provide good support. Properly fitting shoes can prevent lower back fatigue and tired feet.

Oral hygiene. Encourage the pregnant patient to have a thorough dental examination at the beginning of the pregnancy. She should tell the dentist that she is pregnant at the time of the examination. Encourage thorough daily brushing and flossing.

Sexual activity. Refer to an obstetrics textbook for discussion of alterations in sexuality during pregnancy. The wide range of feelings, needs, and intervention deserve more consideration than can be presented in this text.

Smoking and alcohol. The pregnant woman should be encouraged to abstain from smoking and/or drinking alcohol during pregnancy. Numerous data indicate that smoking and drinking are dangerous to the fetus. Increased incidences of neonatal mortality, low birth weight, and prematurity have been well reported (see Chapter 48).

Nutritional needs. Balanced nutrition is always to be encouraged, but it is especially important throughout the course of the pregnancy. Recommended daily allowances vary based on the individual's age, weight at the time of pregnancy, and daily activity level. At all times, allowances must be made to maintain the nutritional needs of the mother and fetus. Refer to a nutrition textbook for specific recommendations.

Encourage eliminating caffeine from the diet during pregnancy. Limit the consumption of coffee, tea, cola beverages, and cocoa. Tell the pregnant woman to check labels for specific caffeine content because many soft drinks contain a significant amount of caffeine. Tell the woman to avoid highly spiced foods and any foods that she knows have caused heartburn and to eat all foods in moderation.

Usual weight gain is 3.5 to 5 pounds during the first trimester, followed by an average gain of 1 pound per week during the second and third trimesters. The rate of weekly weight gain may be slightly higher for an underweight woman and slightly lower for overweight women. Stress the need to report a weight gain of 2 or more pounds in any 1 week for further evaluation.

Bowel habits. Assess the individual's usual pattern of elimination and anticipate its continuance until later in pregnancy. Pressure on the lower bowel from the presenting part of the fetus may cause constipation and hemorrhoids. Stool softeners or a bulk laxative may be prescribed if problems persist. Encourage the consumption of fresh fruits and vegetables as well as whole-grain and bran products and an adequate intake of six to eight 8-ounce glasses of fluid daily.

Douching. Discourage any type of douching because it is contraindicated during pregnancy.

Discomforts of pregnancy. Use assessment data as pregnancy progresses to determine individualized teaching needed to deal with discomforts such as backache, leg cramps, hemorrhoids, and edema.

Complications of pregnancy. Individualize health teaching to deal with complications as they arise. The woman should always immediately report loss of fluid vaginally; decreased fetal movement; dizziness; double or blurred vision; severe headache; abdominal pain or persistent vomiting; fever; edema of the face, fingers, legs, or feet; and weight gain in excess of 2 pounds weekly.

At discharge
- Review instructions on self-care (e.g., breast care, fundal height, lochia, incisional or perineal care, bowel and bladder expectations, nutritional and fluid intake, activity). Stress signs of problems that should be reported to the healthcare provider.
- *Contraceptives:* Discuss appropriate sexual activity and limitations. Remind the woman that breastfeeding is not a form of contraception. Alternative methods of contraception should be used if the patient does not wish to become pregnant immediately.
- Review infant care needs, bathing, vital signs, fontanel assessment, care of the umbilical cord and circumcision, normal sleep pattern, and feeding. Assess the breastfeeding process and assist with education and a public health nurse referral as needed.
- Stress the need for follow-up care of the mother and infant. Provide the specific date and time of healthcare provider appointments. The mother usually returns for a follow-up examination at the healthcare provider's office 6 to 8 weeks after delivery.

Fostering health maintenance
- Discuss any medications prescribed for the mother or infant and how they will benefit the course of treatment to produce optimal response.
- Seek cooperation and understanding of the following points so that medication adherence is increased: name of medication; dosage, route, and times of administration; and common and serious adverse effects.

Patient self-assessment. Enlist the mother's help in developing and maintaining a written record of monitoring parameters (e.g., blood pressure, pulse, daily weight, presence and relief of discomfort, exercise tolerance, fetal movement). See Patient Self-Assessment Forms for Prenatal Care and Postpartum Care on the Evolve website. Complete the Premedication Data column for

use as a baseline to track response to drug therapy, progression of the pregnancy, and postpartum recovery. Ensure that the patient understands how to use the form, and instruct the patient to take the completed form to follow-up visits. During follow-up visits, focus on issues that will foster adherence with the therapeutic interventions prescribed.

DRUG THERAPY IN PREGNANCY
DRUG CLASS: UTERINE STIMULANTS

Uses
There are four primary clinical indications for the use of uterine stimulants: (1) induction or augmentation of labor; (2) control of postpartum atony and hemorrhage; (3) control of postsurgical hemorrhage (as in cesarean birth); and (4) induction of therapeutic (induced) abortion.

Induction of labor. Uterine stimulants, primarily oxytocin, may be prescribed in cases in which, in the healthcare provider's judgment, continuation of the pregnancy is considered to be a greater risk to the mother or fetus than the risk associated with drug-induced induction of labor. A history of **precipitous labor and delivery** (rapid labor and delivery lasting less than 3 hours), postterm pregnancy (pregnancy lasting longer than 40 weeks), prolonged pregnancy with placental insufficiency, PROM, or preeclampsia may indicate the need to induce labor. Vaginal inserts and gels and oral dosage forms of prostaglandins are being tested as adjunctive therapy to help ripen the cervix.

Augmentation of labor. With regard to **augmentation** of labor, in general, oxytocin should not be used to hasten labor. The type and force of contraction induced by the oxytocin may be harmful to the mother and fetus. In occasional cases of **dysfunctional labor**, there is a prolonged latent phase of cervical dilation or arrest of descent through the birth canal. Oxytocin infusions starting with low dosages and continuous fetal monitoring may be beneficial in these cases.

Postpartum atony and hemorrhage. After delivery of the fetus and the placenta, the uterus sometimes remains flaccid and "boggy." Continued IV infusions of low-dose oxytocin or IM injections of methylergonovine may be used to stimulate firm uterine contractions to reduce the risk of postpartum hemorrhage from an atonic uterus or postsurgical hemorrhage.

Occasionally, doses of methylergonovine are administered orally for a few days after delivery to assist in uterine involution.

Therapeutic (induced) abortion. Pharmacologic agents are usually not effective in evacuating uterine contents until several weeks into the second trimester of pregnancy. Various dosage forms of prostaglandins and hypertonic sodium chloride (20%) may be effective. Uterine smooth muscle is not very responsive to oxytocin stimulation until late in the third trimester, so even large doses of oxytocin are not indicated in therapeutic abortion. Regardless of the stage of pregnancy, stimulants such as methylergonovine may be prescribed after the uterus is emptied to control bleeding and maintain uterine muscle tone.

---

dinoprostone (dī-nō-PRŎS-tōn)
Prostin E2, Prepidil, Cervidil

Actions

Dinoprostone (prostaglandin E_2) is a natural chemical in the body that causes uterine and gastrointestinal smooth muscle stimulation. It also plays an active role in cervical softening and dilation (cervical ripening) unrelated to uterine muscle stimulation. When used during pregnancy, it produces cervical softening and dilation and, in higher doses, increases the frequency and strength of uterine contractions.

Uses

Dinoprostone is used to start and continue cervical ripening at term. In larger doses, it is also used to expel uterine contents in cases of intrauterine fetal death, benign hydatidiform mole, missed spontaneous miscarriage, and second-trimester abortion. Occasionally, oxytocin and dinoprostone are used together to shorten the duration of time required to expel uterine contents.

Therapeutic Outcomes

The primary therapeutic outcomes associated with dinoprostone therapy are as follows:
1. Cervical softening and dilation before labor
2. Evacuation of uterine contents

❖ Nursing Implications for dinoprostone

◆ *Premedication assessment*
1. Ask the patient whether she has had a cesarean section or uterine surgery; cephalopelvic disproportion; previous traumatic deliveries; placenta previa; unexplained vaginal bleeding; hypertension or hypotension; a seizure disorder; diabetes; anemia; asthma; glaucoma; or heart, liver, or kidney disease.
2. Obtain baseline vital signs. Temperature and vital signs should be monitored every 30 minutes after initiation of therapy.
3. Assess the state of hydration.
4. Assess uterine activity, including amount and characteristics of any vaginal discharge.
5. Check for antiemetic and antidiarrheal medications ordered at prescribed times or PRN.

◆ *Availability.* **Intravaginal:** *Vaginal insert:* 10 mg (Cervidil); *Cervical gel:* 0.5 mg/3 g in a prefilled applicator (Prepidil); *Vaginal suppository:* 20 mg (Prostin E2).

◆ *Dosage and administration*
Adult: For cervical ripening:
- *Intravaginal insert administration:* The slab (Cervidil) is placed transversely in the posterior fornix of the vagina after removal from foil wrap. The patient should remain supine for 2 hours after insertion but may be ambulatory thereafter. Cervidil is removed at the onset of labor or 12 hours after insertion. The product does not need to be warmed before insertion. Sterile vaginal examinations will indicate whether the cervix is softening or not.
- *Intracervical gel:* Allow the prefilled syringe of gel (Prepidil, 0.5 mg) to warm to room temperature. Do not force the warming process with a water bath or other external source of heat (e.g., microwave oven). A catheter is attached to the syringe (20 mm if the cervix is less than 50% effaced, 10 mm if more than 50% effaced). The patient is placed in a dorsal position, and the cervix is visualized with a speculum. Using sterile technique, the gel is introduced through the catheter into the cervical canal just below the level of the internal os. The catheter is removed after placement of the gel. After administration, the patient should remain supine for 15 to 30 minutes to minimize leakage from the cervical canal. The dose may be repeated in 6 hours. The maximum recommended cumulative dosage for a 24-hour period is 1.5 mg (7.5 mL of dinoprostone gel).

For evacuation of uterine contents:
- *Intravaginal suppository:* Before removing the foil, allow the suppository (Prostin E2) to warm to room temperature. Insert one suppository high into the posterior vaginal fornix. Patients should remain supine for at least 10 minutes after each insertion. Suppositories should be inserted every 2 to 5 hours, depending on uterine activity and tolerance to adverse effects.

◆ *Common adverse effects*
Gastrointestinal
Nausea, vomiting, diarrhea. The most frequently observed gastrointestinal adverse effects are nausea, vomiting, and diarrhea. Premedication with an antiemetic such as prochlorperazine and an antidiarrheal agent (loperamide or diphenoxylate) will reduce, but usually not completely eliminate, these adverse effects.

Thermoregulation
Fever. Chills and shivering may occur in patients receiving dinoprostone. Temperature elevations to approximately 100.6°F (38°C) occur within 15 to 45 minutes and continue for up to 6 hours. Sponge baths with water and maintaining fluid intake may provide symptomatic relief. Aspirin does not inhibit dinoprostone-induced fever.

Patients should be observed for clinical indications of intrauterine infection. Monitor temperature and vital signs every 30 minutes.

◆ *Serious adverse effects*
Cardiovascular
Orthostatic hypotension. Transient hypotension with a drop in diastolic pressure of 20 mm Hg, dizziness, flushing, and dysrhythmias have all been reported. Although these effects are infrequent and generally mild, dinoprostone may cause some degree of orthostatic hypotension manifested by dizziness, flushing, and weakness, particularly when therapy is initiated. Monitor blood pressure in the supine and standing positions. Anticipate the development of orthostatic hypotension and take measures to prevent it. For ambulatory patients, teach the patient to rise slowly from a supine or sitting position and encourage her to sit or lie down if feeling faint. Report rapidly falling blood pressure, bradycardia, paleness, and other alterations in vital signs.

◆ *Drug interactions.* No clinically significant interactions have been reported.

---

misoprostol (mĭ-sō-PRŎS-tōl)
⇄ *Do not confuse misoprostol with metoprolol.*
Cytotec (SĪ-tō-tĕk)
mifepristone (mih-fee-pris tone')
Mifeprex (mih-fee-prex')

Actions
Misoprostol is a synthetic prostaglandin E used to prevent nonsteroidal antiinflammatory drug–induced ulcer disease. The prostaglandin E analogues also induce uterine contractions in the pregnant uterus.

Mifepristone (also known as RU 486) is a steroid that binds to the progesterone receptors of the pregnant uterus, blocking the effects of the hormone progesterone. Blocking this receptor during pregnancy leads to contractions of the uterine muscle with expulsion of fetal contents.

Uses
Misoprostol is used as a cervical ripening agent, for induction of labor, and for treatment of serious postpartum hemorrhage in the presence of uterine atony. Misoprostol should not be used to induce labor in women who have had a previous cesarean delivery. Mifepristone followed by misoprostol may be used to terminate an intrauterine pregnancy through 70 days of gestation.

Therapeutic Outcomes
The primary therapeutic outcomes associated with misoprostol therapy in pregnancy are as follows:
1. Cervical softening and dilation before labor
2. Induction of active labor
3. Reduction in postpartum hemorrhage in the presence of uterine atony
Therapeutic outcomes of misoprostol and mifepristone
4. Evacuation of uterine contents

❖ **Nursing Implications for misoprostol and mifepristone**
◆ *Premedication assessment*
1. Obtain baseline vital signs. Monitor temperature and vital signs every 30 minutes after initiation of therapy.
2. Assess the state of hydration.
3. Assess uterine activity, including amount and characteristics of any vaginal discharge.
4. Check for antiemetic, anticramping and antidiarrheal medications ordered at prescribed times or PRN.

◆ *Availability.* misoprostol: *PO:* 100- and 200-mcg tablets. mifepristone: *PO:* 200-mg tablets.

◆ *Dosage and administration*
Termination of an intrauterine pregnancy
Day 1: mifepristone PO 200 mg as a single dose.
Day 2 or 3: misoprostol 800 mcg buccally 24 to 48 hours after mifepristone administration. Administer as two 200-mcg tablets in each cheek pouch, held in place for 30 minutes. Any tablet fragments may be rinsed with water and swallowed. Most women will expel the uterine contents within 2 to 24 hours after taking the misoprostol. Discuss with the patient an appropriate location for her to be when she takes the misoprostol.
Day 7 to 14: Patients should follow up with their healthcare provider 1 to 2 weeks after the administration of the mifepristone to confirm that complete termination of pregnancy has occurred and to evaluate degree of bleeding. If the pregnancy is not ongoing but complete expulsion has not occurred, another dose of 800 mcg of misoprostol in the buccal pouches may be administered. The patient should follow up with the healthcare provider in approximately 7 days for assessment.

◆ *Common and serious adverse effects.* Misoprostol for short-term obstetric use has not been studied in large, well-controlled trials, so the type and frequency of adverse effects are not well documented. Because it is a member of the prostaglandin E family, it may have adverse effects similar to those of dinoprostone. (See the dinoprostone monograph immediately preceding the misoprostol/mifepristone monograph.)
Infection. Patients undergoing an intrauterine evacuation should be monitored closely for the development of infection. A temperature of 100.4°F or higher for 4 hours or longer, severe abdominal pain, or pelvic tenderness in the days following evacuation should be assessed by their healthcare provider.

◆ *Drug interactions.* No significant drug interactions have been reported.

---

methylergonovine maleate (mĕth-ĭl-ŭr-GŎN-ō-vēn MĂL-ē-āt)

Actions
Methylergonovine directly stimulates uterine contractions. Small doses produce contractions with normal

resting muscle tone, intermediate doses cause more forceful and prolonged contractions with an elevated resting muscle tone, and large doses cause severe, prolonged contractions. Because of this sudden, intense uterine activity, which is dangerous to the fetus, this agent cannot be used for induction of labor.

Uses

Methylergonovine produces more sustained contractions than oxytocin and is used in small doses in postpartum patients to control bleeding and maintain uterine firmness. Methylergonovine may be used in patients who wish to breastfeed because it will not inhibit stimulation of milk production by prolactin. Hypertension and headaches may develop in patients who have received caudal or spinal anesthesia followed by a dose of methylergonovine. Monitor the patient's blood pressure and heart rate and rhythm.

Therapeutic Outcome

The primary therapeutic outcome associated with methylergonovine therapy is reduced postpartum blood loss.

❖ Nursing Implications for methylergonovine

◆ *Premedication assessment*

1. Ask for a medical history, especially of kidney disease, liver disease, high blood pressure, heart disease (such as venoatrial shunts, mitral valve stenosis, chest pain, recent heart attack), diabetes, high cholesterol, smoking/tobacco use, blood vessel disease (such as Raynaud's disease), or complications during pregnancy (such as preeclampsia or eclampsia).
2. Obtain baseline vital signs, especially blood pressure and pulse.
3. Assess amount and characteristics of vaginal discharge and fundal height and contractility.

◆ *Availability. PO:* 0.2-mg tablets.
   Injection: 0.2 mg/mL in 1-mL ampules.

◆ *Dosage and administration.* **Adult:** *PO:* 0.2 mg 3 or 4 times daily for up to 1 week.
   IM: 0.2 mg; repeat as necessary every 2 to 4 hours.

> **Medication Safety Alert**
>
> Use methylergonovine with extreme caution in patients with hypertension, preeclampsia, heart disease, venoatrial shunts, mitral valve stenosis, sepsis, or hepatic or renal impairment.

◆ *Common adverse effects*
   Gastrointestinal
   Nausea, vomiting. These adverse effects are usually mild and tend to resolve with continued therapy. Encourage the patient not to discontinue therapy without first consulting the healthcare provider.

Abdominal cramping. This is normally an indication of therapeutic activity, but, if severe, reduction or discontinuation of medication may be necessary.

◆ *Serious adverse effects*
   Cardiovascular
   Hypertension. Certain patients, especially those who are eclamptic or were previously hypertensive, may be particularly sensitive to the hypertensive effects of this agent. These patients have a higher incidence of developing generalized headaches, severe dysrhythmias, and strokes. Monitor the patient's blood pressure and pulse rate and rhythm. Inform the healthcare provider immediately if the patient complains of headache or palpitations.

◆ *Drug interactions*

Drugs that may enhance therapeutic and toxic effects of methylergonovine include macrolide antibiotics (e.g., erythromycin, clarithromycin), HIV protease or reverse transcriptase inhibitors (e.g., delavirdine, indinavir, nelfinavir, ritonavir), and azole antifungal agents (e.g., ketoconazole, itraconazole, voriconazole). The dose of methylergonovine should be reduced to prevent toxicity.

---

oxytocin (ŏk-sē-TŌ-sĭn)
   Pitocin (pĭ-TŌ-sĭn)

Actions

Oxytocin is a hormone produced in the hypothalamus and stored in the pituitary gland. When released, it stimulates the smooth muscle of the uterus, blood vessels, and the mammary glands. When administered during the third trimester of pregnancy, active labor may be initiated.

Uses

Oxytocin is the drug of choice for inducing labor at term and for augmenting uterine contractions during the first and second stages of labor. Oxytocin is routinely administered immediately postpartum to control uterine atony and hemorrhage.

Therapeutic Outcomes

The primary therapeutic outcomes associated with oxytocin therapy are as follows:

1. Initiation of labor
2. Support of uterine contractions during the first and second stages of labor
3. Control of postpartum bleeding

❖ Nursing Implications for oxytocin

◆ *Premedication assessment.* Never leave a patient receiving an oxytocin infusion unattended. Ensure that the IV site is functional before adding oxytocin; use an infusion pump.

1. Monitor maternal vital signs, especially blood pressure and pulse rate.
2. Obtain baseline assessment data of the mother's hydration status. Continue to monitor intake and output throughout drug therapy.
3. Monitor characteristics of uterine contractions (e.g., frequency, rate, duration, and intensity).
4. Monitor fetal heart rate and rhythm. Be alert for signs of fetal distress.
5. Check amount and characteristics of vaginal discharge.

◆ *Availability.* *IV:* 10 units/mL in 1-mL and 30-mL vials.

◆ *Dosage and administration*

- *Starting the infusion:* Establish records of baseline vital signs and intake and output. Oxytocin administered IV should be added to the solution after the IV is shown to be patent and running.
- *Rate:* Careful monitoring of the prescribed rate of infusion is imperative. Should the IV line suddenly open, the resulting severe contractions could be extremely dangerous to the mother and fetus.
- *Infusion pump:* A constant infusion pump is essential to controlling the rate of administration. Keep in mind that a pump can fail. Continue to monitor the number of drops per minute from the drip chamber.
- *Induction of labor: IV:* Initial rate: 0.5 to 1 milliunit (mU). May increase by 1 to 2 mU/min every 15 to 60 minutes. It is absolutely necessary that an infusion pump be used to help control the rate of oxytocin infusion. Most pregnancies that are close to term will respond well to 2 to 10 mU/min. Rarely will a patient require more than 20 mU/min. Those patients at 32 to 36 weeks' gestation often require 20 to 30 mU/min or more to develop a laborlike contraction pattern. Rates of infusion should not be altered more frequently than every 15 to 30 minutes. It is frequently necessary to reduce or discontinue the infusion as spontaneous uterine activity develops and labor progresses.
- *Augmentation of labor: IV:* Occasionally, labor that started spontaneously may not progress satisfactorily. Labor may be augmented by oxytocin infusions at rates of 0.5 to 2 mU/min.
- *Postpartum hemorrhage: IM:* 3 to 10 units given after delivery of the placenta. *IV:* 10 to 40 units may be added to 1000 mL of normal saline solution and run at a rate necessary to control uterine atony.

> **Medication Safety Alert**
>
> Before starting an oxytocin infusion, establish records of baseline vital signs and intake and output. A constant infusion pump is recommended for controlling the rate of administration. If the infant develops sudden distress, reduce the oxytocin infusion to the slowest possible rate according to hospital policy, turn the mother to the left lateral position, administer oxygen by nasal cannula or face mask, and call the healthcare provider immediately.

◆ *Common adverse effects*
Gynecologic
Uterine contractions. Oxytocin infusions should be monitored by both a tocodynamometer, or "toco" (an instrument that measures uterine contractions), and a fetal heart monitor. Maintain an ongoing record of the frequency, duration, and intensity of uterine contractions. Contractions longer than 90 seconds require that the flow rate of the oxytocin be slowed or discontinued.

Gastrointestinal
Nausea, vomiting. Although uncommon, these adverse effects may occur. Reduction in dosage may control symptoms.

◆ *Serious adverse effects*
Fetal heart rate
Fetal distress. Fetal heart rate should be monitored continuously and especially closely during uterine contractions. Normal fetal heart rate is 120 to 160 beats/min. Indications of fetal distress may be manifested by tachycardia (>160 beats/min) followed by bradycardia (<120 beats/min). As the degree of distress progresses, bradycardia occurs more frequently and lasts longer than 15 seconds after contractions. If the infant develops sudden distress, reduce the oxytocin infusion to the slowest possible rate according to hospital policy, turn the mother to the left lateral position, administer oxygen by nasal cannula or face mask, and call the healthcare provider immediately.

Cardiovascular
Hypertension, hypotension. Check the mother's blood pressure and pulse rate at least every 30 minutes during oxytocin infusion. Report trends upward or downward to the healthcare provider, because oxytocin may cause hypertension or hypotension.

Endocrine
Water intoxication. Oxytocin can alter fluid balance by stimulating antidiuretic hormone, causing the body to accumulate water. This is particularly likely to occur if oxytocin is administered with electrolyte solutions. Symptoms of water intoxication include drowsiness, listlessness, headache, confusion, anuria, edema, and, in extreme cases, seizures.

Metabolic
Dehydration. Because mothers are routinely placed on nothing by mouth (NPO) status during labor, an occasional patient may develop dehydration, even though an IV is running. Monitor urine output; dry, crusted lips; and requests for water. Report to the healthcare provider and request ice chips and additional IV fluids if appropriate.

> ! **Medication Safety Alert**
>
> Overdosage of oxytocin may cause hyperstimulation of the uterus, resulting in severe contractions with possible abruptio placentae, cervical lacerations, impaired uterine blood flow or rupture, and fetal trauma.

Postpartum hemorrhage. Early postpartum hemorrhage occurs within the first 24 hours after delivery and is usually defined as a blood loss of 500 mL or more. The hemorrhage may be caused by uterine atony, retained fragments of placenta, or lacerations of the vaginal tract. Less common causes include defective blood clotting mechanisms, uterine eversion, and uterine infections.

Oxytocin is routinely administered after delivery of the placenta to cause the uterus to contract and to decrease blood loss. Always check the height of the fundus of the uterus (usually at umbilical level) every 5 minutes after delivery. Report if the uterus is not firm or the height is rising. (This may be an indication of urinary retention or a uterus filling with blood.) When the uterus becomes boggy, uterine massage is necessary until it becomes firm.

Check the vaginal flow rate on each perineal pad at least every 30 minutes. With uterine atony or retained placental fragments, the uterus becomes boggy and *dark* vaginal bleeding is present; with a laceration of the cervix or vagina, the bleeding is *bright* red and the uterus is firm. Regardless of the cause of postpartum hemorrhage, the woman must be observed carefully for signs of hypovolemic shock.

Monitor vital signs as ordered by the healthcare provider or every 15 minutes until stable, every 30 minutes for 2 hours, and then every hour until definitely stable. Report an increasing respiratory rate; pulse rate that increases and becomes thready; a pulse deficit; blood pressure that indicates hypotension; skin that is pale, cold, and clammy; or nail beds, lips, and mucous membranes that are pale or cyanotic. Monitor urine output and report an output of 30 mL/hr or less. Observe for restlessness and complaints of thirst and for any decrease in level of consciousness.

◆ *Drug interactions*

Anesthetics. Monitor the blood pressure and heart rate and rhythm closely. Report significant changes. For those patients receiving a local anesthetic containing epinephrine, immediately report any complaints of diaphoresis, fever, chest pain, palpitations, or severe throbbing headache.

DRUG CLASS: UTERINE RELAXANTS

Uterine relaxants, also known as tocolytic agents, are used primarily to delay or prevent preterm labor and delivery in selected patients (see the section Assessment of the Pregnant Patient at Risk earlier in the chapter). Tocolytic agents act by inhibiting uterine muscle contractions. According to the American College of Obstetricians and Gynecologists, they are used to inhibit labor up to 48 hours, enabling corticosteroids to be administered to mature fetal lungs and transport of the mother to a hospital with a neonatal intensive care unit. Agents used are beta-2 agonists (e.g., terbutaline), calcium channel blockers (e.g., nifedipine), magnesium sulfate, and nonsteroidal antiinflammatory drugs (e.g., indomethacin).

---

magnesium sulfate ⓘ

Actions

Magnesium is an ion normally found in the blood in concentrations of 1.8 to 3 mEq/L. When administered parenterally in doses sufficient to produce levels higher than 4 mEq/L, the drug may depress the central nervous system and block peripheral nerve transmission, producing anticonvulsant effects and smooth muscle relaxation.

Uses

Magnesium sulfate is used in obstetrics to inhibit premature labor. It may also be used to control seizure activity associated with preeclampsia or eclampsia. When used as an anticonvulsant or to inhibit labor, blood levels should be maintained at 4 to 8 mEq/L. Clinical trials have not demonstrated that use of magnesium sulfate for tocolysis is any more effective than placebo, and calls are being made for discontinuation of its use for inhibiting preterm labor. It is recommended that magnesium sulfate not be used beyond 5 to 7 days for the treatment of preterm labor because it has been shown to cause low calcium levels and bone changes (osteopenia) in the baby. There is positive evidence of human fetal risk, but the potential benefits from using the drug in pregnant women may be acceptable in certain situations despite its risks.

Patients maintained at a magnesium serum level between 3 and 5 mEq/L rarely show any adverse effects from hypermagnesemia. At a level of approximately 5 to 8 mEq/L, patients begin to show increasing signs of toxicity that correlate fairly well to serum levels. Early signs of maternal toxicity are complaints of "feeling hot all over" and "being thirsty all the time," flushed skin, and diaphoresis. Patients may then become hypotensive and have depressed patellar, radial, and biceps reflexes and flaccid muscles. Later signs of hypermagnesemia are central nervous system depression shown first by anxiety and then confusion, lethargy, and drowsiness. If serum levels continue to increase, cardiac depression and respiratory paralysis may result. Magnesium sulfate should be administered with extreme caution to patients with impaired renal function and whose urine output is less than 100 mL over the past 4 hours.

Therapeutic Outcomes

The primary therapeutic outcomes associated with magnesium sulfate therapy are as follows:
1. Arrest of preterm labor
2. Elimination of seizure activity

❖ **Nursing Implications for magnesium sulfate**
◆ *Premedication assessment*
1. Obtain baseline vital signs, especially blood pressure, pulse, and respirations.

2. Perform a mental status examination: level of consciousness, orientation, and anxiety level.
3. Check deep tendon reflexes; report hyporeflexia or absence of reflexes.
4. Review intake and output record; report declining output.
5. Have calcium gluconate or calcium chloride and equipment for IV administration available in case they are needed.
6. Obtain baseline laboratory values (e.g., serum magnesium level).
7. Monitor fetal heart rate and uterine activity; report distress.

◆ *Availability. Injection:* solutions: 1% (0.081 mEq/mL), 2% (0.162 mEq/mL), 4% (0.325 mEq/mL), 8% (0.65 mEq/mL), and 50% (4 mEq/mL).

◆ *Dosage and administration.* **IM:** Intramuscular injection is extremely painful. Avoid, if possible, or administer in conjunction with a local anesthetic.

IV: It is essential that an infusion pump be used to help control infusion of the loading dose and continuous drip.

Anticonvulsant. IV: *Loading dose:* 4 g of magnesium sulfate is added to 250 mL of 5% dextrose in water (D5W) and infused slowly at a rate of 10 mL/min. (The IV loading dose is usually administered at the same time as a 10-g IM loading dose.) *Maintenance dose:* 1 to 2 g/hr by continuous infusion.

Preterm labor. IV: *Loading dose:* 4 g of magnesium sulfate is added to 250 mL of D5W or 0.9% sodium chloride solution and infused IV over 30 minutes. *Maintenance dose:* 1 to 3 g/hr by continuous infusion.

> **⚠ Medication Safety Alert**
>
> Deep tendon reflexes, intake and output, vital signs, and orientation to the environment must be monitored on a regular, ongoing basis during the administration of magnesium sulfate.

◆ *Serious adverse effects*
Neurologic
Deep tendon reflexes. The presence or absence of the patellar reflex (knee-jerk reflex), biceps reflex, or radial reflex is a primary monitoring parameter for magnesium sulfate therapy.

The patellar reflex should be monitored hourly if the patient is receiving a continuous IV infusion or before every dose if being administered intermittently IM or IV. If the reflex is absent, further doses should be withheld until it returns. If the patellar reflex cannot be used because of epidural anesthesia, the biceps or radial reflex may be used.

Confusion. Perform a baseline assessment of the patient's degree of alertness and orientation to name, place, and time before initiating therapy. Make regularly

scheduled mental status evaluations to ensure that the patient is oriented.
Metabolic
Intake and output. Magnesium toxicity is more likely to occur in patients with reduced renal output. Report urine outputs of less than 30 mL/hr or less than 100 mL over 4 hours. Observe the urine color and measure the specific gravity. Note any other fluid and electrolyte loss, such as vaginal bleeding, diarrhea, or vomiting.
Cardiovascular
Vital signs. Vital signs (blood pressure, heart rate and rhythm) should be measured every 15 to 30 minutes when a patient is receiving a continuous IV infusion. Take vital signs before and after each administration for patients receiving intermittent therapy. The respiratory rate should be at least 16 breaths/min before the administration of further doses of magnesium sulfate. Do not administer additional doses if there is a reduced respiratory rate, a drop in blood pressure or fetal heart rate, or other signs of fetal distress.

Overdose. The antidote for magnesium intoxication (shown by respiratory depression and heart block) is calcium gluconate. A 10% solution of calcium gluconate should be kept ready for use at the patient's bedside. The dosage is 5 to 10 mEq (10 to 20 mL) IV over 3 minutes or 0.5 to 2 g (5 to 20 mL) of a 10% solution of calcium gluconate IV at 200 mg/min. Administer cardiopulmonary resuscitation until the patient responds appropriately.

◆ *Neonatal effects.* Infants born of mothers who receive magnesium sulfate must be monitored for hypotension, hyporeflexia, and respiratory depression.

◆ *Drug interactions*
Central nervous system depressants. Central nervous system depressants, including barbiturates, analgesics, general anesthetics, and alcohol, will potentiate the central nervous system depressant effects of magnesium sulfate.

> **Medication Safety Alert**
>
> Periodically check orientation to make sure the patient is not suffering from magnesium toxicity. Early signs of maternal toxicity are complaints of "feeling hot all over" and "being thirsty all the time," flushed skin color, and diaphoresis. Patients may then become hypotensive; have depressed patellar, radial, and biceps reflexes; and have flaccid muscles. Later signs of hypermagnesemia are central nervous system depression, shown first by anxiety, followed by confusion, lethargy, and drowsiness. If serum levels continue to increase, cardiac depression and respiratory paralysis may result. The patellar reflex should be monitored hourly if the patient is receiving a continuous IV infusion or before every dose if administered intermittently IM or IV. If the reflex is absent, further doses should be withheld until it returns. If the patellar reflex cannot be used because of epidural anesthesia, the biceps or radial reflex may be used.

Neuromuscular blockade. Concurrent use of neuromuscular blocking agents and magnesium sulfate will further depress muscular activity. Monitor the patient closely for depressed reflexes and respiration.

DRUG CLASS: OTHER AGENTS

---

clomiphene citrate (KLŎ-mă-fēn SĬ-trāt)
   Clomid (KLŎ-mĭd) ♣
   ⇄ *Do not confuse clomiphene with clomipramine.*

Actions

Clomiphene is a chemical compound that is structurally similar to natural estrogens. When administered, it binds to estrogen receptor sites, reducing the number of sites available for circulating estrogens. The receptors send back signals to the hypothalamus and pituitary gland, indicating a lack of circulating estrogens. The hypothalamus responds by increasing the secretion of hypothalamic releasing factor. This stimulates the pituitary gland to release luteinizing hormone and follicle-stimulating hormone, which in turn stimulate the ovaries to release ova for potential fertilization.

Uses

Clomiphene is used to induce ovulation in women who are not ovulating because of reduced circulating estrogen levels. Studies indicate that pregnancy occurs in 25% to 30% of patients treated. Ovulation of more than one ovum per cycle with potential fertilization of multiple ova may occur in 5% to 10% of patients treated.

Therapeutic Outcome

The primary therapeutic outcome associated with clomiphene therapy is ovulation, followed by fertilization and pregnancy.

❖ Nursing Implications for clomiphene
♦ *Premedication assessment*
   1. Check to ensure that the patient has had a complete physical examination, including pregnancy testing, before initiating therapy.
   2. Obtain baseline data regarding any gastrointestinal or visual disturbances present before initiating therapy.

♦ *Availability. PO:* 50-mg tablets.

♦ *Dosage and administration.* **Adult:** *PO:* 50 mg daily for 5 days. Start therapy at any time if there has been no recent bleeding. If spontaneous bleeding occurs before therapy, start on or about the fifth day for 5 days. If ovulation does not occur after the first course, give a second course of 100 mg/day for 5 days. Start this course no earlier than 30 days after the previous course. A third course may be administered at 100 mg/day for 5 days. However, most patients who respond will have done so in the first two courses. Reevaluation of the patient is necessary.

It is mandatory that patients have a complete physical examination to rule out other pathologic causes for lack of ovulation before initiating clomiphene therapy. Patients must be informed of the possibility of multiple fetuses with clomiphene treatment and must be instructed to follow the prescriber's recommendations regarding dose and amount.

Possible pregnancy. Clomiphene should not be administered if pregnancy is suspected. Basal temperatures should be followed for 1 month after therapy. Instruct the patient on how to take and record basal temperatures and how to report a biphasic temperature distribution. If the body temperature follows a biphasic distribution (peaks twice within a few days) and is not followed by menses, the next course of clomiphene therapy should not be scheduled until pregnancy tests have been completed.

Timing of intercourse. Timing of intercourse is important to the therapy's success. Make sure that the patient understands the importance of having intercourse during the time of ovulation, usually 6 to 10 days after the last dose of medication.

♦ *Common adverse effects*
   Hormonal
   Nausea, vomiting, diarrhea, constipation, "hot flashes," abdominal cramps. These adverse effects are usually mild and tend to resolve with continued therapy. Encourage the patient not to discontinue therapy without first consulting the healthcare provider.

♦ *Serious adverse effects*
   Gastrointestinal
   Severe abdominal cramps. Patients should be told to report significant abdominal or pelvic pain and bloating that develop during therapy.
   Neurologic
   Visual disturbances. Patients developing visual blurring, spots, or double vision should report for an eye examination. The drug is usually discontinued, and visual disturbances pass within a few days to weeks after discontinuation. Caution the patient to avoid temporarily tasks that require visual acuity, such as driving or operating power machinery.
   Dizziness. Provide for patient safety during episodes of dizziness; report to the healthcare provider for further evaluation.

♦ *Drug interactions.* No clinically significant drug interactions have been reported.

Rh₀(D) immune globulin (human) IM [Rh₀(D) IGIM]
   HyperRHO S/D Full Dose; RhoGAM Ultra-Filtered Plus
Rh₀(D) immune globulin microdose [Rh₀(D) IG microdose]
   MICRhoGAM Ultra-Filtered Plus
Rh₀(D) immune globulin (human) IV [Rh₀(D) IGIV]
   WinRho SDF; Rhophylac

Actions

Rh$_o$(D) immune globulin (human) suppresses the stimulation of active immunity by Rh-positive foreign RBCs that enter the maternal circulation at the time of delivery, at the termination of a pregnancy, or during a transfusion of inadequately typed blood.

Rh hemolytic disease of the newborn can be prevented in subsequent pregnancies by administering Rh$_o$(D) immune globulin [Rh$_o$(D) antibody] to the Rh-negative mother shortly after delivery of an Rh-positive infant.

Uses

Rh$_o$(D) immune globulin (human) is used to prevent Rh immunization of the Rh-negative patient exposed to Rh-positive blood as the result of a transfusion accident, during termination of a pregnancy, or as the result of a delivery of an Rh-positive infant. Full-dose Rh$_o$(D) IGIM and Rh$_o$(D) IGIV are used when there has been a transfusion accident, during termination of a pregnancy more than 12 weeks' gestation, or as the result of a delivery of an Rh-positive infant. Rh$_o$(D) IGIM microdose is used to prevent Rh immunization of the Rh-negative patient exposed to Rh-positive RBCs at the time of spontaneous or induced abortion of up to 12 weeks' gestation.

In addition to preventing Rh immunization of the Rh-negative patient for these causes, Rh$_o$(D) IGIV is used to treat idiopathic thrombocytopenic purpura (ITP), a condition of spontaneous destruction of platelets. The mechanism whereby Rh$_o$(D) IGIV reduces spontaneous rupture of platelets is unknown.

Therapeutic Outcomes

The primary therapeutic outcome associated with Rh$_o$(D) immune globulin (human) therapy is prevention of Rh hemolytic disease. The primary therapeutic outcome associated with Rh$_o$(D) IGIV therapy is prevention of Rh hemolytic disease and platelet destruction in acute cases of ITP.

❖ Nursing Implications for Rh$_o$(D) Immune Globulin (Human)

◆ *Premedication assessment*

1. Check the Rh status of the mother; she must be Rh negative. Has the mother previously been sensitized to Rh factor through blood transfusion or previous pregnancy?
2. Check the platelet count of those patients being treated for ITP.

◆ *Availability.* **IM:**

-Rh$_o$(D) immune globulin microdose (MICRhoGAM Ultra-Filtered Plus): prefilled syringe, 250 units;

-Rh$_o$(D) immune globulin full dose (HyperRHO S/D Full Dose, RhoGAM Ultra-Filtered Plus): prefilled syringe, 250 units and 1500 units.

IV:

-WinRho SDF: 1500, 2500, 5000, and 15,000 units in single-dose vials;

-Rhophylac: 1500 units in prefilled syringe.

◆ *Dosage and administration.* Although there is no need to administer Rh$_o$(D) immune globulin to a woman who is already sensitized to the Rh factor, the risk is no greater than when given to a woman who is not sensitized. When in doubt, administer Rh$_o$(D) immune globulin.

> **❗ Medication Safety Alert**
>
> - *Never* administer the Rh$_o$(D) IGIM full-dose or microdose products intravenously. (However, the Rh$_o$(D) IGIV full-dose product may be administered intramuscularly or intravenously.)
> - *Never* administer to a neonate.
> - *Confirm* that the mother is Rh negative.

Postpartum prophylaxis. One standard-dose vial of Rh$_o$(D) IGIM given IM, or one standard-dose vial of Rh$_o$(D) IGIV administered IM or IV. Additional vials may be necessary if there was unusually large fetal-maternal hemorrhage.

Antepartum prophylaxis. One standard-dose vial IM at about 28 weeks' gestation. This must be followed by another vial administered within 72 hours of delivery. After amniocentesis, miscarriage, abortion, or ectopic pregnancy and less than 13 weeks' gestation: one microdose vial IM within 72 hours; 13 or more weeks of gestation: one standard-dose vial IM within 72 hours.

Transfusion accident. Rh-negative, premenopausal women who receive Rh-positive red cells by transfusion should receive one standard-dose vial IM for each 15 mL of transfused packed red cells.

Idiopathic thrombocytopenic purpura. Before administration:

1. Confirm that the person is Rh positive.
2. Follow manufacturer's instructions on dilution and administration of Rh$_o$(D) IGIV.

IV: Initial dose: 250 units/kg as a single injection. Additional doses depend on response.

◆ *Common adverse effects*

Inflammatory, immune system

Localized tenderness. Inform the patient that she may experience stiffness at the site of injection for a few days.

Fever, arthralgias, generalized aches, pains. Monitor on a regular basis for these symptoms. Follow routine orders of the healthcare provider or hospital concerning the use of analgesics (usually acetaminophen; do not use aspirin or other antiinflammatory agents) for patient discomfort.

Hypersensitivity, immune system

Urticaria, tachycardia, hypotension. Allergic reactions require immediate treatment. Monitor patients for 20 to 30 minutes after administration. Have emergency supplies readily available.

◆ *Drug interactions.* No significant drug interactions have been reported.

erythromycin ophthalmic ointment (ĕ-rĭth-rō-MĪ-sĭn)
phytonadione (fī-tō-nă-DĪ-ōn)

Actions and Uses

Erythromycin is a macrolide antibiotic used prophylactically to prevent ophthalmia neonatorum caused by *N. gonorrhoeae* and chlamydial ophthalmia caused by *C. trachomatis.*

Therapeutic Outcome

The primary therapeutic outcome associated with erythromycin ophthalmic ointment therapy is prevention of postpartum gonorrhea or chlamydia eye infection.

❖ Nursing Implications for erythromycin Ophthalmic Ointment

◆ *Premedication assessment.* Describe any drainage present in the eye or on the lids; cleanse thoroughly.

◆ *Availability.* **Ophthalmic ointment:** 5 mg/gram in 1-g tube.

◆ *Dosage and administration*
  * *Ointment:* A new tube should be started for each infant.
  * *Wash hands:* Wash hands immediately before administration to prevent bacterial contamination. Apply clean gloves.
  * *Cleanse the eyes:* Using a separate sterile absorbent cotton or gauze pad for each eye, wash the unopened lids from the nose outward until free of blood, mucus, or meconium.
  * *Open the eyes and instill medication:* For each eye, separate the eyelids and instill a ¼-inch ribbon of erythromycin ointment along the lower conjunctival surface; begin at the inner canthus and move to the outer aspect of the eye. Administer medication within 2 hours of birth.
  * *Irrigation:* DO NOT irrigate the eyes after instillation.

◆ *Common adverse effects*
  Sensory
  Mild conjunctivitis. Mild conjunctival inflammation occurs in the neonate and may interfere with the ability to focus. This adverse effect generally disappears in 1 to 2 days. Assure the family that the redness is temporary.

◆ *Drug interactions.* No significant drug interactions have been reported.

Actions

Vitamin K is a fat-soluble vitamin necessary for the production of the blood-clotting factors prothrombin (factor II), proconvertin (factor VII), plasma thromboplastin component (factor IX), and Stuart factor (factor X) in the liver. Vitamin K is absorbed from the diet and is normally produced by the bacterial flora in the gastrointestinal tract, from which it is absorbed and transported to the liver for clotting factor production. Because bacteria have not yet colonized the colon, newborns are often deficient in vitamin K. They also may be deficient in these clotting factors and are therefore more susceptible to hemorrhagic disease in the first 5 to 8 days after birth.

Uses

Phytonadione is routinely administered prophylactically to protect against vitamin K deficiency bleeding (VKDB) of the newborn (formerly known as *hemorrhagic disease of the newborn*).

Therapeutic Outcome

The primary therapeutic outcome associated with phytonadione therapy is prevention of VKDB of the newborn.

❖ Nursing Implications for phytonadione
◆ *Premedication assessment.* No assessment is required.

◆ *Availability.* **Injection:** 1 mg in 0.5-mL ampule and prefilled syringe.

◆ *Dosage and administration.* **IM:** 0.5 to 1 mg in the lateral aspect of the thigh within 1 hour of birth.

 Medication Safety Alert

DO NOT administer phytonadione intravenously! Severe reactions, including hypotension, cardiac dysrhythmias, and respiratory arrest, have been reported.

◆ *Serious adverse effects*
  Hematologic
  Bruising, hemorrhage. Observe for bleeding (usually occurring on the second or third day). Bleeding may be seen as petechiae; generalized ecchymoses; or bleeding from the umbilical stump, circumcision site, nose, or gastrointestinal tract. Assess results of serial prothrombin times.

◆ *Drug interactions.* No significant drug interactions have been reported.

Get Ready for the NCLEX® Examination!

Key Points

- Today's healthcare system is placing more emphasis on self-care for the mother and her newborn. Shortened hospital stays have heightened the healthcare professional's awareness of the need to provide more education to the mother and significant others, not only for the care needs of the mother but also for those of the newborn.
- Every encounter with the mother is an opportunity to enhance her learning and preparation for parenting. Use of community resources for prenatal and parenting classes should be encouraged.
- The prenatal examination provides a basis for establishing the future healthcare needs of the mother and infant. Psychosocial and cultural aspects of care must be incorporated into the assessments and interventions planned for self-care. At subsequent prenatal visits, relevant information must be provided on all aspects of self-care to enhance the normal growth and development of the fetus and to prevent or manage potential complications of pregnancy.
- After delivery, the mother should be provided with the pertinent discharge information through one-on-one teaching or through discharge classes and be provided with telephone follow-up, home visitations, and referrals to available community resources to meet the care needs of the mother and newborn at home.

Additional Learning Resources

SG Go to your Study Guide for additional Review Questions for the NCLEX® Examination, Critical Thinking Clinical Situations, and other learning activities to help you master this chapter content.

Go to your Evolve website (https://evolve.elsevier.com/Clayton) for additional online resources.

Review Questions for the NCLEX® Examination

1. The nurse's assessment of a pregnant patient who is in the early stages of labor includes which of the following? (Select all that apply.)
   1. Vital signs
   2. Apgar score
   3. Frequency of uterine contractions
   4. A history of the pregnancy
   5. Checking the fundus

2. High-risk pregnancy refers to women who develop which of the following signs and symptoms? (Select all that apply.)
   1. Elevated blood pressure
   2. Proteinuria
   3. Persistent, severe vomiting
   4. Presence of colostrum
   5. Absence of patellar reflex

3. A pregnant woman with an estimated gestational age of 28 weeks presents to the hospital with contractions. The nurse expects that in addition to starting an IV for hydration and ruling out any complications, in order to delay delivery, which of the following medications may be administered? (Select all that apply.)
   1. Magnesium sulfate
   2. Nifedipine
   3. Dinoprostone
   4. Indomethacin
   5. Misoprostol

4. A mother in active labor was given the uterine stimulant oxytocin. She developed dry lips and requested water. What would be an appropriate response by the nurse?
   1. "You can have water while you are in labor, but I need to check your urine output."
   2. "You have an IV running so you should not need any water. I will check your urine output."
   3. "You are having signs of water intoxication; I will notify your physician and check your urine output."
   4. "Let me call the physician and get you some ice chips. I need to check your urine output."

5. The nurse understands that misoprostol (Cytotec), a prostaglandin E analogue, is used for which purpose? (Select all that apply.)
   1. Cervical softening and dilation before labor
   2. Induction of active labor
   3. Reduction in postpartum hemorrhage in the presence of uterine atony
   4. Evacuation of uterine contents
   5. Prevention of uterine cramping

6. The nurse was assessing a postpartum mother and noted that the perineal pads were being changed every 15 minutes. What further assessments need to be made to manage postpartum hemorrhage? (Select all that apply.)
   1. Observe the color of the bleeding
   2. Take vital signs frequently
   3. Assess fundal height and position
   4. Observe for restlessness
   5. Report urine output of 50 mL/hr or higher

7. A nurse taking care of a mother who is Rh negative knows that the timing of the $Rh_o(D)$ immune globulin is critical and that it needs to be administered when? (Select all that apply.)
   1. Immediately after delivery
   2. At 28 weeks' gestation
   3. Within 72 hours of delivery
   4. 3 weeks after delivery
   5. When the infant has started nursing

8. The nurse giving instructions to a new mother prior to discharge realizes further teaching is needed after the mother made which statement?
   1. "I understand that I need to get rest throughout the day so I don't get exhausted, which is why my mother will be staying with me for a few weeks."
   2. "If I have any trouble with breastfeeding, I can call the lactation consultant."
   3. "You gave my baby that shot of vitamin K, so I don't have to worry about any brain injury that might have happened during birth."
   4. "I know I need to come back for a checkup in 6 weeks."

Objectives

1. Identify important personal hygiene measures to educate women and men regarding prevention of the spread of sexually transmitted infections.
2. Describe the major adverse effects and contraindications to the use of oral contraceptive agents.
3. Identify the patient teaching necessary with the administration of the transdermal contraceptive and the intravaginal hormonal contraceptive.
4. Discuss osteoporosis and its risk factors as well as preventative measures and the pharmacologic treatment used.
5. Describe pharmacologic treatments of benign prostatic hyperplasia.
6. Describe the pharmacologic treatment of erectile dysfunction.

Key Terms

leukorrhea (lŭ-kō-RĒ-ă) (p. 616)
sexually transmitted infections (SĔK-shū-ăl-ē trănz-MĬT-ĕd ĭn-FĔK-shŭnz) (p. 616)
dysmenorrhea (dĭs-mĕn-ō-RĒ-ă) (p. 623)

osteoporosis (ŏs-tē-ō-pō-RŌ-sĭs) (p. 628)
benign prostatic hyperplasia (bē-NĪN prō-STĂT-ĭc hī-pŭr-PLĀ-zhă) (p. 632)
erectile dysfunction (ĕ-RĔK-tīl dĭs-FŬNK-shŭn) (p. 635)

VAGINITIS

Secretions from the vagina usually represent a normal physiologic process, but if the discharge becomes excessive, it is known as leukorrhea, an abnormal, usually whitish, vaginal discharge that may occur at any age. It affects almost all females at some time in their lives. Leukorrhea is not a disease but a symptom of an underlying disorder. The most common cause is an infection of the lower reproductive tract, but other physiologic and noninfectious causes of vaginal discharge are well known (Box 40.1).

The most common organisms causing the infectious type of leukorrhea are *Candida albicans, Trichomonas vaginalis,* and *Gardnerella vaginalis* (Box 40.2). Occasionally, *C. albicans* infections of the mouth, gastrointestinal tract, or vagina may develop as secondary infections during the use of broad-spectrum antibiotics, such as penicillins, tetracyclines, and cephalosporins.

Pathogens that are commonly transmitted by sexual contact are called sexually transmitted infections (STIs). In some diseases, such as gonorrhea, syphilis, chlamydia, and genital herpes simplex virus, and in human papillomavirus (HPV) infection, sexual transmission is the primary mode of transmission. The medications used to treat these infections are found in Table 40.1. In other diseases, such as giardiasis, shigellosis, and infections with the hepatitis viruses, other important nonsexual means of transmission also exist. Unfortunately, the true incidence of STIs is not known in the United States because of large numbers of unreported cases.

DRUG THERAPY FOR LEUKORRHEA AND GENITAL INFECTIONS

See Table 40.1.

❖ NURSING IMPLICATIONS FOR MEN'S AND WOMEN'S HEALTH

◆ Assessment
The following assessment questions apply to all age groups.

Female reproductive history. Assess for the following:
- Age of menarche
- Usual pattern of menses: duration, number of pads used, last menstrual period
- Pain, discomfort, spotting between periods, or extended time of menstrual flow
- Number of pregnancies, live births, miscarriages, or abortions
- Vaginal discharges, infections, genital lesions, or warts. Describe color, odor, and amount of discharge; describe lesions or any itching. Is there pain with urination or sexual intercourse?

Box 40.1   Causes of Vaginal Discharge

PHYSIOLOGIC
- Ovulation
- Coitus
- Oral contraceptives
- Pregnancy
- Premenstruation
- Premenarche
- Intrauterine device

INFECTIOUS
- Vaginal
  - Candida
  - Trichomonas
  - Gardnerella
  - Toxic shock syndrome
- Vulvar
  - Herpes
  - Condylomata acuminata
  - Syphilis
  - Bartholinitis
  - Lymphogranuloma venereum
  - Granuloma inguinale
  - Urethritis
  - Pyoderma
- Cervical
  - Gonorrhea
  - Chlamydial or bacterial cervicitis
  - Chronic cervicitis
  - Pelvic inflammatory disease

NONINFECTIOUS
- Atrophic vaginitis
- Foreign body
- Vaginal adenosis
- Allergic vulvovaginitis
- Vulvar, vaginal carcinoma
- Cervical polyps
- Cervical erosions, ulcers
- Uterine carcinoma
- Endometrial myoma
- Vesicovaginal fistula
- Enterovaginal fistula

Box 40.2   Sexually Transmitted Infections

BACTERIA
- *Neisseria gonorrhoeae*
- *Gardnerella vaginalis*
- *Treponema pallidum*
- *Calymmatobacterium granulomatis*

CHLAMYDIAE
- *Chlamydia trachomatis*

ECTOPARASITES
- *Sarcoptes scabiei*
- *Phthirus pubis*

FUNGUS
- *Candida albicans*

MYCOPLASMA
- *Ureaplasma urealyticum*
- *Mycoplasma hominis*

PROTOZOA
- *Trichomonas vaginalis*
- *Entamoeba histolytica*
- *Giardia lamblia*

VIRUSES
- Herpes simplex virus
- Hepatitis A, B, C
- Cytomegalovirus
- Human papillomavirus (HPV)
- Poxvirus
- Human immunodeficiency virus (HIV)

- History and frequency of Papanicolaou (Pap) smears
- Reproductive problems (e.g., endometriosis, ovarian cysts, and uterine fibroids)
- History of STIs (e.g., chlamydia, syphilis, gonorrhea, yeast infections, genital herpes, human immunodeficiency virus [HIV], genital warts [HPV]). If so, when and what was the treatment?
- If a prescription for oral contraceptive therapy is being requested, ask about any indication of hypertension, heart or liver disease, thromboembolic disorders, smoking history, or cancer of the reproductive organs.

Male reproductive history.   Assess for the following:
- Pattern of urination. Has there been a recent change in the pattern of urination (e.g., difficulty initiating urine stream, need to strain to empty the bladder, frequency of nocturia, pain on urination, frequency, urgency, hematuria, incontinence, dribbling, or urinary retention)?
- Presence of a urethral discharge or genital or perianal lesions. Is there any swelling of the penis?
- Is there pain in the lower back, perineum, or pelvis?
- History of prostatitis, benign prostatic hyperplasia, or prostatic cancer
- Is testicular self-examination performed regularly? Have any abnormal findings been noted, such as lumps or masses?

- Contraceptive methods used (e.g., oral contraceptives, intrauterine device, condoms, or spermicidal products)
- If taking oral contraceptives, what types? How long have oral contraceptives been used? Are they taken regularly? What, if any, adverse effects have been experienced?
- History of multiple sexual partners—male, female, or both. What type of protection is used during sexual intercourse?
- Is breast self-examination performed regularly? Have any abnormal findings been noted, such as lumps or discharge?
- Age of menopause
- Postmenopausal women: Has there been any vaginal bleeding?

Table **40.1**	Causative Organisms and Products Used to Treat Genital Infections[a]		
CAUSATIVE ORGANISM	**GENERIC NAME**		**BRAND NAME**
Vulvovaginitis			
Candida albicans (fungus)	butoconazole vaginal cream		Gynazole-I
	clotrimazole vaginal cream, vaginal tablets		Gyne-Lotrimin
	fluconazole oral tablets		Diflucan
	itraconazole oral capsules		Sporanox
	miconazole vaginal cream, suppositories		Monistat 3, Monistat 7
	terconazole vaginal cream, suppositories		—
Trichomonas vaginalis (protozoa)	metronidazole oral tablets		Flagyl
	tinidazole oral tablets		Tindamax
Bacterial vaginosis (formerly known as *Gardnerella vaginalis* [bacteria])	metronidazole oral tablets, vaginal gel		Flagyl; MetroGel-Vaginal
	tinidazole oral tablets		Tindamax
	clindamycin vaginal cream		Cleocin
Gonorrhea			
Neisseria gonorrhea (bacteria)	ceftriaxone (+ azithromycin or doxycycline)		
	cefixime (+ azithromycin)		Suprax
	Cefixime should only be used if ceftriaxone is unavailable		
	azithromycin		Zithromax
	doxycycline		Vibramycin
Syphilis			
Treponema pallidum (spirochete)	penicillin G benzathine		Bicillin L-A
	tetracycline		Tetracycline
	doxycycline		Vibramycin
	azithromycin (resistance reported)		Zithromax
Genital Herpes			
Herpes simplex genitalis (virus)	acyclovir oral capsules		Zovirax
	famciclovir oral tablets		—
	valacyclovir oral tablets		Valtrex
Chlamydiae			
Chlamydia trachomatis (chlamydia)	azithromycin		Zithromax
	doxycycline		Vibramycin
	erythromycin		Erythromycin
	levofloxacin		
	ofloxacin		

Data from Workowski KA, Bolan GA; Centers for Disease Control and Prevention. Sexually transmitted diseases treatment guidelines, 2015. *MMWR Recomm Rep.* 2015;64(No. RR-3):1-137; Gilbert DN, Chambers HF, Eliopoulos GM, et al. *The Sanford Guide to Antimicrobial Therapy 2014*, 44th ed. Sperryville, VA: Antimicrobial Therapy, Inc.; 2014.
[a]See Chapter 45 for individual drug monographs.

- History of STIs (e.g., chlamydia, syphilis, gonorrhea, yeast infections, genital herpes, HIV, genital warts [HPV]). If so, when and what was the treatment?
- History of multiple sexual partners—male, female, or both. What type of protection is used during sexual intercourse?
- History of arthralgia, fever, chills, malaise, pharyngitis, or oral lesions
- History of prior illnesses
- History of erectile dysfunction and description of pattern of altered erectile functioning
- If erectile dysfunction has occurred, ask specifically about vascular disorders that may lead to changes in blood flow to the penis (e.g., stroke). Ask about smoking and the use of drugs that may affect the vascular system (e.g., antihypertensive agents).

- Has the individual had prostate surgery? If so, was the onset of the erectile dysfunction before or after the surgery?
- Other neurologic disorders (e.g., Parkinson's disease and spinal cord injuries) may cause problems with sexual functioning.
- Has the individual had any other genitourinary conditions (e.g., testicular injury) that may be associated with sexual dysfunction?
- Endocrine disorders such as thyroid disease, adrenal disorders, and diabetes mellitus are also associated with sexual dysfunction. Does the patient have any of these illnesses?

History of current symptoms. Ask the patient to describe the current problem or problems that initiated this visit.

How long have the symptoms existed? Is there a recurrence of symptoms that were treated previously?

Medication history
- Has the individual taken steroids or antibiotics recently? If so, what condition was being treated and for how long? How long ago was therapy discontinued?
- Are over-the-counter, herbal, prescribed, or recreational drugs being taken? If so, what, why, and for how long?
- Are there any allergies to medications (e.g., antibiotics)?
- If having a recurrence of an STI, what was the previous treatment?
- In the presence of erectile dysfunction, a number of drugs may contribute to the problem (e.g., antihypertensives, antipsychotics, tricyclic antidepressants, monoamine oxidase inhibitors, hormones, sedative-hypnotics, stimulants, hormonal chemotherapeutics, opiates, steroids, and recreational drugs); therefore a medication history is extremely important.

Psychosocial. Sexually transmitted infections cause a high degree of anxiety. The intimate nature of the questioning required to obtain a sexual history may be embarrassing. Vaginal or urethral discharge may also be alarming to the patient seeking healthcare. When an STI diagnosis is suspected, explain the confidentiality policy of the facility before asking about sexual partners. (Many individuals do not return for follow-up appointments; there may be only one chance to obtain relevant information about contacts.)

Ask about lifestyle orientation (e.g., heterosexual, bisexual, or homosexual and number of partners). Has there been known contact with people with STIs? Are precautions used during sexual contacts?

Assess the level of anxiety present and adaptive responses and coping mechanisms used.

Laboratory and diagnostic studies
- Review reports on Gram stains and cultures from the anus, throat, and urethra for gonorrhea; Venereal Disease Research Laboratory, rapid plasma reagin, and fluorescent treponema antibody absorption tests for syphilis; tissue cultures for herpes simplex virus type 2; HIV testing (antibodies against HIV-1 and HIV-2 starting with enzyme immunoassay; confirm by using the Western blot test or an immunofluorescence assay). HIV testing should be offered to everyone evaluated for any type of STI.
- Diagnostic studies are individualized to the suspected cause of the signs and symptoms (e.g., complete blood count, cultures of prostate secretions, urine cultures, levels of prostate-specific antigen, blood urea nitrogen, creatinine) for prostatic disorders.

Physical examination
- Perform routine physical examination of the woman, including pelvic examination, Pap smear, cultures, and breast examination.
- Perform routine physical examination of the man, including testicular examination (rectal examination with palpation of prostate after age 40). An anorectal examination and examination of throat, tonsils, and mouth should be completed for men of homosexual or bisexual orientation.

◆ Implementation
- Record basic patient data (e.g., height, weight, vital signs).
- Prepare the patient for, and assist with, a physical examination.
- Observe distribution of body hair and presence of any scars, lesions, body rashes, pubic lice, or mites.
- Assist with specimen collection (e.g., vaginal smears, cultures of discharge).
- Inspect the penis and scrotum for swelling or abnormalities; observe for urethral discharge.
- Provide psychological support and refer for available counseling, as appropriate.

◆ Patient Education
Instructions for adolescents. The rate of STIs is high in this age group, so it is important to do a thorough assessment of sexual activity and practices. For those who are sexually active, counseling regarding safe sex practices and voluntary testing and treatment should be offered. Medical care for STIs can be provided without parental consent or knowledge. Check individual state laws for those that allow testing and counseling for HIV. All adolescents should be taught thoroughly about alternatives for abstinence and about safe sex practices.

Instructions for women
- Refrain from using irritating substances such as deodorants, scented toilet paper, and perfumed soaps or sprays.
- Warm sitz baths may help relieve vaginal or perineal irritation.
- Douching should be avoided unless specifically prescribed by the healthcare provider. Douching alters the pH of the vagina and may encourage the growth of opportunistic organisms.
- Personal hygiene should include wiping from front to back after voiding and defecation, voiding before and after intercourse, cleansing genitals thoroughly before and after intercourse, and changing menstrual tampons or pads frequently. Avoid wearing underwear made of synthetic materials; cotton materials help prevent moisture accumulation.
- Contraceptive methods (e.g., oral and other hormonal contraceptives, intrauterine devices) or surgical procedures such as hysterectomy do not provide any protection against HIV or other STIs. It is necessary to use physical and chemical barriers (e.g., condoms, foam spermicides).
- Stress the need for an annual Pap smear to detect cervical cancer that originates from cervical intraepithelial neoplasia.

Instructions for men

- Practice good personal hygiene. Keep the penis, scrotum, and perianal area thoroughly cleansed. Wash areas before and after intercourse. Urinate after intercourse. Wash hands well.
- Prostatitis is treated with antibiotics, antiinflammatory agents, and stool softeners. The local application of heat with a sitz bath, drinking plenty of fluids, and adequate rest are also usually used for relief of the symptoms of prostatitis.
- Men need annual physical examinations after age 40, which includes a rectal examination to palpate the prostate.
- Discuss appropriate interventions for men with altered sexual function that may be treated with medications such as phosphodiesterase inhibitors (e.g., Viagra, Cialis) or surgical intervention (e.g., penile prosthesis). Remind the patient of the need for consultation with a healthcare provider before using phosphodiesterase inhibitors. Although these drugs are readily available over the Internet, people with cardiovascular disorders are particularly susceptible to life-threatening consequences with their use.
- Latex condoms can be effective in reducing sexual transmission of HIV and some other STIs (e.g., gonorrhea, trichomonas, chlamydia), but condoms are not as effective against STIs transmitted by skin-to-skin contact, such as herpes simplex virus, HPV, and syphilis.
- Men having homosexual relationships and people who inject drugs should be vaccinated for hepatitis A virus. The frequent use of nonoxynol-9 spermicide during anal intercourse irritates the epithelial lining of the rectum, providing a portal of entry for HIV and other STIs.

Instructions for women and men

- When infections are present, abstain from sexual intercourse. Stress the need to prevent reinfection. When sexual practices are resumed, use latex condoms. Recent research demonstrates that vaginal spermicides containing nonoxynol-9 may not be effective in preventing cervical gonorrhea, chlamydia, or HIV infection. According to the Centers for Disease Control and Prevention, the role of spermicides, sponges, and diaphragms for preventing transmission of HIV has not been evaluated. A recent study indicates that the frequent use of nonoxynol-9 may actually increase the risk of HIV infection during vaginal intercourse because of irritation of vaginal tissues.
- Use sexual abstinence during the communicable phase of any disease. Remember that when having sex with an individual, one is also having sex with all previous sexual partners, and thus the infectious possibilities should be considered.
- If having sex with a partner with an unknown status or one infected with HIV or another STI, a new condom should be used for each insertive intercourse.

- It is advised that both partners be tested for STIs, including HIV, before the first sexual encounter.
- Practice safe sex, if not abstinence. Use latex condoms. Discuss proper techniques for applying, using, removing, and discarding condoms.
- Arrange for follow-up appointments with the healthcare provider and appropriate referrals for counseling or with the social services department as needed.
- All sexual partners need to understand the importance of "partner services," the documentation of all sexual partners for the purpose of providing evaluation and treatment to anyone who may have been exposed to an STI before the infected individual became clinically symptomatic. Cases of syphilis, gonorrhea, chlamydia, and acquired immunodeficiency syndrome are reported in every state.

Medications

For women. Teach the patient the proper way to apply medications topically or intravaginally using ointments or suppositories. It is imperative that proper cleansing of the genital area be done regularly using soap and water; rinse and dry well. Hands should be washed before and after the application or insertion of medications and before and after toileting. After every use, the vaginal applicator should be thoroughly washed with soap and water and then dried. After inserting a vaginal medication (cream or suppository), the woman should remain in a recumbent position for 30 minutes to allow time for drug absorption. A minipad can be worn to catch remaining drainage. (See Fig. 7.13 for proper administration of vaginal medication.)

With oral contraceptive therapy, teach not only the medication schedule and dosage, but also what to do if a dose is missed, frequency of follow-up care, and common and serious adverse effects.

For men and women. Teach the medication regimen and who must take the medications—both partners in a sexual relationship.

Fostering health maintenance

- Throughout the course of treatment, discuss medication information and how it will benefit the patient. Stress the importance of nonpharmacologic interventions such as maintaining general health and proper nutrition and hygiene. Stress the need for adherence with the treatment regimen.
- Provide the patient and significant others with important information contained in the specific drug monographs for the drugs prescribed. Additional health teaching and nursing interventions for common and serious adverse drug effects are found in each monograph.
- Seek cooperation and understanding of the following points so that medication adherence is increased: name of medication; dosage, route, and times of administration; and common and serious adverse drug effects.

Patient self-assessment. Enlist the patient's help in developing and maintaining a written record of monitoring parameters (e.g., blood pressure, pulse, weight, degree of relief from menstrual pain, menstrual cycle information for women on oral contraceptives). See Appendix B: Template for Developing a Written Record for Patients to Monitor Their Own Therapy. For patients with STIs, a listing of the symptoms present and degree of relief obtained may be appropriate. Complete the Premedication Data column for use as a baseline to track response to drug therapy. Ensure that the patient understands how to use the form, and instruct the patient to bring the completed form to follow-up visits. During follow-up visits, focus on issues that will foster adherence with the therapeutic interventions prescribed.

Health Promotion

The consistent use of male latex condoms significantly reduces the risk of HIV infection, gonorrhea and chlamydia, herpes simplex virus in men and women, and HPV in women, but male condoms may be less effective in protecting against STIs transmitted by skin-to-skin contact (e.g., genital herpes, syphilis) because the infected areas may not be covered by the condom.

DRUG THERAPY FOR CONTRACEPTION

Oral (hormonal) contraceptives (birth control pills) became available in 1960. They now represent one of the most common forms of artificial birth control in the United States. It is estimated that approximately one-third of all women between 18 and 44 years of age use oral contraceptives.

DRUG CLASS: ORAL CONTRACEPTIVES

Actions

Estrogens, and progestins to some extent, induce contraception by inhibiting ovulation. The estrogens block pituitary release of follicle-stimulating hormone (FSH), preventing the ovaries from developing a follicle from which the ovum is released. Progestins inhibit pituitary release of luteinizing hormone (LH), the hormone responsible for releasing an ovum from a follicle. Other mechanisms play a contributory role in preventing conception. Estrogens and progestins alter cervical mucus by making it thick and viscous, inhibiting sperm migration. Hormones also change the endometrial wall, impairing implantation of the fertilized ovum.

Uses

There are two types of oral contraceptives: the combination pill, which contains both an estrogen and a progestin, and the minipill, which contains only a progestin. The combination pills are subdivided into fixed combination or monophasic (Table 40.2), biphasic (Table 40.3), triphasic (Table 40.4), and quadriphasic (Table 40.5)

Table 40.2 Monophasic Oral Contraceptives[a]

PRODUCT	PROGESTIN	ESTROGEN
Aviane	levonorgestrel (0.1 mg)	ethinyl estradiol (20 mcg)
Apri	desogestrel (0.15 mg)	ethinyl estradiol (30 mcg)
Yaz	drospirenone (3 mg)	ethinyl estradiol (20 mcg)
Brevicon	norethindrone (0.5 mg)	ethinyl estradiol (35 mcg)
Cryselle	norgestrel (0.3 mg)	ethinyl estradiol (30 mcg)
Altavera	levonorgestrel (0.15 mg)	ethinyl estradiol (30 mcg)
Junel 1/20	norethindrone acetate (1 mg)	ethinyl estradiol (20 mcg)
Kelnor 1/35	ethynodiol diacetate (1 mg)	ethinyl estradiol (35 mcg)
Ortho-Cyclen	norgestimate (0.25 mg)	ethinyl estradiol (35 mcg)
Quasense[b] (91 tablets)	levonorgestrel (0.15 mg)	ethinyl estradiol (30 mcg)

[a]There are over 80 monophasic oral contraceptive products available. This table is a representative list of estrogen-progestin combinations available under a variety of brand names. Unless otherwise listed, monophasic contraceptives contain 21 active tablets followed by 7 inactive tablets.
[b]Extended- or continuous-cycle oral contraceptive. Contains 84 active tablets and 7 inert tablets. A menstrual period occurs only during the time the inert tablets are taken.

products. The monophasic combination pills contain a fixed ratio of estrogen and progestin given daily for 21 days, beginning on day 5 of the menstrual cycle. The biphasic product contains a fixed dose of estrogen and a progestin dose on days 1 to 10 that is lower than that on days 11 to 21 of the menstrual cycle. The triphasic combination pills provide three concentrations of estrogen and progestin, and the quadriphasic pills provide four concentrations of hormones. The purpose of the variable concentrations is to provide contraception with the lowest necessary dose of hormones. Most of the combination pills are also packaged in 28-tablet containers. The last 7 tablets are inert but are supplied so that there is no break in the routine of taking 1 tablet daily. The progestin-only products (Box 40.3) are packaged in units of 28 tablets. All tablets contain active hormone; 1 tablet should be taken daily at approximately the same time each day. There is no cyclic break.

The progestin-only pills, or minipills, represent a common form of oral contraceptive therapy. Many adverse effects of combination-type contraceptives are caused by the estrogen component of the tablet. For those women particularly susceptible to adverse effects of estrogen therapy, the minipill provides an alternative. Women who might prefer the minipill are those with

Table 40.3 Biphasic Oral Contraceptives[a]

PRODUCT	PROGESTIN	ESTROGEN	OTHER INGREDIENTS
Amethia (91 tablets)[b]	levonorgestrel 84 white tablets (0.15 mg)	ethinyl estradiol 84 white tablets (30 mcg) 7 blue tablets (10 mcg)	—
Lo Loestrin FE (28 tablets)	norethindrone 24 blue tablets (1 mg)	ethinyl estradiol 24 blue tablets (10 mcg) 2 white tablets (10 mcg)	ferrous fumarate (75 mg) (2 brown tablets)
Mircette (28 tablets)[c]	desogestrel 21 white tablets (0.15 mg)	ethinyl estradiol 21 white tablets (20 mcg) 5 yellow tablets (10 mcg)	—
Necon 10/11 (28 tablets)	norethindrone 10 tablets (0.5 mg) 11 tablets (1 mg)	ethinyl estradiol 35 mcg 35 mcg	—

[a]There are over 13 biphasic oral contraceptive products available. This table is a representative list of estrogen-progestin combinations available under a variety of brand names.
[b]Active for 84 days, followed by a menstrual period.
[c]One white tablet is taken daily for 21 days, followed by one green (inert) tablet for 2 days, then one yellow (active) tablet daily for 5 days.

Table 40.4 Triphasic Oral Contraceptives[a]

PRODUCT	PROGESTIN	ESTROGEN (MCG)	OTHER INGREDIENTS
Aranelle[b]	norethindrone 7 tablets (0.5 mg) 9 tablets (1 mg) 5 tablets (0.5 mg)	ethinyl estradiol 35 mcg 35 mcg 35 mcg	—
Caziant[b]	desogestrel 7 tablets (0.1 mg) 7 tablets (0.125 mg) 7 tablets (0.15 mg)	ethinyl estradiol 25 mcg 25 mcg 25 mcg	—
Enpresse-28[b]	levonorgestrel 6 tablets (0.05 mg) 5 tablets (0.075 mg) 10 tablets (0.125 mg)	ethinyl estradiol 30 mcg 40 mcg 30 mcg	—
Estrostep Fe (28 tablets)	norethindrone acetate 5 tablets (1 mg) 7 tablets (1 mg) 9 tablets (1 mg)	ethinyl estradiol 20 mcg 30 mcg 35 mcg	ferrous fumarate (75 mg) 7 brown tablets
Ortho Tri-Cyclen Lo (28 tablets)[b]	norgestimate 7 tablets (0.180 mg) 7 tablets (0.215 mg) 7 tablets (0.250 mg)	ethinyl estradiol 25 mcg 25 mcg 25 mcg	—

[a]There are over 30 triphasic oral contraceptive products available. This table is a representative list of estrogen-progestin combinations available under a variety of brand names.
[b]Seven inert tablets.

Table 40.5 Quadriphasic Oral Contraceptive[a]

PRODUCT	PROGESTIN	ESTROGEN
Natazia	Phase 1: 2 dark yellow tablets (no progestin)	estradiol valerate (3 mg)
	Phase 2: 5 medium red tablets dienogest (2 mg)	estradiol valerate (2 mg)
	Phase 3: 17 light yellow tablets dienogest (3 mg)	estradiol valerate (2 mg)
	Phase 4: 2 dark red tablets (no progestin)	estradiol valerate (1 mg)

[a]Other quadriphasic oral contraceptives are: Fayosim, Quartette and Rivelsa.

Box 40.3 Progestin-Only Contraceptives

The progestin-only contraceptives contain 0.35 mg of norethindrone (progestin):

- Camila
- Errin
- Heather
- Jolivette
- Ortho-Micronor
- Nora-BE
- Norlyda
- Sharobel
- Tulana

a history of migraine headaches, hypertension, mental depression, weight gain, and breast tenderness and those who want to breastfeed postpartum. The minipill is not without its disadvantages, however. Between 30% and 40% of women taking the minipill continue to ovulate. **Dysmenorrhea**, manifested by irregular periods, infrequent periods, and spotting between periods, is common in women taking the minipill. Birth control is maintained by progestin activity on cervical mucus, uterine and fallopian transport, and implantation. There is a slightly higher incidence of both uterine and tubal pregnancies.

New dosage forms for oral contraceptives have become available that are known as extended-cycle and continuous-cycle oral contraceptives. These new monophasic combination oral contraceptives are given in the following regimens: 24 days, followed by placebo for 4 days (24/4 regimen; e.g., Yaz, Loestrin 24 Fe, Gianvi); 84 days, followed by placebo for 7 days (84/7 regimen; e.g., Jolessa, Quasense,); or continuously (without placebo; Amethyst). A primary purpose for these contraceptive products is to shorten the duration of menses, decreasing the frequency to four times per year, or completely eliminating menses. With sustained hormone use, there is greater suppression of endometrial growth, reducing pregnancy risk, and a lighter period, if any, lasting about 2 days during the 7 days off the active tablets (84/7 regimen). Other advantages to these products, in addition to fewer periods, is a lower cumulative dose of hormones taken compared with oral contraceptives cycled monthly, and the alleviation of symptoms of coexisting medical conditions that may be exacerbated during menses (e.g., anemia).

Clinical trials indicate that extended- and continuous-cycle oral contraceptives are as effective in preventing pregnancy as monthly oral contraceptives. These products have similar adverse effect profiles; the only significantly different adverse effect compared with monthly oral contraceptives is a change in bleeding pattern. These oral contraceptives are associated with more breakthrough bleeding and spotting than the monthly oral contraceptive pills.

Cigarette smoking increases the risk of serious adverse cardiovascular effects (e.g., blood clots) in persons who both smoke and use combination oral contraceptives. This risk increases with age and heavy smoking (at least 15 cigarettes daily) and is quite significant in women older than 35 years. Women who use oral contraceptives are strongly encouraged not to smoke.

Therapeutic Outcome

The primary therapeutic outcome associated with oral contraceptive therapy is prevention of pregnancy.

❖ **Nursing Implications for Oral Contraceptives**
◆ *Premedication assessment*
1. Review the medical history. If there is a history of obesity, smoking, hypertension, gallbladder disease,

diabetes mellitus, severe varicose veins, seizure disorders, oligomenorrhea or amenorrhea, rheumatic heart disease, thromboembolic disease, stroke, malignancy of breast or the reproductive system, renal or liver disease, severe mental depression, suspected pregnancy, or repeated contraceptive failure, consult with a healthcare provider before dispensing birth control pills.
2. Take a baseline body weight measurement, along with blood pressure measurement in the supine and sitting positions.
3. Ensure that a pregnancy test has been given and that the patient is not pregnant.

◆ *Availability.* See Tables 40.2, 40.3, 40.4, and 40.5 and Box 40.3.

◆ *Dosage and administration.* The estrogenic component of the combination-type pills is responsible for most of the adverse effects associated with therapy. The US Food and Drug Administration (FDA) has recommended that therapy be initiated with a product containing a low dose of estrogen. Adverse effects must be reviewed in relation to individual case histories and may be adjusted based on the incidence and type of adverse effects.

Before initiating therapy. The patient should have a complete physical examination that includes blood pressure, body weight, pelvic and breast examinations, Pap smear, urinalysis, and hemoglobin or hematocrit.

Instructions for using combination oral contraceptives. Start the first pill on the first Sunday after the menstrual period begins. Take one pill daily, at the same time, until the pack is gone. If using a 21-day pack, wait 1 week and restart on the next Sunday. If using a 28-day pack, start a new pack the day after finishing the last pack. Full protection by the pill during the first month may not occur, so the use of an additional form of birth control (condoms, foam) during the first month is advised. If the product prescribed also contains an iron supplement, be sure to take the 7 inert tablets monthly. The iron supplement is in the 7 inert tablets, not the 21 tablets containing hormones. (Many women skip the inert tablets each month, thinking that they have no benefit.)

- *Severe diarrhea or vomiting:* If severe diarrhea or vomiting occur within 3 to 4 hours after taking an active tablet, it should be considered a missed dose; additional contraceptive measures are recommended
- *Missed pills:* Take the pill as soon as a missed pill is remembered; take the next pill at the regularly scheduled time. If two pills are missed, take two pills as soon as remembered and two pills the next day. Spotting may occur when two pills are missed. Use another form of birth control (condoms, foam) until the pack of pills is finished. If *three or more pills* are missed, start using another form of birth control immediately. Start a new pack of pills on the next Sunday even if menstruating. Discard the old pack

of pills. Use other forms of birth control through the next month after missing three or more pills.

- *Missed pills and skipped periods:* Return to the healthcare provider for a pregnancy test.
- *Skipping one period but not missing a pill:* It is not uncommon for a woman to miss a period occasionally when on the pill. Start the next pack on the appropriate Sunday.
- *Spotting for two or more cycles:* See the healthcare provider. A dosage adjustment may be necessary.
- *Periodic examinations:* A yearly examination should include blood pressure tests, pelvic examination, urinalysis, breast examination, and Pap smear.
- *Discontinuing the pill for conception:* Because of a possibility of birth defects, the pill should be discontinued 3 months before attempting pregnancy. Use other methods of contraception for these 3 months.
- *Duration of oral contraceptive therapy:* Many healthcare providers prefer to have patients discontinue the pill for 3 of every 28 months. This allows the body to return to a normal cycle. Be sure to use other forms of contraception during this time. Long-term use (3 or more years) must be determined on an individual basis.
  - *Serious adverse effects to be reported as soon as possible:* Severe headaches, dizziness, blurred vision, leg pain, shortness of breath, chest pain, and acute abdominal pain. Although these adverse effects are usually of minor consequence, a more serious condition must be ruled out.

NOTE: When being seen by a healthcare provider or a dentist for other reasons, be sure to mention taking oral contraceptives.

Instructions for using the minipill. Start using the minipill on the first day of menstruation. Take one tablet daily, every day, regardless of when the next period is. Tablets should be taken at approximately the same time every day.

- *Missed pills:* If one pill is missed, take it as soon as remembered, and take the next pill at the regularly scheduled time. Use another form of birth control until the next period. If two pills are missed, take one of the missed pills immediately and take the regularly scheduled pill for that day on time. The next day, take the regularly scheduled pill and the other missed pill. Use another method of birth control until the next period.
- *Missed periods:* Some women note changes in the time as well as duration of their periods while using minipills. This is to be expected. If menses is every 28 to 30 days, ovulation may still be occurring. For maximal safety, use alternative forms of contraception on days 10 through 18. If irregular bleeding occurs every 25 to 45 days, ovulation is probably not regular. If all tablets are taken correctly but no period has resulted for more than 60 days, speak to the healthcare provider about a pregnancy test.
- NOTE: Report sudden, severe abdominal pain, with or without nausea and vomiting, to the healthcare

provider immediately. There is a higher incidence of ectopic pregnancy with the minipill because it does not inhibit ovulation in all women.

- *Serious adverse effects to be reported as soon as possible:* Severe headaches, dizziness, blurred vision, leg pain, shortness of breath, chest pain, and acute abdominal pain. Although these adverse effects are usually of minor consequence, a more serious condition must be ruled out.
- *Duration of oral contraceptive therapy:* Many healthcare providers prefer to have their patients discontinue the pill for 3 of every 28 months. This allows the body to return to a normal cycle. Be sure to use other forms of contraception during this time. Long-term use (3 or more years) must be determined on an individual basis.
- *Discontinuing the pill for conception:* Because of a possibility of birth defects, discontinue the pill 3 months before attempting pregnancy. Use other methods of contraception for these 3 months.

◆ **Common adverse effects.** These are the most common adverse effects of hormonal contraceptive therapy. If these symptoms are not resolved after 3 months of therapy, the woman should return to her healthcare provider for reevaluation and a possible change in prescription.

Gastrointestinal. Nausea.

Gynecologic, hormonal. Weight gain, spotting, changed menstrual flow, missed periods, chloasma (facial pigmentation).

Psychological, neurologic. Depression, mood changes, headaches.

◆ **Serious adverse effects.** The following symptoms represent the development of secondary disorders. Examination, a change in oral contraceptive, and possible treatment with other medications may be necessary.

Gynecologic. Vaginal discharge, breakthrough bleeding, yeast infection.

Neurologic

Blurred vision, severe headaches, dizziness. Report as soon as possible. These adverse effects are usually of minor consequence, but they may be early indications of serious adverse effects.

Cardiovascular

Leg pain, chest pain, shortness of breath. Report as soon as possible; these may be early indications of serious adverse effects.

Gastrointestinal

Acute abdominal pain. Report as soon as possible; this may be an early indication of serious adverse effects.

◆ **Drug interactions**

Drugs that reduce therapeutic effects

- Barbiturates, carbamazepine, oxcarbazepine, felbamate, phenytoin, primidone, topiramate, St. John's wort, and the antiviral protease inhibitors (e.g., saquinavir, ritonavir, indinavir, nelfinavir, amprenavir) may increase the rate of metabolism of the oral contraceptive hormones in the liver, possibly decreasing their contraceptive effect. An alternative or additional form of birth control is advisable during concurrent use.

- Antibacterial agents (e.g., penicillins, tetracyclines, rifampin, isoniazid, griseofulvin) apparently alter metabolism of hormones in the gut, making the contraceptive less effective. An alternative or additional form of birth control is advisable during concurrent use.

Herbal Interactions

St. John's Wort

St. John's wort may increase the liver's metabolism of oral contraceptive hormones, possibly resulting in decreased contraceptive effect. An alternative or additional form of birth control is advisable during concurrent use.

Drugs that enhance therapeutic and toxic effects. Itraconazole and ketoconazole may inhibit the metabolism of oral contraceptives. Menstrual irregularities also may be noted. Adjustment of hormone dosage may be necessary.

Warfarin. Oral contraceptives may diminish or enhance the anticoagulant effects of warfarin. Monitor the prothrombin time and the international normalized ratio, and adjust the dosage of warfarin if necessary.

Phenytoin. Monitor patients with concurrent therapy for signs of breakthrough seizures or phenytoin toxicity—nystagmus, sedation, and lethargy. Serum levels may be ordered, and a change in dosage of phenytoin may be required.

Thyroid hormones. Patients who have no thyroid function and who start estrogen therapy may require an increase in thyroid hormone dosage. Estrogens increase thyroid-binding globulin levels, which reduce the level of circulating free thyroxine (T_4). The total level of T_4 is either normal or increased. Do not adjust the thyroid hormone dosage until the patient shows clinical signs of hypothyroidism.

Benzodiazepines. Oral contraceptives appear to have a variable effect on the metabolism of benzodiazepines. Those that have reduced metabolism with an increase in therapeutic response and toxic effect are alprazolam, clorazepate, chlordiazepoxide, diazepam, and flurazepam. Benzodiazepines that have enhanced metabolism and reduced therapeutic activity when taken with oral contraceptives are lorazepam, oxazepam, and temazepam. Adjust the dosage of the benzodiazepine accordingly.

DRUG CLASS: TRANSDERMAL CONTRACEPTIVES

norelgestromin–ethinyl estradiol transdermal system
(nōr-ĕl-JĔS-trō-mĭn–ĔTH-ĭ-nĕl ĕs-trĕ-DĪ-ŏl)
Xulane (ZŪ-lān)

Actions

Ethinyl estradiol, an estrogen, and norelgestromin, a progestin, work together as a contraceptive by inhibiting ovulation. Estrogens block pituitary release of FSH, preventing the ovaries from developing a follicle that releases an ovum. Progestins inhibit pituitary release of LH, the hormone responsible for releasing an ovum from a follicle. Other mechanisms play a contributory role in preventing conception. Estrogens and progestins alter cervical mucus by making it thick and viscous, inhibiting sperm migration. Hormones also change the endometrial wall, impairing implantation of the fertilized ovum.

Uses

The transdermal contraceptive system works very much like the combination oral contraceptives, except that the estrogen and progestin hormones are in a transdermal patch dosage form that is applied weekly for 3 weeks. During the fourth week of the menstrual cycle, no patch is worn and withdrawal bleeding (menses) should begin.

In November 2005, the FDA issued a cautionary note about concern for greater exposure to estrogens from the patch compared with taking a similar oral contraceptive tablet product. In general, increased estrogen exposure increases the risk of blood clots. Although the FDA believes that the transdermal contraceptive system is a safe and effective method of contraception, the FDA encourages women to discuss the issue with their healthcare provider, particularly if they are at higher risk for cardiovascular diseases based on the presence of hypertension, obesity, diabetes, smoking, and/or older age.

Cigarette smoking increases the risk of serious adverse cardiovascular effects (e.g., blood clots) in those who both smoke and use combination contraceptives. This risk increases with age and heavy smoking (at least 15 cigarettes per day) and is significant in women older than 35 years. Women who use combination contraceptives such as the transdermal patch are strongly encouraged not to smoke.

Therapeutic Outcome

The primary therapeutic outcome associated with transdermal contraceptive therapy is prevention of pregnancy.

❖ Nursing Implications for Transdermal Contraceptives

◆ Premedication assessment

1. Review the medical history. If there is a history of hypertension, gallbladder disease, diabetes mellitus, severe varicose veins, seizure disorders, oligomenorrhea or amenorrhea, rheumatic heart disease, thromboembolic disease, stroke, malignancy of breast or the reproductive system, renal or liver disease, severe mental depression, suspected pregnancy, or repeated contraceptive failure, or if the patient

smokes, consult with the healthcare provider before dispensing birth control patches.

2. Take a baseline blood pressure in the supine and sitting positions.
3. Ensure that a pregnancy test has been given and that the patient is not pregnant.

◆ *Availability. Transdermal patch:* 4.86 mg norelgestromin and 0.53 mg ethinyl estradiol per patch. The patch releases 150 mcg of norelgestromin and 35 mcg of ethinyl estradiol per 24 hours.

◆ *Implementation*

Before initiating therapy. The patient should have a complete physical examination that includes blood pressure, pelvic and breast examinations, Pap smear, urinalysis, and hemoglobin or hematocrit. A pregnancy test should be performed on sexually active female patients.

Instructions for using transdermal contraceptives. A new patch should be applied on the same day of the week. This day is known as "patch change day." The patch should be applied to clean, dry, intact, healthy skin on the buttock, abdomen, upper outer arm, or upper torso in a place where it will not be rubbed by tight clothing. Patches should not be placed on red irritated skin or on the breasts. Patches should not be cut. Topical products such as makeup, powder, lotions, or creams should not be applied to the skin or to the patch area because the patch may not adhere properly and absorption of the hormones may be impaired.

Select one of the following methods to start contraception:

- *First day start:* Apply the first patch during the first 24 hours of the menstrual period. Note on a calendar the day of the week as a reminder of patch change day. If the patch is started after the first 24 hours of the menstrual cycle, a nonhormonal backup contraceptive (condoms, spermicidal foam, diaphragm) should be used concurrently for the first 7 consecutive days of the first cycle.
- *Sunday start:* Start the first patch on the first Sunday after menses begins. A nonhormonal backup contraceptive (condoms, spermicidal foam, diaphragm) should be used concurrently for the first 7 consecutive days of the first cycle.
- *Switching from oral contraceptives to the patches:* Apply a patch on the first day of the menses. If there is no withdrawal bleeding within 5 days of the last active hormone tablet (after day 21), a pregnancy test should be completed to ensure that there is no pregnancy before the patch is started.

> **! Medication Safety Alert**
>
> When removing the patch, dispose of it properly. Fold the used patch over on itself and place in a sturdy container, preferably with a child-resistant cap, and discard in a waste receptacle out of reach of children and pets. It still contains active hormone residual. Do not flush down the toilet.

If a patch is partially or completely detached:

- *For less than 24 hours:* Try to reapply the patch in the same place or replace it with a new patch immediately. No backup contraception is necessary. Patch change day will remain the same. Do not try to reapply the patch if the adhesive will not adhere to the skin. Do not use other adhesives or tape to hold a patch in place. Apply a new patch in a different location.
- *For more than 24 hours or if not sure how long since detachment:* Because there may be a lack of protection from pregnancy, stop the current contraceptive cycle and start a new cycle immediately by applying a new patch. This is a "new day 1" and a new patch change day. A nonhormonal backup contraceptive (condoms, spermicidal foam, diaphragm) should be used concurrently for the first 7 consecutive days of the new cycle.

If a woman forgets to change the patch:

- *At the start of any patch cycle (week 1/day 1):* There may be a lack of protection from pregnancy. Apply the new patch as soon as it is remembered. This is a new day 1 and a new patch change day. A nonhormonal backup contraceptive (condoms, spermicidal foam, diaphragm) should be used concurrently for the first 7 consecutive days of the new cycle.
- In the middle of the patch cycle (week 2/day 8 or week 3/day 15):
    - *For up to 48 hours:* Apply a new patch immediately. The next patch should be applied on the usual patch change day. No backup contraception is needed.
    - *For more than 48 hours:* Because there may be a lack of protection from pregnancy, stop the current contraceptive cycle and start a new 4-week cycle immediately by applying a new patch. This is a new day 1 and a new patch change day. A nonhormonal backup contraceptive (condoms, spermicidal foam, diaphragm) should be used concurrently for the first 7 consecutive days of the new cycle.
- *At the end of the patch cycle (week 4/day 22):* The patch should be removed as soon as the woman remembers to remove it. The new cycle should be started on the usual patch change day, which is the day after day 28. No backup contraception is needed.

Other important points:

- *Missed patches and skipped periods:* Return to the healthcare provider for a pregnancy test.
- *Skipping one period but not missing a patch:* It is not uncommon for a woman to occasionally miss a period when receiving hormone therapy. Start the next cycle on the same patch change day. If two consecutive periods are missed, a pregnancy test is in order. Contraceptive therapy should be discontinued if pregnancy is confirmed.
- *Spotting for two or more cycles:* See the healthcare provider to have other causes of bleeding assessed.
- *Periodic examinations:* A yearly examination should include blood pressure tests, pelvic examination, urinalysis, breast examination, and Pap smear.

- *Serious adverse effects to be reported as soon as possible:* Severe headaches, dizziness, blurred vision, leg pain, shortness of breath, chest pain, and acute abdominal pain. Although these adverse effects are usually of minor consequence, absence of serious adverse effects such as thromboembolism or ectopic pregnancy must be confirmed.

  NOTE: When being seen by a healthcare provider or a dentist for other reasons, be sure to mention that hormonal contraceptives are being taken.

◆ *Common and serious adverse effects.* See Common Adverse Effects and Serious Adverse Effects for Oral Contraceptives earlier in this section.

◆ *Drug interactions.* See Drug Interactions for Oral Contraceptives earlier in this section.

DRUG CLASS: INTRAVAGINAL HORMONAL CONTRACEPTIVES

etonogestrel–ethinyl estradiol vaginal ring (ē-tŏn-ō-GĔS-trĕl–ĔTH-ĭ-nĕl ĕs-trĕ-DĪ-ŏl VĂ-gĭ-năl RĬNG)
  NuvaRing (NŪ-vă-rĭng)
segestrone–ethinyl estradiol vaginal ring (sedg-est-rohn)
  Annovera (ahn-ov-rah)

Actions

An estrogen (ethinyl estradiol) and a progestin (etonogestrel or segestrone) work together as a contraceptive by inhibiting ovulation. Estrogens block pituitary release of FSH, preventing the ovaries from developing a follicle that releases an ovum. Progestins inhibit pituitary release of LH, the hormone responsible for releasing an ovum from a follicle. Other mechanisms play a contributory role in preventing conception. Estrogens and progestins alter cervical mucus by making it thick and viscous, inhibiting sperm migration. Hormones also change the endometrial wall, impairing implantation of the fertilized ovum.

Uses

The NuvaRing and Annovera vaginal rings work very much like the combination oral contraceptives, except that the estrogen and progestin hormones are in a plastic ring dosage form that the woman inserts into her vagina for 3 weeks. The ring is removed for a 1-week break, during which withdrawal bleeding (menses) should begin.

Cigarette smoking increases the risk of serious adverse cardiovascular effects (e.g., blood clots) in persons who both smoke and use combination contraceptives. This risk increases with age and heavy smoking (at least 15 cigarettes per day) and is quite significant in women older than 35 years. Women who use hormone contraceptives are strongly encouraged not to smoke.

Therapeutic Outcome

The primary therapeutic outcome associated with intravaginal hormone contraceptive therapy is prevention of pregnancy.

❖ **Nursing Implications for Intravaginal Hormonal Contraceptive**

◆ *Premedication assessment*

1. Review the medical history. If there is a history of hypertension, gallbladder disease, diabetes mellitus, severe varicose veins, seizure disorders, oligomenorrhea or amenorrhea, rheumatic heart disease, thromboembolic disease, stroke, malignancy of breast or the reproductive system, renal or liver disease, severe mental depression, suspected pregnancy, or repeated contraceptive failure, or if the patient smokes, consult with the healthcare provider before dispensing the birth control ring.
2. Take a baseline blood pressure in the supine and sitting positions.
3. Ensure that a pregnancy test has been given and that the patient is not pregnant.

◆ *Availability.* NuvaRing releases 0.12 mg etonogestrel and 0.015 mg ethinyl estradiol per day.

  Annovera releases 0.15 mg segesterone and 0.015 mg ethinyl estradiol per day.

◆ *Implementation*

  Before initiating therapy. The patient should have a complete physical examination that includes blood pressure, pelvic and breast examinations, Pap smear, urinalysis, and hemoglobin or hematocrit.
  Instructions for using the intravaginal hormonal contraceptive

- *Insertion:* Selecting a comfortable position, compress the ring and insert into the vagina. The exact position inside the vagina is not critical for its function but should be behind the pelvic bone. Insert on the appropriate day, as described later, and leave in place for 3 consecutive weeks. Check regularly (such as before and after intercourse) to ensure that the ring is in place to provide optimal protection.
- *Removal:* Remove the ring 3 weeks later on the same day of the week as it was inserted and at about the same time. Remove by hooking the index finger under the forward rim or by grasping the rim between the index and middle fingers and pulling it out.
  - NuvaRing: Place the used ring in the foil pouch and discard in a waste receptacle out of reach of children and pets. It still contains active hormone residual. Do not flush down the toilet. Insert a new ring on day 7 (the same day and time of the week) that the old ring was removed.
  - Annovera: After removal, wash with warm water and mild soap, dry with a clean cloth or paper towel, and store in the case provided. Reinsert the same ring on day 7 (the same day and time of the week) that the ring was removed, washed, and stored).

Select one of the following methods to start contraception:

- *If no hormonal contraceptive was in use in the past month:* Counting the first day of menstruation as day 1, insert the contraceptive ring on or prior to day 5 of the cycle, even if menses is continuing. Note on a calendar the day of the week as a reminder of the removal day 3 weeks later. A nonhormonal backup contraceptive (e.g., condoms, spermicidal foam, diaphragm) should be used concurrently for the first 7 consecutive days of continuous ring use.

- *Switching from a combination oral contraceptive:* Insert the ring any time within 7 days after the last active combined oral contraceptive tablet and no later than the day that a new cycle of pills would have been started. No backup contraception is necessary.

- *Switching from a progestin-only minipill:* Insert the ring the following day after discontinuing the minipill. A nonhormonal backup contraceptive (e.g., condoms, spermicidal foam, diaphragm) should be used concurrently for the first 7 consecutive days of continuous ring use.

If the ring is expelled or removed, or there is a prolonged ring-free interval during the active 3 weeks:

- *For less than 2 hours:* Rinse the ring in cool or lukewarm (not hot) water and reinsert as soon as possible.

- *For longer than 2 hours or if not sure how long since expelled:* If the ring has been out for longer than 2 hours, there may be a lack of protection from pregnancy. Reinsert the ring, but use a nonhormonal backup contraceptive (e.g., condoms, spermicidal foam, diaphragm) for the next 7 consecutive days of continuous ring use.

If a woman forgets to change the ring:

- *If left in place for up to 1 extra week (4 weeks total):* Remove it and insert a new ring after a 1-week ring-free interval. Use a nonhormonal backup contraceptive (e.g., condoms, spermicidal foam, diaphragm) for the next 7 consecutive days of continuous ring use.

- *If left in place for more than 4 weeks:* Remove the ring. Rule out pregnancy. Insert a new ring after a 1-week ring-free interval if not pregnant. Use a nonhormonal backup contraceptive (e.g., condoms, spermicidal foam, diaphragm) for the next 7 consecutive days of continuous ring use.

Other important points:

- *Missing one period but being adherent to the program:* It is not uncommon for a woman to occasionally miss a period when receiving hormone therapy. Start the next cycle on the same insertion day (i.e., on the 29th day). If two consecutive periods are missed, a pregnancy test is in order. Contraceptive therapy should be discontinued if pregnancy is confirmed.

- *Missed one period and the ring was out for more than 2 hours or was left in for more than 4 weeks:* Return to the healthcare provider for a pregnancy test.

- *Spotting for two or more cycles:* See the healthcare provider to have other causes of bleeding assessed.

- *Periodic examinations:* A yearly examination should include blood pressure tests, pelvic examination, urinalysis, breast examination, and Pap smear.

- *Serious adverse effects to be reported as soon as possible:* Severe headaches, dizziness, blurred vision, leg pain, shortness of breath, chest pain, and acute abdominal pain. Although these adverse effects are usually of minor consequence, absence of serious adverse effects such as thromboembolism or ectopic pregnancy must be confirmed.

NOTE: When being seen by a healthcare provider or a dentist for other reasons, be sure to mention that hormonal contraceptives are being taken.

◆**Common and serious adverse effects.** See Common Adverse Effects and Serious Adverse Effects for Oral Contraceptives earlier in this section.

◆**Drug Interactions.** See Drug Interactions for Oral Contraceptives earlier in this section.

OSTEOPOROSIS

Osteoporosis is the most common bone disease. It is characterized by low bone mineral density (BMD) (i.e., low bone mass) and microarchitectural alterations that result in bone fragility and increased risk of fractures. The bones most commonly affected by osteoporosis include the hip, spine, and wrist. Over 50 million men and women in the United States have osteoporosis or osteopenia (low BMD). About one of every two people in the United States older than 50 years is at risk for an osteoporotic fracture.

Bone is living tissue that is constantly being broken down and replaced (bone remodeling). The process of bone remodeling maintains a healthy skeleton. Bone remodeling occurs at specific sites within the skeleton and proceeds in an orderly fashion; bone resorption is always followed by bone formation. Osteoclasts are responsible for bone resorption, whereas osteoblasts are responsible for bone formation. Both types of cells are dependent on each other for the process of bone remodeling. In osteopenia and osteoporosis, the balance is altered between osteoclasts and osteoblasts, resulting in greater bone removal than replacement. Osteoclasts require weeks to resorb bone, whereas osteoblasts need months to produce new bone. Therefore any process that increases the rate of bone remodeling results in net bone loss over time.

Risk factors associated with osteoporosis and fractures include (but are not limited to) increasing age, female sex, postmenopausal women, hypogonadism (decreased sex hormones), low body weight, history of parental hip fracture, ethnic background (white persons are at higher risk than black persons), rheumatoid arthritis, current smoking, alcohol intake (3 or more drinks daily), low BMD, vitamin D deficiency, and low calcium intake. Another risk factor for osteoporotic fracture is long-term use of certain medications; the most commonly implicated drugs are glucocorticoids, anticoagulants, anticonvulsants, aromatase inhibitors, anticancer drugs, and gonadotropin-releasing hormone agonists.

Osteoporosis is often diagnosed after the occurrence of fragility fracture (a type of fracture that occurs as result of normal activities, such as a fall from standing height or less). In patients without fragility fracture, osteoporosis is often diagnosed by low BMD. Dual-energy x-ray absorptiometry (DEXA) is the current gold standard test for diagnosing osteoporosis in people without an osteoporotic fracture. Results of DEXA are scored as the number of standard deviations (SDs) from a young, healthy norm (usually female) and reported as T scores. For example, a T score of −2 indicates a BMD that is 2 SDs below the comparative norm. A T score of −2.5 or below indicates the presence of osteoporosis. The international reference standard for the description of osteoporosis in postmenopausal women and in men age 50 years or older is a femoral neck BMD of 2.5 SDs or more below the young female adult mean T score of 2. However, low BMD as measured by DEXA is an imperfect predictor of fracture risk, identifying less than one-half of the people who go on to have an osteoporotic fracture.

Several interventions to preserve bone strength are recommended to the general population. These include an adequate intake of calcium and vitamin D, lifelong participation in regular weight-bearing and muscle-strengthening exercises, cessation of tobacco use, identification and treatment of alcoholism, and identification of risk factors for falling.

DRUG THERAPY FOR OSTEOPOROSIS

According to the guidelines of the American College of Physicians and of the American Association of Clinical Endocrinologists and American College of Endocrinologists, the bisphosphonates (alendronate, risedronate, and zoledronic acid) and denosumab are appropriate as initial therapy for most patients with osteoporosis. They all reduce hip, nonvertebral, and vertebral (spine) fractures. Other treatments include abaloparatide, ibandronate, raloxifene, and teriparatide. Dietary and supplemental calcium and vitamin D are also used for treatment.

❖ NURSING IMPLICATIONS FOR OSTEOPOROSIS

◆ Assessment

History of risk factors

Smoking. Obtain a history of the number of cigarettes or cigars that the patient smokes daily; include other sources of nicotine, such as chewing tobacco and replacement therapy. How long has the person smoked? Has the person ever tried to stop smoking? Ask if the patient understands the effect of smoking on bone health. How does the individual feel about modifying his or her smoking habit?

Dietary habits. Obtain a dietary history. Ask specific questions to obtain data relating to the amount of calcium- and vitamin D–rich foods, such as milk, that are consumed on a daily basis.

Psychomotor functions

- Determine the patient's type of lifestyle. Have the patient describe exercise level in terms of amount (e.g., walking 3 miles), intensity (e.g., walking 3 mph), and frequency (e.g., walking every other day). Is the patient's job physically demanding or of a sedentary nature?
- Determine the patient's level of psychological stress. Ask the individual to estimate the amount of stress in his or her life. How does the person cope with stressful situations at home and in the workplace?

Alcohol. Determine if the patient consumes alcohol greater than 3 drinks daily, and counsel the need to decrease consumption or stop altogether.

Dentition. Nurses should provide education regarding the need for dental examination prior to initiation of medication. Complications from the use of these drugs have been associated with dental work, such as tooth extractions, dental implants, dental surgery, and poor oral hygiene. Good oral hygiene needs to be stressed.

Pain. Assess for and report increased pain in hips, groin, or thighs with long-term use of medication.

◆ Implementation

- Perform nursing assessments on a scheduled basis.
- Make referrals as indicated for stress management, smoking cessation, and dietary counseling and for an exercise program appropriate for the individual's needs.
- Protect the patient from possible falls by assisting during ambulation.

◆ Patient Education

Suggest that patients stop smoking if they do smoke. Provide educational materials for smoking cessation. Smoking has been linked to osteoporosis because studies have indicated that nicotine interferes with the function and growth of the osteoblasts. Therefore encourage a drastic reduction in—and preferably total abstinence from—smoking. Include information about smoking cessation and available support resources.

Fostering health maintenance

- Throughout the course of treatment, discuss medication information and how it will benefit the patient.
- Teach patient how to manage symptoms of osteoporosis, specifically pain.

- Explain the need to maintain an exercise program and modify dietary habits to increase calcium and vitamin D in the diet. Cessation of smoking and minimal alcoholic intake are strongly recommended.
- Provide the patient and significant others with the important information contained in the specific drug monographs for the drugs prescribed. Additional health teaching and nursing interventions for common and serious adverse effects will be found in each drug monograph.
- Seek cooperation and understanding of the following points so that medication compliance is increased: name of medication; dosage, routes, and times of administration; and common and serious adverse effects.

Patient self-assessment. Enlist the patient's help in developing and maintaining a written record of monitoring parameters (e.g., blood pressures, weight, exercise). See the Patient Self-Assessment Form for Osteoporosis Agents on the Evolve website. Complete the Premedication Data column for use as a baseline to track response to drug therapy. Ensure that the patient understands how to use the form, and instruct the patient to bring the completed form to follow-up visits. During follow-up visits, focus on issues that will foster adherence with the therapeutic interventions prescribed.

DRUG CLASS: BISPHOSPHONATES

Actions

Bisphosphonates (alendronate, risedronate, and zoledronic acid) inhibit bone resorption by actions on osteoclasts. Decreasing the rate of bone resorption leads to an indirect increase in BMD.

Uses

Alendronate is used in the treatment and prevention of osteoporosis in postmenopausal women, the treatment of osteoporosis in men, and the treatment of glucocorticoid-induced osteoporosis in men and women with low BMD who are receiving a daily dosage of 7.5 mg or more of prednisone.

Risedronate is used in the treatment and prevention of osteoporosis in postmenopausal women, the treatment of osteoporosis in men, and the treatment and prevention of glucocorticoid-induced osteoporosis.

Zoledronic acid is used in the treatment and prevention of osteoporosis in postmenopausal women, the treatment of osteoporosis in men, and the treatment and prevention of glucocorticoid-induced osteoporosis in men and women who are initiating or continuing systemic glucocorticoids in a daily dosage equivalent to 7.5 mg or more of prednisone and who are expected to remain on glucocorticoids for at least 12 months.

Therapeutic Outcome

The primary therapeutic outcome for bisphosphonates is to reduce fractures in patients with osteoporosis.

❖ Nursing Implications for Bisphosphonates

◆ *Premedication assessment*

1. Obtain the patient's baseline vital signs and note any bone pain present prior to treatment.
2. Encourage an adequate calcium and vitamin D intake in the diet while taking these drugs.
3. Provide education regarding the need for a dental examination prior to initiation of medication.
4. Check laboratory values for calcium, magnesium, and phosphate.

◆ *Availability, dosage, and administration*
See Table 40.6.

 Medication Safety Alert

Administer bisphosphonates in the morning 30 minutes or more before the first food, beverage (except plain water), or other medication(s) of the day. Do not take with mineral water or with other beverages. Patients should be instructed to sit or stand upright (not to lie down) for at least 30 minutes after administration and until after first food of the day (to reduce esophageal irritation).

Oral solution: Must be followed with at least 2 ounces of plain water.

Tablets: Must be taken with 6 to 8 ounces of plain water. The tablet should be swallowed whole.

Effervescent tablet: Dissolve one tablet in 4 ounces of room-temperature plain water only; once effervescence stops, wait 5 minutes or more and stir the solution for approximately 10 seconds to remove bubbles and then drink.

◆ *Common adverse effects*

Neurologic

Headache. Tell the patient that a headache may occur but tends be self-limiting.

Gastrointestinal

Abdominal pain, gastroesophageal reflux disease, dyspepsia, constipation, diarrhea. These adverse effects are most common and are usually mild and tend to resolve with continued therapy. If adverse effects become more severe, the patient should contact the healthcare provider.

Musculoskeletal pain. This is a common adverse effect. It is usually mild and tends to resolve with continued therapy. If adverse effects become more severe, the patient should contact the healthcare provider

◆ *Serious adverse effects*

Dysphagia, gastritis, gastric ulcers. Bisphosphonates given orally may cause local irritation of the upper gastrointestinal mucosa. Use caution in patients with active upper gastrointestinal problems such as dysphagia, gastritis, or ulcers. Patients should be instructed to discontinue therapy and alert the healthcare provider if difficulty in swallowing, pain on swallowing, chest pain, or new or worsening heartburn develops.

Table 40.6 Bisphosphonates

GENERIC NAME	BRAND NAME	AVAILABILITY	DOSAGE
alendronate	Fosamax Binosto	Solution: 70 mg/75 mL Tablets: 5, 10, 35, 70 mg Effervescent tablet: 70 mg	Glucocorticoid-induced osteoporosis: PO: 5 mg once daily; Postmenopausal women not receiving estrogen PO: 10 mg once daily Osteoporosis in men: PO: 70 mg once weekly or 10 mg once daily Osteoporosis in postmenopausal women: *Prevention:* PO: 35 mg once weekly or 5 mg once daily *Treatment:* PO: 70 mg once weekly or 10 mg once daily
risedronate	Actonel	Tablets: 5, 35, 150 mg	Glucocorticoid-induced osteoporosis: PO: 5 mg daily Osteoporosis in men: PO: 35 mg once weekly Osteoporosis in postmenopausal women: PO: 5 mg daily or 35 mg once weekly or 150 mg once a month
zoledronic acid	Reclast Aclasta ♣	IV Solution: 5 mg/100 mL	Osteoporosis treatment: 5 mg IV infusion over no less than 15 min once a year Osteoporosis prevention: Reclast: IV: 5 mg once every 2 yr Aclasta: IV: 5 mg as a single (one-time) dose Glucocorticoid-induced osteoporosis: 5 mg IV infusion over no less than 15 min once a year

♣ Available in Canada.

Musculoskeletal pain. Incapacitating bone, joint, and or muscle pain has been reported. The onset of symptoms varies from 1 day to several months. Patients should be instructed to discontinue therapy and contact the healthcare provider if severe symptoms develop.

Nephrotoxicity. Bisphosphonates are contraindicated in patients with a creatinine clearance of less than 35 mL/min.

Zoledronic acid should be used with caution in patients with chronic renal impairment, especially in patients with preexisting renal compromise, as well as patients with advanced age, concomitant nephrotoxic medications, concomitant diuretic therapy, or severe dehydration.

Osteonecrosis of the jaw. Osteonecrosis of the jaw is generally associated with tooth extraction. Risk factors include tooth extractions, dental implants, dental surgery, diagnosis of cancer, and poor oral hygiene. The risk increases with duration of treatment.

Atypical femoral fractures. Atypical femoral fractures may occur with minimal or no trauma to the affected area. Patients should report any thigh or groin pain. Stopping the bisphosphonates should be considered after discussion with the healthcare provider.

◆ *Drug interactions*

Calcium supplements/antacids. Coadministration with calcium and antacids will interfere with the absorption of oral bisphosphonates. Patients should wait at least 30 minutes after taking bisphosphonates before taking calcium or antacids.

Aspirin and nonsteroidal antiinflammatory drugs. The incidence of upper gastrointestinal adverse effects is increased with daily oral doses of aspirin or nonsteroidal antiinflammatory drugs while taking bisphosphonates. Use caution because administration of nonsteroidal antiinflammatory drugs is associated with gastrointestinal irritation.

Nephrotoxic drugs. Use caution when taking zoledronic acid with other potentially nephrotoxic drugs such as nonsteroidal antiinflammatory drugs and aminoglycosides.

denosumab (dĕn-Ō-sū-măb)
Prolia

Actions

Denosumab is a monoclonal antibody that prevents osteoclast formation, leading to decreased bone resorption and increased bone mass in patients with osteoporosis.

Uses

Denosumab is used in the treatment of osteoporosis in postmenopausal women and men at high risk of fracture and in glucocorticoid-induced osteoporosis.

It is also used as treatment for bone loss in men receiving androgen deprivation therapy (e.g., leuprolide) for nonmetastatic prostate cancer and treatment of bone loss in women receiving aromatase inhibitor therapy (e.g., anastrozole) for breast cancer.

Therapeutic Outcome

The therapeutic outcomes for denosumab are a reduction in fractures in patients with osteoporosis and prevention of bone loss in men receiving androgen deprivation therapy and women receiving aromatase inhibitors for breast cancer.

❖ Nursing Implications for denosumab

◆ Premedication assessment

1. Obtain baseline temperature, blood pressure, and heart rate.
2. Check laboratory values for calcium, magnesium, and phosphate.

◆ Availability. *Subcutaneous solution:* 60 mg/mL in 1-mL prefilled syringe; 120 mg/1.7 mL in 1.7-mL vial.

◆ Dosage and administration. Denosumab should be administered subcutaneously in the upper arm, upper thigh, or abdomen by a healthcare professional.

Instruct patients to take calcium 1000 mg daily and at least 400 IU vitamin D daily.

Treatment of androgen deprivation–induced bone loss in men with prostate cancer: **Subcutaneous:** 60 mg as a single dose, once every 6 months.

Treatment of aromatase inhibitor–induced bone loss in women with breast cancer: **Subcutaneous:** 60 mg as a single dose, once every 6 months.

Treatment of osteoporosis in men or in postmenopausal women: **Subcutaneous:** 60 mg as a single dose, once every 6 months.

Treatment of glucocorticoid-induced osteoporosis: Subcutaneous: 60 mg as a single dose, once every 6 months.

◆ Common adverse effects

Dermatologic. Dermatitis (4% to 11%), eczema (4% to 11%), skin rash (3% to 11%).

Cardiovascular. Hypertension, hypercholesterolemia in women.

Musculoskeletal. Arthralgia (7% to 14%), limb pain (10% to 12%), back pain (8% to 12%).

Urinary. Cystitis may occur in women. Instruct the patient to contact the healthcare provider.

◆ Serious adverse effects. Instruct the patient to contact the healthcare provider regarding the following symptoms or conditions.

Hypersensitivity. Anaphylactic reactions may occur. Denosumab may be discontinued permanently if a significant reaction occurs.

Hypocalcemia. Obtain calcium level before initiating therapy; a deficient level must be corrected before initiating denosumab therapy. Adequately supplement patients with calcium and vitamin D.

Osteonecrosis of the jaw. Monitor for symptoms of jaw pain, difficulty in chewing.

Atypical femoral fractures. Evaluate patients with thigh or groin pain to rule out a femoral fracture.

Infections. The patient may develop signs or symptoms of infection such as fever, tenderness and inflammation, or muscle or joint pain.

Dermatologic reactions. Severe symptoms of dermatitis, rashes, and eczema may develop.

◆ Drug interactions. No drug interactions have been reported.

BENIGN PROSTATIC HYPERPLASIA

The prostate gland functions as part of the male reproductive system. It is a firm organ, weighing about 20 g, the size of a walnut. It is located at the base of the urinary bladder and completely surrounds the proximal urethra. As part of the male reproductive system, it produces a fluid during ejaculation that mixes with sperm from the testes and fluid from the seminal vesicles to form semen. The gland may also protect against urinary tract infections through secretion of prostatic antibacterial factor. Two other chemicals secreted by the prostate gland are acid phosphatase and prostate-specific antigen (PSA). An elevated PSA level may indicate the presence of prostate cancer.

Enlargement of the prostate gland as men age is an almost universal phenomenon. A condition called *enlarged prostate, prostatism,* or **benign prostatic hyperplasia** *(BPH)* is common later in life, affecting more than 50% of men in their 60s and as many as 90% in their 70s and 80s. Many men with BPH will need some type of treatment. Although an enlarged prostate is an apparently normal part of aging, problems with urination that often accompany this enlargement are not normal.

Benign prostatic hyperplasia is much more common than prostate cancer; however, an enlarged prostate gland can be caused by prostate cancer. Because the signs of enlarged prostate are often the same as the signs and symptoms of prostate cancer, it is important to obtain a healthcare provider's opinion so that the proper diagnosis can be made. The healthcare provider may also need to rule out prostate infection and other possible causes of the patient's symptoms.

The pathogenesis of BPH is not well understood, but it appears to involve the presence of increasing levels of dihydrotestosterone (DHT), caused by a slow increase in production, reduced metabolism, or both, that stimulate the growth of new prostate cells. Dihydrotestosterone is formed in the prostate gland from testosterone produced in the testes. The conversion of testosterone to DHT is catalyzed by the enzyme 5-alpha reductase.

The symptoms of BPH are highly variable and patient specific and are divided into two categories: obstructive and irritative (Box 40.4). Obstructive symptoms result directly from narrowing of the bladder neck and urethra. Irritative symptoms result from incomplete bladder emptying or urinary tract infection secondary to prostatic obstruction. As the prostate gland enlarges, it compresses the urethra, partially or completely obstructing urine flow from the bladder. Over time, symptoms become progressively worse, requiring medical attention. When necessary the hyperplastic tissue may be removed surgically to reduce the urinary obstruction. Transurethral resection or laser therapy may be used to treat glands smaller than 60 g, whereas larger glands are removed surgically (prostatectomy). Intermittent catheterization several times daily or placement of a permanent indwelling catheter may be used if the patient is not a candidate for surgery.

Box 40.4	Symptoms of Benign Prostatic Hyperplasia

OBSTRUCTIVE
- Reduced force of urinary stream
- Resistance to initiation of voiding
- Prolonged dribbling after urination
- Sensation of incomplete bladder emptying
- Decreased or interrupted stream
- Double voiding
- Straining or pushing to urinate

IRRITATIVE
- Increased frequency
- Nocturia
- Difficult or painful urination (dysuria)
- Sudden urgency
- Urge incontinence

DRUG THERAPY FOR BENIGN PROSTATIC HYPERPLASIA

Benign prostatic hyperplasia may also be treated successfully with medicines. The alpha-1 adrenergic blocking agents alfuzosin or tamsulosin are used to relax the smooth muscle of the bladder and prostate. Other alpha-1 adrenergic blocking agents (e.g., doxazosin, terazosin) are also used to treat hypertension (see Chapter 22). Antiandrogen agents, such as finasteride and dutasteride, selectively block androgens at the prostate cellular level and cause the prostate gland to shrink. Studies indicate that a combination of an alpha blocker with a 5-alpha reductase inhibitor is more effective in slowing the progression of BPH than either agent alone. The phosphodiesterase inhibitor tadalafil has also been approved for the treatment of BPH.

DRUG CLASS: ALPHA-1 ADRENERGIC BLOCKING AGENTS

Actions
Alpha-1 adrenergic blocking agents have selectivity for the alpha-1A receptor subtype found on the prostate gland. Approximately 70% of the alpha-1 receptors in the human prostate are of the alpha-1A subtype. Alfuzosin, silodosin, and tamsulosin are alpha-1A–specific adrenergic blocking agents, whereas doxazosin and terazosin are nonspecific alpha-1 blocking agents. These agents block alpha-1 receptors on the prostate gland and certain areas of the bladder neck, causing muscle relaxation and allowing greater urinary outflow in men with an enlarged prostate gland. Alpha-1 blocking agents do not reduce prostate size or inhibit testosterone synthesis as do the 5-alpha reductase inhibitors, nor do they affect PSA levels.

Uses
Alpha-1 blocking agents are used to reduce mild to moderate urinary obstruction manifestations (e.g., hesitancy, terminal urine dribbling, interrupted stream, impaired size and force of stream, sensation of incomplete bladder

emptying) in men with BPH. They produce a 20% to 30% increase in urine flow rate in up to 50% of men with urinary symptoms. Symptoms show improvement after 1 week of therapy, but 2 to 3 months of continued therapy are required to assess full effect. Alpha-1A–specific drugs (i.e., alfuzosin, tamsulosin, silodosin) are not used to treat hypertension.

Therapeutic Outcomes
The primary therapeutic outcomes expected from alpha-1 blocker therapy are reduced symptoms and improvement in urine flow associated with prostate gland enlargement.

❖ **Nursing Implications for Alpha-1 Adrenergic Blocking Agents**

◆ *Premedication assessment*
1. Obtain baseline blood pressure readings in supine and standing positions.
2. Check if the patient has a history of severe cerebral or coronary arteriosclerosis, gastritis, or peptic ulcer disease. (Reduction of blood pressure may diminish blood flow to these regions, causing therapy to worsen the condition.)

◆ *Availability, dosage, and administration*
See Table 40.7.

 Medication Safety Alert

The initial doses of the alpha-1 blocking agents may cause dizziness (6% to 7%) and hypotension with tachycardia and fainting (<0.5%) in patients starting therapy. This effect may be minimized by giving the first doses with food. Patients should be warned that this adverse effect might occur, it is transient, and they should lie down immediately if symptoms develop.

◆ *Common adverse effects*
Neurologic
Drowsiness, headache, dizziness, weakness, lethargy. Tell the patient that these adverse effects may occur but tend to be self-limiting. The patient should not stop taking the medication and should consult the healthcare provider if the problem becomes unacceptable.
Cardiovascular
Dizziness, tachycardia, fainting. Dizziness may occur in more than 2% of patients, and orthostatic hypotension occurs in less than 0.5% of patients when therapy is initiated. Symptoms develop 15 to 90 minutes after the first dose is taken. To decrease the incidence, administer the first dose with food. Instruct the patient to lie down immediately if these symptoms occur. Provide for the patient's safety.

◆ *Drug interactions*
Drugs that enhance therapeutic and toxic effects. Diuretics, cimetidine, tranquilizers, alcohol, barbiturates, antihistamines, beta-adrenergic blocking agents (e.g., propranolol, atenolol), and other antihypertensive agents should not be used with alfuzosin. Monitor the blood

Table 40.7   Alpha-1 Blocking Agents Used for Benign Prostatic Hyperplasia

GENERIC NAME	BRAND NAME	AVAILABILITY	DOSAGE
alfuzosin	Uroxatral	Tablets, extended-release (24 hr): 10 mg	PO: 10 mg daily to be taken immediately after the same meal each day Tablets should not be crushed or chewed
doxazosin	Cardura Cardura XL	Tablets: 1, 2, 4, 8 mg Tablets, extended-release (24 hr): 4, 8 mg	PO: 1-8 mg once daily
silodosin	Rapaflo	Capsules: 4, 8 mg	PO: 8 mg daily; 4 mg daily for patients with renal impairment
tamsulosin	Flomax	Capsules: 0.4 mg	PO: 0.4 mg daily, taken approximately 30 min following the same meal each day If symptoms are not adequately controlled after 2-4 wk of therapy, the dose may be increased to 0.8 mg once daily If administration is discontinued or interrupted for several days, at either the 0.4- or 0.8-mg dose, start therapy again with the 0.4-mg once-daily dose
terazosin	—	Capsules: 1, 2, 5, 10 mg	PO: Initial: 1 mg daily at bedtime Increase stepwise to 2 mg, 5 mg, or 10 mg daily to achieve desired response of symptoms and flow rate Maximum dose is 20 mg divided twice daily

pressure response to the cumulative effects of antihypertensive agents. Take the patient's blood pressure in supine and erect positions.

Ketoconazole, itraconazole, ritonavir, diltiazem, and other potent cytochrome P-450 component 3A4 inhibitors inhibit the metabolism of alfuzosin and should not be used concurrently with alfuzosin.

Monitor for an increase in severity of adverse side effects such as sedation, hypotension, and bradycardia or tachycardia.

Avanafil, sildenafil, tadalafil, vardenafil. These drugs are used to treat erectile dysfunction. They may aggravate hypotensive effects of doxazosin and terazosin, causing dizziness and tachycardia. Adjust by reducing the dose of the drugs used to treat erectile dysfunction.

DRUG CLASS: ANTIANDROGEN AGENTS

dutasteride (dŭ-TĂS-tĕr-īd)
  Avodart (ĂV-ō-dărt)

Actions
Dutasteride is an androgen hormone inhibitor that acts by inhibiting the enzyme 5-alpha reductase. The conversion of testosterone to DHT is catalyzed by 5-alpha reductase types 1 and 2. Reduction in DHT levels reduces the hyperplastic cell growth associated with prostatic hyperplasia.

Uses
Dutasteride inhibits 5-alpha reductase types 1 and 2. It is used to treat the symptoms associated with BPH, reduce the risks associated with urinary retention, and minimize the need for surgery associated with BPH. More than 6 to 12 months of treatment may be

necessary to assess whether a therapeutic response has been achieved. Patients who respond to therapy have fewer symptoms associated with partial obstruction, improved urinary flow rates, and a smaller prostate gland. Dutasteride is not approved by the FDA to treat male pattern baldness.

Therapeutic Outcomes
The primary therapeutic outcomes expected from dutasteride therapy are as follows:
- Reduced symptoms and improvement in urine flow associated with prostatic enlargement
- Reduced need for surgery for BPH

❖**Nursing Implications for dutasteride**
◆*Premedication assessment.* Obtain a baseline PSA blood level. Dutasteride causes a decrease in serum PSA levels by about 50% in patients with BPH, even in the presence of prostate cancer. Any sustained increase in PSA levels while a patient is receiving dutasteride should be investigated, including consideration of prostate cancer and noncompliance with therapy.

◆*Availability.* *PO:* 0.5-mg capsules.

 Medication Safety Alert

Dutasteride is contraindicated in women who are or may become pregnant because it may cause abnormalities of the external genitalia of a male fetus of a pregnant woman who received the drug. Dutasteride is absorbed through human skin. A woman who is pregnant or who may become pregnant should not handle crushed or broken dutasteride capsules.

Men treated with dutasteride should not donate blood until at least 6 months after stopping therapy to avoid introducing the drug to a pregnant woman.

◆ *Dosage and administration.* *PO:* 0.5 mg once daily, with or without food.

◆ **Common adverse effects**

Reproductive

Impotence, decreased libido, decreased volume of ejaculate. These adverse effects appear in small numbers of men receiving higher doses of dutasteride. Tell the patient that these adverse effects may occur but tend to be self-limiting. The incidence of impotence, decreased libido, and ejaculation disorder decreases with increasing duration of treatment. Decreased volume of ejaculate does not appear to interfere with normal sexual function. The patient should not stop taking the medication and should consult his healthcare provider if the problem becomes unacceptable.

◆ *Drug interactions*

Drugs that enhance toxic effects. Ketoconazole, itraconazole, ritonavir, diltiazem, verapamil, cimetidine, and ciprofloxacin inhibit the metabolism of dutasteride. Dutasteride should be given with extreme caution to men taking any of these medications.

---

finasteride (fĭn-ĂS-tĕr-īd)
  Proscar (PRŌ-skăr), **Propecia** (prō-PĒ-shē-ă)

Actions

Finasteride is an androgen hormone inhibitor that acts by inhibiting the enzyme 5-alpha reductase. The conversion of testosterone to DHT is catalyzed by 5-alpha reductase. Reduction in DHT levels reduces the hyperplastic cell growth associated with prostatic hyperplasia. Elevated DHT levels also induce androgenetic alopecia, more commonly known as *male pattern baldness* (vertex and anterior midscalp).

Uses

Finasteride inhibits 5-alpha reductase type 2. Proscar is used to treat the symptoms associated with BPH, reduce the risks associated with urinary retention, and minimize the need for surgery associated with BPH. More than 6 to 12 months of treatment may be necessary to assess whether a therapeutic response has been achieved. Patients who respond to therapy have fewer symptoms associated with partial obstruction, improved urinary flow rates, and a smaller prostate gland.

Propecia is used to treat androgenetic alopecia. After at least 3 months of daily use, finasteride maintains hair count and stimulates new hair growth in those who respond. Continued use is necessary to sustain the results. With discontinuation of treatment, the effects are reversed within 1 year. Finasteride does not appear to affect nonscalp body hair.

Therapeutic Outcomes

The primary therapeutic outcomes expected from finasteride therapy are as follows:

- Reduced symptoms and improvement in urine flow associated with prostatic enlargement
- Reversal of male pattern hair loss

❖ **Nursing Implications for finasteride**

◆ *Premedication assessment.* Obtain a baseline PSA blood level. Finasteride causes a decrease in serum PSA levels by about 50% in patients with BPH, even in the presence of prostate cancer. Any sustained increase in PSA levels while receiving finasteride should be investigated, including consideration of prostate cancer and noncompliance with therapy.

◆ *Availability.* *PO:* Proscar: 5-mg tablets; Propecia: 1-mg tablets.

◆ *Dosage and administration.* *BPH: PO:* 5 mg once daily, with or without food.

Androgenetic alopecia: PO: 1 mg once daily, with or without food.

> ⚠ **Medication Safety Alert**
>
> Finasteride is contraindicated in women who are or may become pregnant because it may cause abnormalities of the external genitalia of a male fetus of a pregnant woman who received the drug. Finasteride is absorbed through human skin. A woman who is pregnant or who may become pregnant should not handle crushed or broken finasteride tablets. Tablets are coated and will prevent contact with the active ingredient during normal handling.

◆ **Common adverse effects**

Reproductive

Impotence, decreased libido, decreased volume of ejaculate. These adverse effects appear in small numbers of men receiving higher doses of finasteride. Tell the patient that these adverse effects may occur but tend to be self-limiting. The decreased volume of ejaculate does not appear to interfere with normal sexual function. The patient should not stop taking the medication and should consult his healthcare provider if the problem becomes unacceptable.

◆ *Drug interactions.* No clinically significant drug interactions have been reported to date.

ERECTILE DYSFUNCTION

Erectile dysfunction (ED) is the consistent inability to achieve or maintain an erection sufficient for satisfactory sexual activity. There has been a significant increase in discussion about ED, sometimes called *impotency*, because of the availability and high efficacy of oral medicine used to treat certain types of cases of ED. The prevalence of ED increases with age, although it is not an inevitable outcome of aging. Approximately 5% of men experience the problem at the age of 40, and 15% to 25% of men age 65 years or older are affected.

Erectile dysfunction usually is the result of a combination of vascular, neurologic, and psychological factors. Vascular and neurogenic causes of ED increase with age. Risk factors include cigarette smoking, hyperlipidemia, hypertension, diabetes mellitus, coronary artery disease, and peripheral vascular disease. Other causes of ED are psychological (e.g., stress, depression, interpersonal relationships), damage to neurologic pathways (e.g., trauma from bicycle seats, prostatectomy, transurethral resection of the prostate, diabetes mellitus, alcohol abuse). A common cause of ED is the use of medicines for other medical conditions (Box 40.5). It is often difficult to determine whether ED is caused by medicines, the condition for which the medicine is used, or both.

The diagnosis of ED is based on a medical and sexual history, physical examination, and laboratory studies. An abrupt onset and intermittent pattern of difficulty achieving or maintaining an erection may suggest a psychological cause, whereas a gradual onset in ED is more likely the result of a vascular or neurologic cause. The cause of ED is usually multifactorial. A variety of treatments have been developed for ED, each with advantages and disadvantages—psychotherapy, intracavernosal injection with prostaglandins, intraurethral prostaglandin, vacuum constriction devices, vascular surgery, hormonal therapy, penile prostheses, and oral phosphodiesterase inhibitor therapy.

DRUG THERAPY FOR ERECTILE DYSFUNCTION

DRUG CLASS: PHOSPHODIESTERASE INHIBITORS

Actions

Phosphodiesterase inhibitors are selective inhibitors of the phosphodiesterase 5 (PDE5) enzyme. Research indicates that nitric oxide, a naturally occurring neurotransmitter found in nerve endings and endothelial cells, activates the enzyme guanylate cyclase, which converts guanosine triphosphate to cyclic guanosine monophosphate (cGMP) in smooth muscle cells. The increase in cGMP causes smooth muscle relaxation. In the corpus cavernosum of the penis, smooth muscle relaxation allows blood inflow to fill the many small sinusoidal spaces, resulting in an erection. In the corpus cavernosum, the enzyme PDE5 inactivates cGMP. The phosphodiesterase inhibitors enhance the relaxant effect of nitric oxide released in response to sexual stimulation by increasing cGMP concentration in the corpus cavernosum, resulting in smooth muscle relaxation and greater blood flow into the corpus cavernosum, which produces an erection.

Uses

Sildenafil was approved in 1998 as the first oral therapy to treat male ED. Three other products, vardenafil, tadalafil, and avanafil, have since been approved. Sexual stimulation is required for an erection because the phosphodiesterase inhibitors do not have a direct relaxant effect on the smooth muscle of the corpus cavernosum. In the absence of sexual stimulation, these agents have no pharmacologic effect. They are not an aphrodisiac; they do not increase sexual desire or sexual stimulation or affect the frequency of sexual intercourse. Sildenafil and vardenafil are taken at any point from 30 minutes to 4 hours before sexual activity. Avanafil is approved to be taken 15 minutes before sexual activity. Tadalafil also starts to work within 30 minutes, but may last for up to 36 hours. Tadalafil has also been approved as a once-daily dose that, when taken daily, may significantly reduce the onset of action, allowing more spontaneity in sexual relations. Tadalafil is also approved for the treatment of BPH.

Sexual stimulation is required with all four agents for erection. The erection lasts for an hour or so, although it is highly variable, based on continued sexual

Box 40.5 Drugs That May Cause Erectile Dysfunction

ANTIHYPERTENSIVE AGENTS
- Thiazide diuretics (most common)
- Beta-adrenergic blocking agents (especially propranolol and nonselective agents; less so with beta-1 selective agents)
- Alpha-adrenergic blocking agents (e.g., prazosin, terazosin)
- Sympatholytic agents (e.g., clonidine, methyldopa, reserpine)
- Spironolactone (antiandrogen effect)

CENTRAL NERVOUS SYSTEM DEPRESSANTS
- Phenothiazine antipsychotic agents (e.g., fluphenazine, thioridazine)
- Butyrophenones (e.g., haloperidol)
- Monoamine oxidase inhibitors
- Tricyclic antidepressants
- Selective serotonin reuptake inhibitors (e.g., sertraline, paroxetine)
- Lithium

CARDIOVASCULAR AGENTS
- Digoxin (estrogen effect)
- Clofibrate
- Gemfibrozil

MISCELLANEOUS AGENTS
- Substances of abuse (e.g., smoking, alcohol, cocaine, marijuana)
- Chemotherapy agents (e.g., chlorambucil, cyclophosphamide, methotrexate)
- Anabolic steroids
- Estrogens
- Corticosteroids
- Cimetidine (antiandrogen effect)
- 5-Alpha reductase inhibitors (finasteride, dutasteride)
- Interferon-α

Data from Koeneman KS, Mulhall JP, Goldstein I. Sexual health for the man at midlife: in-office workup. *Geriatrics.* 1997;52:76-86; Brock GB, Lue TF. Drug-induced male sexual dysfunction, an update. *Drug Saf.* 1993;8:414-426; and McVary KT. Erectile dysfunction. *N Engl J Med.* 2007;357:2472-2481, 2007.

stimulation, attainment of orgasm, and the individual patient. The phosphodiesterase inhibitors should not be taken more often than once every 24 hours. The phosphodiesterase inhibitors have been tested in women to treat sexual dysfunction, but the results to date have been inconclusive, so phosphodiesterase inhibitors are not recommended for women.

Phosphodiesterase inhibitors are also finding a new therapeutic use in a rare lung condition known as *pulmonary arterial hypertension.* By mechanisms in lung tissue similar to those in penile tissue as described earlier, phosphodiesterase inhibitors cause an increase in cGMP in pulmonary tissue, leading to relaxation of smooth muscle and vasodilation of the pulmonary arterial bed, reducing hypertension. Sildenafil (Revatio) and tadalafil (Adcirca) have been approved for use in pulmonary arterial hypertension.

Therapeutic Outcome

The primary therapeutic outcome expected from phosphodiesterase inhibitor therapy is improved erectile function and overall sexual satisfaction in men with ED. Tadalafil may also be used to reduce symptoms and improve urinary flow associated with prostatic enlargement.

❖ Nursing Implications for Phosphodiesterase Inhibitors

◆ *Premedication assessment.* Obtain baseline vital signs and a history of recent use of medicines, including recreational drugs. Patients with cardiovascular disease should seek their healthcare provider's approval before starting phosphodiesterase inhibitor therapy.

◆ *Availability, dosage, and administration.* See Table 40.8. Phosphodiesterase inhibitors do not protect against STIs or pregnancy. Use of a condom and a spermicide containing nonoxynol-9 will help protect against some STIs and unwanted pregnancy. Phosphodiesterase inhibitors do not affect sperm count or motility and do not reduce fertility.

◆ *Common adverse effects*
   Vascular

   Headache, flushing of the face and neck. These adverse effects appear in small numbers of men receiving higher doses of phosphodiesterase inhibitors. Tell the patient that these adverse effects may occur but tend to be self-limiting. If they continue to be a problem, a reduced dosage may eliminate the adverse effects. The patient should consult his healthcare provider if the problem becomes unacceptable.

   Sensory

   Color vision impairment. Mild, transient reversible impairment of blue or green color interpretation may occur. This is thought to be caused by inhibition of the phosphodiesterase 6 enzyme, which plays a role in phototransduction in the retina. If this continues to be problem, a reduced dosage may eliminate the adverse effect. Tell the patient to consult a healthcare provider if the problem becomes unacceptable.

◆ *Serious adverse effects*
   Cardiovascular

   Hypotension, dizziness, angina. Patients with heart disease, angina, diabetes mellitus, and hypertension should seek their healthcare provider's approval before using phosphodiesterase inhibitors. Patients receiving nitroglycerin or isosorbide should not take phosphodiesterase inhibitors because of a potentially fatal interaction. If hypotension, dizziness, or angina develops, the patient should lie down, discontinuing sexual activity. **Do not take nitroglycerin for angina.** It may worsen the symptoms. Seek medical attention, as needed.

Table 40.8 Phosphodiesterase Inhibitors Used for Erectile Dysfunction

GENERIC NAME	BRAND NAME	AVAILABILITY	DOSAGE
avanafil	Stendra	Tablets: 50, 100, 200 mg	Initial: 100 mg Maintenance: 50-100 mg Maximum: 200 mg/24 hr
sildenafil	Viagra	Tablets: 25, 50, 100 mg	Initial: 50 mg Maintenance: 25-50 mg Maximum: 100 mg/24 hr
tadalafil[a]	Cialis	Tablets: 2.5, 5, 10, 20 mg	Intermittent use: initial, 10 mg Maintenance: 5-10 mg Maximum: 20 mg/24 hr Daily use: initial, 2.5 mg; maximum for daily use, 5 mg
vardenafil	Levitra[b]	Tablets: 2.5, 5, 10, 20 mg	Initial: 10 mg; older than 65 yr, 5 mg Maintenance: 5-10 mg Maximum: 20 mg/24 hr
	Staxyn[b]	Tablet, dispersible: 10 mg	Initial: 10 mg Maximum: 10 mg; if dosage adjustment is needed, switch to Levitra

[a]Tadalafil is also approved for treatment of benign prostatic hyperplasia (5 mg once daily).
[b]Staxyn and Levitra are not interchangeable.

Sensory

Loss of vision. A small number of cases of sudden vision loss caused by nonarteritic ischemic optic neuropathy (NAION) have been reported. This is a condition in which blood flow to the optic nerve is blocked. People suffering sudden reduction in vision or vision loss should stop taking these medicines and seek medical attention quickly. Patients who are considering taking these medicines should inform their healthcare provider if they have ever had severe loss of vision, which might reflect a prior episode of NAION. At this time, it is not known whether these medicines for erectile dysfunction are the cause of the loss of vision or whether the problem is related to other medical conditions, such as high blood pressure, diabetes, or a combination of these problems.

Sudden decrease or loss of hearing. Sudden decrease or loss of hearing has been reported rarely; hearing changes may be accompanied by tinnitus and dizziness. Instruct patients to seek medical assistance for sudden decrease in hearing or loss of hearing

Reproductive

Sustained erection. Priapism is an erection that will not go away. If an erection lasts more than 4 hours, medical attention should be sought quickly. Priapism must be treated as soon as possible or lasting damage can happen to the penis, including the inability to have erections.

◆ *Drug interactions*

Nitroglycerin patches, nitroglycerin ointment, amyl nitrate. Nitrates increase the production of nitric oxide, potentially causing hypotension and arrhythmias. It is thought that nitrates inhaled for recreational use during sexual activity (e.g., "poppers" such as butyl nitrate, amyl nitrate, or amyl nitrite) will have the same effect when combined with phosphodiesterase inhibitors. Nitrates from food sources do not react with phosphodiesterase inhibitors.

Cimetidine, erythromycin, ketoconazole, itraconazole, ritonavir, indinavir, saquinavir. These agents inhibit the metabolism of phosphodiesterase inhibitors, potentially causing an increased incidence of adverse effects such as flushing, hypotension, and dizziness. A lower dosage of the phosphodiesterase inhibitor may be necessary.

Alcohol. Alcohol and phosphodiesterase inhibitors are both mild vasodilators. Excessive consumption of alcohol in combination with phosphodiesterase inhibitors may cause decreased blood pressure, dizziness, and orthostatic hypotension. Use caution when combining phosphodiesterase inhibitors and alcohol.

Alpha-adrenergic blocking agents. Use of alpha-adrenergic blocking agents (e.g., tamsulosin, alfuzosin, terazosin, doxazosin, prazosin) and vardenafil or tadalafil is **contraindicated.** Significant hypotension may result. Use with sildenafil is not contraindicated but a lower dose of sildenafil may be required to prevent hypotension.

There are no recommendations for the use of avanafil and alpha-adrenergic blocking agents.

Rifampin. This drug may enhance the metabolism of sildenafil and tadalafil, reducing their duration of action. An increase in dosage or earlier sexual activity may resolve the problem.

Get Ready for the NCLEX® Examination!

Key Points

- There is a great need for counseling about contraception and about modes of transmission of STIs for all those who are sexually active. One age group that is frequently not receiving adequate counseling on safe sex practices is adolescents, many of whom are sexually active.
- Nurses must be leaders in encouraging people to report STIs and seek healthcare as soon as an STI is suspected.
- Nurses must be leaders in promoting health and wellness, encouraging men and women to complete annual physical examinations that could detect the early onset of disease.
- It is important for the consumer to be aware that hormonal contraceptives have reduced effectiveness when taken in combination with many other medications or when doses are missed, thus requiring an alternative form of contraception.
- Osteoporosis effects both men and women and is considered a part of aging. Bone loss can be managed with proper exercise, diet, and pharmacologic agents.
- Benign prostatic hyperplasia and erectile dysfunction are the two most common male reproductive system conditions that are treated successfully with pharmacotherapy.

Additional Learning Resources

SG Go to your Study Guide for additional Review Questions for the NCLEX® Examination, Critical Thinking Clinical Situations, and other learning activities to help you master this chapter content.

Go to your Evolve website (https://evolve.elsevier.com/Clayton) for additional online resources.

Review Questions for the NCLEX® Examination

1. The nurse educating a patient being treated for chlamydia about personal hygiene will include which of these statements during the discussion? *(Select all that apply.)*
   1. "It is advisable to urinate before and after intercourse and to clean your private area thoroughly."
   2. "Remember that oral contraceptives do not protect you against sexually transmitted infections, but condoms provide a physical barrier against STIs."
   3. "Since you have an infection, you need to have your partner tested and treated."
   4. "Now that you have an infection, it is not necessary to practice safe sex."
   5. "I know this information can be overwhelming, so we can go over the rest of this when you return for your checkup."

2. Which type of oral contraceptive reduces the number of yearly menstrual periods from 13 to 4?
   1. Monophasic
   2. Biphasic
   3. Triphasic
   4. Quadriphasic

3. It is important to get a thorough history on a woman who wishes to start oral contraceptives because the increased estrogen exposure may increase the risk for developing which complication?
   1. Blood clots
   2. Kidney disease
   3. Leukorrhea
   4. Chlamydia

4. The nurse giving instructions to a patient about the use of the minipill realizes that further education is needed after the patient made which statement?
   1. "I will need to use condoms for the first month while on the pill to provide birth control."
   2. "I know that if I get a bad headache, dizziness, or blurred vision, I will need to contact this clinic as soon as possible."
   3. "I know I should switch to some other form of birth control for 3 months before I try to get pregnant."
   4. "I think I can remember to take the pill every day, but if I do forget, I can simply skip it and wait until the next day to take the pill again."

5. Which drugs are approved for use to reduce the symptoms of benign prostatic hyperplasia? *(Select all that apply.)*
   1. avanafil (Stendra)
   2. alfuzosin (Uroxatral)
   3. tamsulosin (Flomax)
   4. dutasteride (Avodart)
   5. finasteride (Proscar)

6. The nurse is completing a patient history on a man who presents with erectile dysfunction and is requesting a prescription for sildenafil (Viagra). Which conditions, if present, require the healthcare provider's assessment and approval prior to starting sildenafil? *(Select all that apply.)*
   1. STIs
   2. Diabetes mellitus
   3. Gastritis or peptic ulcer disease
   4. Cardiovascular disease
   5. Asthma

7. The patient taking denosumab (Prolia) for osteoporosis asks the nurse how it works. What is the most appropriate response by the nurse?
   1. "This medication decreases the rate at which bone is broken down and reabsorbed into the bloodstream."
   2. "This medication increases the rate at which bone is remodeled or new bone is laid down."
   3. "This medication increases the rate at which bone is broken down and reabsorbed into the bloodstream."
   4. "This medication works with the calcium in your body to build new bone."

41 Drugs Used to Treat Disorders of the Urinary System

https://evolve.elsevier.com/Clayton

Objectives

1. Explain the major actions of drugs used to treat disorders of the urinary tract.
2. Identify baseline data that the nurse should collect for comparison and evaluation of drug effectiveness.
3. Identify important nursing implementations associated with the drug therapy and treatment of diseases of the urinary system.
4. Identify the symptoms, treatment, and medications used for overactive bladder syndrome.

Key Terms

pyelonephritis (pī-ă-lō-ně-FRĪ-tĭs) (p. 640)
cystitis (sĭs-TĪ-tĭs) (p. 640)
prostatitis (prŏs-tă-TĪ-tĭs) (p. 640)
urethritis (yū-rě-THRĪ-tĭs) (p. 640)
acidification (ă-sĭd-ĭ-fĭ-KĀ-shŭn) (p. 643)
overactive bladder (OAB) syndrome (ō-věr-ĂK-tĭv BLĂ-děr SĬN-drōm) (p. 645)
frequency (FRĒ-kwěn-sē) (p. 645)

urgency (ĔR-jěn-sē) (p. 645)
incontinence (ĭn-KŌN-tĭ-něns) (p. 645)
urge incontinence (ĔRJ ĭn-KŌN-tĭ-něns) (p. 645)
stress incontinence (p. 646)
overflow incontinence (p. 646)
nocturia (nŏk-TŪ-rē-ă) (p. 646)
urinary antispasmodic agents (YĔR-ĭn-ăr-ē ăn-tī-spăz-MŎD-ĭk Ā-jěnts) (p. 646)

URINARY TRACT INFECTIONS

Urinary tract infections (UTIs) are among the most common infectious diseases in humans, accounting for more than 11 million healthcare providers' office visits yearly. Urinary tract infections are second only to upper respiratory tract infections as a cause of morbidity from infection. Urinary tract infections encompass several different types of infection of local tissue: pyelonephritis (the kidneys), cystitis (the bladder), prostatitis (the prostate gland), and urethritis (the urethra) (Fig. 41.1).

The incidence of UTIs in women is approximately 10 times higher than in men. The urethra is shorter in females than it is in males, so bacteria have a shorter distance to travel to the bladder. Proximity of the urethral meatus to the vagina and rectum can also make it easier for bacteria to cause an infection. The incidence increases in women with age, so that by 60 years of age, up to 20% of women will have suffered from at least one UTI in their lives.

Gram-negative aerobic bacilli from the gastrointestinal tract cause most UTIs. *Escherichia coli* accounts for about 80% of non–institutionally acquired uncomplicated UTIs.

Other common infecting organisms are *Staphylococcus saprophyticus, Klebsiella pneumoniae, Enterobacter* species, *Proteus mirabilis,* and *Pseudomonas aeruginosa.* Healthcare-associated UTIs and those associated with urinary tract pathologic abnormalities are considered to be complicated UTIs. The pathogens tend to be the same types of bacteria, but they are frequently more resistant to the antibiotics commonly used. This requires the use of more potent antibiotics for longer courses of therapy, placing the patient at a greater risk for complications secondary to drug therapy.

The use of an indwelling urinary catheter should be avoided if possible. When used, adherence to strict aseptic technique and attachment to a closed drainage system are necessary to reduce the rate of infection.

❖NURSING IMPLICATIONS FOR URINARY SYSTEM DISEASE

The information the nurse gains through assessment of the patient's clinical signs and symptoms is important to the healthcare provider when analyzing data for diagnosis and for evaluation of the patient's response to prescribed treatment.

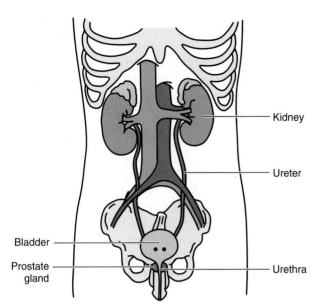

Fig. 41.1 The urinary system. (Modified from Gould B. *Pathophysiology for the Health Professions.* 3rd ed. Philadelphia: Saunders; 2006.)

◆ **Assessment**

History of urinary tract symptoms

- Does the individual have a history of a congenital disorder of the urinary tract, sexually transmitted infections, recent delivery of a baby, prostatic disease, recent catheterization, urologic instrumentation or surgical procedure, renal calculi, gout, UTI, or bladder dysfunction of neurologic origin? Obtain details applicable to the patient's responses.
- Is there a problem with defecation? When was the last bowel movement?

History of current symptoms

- Has the individual had any chills, fever, general malaise, or a change in mental status? New confusion in an older patient may be the only sign of a UTI. Ask questions relating to personal hygiene practices and sexual intercourse to evaluate for the possibility of bacterial contamination as an underlying cause of cystitis. Has the person been catheterized or on prolonged bed rest for any reason?
- *Pattern of urination:* Ask the individual to describe the symptoms that affect his or her ability to void. What is the current urination pattern, and have there been recent changes? Such details as frequency, dysuria (painful urination), changes in the urine stream, hesitancy in starting to void, hematuria (blood in the urine), nocturia (awaken at night with the desire to urinate and, if so, how many times does this occur during an average night?), and urgency are all of significance. Ask about the ability to sit through a 2-hour meeting or ride in a car for 2 hours without urinating. State the onset, course of progression of the symptoms, and any self-treatment that has been attempted and response achieved. Is it difficult to postpone urination when the urge to urinate is felt? Is there incontinence (leaking) of urine? If so, when does this happen and what causes it? Does the incontinence occur when coughing, walking, running, lifting a heavy object, or if one is unable to reach a toilet immediately?
- *Pattern of pain:* Record the details of any pain the patient describes—frequency, intensity, duration, and location. Use a pain rating scale (0 to 10: 0 for no pain; 10 for severe pain). Pain associated with renal pathology usually occurs at the groin, back, flank, and suprapubic area, and upon urination (dysuria). Does the pain radiate? If so, obtain details.
- *Intake and output:* Ask specifically about the individual's usual daily fluid intake. How frequently does the patient usually void? What is the amount of each voiding?

🌿 **Life Span Considerations**

Urinary Tract Infections

In children and men, UTIs may have a serious underlying cause and must be thoroughly investigated to identify the cause.

Medication history. Ask for a list of all prescribed over-the-counter medicines and herbal supplements being taken. Many pharmacologic agents (e.g., anticholinergic agents, cholinergic agents, antihistamines, antihypertensives, chemotherapeutic agents, and immunosuppressants) can induce urinary retention, an altered urinary elimination pattern, or urologic symptoms. Has the person recently been on medications to prevent or treat a UTI?

Nutritional history

- Has the individual been fasting for any prolonged period?
- How much alcoholic beverage has been consumed?
- Are vitamins, minerals, or other dietary supplements taken regularly?
- What kinds of fluids are taken daily: water, coffee, soft drinks, energy drinks?
- How many dairy products, chocolate foods, spicy foods, or meat products are consumed daily?

Laboratory and diagnostic studies. Review diagnostic and laboratory reports, such as urinalysis, renal function tests, voiding evaluatory procedures (e.g., urodynamic studies), cystoscopy, and complete blood count with differential, urine culture, and sensitivity results.

Urinalysis is a physical, chemical, and microscopic examination of the urine and is the most routine test that the nurse encounters. The color, appearance (e.g., clear, foamy, cloudy), and odor of the urine are noted, and the pH, protein, glucose, and ketones are determined with reagent dipsticks. Specific gravity is measured with a refractometer, and a microscopic examination of the urinary sediment is performed to detect the presence of red and white blood cells, bacteria, casts, and crystals. An understanding of the significant data that this basic test can reveal is imperative to monitoring the patient. Refer to Table 41.1 for a description of the data. See a general medical-surgical text for details of collecting urine samples correctly.

◆ **Implementation**
- Individualize the care plan to address the type of urinary tract disorder (e.g., retention, incontinence, or cystitis).
- Administer medications prescribed and listed on the medication administration record or in the electronic medical record.
- Monitor laboratory studies (e.g., urinalysis, complete blood count with differential, and creatinine clearance).

- Note dietary orders; indicate the amount of fluid to be taken every shift to maintain an adequate intake.
- Note daily weights as appropriate to diagnosis; indicate whether bladder training, Kegel exercises, or other measures should be taught and encouraged.
- Indicate the level of activity or exercise permitted.
- Perform focused assessment of symptoms (e.g., retention, urinary frequency, and pain).
- Monitor the pain level and provide appropriate supportive and pharmacologic interventions.
- Administer prescribed medications; monitor response and adverse effects.
- Maintain adequate fluid intake and an accurate intake and output record. Instruct the patient to avoid foods known to be bladder irritants, such as spicy foods, citrus juices, alcohol, and caffeine.
- For inability to void, institute techniques to stimulate voiding (e.g., proper positioning to void,

Table 41.1   Urinalysis

PROPERTY	NORMAL DATA	ABNORMAL DATA
Color, appearance	Straw, clear yellow, or amber	Dark smoky color, reddish, or brown may indicate blood; white or cloudy may indicate UTI or chyluria; dark yellow to amber may indicate dehydration; green, deep yellow, or brown may indicate liver or biliary disease. Some drugs or foods also alter urine color: red or red-brown (beets, rhubarb), reddish orange (phenazopyridine [Pyridium]), dark yellow or brown (nitrofurantoin), blue (methylene blue), bright yellow (vitamin B complex), reddish orange (rifampin)
Odor	Ammonia-like on standing	Foul smell may indicate infection; dehydrated patient's urine is concentrated, with ammonia smell resulting from urea breakdown by bacteria; sweet or fruity odor associated with starvation or diabetic acidosis (ketoacidosis)
Protein	0 to trace	Foamy or frothy-appearing urine may indicate protein in urine; proteinuria associated with kidney disease, toxemia of pregnancy; also found in leukemia, lupus erythematosus, cardiac disease
Glucose	0 to trace	Presence usually associated with diabetes mellitus or low renal threshold with glucose "spillage"; also seen at times of severe stress (e.g., major infection) or after high carbohydrate intake
Ketones	0	Associated with dehydration, starvation, ketoacidosis, diet high in protein and low in carbohydrates
pH	4.5-8.0	pH <4.5 indicates metabolic acidosis, respiratory acidosis, diet high in meat protein and/or cranberries. Medications can be prescribed to produce alkaline or acidic urine. pH >8.0 associated with bacteriuria (UTI from *Klebsiella* or *Proteus*), diet high in fruits and/or vegetables
Red blood cell count	0-3/HPF	Indicative of bleeding at some location in the urinary tract; infection, obstruction, calculi, renal failure, tumors, anticoagulants, excess aspirin, menstrual contamination
White blood cell count	0-5/HPF	Increase indicates infection somewhere in urinary tract; may also be associated with lupus nephritis, strenuous exercise
Casts	0	May indicate dehydration, possible infection within renal tubules, other types of renal disease
Bacteria	0	May indicate UTI or contaminated specimen collection
Specific gravity (sp gr)	1.003-1.029	Used as indicator of hydration (in absence of renal pathology); sp gr >1.018 is early sign of dehydration; sp gr <1.010 is "dilute urine" and may indicate fluid accumulation; fixed sp gr ≅1.010 may indicate renal disease; sp gr <1.005 may indicate diabetes insipidus, excess fluid intake, overhydration; sp gr >1.026 may indicate decreased fluid intake, vomiting, diarrhea, diabetes mellitus

HPF, High-power field; *UTI*, urinary tract infection.

running water in sink, and pouring warm water over perineum).

- For incontinence, establish a regular toileting schedule and initiate bladder training measures as appropriate and as ordered. Start measures to prevent perineal irritation. Apply external urinary diversion devices as ordered, such as an external condom catheter. Use incontinence pads as needed. Keep the urinal or bedpan readily available.
- Facilitate modifications of the environment that promote regular, easy access to toilet facilities, and promote the patient's safety with features such as better lighting, ambulatory assistance equipment, clothing alterations, timed voiding, and toileting equipment, such as an elevated toilet seat or commode.
- Implement measures to maintain the individual's dignity and privacy and to prevent embarrassment when incontinence is present.
- Maintain the activity and exercise level prescribed.

◆ Patient Education
For incontinence
- Teach personal hygiene measures to keep the skin clean and dry and prevent perineal breakdown. Explore appliances and incontinence products available for personal use.
- Teach Kegel exercises and bladder training, and stress the importance of responding to the urge to void.

For urinary tract infections
- Teach women the following measures to avoid future UTIs: avoid nylon underwear (use cotton) and tight, constrictive clothing in the perineal area; avoid frequent use of bubble baths; wash the perineal area immediately before and after sexual intercourse; and urinate immediately after intercourse.
- Teach women the proper method of wiping after defecation or urination (front to back) to prevent bacterial contamination. Explain the correct procedure for obtaining a clean-catch urine sample and the importance of having follow-up urine cultures collected as requested by the healthcare provider.
- Teach comfort measures, such as the use of a sitz bath.
- Stress the importance of adequate fluid intake and its effect of diluting the urine, decreasing bladder irritability, and helping remove organisms present in the bladder. Define "adequate intake of fluid" to the individual in terms of the number and size of glasses of liquid to be consumed during the day.
- Explain the signs of improvement or worsening of the urinary condition appropriate to the individual's diagnosis. Emphasize symptoms that should be reported to the healthcare provider.

For urinary retention. Teach self-examination to assess for bladder distention, Credé's maneuver (manual compression of the bladder through pressure on the lower abdomen) to aid in emptying the bladder, and, as appropriate, self-catheterization.

Medications
- For urinary retention, explain adverse effects to anticipate with the prescribed medications.
- For the urinary analgesic phenazopyridine hydrochloride, explain that the urine will be reddish orange. If discoloration of the skin or sclera occurs, the patient should contact the healthcare provider.
- For UTIs, instruct patients to take the medicines exactly as prescribed for the entire course of medication. Discontinuing the antimicrobial agent when the symptoms improve may result in another infection after approximately 2 weeks that will be resistant to antimicrobial treatment. **Acidification** of the urine is another way to prevent repeated UTIs. Ascorbic acid (vitamin C) is often prescribed to help maintain the acidity of the urine.
- See individual drug monographs regarding treatment of acute attacks and how long before response can be anticipated. Stress the need for follow-up laboratory results to evaluate response to therapy.

Fostering health maintenance
- Discuss medication information and how it will benefit the course of treatment to produce an optimal response. Stress maintenance of adequate urine volume as a part of the overall treatment of urinary tract disorders.
- Seek cooperation and understanding of the following points so that medication adherence is increased: name of medication; dosage, route, and times of administration; and common and serious adverse effects. See individual drug monographs for additional teaching.

Patient self-assessment. Enlist the patient's help in developing and maintaining a written record of monitoring parameters for urinary antimicrobial agents. See the Patient Self-Assessment Form for Urinary Antibiotics on the Evolve website. Complete the Premedication Data column for use as a baseline to track response to therapy. Ensure that the patient understands how to use the form, and instruct the patient to take the completed form to follow-up visits. During follow-up visits, focus on issues that will foster adherence with the therapeutic interventions prescribed.

DRUG THERAPY FOR URINARY TRACT INFECTIONS

DRUG CLASS: URINARY ANTIMICROBIAL AGENTS

Actions
Urinary antimicrobial agents are substances that are secreted and concentrated in the urine in sufficient amounts to have an antiseptic effect on the urine and urinary tract.

Uses

Selection of the product to be used is based on identification of the pathogens by Gram staining or by urine culture in severe, recurrent, or chronic infections.

Fosfomycin and nitrofurantoin are used only for UTIs. Examples of other antibiotics that are also used to treat urinary infections are cotrimoxazole, ciprofloxacin, levofloxacin, ceftriaxone, cephalexin, and gentamicin. These agents are effective in a variety of tissue infections against many different microorganisms. Because of their use in multiple organ systems, they are discussed in detail (with nursing processes) in Chapter 45.

Fluid intake should be encouraged so that there will be at least 2000 mL of urinary output daily. Duration of treatment depends on whether the infection is uncomplicated or complicated; whether the infection is acute, chronic, or recurrent; the pathogen being treated; the antimicrobial agent being used for treatment; and whether a follow-up culture can be collected to assess the success of the therapy.

DRUG CLASS: FOSFOMYCIN ANTIBIOTICS

fosfomycin (fŏs-fō-MĪ-sĭn)
Monurol (MŎN-ĕr-ŏl)

Actions

Fosfomycin is the first of the class of fosfomycin antibiotics. Fosfomycins act by inhibiting bacterial cell wall synthesis and by reducing adherence of bacteria to epithelial cells of the urinary tract.

Uses

Fosfomycin is the first antibiotic agent to be approved as a single-dose treatment for UTIs. It is used to treat uncomplicated acute cystitis in women caused by susceptible strains of *E. coli* and *Enterococcus faecalis*. It is not indicated for the treatment of kidney infections such as pyelonephritis.

Therapeutic Outcome

The primary therapeutic outcome associated with fosfomycin therapy is resolution of the UTI.

❖ Nursing Implications for fosfomycin

◆ *Premedication assessment*

1. Record voiding characteristics (e.g., frequency, amount, color, odor, and associated symptoms such as burning and pain) to serve as a baseline for monitoring therapy.
2. Assess for and record any existing gastrointestinal complaints before initiating therapy.
3. Record baseline vital signs.

◆ *Availability.* **PO:** Single-dose 3-g packets of fosfomycin granules.

◆ *Dosage and administration.* **Adult:** *PO:* Pour the entire contents of a single-dose packet of fosfomycin into 90 to 120 mL (3 to 4 ounces) of water and stir to dissolve. Do not use hot water. Take immediately after dissolving in water. Fosfomycin may be taken with or without food. Do not take additional packets of medicine without approval from the healthcare provider. Additional adverse effects develop with multiple doses, but there is little therapeutic gain. Do not take in its dry form; always mix fosfomycin with water before ingesting.

◆ *Common adverse effects*
Gastrointestinal
Nausea, diarrhea, abdominal cramps, flatulence. These adverse effects are usually mild and tend to resolve without need for therapy because only one dose of fosfomycin is administered.

◆ *Serious adverse effects*
Genitourinary
Perineal burning, dysuria. Burning with urination may be produced by the infection itself. Symptoms should improve in 2 to 3 days after taking fosfomycin; if not improved, the patient should contact his or her healthcare provider.

◆ *Drug interactions*
Metoclopramide. Metoclopramide has been reported to lower the serum concentration and urinary excretion of fosfomycin by enhancing gastric motility.

DRUG CLASS: OTHER URINARY ANTIBACTERIAL AGENTS

nitrofurantoin (nī-trō-fŭ-RĂN-tō-ĭn)
Furadantin (fŭr-ă-DĂN-tĭn)
Macrodantin (măk-rō-DĂN-tĭn)
Macrobid (MĂK-rō-bĭd)

Actions

Nitrofurantoin is an antibiotic that acts by interfering with several bacterial enzyme systems.

Uses

This antibiotic is not effective against microorganisms in the blood or in tissues outside the urinary tract. It is active against many gram-positive and gram-negative organisms, such as *E. faecalis*, *E. coli*, and *Proteus* species. It is not active against *P. aeruginosa* or *Serratia* species.

Therapeutic Outcome

The primary therapeutic outcome associated with nitrofurantoin therapy is resolution of the UTI.

❖ Nursing Implications for nitrofurantoin

◆ Premedication assessment

1. Record voiding characteristics (e.g., frequency, amount, color, odor, and associated symptoms such as burning and pain) to serve as a baseline for monitoring therapy.
2. Assess for and record any gastrointestinal complaints present before initiating drug therapy.
3. When using nitrofurantoin, check for history of glucose-6-phosphate dehydrogenase deficiency; if present, withhold the drug and contact the healthcare provider.
4. To serve as a baseline, assess the patient for the presence of peripheral neuropathies before initiating therapy.
5. Record baseline vital signs.

◆ Availability. PO: 25-, 50-, and 100-mg capsules; 25-mg/5-mL suspension.

◆ Dosage and administration. Adult: PO: Furadantin or Macrodantin 50 to 100 mg four times daily; or Macrobid 100 mg two times a day for 7 days or at least 3 days after obtaining sterile urine. Administer with food or milk to reduce gastrointestinal adverse effects. To maintain adequate urine concentrations, space the doses at even intervals around the clock. According to the Infectious Diseases Society of America, nitrofurantoin monohydrate/macrocrystals can be dosed 100 mg twice daily for 5 days in women.

Pediatric: Do not administer to infants younger than 1 month of age. *PO:* 5 to 7 mg/kg/24 hr in four divided doses. *Suspension:* Store in a dark amber container away from bright light.

> **[!] Medication Safety Alert**
>
> Nitrofurantoin must be in the bladder in a sufficient concentration to be therapeutically effective. Nitrofurantoin therapy is *not* recommended for use in patients who have a creatinine clearance lower than 60 mL/min. However, according to the 2015 Beers Criteria, nitrofurantoin can be used in individuals with a creatinine clearance of 30 mL/min or greater, but prolonged use should be avoided.

◆ Common adverse effects

Gastrointestinal

Nausea, vomiting, anorexia. Administer with food or milk to reduce gastric irritation.

Urinary

Urine discoloration. Tell the patient that urine may be tinted rust brown to yellow and that this discoloration should not be a cause for alarm.

◆ Serious adverse effects

Hypersensitivity, immune system

Dyspnea, chills, fever, erythematous rash, pruritus. These symptoms are the early indications of an allergic reaction to nitrofurantoin. Acute reactions usually occur within 8 hours in previously sensitized individuals and within 7 to 10 days in patients who develop sensitivity during the course of therapy. Discontinue the drug and notify the healthcare provider.

Neurologic

Peripheral neuropathies. Nitrofurantoin may cause peripheral neuropathies, particularly in patients with renal impairment, anemia, diabetes, electrolyte imbalance, or vitamin B deficiency. Nitrofurantoin should be discontinued at the first sign of numbness or tingling in the extremities.

Inflammation, immune system

Second infection. Inform the healthcare provider immediately if dysuria, pungent-smelling urine, or fever develops. These symptoms may be the early indication of a second infection by an organism resistant to nitrofurantoin.

◆ Drug interactions

Probenecid. Probenecid may inhibit the excretion of nitrofurantoin from the renal tubules. Monitor patients for the development of adverse effects of nitrofurantoin and for signs of incompletely treated UTI.

Eplerenone, spironolactone. Nitrofurantoin may enhance the hyperkalemic effects of these two agents. Monitor serum potassium levels and for the development of dysrhythmias.

Antacids. Discourage the patient from taking products containing magnesium trisilicate (e.g., Gaviscon-2) concurrently with nitrofurantoin because the antacid may inhibit absorption of the nitrofurantoin.

DRUG THERAPY FOR OVERACTIVE BLADDER SYNDROME

Overactive bladder (OAB) syndrome is a common problem affecting many adults, especially those older than 65 years. It is defined by the International Continence Society as "urgency, with or without urge incontinence, usually with frequency and nocturia" (Urology, 2001). These symptoms are thought to be due to detrusor muscle [of the bladder] becoming overactive but can also be due to other urinary problems. The diagnosis of OAB can be made if there is no proven infection or other obvious pathology. Overactive bladder without urge incontinence is more common in men than in women. However, it is not uncommon for patients with OAB also to have stress incontinence.

The three primary symptoms of OAB syndrome are frequency, urgency, and urinary incontinence. **Frequency** is the need to void eight or more times daily. **Urgency,** the most common symptom associated with OAB, is a sudden, compelling desire to pass urine that is very difficult to ignore. **Incontinence** is the inability to control urine from passing from the bladder. Incontinence can be subdivided into urge incontinence, stress incontinence, and overflow incontinence. **Urge incontinence is the** involuntary leakage of urine accompanied or immediately preceded by urgency. **Stress incontinence** is the brief burst of incontinence brought on by exercise, running, lifting, sneezing, or coughing. Predisposing factors are age, pregnancy, childbirth, cognitive impairment, and obesity. **Overflow incontinence**, also known as *chronic urinary retention*, is urinary leakage resulting from an overfilled and distended bladder that is unable to empty, causing urine to leak from the distended bladder. This may be caused by the inability to feel the urge to urinate, and therefore the bladder is never emptied. This occurs in men with benign prostatic hyperplasia (BPH). **Nocturia** is the need to void at night. Nocturia usually accompanies urgency, with or without urge incontinence, and is the complaint that the individual has to wake at night one or more times to void.

In males, an overlapping and often confusing problem is BPH (see Chapter 40). Patients with BPH are also susceptible to frequent urination but, unlike OAB, BPH can cause hesitancy and decreased flow during urination. Many men have symptoms of OAB and BPH and can be treated for both at the same time.

Overactive bladder syndrome cannot be cured, but a variety of nonpharmacologic and pharmacologic treatments can be used to reduce the symptoms associated with the disease. The goals of therapy are to decrease frequency by increasing voided volume, to decrease urgency, and to reduce incidents of urinary urge incontinence. A diary to record the pattern and type of urinary leakage and frequency and the volume of fluid consumption ("ins and outs") can be very helpful in developing an awareness of contributors and improvement or deterioration of symptoms over time. Lifestyle changes—such as spacing fluid consumption throughout the day instead of a large intake at one time; avoiding diuretic-like stimulants, such as alcohol, caffeine, and spicy foods; and avoiding fluid intake after 6 PM—can help with symptoms.

Sources of caffeine that are present in drugs such as Excedrin, Midol, Vanquish, and Anacin should be noted. Kegel exercises are recommended to strengthen external sphincter function and increase resistance when there is sudden urinary urgency. Bladder training—the patient is initially taught to void every hour on the hour, then asked to increase the duration between voids by 15 minutes each week—can help increase volume and control urgency. A combination of bladder training and Kegel exercises helps the patient regain bladder control, increasing voided volumes and the time interval between voids. Absorbent undergarment products are helpful in allowing social mobility and maintaining dry skin. They also help promote self-confidence and dignity.

The first lines of pharmacologic treatment of OAB are anticholinergic agents and mirabegron (Myrbetriq), a beta-3 adrenergic agonist. Anticholinergic agents with more selective action on the bladder are darifenacin, fesoterodine, oxybutynin, solifenacin, tolterodine, and trospium.

DRUG CLASS: ANTICHOLINERGIC AGENTS FOR OVERACTIVE BLADDER SYNDROME

Actions
Anticholinergic agents, also known as *urinary antispasmodic agents*, block the cholinergic (muscarinic) receptors of the detrusor muscle of the bladder, causing relaxation. They decrease involuntary contractions of the detrusor muscle and improve bladder volume capacity.

Uses
The anticholinergic agents are used to reduce the urgency and frequency of bladder contractions and delay the initial desire to void in patients with overactive bladder. Cholinergic receptors are found throughout the body, particularly in the salivary glands, eyes, colon, and brain. Thus inhibition of these receptors can lead to adverse effects, including dry mouth, blurred vision, constipation, confusion, and sedation. Each of these agents has some degree of selectivity for the cholinergic receptors in the bladder, but the agents are variable in whether they also block receptors in other parts of the body, leading to more adverse effects. They should not be used for patients with narrow-angle glaucoma, myasthenia gravis, gastric retention, or bowel disease such as ulcerative colitis, or patients with urinary retention caused by an obstructive uropathy such as prostatitis.

Therapeutic Outcome
The primary therapeutic outcome expected from urinary anticholinergic agents is control of incontinence associated with OAB.

❖ **Nursing Implications for Urinary Anticholinergic Agents**

◆ *Premedication assessment*
1. Record voiding characteristics (e.g., frequency, amount, color, odor, associated symptoms such as burning and pain) to serve as a baseline for monitoring therapy.
2. Obtain baseline vital signs.

◆ *Availability, dosage, and administration*
See Table 41.2.

◆ *Common adverse effects*
Neurologic
Dry mouth, urinary hesitancy, retention, sedation. These adverse effects are usually dosage related and respond to a reduction in dosage. Sedation often resolves with continued use. Instruct the patient to relieve dry mouth by sucking on ice chips or hard candy or by chewing gum.

Gastrointestinal
Constipation, bloating. Encourage balanced nutrition and inclusion of fresh fruits and vegetables for fiber and an adequate fluid intake to help alleviate these

Table 41.2 Urinary Anticholinergic Agents

GENERIC NAME	BRAND NAME	AVAILABILITY	DOSAGE
darifenacin	Enablex ⇄ Do not confuse Enablex with Enbrel.	Tablets, extended release (24 hr): 7.5, 15 mg	Initial dose: 7.5 mg once daily Based on individual response, the dosage may be increased to 15 mg once daily as early as 2 wk after starting therapy May be taken without regard to food
oxybutynin ⇄ Do not confuse oxybutynin with OxyContin.		Tablets: 5 mg Syrup: 5 mg/5 mL	Initial dose: 5 mg (tablets or syrup) two or three times/day Maximum dose: 20 mg daily
	Ditropan XL	Tablets, extended release (24 hr): 5, 10, 15 mg	Initial dose: 5 mg once daily Dosage may be adjusted at weekly intervals in 5-mg increments Maximum dose: 30 mg daily May be administered with or without food and must be swallowed whole with the aid of liquids; do not crush or chew Pediatric (6 yr and older): PO: 5 mg once daily; adjust dose as needed in 5 mg increments at weekly intervals; maximum dose, 20 mg daily
	Gelnique	Topical gel: 10%	Apply the contents of one sachet once daily to clean, dry, intact skin on abdomen, thighs, or upper arms/shoulder Rotate site; do not apply to same site on consecutive days Wash hands after use Cover treated area with clothing after gel has dried to prevent transfer of medication to others Do not bathe, shower, or swim until 1 hr after gel is applied
	Oxytrol	Transdermal patch: 36 mg (3.9 mg/day release)	Initial dose: Apply one patch every 3 to 4 days to dry, intact skin on abdomen, hip, or buttock Select a new application site with each new patch to avoid reapplication to the same site within 7 days
fesoterodine	Toviaz	Tablets, extended release (24 hr): 4, 8 mg	4-8 mg daily; 4 mg daily for patients taking potent CYP3A4 inhibitors or with renal impairment
solifenacin	VESIcare	Tablets: 5, 10 mg	Initial dose: 5 mg once daily If well tolerated, dosage may be increased to 10 mg once daily May be taken without regard to food.
tolterodine ⇄ Do not confuse tolterodine with tolcapone.	Detrol ⇄ Do not confuse Detrol with Datril. Detrol LA	Tablets: 1, 2 mg Capsules, extended release (24 hr): 2, 4 mg	Initial dose: 1-2 mg twice daily based on individual response and tolerance Initial dose: 2-4 mg once daily taken with liquids and swallowed whole
trospium	—	Tablets: 20 mg	Initial dose: 20 mg twice a day at least 1 hr before meals on an empty stomach For patients with renal impairment (CrCl <30 mL/min), recommended dose is 20 mg once daily at bedtime
	—	Capsules, extended release (24 hr): 60 mg	Initial dose: 60 mg daily in the morning; should be taken with water on an empty stomach at least 1 hr before food Not recommended for patients with renal impairment (CrCl <30 mL/min)

CrCl, Creatinine clearance; CYP3A4, cytochrome P450 component 3A4.

complications. If this approach is unsuccessful, suggest a stool softener or bulk-forming supplement. Avoid stimulant laxatives, which may have cholinergic effects, counteracting the anticholinergic properties.

Sensory

Blurred vision. Caution patients not to drive or operate power equipment until they have adjusted to this adverse effect.

◆ **Serious adverse effects.** If any of the aforementioned adverse effects intensifies, it should be reported to the prescribing healthcare provider for evaluation.

◆ **Drug interactions**

Anticholinergic agents. The concurrent use of the urinary anticholinergic agents with other anticholinergic agents may increase the frequency and severity of dry mouth, blurred vision, constipation, and other anticholinergic pharmacologic effects.

Fluoxetine, erythromycin, clarithromycin, ketoconazole, itraconazole, vinblastine, ritonavir. These agents inhibit the metabolism of tolterodine, darifenacin, and solifenacin. It is recommended that dosages not be raised above the initial starting dosage in patients taking these medicines concurrently.

DRUG CLASS: BETA-3 ADRENERGIC AGENT FOR OVERACTIVE BLADDER SYNDROME

> **mirabegron** (mĭr-ă-BĔG-rŏn)
> **Myrbetriq** (mĕr-BĔH-trĭk)

Actions

Mirabegron is a beta-3 adrenergic agonist. It relaxes the detrusor muscle during the storage phase of bladder filling, which increases bladder capacity.

Uses

Mirabegron is used for the treatment of OAB with symptoms of urge incontinence, urgency, and urinary frequency. Because mirabegron relaxes the detrusor muscle, patients with bladder outlet obstruction (e.g., enlarged prostate) and patients taking anticholinergic drugs for OAB may be at risk of urinary retention.

Therapeutic Outcome

The primary therapeutic outcome expected from mirabegron is control of incontinence associated with OAB.

❖ **Nursing Implications for mirabegron**

◆ *Premedication assessment*

1. Record voiding characteristics (e.g., frequency, amount, color, odor, associated symptoms such as burning and pain) to serve as a baseline for monitoring therapy.
2. Obtain baseline vital signs.

◆ *Availability.* **PO:** 25- and 50-mg tablets, extended release (24 hr).

◆ *Dosage and administration.* **PO:** Initial: 25 mg once daily; efficacy is observed within 8 weeks for 25-mg dose. May increase to 50 mg once daily based on individual patient efficacy and tolerability.

◆ *Common adverse effects*

Gastrointestinal

Constipation, diarrhea, dry mouth. About 1.5% of patients being treated with mirabegron reported constipation or diarrhea. Therapy usually does not need to be discontinued, but eating foods that add bulk to the diet may be helpful for both constipation and diarrhea. Patients with constipation may also benefit from the use of a stool softener. Encourage adequate fluid intake.

Mouth dryness may be alleviated by sucking hard candy or ice chips or by chewing gum. Encourage adequate fluid intake.

Urinary

Urinary retention. Urinary retention is more likely to be reported by patients who already have some degree of bladder outlet obstruction (most commonly prostatic enlargement) and in those patients already taking anticholinergic agents for OAB. Start therapy with the lower dose available.

Urinary tract infection. Approximately 4% of patients being treated with mirabegron developed a UTI. If symptoms of OAB become more severe, or burning on urination is reported, inform the healthcare provider. Mirabegron usually does not need to be discontinued but the UTI should be treated.

◆ *Serious adverse effects*

Hypertension. Monitor the patient's blood pressure periodically. Notify the healthcare provider if this effect starts to occur, because this happens primarily with individuals already being treated for hypertension.

◆ *Drug interactions*

Metoprolol, digoxin, nebivolol, fesoterodine. Mirabegron inhibits the metabolism of metoprolol, digoxin, nebivolol, and fesoterodine. When any of these drugs is administered with mirabegron, start the drug with the lowest dose available to determine the impact of the alteration of its metabolism by mirabegron. Alternatively, change to medicines whose metabolism is not inhibited by mirabegron.

Anticholinergic agents. The concurrent use of mirabegron with anticholinergic agents used for OAB may enhance the risk of urinary retention and other anticholinergic adverse/toxic effects (e.g., constipation, dry mouth). Initiate anticholinergic agent therapy with low doses to assess tolerance of the patient to potential adverse effects.

MISCELLANEOUS URINARY AGENTS

bethanechol chloride (bĕ-THĂN-ĕ-kŏl)
   Urecholine (yŭr-ĕ-KŌL-ēn)

Actions
Bethanechol is a parasympathetic nerve stimulant that causes contraction of the detrusor urinae muscle in the bladder, usually resulting in urination. It may also stimulate gastric motility, increase gastric tone, and restore impaired rhythmic peristalsis.

Uses
Bethanechol is used in cases of nonobstructive urinary retention, particularly in postoperative and postpartum patients, to restore bladder tone and urination.

Therapeutic Outcome
The primary therapeutic outcome associated with bethanechol therapy is restoration of bladder tone and urination.

❖ Nursing Implications for bethanechol
◆ *Premedication assessment*
1. Record voiding characteristics (e.g., frequency, amount, color, odor, and associated symptoms such as burning and pain) to serve as a baseline for monitoring therapy.
2. Record any gastrointestinal symptoms present to serve as a baseline for monitoring therapy.

◆ *Availability.* *PO:* 5-, 10-, 25-, and 50-mg tablets.

◆ *Dosage and administration.* **Adult:** *PO:* 10 to 50 mg two to four times daily. The maximum daily dosage is 120 mg.

◆ *Common adverse effects*
   Vascular
   Flushing of skin, headache. A pharmacologic property of the drug results in dilated blood vessels.

◆ *Serious adverse effects*
   Gastrointestinal
   Nausea, vomiting, sweating, colicky pain, abdominal cramps, diarrhea, belching, involuntary defecation. These effects are caused by a pharmacologic property of the drug. Consult the healthcare provider; a dosage adjustment may control these adverse effects. Provide support for the patient who develops diarrhea or involuntary defecation.

◆ *Drug interactions*
   Quinidine. Do not use quinidine concurrently with bethanechol. The pharmacologic properties of quinidine counteract those of bethanechol.

phenazopyridine hydrochloride (fĕn-ā-zō-PĬR-ă-dēn)
   Pyridium (pī-RĬD-ē-ŭm)

Actions
Phenazopyridine is an agent that, as it is excreted through the urinary tract, produces a local anesthetic effect on the mucosa of the ureters and bladder. It acts within about 30 minutes after oral administration.

Uses
Phenazopyridine relieves burning, pain, urgency, and frequency associated with UTIs. It also reduces bladder spasm, which relieves the resulting urinary retention and urgency. Phenazopyridine is also used for preoperative and postoperative surface analgesia in urologic surgical procedures and after diagnostic tests in which instrumentation is necessary. It is occasionally used to relieve the discomfort caused by an indwelling catheter.

Therapeutic Outcome
The primary therapeutic outcome associated with phenazopyridine therapy is relief of burning, frequency, pain, and urgency associated with UTI.

❖ Nursing Implications for phenazopyridine
◆ *Premedication assessment*
1. Record voiding characteristics (e.g., frequency, amount, color, odor, and associated symptoms such as burning and pain) to serve as a baseline for monitoring therapy.
2. Record skin color before initiating therapy.

◆ *Availability.* *PO:* 95-, 100-, and 200-mg tablets.

◆ *Dosage and administration.* **Adult:** *PO:* 200 mg three times daily.

◆ *Common adverse effects*
   Urinary
   Reddish-orange urine discoloration. Be certain that the patient understands that the color of the urine will become reddish orange when this drug is used and that this discoloration is no cause for alarm.

◆ *Serious adverse effects*
   Integumentary, sensory
   Yellow sclera or skin. The patient should report any yellowish tinge developing in the sclera (white portion) of the eye.

◆ *Drug interactions*
   Urine colorimetric procedures. Phenazopyridine interferes with colorimetric diagnostic tests performed on urine. Consult the hospital laboratory for alternative measures.

Get Ready for the NCLEX® Examination!

Key Points

- Urinary tract infections are some of the most common types of infections and are found in all patient care settings.
- For UTIs, instruct patients to take the medicines exactly as prescribed for the entire course of medication. Discontinuing the antimicrobial agent when the symptoms improve may result in another infection that may be resistant to antimicrobial treatment.
- The nurse can provide significant care by understanding and reporting the early symptoms associated with acute and chronic infections, and assisting patients who have difficulty with urinary retention and incontinence.
- Overactive bladder syndrome has three primary symptoms. A combination of bladder training and Kegel exercises helps the patient regain bladder control, increasing voided volumes and the time interval between voids. Anticholinergic agents are used to reduce the symptoms of OAB.

Additional Learning Resources

SG Go to your Study Guide for additional Review Questions for the NCLEX® Examination, Critical Thinking Clinical Situations, and other learning activities to help you master this chapter content.

Go to your Evolve website (https://evolve.elsevier.com/Clayton) for additional online resources.

Review Questions for the NCLEX® Examination

1. The nurse is providing education to a patient who has been prescribed phenazopyridine hydrochloride (Pyridium). Which common adverse effect is explained by the nurse to the patient?
   1. "You can expect some urinary retention with this drug."
   2. "Since it is common to get a dry mouth with this medication, you can suck on candy to counteract that effect."
   3. "Unfortunately, some patients experience colicky pain when taking this; please call us if that happens."
   4. "There is no cause for concern, but this drug will turn your urine a reddish-orange color."

2. Nurses caring for patients with cerebral palsy and known neurogenic bladder can expect which medication to be ordered?
   1. nitrofurantoin (Macrodantin)
   2. fosfomycin (Monurol)
   3. tolterodine (Detrol)
   4. mirabegron (Myrbetriq)

3. The nurse was teaching health promotion to a female patient with stress incontinence and realized that the patient needed further education after she made which statement?
   1. "I know that I need to keep my skin clean and dry and prevent skin breakdown so I don't get an infection."
   2. "I know that when I get the urge to urinate that it is okay to wait."
   3. "I understand that I can use some incontinence products so I am not embarrassed in public."
   4. "I will practice those Kegel exercises you taught me so that I have better control."

4. Anticholinergic agents will cause which side effects because of the many cholinergic receptors found throughout the body? *(Select all that apply.)*
   1. Dry mouth
   2. Blurred vision
   3. Constipation
   4. Urinary frequency
   5. Diarrhea

5. Bethanechol chloride (Urecholine) is used for the treatment of which disorder?
   1. Overactive bladder syndrome
   2. Acute cystitis
   3. Nonobstructive urinary retention
   4. Urinary tract infection

6. The nurse explaining ways to prevent UTIs to a female patient knows that further teaching is needed after the patient makes which statement?
   1. "I know that it is important to wipe front to back after voiding."
   2. "I will remember to drink more fluids so I will not be so prone to getting an infection."
   3. "I know I need to report any change in my urine; it should be clear and yellow."
   4. "I will remember to use the Credé maneuver to prevent infections."

Drugs Used to Treat Glaucoma and Other Eye Disorders

42

Objectives

1. Describe the anatomy and physiology of the eye and the normal flow of aqueous humor.
2. Identify the changes in normal flow of aqueous humor caused by open-angle and closed-angle glaucoma.
3. Explain patient assessments needed for eye disorders.
4. Review the correct procedure for instilling eyedrops or eye ointments and discuss patient teaching needs for glaucoma medication use.

Key Terms

cornea (KŎR-nē-ă) (p. 651)
sclera (SKLĀR-ă) (p. 651)
iris (Ī-rĭs) (p. 651)
sphincter muscle (SFĬNK-tĕr MŬS-ŭl) (p. 651)
miosis (mī-Ō-sĭs) (p. 651)
dilator muscle (DĪ-lā-tŭr) (p. 651)
mydriasis (mī-DRĪ-ă-sĭs) (p. 651)
lens (LĔNZ) (p. 651)

near point (NĒR PŌYNT) (p. 651)
zonular fibers (ZŎN-yū-lăr) (p. 651)
cycloplegia (sī-klō-PLĒ-jē-ă) (p. 652)
lacrimal canaliculi (LĂ-krĭ-măl kăn-ă-LĬK-yū-lī) (p. 652)
intraocular pressure (IOP) (ĭn-tră-ŎK-yū-lăr) (p. 653)
closed-angle glaucoma (KLŌZD ĂN-gŭl glŏ-KŌ-mă) (p. 653)
open-angle glaucoma (ō-PĔN ĂN-gŭl glŏ-KŌ-mă) (p. 653)

ANATOMY AND PHYSIOLOGY OF THE EYE

The eyeball has three coats, or layers: the protective external, or corneoscleral coat; the nutritive middle vascular layer, called the *choroid;* and the light-sensitive inner layer, or retina (Fig. 42.1).

The cornea, or outermost sheath of the anterior eyeball, is transparent so that light can enter the eye. The cornea has no blood vessels; it receives its nutrition from the aqueous humor and its oxygen supply by diffusion from the air and surrounding vascular structures. There is a thin layer of epithelial cells on the external surface of the cornea that is resistant to infection. An abraded cornea, however, is highly susceptible to infection. The cornea has sensory fibers, and any damage to the corneal epithelium will cause pain. Seriously injured corneal tissue is replaced by scar tissue that is usually not transparent. The sclera is the eye's white portion that is continuous with the cornea and is not transparent. The pupil is the center black portion of the eye, which is actually a hole in the iris that allows light to reach the retina.

The iris is a diaphragm that surrounds the pupil and gives the eye its color—blue, green, hazel, brown, or gray. The sphincter muscle within the iris encircles the pupil and is innervated by the parasympathetic nervous system. Miosis is contraction of the iris sphincter muscle, which causes the pupil to narrow. The dilator muscle, which runs radially from the pupillary margin to the iris periphery, is sympathetically innervated. Mydriasis is contraction of the dilator muscle and relaxation of the sphincter muscle, which causes the pupil to dilate (Fig. 42.2).

Constriction of the pupil normally occurs with light or when the eye is focusing on nearby objects. Dilation of the pupil normally occurs in dim light or when the eye is focusing on distant objects.

The lens is a transparent gelatinous mass of fibers encased in an elastic capsule situated behind the iris. Its function is to ensure that the image on the retina is in sharp focus. It does this by changing shape (accommodation). This occurs readily in youth, but with age the lens becomes more rigid and the ability to focus close objects is lost. The near point, the closest point that can be seen clearly, recedes. With age, the lens may lose its transparency and become opaque, forming a cataract. Blindness can occur unless the cataract can be treated or surgically removed.

The lens has ligaments around its edge, called zonular fibers, that connect with the ciliary body. Tension on the zonular fibers helps change the shape of the lens. In the unaccommodated eye, the ciliary muscle is relaxed and the zonular fibers are taut. For near vision, the ciliary muscle fibers contract, relaxing the pull on the ligaments and allowing the lens to become thick. Accommodation depends on two factors: (1) the ability of the lens to assume a more biconvex shape when tension on the ligaments is relaxed, and (2) ciliary muscle

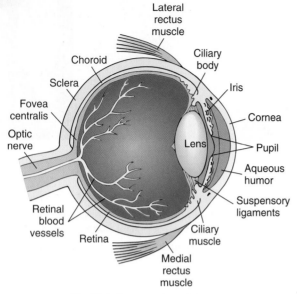

Fig. 42.1 Cross-section of the eye.

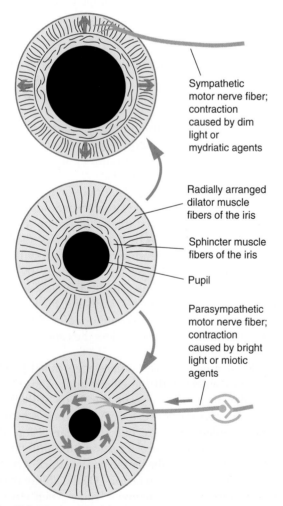

Fig. 42.2 Effect of light or ophthalmic agents on the iris of the eye.

contraction. Paralysis of the ciliary muscle is termed *cycloplegia*. The ciliary muscle is innervated by parasympathetic nerve fibers.

The ciliary body secretes aqueous humor, which bathes and feeds the lens, posterior surface of the cornea, and iris. After it is formed, the fluid flows forward between the lens and the iris into the anterior chamber. It drains out of the eye through drainage channels located near the junction of the cornea and sclera into a meshwork that leads into Schlemm's canal and into the venous system of the eye.

Eyelids, eyelashes, tears, and blinking all protect the eye. There are about 200 eyelashes for each eye. The eyelashes cause a blink reflex whenever a foreign body touches them, closing the lids for a fraction of a second to prevent the foreign body from entering the eye. Blinking, which is bilateral, occurs every few seconds during waking hours. It keeps the corneal surface free from mucus and spreads the lacrimal fluid evenly over the cornea. Tears are secreted by lacrimal glands and contain lysozyme, a mucolytic lubrication for lid movements. They wash away foreign objects and form a thin film over the cornea, providing it with a good optical surface. Tear fluid is lost by drainage into two small ducts, the lacrimal canaliculi, at the inner corners of the eyelids and by evaporation.

GENERAL CONSIDERATIONS FOR TOPICAL OPHTHALMIC DRUG THERAPY

The most common route of administration for ophthalmic drugs is topical application. Advantages include convenience, simplicity, noninvasive nature, and the ability of the patient to self-administer. Topically administered medications do not penetrate adequately for use with posterior eye diseases, such as diseases of the optic nerve or retina, so topical administration is not used for such diseases.

Proper administration of ophthalmic drugs is essential to optimal therapeutic response. The administration technique used often determines drug safety and efficacy (see Chapter 7, Figs. 7.6 and 7.7).

- Based on the volume that the eye can retain, use of more than 1 drop per administration is questionable.
- If more than one drug is to be administered at about the same time, separate the administration of the different medications by at least 5 minutes. This ensures that the first medication is not washed away by the second, or that the second medication is not diluted by the first.
- Minimize systemic absorption of ophthalmic drops by compressing the tear duct at the inner canthus of the eye for 3 to 5 minutes after instillation. This reduces the passage of medication via the nasolacrimal duct into areas of absorption, such as the nasal and pharyngeal mucosa.
- Eyecup use is discouraged because of the risk of contamination, which can cause infection.

- Ophthalmic ointments may impede delivery of other ophthalmic drugs to the affected site by serving as a barrier to contact. Administer drops *before* applying ointments. Try not to administer drops for a few hours after the use of ointment. The ointment should be administered beginning at the inner canthus and moving to the outer aspect of the eye.
- Ointments may blur vision during the waking hours. Use with caution in conditions in which visual clarity is critical (e.g., operating motor equipment, reading).
- Observe expiration dates closely. Do not use outdated medication.
- Solutions and ointments are frequently misused. Do not assume that patients know how to effectively use these agents.
- In an effort to enhance safety of ophthalmic medications, the ophthalmic medicine industry recommends the use of standard colors for drug labels and bottle caps (see the following chart). Ophthalmic drug labels include "For Ophthalmic Use." The nurse should become familiar with these colors and types of ophthalmic medications to help prevent inadvertently picking up and administering the wrong solution.

THERAPEUTIC CLASS	CAP AND LABEL COLOR
Antiinfectives	Brown or tan
Beta-adrenergic blocking agents	Yellow, blue, or both
Miotics	Green
Mydriatics and cycloplegics	Red
Nonsteroidal antiinflammatory agents	Gray

GLAUCOMA

Glaucoma is an eye disease characterized by abnormally elevated **intraocular pressure (IOP)**, which may result from excessive production of the aqueous humor or from diminished ocular fluid outflow. Increased pressure, if persistent and sufficiently elevated, may lead to permanent blindness. There are three major types of glaucoma: primary, secondary, and congenital. Primary includes **closed-angle glaucoma** (also known as narrow-angle glaucoma) and **open-angle glaucoma**. These are diagnosed by determination of the iridocorneal angle of the anterior chamber, where aqueous humor reabsorption takes place. Secondary glaucoma may result from previous eye disease or may occur after a cataract extraction and may require drug therapy for an indefinite period. Congenital glaucoma requires surgical treatment.

Open-angle glaucoma develops insidiously over the years as pathologic changes at the iridocorneal angle prevent the outflow of aqueous humor through the trabecular network to Schlemm's canal and into the veins of the eye (Fig. 42.3). In cases of open-angle glaucoma, there is reduced outflow of aqueous humor through the trabecular network and Schlemm's canal because of resistance of the aqueous humor outflow; the iridocorneal angle is open (Fig. 42.4).

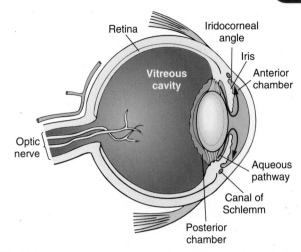

Fig. 42.3 Anterior and posterior chambers of the eye. *Arrows* indicate the pathway of aqueous flow.

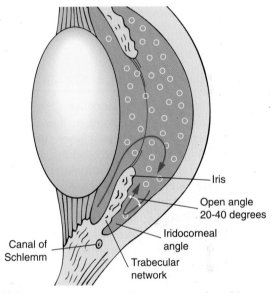

Fig. 42.4 Open-angle glaucoma. Obstruction to the flow of the aqueous humor is caused by reduced outflow at Schlemm's canal in the trabecular network. There is no obstruction from closure of the iridocorneal angle.

Intraocular pressure builds up and, if not treated, will damage the optic disk. Initially the patient has no symptoms, but over the years there is a gradual loss of peripheral vision. If untreated, total blindness may result.

Acute closed-angle glaucoma occurs when there is a sudden increase in IOP caused by a mechanical obstruction of the trabecular network in the iridocorneal angle (Fig. 42.5). This occurs in patients who have narrow anterior chamber angles. Symptoms develop gradually and appear intermittently for short periods, especially when the pupil is dilated. (Dilation of the pupil pushes the iris against the trabecular meshwork, causing the obstruction.) Symptoms often reported are blurred vision, halos around white lights, frontal headache, and eye pain. Patients often associate the symptoms with stress or fatigue. An attack can also be precipitated by administration of a mydriatic agent, such as atropine or scopolamine, for eye examination.

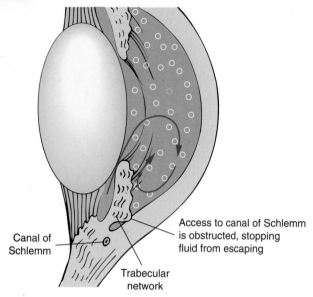

Canal of Schlemm

Access to canal of Schlemm is obstructed, stopping fluid from escaping

Trabecular network

Fig. 42.5 Closed-angle glaucoma. Obstruction to the flow of aqueous fluid to Schlemm's canal causes closed-angle glaucoma.

DRUG THERAPY FOR GLAUCOMA

The treatment of open-angle glaucoma is maintenance of IOP at normal levels to prevent further blindness. Treatment options include surgery, laser surgery, and drug therapy. A beta-adrenergic blocking agent (e.g., timolol maleate) has become the initial drug of choice. Other agents that may also be used are prostaglandins (e.g., latanoprost), sympathomimetic agents (e.g., brimonidine), and carbonic anhydrase inhibitors (e.g., acetazolamide). The selection of the drug is determined to a great extent by the requirements of the individual patient and response to therapy.

Acute closed-angle glaucoma requires immediate treatment to reduce IOP. Intravenous mannitol, an osmotic diuretic, may be administered to draw aqueous humor from the eye. Topical corticosteroids may be used to reduce ocular inflammation. Other medications used to reduce formation of aqueous humor include beta blockers, prostaglandins, a sympathomimetic agent, or a carbonic anhydrase inhibitor. After IOP has been reduced, pilocarpine may be used to induce miosis, relieving the pressure of the iris against the trabecular network and allowing drainage of the aqueous humor. Analgesics and antiemetics may be administered if pain and vomiting persist. Surgery is then required to correct the abnormality.

❖ NURSING IMPLICATIONS FOR GLAUCOMA AND OTHER EYE DISORDERS

The nurse has an important role in educating the public and promoting safety measures to protect the eye from potential sources of injury. Healthcare professionals can participate in this role during their daily contacts with people in the community. The use of safety glasses in potentially hazardous situations, prevention of chemical burns from common household cleaning items or other agents at home or work, proper cleaning and wearing of contact lenses or glasses, and selection of safe toys and play activities for children are some areas about which the nurse can teach the public. These safety measures can significantly reduce the number of injuries that occur annually.

Nurses play an important role in detecting eye disorders and implementing treatment plans. An example of this is in patients with diabetes mellitus. Encourage annual, or more frequent, eye examinations to detect and prevent complications associated with the disease.

The primary delivery of eye care is through self-administration of drugs. One of the greatest challenges in the care of chronic eye disorders such as glaucoma is convincing the patient of the need for long-term treatment and adherence to the therapeutic regimen.

◆ Assessment

Eye examination

- When an eye injury has occurred, document visual acuity by screening vision with the Snellen chart. Comparison screenings should be performed at each subsequent visit.
- Observe for eyelid edema. It may be an indication of a systemic disease process or tumor. Report if present.
- Assess pupils for equality of size, roundness, and response to light. Report irregular contour, unequal size, or decreased response to light.
- Observe for and report nystagmus.
- Observe for any redness or drainage in the eyes.
- Observe for complete closure of the eyelid. This is essential for protection of the cornea. Patients who have received corneal anesthesia, have had fifth cranial nerve surgery, have exophthalmos, or are unconscious must have the cornea protected to prevent damage.
- Ask whether glasses or contact lenses are worn.
- Inspect the eye dressings and report immediately for evaluation if any drainage is observed. Never remove the surgical dressing after surgery to inspect the eye.

History of symptoms

- Ask the patient to describe the symptoms for which treatment is being sought. How do symptoms affect daily life? Do visual problems affect ability to read?
- Is there a family history of cataracts, glaucoma, or macular degeneration?
- Are activities limited in any way by any vision problem?
- Do any leisure activities have the potential for eye injury?
- Has the person had any noticeable pain, burning, foreign body sensation, blurred or halo vision, or loss of vision?

- Ask whether there is any difficulty in adjusting vision when going from a dark to a brightly lighted area or vice versa.
- Are colors clear and crisp, or do they lack clarity?
- Has there been an increase in tearing or discharge from the eye? If so, ask for details of appearance and amount of drainage.
- Has there been any recent nausea or vomiting?

Psychological. What type of response is the patient exhibiting to the disturbance in visual acuity? Is the patient withdrawing socially? Identify a support system available for at-home care and assistance. Plan a specific time to meet with the patient and significant others to discuss at-home care and community resources available if assistance is indicated.

 Life Span Considerations

Diminished Visual Acuity

Diminished visual acuity affects most aspects of a person's life, so it is imperative to evaluate an individual's ability to perform the usual activities of daily living when visual impairment develops. Many medications used to treat other disorders can reduce visual acuity; this adverse effect should be anticipated and its consequences monitored. Every attempt must be made to help the patient adapt to the visual impairment and provide for personal safety.

Diagnostics. Ask the patient to describe what eye diagnostic procedures have been completed before admission (e.g., visual acuity measurement, tonometry, slit-lamp examination, visual fields). A tonometer is used to measure the IOP inside the eye to evaluate a patient's risk for glaucoma and to assess the success or failure of ongoing treatment. There are several types of tonometers available (e.g., applanation, Goldmann, noncontact, ocular response analyzer), the use of which ranges from quick screening for increased IOP to very precise measurement of IPO. Most tonometers measure pressure in units of millimeters of mercury (mm Hg).

Medications. Ask for a list of all prescribed and over-the-counter medications and herbal products being taken. Ask for details on medications, dosage, schedule, and degree of compliance. List all ordered medications on the medication administration record (MAR). If beta blockers are being taken, list the pulse and blood pressure on the MAR as a preassessment to administration of the ophthalmic drops. Note parameters relating to the prevention of injury, the activity and exercise level permitted, and diet orders.

◆ **Implementation**
- Perform assessments every shift consistent with the patient's status and diagnosis.
- Prepare the patient for eye examinations, diagnostics, or eye surgery.

- Administer cycloplegic and mydriatic medications prescribed for dilation of the eye before an eye examination or ophthalmic surgery.
- Administer miotic medication to produce constriction of the eye after eye examination or diagnostic procedures, as prescribed.
- Administer all ophthalmic medications prescribed while maintaining aseptic technique to prevent the transfer of infection from one eye to the other.
- Protect the cornea from damage during anesthesia or in an unconscious patient through the use of ophthalmic ointment or artificial tears to prevent corneal drying.
- Assist with diagnostic procedures (e.g., visual fields, tonometry, visual acuity).
- Take baseline vital signs.
- Institute appropriate comfort measures.
- If eye surgery has been performed (e.g., trabeculectomy), institute routine postoperative care measures. Position the patient as ordered, usually on the back or on the unoperated side. With the scleral buckling procedure, positioning orders may be extremely specific.
- Ensure that an eye patch and shield are applied properly to protect the eye from further injury.
- Explain and enforce activity and exercise restrictions. To prevent an increase in IOP, instruct the patient to avoid heavy lifting, straining on defecation, coughing, or bending and placing the head in a dependent position.
- A blind or disoriented patient or a patient with both eyes patched may experience effects of sensory deprivation.
- Always speak before touching a person with impaired vision.

 Health Promotion

- Perform hand hygiene thoroughly each time the area is touched (before or after eye treatments or instillation of medications).
- Use only sterile medications or dressings on the eye.
- Wipe the eye from the inner canthus outward; discard the tissue used; perform hand hygiene before proceeding to the second eye.
- When an infection is present, prevent cross-contamination; always use a separate source of medication and dropper for each eye.
- Never touch the eyeball or face with the tip of the dropper or opening of the ointment container. Demonstrate the proper way to set the medication lid down so that the inside is not contaminated.
- When inserting or removing contact lenses, perform hand hygiene first and then follow the manufacturer's instructions regarding the cleansing and care of the lenses.
- Report any persistent redness or drainage from the eyes.

- Check on the patient at frequent intervals; initiate conversations and regularly orient the patient to date, time, and place.
- If the patient is agitated, contact the prescribing healthcare provider; it may be necessary to obtain an order to remove one eye patch or sedate the patient.
- Provide emotional support.

◆ Patient Education

After eye surgery

- Teach the patient and family proper hygiene and eye care techniques to ensure that medications, dressings, and/or surgical wounds are not contaminated during necessary eye care.
- Teach the patient and family about signs and symptoms of infections and when and how to report them to allow early recognition and treatment of possible infection.
- Instruct the patient to comply with postoperative restrictions on head positioning, bending, coughing, and the Valsalva maneuver to optimize visual outcomes and prevent increased IOP.
- Instruct the patient to instill the eye medications using aseptic techniques and to comply with the prescribed eye medication routine to prevent infection (see Chapter 7, Figs. 7.6 and 7.7). In general, using more than 1 drop per dose of medication does not improve response but increases the frequency of adverse effects and the cost of therapy. Instruct the patient on how to block the nasolacrimal duct during instillation to minimize systemic effects.
- When using more than one medication, separate drop instillation of each agent by at least 5 minutes to provide optimal ocular contact for each medication.
- Instruct the patient to monitor pain and take prescribed pain medication as directed; report pain not relieved by prescribed medications.
- Instruct the patient about the importance of continued follow-up as recommended to maximize potential visual outcomes.

Disease or disorder

- Reinforce the teaching of pertinent facts regarding the diagnosis and disease process.
- If the patient is being treated for glaucoma, stress the need for lifelong treatment and use of medications. Explain that adherence with the drug regimen can help prevent blindness.
- If an infectious process is present, teach personal hygiene measures to prevent introduction of an infection.

Visual acuity

- Provide for patient safety.
- Assess whether diminished visual acuity will reduce the ability of the patient to perform his or her usual activities of daily living. Teach adaptation methods appropriate to the situation.

- Restrict the operation of tools or power equipment as appropriate to the degree of alteration present.

Medications

- Review the details of medication administration.
- Ensure that directions are printed in large, bold print that the individual can read.
- Have the patient store all medications in an area separate from other containers so that she or he cannot inadvertently put things other than medication into the eye.
- Have the person demonstrate the ability to self-administer the eye medications to ensure manual dexterity to perform the procedures.
- Keep an extra bottle of eye medications on hand, particularly those used to reduce IOP.

Fostering health maintenance

- Discuss medication information and how it will benefit the course of treatment (e.g., reduction of IOP, elimination of an infection).
- Seek cooperation and understanding of the following points so that medication compliance is increased: name of medication; dosage, route, and times of administration; and common and serious adverse effects. Verify ability to self-administer all medications. Additional health teaching is included in the individual drug monographs.
- Encourage the patient to discuss any adverse effects that the medications may produce with the healthcare provider to plan mutually for ways to minimize these effects or make adaptations rather than reduce the frequency or eliminate the use of the medications.

Patient self-assessment. Enlist the patient's help in developing and maintaining a written record of monitoring parameters (e.g., blood pressure and pulse with adrenergic and beta-adrenergic blocking agents, degree of visual disturbance, progression of impairment) and response to prescribed therapies for discussion with the physician. See Patient Self-Assessment Form for Eye Medications on the Evolve website. Complete the Premedication Data column for use as a baseline to track response to therapy. Ensure that the patient understands how to use the form and instruct the patient to take the completed form to all follow-up visits. During follow-up visits, focus on issues that will foster adherence with the therapeutic interventions prescribed.

DRUG CLASS: CARBONIC ANHYDRASE INHIBITORS

Actions

These agents are inhibitors of the enzyme carbonic anhydrase. Inhibition of this enzyme results in a decrease in the production of aqueous humor, thus lowering IOP.

Table 42.1   Carbonic Anhydrase Inhibitors

GENERIC NAME	BRAND NAME	AVAILABILITY	DOSAGE
acetazolamide	— Diamox Sequels	Tablets: 125, 250 mg Capsules, extended release (12 hr): 500 mg Powder for injection: 500 mg	PO: 250 mg one to four times daily or 500 mg extended release twice daily
brinzolamide	Azopt	Ophthalmic solution: 1% in 10- and 15-mL dropper bottles	Intraocular: 1 drop in affected eye(s) three times daily If more than one ophthalmic agent is to be administered in the same eye, separate the administration by at least 10 min
dorzolamide	Trusopt	Ophthalmic solution: 2% in 10-mL dropper bottle	Intraocular: 1 drop in affected eye(s) three times daily If more than one ophthalmic agent is to be administered in the same eye, separate the administration by at least 10 min
methazolamide	Neptazane	Tablets: 25, 50 mg	PO: 50-100 mg, two or three times daily

Uses

These agents are used in conjunction with other treatments to control IOP in cases of intraocular hypertension and closed-angle and open-angle glaucoma. Dorzolamide has the advantage of intraocular administration, with less potential for systemic adverse effects.

Therapeutic Outcome

The primary therapeutic outcome expected from carbonic anhydrase inhibitors is reduced IOP.

❖ Nursing Implications for Carbonic Anhydrase Inhibitors

◆ Premedication assessment

1. Establish whether the patient is pregnant; if pregnancy is suspected, withhold the medication and contact the healthcare provider.
2. Check for allergy to sulfonamide antibiotics; withhold the medication and contact the healthcare provider if allergy is present.
3. Ensure that contact lenses have been removed before the instillation of dorzolamide drops.
4. Ensure that baseline electrolyte laboratory studies have been drawn as ordered.
5. Assess and record baseline weight, hydration data, vital signs, and mental status.
6. Record premedication IOP readings and visual acuity data.
7. Assess for signs of gastric symptoms before initiating drug therapy. If present, schedule medications for administration with milk or food.

◆ Availability, dosage, and administration
See Table 42.1.

◆ Common adverse effects
Gastric irritation. If gastric irritation occurs, administer the medication with food or milk. If symptoms persist or increase in severity, report to the healthcare provider for evaluation.

◆ Serious adverse effects
Hematologic
Electrolyte imbalance, dehydration. Although infrequent, treatment with carbonic anhydrase inhibitors may lead to excessive diuresis, resulting in water dehydration and electrolyte imbalance. The electrolytes most commonly altered are K^+, Na^+, and Cl^-. Hypokalemia is most likely to occur. Many symptoms associated with altered fluid and electrolyte balance are subtle and resemble general symptoms of drug toxicity or the disease process itself. Gather data about changes in the patient's mental status (e.g., alertness, orientation, confusion), muscle strength, muscle cramps, tremors, nausea, and general appearance (e.g., drowsy, anxious, lethargic). Always check the electrolyte reports for early indications of electrolyte imbalance. Keep accurate records of intake and output, daily weight, and vital signs.

Sulfonamide-like reactions
Dermatologic, hematologic, neurologic reactions. Carbonic anhydrase inhibitors are sulfonamide derivatives and thus have the potential to cause adverse effects similar to those associated with sulfonamide antimicrobial therapy. These adverse effects, although rare, include dermatologic, hematologic, and neurologic reactions. (For further discussion, see the section on sulfonamides in Chapter 45.) Do not administer to patients who are allergic to sulfonamide antibiotics without healthcare provider approval. Observe closely for the development of hypersensitivity.

Neurologic
Confusion. Perform a baseline assessment of the patient's degree of alertness and orientation to name, place, and time before initiating therapy. Make regularly scheduled subsequent mental status evaluations and compare findings. Report changes in the patient's mental status.

Drowsiness. This adverse effect is usually mild and tends to resolve with continued therapy. Encourage the patient not to discontinue therapy without first consulting the healthcare provider. The patient who works with machinery, operates a motor vehicle, administers medications, or performs other duties that require mental alertness should not take these medications while working.

◆ *Drug interactions*

Digoxin. Patients receiving these diuretic drugs may excrete excess potassium, which leads to hypokalemia. If the patient is also receiving digoxin, monitor closely for signs of digoxin toxicity (e.g., anorexia, nausea, fatigue, blurred or colored vision, bradycardia, dysrhythmias).

Corticosteroids (prednisone, others). Corticosteroids may enhance the loss of potassium. Check potassium levels and monitor more closely for hypokalemia when these two agents are used concurrently.

DRUG CLASS: CHOLINERGIC AGENTS

Actions
Cholinergic agents produce strong contractions of the iris (miosis) and ciliary body musculature (accommodation).

Uses
Cholinergic agents lower IOP in patients with glaucoma by widening the filtration angle, which permits outflow of aqueous humor. They also may be used to counter the effects of mydriatic and cycloplegic agents after surgery or ophthalmoscopic examination.

Cholinergic agents have several advantages: they are effective in many cases of chronic glaucoma, the adverse effects are less severe and occur less frequently than those of anticholinesterase agents, and they give better control of IOP with fewer fluctuations in pressure.

Therapeutic Outcomes
The primary therapeutic outcomes expected from cholinergic agents are as follows:
1. Reduced IOP in patients with glaucoma
2. Reversal of the mydriasis and cycloplegia secondary to ophthalmic agents used in surgery or ophthalmic examination

❖ **Nursing Implications for Cholinergic Agents**
◆ *Premedication assessment*
1. Obtain baseline vital signs.
2. Record premedication IOP readings and visual acuity data.

◆ *Availability, dosage, and administration*
See Table 42.2.

◆ *Common adverse effects*
   Sensory
   Reduced visual acuity. A common adverse effect of cholinergic agents is difficulty in adjusting quickly to changes in light intensity. Reduced visual acuity may be most notable at night, particularly in areas of poor lighting, as well as in older patients and those developing lens opacities. Advise patients to use caution while driving at night or performing hazardous tasks in poor light. Blurred vision can occur, particularly during the first 1 to 2 hours after instilling the medication. Be sure to keep eye medications separate from other solutions.

The ability to read for long periods is decreased because of impairment of near-vision accommodation. Provide for patient safety when visual impairment exists. In hospitals, orient the patient to the hospital unit, furniture placement, and call light; place the bed in a low position. At home, do not move furniture or the individual's household or personal belongings.

   Conjunctival irritation, erythema, headache. These adverse effects are usually mild and tend to resolve with continued therapy. Encourage the patient not to discontinue therapy without first consulting the healthcare provider.

   Pain, discomfort. Because of pupillary constriction, an increase in pain or discomfort may occur, particularly in bright light. Stress the need for adherence and assure the patient that this adverse effect will diminish with continued use.

   Neurologic
   Headache. This adverse effect is usually mild and tends to resolve with continued therapy. Encourage the patient not to discontinue therapy without first consulting the healthcare provider.

◆ *Serious adverse effects*
   Systemic adverse effects. Rarely, a patient may develop signs of systemic toxicity manifested by diaphoresis, salivation, abdominal discomfort, diarrhea, bronchospasm, muscle tremors, hypotension, dysrhythmias, and/or bradycardia. These symptoms are indications of excessive administration. Report to the healthcare provider for dosage adjustment. The adverse effects themselves usually do not need to be treated because they will resolve by withholding cholinergic therapy. Prevent systemic effects by carefully blocking the inner canthus for 3 to 5 minutes after instilling the medication to prevent absorption via the nasolacrimal duct. During drug therapy, assess the blood pressure every shift and report significant changes from the baseline data. If accidental overdose occurs during instillation, flush the affected eye with water or normal saline.

◆ *Drug interactions*
   Carbamate and/or organophosphate insecticides and pesticides. Gardeners, farmers, manufacturing employees, and others who are exposed to these pesticides and insecticides and who are receiving cholinergic agents should be warned of the added risk of systemic symptoms from absorption of these chemicals through the skin and respiratory tract. Respiratory masks, frequent washing, and clothing changes are advisable.

Table 42.2 Cholinergic Agents

GENERIC NAME	BRAND NAME	AVAILABILITY	DOSAGE	COMMENTS
acetylcholine chloride, intraocular	Miochol-E	20 mg in 2-mL vial for reconstitution, making a 1:100 solution	0.5-2 mL instilled into the eye during surgery	Used only during surgery to produce complete miosis within seconds; duration of action is only a few minutes, so pilocarpine may be added to maintain miosis
carbachol, intraocular	Miostat	Solution: 0.01%	0.5 mL	Used only during surgery to produce complete miosis within 2-5 min
pilocarpine	Isopto Carpine	Solution: 1%, 2%, 4%	1 drop up to four times daily; 1%-4% solutions used most frequently	Safest, most commonly used miotic for glaucoma; also used to reverse mydriasis after eye examination; onset is 10-30 min; lasts for 4-8 hr

DRUG CLASS: ALPHA-ADRENERGIC AGENTS

Actions

Alpha-adrenergic agents have several uses in ophthalmology. Sympathomimetic agents cause pupil dilation, increased outflow of aqueous humor, vasoconstriction, relaxation of the ciliary muscle, and a decrease in the formation of aqueous humor.

Uses

Alpha-adrenergic agents are used to lower IOP in open-angle glaucoma, relieve congestion and hyperemia, and produce mydriasis for ocular examinations. Use with caution in patients with hypertension, diabetes mellitus, hyperthyroidism, heart disease, arteriosclerosis, or long-standing bronchial asthma.

Therapeutic Outcomes

The primary therapeutic outcomes expected from alpha-adrenergic agents are as follows:

1. Mydriasis for ophthalmic examination
2. Reduced IOP in open-angle glaucoma
3. Reduced redness of the eyes from irritation

❖ Nursing Implications for Alpha-Adrenergic Agents

◆ *Premedication assessment*

1. Obtain baseline vital signs, including blood pressure and pulse.
2. Record premedication IOP readings and visual acuity data.

◆ *Availability, dosage, and administration*
See Table 42.3.

◆ *Common adverse effects*
  Sensory
  Sensitivity to bright light. The mydriasis produced allows excessive amounts of light into the eyes, which causes the patient to squint. Sunglasses will help reduce the brightness. Caution the patient to temporarily avoid tasks that require visual acuity, such as driving or operating power machinery.

  Conjunctival irritation, lacrimation. These adverse effects are usually mild and tend to resolve with continued therapy. Encourage the patient not to discontinue therapy without first consulting the healthcare provider.

◆ *Serious adverse effects*
  Cardiovascular
  Systemic adverse effects. Systemic effects from ophthalmic instillation are uncommon and minimal; however, systemic absorption may occur via the lacrimal drainage system into the nasopharyngeal passages. Systemic effects are manifested by palpitations, tachycardia, dysrhythmias, hypertension, faintness, trembling, and diaphoresis. These are indications of overdose or excessive administration. Report to the healthcare provider for treatment and dosage adjustment. Prevent systemic effects by carefully blocking the inner canthus for 3 to 5 minutes after instilling the medication to prevent absorption via the nasolacrimal duct. Monitor the pulse rate and blood pressure, and instruct the patient to continue to do this at home; report significant changes from the baseline data.

  Diaphoresis, trembling. Touch the patient and bedding to assess for diaphoresis, particularly when these medications are used in surgery in which the patient is under sterile drapes, anesthetized, and unable to respond to verbal questioning.

◆ *Drug interactions*
  Tricyclic antidepressants. Tricyclic antidepressants (e.g., amitriptyline, imipramine, doxepin) may cause additive hypertensive effects. Monitor carefully for poor blood pressure control or a gradually increasing blood pressure.

Table 42.3 Alpha-Adrenergic Agents

GENERIC NAME	BRAND NAME	AVAILABILITY	DOSAGE	COMMENTS
apraclonidine	Iopidine	Solution: 0.5%, 1%	1 drop 1 hr before surgery and 1 drop immediately after surgery	An alpha-2 adrenergic agent used to control IOP after laser surgery
brimonidine	Alphagan P	Solution: 0.1%, 0.15%, 0.2%	1 drop q8h in affected eye(s)	An alpha-2 adrenergic agent used to lower IOP in open-angle glaucoma or ocular hypertension
naphazoline hydrochloride	Clear Eyes	Solution: 0.0125%	1-2 drops q3-4h (up to four times daily)	Used as a topical vasoconstrictor; therapy should not exceed 3 days
phenylephrine	Altafrin	Solution: 2.5%, 10%	1-2 drops two or three times daily	2.5% and 10% solutions used for pupil dilation in uveitis, open-angle glaucoma, and diagnostic procedures
tetrahydrozoline hydrochloride	Opti-Clear; Good Sense Eye Drops	Solution: 0.05%	1-2 drops two to four times daily	Used as a topical vasoconstrictor

IOP, Intraocular pressure.

DRUG CLASS: BETA-ADRENERGIC BLOCKING AGENTS

Actions

Beta-adrenergic blocking agents are used in ophthalmology to reduce elevated IOP. Their exact mechanism of action is not known, but it is thought that they reduce the production of aqueous humor.

Uses

Beta blockers are used to reduce IOP in patients with chronic open-angle glaucoma or ocular hypertension. Unlike anticholinergic agents, there is no blurred or dim vision or night blindness because IOP is reduced with little or no effect on pupil size or visual acuity.

Therapeutic Outcome

The primary therapeutic outcome expected from beta-adrenergic blocking agents is reduced IOP.

❖ **Nursing Implications for Beta-Adrenergic Blocking Agents**

◆ *Premedication assessment*
1. Obtain baseline vital signs, including pulse and blood pressure; hold the medication and contact the healthcare provider if bradycardia, hypertension, or respiratory disorders are present.
2. Record the premedication IOP readings and visual acuity data.

◆ *Availability, dosage, and administration*
See Table 42.4.

◆ *Common adverse effects*
Sensory
Conjunctival irritation, lacrimation. These adverse effects are usually mild and tend to resolve with continued

therapy. Encourage the patient not to discontinue therapy without first consulting the healthcare provider.

◆ *Serious adverse effects*
Cardiovascular
Bradycardia, hypotension. Systemic effects are uncommon but may be manifested by bradycardia, dysrhythmias, hypotension, faintness, and bronchospasm. These adverse effects are more frequently observed in patients requiring higher dosages of beta-adrenergic blocking agents and in patients with hypertension, diabetes mellitus, heart disease, arteriosclerosis, or long-standing bronchial asthma. Report to the healthcare provider for treatment and dosage adjustment. Record the blood pressure and pulse rate at specific intervals.

◆ *Drug interactions*
Nonophthalmic beta-adrenergic blocking agents. Nonophthalmic beta blockers (e.g., propranolol, atenolol, metoprolol) may enhance the systemic therapeutic and toxic effects of ophthalmic beta-adrenergic blocking medications. Monitor for an increase in severity of adverse effects such as fatigue, hypotension, bronchospasm, and bradycardia.

DRUG CLASS: PROSTAGLANDIN AGONISTS

Actions

Prostaglandin agonists reduce IOP by increasing the outflow of aqueous humor.

Uses

The prostaglandin agonists are used to reduce IOP in patients with chronic open-angle glaucoma or ocular hypertension who have not responded well to other IOP-lowering agents.

Table 42.4   Beta-Adrenergic Blocking Agents

GENERIC NAME	BRAND NAME	AVAILABILITY	INITIAL DOSAGE	COMMENTS
betaxolol hydrochloride	Betoptic S	Solution: 0.25%, 0.5% in 5-, 10-, 15-mL dropper bottles	1-2 drops twice daily	Beta-1 blocking agent; onset in 30 min, duration is 12 hr; several weeks of therapy may be required to determine optimal dosage
carteolol	—	Solution: 1% in 5-, 10-, 15-mL dropper bottles	1 drop twice daily	Beta-1, beta-2 blocking agent; duration is up to 12 hr
levobunolol hydrochloride	Betagan	Solution: 0.5% in 5-, 10-, 15-mL dropper bottles	1 drop once or twice daily	Beta-1, beta-2 blocking agent; onset within 60 min, duration is up to 24 hr
metipranolol	—	Solution: 0.3% in 5-, 10-mL dropper bottles	1 drop twice daily in affected eye(s)	Beta-1, beta-2 blocking agent; onset within 30 min, duration is 12-24 hr
timolol maleate	Timoptic	Solution: 0.25%, 0.5% in 5-, 10-, 15-mL dropper bottles Solution, gel-forming: 0.25%, 0.5%	1 drop of 0.25% solution twice daily; 1 drop of gel solution once daily	Beta-1, beta-2 blocking agent; onset within 30 min, duration is up to 24 hr; gel may be used once daily

Therapeutic Outcome

The primary therapeutic outcome expected from prostaglandin agonists is reduced IOP.

❖ Nursing Implications for Prostaglandin Agonists

◆ *Premedication assessment*

1. Obtain baseline vital signs.
2. Record the premedication IOP readings and visual acuity data.

◆ *Availability, dosage, and administration.* See Table 42.5. If more than one drug is to be instilled in the same eye, administer the drugs at least 5 minutes apart.

> **⚠ Medication Safety Alert**
>
> Do not administer prostaglandin agonists into the eyes when the patient is wearing contact lenses. Lenses may be reinserted 15 minutes following administration.

◆ *Common and serious adverse effects*

Sensory

Conjunctival irritation, burning and stinging, lacrimation. These adverse effects are usually mild and tend to resolve with continued therapy. Encourage the patient not to discontinue therapy without first consulting the healthcare provider.

Eye pigment changes. The prostaglandin agonists may gradually cause changes to pigmented tissues, including change to eye color, increasing the amount of brown pigment in the iris. The change may take several months to years to develop and is thought to be permanent. Iris pigmentation changes may be more evident in patients with green-brown, blue-brown, gray-brown, or yellow-brown irises. The eyelids may also develop color changes. There may also be an increased growth of eyelashes.

◆ *Drug interactions*

Thimerosal. A precipitate occurs when eyedrops containing thimerosal (a commonly used preservative in ophthalmic solutions) are mixed with latanoprost. Administer eyedrops at least 5 minutes apart.

OTHER OPHTHALMIC AGENTS

DRUG CLASS: ANTICHOLINERGIC AGENTS

Actions

Anticholinergic agents cause the smooth muscle of the ciliary body and iris to relax, producing mydriasis (extreme dilation of the pupil) and cycloplegia (paralysis of the ciliary muscle).

Uses

Ophthalmologists use anticholinergic agents for their pharmacologic effects to examine the interior of the eye, measure the proper strength of lenses for eyeglasses (refraction), and rest the eye in inflammatory conditions of the uveal tract.

Table 42.5 Prostaglandin Agonists

GENERIC NAME	BRAND NAME	AVAILABILITY	DOSAGE	COMMENTS
bimatoprost	Lumigan	Solution: 0.01%, 0.03% in 2.5-, 5-, 7.5-mL dropper bottles	1 drop in each affected eye in the evening	Do not exceed dosage because it may reduce IOP-lowering effect
latanoprost	Xalatan	Solution: 0.005% in 2.5, 7.5-mL dropper bottle	1 drop in each affected eye in the evening	Do not exceed dosage because it may reduce IOP-lowering effect
tafluprost	Zioptan	Solution: 0.0015% in 0.3-mL pouch	1 drop in each affected eye in the evening	Do not exceed dosage because it may reduce IOP-lowering effect. If used with other ophthalmic agents, separate administration by at least 5 min
travoprost	Travatan Z	Solution: 0.004% in 2.5-, 5-mL dropper bottles	1 drop in each affected eye in the evening	Do not exceed dosage because it may reduce IOP-lowering effect

IOP, Intraocular pressure.

Therapeutic Outcomes

The primary therapeutic outcomes expected from anticholinergic ophthalmic use are as follows:

1. Visualization of intraocular structures
2. Reduced uveal tract inflammation

❖ Nursing Implications for Anticholinergic Agents

◆ Premedication assessment

1. Check for the diagnosis of increased IOP. If present, hold the medication and contact the healthcare provider for approval before instillation of the anticholinergic agent.
2. Take vital signs; if the patient has hypertension, contact the healthcare provider for approval before instilling the anticholinergic agent.

◆ Availability, dosage, and administration

See Table 42.6.

> **! Medication Safety Alert**
>
> The pharmacologic effects of anticholinergic agents cause an increase in IOP. Use these agents with extreme caution in patients with narrow anterior chamber angle; in infants, children, and older adults; and in patients with hypertension, hyperthyroidism, and diabetes. Discontinue therapy if signs of increased IOP (i.e., blurred vision, halos around white lights, frontal headaches and eye pain) or systemic effects develop.

◆ Common adverse effects

Sensory

Sensitivity to bright light. The mydriasis produced allows excessive light into the eyes, causing the patient to squint. Sunglasses will help reduce the brightness. Caution the patient to temporarily avoid tasks that require visual acuity, such as driving or operating power machinery.

Conjunctival irritation, lacrimation. These adverse effects are usually mild and tend to resolve with continued therapy. Encourage the patient not to discontinue therapy without first consulting the healthcare provider.

◆ Serious adverse effects

Neurologic

Systemic adverse effects. Prolonged use may result in systemic effects manifested by flushing and dryness of the skin, dry mouth, blurred vision, tachycardia, dysrhythmias, urinary hesitancy and retention, vasodilation, and constipation. These are indications of overdose or excessive administration. Report to the healthcare provider for treatment and dosage adjustment. Prevent systemic effects by carefully blocking the inner canthus for 3 to 5 minutes after instilling the medication to prevent absorption via the nasolacrimal duct. Monitor the pulse rate and blood pressure, and instruct the patient to continue to do this at home; report significant changes from the baseline data. Children are particularly prone to developing systemic reactions.

◆ Drug interactions

No clinically significant drug interactions have been reported.

DRUG CLASS: ANTIFUNGAL AGENTS

natamycin (nă-tă-MĪ-sĭn)
  Natacyn (NĂT-ă-sĭn)

Actions

Natamycin acts by altering the cell wall of the fungus to prevent it from serving as a selective barrier, therefore causing loss of fluids and electrolytes.

Uses

Natamycin is an antifungal agent that is effective against a variety of yeasts, including *Candida* species, *Aspergillus*

Table 42.6 Anticholinergic Agents

GENERIC NAME	BRAND NAME	AVAILABILITY	DOSAGE	COMMENTS
atropine sulfate		Ointment: 1% Solution: 1%	Uveitis: 1-2 drops up to three times daily	Onset of mydriasis and cycloplegia is 30-40 min, duration is 7-12 days Do not use in infants
cyclopentolate hydrochloride	Cyclogyl	Solution: 0.5%, 1%, 2%	Refraction: 1 drop followed by another drop in 5-10 min	For mydriasis and cycloplegia necessary for diagnostic procedures; 1-2 drops of 1%-2% pilocarpine allows full recovery within 6-24 hr CNS disturbances of hallucinations, loss of orientation, restlessness, and incoherent speech have been reported in children
homatropine hydrobromide		Solution: 5%	Uveitis: 1-2 drops q3-4h	Onset of mydriasis and cycloplegia is 40-60 min; duration is 1-3 days
Tropicamide	Mydriacyl	Solution: 0.5%, 1%	Refraction: 1-2 drops, repeated in 5 min	Onset of mydriasis and cycloplegia is 20-40 min; duration is 6 hr CNS disturbances such as hallucinations, loss of orientation, restlessness, and incoherent speech have been reported in children

CNS, Central nervous system.

species, and *Fusarium* species. It is effective in treating fungal blepharitis, conjunctivitis, and keratitis caused by susceptible organisms. If little or no improvement is noted after 7 to 10 days of treatment, resistance to the antifungal agent may have developed. Topical administration does not appear to result in systemic effects.

Therapeutic Outcome

The primary therapeutic outcome expected from natamycin is eradication of fungal infection.

❖ Nursing Implications for Natamycin

◆ *Premedication assessment*
1. Collect ordered cultures or smears before initiating drug therapy.
2. Record baseline data relating to symptoms accompanying the fungal infection and the degree of visual impairment.

◆ *Availability. Ophthalmic:* 5% suspension.

◆ *Dosage and administration. Fungal keratitis:* One drop in the conjunctival sac at 1- or 2-hour intervals for the first 3 to 4 days. The dosage may then be reduced to 1 drop every 3 to 4 hours. Continue therapy for 14 to 21 days.

Fungal blepharitis or conjunctivitis: One drop in the conjunctival sac every 4 to 6 hours.

◆ *Common adverse effects*
  Sensory
  Sensitivity to bright light. The slight mydriasis produced allows an excessive amount of light into the eyes, causing the patient to squint. Sunglasses will help reduce the brightness. Caution the patient to avoid tasks temporarily

that require visual acuity, such as driving or operating power machinery.

Blurred vision, lacrimation, redness. Provide for patient safety during temporary visual impairment. Instruct the patient not to rub the eyes forcefully while tearing. These adverse effects are usually mild and tend to resolve with continued therapy. Encourage the patient not to discontinue therapy without first consulting the healthcare provider.

◆ *Serious adverse effects*
  Sensory
  Eye pain. If eye pain develops, discontinue use and consult an ophthalmologist immediately.
  Therapeutic effect. If, after several days of therapy, the symptoms do not improve or if they gradually worsen, consult the prescribing healthcare provider treating the patient.

◆ *Drug interactions.* No significant drug interactions have been reported.

DRUG CLASS: ANTIVIRAL AGENTS

Actions

The ophthalmic antiviral agents act by inhibiting viral replication.

Uses

Trifluridine is used to treat keratitis caused by herpes simplex virus types 1 and 2. Ganciclovir is used to treat cytomegalovirus retinitis for patients with acquired immunodeficiency syndrome. These antiviral agents are not effective against infections caused by bacteria, fungi, or *Chlamydia* organisms.

Therapeutic Outcome

The primary therapeutic outcome expected from antiviral agents is eradication of the viral infection.

❖ **Nursing Implications for Antiviral Agents**

◆ *Premedication assessment.* Record baseline data concerning the symptoms and the degree of visual impairment.

◆ *Availability, dosage, and administration*

See Table 42.7.

  Storage. Trifluridine should be stored in the refrigerator.

> ❗ **Medication Safety Alert**
>
> If significant improvement has not occurred 7 to 14 days after initiating treatment with trifluridine, other therapy should be considered. Do not exceed 21 days of continuous therapy because of potential ocular toxicity.

◆ *Common adverse effects*

  Sensory

  Visual haze, lacrimation, redness, burning. Patients may notice a mild, transient stinging, burning, and redness of the conjunctiva and sclera on instillation. Provide for patient safety during temporary visual impairment. Instruct the patient not to rub the eyes forcefully while tearing. These adverse effects are usually mild and tend to resolve with continued therapy. Encourage the patient not to discontinue therapy without first consulting the healthcare provider.

  Sensitivity to bright light. The slight mydriasis produced allows excessive light into the eyes, causing the patient to squint. Sunglasses will help reduce the brightness. Caution the patient to temporarily avoid tasks that require visual acuity, such as driving or operating power machinery.

◆ *Serious adverse effects*

  Immune system

  Allergic reactions. Discontinue therapy and consult an ophthalmologist immediately.

◆ *Drug interactions.* No significant drug interactions have been reported.

DRUG CLASS: OPHTHALMIC ANTIBIOTICS

Uses

Ophthalmic antibiotics (Table 42.8) are used to treat superficial eye infections and for prophylaxis against gonorrhea infection in the eyes of newborn infants (ophthalmia neonatorum). Prolonged or frequent intermittent use of topical antibiotics should be avoided because of the possibility of hypersensitivity reactions and the development of resistant organisms, including fungi. If hypersensitivities or new infections appear during use, consult an ophthalmologist immediately. Refer to Chapter 45 for a discussion of these antibiotics.

DRUG CLASS: CORTICOSTEROIDS

Uses

Corticosteroid therapy (Table 42.9) is used for allergic reactions of the eye and other acute, noninfectious inflammatory conditions of the conjunctiva, sclera, cornea, and anterior uveal tract. Corticosteroid therapy must not be used for bacterial, fungal, or viral infections of the eye because corticosteroids decrease defense mechanisms and reduce resistance to pathologic organisms. This therapy should be used only for a limited time and the eye should be checked frequently for an increase in IOP. Prolonged ocular steroid therapy may cause glaucoma and cataracts. Refer to Chapter 37 for further discussion of the corticosteroids.

DRUG CLASS: OPHTHALMIC ANTIINFLAMMATORY AGENTS

Flurbiprofen sodium, ketorolac tromethamine, bromfenac, nepafenac, and diclofenac sodium are topical nonsteroidal antiinflammatory drugs for ophthalmic use. These agents have been shown to have antiinflammatory, antipyretic, and analgesic activity by inhibiting the biosynthesis of prostaglandins that are responsible for an increase in intraocular inflammation and pressure. They also inhibit prostaglandin-mediated constriction of the iris (miosis) that is independent of cholinergic mechanisms. Flurbiprofen is used primarily to inhibit miosis during cataract surgery. Diclofenac sodium, nepafenac, and bromfenac are used to treat postoperative inflammation after cataract extraction.

 Table 42.7 Antiviral Agents

GENERIC NAME	BRAND NAME	AVAILABILITY	DOSAGE
ganciclovir	Zirgan	Gel: 0.15%	Initial dosage: 1 drop in affected eye five times daily (about q3h while awake) until the corneal ulcer heals Maintenance dosage: 1 drop three times daily for 7 days
trifluridine	Viroptic	Solution: 1% in 7.5-mL dropper bottle	Intraocular: Place 1 drop onto the cornea of the affected eye q2h during waking hours; do not exceed 9 drops daily Continue for 7 more days to prevent recurrence, using 1 drop q4h (5 drops daily)

Table 42.8   Ophthalmic Antibiotics

Antibiotic	Brand Name	Availability
azithromycin	AzaSite	Drops
bacitracin	Bacitracin ophthalmic	Ointment
besifloxacin	Besivance	Drops
ciprofloxacin	Ciloxan	Drops, ointment
erythromycin		Ointment
gatifloxacin	Zymaxid	Drops
gentamicin	Gentak	Drops, ointment
levofloxacin	—	Drops
moxifloxacin	Moxeza, Vigamox	Drops
ofloxacin	Ocuflox	Drops
sulfacetamide	Bleph-10	Drops
tobramycin	Tobrex ophthalmic	Drops, ointment
Combinations		
trimethoprim-polymyxin B	Polytrim ophthalmic	Drops
polymyxin B-bacitracin	Polycin	Ointment
neomycin-polymyxin B-bacitracin	Neo-Polycin ophthalmic	Ointment
neomycin-polymyxin B-gramicidin	Neosporin ophthalmic	Solution

Table 42.9   Corticosteroids

Generic Name	Brand Name	Availability
dexamethasone	Maxidex — Ozurdex	Suspension Solution Implant
difluprednate	Durezol	Suspension
fluocinolone	Retisert	Implant
fluorometholone	FML FML Liquifilm	Ointment Suspension
loteprednol	Lotemax	Suspension; ointment; gel
prednisolone	Omnipred	Suspension
triamcinolone	Triesence	Suspension for intravitreal injection

Flurbiprofen is available as a 0.03% solution, which should be used by instilling 1 drop in the appropriate eye every 30 minutes, beginning 2 hours before surgery (for a total of 4 drops). Diclofenac sodium is available as a 0.1% solution. One drop is applied to the affected eye four times daily beginning 24 hours after surgery and continuing for 2 weeks. Ketorolac tromethamine is available as a 0.4% solution (Acular LS) and a 0.5% solution (Acular). One drop is applied to each eye four times daily to relieve ocular itching associated with seasonal allergic conjunctivitis. This same dose may be applied to the operated eye for pain and photophobia for up to 3 days after surgery. Bromfenac is available as a 0.07% solution (Prolensa), a 0.075% solution (BromSite), and a 0.09% solution. One drop is instilled in the operated eye once or twice daily (depending on product) beginning 24 hours after cataract surgery for up to 2 weeks to treat postoperative pain and inflammation. Nepafenac is available as a 0.1% suspension (Nevanac) and a 0.3% suspension (Ilevro). One drop is instilled in the affected eye(s) one time daily (Ilevro) or three times daily (Nevanac) beginning 1 day before cataract surgery; continue the day of surgery and through the first 2 weeks of the postoperative period for pain and inflammation.

DRUG CLASS: ANTIHISTAMINES

Alcaftadine, azelastine, bepotastine, cetirizine, emedastine, epinastine, ketotifen, and olopatadine are histamine-1 antagonists that act by inhibiting release of histamine from mast cells. They are used for relief of signs and symptoms and prevention of itching associated with allergic conjunctivitis. For best results, they should be instilled in the eyes before exposure to allergens such as pollen (Table 42.10).

DRUG CLASS: ANTIALLERGENIC AGENTS

Uses

Cromolyn sodium, lodoxamide, and nedocromil are stabilizing agents that inhibit the release of histamine and the slow-reacting substance of anaphylaxis from mast cells after exposure to specific antigens. They are used to treat allergic ocular disorders such as vernal keratoconjunctivitis, vernal keratitis, and allergic keratoconjunctivitis. Cromolyn sodium is available as a 4% solution; 1 or 2 drops are applied in each eye four to six times daily at regular intervals. Lodoxamide (Alomide) is available as a 0.1% solution; 1 or 2 drops are applied in each affected eye four times daily. Nedocromil (Alocril) is available as a 2% solution; 1 or 2 drops are applied in each eye twice daily at regular intervals.

DRUG CLASS: DIAGNOSTIC AGENT

fluorescein (flŭ-RĔS-ēn)

Uses

Fluorescein is used in fitting hard contact lenses and as a diagnostic aid in identifying foreign bodies in the eye and abraded or ulcerated areas of the cornea. It is also useful for evaluating retinal vasculature for abnormal circulation.

Table 42.10 Ophthalmic Antihistamines

GENERIC NAME	BRAND NAME	AVAILABILITY	DOSAGE
Alcaftadine	Lastacaft	Solution: 0.25% in 3-mL dropper bottle	Instill 1 drop in each eye once daily
Azelastine	—	Solution: 0.05% in 6-mL dropper bottle	Instill 1 drop in each affected eye twice daily
Bepotastine	Bepreve	Solution: 1.5% in 5 and 10-mL dropper bottle	Instill 1 drop in each affected eye twice daily
cetirizine	Zerviate	Solution: 0.24% in 7.5-, 10-mL dropper bottle	Instill 1 drop in affected eye twice daily (~8 hr apart)
emedastine	Emadine	Solution: 0.05% in 5-mL dropper bottle	Instill 1 drop in each eye up to four times daily
epinastine	Elestat	Solution: 0.05% in 5-mL dropper bottles	Instill 1 drop in each eye twice daily
ketotifen	Zaditor	Solution: 0.025% in 5-, 10-mL dropper bottles	Instill one drop in each eye q8-12h
olopatadine	Patanol	Solution: 0.1% in 5-mL dropper bottle	Instill 1-2 drops in each affected eye twice daily at interval of 6-8 hr
olopatadine	Pataday	Solution: 0.2% in 2.5-mL dropper bottle	Instill 1 drop in each affected eye once daily
olopatadine	Pazeo	Solution: 0.7% in in 2.5-mL dropper bottle	Instill 1 drop in each affected eye once daily

When fluorescein is instilled in the eye, it stains the pathologic tissues green if observed under normal light and bright yellow if viewed under cobalt blue light. Fluorescein is available in 0.6- and 1-mg strips for topical application, and 10% and 25% solutions for injection into the aqueous humor. The strips have the advantage of being used once and then discarded. Product names include Fluorescite, AK-Fluor, BioGlo, and Ful-Glo.

DRUG CLASS: ARTIFICIAL TEAR SOLUTIONS

Uses

Artificial tear solutions mimic natural secretions of the eye. They provide lubrication for dry eyes and may be used as lubricants for artificial eyes. Most products contain variable concentrations of methylcellulose, polyvinyl alcohol, and polyethylene glycol. The dosage is 1 to 3 drops in each eye three or four times daily, as needed. Product names include Systane Ultra, Refresh, Tears Naturale Free, Artificial Tears, and HypoTears.

DRUG CLASS: VASCULAR ENDOTHELIAL GROWTH FACTOR ANTAGONIST

Macular degeneration is a deterioration of the macula, a small area in the retina at the back of the eye that is required to see fine details clearly (e.g., reading or threading a needle) or to judge distances (e.g., when driving an automobile). With macular degeneration, central vision is affected by blurriness, dark areas, and distortion. Peripheral vision is usually not affected.

Many older people develop macular degeneration as part of the body's natural aging process. The most common is age-related macular degeneration (AMD). Why it develops is unknown. Macular degeneration is the leading cause of severe vision loss in whites older than 65 years.

The two most common types of AMD are "dry" (atrophic) and "wet" (exudative).

- *Dry macular degeneration* (atrophic) is caused by the aging and thinning of the tissues of the macula. Vision loss is usually gradual. Most people have the dry form of AMD.
- *Wet macular degeneration* (exudative) accounts for about 10% of all AMD cases. It results when abnormal blood vessels form underneath the retina at the back of the eye. These new blood vessels leak fluid or blood and blur central vision. Vision loss may be rapid and severe.

Pegaptanib (Macugen), aflibercept (Eylea), and ranibizumab (Lucentis) are selective vascular endothelial growth factor (VEGF) antagonists. Vascular endothelial growth factor is secreted and binds to its receptors, which are located primarily on the surface of endothelial cells of blood vessels. Vascular endothelial growth factor induces new blood vessel growth and increases vascular permeability and inflammation, all of which are thought to contribute to the progression of the wet form of AMD. Pegaptanib, aflibercept, and ranibizumab are antagonists that bind to extracellular VEGF, preventing it from binding to VEGF receptors and thus preventing it from forming new blood vessels. Pegaptanib is injected into the vitreous humor of the affected eye once every 6 weeks; aflibercept is administered every 4 weeks for the first 12 weeks, then every 8 weeks thereafter. Ranibizumab is administered once monthly. In the days following administration of either agent, patients are at risk for the development of endophthalmitis. Instruct the patient to seek immediate care from his or her ophthalmologist if the eye becomes red, sensitive to light, or painful or if a deterioration of vision is noted.

Get Ready for the NCLEX® Examination!

Key Points

- The nurse has an important role to educate the patient about glaucoma management.
- The nurse is instrumental in educating the public and promoting safety measures to protect the eyes from sources of injury.
- Examples of areas in which the nurse can teach the public are the use of safety glasses in hazardous situations, prevention of chemical burns from common household cleaning items or other agents at home or work, proper cleaning and wearing of contact lenses or glasses, and the selection of safe toys and play activities for children. These safety measures can significantly reduce the number of injuries that occur annually.
- Nurses instruct patients on proper administration of eye medications.
- Nurses need to determine that the patient understands how to prevent eye infections as well as how eye infections are treated.

Additional Learning Resources

SG Go to your Study Guide for additional Review Questions for the NCLEX® Examination, Critical Thinking Clinical Situations, and other learning activities to help you master this chapter content.

Go to your Evolve website (https://evolve.elsevier.com/Clayton) for additional online resources.

Review Questions for the NCLEX® Examination

1. The nurse was explaining the difference between open-angle glaucoma and closed-angle glaucoma to a patient who was recently diagnosed with open-angle glaucoma. Which statement by the patient would indicate further education is needed?
   1. "As I understand it, this type of glaucoma develops slowly over many years."
   2. "This would have been prevented if I had not worn contact lenses when I was a teen."
   3. "The symptoms of blurred vision, halos around white lights, frontal headache, and eye pain indicate that there is an obstruction of the fluid in my eyeball."
   4. "When my eyes are dilated, the symptoms of glaucoma can occur."

2. After the nurse uses the proper technique for instilling eyedrops, further patient education is needed to ensure absorption of the drug by explaining what to the patient?
   1. Tilting his or her head to the side that the eyedrop was administered is necessary.
   2. He or she will need to keep the eyes open after administration.
   3. Gentle pressure at the inner canthus to block the tear duct for several minutes will be needed.
   4. He or she will need to wear contact lenses prior to administration.

3. The nurse is instructing the patient on the use of pilocarpine. Which statement by the nurse is correct?
   1. "This medication will inhibit the release of histamine so you will not have itchy eyes."
   2. "These eyedrops are used to treat your glaucoma."
   3. "When these drops are used, they cause a stain on the eye for examination purposes."
   4. "This medication prevents production of aqueous humor so increased intraocular pressure is reduced."

4. Before administering a beta-adrenergic blocking agent for reduction of intraocular pressure, the nurse should assess the patient for a history of which disorders? *(Select all that apply.)*
   1. Respiratory disorders
   2. Diabetes mellitus
   3. Hypertension
   4. Urinary retention
   5. Rheumatoid arthritis

5. The nurse instructs the patient on which precaution to use after insertion of ophthalmic ointment?
   1. "You need to compress the tear duct for 3 to 5 minutes after I have applied this."
   2. "The ointment may cause some visual blurriness for a while. Blinking will help disperse the ointment, reducing the blurred vision."
   3. "After I give this to you, please look up at the ceiling for a few minutes."
   4. "It does not matter which order you apply the eyedrops or eye ointment."

6. The nurse providing postoperative instructions for a patient following eye surgery will include which of these statements? *(Select all that apply.)*
   1. "You will need to notify your healthcare provider when any eye pain is not relieved by pain medication."
   2. "You can resume normal activities without restriction."
   3. "You need to use aseptic technique when changing dressings or administering medications."
   4. "Please be sure to call your healthcare provider with any signs of infection in your eye."
   5. "Remember to store your eyedrops with other containers that look alike, so you do not lose them."

7. The patient asked the nurse what the eye medication timolol (Timoptic) was given for. Which statement by the nurse is the most appropriate?
   1. "This medication will be effective in preventing any eye infection."
   2. "This medication is for glaucoma and will increase the outflow of aqueous humor in your eye so that the pressures are decreased."
   3. "This medication is considered an antiinflammatory agent used to help any itching you have."
   4. "This medication is for glaucoma and will lower the pressures in your eye by reducing the production of aqueous humor."

43

Drugs Used to Treat Cancer

Objectives

1. Cite the goals of chemotherapy.
2. Describe the role of targeted anticancer agents in treating cancer.
3. Identify how chemoprotective agents are used in treating cancer.
4. Discuss bone marrow stimulants and their effect and use.
5. Describe the nursing assessments and interventions needed to help alleviate the adverse effects of chemotherapy.

Key Terms

cancer (KĂN-sŭr) (p. 668)
metastases (mĕ-TĂS-tă-sēz) (p. 668)
neoplastic disease (nē-ō-PLĂS-tĭk dĭs-ĒZ) (p. 668)
malignant (mă-LĬG-nănt) (p. 668)
palliation (păl-ē-Ā-shŭn) (p. 669)

combination therapy (kŏm-bĭ-NĀ-shŭn THĀR-ŭ-pē) (p. 670)
targeted anticancer agents (TĂR-gĕt-ĕd ăn-tē-KĂN-sŭr) (p. 671)
chemoprotective agents (kē-mō-prō-TĔK-tĭv) (p. 671)

CANCER AND THE USE OF ANTINEOPLASTIC AGENTS

Cancer is a group of more than 100 different diseases that are characterized by uncontrolled cellular growth, local tissue invasion, and distant metastases (Chabner, 2010). It is a group of once-normal cells that have mutated to abnormal cells that generally multiply more rapidly than normal cells, lose the ability to perform specialized functions, invade surrounding tissues, and develop growths in other tissues distant to the site of original growth (metastases). Cancer is also referred to as a *neoplasm, neoplastic disease,* or *new growth.* The new growth may be subdivided into benign or malignant cells. Since benign cells do not metastasize, they are generally not as life threatening as the malignant cells. Malignant cells often metastasize to other organs of the body, making treatment and survival substantially less likely.

The American Cancer Society reported that the rates of cancer occurrences and deaths have decreased since an all-time high in the year 1991. As of 2014 the rate has dropped by 25% due to reduction in smoking as well as improvements in detection and treatment. Cancer is the second most common cause of death in the United States, exceeded only by heart disease (Fig. 43.1). Estimates indicated that, in 2017, there would be almost 1.7 million new cancer cases and almost 601,000 deaths from cancer, which is about 1650 deaths per day.

Cancers can occur anywhere in the body: within organs (e.g., liver, colon, lungs); within blood components (e.g., lymphatic system) causing lymphoma; and within bone marrow, causing leukemias. Treatment of cancer often requires a combination of surgery, radiation, chemotherapy, targeted drug therapy, and biologic therapy. Biologic therapies are made from a living organism or its by-products and include antibodies, vaccines, growth factors, and cytokines. Surgery and radiation are considered to be local therapy, whereas chemotherapy, targeted drug therapy, and biologic therapies use the systemic circulation to treat the primary tumor and metastases. Recent advancements in understanding carcinogenesis, cellular and molecular biology, genetics, and tumor immunology have enhanced the role that antineoplastic agents may play in treatment. It is beyond the scope of this chapter to delve into the interrelationships of chemotherapy and neoplastic disease; however, a short discussion of the concepts of cancer chemotherapy will be presented. As a result of rapidly changing approaches to the treatment of specific malignancies and the changing nature of chemotherapeutic regimens, specific agents and dosages will not be discussed.

All cells, whether normal or malignant, pass through a similar series of phases during their lifetime, although duration of time spent in each phase differs with the type of cell (Fig. 43.2). The cell cycle involves five stages: DNA replication (S phase), cell division (M phase), two

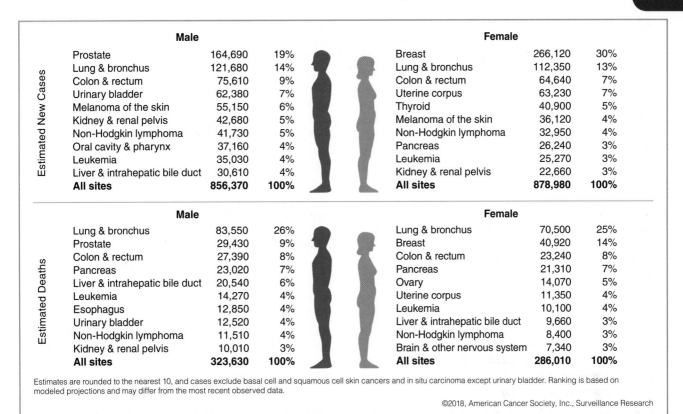

	Male				**Female**		
Estimated New Cases	Prostate	164,690	19%	Breast	266,120	30%
	Lung & bronchus	121,680	14%	Lung & bronchus	112,350	13%
	Colon & rectum	75,610	9%	Colon & rectum	64,640	7%
	Urinary bladder	62,380	7%	Uterine corpus	63,230	7%
	Melanoma of the skin	55,150	6%	Thyroid	40,900	5%
	Kidney & renal pelvis	42,680	5%	Melanoma of the skin	36,120	4%
	Non-Hodgkin lymphoma	41,730	5%	Non-Hodgkin lymphoma	32,950	4%
	Oral cavity & pharynx	37,160	4%	Pancreas	26,240	3%
	Leukemia	35,030	4%	Leukemia	25,270	3%
	Liver & intrahepatic bile duct	30,610	4%	Kidney & renal pelvis	22,660	3%
	All sites	**856,370**	**100%**	**All sites**	**878,980**	**100%**

	Male				**Female**		
Estimated Deaths	Lung & bronchus	83,550	26%	Lung & bronchus	70,500	25%
	Prostate	29,430	9%	Breast	40,920	14%
	Colon & rectum	27,390	8%	Colon & rectum	23,240	8%
	Pancreas	23,020	7%	Pancreas	21,310	7%
	Liver & intrahepatic bile duct	20,540	6%	Ovary	14,070	5%
	Leukemia	14,270	4%	Uterine corpus	11,350	4%
	Esophagus	12,850	4%	Leukemia	10,100	4%
	Urinary bladder	12,520	4%	Liver & intrahepatic bile duct	9,660	3%
	Non-Hodgkin lymphoma	11,510	4%	Non-Hodgkin lymphoma	8,400	3%
	Kidney & renal pelvis	10,010	3%	Brain & other nervous system	7,340	3%
	All sites	**323,630**	**100%**	**All sites**	**286,010**	**100%**

Estimates are rounded to the nearest 10, and cases exclude basal cell and squamous cell skin cancers and in situ carcinoma except urinary bladder. Ranking is based on modeled projections and may differ from the most recent observed data.

©2018, American Cancer Society, Inc., Surveillance Research

Fig. 43.1 Leading sites of new cancer cases and deaths—2018 estimates. (Data from American Cancer Society. *Cancer Facts & Figures 2015.* Atlanta: American Cancer Society; 2019. Retrieved from https://www.cancer.org/content/dam/cancer-org/research/cancer-facts-and-statistics/annual-cancer-facts-and-figures/2018/leading-sites-of-new-cancer-cases-and-deaths-2018-estimates.pdf.)

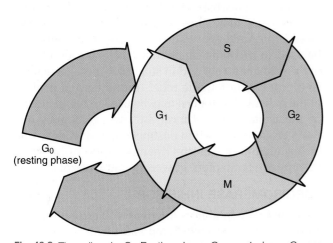

Fig. 43.2 The cell cycle. G_0, Resting phase; G_1, gap 1 phase; G_2, gap 2 phase; M, mitosis; S, synthesis.

resting phases (G_1 and G_2), and a resting (nondividing state [G_0]) phase. The cell cycle begins again when the cell is divided into two daughter cells. The daughter cells may advance again into the same cycle. The time required to complete one cycle is termed the *generation time.*

Many antineoplastic agents are cell cycle specific (i.e., the drug is selectively toxic when the cell is in a specific phase of growth and therefore is schedule dependent). Malignancies most amenable to cell cycle–specific chemotherapy are those that proliferate or grow very rapidly. Cell cycle–nonspecific drugs are active throughout the cell cycle and may be more effective against slowly proliferating neoplastic tissue. These agents are not schedule dependent but are dose dependent. One implication of cell cycle specificity is the importance of correlating the dosage schedule of anticancer therapy with the known cellular kinetics of that type of neoplasm. Drugs are usually administered when the cell is most susceptible to the cytotoxic effects of the agent for a higher "kill rate" of neoplastic cells.

DRUG THERAPY FOR CANCER

The overall goal of cancer chemotherapy is to give a dose large enough to be lethal (cytotoxic) to the cancer cells but small enough to be tolerable for normal cells. It is hoped that a long-term survival or cure can be achieved by this means. A second goal may be control of the disease (arresting tumor growth). When a cancer is beyond control, the goal of treatment may be **palliation** (alleviation) of symptoms (e.g., administration of chemotherapy to reduce tumor size for easier breathing in a patient with lung cancer). Finally, in some types of cancer in which no tumor is detectable yet the patient is known to be at risk of developing a particular cancer or having recurrence of a cancer, prophylactic surgery and/or chemotherapy may be administered.

Chemotherapy is most effective when the tumor is small and the cell replication is rapid. Cancer cells are the most sensitive to chemotherapy when the cells are dividing rapidly. This is when phase-specific drugs are most effective. As a tumor enlarges, more of the cells are in the resting phase. These cells respond better to phase-nonspecific chemotherapeutic agents. **Combination therapy**, using cell cycle–specific and cell cycle–nonspecific agents, is superior in therapeutic effect than the use of single-agent chemotherapy. The use of combination drug therapy allows for cell death during different phases of the cell cycle, but the agents often have toxic effects on different organs at different time intervals after administration. The choice of chemotherapeutic agents depends on the type of tumor cells, their rate of growth, and the size of the tumor.

The traditional major groups of chemotherapeutic agents have been classified as alkylating agents, antimetabolites, natural products, antineoplastic antibiotics, and hormones but now include the topoisomerase inhibitors, tyrosine kinase inhibitors, polyadenosine diphosphate ribose polymerase (PARP) inhibitors, cyclin-dependent kinases 4 and 6 inhibitors, proteasome inhibitors, and biologic therapies. (For information on specific drugs, refer to the Antineoplastic Agents section on the Evolve website.)

ALKYLATING AGENTS

Alkylating agents are highly reactive chemical compounds that bond with DNA molecules, causing cross-linking of DNA strands. The interstrand binding prevents the separation of the double-coiled DNA molecule that is necessary for cellular division. Alkylating agents are cell cycle nonspecific, which means that they are capable of combining with cellular components at any phase of the cell cycle. Generally, the development of resistance to one alkylating agent imparts cross-resistance to other alkylators. Examples of alkylating agents are busulfan, cisplatin, and cyclophosphamide.

ANTIMETABOLITES

Antimetabolites (subclassified as folic acid, purine, and pyrimidine antagonists) inhibit key enzymes in the biosynthetic pathways of DNA and RNA synthesis. These agents interfere with the ability of the neoplastic cell to multiply. Many of the antagonists are cell cycle specific, killing cells during the S phase of cell maturation. Unfortunately, these agents are not selective to cancer cells, killing rapidly growing normal cells as well. Their most common side effects are secondary to injury to normal cells, such as bone marrow cells and hair follicle cells. Examples of antimetabolites are 6-mercaptopurine, capecitabine, methotrexate, and fluorouracil.

NATURAL PRODUCTS

Natural products are derived from living tissue. As examples, vincristine and vinblastine are natural derivatives of the periwinkle plant. They are cell cycle–specific agents that block the formation of the mitotic spindle during mitosis, thus inhibiting cell division. Even though there is close structural similarity, cross-resistance does not usually develop between the two agents. Other natural products include docetaxel, etoposide (also a topoisomerase inhibitor), and paclitaxel.

ANTINEOPLASTIC ANTIBIOTICS

Antineoplastic antibiotics bind to DNA, inhibiting DNA or RNA synthesis; this eventually inhibits protein synthesis, preventing cell replication. Dactinomycin, daunorubicin, and doxorubicin are cell cycle–nonspecific antineoplastic antibiotics.

HORMONES

Hormones play a major role in cancer chemotherapy. Corticosteroids (usually prednisone) may be beneficial in treating lymphomas and acute leukemia because of their lympholytic effects and ability to suppress mitosis in lymphocytes. Steroids are also used to help reduce inflammation and edema secondary to radiation therapy. As palliative therapy, corticosteroids are used to temporarily suppress fever, diaphoresis, and pain and to restore—to some degree—appetite, weight, strength, and a sense of well-being in critically ill patients. With symptomatic relief, it is hoped that the patient's general physical condition may be improved sufficiently to permit further definitive therapy.

Estrogens and androgens are used for malignancies of sexual organs based on the assumption that these malignancies have hormonal requirements similar to those of nonmalignant sexual organs. Estrogens may be used in prostatic carcinoma. There are regressions in the primary tumor and in soft tissue metastases, with significant symptomatic relief from the point of view of the patient. Androgens may be used in the treatment of metastatic breast cancer in any age group, and estrogens may be used in postmenopausal women with metastatic breast cancer. Other examples of hormone therapy are tamoxifen, goserelin, and letrozole.

TOPOISOMERASE INHIBITORS

Topoisomerase inhibitors interfere with enzymes called topoisomerases, which help separate the strands of DNA so they can be copied. (Enzymes are proteins that cause chemical reactions in living cells.) Irinotecan is a topoisomerase inhibitor.

TYROSINE KINASE INHIBITORS

Tyrosine kinase inhibitors compete with adenosine 5-triphosphate (ATP) and inhibit tyrosine kinase, an enzyme that can transfer a phosphate group from ATP to a protein in a cell. There are several examples of these drugs such as gefitinib, erlotinib, and sorafenib.

POLYADENOSINE DIPHOSPHATE RIBOSE POLYMERASE INHIBITORS

PARP inhibitors are the enzymes responsible for cell activity such as DNA repair, genomic stability, and programmed cell death. These inhibitors are currently targeted for ovarian and breast cancer.

CYCLIN-DEPENDENT KINASES 4 AND 6 INHIBITORS

Cyclin-dependent kinases 4 and 6 are enzymes important in the cell cycle as it moves from the G1 to the S phase. The inhibitor drugs stop the cell cycle from progressing. These inhibitors are used for metastatic breast cancer.

PROTEASOME INHIBITORS

Proteasome inhibitors are drugs that block the action of proteasomes, which are part of cellular complexes that break down proteins. Three of these drugs have been approved to treat multiple myeloma.

BIOLOGIC THERAPIES

Biologic therapies, also known as **targeted anticancer agents**, include cytokines, monoclonal antibodies, growth factors, and vaccines. They evolved from research indicating that cell membrane receptors control cell proliferation, cell migration, angiogenesis (new blood vessel growth), and cell death that are integral to the growth and spread of cancer. Many of the biologic therapies act on receptors, such as epidermal growth factor receptors (EGFRs) (e.g., human epidermal growth factor receptor-2 [HER-2]), platelet-derived growth factor,

and vascular endothelial growth factor (VEGF). Targeted anticancer agents are noncytotoxic drugs that target the key pathways (e.g., EGFR, VEGF) that provide growth and survival advantages for cancer cells, while not assaulting normal cells. These pathways are relatively specific for cancer cells; theoretically, targeted agents are not associated with the severe toxicities common with cytotoxic chemotherapy, but allergic reactions are more common since many of the products are derived from foreign proteins.

OTHER AGENTS

As new pathways of tumor cell metabolism are identified, however, not all agents will fit into these classes. The mechanisms whereby these agents cause cell death have not been fully determined in all cases.

Two other groups of medicines—chemoprotective agents and bone marrow stimulants—have become available to help protect normal human cells from chemotherapy and help stimulate the normal body defense mechanism. **Chemoprotective agents** (Table 43.1) help reduce the toxicity of chemotherapeutic agents to normal cells. Both targeted agents (described earlier) and chemoprotective agents allow the use of full therapeutic doses of chemical chemotherapies to attack the cancer. Bone marrow stimulants (Table 43.2) are also used in supporting persons undergoing cancer

Table 43.1 Chemoprotective Agents

GENERIC NAME	BRAND NAME	MAJOR INDICATIONS
amifostine	Ethyol	Amifostine is a prodrug that is metabolized by enzymes in tissues to a free thiol metabolite that can reduce the toxic effects of cisplatin. Normal tissue has a higher affinity for the free thiol. The higher concentration of free thiol in normal tissues is available to bind to and detoxify the reactive metabolites of cisplatin, reducing damage to normal tissues. Amifostine is used to reduce the cumulative renal toxicity associated with the repeated administration of cisplatin in patients with advanced ovarian cancer and non–small cell lung cancer. It is also used to reduce the incidence of xerostomia in patients undergoing postoperative radiation treatment for head and neck cancer.
dexrazoxane	Zinecard	Dexrazoxane is an intracellular chelating agent used in conjunction with doxorubicin. It is used to reduce the incidence and severity of cardiomyopathy associated with doxorubicin in women with metastatic breast cancer who have received a cumulative doxorubicin dose of 300 mg/m^2 and who would benefit from continuing doxorubicin therapy.
glucarpidase	Voraxaze	Glucarpidase is used in the treatment of toxic plasma methotrexate concentrations. It breaks down methotrexate into inactive metabolites that are then eliminated from the body.
leucovorin	–	Leucovorin is administered hours after high-dose methotrexate chemotherapy to prevent methotrexate toxicity (commonly referred to as *leucovorin rescue*). Leucovorin may also be administered as an antidote to an inadvertent overdose of methotrexate, pemetrexed, or pralatrexate chemotherapy.
mesna	Mesnex	Mesna is a prodrug that is metabolized by enzymes in kidney tissue to a free thiol metabolite that can reduce the toxic effects of ifosfamide and cyclophosphamide. The free thiol binds and deactivates the toxic metabolites of ifosfamide and cyclophosphamide. Mesna is used as a prophylactic agent to reduce the incidence of ifosfamide- and cyclophosphamide-induced hemorrhagic cystitis.

Table 43.2   **Bone Marrow Stimulants**

GENERIC NAME	BRAND NAME	MAJOR INDICATIONS
darbepoetin	Aranesp ⇄ *Do not confuse Aranesp with Aricept or Arimidex.*	Darbepoetin stimulates erythropoiesis (production of red blood cells [RBCs]). It is used to treat anemia in patients receiving chemotherapy and anemia associated with chronic kidney disease. Increased hemoglobin levels are not generally observed until 2-6 wk after initiating treatment with darbepoetin. Darbepoetin is administered by weekly subcutaneous injection.
epoetin alfa	Procrit, Epogen	Epoetin alfa stimulates production of RBCs. It is used to treat anemia in patients with chronic renal failure or those receiving chemotherapy. Epoetin is administered by subcutaneous or IV injection three times weekly.
filgrastim	Neupogen	Filgrastim is also known as a human granulocyte colony-stimulating factor (G-CSF). It stimulates production of neutrophilic white blood cells. It is used to reduce the neutropenia interval in bone marrow transplantation, to stimulate white blood cell production in patients receiving myelosuppressive chemotherapy, and to treat neutropenia in acute myelogenous leukemia. It is also used to increase the yield of peripheral blood progenitor cells prior to bone marrow ablation; filgrastim is administered, and peripheral progenitor cells are harvested and then readministered after bone marrow ablation for a more rapid recovery of the bone marrow.
pegfilgrastim	Neulasta	Pegfilgrastim and filgrastim have the same mechanism of action. Pegfilgrastim has reduced renal clearance and prolonged duration of action compared with filgrastim.
sargramostim	Leukine	Sargramostim is also known as granulocyte macrophage colony-stimulating factor (GM-CSF). It stimulates production of granulocytes and macrophages, increases the cytotoxicity of monocytes toward certain neoplastic cell lines, and activates polymorphonuclear neutrophils to inhibit the growth of tumor cells. Sargramostim is used to accelerate bone marrow transplant recovery, correct neutropenia in patients with aplastic anemia, and stimulate bone marrow recovery in patients receiving myelosuppressive chemotherapy.

treatment as well as bone marrow transplantation of healthy cells. Several types of cancer (e.g., leukemias, lymphomas) are treated by chemotherapeutic agents that kill bone marrow cells while killing the cancer cells. The bone marrow stimulants trigger the recovery of the bone marrow cells several days earlier than would happen in the natural course of recovery. The major benefit to this earlier recovery is that patients' immune systems are able to respond to and stop infections from being so pathologic, and thus patients can be released from isolation rooms several days earlier. Cancers and other diseases (chronic renal failure, anemia of chronic disease) also cause anemia, which can be very debilitating to the patient. Darbepoetin and epoetin stimulate the bone marrow to produce red blood cells to treat anemia.

A routine complication of chemotherapy is nausea and vomiting. See Chapter 33 for more information.

SAFETY WHEN USING CHEMOTHERAPY

Guidelines for the safe handling of chemotherapeutic agents by healthcare providers include measures to prevent inhalation of aerosols, prevention of drug absorption through the skin, safe disposal, and prevention of contamination of body fluids. Many chemotherapeutic agents may induce cancers in healthy individuals. Chemotherapy should only be mixed in the pharmacy department using vertical-flow laminar hoods and other sterile precautions.

Chemotherapy is individualized to the patient and is often prescribed according to the patient's calculated body surface area (m²) and type of cancer.

❖ NURSING IMPLICATIONS FOR CHEMOTHERAPY

◆ Assessment

History of risk factors

- Ask for age, gender, and race. Take a family history of the incidence of cancer.
- Ask about job-related exposure to known chemical carcinogens (e.g., benzene, vinyl chloride, asbestos, soot, tars, oils).
- Ask about exposure to tobacco and tobacco smoke. Obtain a history of the use of smokeless tobacco or the number of cigarettes or cigars smoked daily. How long has the person smoked? Has the person ever tried to stop smoking? How does the person feel about modifying the smoking habit? Is there chronic exposure to secondhand smoke at home or at work?
- Ask about a drug history to obtain information on pharmacologic agents that have the potential to become carcinogens (e.g., diethylstilbestrol, cyclophosphamide, melphalan, azathioprine).
- Ask about a history of viral diseases suspected of being associated with carcinogenesis (e.g., Epstein-Barr

virus, hepatitis B virus, human immunodeficiency virus, human papillomavirus).

- Is there a history of exposure to, or treatment with, radiation?

Dietary habits

- Take a dietary history. Ask specific questions to obtain data relating to foods eaten that are high in fat or in animal protein (especially red meats; salt-cured, smoked, or charcoaled foods; and nitrate and nitrite additives). Are whole grains included in the diet? How many servings of fruits and vegetables are eaten daily? What types of vegetables are eaten daily? Estimate the number of calories consumed per day.
- Ask the patient about normal eating patterns, food likes and dislikes, and elimination pattern.
- Ask whether certain foods cause bloating, indigestion, or diarrhea, and how much seasoning and spices are put on food.
- What is the usual fluid intake daily? How much coffee, tea, soda (soft drinks), and fruit juice is consumed? Determine the frequency and volume of alcoholic beverages consumed.
- Is the person experiencing anorexia, nausea, and vomiting? If so, what measures are being used to control these symptoms?
- Obtain a baseline height and weight. Has there been a weight gain or loss in the past year?
- Obtain details of any symptoms that are affecting the individual's ability to eat (e.g., anorexia, vomiting, diarrhea, smells that deter eating, pain).

Preexisting health problems. Ask about any preexisting health problems for which the patient is, or has been, receiving treatment. Continue treatment of any preexisting health problems (e.g., angina, heart failure, asthma).

Understanding of the diagnosis

- Ask the patient to explain his or her understanding of the current diagnosis and plan of treatment.
- Review the admission notes or old charts to determine the details relating to the diagnostic test data, type of cancer, staging of the disease, laboratory values, and treatments to date (Box 43.1).

Adaptation to the diagnosis

- Determine whether this is the initial or a subsequent cycle of chemotherapy. Gather data regarding the patient's and significant others' understanding of the disease and the planned course of treatment.
- Ask how the patient normally copes with stressful situations. Does the patient have a confidante who is supportive and understanding?
- Observe both the verbal and nonverbal messages conveyed during the interview. Take note of the patient's general appearance, tone of voice, inflections, and gestures. Try to pick up on subtle clues and confirm their meanings with the patient.

Box 43.1   Cancer Care

Nursing assessments that apply to the patient undergoing chemotherapy:

1. *Pain management:* Work with the healthcare provider to manage pain.
2. *Ability to perform activities of daily living:* Encourage self-care as tolerated.
3. *Activity tolerance:* Whether bedbound or chairbound.
4. *Appetite:* Encourage small amounts and favorite foods.
5. *Oral care:* Use soft brush or soft cloth, mouthwash with viscous lidocaine. Use a mucositis scale for oral assessment. If dry mouth is present, consider lubricating and moisturizing agents, sugarless gum, Blistex, and protect from trauma (see Chapter 31 for further discussion).
6. *Allow rest periods:* Fatigue is common with normal activities.
7. *Determine IV access:* Implanted infusion ports such as tunneled Hickman catheter or Port-a-Cath implantable infusion port (see Chapter 11 for further discussion).
8. *Observe for any impaired skin integrity:* From pressure ulcers to excoriation from diarrhea.

- Inquire regarding psychological issues that the patient is perceiving, such as loss of control, loss of self-esteem, loss of body parts, change in lifestyle, and/or guilt.
- Review the healthcare provider's progress notes for information being given to the patient and family throughout the course of treatment.

Psychomotor functions

- Ask the patient to describe exercise levels in terms of amount tolerated, the degree of fatigue present, and the ability to perform activities of daily living.
- Is the patient having difficulty performing normal roles (e.g., homemaker, provider, mother, father)?
- Refer the patient and family to social services for needed guidance and support personnel to assist in the management of problems such as inability to work and need for home care.

Safety. Assess for weakness, confusion, orthostatic hypotension, or similar symptoms that could signal impending potential for injury.

Symptoms of pharmacologic adverse effects. Ask specific questions to determine whether the individual has been or is experiencing symptoms associated with the type of drugs being administered, such as myelosuppression, anemia, bleeding, stomatitis (mucositis), altered bowel patterns (e.g., diarrhea, constipation), alopecia, neurotoxicity, anorexia, nausea, or vomiting.

Physical assessment

- Perform a baseline physical, psychosocial, and spiritual assessment of the individual to serve as the database for ongoing assessments throughout the course of care.

- Throughout the course of therapy, perform daily assessments of the physical, psychosocial, and spiritual needs of the individual and family. Perform a focused assessment on the body systems affected by the disease process and those likely to be affected by metastasis (e.g., lungs, brain, bone, liver).

Sexual assessment. Discuss birth control and reproductive counseling issues at the time of initiation of therapy. Male patients may wish to use a sperm bank. Female patients may wish to harvest eggs. A contraceptive method should be discussed.

Smoking. Discuss tobacco use with the patient and plan a mutually agreeable way to handle this habit, both while hospitalized and when at home. Does the patient wish to modify the habit? Provide smoking cessation education.

Pain. Ask whether the person is having any pain and what interventions are being used to manage the pain. Obtain a rating of pain level and the degree of relief being gained from current medications and supportive practices (e.g., relaxation or guided imagery).

◆ **Implementation**
- Implement planned interventions consistent with assessment data and identified individual needs of the patient (e.g., nutritional support, blood component therapy, growth factor therapy, fatigue, alopecia, anemia, constipation, diarrhea, nausea and vomiting, neutropenia, pain, and thrombocytopenia).
- Assess body weight and height, because dosages of many chemotherapeutic agents are based on body surface area.
- Examine laboratory data on a continuum. Monitor for the development of cancer emergencies (e.g., hypercalcemia, superior vena cava syndrome, disseminated intravascular coagulation).
- Administer intravenous (IV) medications (see Chapter 11 for IV administration principles, administration of drugs via venous access devices, and care and handling of venous catheters). It is essential to wear nitrite gloves and disposable nonpermeable fabric when handling any body fluids.
- Monitor vital signs, including temperature, pulse, respirations, and blood pressure, at least every shift or more frequently depending on recommended monitoring parameters of specific drugs prescribed.
- *Hydration:* Monitor the patient's state of hydration. Check skin turgor, mucous membranes, and softness of the eyeballs. Electrolyte reports require vigilant observation; report abnormal findings to the healthcare provider. Fluid replacement via IV administration or total parenteral nutrition may be appropriate in some cases. Some chemotherapeutic agents require

hydration before administration to prevent damage to the kidneys or bladder. Prehydration is also planned for highly emetogenic chemotherapy (see Chapter 33, Table 33.1) to prevent dehydration from vomiting. Regardless of the agents administered, always monitor 24-hour urine output and read the urinalysis to detect abnormalities. Chemotherapy administration should be performed by qualified registered nurses or prescribers with specific skills in the correct handling and administration techniques for chemotherapeutic agents. For more information on advanced education required for administering chemotherapeutic agents, consult Oncology Nursing Society guidelines, available at https://www.ons.org/.
- *Infection:* Report even the slightest sign of infection for evaluation (e.g., elevating temperature, chills, malaise, hypotension, pallor).
- *Nausea, vomiting:* There are three patterns of emesis associated with antineoplastic therapy: acute, delayed, and anticipatory. (See Chapter 33 for the treatment of nausea and vomiting associated with chemotherapy.) The goal of treatment is to prevent nausea and vomiting. Many chemotherapy regimens require prechemotherapy administration of an antiemetic followed by as-needed (PRN) orders for breakthrough nausea and vomiting.
  1. Chart the degree of effectiveness achieved when antiemetics are given.
  2. Report poor control to the prescriber.
  3. Changing the antiemetic medication ordered or the route of administration may improve control.
  4. Patients experiencing nausea and vomiting must be weighed daily and monitored for electrolyte values and accurate intake and output.
- *Positioning:* Position changes should be scheduled to prevent alterations in skin integrity.
- *Diarrhea:* Record the color, frequency, and consistency of stool. Include an estimate of the volume of watery stools in the output record. Check for occult blood. Provide for adequate hydration and administer any drugs ordered to relieve the symptoms.
  1. Encourage adequate fluid intake and dietary alterations, such as eliminating spicy foods and foods high in fat content. It may be necessary to switch to a clear liquid diet followed by a diet low in roughage. Diarrhea may require high-protein foods with high caloric value and vitamin and mineral supplements. Patients with diarrhea should be weighed daily and monitored for fluid intake and output and electrolyte values.
  2. Check the anal area for irritation, provide for hygiene measures, and protect from excoriation with products such as A+D Ointment or zinc oxide ointment.
- *Constipation:* Compare this symptom with the patient's usual pattern of elimination. Many people do not normally defecate daily. Perform daily assessment of bowel sounds when the patient is hospitalized.

When a patient is constipated, the prescriber usually orders stool softeners or laxatives, fluids, and a diet that enhances normal defecation. Observe carefully for signs of an impaction (the urge to defecate with little to no stool or seepage of watery stool).

- *Stomatitis (mucositis):* Use meticulous oral hygiene measures (see Chapter 31). Schedule oral hygiene measures using prescribed local anesthetic and antimicrobial solutions. Perform oral hygiene before and after meals and at bedtime if symptoms are mild. With moderate lesions, increase the frequency to every 2 hours. In patients with severe symptoms, the mouth is rinsed hourly while the patient is awake.
- *Bleeding:* Observe and report signs and symptoms of bleeding (e.g., epistaxis; hematuria; bruises; petechiae; dark, tarry stools; coffee-ground emesis; or blurred vision). Instruct female patients to report menstrual flow that is excessive, is bright colored, or lasts for a prolonged period. Check laboratory reports for indications of, for example, changes in hematologic status and electrolytes; report abnormal or changing values to the healthcare provider.
- *Pain:* Administer pain medications prescribed at scheduled intervals to maintain a constant blood level of the analgesic and thereby promote maximum pain control. Maintain a record of pain medications administered and the patient's rating of the degree of pain relief achieved (see Chapter 19).
  1. Report insufficient pain relief.
  2. Obtain orders for the treatment of the pain, or institute PRN analgesics prescribed for breakthrough pain episodes.
- *Neurotoxicity:* Monitor for disorientation, confusion, fine-motor activity alterations, gait alterations, and paresthesias.
- *Anxiety:* Monitor the degree of anxiety being exhibited and intervene appropriately to alleviate. Give prescribed medications; discuss issues about which the patient or significant others are concerned. Keep the patient involved in making appropriate decisions regarding self-care to give some degree of control over the situation; discuss when prescribed treatments are to be performed.
  1. Implement relaxation techniques (use of biofeedback, visual imagery) as prescribed.
  2. Deal with stress-related issues that arise in the support or family group.

◆ Patient Education
Nutrition
- Teach the patient specific ways to implement dietary needs (e.g., ways to support increased protein and caloric intake, such as adding powdered milk to puddings, creamed soups). Suggest using nutritional supplements such as Ensure or Boost (see Chapter 46). Suggest the patient try different brands and add freshly squeezed orange or lemon juice to help alter the aftertaste frequently cited by postchemotherapy patients who are using nutritional supplements.
- If the patient is receiving enteral tube feedings, peripheral parenteral nutrition, or total parenteral nutrition, arrange for necessary at-home support for administration and monitoring of therapy. Suggest obtaining educational materials from the American Cancer Society on dietary interventions during the treatment of cancer.

Diagnosis and adaptation to diagnosis
- Encourage the patient and support group to discuss concerns about the disease, prognosis, and treatment.
- Present the patient with appropriate choices that allow involvement in the decisions concerning selection of care. Encourage the patient to maintain the best health possible. Include the patient in selecting the diet, planning activities, scheduling rest periods, and attending to personal care. Stress what the patient *can* do, not what the patient cannot do.
- Emphasize the prevention of complications through maintenance of nutrition and hydration and commitment to hygiene practices.

Sexual needs. Patients should discuss methods of birth control to be used during chemotherapy and/or sperm storage and fertilization counseling.

Vascular access devices. The need for frequent injection of chemotherapeutic agents intravenously necessitates the use of implanted vascular access devices, which include Hickman catheters, Port-A-Cath implantable infusion ports, and peripherally inserted central catheter (PICC) lines (see Chapter 11 for more information regarding care of these devices). Instruction should be provided on the self-care and frequency of required follow-up care for central lines or ports.

Skin care
- Have the patient bathe in lukewarm water and use mild soap. Gently pat the skin dry. Discuss the use of skin moisturizer with the prescriber.
- Instruct the patient to report rashes or areas that appear sunburned or blistered.
- Stress the need to avoid sunlight for patients receiving drugs that may produce a photosensitivity reaction.
- Teach personal hygiene measures to provide for skin care and to prevent skin breakdown.

Psychomotor
- Discuss activities the patient is able to perform independently and those requiring assistance.
- Provide for patient safety on a continuum.
- Include the support group in the development of a plan to provide for self-care at home.
- Arrange appropriate referrals to support the self-care needs of the person in the home environment.

Nausea and vomiting

- Teach the patient when and how to take prescribed antiemetics. Have the patient verbalize his or her understanding with teach-back.
- Make suggestions for comfort measures to minimize nausea (e.g., rinsing the mouth frequently, using a cool cloth to wash the face, employing relaxation and distraction techniques).
- Teach the patient to take his or her weight daily and explain parameters of weight loss that must be reported to the healthcare provider.

Diarrhea or constipation

- Teach the patient the proper use of PRN medications prescribed to treat constipation or diarrhea.
- Explain measures to prevent constipation, such as drinking sufficient fluids daily, eating high-fiber foods, and avoiding foods that cause constipation. Instruct the individual to report failure to have stools in a usual pattern of elimination or the presence of seeping, loose, watery stools while feeling the need to defecate (may be an indication of an impaction).
- When diarrhea is present, instruct the patient to avoid foods that irritate or stimulate peristalsis—for example, coffee, tea, and hot or cold beverages. Encourage the increased intake of potassium-containing foods.

Neutropenia

- Explain the measures that the individual should initiate to minimize the chance of infection when neutropenia is present (e.g., handwashing; avoidance of exposure to individuals known to have an infection; no fresh flowers, vegetables, or receptacles with free-standing water such as denture cups or humidifiers; and avoidance of pets and patients receiving immunizations).
- Teach signs and symptoms of infection and when to report symptoms. Be certain that the person understands how to take her or his temperature and that even minor elevations should be reported.
- Teach self-care of central lines, when present, consistent with the patient's or significant others' ability to perform the procedure while maintaining strict aseptic technique. Arrange for referral to a community or home care agency as indicated.
- See Table 43.2 for bone marrow stimulants used to treat neutropenia.

Pain

- Discuss beliefs about pain with the patient and significant others as a baseline for health teaching needed.
- Instruct the patient to record the intensity of the pain experienced and degree of pain relief obtained from prescribed medications (see Chapter 19 for a pain scale).
- Emphasize the need to report both pain that is not being controlled and new symptoms of pain being felt.

- Stress the importance of taking pain medications at prescribed intervals to obtain maximum relief.
- Determine whether the patient has access to medications for pain. (Does the patient have sufficient money to purchase or obtain prescribed medication?)
- Stress the need for the patient to start stool softeners and to take them regularly to prevent constipation when narcotics are used.
- Oral medications are often used to provide pain relief. Several analgesics are also available as rectal suppositories. Pain control must be achieved. When oral and rectal forms of pain management no longer suffice, patients may require hospitalization for stabilization on parenteral forms of narcotic analgesics. Infusion pumps are frequently used, and spinal morphine may be delivered effectively via epidural or intrathecal catheters; transdermal and sublingual pain control methods may also be used. Patients must understand that they can be kept comfortable.

Anemia

- Teach the patient the possible causes and related self-care needed when anemia is present (e.g., management of fatigue by spacing of activities and prevention of orthostatic hypotension by rising slowly, sitting and resting, and then standing).
- Instruct the patient not to drive or operate power equipment for safety reasons.
- See Table 43.2 for bone marrow stimulants used to treat anemia.

Thrombocytopenia

- Teach self-monitoring for other blood-related symptoms (e.g., bleeding, bruising, hematuria, epistaxis, coffee-ground emesis, or excessive or prolonged menstrual flow).
- Suggest safety measures when at home (e.g., avoiding use of sharp knives, shaving with an electric razor, wearing a thimble when sewing).
- Stress that the patient should not take any aspirin or aspirin-containing products that may increase bleeding should it occur.

Home care

- While the patient is receiving chemotherapy, soiled linens should be washed separately from other household linens; the soiled linens should be placed in washable pillowcases and washed twice.
- Because most chemotherapeutic agents are excreted in the urine and feces, it is best to flush the toilet two or three times after each voiding or defecation.
- If emesis occurs, dump waste in toilet and flush two or three times.

Anxiety

- Assist the patient to practice stress reduction techniques, and make the patient aware of cancer support resources available, such as the American Cancer Society (https://www.cancer.org/).

Fostering health maintenance

- Throughout the course of treatment, discuss medication information and how the medication will benefit the patient.
- Drug therapy will be individualized for the patient and type of cancer being treated. The need to follow the established regimen precisely must be emphasized to obtain maximum cytotoxic effects while minimizing adverse effects. Adverse effects to the drug therapy should be expected, and the patient and significant others must be educated in the management of the common and serious adverse effects. Additional teaching must be individualized to the patient for equipment used to administer drug therapy or nutritional support.
- Seek cooperation and understanding of the following points so that medication compliance is increased: name of medication; dosage, route, and times of administration; and common and serious adverse effects. Patients should be encouraged to maintain basic good health practices throughout treatment (e.g., adequate rest, exercise consistent with abilities, stress management or stress reduction techniques, and maintenance of usual spiritual beliefs).

Patient self-assessment. Enlist the patient's help in developing and maintaining a written record of monitoring parameters (e.g., nausea, vomiting, pain relief, constipation, diarrhea). See Patient Self-Assessment Form for Antineoplastic Agents on the Evolve website. Complete the Premedication Data column for use as a baseline to track response to drug therapy. Ensure that the patient understands how to use the form, and instruct the patient to take the completed form to follow-up visits. During follow-up visits, focus on issues that will foster adherence with the therapeutic interventions prescribed.

Get Ready for the NCLEX® Examination!

Key Points

- Nurses play a crucial role in the treatment of patients with cancer. No other disease seems to evoke fear and anxiety in the same way that the diagnosis of cancer has on the patient and family. Nurses are often the contact between the healthcare provider, patient, and family in helping with adaptation to the diagnosis and entry into the healthcare system for treatment.
- Nurses are often the first to identify complications of therapy; for example, they are often the first to recognize and report early symptoms of infection in an immunocompromised patient. Early recognition and prompt action often reduce the severity of the complications.
- It is important for nurses caring for cancer patients to research all drugs prescribed for the patient and to perform focused assessments on body systems known to be affected by the specific agents administered.
- Health teaching for the patient and significant others is essential to achieving the best response to the therapeutic regimen prescribed. Everyone involved in the patient's care needs to understand the purpose of the medications prescribed and when to contact the physician for any problems encountered. The patient and significant others must feel like integral parts of the team, whose members desire the best possible quality of life for those affected by the disease.
- Nurses are active providers of public information on wellness. They also coordinate screening programs for the early detection of cancer.

Additional Learning Resources

SG Go to your Study Guide for additional Review Questions for the NCLEX® Examination, Critical Thinking Clinical Situations, and other learning activities to help you master this chapter content.

Go to your Evolve website (https://evolve.elsevier.com/Clayton) for additional online resources.

Review Questions for the NCLEX® Examination

1. The nurse understands that the goals of chemotherapy may be different for individual patients and include which of the following? *(Select all that apply.)*
   1. Giving a dose large enough to kill cancer cells but preserve normal cells
   2. Killing all fast-growing cells without harmful adverse effects
   3. Controlling the progression of the disease
   4. Alleviating symptoms of cancer in cases in which no cure is available
   5. Preventing cancer from developing in patients at risk for it

2. The nurse is caring for a 43-year-old patient with lymphoma who is receiving prednisone and asks what effects it has. What would be an appropriate response by the nurse?
   1. "You are taking prednisone to prevent further occurrence of your cancer."
   2. "Prednisone is used to suppress fever, sweating, and pain."
   3. "The mechanism of action is unknown, but it seems to work by reducing the need for more chemotherapy."
   4. "Prednisone has a lympholytic effect, which means it will cause the cancerous lymphocytes to die."

3. The nurse is teaching a patient who is taking methotrexate, which can cause thrombocytopenia. What must the nurse include in the teaching? *(Select all that apply.)*
   1. Avoid fresh flowers, vegetables, or fruit.
   2. Use an electric shaver and practice safe handling of sharp objects, such as kitchen knives.
   3. Report coffee-ground emesis, hematuria, or epistaxis.
   4. Obtain adequate daily exercise.
   5. Avoid taking any aspirin or aspirin-containing products.

4. The nurse is administering epoetin alfa (Procrit) to a patient receiving chemotherapy. What is the best explanation to the patient of why this medication is used?
   1. To stimulate white blood cell production
   2. To stimulate red blood cell production
   3. To prevent thrombocytopenia
   4. To protect the kidneys from toxic chemotherapy

5. What are the drugs that are used in conjunction with chemotherapy to reduce the toxic effects?
   1. Chemoprotective agents
   2. Targeted anticancer agents
   3. Bone marrow stimulants
   4. Alkylating agents

6. When teaching a patient about what to report to the healthcare provider, the nurse includes which of the following? *(Select all that apply.)*
   1. Any increase in pain
   2. Nasal stuffiness
   3. Bleeding
   4. Development of a fever
   5. Dry skin over heels

7. The nurse is discussing ways to counteract the effects of diarrhea caused by chemotherapy. Which suggestions should be included in the discussion? *(Select all that apply.)*
   1. Use products that protect the skin around the anus from excoriation (such as A&D Ointment).
   2. Drink more coffee or tea.
   3. Increase intake of potassium-containing foods depending upon other medications being taken.
   4. Obtain daily weights as an indicator of maintenance of hydration.
   5. Take frequent walks, which should alleviate the symptoms.

8. Cancer care involving nursing assessments includes which aspects?
   1. Pain management, activity tolerance, appetite, oral care, and rest periods
   2. Pain management, rest periods, laboratory analysis, and restricting fluids
   3. Pain management, exercise periods, oral care, and daily weights
   4. Pain management, oral care, exercise periods, restricting fluids, and vital signs

Drugs Used to Treat the Musculoskeletal System

44

Objectives

1. Describe the nursing assessment data needed to evaluate a patient with a skeletal muscle disorder.
2. Identify the therapeutic response and the common and serious adverse effects from skeletal muscle relaxant therapy.
3. Describe the effect of centrally acting skeletal muscle relaxants on the central nervous system and the safety precautions required during their use.
4. Describe the physiologic effects of neuromuscular blocking agents and assessments needed, as well as the equipment needed in the immediate patient care area when neuromuscular blocking agents are administered.
5. Describe the nursing assessment data needed to evaluate a patient with gout.
6. Identify the therapeutic response and the common and serious adverse effects from gout medications.

Key Terms

cerebral palsy (sĕ-RĒ-brăl PŎL-zē) (p. 679)
multiple sclerosis (MŬL-tĭ-pŭl sklĕ-RŌ-sĭs) (p. 679)
gout (p. 679)
hypercapnia (hī-pĕr-KĂP-nē-ă) (p. 680)

spasticity (spăs-TĬS-ĭ-tē) (p. 682)
muscle spasms (MŬ-sŭl SPĂ-zĭmz) (p. 682)
neuromuscular blocking agents (nyū-rō-MŬS-kyū-lăr BLŎK-ĭng Ā-jĕnts) (p. 685)

The skeletal system includes the bones of the skeleton and the cartilages, ligaments, and other connective tissue that stabilize or connect the bones. In addition to supporting the weight of the body, bones work together with muscles to maintain body position and to produce controlled, precise movements. Without the skeleton to pull against, contracting muscle fibers could not make us sit, stand, walk, or run. Common musculoskeletal disorders are cerebral palsy, multiple sclerosis, and gout. Cerebral palsy is a condition in which movement of the extremities is marked by any combination of the following: exaggerated reflexes, abnormal posture, involuntary movements, and walking difficulties. Cerebral palsy can be caused by an injury or a birth defect.

Multiple sclerosis is an autoimmune disease that affects the brain and spinal cord. Symptoms may be mild, such as numbness in the limbs, or severe, such as paralysis or loss of vision. The progression, severity, and specific symptoms of multiple sclerosis are unpredictable and highly variable between persons.

Gout is a common and treatable form of inflammatory arthritis. Gout develops due to excessive uric acid in the blood (hyperuricemia). Uric acid, the end product of purine metabolism, is a waste product that has no physiologic role. Humans lack uricase, an enzyme that breaks down uric acid into a more water-soluble product (allantoin). The amount of uric acid in the body depends on the balance between dietary intake purines, synthesis, and the rate of excretion. Gout results from overproduction (10% of cases) or underexcretion (90% of cases) of uric acid. Excess uric acid crystallizes in soft tissues and in particularly in joints. This initiates an inflammatory reaction leading to swelling, heat, and intense pain.

Stroke syndrome is a condition of sudden onset of vertigo, numbness, aphasia, and dysarthria, marked by hemiplegia or hemiparesis due to vascular lesions of the brain, embolism, thrombosis, or ruptured aneurysm. The spasticity caused by the syndrome is treatable with muscle relaxants.

MUSCLE RELAXANTS, NEUROMUSCULAR BLOCKING AGENTS, AND GOUT AGENTS

❖ NURSING IMPLICATIONS FOR SKELETAL MUSCLE RELAXANTS, NEUROMUSCULAR BLOCKING AGENTS, AND GOUT AGENTS

◆ Assessment

Assessment for skeletal muscle disorders. Musculoskeletal disorders may produce varying degrees of pain and immobility, impairing the individual's ability to perform the activities of daily living. The nursing assessments performed are individualized to the muscles affected and the underlying disease.

Current history

- What is the reason for seeking treatment now? Request a brief history of any symptoms present.

- What is the degree of impairment present (e.g., strength, gait, conservation effect, compensatory action)? What is the effect on usual daily activities (e.g., dressing, preparing meals, eating, performing basic hygiene, maintaining home)?
- Assess the pain level and extent, frequency of analgesic use, precipitating factors, and any measures the patient has identified that alleviate pain.
- Assess the extent of muscle spasticity and the muscle groups affected. Are there impairments that affect the patient's self-care, activities of daily living, or ability to fulfill work responsibilities?

History

- Ask the patient to describe the degree of disorder caused by the musculoskeletal impairment (e.g., scoliosis, poliomyelitis, rickets, osteoarthritis, cerebral palsy, multiple sclerosis, muscular dystrophy, spinal cord injury, stroke).
- Have there been any injuries to, or surgeries on, the musculoskeletal system (e.g., dislocations, sprains, fractures, joint replacements)? If so, obtain details.
- Ask the patient if there is a family history of difficulties or abnormal responses to neuromuscular blocking agents during anesthesia.

Medication history

- Ask the patient to list all prescribed and over-the-counter medications taken within the past 6 months. Are any herbal medicines being taken? Ask specifically about antiinflammatory or corticosteroid use.
- What has been the response to the medications taken (e.g., antiinflammatories, analgesics, skeletal muscle relaxants)?
- What are the medications most recently taken and when were they taken?
- What nonpharmacologic treatments are being used (e.g., heating pad, massage therapy, acupuncture, cupping)?

Activity and exercise

- What is the extent of usual daily exercise?
- Determine which activities of daily living can be performed independently and which require assistance.
- Ask about any assistive devices used (e.g., cane, walker).

Sleep and rest

- Does the pain of repositioning at night awaken the patient? Seek further information regarding the positions that initiate pain and the type of padding or additional pillows or devices being used for positioning.

Elimination

- Ask specifically about the ability to toilet independently. Does mobility interfere with this function? Is constipation, diarrhea, or incontinence a problem? If so, how is it managed?

Nutrition

- Take a diet history. Is the diet consistent with the recommended diet? Are supplemental vitamins and minerals (e.g., calcium) taken daily?

- Weigh the individual and ask whether there has been a weight gain or loss over the past 6 months. If so, obtain details.

Physical examination

- Gently inspect the affected part for swelling, edema, bruises, redness, localized tenderness, deformities, or malalignments.
- During examination, note differences in circumference, symmetry, or length of limbs.
- Record any abnormalities present (e.g., scoliosis, contractures, atrophy).
- Record range of motion present in joints, gait, and degree of mobility.
- Evaluate capillary refill and check for presence of paresthesia (numbness and tingling).

Laboratory and diagnostic studies

- Review diagnostic studies performed (e.g., radiography, magnetic resonance imaging, computed tomography, arthroscopic reports, bone scan, bone mass measurements, endoscopy).
- Examine laboratory findings associated with the disease process present (e.g., calcium, phosphorus, lupus testing, rheumatoid factor, uric acid level, C-reactive protein, human leukocyte antigen, aldolase [high levels can be a sign of muscle damage], aspartate, creatine kinase).

Assessment for neuromuscular blocking agents

- Assessment of the patient's vital signs, mental status, and in particular, respiratory function is mandatory for people having received neuromuscular blocking agents. The adverse effects associated with these drugs may occur 48 hours or more after administration. Close observation of respiratory function, ability to swallow secretions, and the presence of a cough reflex is necessary. Suction, oxygen, mechanical ventilators, and resuscitation equipment should be available in the immediate area.
- Monitor blood pressure, pulse, and respirations. Review the baseline readings of the patient's vital signs before administration of anesthetic and neuromuscular blocking agents. Generally, changes from the baseline should be reported.
- Monitor the patient closely for clinical signs of hypoxia and **hypercapnia** (symptoms of elevated carbon dioxide levels, including tachycardia, hypotension, and cyanosis). Arterial blood gas levels (see Chapter 30, Table 30.1) may confirm the clinical observations.

Detection of respiratory depression

- Early signs of diminished ventilation are difficult to detect, particularly after the patient leaves the immediate postoperative area when continuous monitoring with pulse oximetry is discontinued. Often the signs of restlessness, anxiety, lethargy, decreased mental alertness, and headache are early subtle clues to respiratory distress.
- Use of the abdominal, intercostal, or neck muscles is an indication of respiratory distress. Flaring of the nostrils may be present in severe cases.

- As respiratory distress progresses, respirations become shallow and rapid. Assess for asymmetric chest movements.
- The development of cyanosis is a late sign of respiratory complications. Respiratory distress should be detected early through close observation before cyanosis develops.
- Assess muscle strength by asking the patient to lift his or her head off the pillow and hold a few seconds.
  Pain assessment. Assess the degree of pain present because neuromuscular blocking agents paralyze the muscles but do *not* relieve pain.

◆ Implementation
Nursing interventions with musculoskeletal disorders

- Assist with physical examination, drawing of blood samples, obtaining vital signs, and weighing in preparation of diagnostic procedures.
- Adapt procedures to meet the self-care abilities of the individual patient.
- Administer prescribed medications (e.g., antiinflammatory drugs, analgesics, muscle relaxants).
- Provide specific instructions on the application of hot or cold packs. Generally, ice packs alleviate swelling for the first 48 hours after muscle injury.
- Elevating the extremity immediately after injury decreases swelling and, to some degree, alleviates pain.
- Maintain the activity level prescribed (e.g., bed rest, immobilization of muscle group or limb). During the initial phase of treatment, immobilizing the affected part will decrease muscle spasms and therefore decrease pain. Maintenance of proper alignment of the affected part will also relieve pain and swelling. Various approaches may be used for immobilization, including elastic bandages, splinting, casts, bed rest, or modified activity levels.
- Range-of-motion exercises may be prescribed to maintain joint function and prevent muscle atrophy and contractures. The activity plan prescribed must be individualized to the diagnosis and should be carefully followed for maximum effectiveness.
- Increased anxiety produces stress on the body's muscles. Implement measures to produce relaxation and provide for the psychological needs of the individual.

Nursing interventions with neuromuscular blocking agents

- Neuromuscular blocking agents are used during anesthesia and surgery to relax muscle groups and during the use of mechanical ventilation to improve airflow and oxygenation of the patient. See a critical care nursing text for a detailed discussion of nursing care while the patient is receiving mechanical ventilation. The patient must be intubated and receiving mechanical ventilation before administration of neuromuscular blocking agents.

- Monitor airway patency, respiratory rate, and tidal volume in accordance with hospital policy.
- The histamine release caused by these drugs may produce increased salivation. In patients who are paralyzed or who have incomplete return of control over swallowing, coughing, and deep breathing, these secretions may obstruct the airway. Have suctioning equipment by the bedside.
- Assess for dyspnea and loud or gurgling sounds with respirations. Suction secretions according to hospital policies and procedures. If qualified, palpate for coarse chest wall vibrations and listen for crackles.
- Deep-breathing exercises can allow the opportunity to assess the patient's cough reflex. Assist the patient by splinting any abdominal or thoracic incisions. Have the patient take three or four deep breaths and then cough. During this process, assess the patient's ability to breathe deeply.
- Patients can usually cough better in a semi-Fowler's or high Fowler's position; therefore depending on the situation and stability of the patient's vital signs, elevating the head of the bed may assist coughing and breathing. For unconscious or semiconscious patients, position on the side, using good body alignment. Keep the bed's side rails up.
- People still paralyzed by the effects of neuromuscular blocking agents may experience pain and be unable to speak to request medication. Ensure that analgesics are scheduled on a regular basis and administered on time.
- Deal calmly with the patient experiencing respiratory dysfunction. The inability to breathe may cause the patient to panic. Provide reassurance while initiating measures to assist the patient.
- Question antibiotic orders that prescribe aminoglycosides or tetracycline when neuromuscular blocking agents have been used. These drugs may potentiate the neuromuscular blocking activity.

◆ Patient Education
Pain relief

- The degree of musculoskeletal pain relief with and without activity must be discussed. Make modifications appropriate to the diagnosis and degree of impairment.
- Teach procedures designed to relieve pain (e.g., application of cold or heat, elevation of body part, proper body alignment).

Activities and exercise. The patient must resume activities of daily living within the boundaries set by her or his healthcare provider. Activities such as regular moderate exercise, meal preparation, resumption of usual sexual activities, and social interaction must be encouraged once specific orders have been obtained.

Psychosocial. For chronic disorders, encourage the patient to express feelings regarding chronic illness.

The adjustment to this situation involves working through great personal fears, frustrations, hostilities, and resentments associated with the loss of personal control in one's life.

Medications. Many of the medications used in the treatment of musculoskeletal disorders produce sedation. Teach the patient about safety precautions such as avoiding using power equipment or driving while taking these medications.

Fostering health maintenance

- Throughout the course of treatment, discuss medication information and the individual's expectations of therapy. Ensure that the individual understands the activity level prescribed, pain relief methods, and safety precautions to ensure personal safety during mobility.
- Seek cooperation and understanding of the following points so that medication compliance is increased: name of medication; dosage, route, and times of administration; and common and serious adverse effects.

Patient self-assessment. Enlist the patient's help in developing and maintaining a written record of monitoring parameters (e.g., level, location, and duration of pain; areas or muscles affected; degree of impairment with improvement in mobility; exercise tolerance). See Patient Self-Assessment Form for Muscle Relaxants on the Evolve website. Complete the Premedication Data column for use as a baseline to track response to drug therapy. Episodes of nausea, vomiting, or diarrhea should also be reported for the prescriber's evaluation if it is a new symptom. Ensure that the patient understands how to use the form, and instruct the patient to take the completed form to follow-up visits. During follow-up visits, focus on issues that will foster adherence with the therapeutic interventions prescribed.

DRUG THERAPY FOR MUSCULOSKELETAL DISORDERS

Skeletal muscle relaxants are used to treat musculoskeletal conditions such as low back pain and spastic muscle conditions associated with cerebral palsy, multiple sclerosis, and spinal cord injuries. Approximately 2,000,000 people in the United States use skeletal muscle relaxants annually, primarily for low back pain. Skeletal muscle relaxants are often divided into antispasticity medicines and antispasmodic medicines. **Spasticity** is defined as an upper motor neuron disorder, possibly caused by a conduction interruption in the nerve pathway. Spasticity is characterized by muscle hypertonicity and involuntary jerks, which produce stiff, awkward movements. Spasticity is often a complication in patients with multiple sclerosis or cerebral palsy. Antispasticity agents include tizanidine, dantrolene, baclofen, and diazepam.

Muscle spasms are often associated with musculoskeletal trauma or inflammation (e.g., strains, sprains, sciatica, herniated disks). Spasms are sudden alternating contractions and relaxations or sustained contractions of muscle. Antispasmodic agents used to treat muscle spasms are the benzodiazepines (diazepam), cyclobenzaprine, carisoprodol, metaxalone, chlorzoxazone, methocarbamol, tizanidine, and orphenadrine. Diazepam and tizanidine have both antispastic and antispasmodic activity. The centrally acting skeletal muscle relaxants act within the brainstem, basal ganglia, and spinal cord to induce muscle relaxation (Table 44.1). Dantrolene is a muscle relaxant that acts directly on the skeletal muscle to reduce the force of muscle contractions.

Medications used in the management of gout vary in their actions. Some agents are used to treat acute attacks to relieve pain and inflammation, such as colchicine. Other drugs alter the production or excretion of uric acid.

DRUG CLASS: CENTRALLY ACTING SKELETAL MUSCLE RELAXANTS

Actions

The centrally acting skeletal muscle relaxants belong to a class of compounds used to relieve acute muscle spasm. The exact mechanism of action of the centrally acting skeletal muscle relaxants is not known, except that they act by central nervous system depression. Baclofen (see next drug monograph), a gamma-aminobutyric acid derivative, works by interrupting polysynaptic reflexes at the spinal cord level.

The centrally acting skeletal muscle relaxants do not have any direct effect on muscles, nerve conduction, or neuromuscular junctions. All of these muscle relaxants produce some degree of sedation, and most healthcare providers think that the benefits of these agents, other than baclofen, come from their sedative effects rather than from actual muscle relaxation.

Uses

The centrally acting skeletal muscle relaxants are used in combination with physical therapy, rest, and analgesics to relieve muscle spasm associated with acute, painful musculoskeletal conditions. They should not be used in muscle spasticity associated with cerebral or spinal cord disease because they may reduce the strength of remaining active muscle fibers, causing further impairment and debilitation.

Therapeutic Outcome

The primary therapeutic outcome expected from centrally acting skeletal muscle relaxant therapy is relief from muscle spasm.

Table 44.1   Centrally Acting Skeletal Muscle Relaxants

GENERIC NAME	BRAND NAME	AVAILABILITY	ADULT DOSAGE RANGE (PO)	COMMENTS
carisoprodol	Soma ⇄ *Do not confuse Soma with Senna.*	Tablets: 250, 350 mg	250-350 mg four times daily	Onset of action: 30 min; duration: 4-6 hr
chlorzoxazone	Lorzone	Tablets: 250, 375, 500, 750 mg	250-750 mg three or four times daily	Commonly causes gastrointestinal discomfort; may be hepatotoxic
cyclobenzaprine ⇄ *Do not confuse cyclobenzaprine with cyproheptadine.*	Amrix	Tablets: 5, 7.5, 10 mg Capsules, extended release (24 hr): 15, 30 mg	10-20 mg three times daily; do not exceed 60 mg 15-30 mg once daily; do not exceed 30 mg daily	Recommended only for short-term treatment (2-3 wk) of painful musculoskeletal conditions; very sedating
metaxalone ⇄ *Do not confuse metaxalone with metolazone.*	Skelaxin	Tablets: 400, 800 mg	800 mg three or four times daily	Use with caution in patients with liver disease
methocarbamol	Robaxin	Tablets: 500, 750 mg Injection: 100 mg/mL in 10-mL vials	1-1.5 g four times daily	Mechanism unknown; does not directly relax tense skeletal muscles
orphenadrine citrate	—	Tablets, extended release (12 hr): 100 mg Injection: 30 mg/mL in 2-mL vials	100 mg two times daily	Also has analgesic properties; do not use in patients with glaucoma or prostatic hyperplasia
tizanidine ⇄ *Do not confuse tizanidine with nizatidine or tiagabine.*	Zanaflex ⇄ *Do not confuse Zanaflex with Xanax or Anaflex.*	Tablets: 2, 4 mg Capsules: 2, 4, 6 mg	4-8 mg q6-8h; do not exceed 36 mg daily	Peak effects at 1-2 hr and dissipates between 3 and 6 hr; used for management of increased muscle tone associated with spasticity

❖ **Nursing Implications for Centrally Acting Skeletal Muscle Relaxants**

◆ *Premedication assessment*
1. Review allergies and obtain baseline vital signs and mental status of patient.
2. Have ordered laboratory studies carried out (e.g., liver function studies, complete blood cell count).

◆ *Availability, dosage, and administration.* See Table 44.1.

◆ *Common adverse effects.* These adverse effects are usually mild and tend to resolve with continued therapy. Encourage the patient not to discontinue therapy without first consulting with the healthcare provider.

Neurologic

Sedation, weakness, lethargy, dizziness. Provide for patient safety for the duration of these symptoms; report to the healthcare provider for further evaluation.

Patients must avoid operating power equipment or driving.

Gastrointestinal. Report any gastrointestinal complaints to the healthcare provider for further evaluation.

◆ *Serious adverse effects*

Gastrointestinal

Hepatotoxicity. The symptoms of hepatotoxicity are anorexia, nausea, vomiting, jaundice, hepatomegaly, splenomegaly, and abnormal liver function test results (e.g., elevated bilirubin, aspartate aminotransferase [AST], alanine aminotransferase [ALT], gamma-glutamyltransferase [GGT], and alkaline phosphatase levels; increased prothrombin time).

Hematologic

Blood dyscrasias. Routine laboratory studies (e.g., red blood cell [RBC], white blood cell [WBC], and differential counts) are scheduled for patients taking these agents for 30 days or longer. Stress the importance of returning for this laboratory work. Monitor for the development of sore throat, fever, purpura, jaundice, and/or excessive progressive weakness.

◆ *Drug interactions*

Central nervous system depressants. Central nervous system depressants, including alcohol, opioid agonists, antiepileptics, sedative-hypnotics, benzodiazepines, phenothiazines, and antidepressants, potentiate the sedative effects of centrally acting skeletal muscle relaxants. People who work around machinery, drive a car, administer medicines, or perform other duties that require mental alertness should not take these medications while working.

---

baclofen (BĂK-lō-fĕn)
   Lioresal (lī-ŌR-ĕ-sŏl)

Actions

Baclofen is a centrally acting skeletal muscle relaxant that acts somewhat differently from the other centrally acting agents. It is a gamma-aminobutyric acid derivative that interrupts polysynaptic reflexes at the level of the spinal cord.

Uses

Baclofen is used in the management of muscle spasticity resulting from multiple sclerosis, spinal cord injuries, cerebral palsy, and other spinal cord diseases. It is not recommended for use in spasticity associated with Parkinson's disease, stroke, or rheumatic disorders. Use of baclofen to treat cerebral palsy usually requires intrathecal infusion using a pump. Use baclofen with caution for all patients who must use spasticity to maintain an upright posture and balance in moving.

Therapeutic Outcome

The primary therapeutic outcome expected from baclofen therapy is relief from muscle spasm.

❖ **Nursing Implications for baclofen**

◆ **Premedication assessment**

1. Check history for any spastic disorders (e.g., Parkinson's disease, stroke, rheumatic disorders). If present, withhold medication and check with healthcare provider.
2. Perform a baseline mental status examination.

◆ *Availability.* *PO:* 5-, 10-, and 20-mg tablets, oral suspension 1 mg/mL and 5 mg/mL.
   Intrathecal: 0.05-, 0.5-, 1-, and 2-mg/mL ampules/vials.

◆ *Dosage and administration.* **Adult:** *PO:* Initially 5 mg three times daily. Increase the dosage by 5 mg every 3 to 7 days based on response. Optimum effects are usually

noted at dosages of 40 to 80 mg daily, but may take several weeks to achieve. Intrathecal administration with the use of a pump has become common.

 Medication Safety Alert

Do not abruptly discontinue baclofen therapy. Severe exacerbation of spasticity and hallucinations may result.

◆ *Common adverse effects.* These adverse effects are usually mild and tend to resolve with continued therapy. Encourage the patient not to discontinue therapy without first consulting with the healthcare provider.
   Gastrointestinal. Nausea.
   Neurologic
   Fatigue, headache, drowsiness, dizziness. Provide for patient safety during episodes of dizziness; report to the healthcare provider for further evaluation.

◆ *Drug interactions*

Central nervous system depressants. Central nervous system depressants, including sleep aids, analgesics, benzodiazepines, and alcohol, potentiate the sedative effects of baclofen. Persons who work around machinery, drive a car, administer medicines, or perform other duties in which they must remain mentally alert should not take these medications while working.

DRUG CLASS: DIRECT-ACTING SKELETAL MUSCLE RELAXANTS

---

dantrolene (DĂN-trō-lēn)
   Dantrium (DĂN-trē-ŭm)

Actions

Dantrolene is a muscle relaxant that acts directly on skeletal muscle. This medication produces generalized mild weakness of skeletal muscles and decreases the force of reflex muscle contractions, hyperreflexia, clonus, muscle stiffness, involuntary muscle movements, and spasticity.

Uses

Dantrolene is used to control the spasticity of chronic disorders such as cerebral palsy, multiple sclerosis, spinal cord injury, and stroke syndrome. Dantrolene is also approved by the US Food and Drug Administration to treat neuroleptic malignant syndrome associated with the use of antipsychotic agents (see Chapter 17) and unusual reactions to neuromuscular agents used with balanced anesthesia.

Therapeutic Outcome

The primary therapeutic outcome expected from dantrolene therapy is relief from muscle spasm.

❖ **Nursing Implications for dantrolene**

◆ *Premedication assessment.*

1. When used for neuroleptic malignant syndrome, perform a baseline assessment of vital signs, especially temperature.
2. Establish a baseline of degree of muscle symptoms present.

◆ *Availability. PO:* 25-, 50-, and 100-mg capsules. *IV:* 20-mg/vial.

◆ *Dosage and administration.* **Adult:** *PO:* Initially, 25 mg daily for 7 days. Increase to 25 mg 3 times daily for 7 days; then increase to 50 mg 3 times daily for 7 days, with a final dosage of 100 mg 3 times daily; some patients may require 100 mg 4 times daily.

   Response to therapy. Tell the patient that effectiveness of the drug may not be apparent for 1 week or longer. Encourage the patient not to discontinue therapy without first consulting with the healthcare provider.

◆ *Common adverse effects.* These adverse effects are usually mild and tend to resolve with continued therapy. They can often be minimized by starting therapy with low doses. Encourage the patient not to discontinue therapy without first consulting with the healthcare provider.

   Neurologic

   Weakness, drowsiness, dizziness, lightheadedness. Provide for patient safety during episodes of dizziness; report to the healthcare provider for further evaluation.

   Gastrointestinal. Diarrhea.

◆ *Serious adverse effects*

   Sensory

   Photosensitivity. The patient should be cautioned to avoid exposure to sunlight and ultraviolet light. Suggest wearing long-sleeved clothing, a hat, and sunglasses while exposed to sunlight. The patient must not use tanning lamps. The patient should not discontinue therapy without notifying the healthcare provider.

   Gastrointestinal

   Hepatotoxicity. The symptoms of hepatotoxicity are anorexia, nausea, vomiting, jaundice, hepatomegaly, splenomegaly, and abnormal liver function test results (e.g., elevated bilirubin, AST, ALT, GGT, and alkaline phosphatase; increased INR).

◆ *Drug interactions*

   Central nervous system depressants. Central nervous system depressants, including sleeping aids, analgesics, benzodiazepines, and alcohol, will potentiate the sedative effects of dantrolene. The patient who works with machinery, operates a motor vehicle, administers medications, or performs other duties that require mental alertness should not take these medications while working.

DRUG CLASS: NEUROMUSCULAR BLOCKING AGENTS

Actions

Neuromuscular blocking agents act by interrupting transmission of impulses from motor nerves to muscles at the skeletal neuromuscular junction. Neuromuscular blocking agents have no effect on consciousness, memory, or the pain threshold. Reassurance by nursing personnel is essential to paralyzed patients (e.g., those on ventilators), and analgesics and sedatives must be administered on schedule. These patients may suffer extreme pain and may be unable to ask for analgesics.

Uses

Neuromuscular blocking agents are important skeletal muscle relaxants. These agents are used to produce adequate muscle relaxation during anesthesia to reduce the use (and adverse effects) of general anesthetics, ease endotracheal intubation and prevent laryngospasm, decrease muscular activity in electroshock therapy, and aid in reducing the muscle spasms associated with tetanus.

Therapeutic Outcome

The primary therapeutic outcome expected from neuromuscular blocking therapy is smooth and skeletal muscle relaxation.

❖ **Nursing Implications for Neuromuscular Blocking Agents**

◆ *Premedication assessment.* 1. These drugs are administered by an anesthetist or anesthesiologist during surgical anesthesia or by a critical care nurse when a patient is placed or being maintained on a ventilator. Check hospital or institutional policy to determine who may administer these drugs and what the specific monitoring parameters are.

2. Check history for hepatic, pulmonary, and renal disease or neurologic disorders such as myasthenia gravis, spinal cord injury, or multiple sclerosis. If present, tag the chart appropriately before administration of anesthesia.

3. Have oxygen, suction, and artificial respiration equipment available in the immediate area whenever these drugs are to be used. Also have antidotes (e.g., neostigmine methylsulfate [Prostigmin], pyridostigmine bromide [Mestinon], edrophonium chloride [Enlon]) available.

◆ *Availability.* See Table 44.2.

◆ *Administration.* These agents are usually given by the intravenous (IV) route, but may also be given by the intramuscular (IM) route. Because they are potent drugs, they should be used only by those thoroughly familiar with their effects, such as an anesthetist or anesthesiologist, and under conditions in which the patient can

Table 44.2 Neuromuscular Blocking Agents

GENERIC NAME	BRAND NAME	AVAILABILITY
atracurium besylate		10 mg/mL in 5- and 10-mL vials
cisatracurium besylate	Nimbex ⇄ *Do not confuse Nimbex with Niferex, Bumex*	2 mg/mL in 5- and 10-mL vials; 10 mg/mL in 20-mL vials
pancuronium bromide		1 mg/mL in 10-mL vials
rocuronium bromide		10 mg/mL in 5- and 10-mL vials
succinylcholine	Anectine, Quelicin	20 mg/mL in 10-mL vials, 5-, 7-, 10-mL syringes
vecuronium bromide ⇄ *Do not confuse vecuronium with vancomycin.*		10, 20 mg/vial; 1 mg/mL in 10-mL syringes

receive constant, close attention for signs of respiratory failure. Adequate equipment for artificial respiration, antidotes, and other measures for prompt treatment of toxicity must be readily available.

Patients with hepatic, pulmonary, or renal disease or neurologic disorders such as myasthenia gravis, spinal cord injury, or multiple sclerosis must be fully evaluated to assess their ability to tolerate neuromuscular blocking agents. Much smaller doses are often necessary when these diseases are present. Neonates and older patients also require adjustments in dosage because of the insensitivity of their neuromuscular junctions.

Treatment of overdose. Treatment of overdose includes artificial respiration with oxygen and antidotes such as neostigmine methylsulfate (Prostigmin), pyridostigmine bromide (Mestinon), and edrophonium chloride (Enlon). Atropine sulfate is usually administered with neostigmine or pyridostigmine to block bradycardia, hypotension, and salivation induced by these agents. Another available antidote, sugammadex (Bridion), is the first selective relaxant binding agent used to reverse neuromuscular blockade after administration of the nondepolarizing neuromuscular blocking agents vecuronium or rocuronium. There is no antidote for the early blockade induced by succinylcholine. Fortunately, it is of short duration and does not require reversal.

◆ *Common adverse effects*

Histamine release. Neuromuscular blocking agents cause histamine release, which may cause bronchospasm, bronchial and salivary secretions, flushing, edema, and urticaria. Ensure that the airway is patent and that secretions are suctioned regularly to prevent obstruction. Report evidence of bronchospasm, edema, and urticaria immediately.

Neurologic

Mild discomfort. Mild to moderate discomfort, particularly in the neck, upper back, and lower intercostal and abdominal muscles, will be noted when the patient first ambulates after use.

◆ *Serious adverse effects*

Respiratory

Signs of respiratory distress. Monitor vital signs for a prolonged period after administration of neuromuscular blocking agents.

Diminished cough reflex, inability to swallow. Assess deep breathing and coughing at regular intervals. Have suction and oxygen equipment available, and be familiar with institutional emergency code practices.

◆ *Drug interactions*

Drugs that enhance therapeutic and toxic effects. General anesthetics (e.g., ether, enflurane), aminoglycoside antibiotics (e.g., gentamicin, neomycin, streptomycin, tobramycin, amikacin), clindamycin, tetracycline, quinidine, quinine, procainamide, lidocaine, beta-adrenergic blocking agents (e.g., propranolol, timolol, pindolol, nadolol), aprotinin, metoclopramide, lithium, and agents that deplete potassium (e.g., thiazide diuretics, furosemide, torsemide, bumetanide, ethacrynic acid, chlorthalidone, amphotericin B, corticosteroids) inhibit neuromuscular transmission, which results in prolonged neuromuscular blockade.

Label charts of patients scheduled for surgery who are taking any of these agents. These combinations may potentiate respiratory depression. Check the anesthetist's records of surgical patients. Monitor postoperative patients for respiratory depression for a prolonged period. This may occur 48 hours or more after drug administration.

Drugs that reduce therapeutic effects. These include neostigmine methylsulfate, pyridostigmine bromide, and edrophonium chloride. These agents are used as antidotes in case of overdosage of the neuromuscular blocking agents.

Carbamazepine. Carbamazepine hastens recovery time from neuromuscular blocking agents. Higher or more frequent doses of the neuromuscular blocking agent may be necessary.

Respiratory depressants. Analgesics, sedatives, and benzodiazepines used in combination with muscle relaxants may potentiate respiratory depression. Check the anesthetist's records of surgical patients. Monitor postoperative patients for respiratory depression for a prolonged period. This may occur 48 hours or more after drug administration.

DRUG CLASS: GOUT AGENTS

colchicine (KŌL-chǐ-sēn)

Actions
The exact mechanism of action is not known, but colchicine interrupts the cycle of urate crystal deposition in the tissues that results in an acute attack of gout. It does not affect the amount of uric acid in the blood or urine; therefore it is not a uricosuric agent.

Uses
Colchicine is an alkaloid that has been used for hundreds of years to prevent or relieve acute attacks of gout. Joint pain and swelling begin to subside within 12 hours and are usually gone within 48 to 72 hours after initiating therapy.

Therapeutic Outcome
The primary therapeutic outcome expected from colchicine therapy is elimination of joint pain secondary to acute gout attack.

❖ Nursing Implications for colchicine
◆ Premedication assessment
1. Assess for and record any gastrointestinal complaints present before initiation of drug therapy.
2. Assess for a history of allergy to colchicine. If present, withhold the drug and consult with the healthcare provider.
3. Obtain baseline complete blood count and differential, uric acid level, blood urea nitrogen (BUN), creatinine, AST, ALT, and other values as requested by the healthcare provider for future comparison and for monitoring for development of blood dyscrasias, renal dysfunction, and liver impairment, as well as tracking progress in control of uric acid level.
4. Assess the patient's level and location of pain using the pain rating scale (0 to 10); assess affected area for signs of inflammation—erythema, edema, and mobility.

◆ *Availability.* *PO:* 0.6-mg tablets and capsules.

◆ *Dosage and administration.* **Adult:** *PO: Acute gout:* 1.2 mg at first sign of gout flare, followed by 0.6 mg 1 hour later; do not exceed 1.8 mg over 1 hour. After the acute attack, 0.6 mg should be administered one to two times daily to prevent relapse. Do not repeat high-dose therapy for at least 3 days.

> ! Medication Safety Alert
>
> Use with extreme caution in older adults or debilitated patients and in patients with impaired renal, cardiac, or gastrointestinal function.

Fluid intake. Monitor intake and output during therapy. Maintain fluid intake at 8 to 12 eight-ounce glasses daily.

◆ *Common adverse effects*
Gastrointestinal
Nausea, vomiting, diarrhea. These are common adverse effects of colchicine therapy. Discontinue therapy when gastrointestinal symptoms develop. Always report bright red blood in vomitus, coffee-ground vomitus, or dark, tarry stools.

◆ *Serious adverse effects*
Hematologic
Blood dyscrasias. Serious, potentially fatal, blood dyscrasias, including anemia, agranulocytosis, and thrombocytopenia, have been associated with colchicine therapy. Although the development of blood dyscrasias is rare, periodic differential blood counts are recommended if the patient requires prolonged treatment. Routine laboratory studies (e.g., RBC, WBC, and differential counts) should be scheduled. Stress to the patient the importance of returning for this laboratory work. Monitor for the development of sore throat, fever, purpura, jaundice, or excessive and progressive weakness and report any such development immediately to the healthcare provider.

◆ *Drug interactions.* No clinically significant drug interactions have been reported.

probenecid (prō-BĚN-ě-sǐd)

Actions
Uricosuric agents act on the tubules of the kidneys to enhance the excretion of uric acid. Probenecid promotes renal excretion of a number of substances, including uric acid. It inhibits the reabsorption of urate in the kidney, which results in reduction of uric acid in the blood.

Uses
Probenecid is used to treat hyperuricemia and chronic gouty arthritis. It is not effective for acute attacks of gout and is not an analgesic.

Therapeutic Outcome
The primary therapeutic outcome expected with probenecid therapy is prevention of acute attacks of gouty arthritis.

❖ **Nursing Implications for probenecid**

◆ *Premedication assessment.*
1. Inquire about the time of onset of the last gout attack; do not administer medication during or within 2 to 3 weeks of an acute attack.
2. Assess for and record any gastrointestinal complaints before initiating drug therapy.
3. Ask about any history of blood dyscrasias or kidney stones; if present, withhold drug and contact a healthcare provider.
4. Obtain baseline blood studies as requested (e.g., uric acid and serum creatinine levels) to assess appropriateness and to monitor response to therapy.

> ⚠ Medication Safety Alert
>
> • Do NOT start probenecid therapy during an acute attack of gout; wait 2 to 3 weeks.
> • Do NOT administer to patients with histories of blood dyscrasias or uric acid kidney stones.
> • Do NOT administer to patients with a creatinine clearance lower than 40 mL/min or a BUN level higher than 40 mg/100 mL.

◆ *Availability.* *PO:* 500-mg tablets.

◆ *Dosage and administration.* **Adult:** *PO:* Initially 250 mg twice daily for 1 week, then 500 mg twice daily. The dosage may be increased by 500 mg every few weeks to goal. Administer with food or milk to diminish gastric irritation. Maintain fluid intake at 2 to 3 L daily.

◆ *Common adverse effects*
   Metabolic
   Acute gout attacks. Patients should be told that the incidence of gout attacks may increase for the first few months of therapy and that they should continue therapy without changing the dosage during the attacks.

◆ *Serious adverse effects*
   Gastrointestinal
   Nausea, anorexia, vomiting. Use probenecid with caution in patients with a history of peptic ulcer disease. Individuals who experience symptoms of ulcers and are still undiagnosed should be encouraged to report gastrointestinal symptoms if they increase in intensity or frequency. Always report bright red blood in vomitus, coffee-ground vomitus, or dark, tarry stools.
   Hypersensitivity, immune system
   Hives, pruritus, rash. These are signs of hypersensitivity; notify the healthcare provider. Therapy may have to be discontinued.

◆ *Drug interactions*
   Oral hypoglycemic agents. Monitor for hypoglycemia (e.g., headache, weakness, decreased coordination, general apprehension, diaphoresis, hunger, blurred or double vision). The dosage of the hypoglycemic agent may need to be reduced. Notify the healthcare provider if any of these symptoms appear.

   Acyclovir, famciclovir, valacyclovir, indomethacin, rifampin, sulfonamides, naproxen, penicillins, cephalosporins, methotrexate. Probenecid blocks the renal excretion of these agents. See individual drug monographs of the drugs listed for serious adverse effects that may indicate development of toxicity.

   Salicylates. Although occasional use of aspirin will not interfere with the effectiveness of probenecid, regular use of aspirin or aspirin-containing products should be discouraged. If analgesia is required, suggest acetaminophen.

   Antineoplastic agents. Because of the potential development of renal uric acid stones, probenecid is not recommended for increased uric acid levels caused by antineoplastic therapy.

DRUG CLASS: XANTHINE OXIDASE INHIBITORS

Actions
Xanthine oxidase inhibitors block the terminal pathways in uric acid formation by inhibiting the enzyme xanthine oxidase. The two drugs currently available are allopurinol and febuxostat.

Uses
Allopurinol is used to treat primary hyperuricemia in patients with gout or gout secondary to antineoplastic therapy. It is not effective for treating acute attacks of gouty arthritis. Allopurinol has an advantage over uricosuric agents (probenecid) in that gouty nephropathy and the formation of urate stones are less likely because the drug inhibits the production of uric acid. It may also be used in patients with renal failure. Uricosuric agents should not be used in this case.

Febuxostat is approved for the chronic management of hyperuricemia in patients with gout. Febuxostat is not approved for use in asymptomatic hyperuricemia.

Therapeutic Outcome
The primary therapeutic outcome associated with xanthine oxidase inhibitor therapy is reduced serum uric acid levels with a lower frequency of acute gout attacks.

❖ **Nursing Implications for Xanthine Oxidase Inhibitors**

◆ *Premedication assessment*
1. Inquire about the time of onset of gout attack; do not start the medication during an acute attack.
2. Assess for and record any gastrointestinal complaints before initiating drug therapy.
3. Obtain baseline blood studies, blood counts, and renal and liver function studies as requested.

◆ *Availability, dosage, and administration.* See Table 44.3.

Table 44.3   Xanthine Oxidase Inhibitors

GENERIC NAME	BRAND NAME	AVAILABILITY	DAILY DOSAGE	MAXIMUM DAILY DOSAGE
allopurinol	Zyloprim	PO: 100-, 300-mg tablets	PO: 300 mg	800 mg
febuxostat	Uloric	PO: 40-, 80-mg tablets	PO: Initially, 40 mg *Dosage adjustment:* If serum uric acid level is not <6 mg/dL after 2 wk therapy, raise the dosage to 80 mg	120 mg

Allopurinol. Chemotherapy-induced tumor lysis syndrome:

Adult: *IV:* 200 to 400 mg/kg/day, maximum dose is 600 mg/day. Infuse at a concentration no greater than 6 mg/mL. When possible, allopurinol therapy should be started 24 to 48 hours before chemotherapy known to cause tumor lysis. Dosage must be reduced in patients with a creatinine clearance of 20 mL/min or lower.

Febuxostat. Dosage must be reduced in patients with a creatinine clearance of 30 mL/min or lower.

Fluid intake. Maintain fluid intake at 8 to 12 eight-ounce glasses daily.

◆ *Common adverse effects*
Metabolic
Acute gout attacks. Patients should be told that the frequency of gout attacks may increase for the first few months of therapy with xanthine oxidase inhibitors. The patient should continue therapy without changing the dosage during the attacks. Patients may be treated with nonsteroidal antiinflammatory agents or colchicine to prevent acute gout flare-ups.
Gastrointestinal
Gastric irritation. If gastric irritation occurs, administer with food or milk. If symptoms persist or increase in severity, report to the healthcare provider for evaluation.

Nausea, vomiting, diarrhea. These adverse effects are usually mild and tend to resolve with continued therapy. Encourage the patient not to discontinue therapy without first consulting with the healthcare provider.
Neurologic
Dizziness, headache. These adverse effects are usually mild and tend to resolve with continued therapy. Encourage the patient not to discontinue therapy without first consulting with the healthcare provider.

◆ *Serious adverse effects*
Gastrointestinal
Hepatotoxicity. The symptoms of hepatotoxicity are anorexia, nausea, vomiting, jaundice, hepatomegaly, splenomegaly, and abnormal liver function test results (e.g., elevated bilirubin, AST, ALT, GGT, and alkaline phosphatase levels; increased prothrombin time). Periodic measurement of liver function tests is appropriate when initiating therapy and in patients with hepatic impairment.

Hematologic
Bone marrow suppression. Routine laboratory studies (RBC, WBC, and differential counts) should be scheduled. Stress the importance of the patient returning for this laboratory work. Monitor for sore throat, fever, purpura, jaundice, or excessive and progressive weakness.
Hypersensitivity
Fever, pruritus, rash. Report symptoms for further evaluation by the healthcare provider. Pruritus may be relieved by adding baking soda to the bathwater.

◆ *Drug interactions*
Theophylline derivatives. Xanthine oxidase inhibitors, when given with theophylline derivatives, may cause theophylline toxicity. Observe for vomiting, dizziness, restlessness, and cardiac arrhythmias. The dosage of theophylline may need to be reduced.

Azathioprine, mercaptopurine. Xanthine oxidase inhibitors inhibit the metabolism of these agents. When initiating therapy with azathioprine or mercaptopurine, start at one-fourth to one-third of the normal dosage and adjust subsequent dosages according to the patient's response.

Ampicillin, amoxicillin. There is a high incidence of rash when patients are taking both allopurinol and ampicillin or amoxicillin. Do not consider the patient allergic to either drug until sensitivity tests identify a hypersensitivity reaction.

Cyclophosphamide. There is a greater incidence of bone marrow depression in patients receiving allopurinol and cyclophosphamide concurrently. Monitor for sore throat, fever, purpura, jaundice, or excessive and progressive weakness.

DRUG CLASS: URIC ACID REABSORPTION INHIBITOR

lesinurad (lē-SĬN-ŭr-ăd)
   Zurampic (zĕr-ĂM-pĭk)

Actions

Uric acid reabsorption inhibitors act on the kidneys by inhibiting transport proteins responsible for reabsorption of urate from the renal tubules of the kidneys. This action increases the excretion of uric acid in the urine.

Uses

Lesinurad is used in combination with a xanthine oxidase inhibitor for the treatment of hyperuricemia associated with gout in patients who have not achieved target serum uric acid levels with a xanthine oxidase inhibitor alone.

Therapeutic Outcome

The primary therapeutic outcome is to achieve lower uric acid levels in combination with xanthine oxidase inhibitors to decrease acute gout attacks.

❖ Nursing Implications For lesinurad

◆ Premedication assessment

1. Inquire about the time of gout attack; do not start the medication during an acute attack.
2. Obtain medication history and check for use of a xanthine oxidase inhibitor.
3. Assess for and record any gastrointestinal complaints before and during drug therapy.
4. Obtain baseline renal function tests.

> **! Medication Safety Alert**
>
> Lesinurad should not be used as monotherapy; it should only be used in combination with a xanthine oxidase inhibitor. Do not administer in patients with a creatinine clearance of less than 30 mL/min or receiving dialysis.

◆ **Availability.** *PO:* 200-mg tablets.

◆ **Dosage and administration. Adult:** *PO:* 200 mg once daily in combination with a xanthine oxidase inhibitor. The maximum dose is 200 mg. Administer in the morning with food and water. Maintain fluid intake at 2 L daily.

◆ **Common adverse effects**

Acute gout attacks. Patients should be told that a gout attack may occur after starting lesinurad, but that they should continue therapy. Patients may be treated with other medicines to prevent a gout flare-up.

Gastrointestinal

Gastroesophageal reflex. This adverse effect is usually mild or moderate and usually resolves. If gastroesophageal irritation persists or increases in severity, report to the healthcare provider for evaluation.

Neurologic

Headache. This adverse effect is usually mild to moderate and usually resolves. Encourage the patient not to discontinue therapy without first consulting with the healthcare provider. Maintain adequate fluid intake.

Renal

Increased serum creatinine. As a consequence of increased uric acid excretion by the kidneys, transiently elevated serum creatinine levels can occur but usually resolve. If serum creatinine levels increase to two times the normal limit, discontinuation is recommended.

◆ **Serious adverse effects**

Renal events. Adverse reactions related to renal functions (acute renal failure) may occur when lesinurad is given as monotherapy. Routine renal laboratory studies should be scheduled at initiation and during treatment, especially in patients with a creatinine clearance of less than 60 mL/min.

◆ **Drug interactions**

Drugs that enhance the toxic effect. Amiodarone and fluconazole inhibit the metabolism of lesinurad. Taking more than 325 mg of aspirin per day will decrease the effectiveness of lesinurad with xanthine oxidase inhibitors.

Get Ready for the NCLEX® Examination!

Key Points

- Skeletal muscular disorders such as cerebral palsy, multiple sclerosis, and gout cause pain and varying degrees of immobility, limiting a patient's ability to perform activities of daily living.
- Nurses can play an important role in providing counseling and guidance to patients and family members in understanding muscle spasticity and pain and how to maintain an appropriate balance between daily activities and timing of analgesics to optimize quality of life.
- Nurses also play a crucial role in providing comfort and monitoring to patients who have received neuromuscular blocking agents. It is mandatory that nurses know how to recognize and respond quickly when respiratory emergencies arise.

Additional Learning Resources

SG Go to your Study Guide for additional Review Questions for the NCLEX® Examination, Critical Thinking Clinical Situations, and other learning activities to help you master this chapter content.

Go to your Evolve website (https://evolve.elsevier.com/Clayton) for additional online resources.

Review Questions for the NCLEX® Examination

1. The nurse is administering a centrally acting skeletal muscle relaxant (other than baclofen) and knows that these drugs are used for patients with which diagnoses? *(Select all that apply.)*
   1. Muscle spasms
   2. Cerebral palsy
   3. Spinal cord injury
   4. Pulled back muscles
   5. Gout

2. The nurse is observing for early signs of respiratory depression after the patient received pancuronium during an elective procedure. The nurse should have which of the following on hand? *(Select all that apply.)*
   1. Suction equipment
   2. Oxygen
   3. Infusion pumps
   4. Artificial airways
   5. Flashlight

3. The nurse understands that the drug baclofen (Lioresal) is used for the management of spasticity for which of these disease processes? *(Select all that apply.)*
   1. Multiple sclerosis
   2. Parkinson's disease
   3. Cerebral palsy
   4. Spinal cord injuries
   5. Generalized clonic-tonic disorder

4. The nurse notes that following surgery during which vecuronium was administered, the antibiotic clindamycin had been ordered for a patient. The nurse knows that the combination can cause what?
   1. Prolonged effects of the vecuronium that may result in respiratory depression
   2. An increase in the metabolism of the vecuronium
   3. Increased toxic effects of the vecuronium
   4. Decreased effectiveness of the clindamycin

5. Dantrolene (Dantrium) is used to treat spasticity associated with which chronic diseases? *(Select all that apply.)*
   1. Cerebral palsy
   2. Multiple sclerosis
   3. Stroke syndrome
   4. Parkinson's disease
   5. Rheumatic disorders

6. The nurse is preparing to administer the medication allopurinol (Zyloprim) to an elderly patient and understands that this is used to treat which condition?
   1. Multiple sclerosis
   2. Stroke syndrome
   3. Gout secondary to antineoplastic therapy
   4. Acute attacks of gouty arthritis

7. When monitoring for adverse effects, the nurse will recognize which of the following as reportable symptoms related to colchicine?
   1. Nausea and vomiting
   2. Nasal congestion
   3. Dark, tarry stools
   4. Diarrhea

8. The nurse is teaching a patient about proper administration for probenecid. What information does the nurse include in the teaching plan? *(Select all that apply.)*
   1. "You will need to wait 2 to 3 weeks after an acute attack before starting the medicine."
   2. "The incidence of acute gout attacks will start to decrease in the first few months of therapy."
   3. "Before you start taking this, we need to get a blood sample for a baseline creatinine and BUN to monitor kidney function."
   4. "You will need to drink 2 to 3 quarts of fluid every day while taking this medicine."
   5. "If you are taking a hypoglycemic agent, be sure to monitor your glucose levels closely, as this may increase your blood sugar."

Objectives

1. Explain the major actions and effects of classes of drugs used to treat infectious diseases.
2. List the signs and symptoms of a secondary infection.
3. Describe the signs and symptoms of the common adverse effects of antimicrobial therapy.
4. Describe the nursing assessments and interventions for the common adverse effects associated with antimicrobial agents: allergic reaction, nephrotoxicity, ototoxicity, and hepatotoxicity.
5. Cite the primary uses for antibiotic, antitubercular, antifungal, and antiviral agents.

Key Terms

pathogenic (păth-ō-JĔN-ĭk) (p. 692)
antibiotics (ăn-tī-bī-Ŏ-tĭks) (p. 692)
gram-negative microorganisms (GRĂM NĔG-ĭ-tĭv) (p. 692)
gram-positive microorganisms (GRĂM PŎ-zĭ-tĭv mī-krō-ŌR-găn-ĭz-ĕmz) (p. 692)
prophylactic antibiotics (prō-fĭ-LĂK-tĭk) (p. 692)

nephrotoxicity (nĕf-rō-tŏks-ĬS-ĭ-tē) (p. 694)
ototoxicity (ō-tō-tŏks-ĬS-ĭ-tē) (p. 695)
hypoprothrombinemia (hī-pō-prō-thrŏm-bĭn-Ē-mē-ă) (p. 700)
penicillinase-resistant penicillins (pĕn-ĭ-SĬL-ĭn-ās rē-ZĬS-tĕnt pĕn-ĭ-SĬL-ĭnz) (p. 708)

ANTIMICROBIAL AGENTS

Antimicrobial agents are chemicals that eliminate living microorganisms that are **pathogenic** (toxic) to the patient. Antimicrobial agents may be of chemical origin, such as the sulfonamides, or they may be derived from other living organisms. Those derived from other living microorganisms are called *antibiotics*; for example, penicillin was first derived from the mold *Penicillium notatum*. Most antibiotics used today are harvested from large colonies of microorganisms, which are then purified and chemically modified into semisynthetic antimicrobial agents. The chemical modification makes the antibiotic more effective against specific pathogenic organisms. Antimicrobial agents are often first classified according to the type of pathogen to be destroyed, such as bacteria (antibacterial agents), fungus (antifungal agents), or virus (antiviral agents). The antimicrobial agents are then subdivided by chemical families into drug classes such as the penicillins, tetracyclines, and aminoglycosides.

The selection of the antimicrobial agent must be based on the sensitivity of the pathogen and the possible toxicity to the patient. If at all possible, infecting organisms should first be isolated and identified. Culture and sensitivity tests should be completed to identify the infective organism and determine the antibiotic to which the infecting organism is most sensitive. Bacteria are classified as **gram-negative microorganisms** (e.g., *Acinetobacter* spp., *Citrobacter* spp., *Enterobacter* spp.,

Escherichia coli, *Klebsiella* spp., *Providencia* spp., *Pseudomonas* spp., *Salmonella* spp., and *Shigella* spp.) or **gram-positive microorganisms** (e.g., *Staphylococcus aureus*, *Staphylococcus epidermidis*, *Streptococcus pyogenes*, *Streptococcus pneumoniae*). However, if clinically indicated, a patient may be started on a broad-spectrum antibiotic regimen until the infecting organism is identified and its drug sensitivity is determined. The antimicrobial therapy is then started based on the sensitivity results and the clinical judgment of the healthcare provider. In the inpatient setting, however, it is routine to obtain specimens of the infecting organism from infected sites (e.g., blood, urine, wound) and then start therapy immediately with one or more antimicrobial agents that are most likely to stop the infection. This is known as *empirical treatment*. When the cultures identify the pathogen and the sensitivity tests indicate which antimicrobial agent will be most effective, that antimicrobial agent is started and all other antimicrobial agents are discontinued. Discontinuation of therapy of unneeded antimicrobial agents helps prevent the development of resistant organisms and reduce healthcare costs.

For patients at risk for developing infective endocarditis (IE), the use of *prophylactic antibiotics* is recommended before dental procedures and procedures on respiratory tract or infected skin, skin structures, or musculoskeletal tissue only for patients with underlying cardiac conditions associated with the highest risk of adverse outcome from IE. The American Heart Association and American

College of Cardiology (Nishimura et al, 2017) guidelines recommend prophylactic antibiotic treatment for patients with cardiac conditions that put them at highest risk for IE and at high risk of experiencing adverse outcomes from IE. These cardiac conditions include prosthetic cardiac valve; previous IE; congenital heart disease; unrepaired, cyanotic congenital heart disease, including palliative shunts and conduits; congenital heart defects completely repaired with prosthetic material or a prosthetic device—whether placed by surgery or by catheter intervention—during the first 6 months after the procedure; repaired congenital heart defects with residual defects at the site or adjacent to the site of a prosthetic patch or prosthetic device; and cardiac transplantation.

NURSING IMPLICATIONS FOR ANTIMICROBIAL THERAPY

Nurses must consider the entire patient when administering and monitoring antimicrobial therapy. It is essential that the nurse be knowledgeable about the drugs, including physiologic parameters for monitoring expected therapeutic activity and adverse effects. It is important to teach the individual with an infection the basic principles of self-care, which will enhance the recovery process, and measures to prevent the spread of infection. With communicable diseases, exposed individuals must be contacted for follow-up testing and appropriate treatment.

◆ **Assessment**

History of current infection. What symptoms are described by the patient? Which of the symptoms described potentially relate to an infectious process? Extend questioning to help the patient focus—for example, when did the symptoms begin? Have they worsened? Is there fever, night sweats, malaise, chronic fatigue, weight loss, arthralgia, cough (type of secretions), diarrhea, painful urination, nausea, vomiting, lesions or skin rash, discharge, or drainage? Is there any swelling, pain, or heat in a particular area or discharge from a site? Has the patient been treated previously for a similar infection? Ask questions specific to the body systems affected by the infection (e.g., pain and burning with urination for a urinary tract infection [UTI]). Determine the patient's current living environment and review the institutional policy. Many patients residing in long-term care facilities are screened for methicillin-resistant *Staphylococcus aureus* (MRSA) and vancomycin-resistant *Enterococcus faecium* (VRE).

Healthcare-associated infections are common reasons for admission to hospitals, as well as reasons for extended stays. These infections occur when patients who are being treated for other conditions develop an additional infection while being cared for by healthcare workers. The common types of healthcare-associated infections are healthcare-associated pneumonia (HCAP) and UTIs.

When treating patients with sexually transmitted infections (STIs), ask about the number of sexual partners, sexual orientation, and use of precautions during intercourse. (See Chapter 40 for further details.)

Medication history
- Ask the patient to list all current prescribed and over-the-counter (OTC) medications or those taken in the past 6 months. Ask specifically about any medicines, such as corticosteroids, chemotherapy, or transplant immunosuppressants, that may affect the immune status of the individual.
- Does the person take any type of allergy injections or medications?
- Is the person immunized against childhood diseases?
- Has the person been treated for an infection recently? If yes, what medications were taken and were there any allergic responses? If so, ask for details of the symptoms of the allergic reaction.
- Has the patient taken this medication before? If so, what symptoms (e.g., nausea, vomiting, diarrhea, rash, itching, or hives) developed when taking it that led the patient to state that there was an allergy? Ask the patient to describe the appearance of a rash, where it started, and the course of recovery. How soon after starting the medication did the symptoms develop?
- Ask if the patient has ever developed a secondary infection (black, hairy tongue; white patches [thrush] in mouth; vaginal infection) when taking an antibiotic. For example, women taking antibiotics may develop a vaginal infection because of suppression of normal flora.

Physical examination
- Perform a head-to-toe body or functional assessment, focusing on the areas pertinent to the admitting diagnosis.
- Assess for risk factors that may contribute to development of infection, such as extensive surgical procedures, obesity, underlying contributory conditions (e.g., chronic obstructive pulmonary disease, diabetes), immunotherapy drugs, malnutrition, and age extremes (infants or older adults).

Psychosocial. For an individual with a serious communicable disease, assess the response and adaptive processes used to cope with the disease and its treatments.

Assessments during antimicrobial therapy. Read each drug monograph for specific common and serious adverse effects, and individualize the assessments for the drugs prescribed. Nausea, vomiting, diarrhea, allergies, anaphylaxis, nephrotoxicity, hepatotoxicity, ototoxicity, hematologic dyscrasias, secondary infection, and photosensitivity are found with recurring frequency in the antimicrobial drug monographs.

Nausea, vomiting, and diarrhea. These conditions are the "big three" adverse effects associated with antimicrobial drug therapy. When they occur, gather data such as the following:

1. Did the patient have a history of nausea, vomiting, or diarrhea before starting the drug therapy?
2. How soon after starting the medication did the symptoms start?
3. Since starting the medication, has the diet or water source changed in any way?
4. Was the patient taking other drugs, either prescription or OTC medications, before initiating antibiotic therapy?
5. How much fluid is the patient consuming when taking medications? Inadequate fluid intake sometimes causes gastritis manifested by nausea.
6. For diarrhea, what was the pattern of elimination before drug therapy? Report diarrhea and the character and frequency of stools, as well as any abdominal pain, promptly. Nausea, vomiting, and diarrhea are often dose related and result from changes in normal bacterial flora in the bowel, irritation, and secondary infection. Symptoms resolve within a few days, and discontinuation of therapy is rarely required.

When drug therapy causes nausea and vomiting, the healthcare provider may elect to give the antibiotic with food to decrease irritation, even though absorption may be slightly decreased, or may choose to switch to a parenteral dosage form. When reporting any incidence of nausea and vomiting, all significant data should be collected and reported. Administer prescribed antiemetics or antidiarrheal agents (see also Chapters 33 and 34).

Secondary infection. Assess for symptoms of secondary infection such as oral infection. Observe for a black, hairy tongue; white patches (thrush) in the oral cavity; cold sores; canker sores; and glossitis. There may be lesions and itching in the vaginal and anal areas. Secondary infection of the intestine, such as *Clostridium difficile*, can produce severe, life-threatening diarrhea. Secondary infection may occur in patients receiving broad-spectrum antibiotic therapy, particularly in those who are immunosuppressed. Monitor for the development of symptoms of secondary infection, and notify the healthcare provider if this occurs. Instruct the patient to minimize exposure to people known to have an infection and to practice good personal hygiene measures.

Allergies and anaphylaxis. The severity of an allergic reaction ranges from a mild rash to fatal anaphylaxis. Allergic reactions may develop within 30 minutes of administration of medications (e.g., anaphylaxis, laryngeal edema, shock, dyspnea, skin reactions) or may occur several days after discontinuing therapy (e.g., skin rashes, fever). All patients must be questioned for previous allergic reactions, and allergy-prone patients must be observed closely. It is important that a patient not be labeled "allergic" to a particular medication without adequate documentation. Patients who report

gastrointestinal (GI) symptoms of nausea, vomiting, and/or diarrhea with no other symptoms (e.g., skin rash, facial edema, dyspnea, hypotension) should not be labeled allergic to the medicine. The medication to which a patient claims an allergy may be a lifesaving drug for that patient in the future.

Closely monitor all patients—particularly those with histories of allergies, asthma, or rhinitis and those who are taking multiple drug preparations—for an allergic response during antimicrobial therapy. All patients should be watched carefully for possible allergic reactions for at least 20 to 30 minutes after administration of a medication. However, some drug reactions may not occur for several days. Hold the prescribed antimicrobial medication if the person reports a possible allergy. In the event of suspected anaphylaxis, summon the healthcare provider and the emergency cart immediately.

Although a serious reaction may occur with the first administration of a drug, repeated exposures to a previously sensitized substance can be fatal. Respond immediately to any signs of reaction, including swelling, redness, or pain at the site of injection; hives; nasal congestion and discharge; wheezing progressing to dyspnea; pulmonary edema; stridor; and sternal retractions.

Nephrotoxicity. Assess **nephrotoxicity** through an increasing blood urea nitrogen (BUN) and creatinine, decreasing urine output, decreasing urine specific gravity, casts or protein in the urine, frank blood or smoky-colored urine, or red blood cells (RBCs) in excess of 0 to 3 RBCs/high-power field (HPF) (see Table 41.1) on the urinalysis report.

> **! Medication Safety Alert**
>
> Maintain an accurate intake and output record; report declining output or output below 30 mL/hr in the adult patient. Many antimicrobial agents are potentially nephrotoxic (e.g., aminoglycosides, tetracyclines, vancomycin). Concomitant therapy with diuretics enhances the likelihood of toxicity, particularly in the older or debilitated patient. When renal function is impaired, most drug dosages must be decreased or alternative drug therapy used.

Hepatotoxicity. Assess for preexisting hepatic disease such as cirrhosis or hepatitis. Review laboratory studies (e.g., bilirubin, aspartate aminotransferase [AST], alanine aminotransferase [ALT], gamma-glutamyltransferase [GGT], and alkaline phosphatase levels; international normalized ratio [INR]) and report abnormal findings to the healthcare provider. Several drugs to be studied in this chapter are potentially hepatotoxic (e.g., isoniazid, sulfonamides). The liver is active in the metabolism of many drugs, and drug-induced hepatitis may occur. The actual liver damage may occur shortly after exposure to the pharmacologic agent, or may not appear for several weeks after initial exposure. The symptoms of hepatotoxicity are anorexia, nausea, vomiting, jaundice, hepatomegaly, splenomegaly, and abnormal liver function test results (e.g., elevated bilirubin, AST,

ALT, GGT, and alkaline phosphatase levels; increased INR). Patients with preexisting hepatic disease such as cirrhosis or hepatitis will require lower dosages of drugs metabolized by the liver.

Ototoxicity. Damage to the eighth cranial nerve (oto-toxicity) can occur from drug therapy, particularly from aminoglycosides. This may initially be manifested by dizziness, tinnitus, and progressive hearing loss. Assess the patient for difficulty in walking unaided, and assess the level of hearing daily. Intentionally speak to patients softly; note if they are aware that you said anything. Take particular notice of the patient who repeatedly asks, "What did you say?" or who starts talking more loudly or progressively increases the volume on the television or radio. Report preexisting hearing impairment or symptoms of developing hearing deficits to the healthcare provider and initiate orders prescribed. Provide for patient safety if tinnitus or dizziness accompanies the symptoms of hearing impairment.

Blood dyscrasias

1. Ask specifically about any history of blood disorders diagnosed and treatments prescribed.
2. Ask specifically about any types of anemia (e.g., aplastic, hemolytic, megaloblastic) or deficiencies of folic acid, vitamin B_{12}, or glucose-6-phosphate dehydrogenase.
3. Ask whether the individual has received chemotherapy, radiation therapy, or transplant therapy, all of which may induce an immunocompromised state and changes in the blood.
4. Has the patient received blood cell stimulator drugs, such as epoetin alfa (Epogen) or filgrastim (Neupogen)?
5. Does the patient have any bleeding disorders, such as hemophilia or thrombocytopenia?
6. Observe for bleeding gums, prolonged bleeding at an injection site, petechiae, and epistaxis (nosebleeds).
7. Review admission laboratory studies and report abnormalities (e.g., complete blood count [CBC] with differential, increased BUN or creatinine levels).
8. Individualize care to the type of blood dyscrasia present. When hypoprothrombinemia is present, the usual treatment is administration of vitamin K. Serious and possibly fatal bone marrow suppression may occur after therapy is initiated with some antibiotics (e.g., chloramphenicol). Monitor for signs and symptoms such as sore throat, fatigue, elevated temperature, small petechial hemorrhages, and bruises on the skin, and if present, report these symptoms immediately.

Photosensitivity. Assess for the development of dermatologic symptoms such as exaggerated sunburn, itching, rash, urticaria, pruritus, and scaling, particularly after exposure to sunlight. Photosensitivity is seldom evident during hospitalization. It is more commonly seen in ambulatory practice.

When the drug monograph lists this as a potential serious adverse effect, the nurse should provide health teaching to prevent its occurrence. Instruct the patient to avoid exposure to sunlight and ultraviolet light (e.g., sun lamps, suntanning beds); wear long-sleeved clothing, a hat, and sunglasses; and apply sunscreen to exposed skin when going out into the sunlight.

◆ **Implementation**

- Routine monitoring of all individuals receiving antimicrobial therapy should include status of hydration, temperature, pulse, respirations, and blood pressure. Monitor at least every 4 hours and more frequently as the patient's clinical status warrants.
- Use the Centers for Disease Control and Prevention (CDC) recommended precautions for infection transmission—universal precautions and appropriate guidelines for isolation. Consult the CDC's website, as well as clinical policies and procedures, to prevent transmission of infection. Always remember the importance of adequate handwashing.
- Always monitor for phlebitis when antimicrobials are administered intravenously.
- Administer antimicrobials as prescribed on the time schedule established.
- In some cases, a second drug (e.g., probenecid) may be administered concurrently to inhibit the excretion of the antibiotic (e.g., penicillin, cephalosporin). When this is done, monitor closely for adverse effects.

Medication history

- Ask the patient to list all prescribed medications, OTC medications, and herbal products being taken. Ask specifically about the recent use of corticosteroids, chemotherapy, or transplant suppressants.
- Does the patient have any allergies? If so, obtain details of medications and actual symptoms that occur during an allergic reaction. What treatment was used for any past allergic responses? What antibiotics have been taken? Were there any problems during antibiotic therapy?

◆ **Patient Education**

The following basic principles of patient care should not be overlooked when treating patients with infections:

- Adequate rest with as little stress as possible. Rest decreases metabolic needs and enhances the physiologic repair process.
- Nutritional management, including attention to hydration, proteins, fats, carbohydrates, minerals, and vitamins, to support the body's needs during an inflammatory response. Adequate nutrients to meet the energy needs, especially during times of fever, are essential so that the body will not break down its protein stores to meet energy requirements. The dietary teaching must be individualized to the patient's diagnosis and point of recovery. Unless contraindicated by coexisting disease, encourage adequate fluid intake of 2000 to 3000 mL/24 hr and simultaneously monitor the

patient for signs and symptoms of fluid volume deficit or fluid volume overload.

- Extensive teaching, individualized to the circumstances and mode of transmission of the disease, should be given to those with communicable infection. This should include contacting exposed individuals in accordance with institutional policies for disease screening, treatment, and follow-up counseling.
- Explain personal hygiene measures, such as handwashing techniques, management of excretions such as sputum, wound care, and the importance of not sharing personal hygiene items with others.
- Instruct the patient to refrain from sexual intercourse during therapy for STIs.

Medications

- Drug therapy specific for the type of microorganism causing the infection should be explained in detail so that the patient will realize the need for adherence to the prescribed regimen.
- Examine each drug monograph to identify suggestions to the patient on how to handle the common adverse effects associated with antimicrobial therapy. The patient also must be taught the signs and symptoms that must be reported to the healthcare provider. Stress to the patient the importance of not discontinuing the prescribed medication until the adverse effects have been discussed with the healthcare provider.
- Develop a medication schedule with the patient for at-home medications prescribed. Make sure that the patient understands why it is important to take antimicrobials for the entire course of drug therapy and not to discontinue them when feeling better. Completing treatment is critical to preventing microbial resistance to antibiotics. In addition, patients must know self-monitoring parameters for the prescribed drug therapy.
- Nursing mothers should remind their healthcare provider that they are breast feeding so that antibiotics may be selected that will have no effect on the infant.
- After an allergic reaction, the patient and family should inform anyone treating the patient in the future of the allergy to a specific drug. Wearing an allergy bracelet or tag may be appropriate. A wallet card describing the type of allergy can be helpful to future healthcare providers.
- Follow recommendations for annual influenza vaccine and pneumococcal vaccine for high-risk individuals (e.g., children; patients with diabetes, asthma, or pulmonary disease; older adults; healthcare workers; people with chronic or debilitating diseases). Always check with the healthcare provider if in doubt about advisability of administering vaccine.

Fostering health maintenance

- Throughout the course of treatment, discuss medication information. Continue to emphasize those factors that the patient can control to alter the progression of the disease: maintenance of general health and nutritional needs, adequate rest and appropriate exercise, and taking the prescribed medication until the entire course of therapy has been completed.
- Discuss expectations of therapy so that the patient understands whether a satisfactory response to drug therapy is being achieved, such as the relief of symptoms for which treatment was sought (e.g., relief of burning with urination and frequency of urination, relief of cough, or end of drainage and healing of a wound).

Patient self-assessment. Enlist the patient's help in developing and maintaining a written record of monitoring parameters (e.g., list presenting symptoms: cough with a large amount of phlegm, wound drainage, temperature, exercise tolerance). See Patient Self-Assessment Form for Antibiotics on the Evolve website. Complete the Premedication Data column for use as a baseline to track response to drug therapy. Ensure that the patient understands how to use the form, and instruct the patient to take the completed form to follow-up visits. During follow-up visits, focus on issues that will foster adherence to the therapeutic interventions prescribed.

DRUG THERAPY FOR INFECTIOUS DISEASE

DRUG CLASS: AMINOGLYCOSIDES

Actions
Aminoglycoside antibiotics kill bacteria primarily by inhibiting protein synthesis. Other mechanisms of action have not yet been fully defined.

Uses
The aminoglycosides are used primarily against gram-negative microorganisms that cause UTIs, meningitis, wound infections, and life-threatening septicemias. They are the mainstays in the treatment of healthcare-associated gram-negative infections (e.g., *Acinetobacter* spp., *Citrobacter* spp., *Enterobacter* spp., *E. coli*, *Klebsiella* spp., *Providencia* spp., *Pseudomonas* spp., *Salmonella* spp., and *Shigella* spp.). Neomycin may also be used before surgery to reduce the normal floral content of the intestinal tract.

Therapeutic Outcome
The primary therapeutic outcome expected from aminoglycoside therapy is elimination of bacterial infection.

❖ **Nursing Implications for Aminoglycosides**
◆ *Premedication assessment*
1. Obtain baseline assessments of the presenting symptoms.
2. Record temperature, pulse, respirations, blood pressure, and hydration status.

3. Assess for any allergies and symptoms of hearing loss or renal disease. If present, withhold drug and report findings to the healthcare provider.
4. If the patient has had anesthesia within the past 48 to 72 hours, check to see if skeletal muscle relaxants were administered. If used, withhold the drug and notify the healthcare provider.
5. Check for scheduled time of laboratory aminoglycoside serum level testing. After levels have been determined, assess whether results are normal or toxic. Contact the healthcare provider as appropriate.
6. Obtain baseline laboratory studies ordered and review results (e.g., CBC with differential, BUN, creatinine, culture and sensitivity).

◆ *Availability, dosage, and administration.* See Table 45.1.

Admixture compatibilities. *Do not* mix other drugs in the same syringe with aminoglycoside antibiotics or infuse together with other drugs. See Drug Interactions later in this section for incompatibilities.

Rate of infusion. Check with the hospital laboratory regarding timing of aminoglycoside blood level tests. The rate of infusion is quite important for aminoglycoside antibiotics, especially if preinfusion and postinfusion serum levels are being measured. Consult with a pharmacist or review the individual package literature for proper infusion rate. After levels have been determined, assess whether results are normal or toxic.

◆ **Serious adverse effects**

Sensory

Ototoxicity. Damage to the eighth cranial nerve can occur as a result of aminoglycoside therapy. Continue to observe patients for ototoxicity after therapy has been discontinued. These adverse effects may appear several days later.

Genitourinary

Nephrotoxicity. Monitor urinalysis and kidney function tests for abnormal results. Report increasing BUN and creatinine levels, decreasing urine output or decreasing specific gravity (despite amount of fluid intake), casts or protein in the urine, frank blood or smoky-colored urine, or RBCs in excess of 0 to 3 RBCs/HPF (see Table 41.1) on the urinalysis report.

◆ **Drug interactions**

Nephrotoxic potential. Cephalosporins, enflurane, vancomycin, and diuretics, when combined with aminoglycosides, may increase the nephrotoxic potential. Monitor the urinalysis and kidney function test findings for abnormal results.

Ototoxic potential. Aminoglycosides, when combined with torsemide, bumetanide, and furosemide, may increase ototoxicity. Therefore nursing assessments for tinnitus, dizziness, and decreased hearing should be done regularly every shift.

Neuromuscular blockade. Taking aminoglycoside antibiotics in combination with skeletal muscle relaxants may produce respiratory depression. Check the anesthesia records of postoperative patients to determine if skeletal muscle relaxants such as succinylcholine or pancuronium bromide were administered during surgery.

The nurse should monitor and assess the respiratory rate, depth of respirations, and chest movement and report apnea immediately. Because these effects may be seen for up to 48 hours after administration of skeletal muscle relaxants, continue monitoring respirations,

Table 45.1 Aminoglycosides

GENERIC NAME	BRAND NAME	AVAILABILITY	ADULT DOSAGE RANGE
amikacin ⇌ Do not confuse amikacin with Anakinra.		Injection: 500 mg/2 mL in 2-mL vial 1 g/4 mL in 4-mL vial	IM, IV: 15 mg/kg/24 hr (max 1.5 g/day)
gentamicin		Injection: -10 mg/mL in 2- and 10-mL vials; -40 mg/mL in 2- and 20-mL vials -40-, 60-, 80-, 100-, 120-mg single-dose containers	IM, IV: 3-5 mg/kg/day in two or three doses or 5-7 mg/kg once daily
neomycin		Tablets: 500 mg	PO: 4-12 g daily in four divided doses
streptomycin		Injection: 1-g vials	IM: 15 mg/kg/day once daily
tobramycin		Injection: 10 mg/mL in 2-mL vials 80 mg/2 mL in 2-mL vials 1.2 g in 30-mL bulk vials 2 g in 50-mL bulk vials Inhalation: 300-mg/5-mL nebulizer solution Inhalation: 28-mg capsules	IM, IV: 3-5 mg/kg/day in two or three doses or 5 mg/kg once daily

pulse, and blood pressure beyond the usual postsurgical vital signs routine.

Heparin. The aminoglycoside gentamicin and heparin are physically incompatible. *Do not* mix together before infusion.

Beta-lactam–type antibiotics (penicillins, cephalosporins). These drugs rapidly inactivate aminoglycoside antibiotics. *Do not* mix together or administer together at the same intravenous (IV) site.

DRUG CLASS: CARBAPENEMS

Actions

The carbapenems are extremely potent broad-spectrum antibiotics resistant to beta-lactamase enzymes secreted by bacteria. They act by inhibiting bacterial cell wall synthesis.

Uses

- Imipenem-cilastatin (Primaxin) is a combination product containing a carbapenem antibiotic called imipenem and cilastatin, an inhibitor of the renal dipeptidase enzyme dehydropeptidase I. Cilastatin has no antimicrobial activity; it prevents the inactivation of imipenem by the renal enzyme. It is used for the treatment of lower respiratory tract and intraabdominal infections; infections of the urinary tract, bones, joints, and skin; gynecologic infections; endocarditis; and bacterial septicemia caused by gram-negative or gram-positive organisms. A primary therapeutic role of imipenem-cilastatin is in the treatment of severe infections caused by multiresistant organisms and in mixed anaerobic-aerobic infections, primarily those involving intraabdominal and pelvic sepsis in which *Bacteroides fragilis* is a common pathogen. It should be used in combination with antipseudomonal agents because of resistance of *Pseudomonas cepacia* and *Pseudomonas aeruginosa* to imipenem.

- Meropenem is a carbapenem antibiotic that has a chemical structure that protects it against dehydropeptidase I, so that cilastatin is not necessary. It has a broad spectrum of activity similar to that of imipenem, but it is more active against Enterobacteriaceae and less active against gram-positive bacteria. It is used alone by the IV route for the treatment of intraabdominal infections caused by *E. coli, Klebsiella pneumoniae, P. aeruginosa, B. fragilis,* and *Peptostreptococcus* spp. It is also used alone intravenously to treat bacterial meningitis caused by *Strep. pneumoniae, Haemophilus influenzae,* and *Neisseria meningitidis.* Vaborbactam is a beta-lactamase inhibitor that protects meropenem from degradation by certain beta lactamases. Vaborbactam is used in combination with meropenem (Vabomere) to treat complicated urinary tract infections, including pyelonephritis caused by *E. coli, K. pneumoniae,* and *Enterobacter cloacae* species in patients at least 18 years of age.

- Ertapenem is a carbapenem antibiotic that has a chemical structure that protects it against dehydropeptidase I, so that cilastatin is not necessary. It has a broad spectrum of activity and is approved to treat infections caused by aerobic and anaerobic gram-positive and gram-negative bacteria causing complicated intraabdominal infections, skin and skin structure infections, community-acquired pneumonia, UTIs (including pyelonephritis), and acute pelvic infections. It is effective against susceptible strains of *S. aureus, S. agalactiae, Strep. pneumoniae, S. pyogenes, E. coli, K. pneumoniae, Moraxella catarrhalis, H. influenzae, Bacteroides* spp., *Clostridium* spp., and *Peptostreptococcus* spp.

- Doripenem is a single agent that has a gram-negative and gram-positive spectrum similar to imipenem and meropenem combined. It is used to treat complicated intraabdominal infections caused by *E. coli, K. pneumoniae, P. aeruginosa, Bacteroides* spp. (*B. caccae, B. fragilis, B. thetaiotaomicron, B. uniformis, B. vulgatus*), *S. intermedius, S. constellatus,* and *Peptostreptococcus micros.* It is also approved for use in complicated UTIs caused by *E. coli* (including cases with concurrent bacteremia), *K. pneumoniae, Proteus mirabilis, P. aeruginosa,* and *Acinetobacter baumannii.*

Therapeutic Outcome

The primary therapeutic outcome expected from carbapenem therapy is elimination of bacterial infection.

❖ Nursing Implications for Carbapenems

◆ Premedication assessment

1. Obtain baseline assessments of presenting symptoms.
2. Record temperature, pulse, respirations, blood pressure, and hydration status.
3. Assess for and record any gastric symptoms before initiating therapy.
4. Assess for any allergies. Ask specifically about penicillin and cephalosporin allergies.
5. Obtain baseline laboratory studies ordered and review results (e.g., CBC with differential, culture and sensitivity).
6. Perform a baseline assessment of the patient's degree of alertness and orientation to name, place, and time before beginning therapy.
7. Ask whether there is a history of seizure activity before initiating therapy.

◆ Availability, dosage, and administration. See Table 45.2.

Hypersensitivity. Although these antibiotics are carbapenems rather than penicillins or cephalosporins, they also contain a beta-lactam nucleus. Cross-hypersensitivity may develop between these classes. Complete a history of hypersensitivity before starting therapy. If an allergic reaction to a carbapenem occurs, discontinue the infusion. Serious reactions may require epinephrine and other emergency measures.

Table 45.2   Carbapenems

GENERIC NAME	BRAND NAME	AVAILABILITY	DOSAGE RANGE
doripenem	—	Injection: 250-, 500-mg vials	IV: 500 mg q8h over 1 hr
ertapenem	Invanz	Injection: 1-g vials	IM, IV: 1 g daily. Infuse IV solution over 30 min for up to 14 days. Limit IM injection to 7 days.
imipenem-cilastatin	Primaxin ⇄ *Do not confuse Primaxin with Premarin.*	Injection: IV: 250-, 500-mg vials	IV: 50 mg/kg/day up to 4 g/day in two to four doses; 125, 250, or 500 mg by IV infusion over 20-30 min. Infuse 750-mg or 1-g dose over 40-60 min. If nausea develops, slow the infusion rate. IM: 500-750 mg q12h, depending on severity of infection. Do not exceed 1500 mg/day.
meropenem	Merrem	Injection: 500-mg, 1-g vials	IV: 1 g IV q8h; infuse over 15-30 min or as a bolus over 3-5 min.
meropenem-vaborbactam	Vabomere	Injection: 2-g vials	IV: 4 g q8h for up to 14 days; infuse over 3 hours.

Admixture compatibilities. *Do not* mix other drugs in the same syringe with carbapenems or infuse together with other drugs. See Drug Interactions later in this section for incompatibilities.

The carbapenems require special care regarding mixing and administration:

- Imipenem-cilastatin should not be mixed with or physically added to other antibiotics, but it may be administered concomitantly with other antibiotics, such as aminoglycosides.
- Meropenem should not be mixed with or physically added to solutions containing other medicines.
- Ertapenem for IV use should be reconstituted with bacteriostatic water or 0.9% sodium chloride (normal saline) for injection. Do not reconstitute or dilute with dextrose solutions.
- Ertapenem for IM use should be reconstituted with 1% lidocaine injection (without epinephrine). Administer the injection within 1 hour of reconstitution.

◆ *Common adverse effects*

Gastrointestinal

Severe diarrhea. Severe diarrhea may develop from using carbapenems. Blood and mucus in the stool may also be present. This may be an indication of drug-induced pseudomembranous colitis and should be reported immediately. Withhold the next dose of antibiotic until the healthcare provider gives approval for administration.

Neurologic

Dizziness. Provide for patient safety during episodes of dizziness; report for further evaluation.

Confusion, seizures. Seizure activity—including myoclonic activity, focal tremors, confusional states, and other seizures—has been reported with the carbapenems. These episodes occur most commonly in patients with histories of previous seizure activity and renal impairment.

Perform a baseline assessment of the patient's degree of alertness and orientation to name, place, and time before initiating therapy. Make regularly scheduled subsequent mental status evaluations, and compare findings. Report alterations in consciousness.

Implement seizure precautions. Make sure that the patient continues with anticonvulsant therapy. If seizures develop, provide for patient safety and then record the exact time of seizure onset and duration of each phase, a description of the specific body parts involved, and any progression in the affected parts. Describe automatic responses during the clonic phase: altered, jerky respirations or frothy salivation, dilated pupils and any eye movements, cyanosis, diaphoresis, or incontinence.

Vascular

Phlebitis. Carefully assess patients for thrombophlebitis. Inspect the IV area frequently when providing care; inspect visually during dressing changes and whenever the IV is changed to a new site. Report redness, warmth, tenderness to touch, and edema in the affected part. Compare the affected limb with the unaffected limb.

◆ *Drug interactions*

Probenecid. Probenecid inhibits the urinary excretion of carbapenems. Do not administer probenecid concurrently.

Valproic acid. Carbapenem antibiotics may produce clinically significant reductions in valproic acid levels, which may lead to a loss of seizure control. If any carbapenem is administered with valproic acid, serum valproic acid levels should be monitored frequently.

Ganciclovir. Concurrent administration of ganciclovir and imipenem-cilastatin has resulted in an increased incidence of seizures. Avoid concurrent use if at all possible.

DRUG CLASS: CEPHALOSPORINS

Actions

The cephalosporins are chemically related to the penicillins and have a similar mechanism of activity. The cephalosporins act by inhibiting cell wall synthesis in bacteria. The cephalosporins may be divided into groups, or "generations," based primarily on antimicrobial activity. The first-generation cephalosporins have effective activity against gram-positive microorganisms (*Staph. aureus, Staph. epidermidis, Strep. pyogenes, Strep. pneumoniae*) and relatively mild activity against gram-negative microorganisms (*E. coli, K. pneumoniae, Proteus mirabilis*). Second-generation cephalosporins have somewhat increased activity against gram-negative bacteria but are much less active than the third-generation agents, which are generally less active than first-generation agents against gram-positive cocci, although they are much more active against penicillinase-producing bacteria. Some of the third-generation cephalosporins also are active against *P. aeruginosa*, a potent gram-negative microorganism. Fourth-generation cephalosporins are broad-spectrum agents with both gram-negative and gram-positive coverage. Ceftaroline, a fifth-generation agent, is the only cephalosporin with activity against MRSA. It is currently approved only to treat susceptible skin infections.

Uses

Cephalosporins may be used with caution as alternatives when patients are allergic to the penicillins unless they are also allergic to the cephalosporins. The cephalosporins are used for certain urinary and respiratory tract infections, abdominal infections, bacteremia, meningitis, and osteomyelitis.

Therapeutic Outcome

The primary therapeutic outcome expected from cephalosporin therapy is elimination of bacterial infection.

❖ Nursing Implications for Cephalosporins

◆ *Premedication assessment*

1. Obtain baseline assessments of presenting symptoms.
2. Record temperature, pulse, respirations, blood pressure, and hydration status.
3. Assess for any allergies, symptoms of renal disease, or bleeding disorders. If present, withhold drug and report findings to the healthcare provider.
4. Obtain baseline laboratory studies ordered and review results (e.g., CBC with differential, culture and sensitivity).

◆ *Availability, dosage, and administration.* See Table 45.3.

◆ *Common adverse effects*

Gastrointestinal

Diarrhea. Cephalosporins cause diarrhea by altering the bacterial flora of the GI tract. The diarrhea is usually not severe enough to warrant discontinuing medication.

Encourage the patient not to discontinue therapy without consulting the healthcare provider. When diarrhea persists, monitor the patient for signs of dehydration.

Hepatotoxicity. Transient elevations of liver function test results (e.g., AST, ALT, alkaline phosphatase) have been reported. Monitor returning laboratory data and report abnormal findings to the healthcare provider.

Immune system (opportunistic infections)

Secondary infections. Oral thrush, genital and anal pruritus, vaginitis, and vaginal discharge may occur with cephalosporin therapy. Report to the healthcare provider promptly because these infections are resistant to the original antibiotic used. Teach the importance of meticulous oral and perineal personal hygiene.

Renal

Nephrotoxicity. Transient elevations of renal test results (e.g., BUN, serum creatinine) have been reported. Renal toxicity, as evidenced by proteinuria, hematuria, casts, decreased creatinine clearance, and decreased urine output, also has been reported. Monitor returning laboratory data and report abnormal findings to the healthcare provider.

Hematologic

Hypoprothrombinemia. Hypoprothrombinemia, a reduction in circulating prothrombin, with and without bleeding, has been reported. This rare occurrence is most frequent in older adult, debilitated, or otherwise compromised patients with borderline vitamin K deficiency. Treatment with broad-spectrum antibiotics eliminates enough GI flora to cause a further reduction in vitamin K synthesis.

Assess the patient for ecchymosis after minimal trauma; prolonged bleeding at an infusion site or from a surgical wound; or the development of petechiae, bleeding gums, or nosebleeds. Notify the healthcare provider of any of the signs of hypoprothrombinemia. The usual treatment is administration of vitamin K.

Electrolyte imbalance. If a patient develops hyperkalemia or hypernatremia, consider the electrolyte content of the antibiotics. Most cephalosporins have a high electrolyte content.

Vascular

Thrombophlebitis. Phlebitis and thrombophlebitis, or inflammation of the vein with a blood clot or thrombus, are recurrent problems associated with IV administration of cephalosporins. Use small IV needles in large veins and alternate infusion sites, if possible, to minimize irritation. Carefully assess patients receiving IV cephalosporins for the development of thrombophlebitis. Inspect the IV infusion area frequently when providing care; inspect during dressing changes and when the infusion is changed to a new site. Always investigate pain at the IV site. Report redness, warmth, tenderness to touch, and edema in the affected part.

◆ *Drug interactions*

Nephrotoxic potential. Patients receiving cephalosporins, aminoglycosides, vancomycin, and loop diuretics

Table 45.3 Cephalosporins

GENERIC NAME	BRAND NAME	GENERATION	AVAILABILITY	ADULT DOSAGE RANGE

cefaclor	Nu-Cefaclor ♣	2	Capsules: 250, 500 mg
			Tablets, extended release (12 hr):
			  500 mg
			Oral suspension: 125, 250,
			  375 mg/5 mL
				PO: 250-500 mg q8h; do not
				  exceed 4 g/day

cefadroxil	–	1	Capsules: 500 mg Tablets: 1000 mg Suspension: 250, 500 mg/5 mL	PO: 1-2 g daily in one or two doses

cefazolin	–	1	Injection: 500-mg and 1-, 2-, 10-,
			  20-, 100-, 300-g vials
				IM, IV: dose depends on
				  organism being treated

cefdinir	–	3	Capsules: 300 mg
			Oral suspension: 125,
			  250 mg/5 mL
				PO: 300 q12h and 600 mg
				  once daily

cefditoren	Spectracef	2	Tablets: 200, 400 mg	PO: 200-400 mg q12h
cefepime	Maxipime	4	Injection: 1-, 2-g vials	IM, IV: 0.5-2 g q8-12h

cefixime	Suprax
	⇄ Do not confuse
	  Suprax with
	  Surfak.
		3	Tablets, chewable: 100, 200 mg
			Capsules: 400 mg
			Suspension: 100, 200,
			  500 mg/5 mL
				PO: 200 mg q12h or 400 mg
				  once daily

cefotaxime	—	3	IV: 500-mg and 1-, 2-, 10-g vials	IV: 1-2 g q4-12h; do not exceed 12 g/day
cefotetan	Cefotan	3	Injection: 1-, 2-, 10-g vials	IM, IV: 1-3 g q12h; do not exceed 6 g/day

cefoxitin	—	2	Injection: 1-, 2-, 10-g vials	IM, IV: 1-2 g q4-6h or 2-3 g
				  q6-8h; do not exceed
				  12 g/day

cefpodoxime	—	3	Tablets: 100, 200 mg Suspension: 50, 100 mg/5 mL	PO: 200 mg q12h for 7-14 days
cefprozil	—	2	Tablets: 250, 500 mg Suspension: 125, 250 mg/5 mL	PO: 250-500 mg q12h for 10 days
ceftaroline	Teflaro	5 (MRSA active)	IV: 400-, 600-mg vials	IV: 600 mg q12h for 5-14 days
ceftazidime	Fortaz, Tazicef	3	Injection: 500-mg and 1-, 2-, 6-g vials	IM, IV: 1-2 g q12h
ceftazidime/ avibactam	Avycaz		Injection: 2 g ceftazidime; 500 mg avibactam	IV: 2.5 mg ceftazidime q8h

ceftibuten	Cedax	3	Capsules: 400 mg
			Suspension: 180 mg/5 mL
				PO: 400 mg once daily 2 hr
				  before or 1 hr after meals
				  for 10 days

ceftolozane/ tazobactam	Zerbaxa		Injection: 1.5 g ceftolozane; 500 mg tazobactam	IV: 1.5 g ceftolozane q8h

ceftriaxone	—	3	Injection: 250-, 500-mg and 1-,
			  2-, 10-, 100-g vials
				IM, IV: 1-2 g once daily; do
				  not exceed 4 g daily

cefuroxime
⇄ Do not confuse
  cefuroxime with
  deferoxamine.
	–	2	Tablets: 250, 500 mg
			IV: 750-mg and 1.5-, 7.5-, 75-,
			  225-g vials
			Suspension: 125, 250 mg/5 mL
				PO: 250-500 mg q12h
				IV: 750 mg-1.5 g q8h

cephalexin	Keflex Daxbia	1	Tablets: 250, 500 mg Capsules: 250, 333, 500, 750 mg Suspension: 125, 250 mg/5 mL	PO: 250-1000 mg q6h or 500 mg q12h

♣ Available in Canada.

concurrently should be assessed for signs of nephrotoxicity. Monitor urinalysis and kidney function tests for abnormal results. Report increasing BUN and creatinine levels, decreasing urine output or decreasing specific gravity (despite amount of fluid intake), casts or protein in the urine, frank blood or smoky-colored urine, or RBCs in excess of 0 to 3 RBCs/HPF (see Table 41.1) on the urinalysis report.

Antacids. Antacids inhibit the absorption of cefaclor, cefdinir, and cefpodoxime. If antacids must be taken, the antibiotic should be taken 2 hours before or after the antacid.

Histamine-2 (H₂) antagonists. Histamine-2 antagonists (e.g., cimetidine, famotidine, nizatidine, ranitidine) inhibit the absorption of cefpodoxime and cefuroxime, decreasing the antibiotic effect. Because of the long duration of action of the H_2 antagonists, it is recommended that they not be administered when these cephalosporins are prescribed.

Iron supplements. Iron supplements and food fortified with iron inhibit the absorption of cefdinir. If iron supplements must be taken, the antibiotic should be taken 2 hours before or after the iron supplement.

Probenecid. Patients receiving probenecid in combination with cephalosporins are more susceptible to toxicity because of the inhibition of excretion of the cephalosporins by probenecid. Monitor closely for adverse effects.

Alcohol. Instruct the patient to avoid alcohol consumption during cefotetan therapy. Patients ingesting alcohol during, and for 24 to 72 hours after, administration of cefotetan will become flushed, tremulous, dyspneic, tachycardic, and hypotensive. Also, tell the patient not to use OTC preparations containing alcohol, such as mouthwash (e.g., Cēpacol, Listerine) or cough preparations.

Oral contraceptives. Cephalosporins may interfere with the contraceptive activity of oral contraceptives. Oral contraceptives should not be discontinued, but counseling regarding use of additional methods of contraception (e.g., condoms and foam) should be planned.

DRUG CLASS: GLYCOPEPTIDES

Actions

Glycopeptides are a class of antibiotics that prevents the synthesis of bacterial cell walls. This site of action is different from the sites of other antibiotics interfering with cell wall synthesis.

Uses

- Dalbavancin is used in the treatment of adult patients with acute bacterial skin and skin structure infections caused by susceptible isolates of the following gram-positive microorganisms: *Staph. aureus* (including methicillin-susceptible and methicillin-resistant strains), *Strep. pyogenes, Streptococcus agalactiae,*
Streptococcus dysgalactiae, Streptococcus anginosus group, and *Enterococcus faecalis* (vancomycin-susceptible strains).

- Oritavancin is used in the treatment of adult patients with acute bacterial skin and skin structure infections caused by susceptible isolates of the following gram-positive microorganisms: *Staph. aureus* (including methicillin-susceptible and methicillin-resistant strains), *Strep. pyogenes, Strep. agalactiae, Strep. dysgalactiae, Strep. anginosus* group, and *Enterococcus faecalis* (vancomycin-susceptible strains).

- Telavancin is used in the treatment of complicated skin and skin structure infections (cSSSIs) caused by susceptible gram-positive organisms including methicillin-susceptible or -resistant *Staph. aureus,* vancomycin-susceptible *Enterococcus faecalis,* and *Strep. pyogenes, Strep. agalactiae,* or *Strep. anginosus* group. It is also used to treat hospital-acquired and ventilator-associated bacterial pneumonia caused by susceptible isolates of *Staph. aureus* when alternative treatments are not appropriate.

- Vancomycin is effective against only gram-positive bacteria such as streptococci, staphylococci, *C. difficile, Listeria monocytogenes,* and *Corynebacterium* that may cause endocarditis, osteomyelitis, meningitis, pneumonia, or septicemia. It may be used orally against staphylococcal enterocolitis and antibiotic-associated pseudomembranous colitis produced by *C. difficile.* Because of potential adverse effects, vancomycin therapy is reserved for patients with potentially life-threatening infections who cannot be treated with less toxic agents such as penicillins or cephalosporins.

Therapeutic Outcome

The primary therapeutic outcome expected from all the glycopeptide therapies is elimination of bacterial infection.

❖ Nursing Implications for Glycopeptides
◆ Premedication assessment
1. Obtain baseline assessments of presenting symptoms.
2. Record temperature, pulse, respirations, blood pressure, and hydration status.
3. Assess for normal renal function and hearing before initiating therapy.
4. Assess for any allergies.
5. Obtain baseline laboratory studies ordered and review results (e.g., CBC with differential, culture and sensitivity).

◆ Availability, dosage, and administration. See Table 45.4.
Serum levels. Serum trough levels of vancomycin should be routinely ordered to minimize adverse effects. Notify the healthcare provider of any abnormal serum levels reported so that dosage adjustments may be made. Consult laboratory reports for normal range. Serum levels are not necessary for telavancin, dalbavancin, or oritavancin.

Table 45.4   Glycopeptides

GENERIC NAME	BRAND NAME	AVAILABILITY	DOSAGE RANGE
dalbavancin	Dalvance	IV: 500 mg/vial	1500 mg as a single dose *or* 1000 mg as a single dose initially, followed by 500 mg as a single dose 1 wk later
oritavancin	Orbactiv	IV: 400 mg/vial	1200 mg as a single dose
telavancin	Vibativ	IV: 750 mg/vial	10 mg/kg q24h
vancomycin ⇄ *Do not confuse vancomycin with vecuronium, vibramycin, azithromycin, or gentamicin.*	Vancocin	PO: 125- and 250-mg capsules; 25-, 50-mg/mL oral solution IV: 0.5-, 0.75-, 1-, 5-, and 10-g powder/vial	Adult: PO: 500-2000 mg daily in divided doses q6h (not appropriate for systemic infections due to low absorption) IV: 15 mg/kg q12h is a usual starting dose in most nonobese patients with normal renal function or 15-20 mg/kg/dose q8-12h with normal renal function Pediatric: PO: 40 mg/kg/day in three or four divided doses for 7-10 days (maximum: 2000 mg/day) IV: 40 mg/kg/day in three or four divided doses for 7-10 days (maximum: 2000 mg/day)

⚠ Medication Safety Alert

Rapid IV administration of vancomycin, telavancin, or dalbavancin may result in a severe hypotensive episode. Patients develop a red neck syndrome, or red man syndrome, characteristic of vancomycin. It is manifested by a sudden and profound hypotension, with or without a maculopapular rash over the face, neck, upper chest, and extremities. The rash generally resolves within a few hours after terminating the infusion. In rare cases, the administration of fluids, antihistamines, or corticosteroids may be necessary. For vancomycin and telavancin, administer the solution over at least 60 minutes. For dalbavancin, administer over 30 minutes. Monitor blood pressure during infusion.

Oritavancin should be infused over 3 hours. If an infusion-related reaction (pruritus, urticaria, flushing) occurs, consider slowing or interrupting the infusion.

◆ Serious adverse effects

Sensory

Ototoxicity. Vancomycin may cause ototoxicity. This may initially be manifested by dizziness, tinnitus, high tone hearing loss, and progressive overall hearing loss. Older patients are particularly susceptible to deafness. Assess patients for difficulty in walking unaided, and assess the level of hearing daily. Intentionally speak to patients softly; note if they are aware that anything was said. Take particular notice of the patient who repeatedly asks, "What did you say?" or who starts talking more loudly or progressively increases the volume on the television or radio.

Urinary

Nephrotoxicity. Monitor urinalysis and kidney function tests for abnormal results. Report increasing BUN and creatinine levels, decreasing urine output or decreasing urine specific gravity (despite amount of fluid intake), casts or protein in the urine, frank blood or smoky-colored urine, or RBCs in excess of 0 to 3 RBCs/HPF (see Table 41.1) on the urinalysis report.

Cardiovascular

Q–T interval prolongation. Avoid telavancin in patients with congenital long QT syndrome, known prolongation of the Q–Tc interval, uncompensated heart failure, or severe left ventricular hypertrophy.

Coagulation. Although telavancin and oritavancin do not interfere with coagulation, they can interfere with certain tests used to monitor coagulation, such as prothrombin time or INR, activated partial thromboplastin time, and activated clotting time.

Hepatic effects. ALT elevations have been reported with dalbavancin.

Immune system (opportunistic infections)

Secondary infections. Oral thrush, genital and anal pruritus, vaginitis, and vaginal discharge may occur. Report promptly because these infections are resistant to the original antibiotic used. Teach the importance of meticulous oral and perineal personal hygiene.

◆ Drug interactions

Nephrotoxicity, ototoxicity. Concurrent and sequential use of vancomycin with other ototoxic or nephrotoxic agents such as the aminoglycosides (e.g., gentamicin, tobramycin, amikacin), cisplatin, furosemide, torsemide, and bumetanide requires careful monitoring.

Neuromuscular blockade. Vancomycin in combination with skeletal muscle relaxants may produce respiratory depression. Check the anesthesia record in postoperative patients to determine if skeletal muscle relaxants such as succinylcholine or pancuronium bromide were administered during surgery. The nurse should monitor and assess the respiratory rate, depth of respirations, and chest movement and report apnea immediately. Because these effects may be seen for up to 48 hours after administration of skeletal muscle relaxants, continue monitoring respirations, pulse, and blood pressure beyond the usual postsurgical vital signs routine.

Heparin. Avoid the use of IV heparin with telavancin and oritavancin. Both may artificially increase the results of laboratory tests commonly used to monitor IV heparin effectiveness (e.g., activated partial thromboplastin time).

DRUG CLASS: GLYCYLCYCLINES

tigecycline (tī-gĕ-SĪ-klēn)
Tygacil (TĪG-ă-sĭl)

Actions

Tigecycline is the first of the antimicrobial agents known as the glycylcyclines. Tigecycline is chemically related to the tetracyclines but is not susceptible to the mechanisms that cause resistance to the tetracyclines. It acts by binding to the 30S ribosome, preventing protein synthesis. It is a bacteriostatic antibiotic effective against a broad spectrum of gram-positive, gram-negative, and anaerobic microorganisms. It is not effective against viruses.

Uses

Tigecycline is used to treat cSSSIs caused by *E. coli, Enterococcus faecalis, Staph. aureus* (methicillin-susceptible and methicillin-resistant isolates), *Strep. agalactiae,* and *B. fragilis.* It may also be used to treat complicated intraabdominal infections caused by *Citrobacter freundii, Enterobacter cloacae, E. coli, Klebsiella oxytoca, K. pneumoniae, Enterococcus faecalis, Staph. aureus* (methicillin-susceptible isolates only), *B. fragilis, B. vulgatus, Clostridium perfringens,* and *Peptostreptococcus micros.* In an effort to slow the development of strains of bacteria resistant to tigecycline, it should be used only when the pathogen is resistant to other available antibiotics.

Tigecycline is not approved for use in people younger than 18 years. As with tetracyclines, tigecycline administered during the ages of tooth development (the last half of pregnancy through 8 years of age) may cause enamel hypoplasia and permanent yellow, gray, or brown staining of the teeth.

Therapeutic Outcome

The primary therapeutic outcome expected from tigecycline therapy is elimination of bacterial infection.

❖ **Nursing Implications for Tigecycline**
◆ *Premedication assessment*
 1. Obtain baseline assessments of presenting symptoms.
 2. Record temperature, pulse, respirations, blood pressure, and hydration status.
 3. Assess for and record any gastric symptoms before initiating therapy.
 4. Assess for any allergies.
 5. Obtain baseline laboratory studies ordered and review results (e.g., CBC with differential, culture and sensitivity).

◆ *Availability.* *IV:* 50-mg vials.

◆ *Dosage and administration.* *IV:* Initial: 100 mg followed by 50 mg every 12 hours. Administer by IV infusion over 30 to 60 minutes. Therapy is continued for 5 to 14 days, depending on the severity and site of the infection and the patient's clinical progress.

◆ *Common adverse effects*
 Gastrointestinal
 Gastric irritation. The most common adverse effects of tigecycline therapy are nausea and vomiting (30% and 20%, respectively). These adverse effects are usually mild to moderate in the first 1 to 2 days of therapy and tend to resolve with continued therapy.
 Severe diarrhea. Rarely, severe diarrhea may develop from the use of tigecycline. Report diarrhea of five or more stools daily to the healthcare provider. This may be an indication of drug-induced pseudomembranous colitis. Blood or mucus in the stool also should be reported to the healthcare provider. **Warn patients not to treat diarrhea themselves when taking this drug.** The use of diphenoxylate, loperamide, or paregoric may prolong or worsen the condition.
 Integumentary
 Photosensitivity. Photosensitivity resulting in an exaggerated sunburn after short exposure has been reported. The patient should be cautioned to avoid exposure to sunlight and ultraviolet light. Suggest wearing long-sleeved clothing, a hat, and sunglasses when outdoors. Discourage the use of tanning lamps. Consult the healthcare provider about the advisability of discontinuing therapy.

◆ *Drug interactions*
 Warfarin. Tigecycline may enhance the anticoagulant effects of warfarin. Observe for petechiae; ecchymoses; nosebleeds; bleeding gums; dark, tarry stools; and bright red or coffee-ground emesis. Monitor the INR and reduce the dosage of warfarin if necessary.
 Oral contraceptives. Tigecycline may interfere with the activity of oral contraceptives. Oral contraceptives should not be discontinued, but counseling regarding use of additional methods of contraception (e.g., condoms and foam) should be planned.

DRUG CLASS: MACROLIDES

Actions

The macrolide antibiotics act by inhibiting protein synthesis in susceptible bacteria. They are bacteriostatic and bacteriocidal, depending on the organism and drug concentration present. Erythromycin is effective against gram-positive microorganisms and gram-negative cocci. Azithromycin is less active against gram-positive organisms than erythromycin but has greater activity against gram-negative organisms that are resistant to erythromycin. Clarithromycin has a spectrum of activity similar to that of erythromycin but has considerably greater potency.

Uses

The macrolides are used for respiratory, GI tract, skin, and soft tissue infections and for STIs, especially when penicillins, cephalosporins, and tetracyclines cannot be used. Fidaxomicin is a macrolide antibiotic used to treat *C. difficile*–associated diarrhea. It should be used only for *C. difficile* infections.

Therapeutic Outcome

The primary therapeutic outcome expected from macrolide therapy is elimination of bacterial infection.

❖ Nursing Implications for Macrolides
◆ Premedication assessment
1. Obtain baseline assessments of presenting symptoms.
2. Record temperature, pulse, respirations, blood pressure, and hydration status.
3. Assess for and record any gastric symptoms before initiating therapy.
4. Assess for any allergies.
5. Obtain baseline laboratory studies ordered and review results (e.g., CBC with differential, culture and sensitivity).

◆ Availability, dosage, and administration. See Table 45.5.
PO: Azithromycin and erythromycin should be administered at least 1 hour before or 2 hours after meals. Clarithromycin may be taken without regard to meals.

IM: Because of pain on injection and the possibility of sterile abscess formation, IM administration of erythromycin is generally not recommended for multiple-dose therapy.

IV: Dilute the dosage of erythromycin in 100 to 250 mL of saline solution or 5% dextrose and administer over 20 to 60 minutes. Thrombophlebitis after IV infusion is a relatively common adverse effect.

◆ Common adverse effects
Gastrointestinal
Gastric irritation. The most common adverse effects of oral macrolide therapy are diarrhea, nausea and vomiting, and abnormal taste. These adverse effects are usually mild and tend to resolve with continued therapy. Encourage the patient not to discontinue therapy without first consulting the healthcare provider.

◆ Serious adverse effects
Gastrointestinal
Severe diarrhea. Severe diarrhea may develop from the use of erythromycin. Report diarrhea of five or more stools daily to the healthcare provider. This may be an indication of drug-induced pseudomembranous colitis. Blood or mucus in the stool should also be reported to the healthcare provider. **Warn patients not to treat diarrhea themselves when taking this drug.** The use of diphenoxylate, loperamide, or paregoric may prolong or worsen the condition.

Vascular
Thrombophlebitis. Carefully assess patients receiving IV erythromycin for thrombophlebitis. Inspect the IV infusion area frequently when providing care; inspect during dressing changes and when the infusion is changed to a new site. Always investigate pain at the IV site. Report redness, warmth, tenderness to touch, and edema in the affected part.

◆ Drug interactions
Toxicity caused by macrolides. Macrolide antibiotics may inhibit the metabolism of several drugs, causing accumulation and potential toxicity. These drugs are alfentanil, benzodiazepines (e.g., alprazolam, diazepam, midazolam, triazolam), buspirone, carbamazepine, cyclosporine, digoxin, felodipine, hydroxymethylglutaryl coenzyme A (HMG-CoA) reductase inhibitors (e.g., atorvastatin, lovastatin, simvastatin), omeprazole, tacrolimus, theophyllines, vinblastine, warfarin, and other drugs metabolized by the cytochrome P450 (CYP) CYP3A enzyme system. Read individual drug monographs for monitoring parameters of toxicity from these agents.

Pimozide. Coadministration of a macrolide antibiotic with pimozide is contraindicated. Death has resulted from this combination of drug therapy.

Rifampin, rifabutin. The coadministration of a macrolide antibiotic with rifampin or rifabutin may cause a reduction in antimicrobial effect while increasing the frequency of GI adverse effects.

Oral contraceptives. Macrolides may interfere with the activity of oral contraceptives. Oral contraceptives should not be discontinued, but counseling regarding use of additional methods of contraception (e.g., condoms and foam) should be planned.

DRUG CLASS: OXAZOLIDINONES

linezolid (lĭn-ā-ZŌ-lĭd)
  Zyvox (ZĪ-vŏks)
  ⇄ *Do not confuse Zyvox with Zosyn or Zovirax.*
tedizolid (tĕd-ī-ZŌ-lĭd)
  Sivextro (siv-EX-troh)

Actions

Linezolid and tedizolid are both *oxazolidinones*. They act by inhibiting protein synthesis in bacterial cells. They are bactericidal in certain strains of bacteria and

Table 45.5 Macrolides

GENERIC NAME	BRAND NAME	AVAILABILITY	ADULT DOSAGE RANGE
azithromycin	Zithromax	Tablets: 250, 500, 600 mg Packets: 1 g Suspension: 100, 200 mg/5 mL Injection: 500 mg in 10-mL vial	PO: 500 mg as a single dose on day 1, followed by 250 mg once daily on days 2-5 for a total dose of 1.5 g IV: 500 mg daily. Dilute powder to a concentration of 1-2 mg/mL; infuse 1-mg/mL concentration over 3 hr or 2-mg/mL concentration over 1 hr *Do not* administer as an IV bolus or IM
clarithromycin	—	Tablets: 250, 500 mg Suspension: 125, 250 mg/5 mL Tablets, extended release (24 hr): 500, mg	PO: 250-500 mg q12h for 7-14 days
erythromycin	Erythrocin Eryc ♣ many others	Tablets: 250, 400, 500 mg Tablets, delayed release: 250, 333, 500 mg Capsules, delayed release particles: 250, 333 mg Suspension: 200, 400 mg/5 mL IV: 500-mg vials for reconstitution	PO: 250 mg four times daily for 10-14 days IV: 15-20 mg/kg/24 hr; up to 4 g/24 hr
fidaxomicin	Dificid	Tablets: 200 mg	200 mg twice daily for 10 days

♣ Available in Canada.

bacteriostatic in others. Unrelated to antibacterial activity, they are reversible monoamine oxidase inhibitors, inhibiting the action of monoamine oxidase type A, an enzyme responsible for metabolizing serotonin in the brain.

Uses

Linezolid is used in the treatment of serious or life-threatening infections caused by gram-positive microorganisms. It is approved for use with VRE bacteria and uncomplicated and cSSSIs caused by methicillin-susceptible and methicillin-resistant *Staph. aureus, Strep. pyogenes,* or *Strep. agalactiae.* It may also be used to treat community-acquired pneumonia caused by penicillin-susceptible *Strep. pneumoniae.* It is not indicated for treatment of gram-negative infections. Other appropriate antibiotics to provide gram-negative coverage should be used concurrently. Linezolid should be reserved for those cases in which other antibiotics such as vancomycin are ineffective, so that resistant strains of bacteria do not rapidly develop.

Tedizolid is used in treatment of adult patients with acute bacterial skin and skin structure infections caused by susceptible isolates of the following gram-positive microorganisms: methicillin-resistant and methicillin-susceptible *Staph. aureus, Strep. pyogenes, Strep. agalactiae, Strep. anginosus* group, and *Enterococcus faecalis.*

Therapeutic Outcome

The primary therapeutic outcome expected from linezolid and tedizolid therapy is elimination of bacterial infection.

❖ Nursing Implications for Linezolid and Tedizolid
◆ Premedication assessment
1. Obtain baseline assessments of presenting symptoms.
2. Record temperature, pulse, respirations, blood pressure, and hydration status.

3. Assess for and record any gastric and visual symptoms before initiating therapy.
4. Assess for any allergies.
5. Obtain baseline laboratory studies ordered and review results (e.g., CBC with differential, platelets, blood glucose, electrolytes, culture and sensitivity).

◆ **Availability.** Linezolid.
PO: 600-mg tablets; 100-mg/5-mL oral suspension in 150 mL. *IV:* 200- and 600-mg prefilled containers at 2 mg/mL.
Tedizolid. *PO:* 200-mg tablets; *IV:* 200 mg/vial.

◆ **Dosage and administration.** Linezolid.
Adults:

TYPE OF INFECTION	DOSE AND ROUTE OF ADMINISTRATION	DURATION (DAYS)
Skin (uncomplicated)	400 mg PO q12h	10-14
Skin (complicated)	600 mg PO or IV q12h	10-14
Community-acquired pneumonia	600 mg PO or IV q12h	10-14
Methicillin-resistant staphylococcal infections (e.g., MRSA)	600 mg PO or IV q12h	Determined clinically
Vancomycin-resistant infections	600 mg PO or IV q12h	14-28
Hospital-acquired pneumonia	600 mg PO or IV q12h	10-14

IV: Infuse the dose over 30 to 120 minutes. Do not administer concurrently with other medicines. If the same IV line is used for sequential infusion of other medicines, flush the line before and after infusion of linezolid with 5% dextrose, normal saline, or lactated Ringer's solution. Keep the linezolid infusion in its wrapper until ready for administration. Linezolid may exhibit a yellow color that may intensify over time but without a loss of potency.

No dosage adjustment is necessary when switching from IV to oral administration using the tablet or oral suspension dosage form.

Tedizolid. **Adults:** *Acute bacterial skin and skin structure infections: PO, IV:* 200 mg once daily for 6 days.

IV: Infuse the dose over 1 hour. If the same intravenous line is to be used for sequential infusion of other drugs or solutions, the line should be flushed with normal saline before and after tedizolid infusion.

◆ *Common adverse effects*
Gastrointestinal
Gastric irritation. The most common adverse effects of both agents are nausea and vomiting (9% and 11%, respectively). These adverse effects are usually mild and moderate in the first few days of therapy and tend to resolve with continued therapy.
Neurologic
Headaches. Headaches were reported in 1% to 11% of patients taking both agents. Headaches were not severe enough to discontinue therapy and tended to resolve with continued therapy.

◆ *Serious adverse effects*
Gastrointestinal
Severe diarrhea. Rarely, severe diarrhea may develop from the use of both agents. Report diarrhea of five or more stools daily to the healthcare provider. This may be an indication of drug-induced pseudomembranous colitis. Blood or mucus in the stool should also be reported to the healthcare provider. **Warn patients not to treat diarrhea themselves when taking this drug.** The use of diphenoxylate, loperamide, or paregoric may prolong or worsen the condition.
Hematologic
Bone marrow suppression. Serious and possibly fatal bone marrow suppression may occur after therapy is initiated with both agents. Early signs include sore throat, fatigue, elevated temperature, and small petechial hemorrhages and bruises on the skin. If patients describe any of these symptoms, report them to the healthcare provider immediately. Routine laboratory studies (RBC and white blood cell counts, differential counts, platelets) are scheduled for patients taking linezolid for 14 days or longer. Stress the importance of returning for this laboratory work. Monitor for the development of sore throat, fever, purpura, jaundice, or excessive or progressive weakness.
Immune system (opportunistic infections)
Secondary infections. Oral thrush, genital and anal pruritus, vaginitis, and vaginal discharge may occur. Report to the healthcare provider promptly because these infections are resistant to the original antibiotic used. Teach the importance of meticulous oral and perineal hygiene.
Metabolic
Lactic acidosis. Lactic acidosis has been reported in conjunction with linezolid therapy. Patients who develop recurrent nausea or vomiting, unexplained acidosis, or a low bicarbonate level should be reported to the healthcare provider as soon as possible.
Neurologic
Seizures. Seizures have been reported in patients receiving both agents. Patients should be monitored for the development of seizures, particularly those with a history of seizure activity or those patients whose clinical condition (e.g., hypoxia) may make them more susceptible to seizures.

Visual neuropathy. Changes in vision from blurred vision to loss of vision have been reported with both agents. Patients should be asked to report, and should be monitored for, changes in visual acuity, color vision, or visual field and blurred vision. These symptoms should be reported to the healthcare provider for further evaluation.

◆ *Drug interactions*
Monoamine oxidase inhibitors. Both agents inhibit monoamine oxidase A and should not be used in patients taking other monoamine oxidase inhibitors (e.g., phenelzine, isocarboxazid, tranylcypromine, meperidine, selegiline, rasagiline, tramadol, methadone) or within 2 weeks of taking such products. Although not reported with either agent, fatal drug interactions have been reported between monoamine oxidase inhibitors and the agents listed here.

Adrenergic agents. Both agents are monoamine oxidase inhibitors that will reduce the metabolism of adrenergic agents (e.g., dopamine, epinephrine, norepinephrine, ephedrine, pseudoephedrine, phenylpropanolamine), potentially resulting in tachycardia and hypertension. Initial doses of the adrenergic agents should be reduced to see how the patient responds before using normal doses.

Serotonergic agents. As monoamine oxidase A inhibitors, both agents have the potential to interact with serotonergic agents (e.g., fluoxetine, paroxetine, sertraline; tricyclic antidepressants; buspirone; triptans) to induce a serotonin syndrome. Patients developing signs and symptoms of serotonin syndrome, such as hyperreflexia (twitching) and incoordination, fever, excessive sweating, shivering or shaking, diarrhea, and confusion, should be reported to the healthcare provider for further evaluation.

DRUG CLASS: PENICILLINS

Actions

Penicillins were the first true antibiotics to be grown and used against pathogenic bacteria in humans. They currently remain one of the most widely used classes of antibiotics.

The penicillins act by interfering with the synthesis of bacterial cell walls. The resulting cell wall is weakened because of defective structure, and the bacteria are subsequently destroyed by osmotic lysis. The penicillins are most effective against bacteria that multiply rapidly. They do not hinder growth of human cells because human cells have protective membranes but no cell wall.

Many bacteria that are initially sensitive to penicillins develop a protective mechanism and become resistant to penicillin therapy. These bacteria produce the enzyme penicillinase (beta-lactamase), which can destroy the antibacterial activity of most penicillins. Penicillinase inactivates the penicillin antibiotics by splitting open the beta-lactam ring of the penicillin molecule. Researchers have developed two mechanisms to prevent this inactivation. The first is to modify the penicillin molecule to "protect" the ring structure while retaining antimicrobial activity. This mechanism culminated in the development of the penicillinase-resistant penicillins (e.g., nafcillin, oxacillin, dicloxacillin). The second method is to add another chemical with a similar structure that will more readily bond to the penicillinase enzymes than the penicillin, leaving the free penicillin to inhibit cell wall synthesis. Potassium clavulanate is now added to amoxicillin (Augmentin) to bond to penicillinases that would normally destroy this antibiotic. Sulbactam has been added to ampicillin (Unasyn) and tazobactam to piperacillin (Zosyn) for similar reasons.

Uses

Penicillins are used to treat middle ear infections (otitis media), pneumonia, meningitis, UTIs, and syphilis, and as a prophylactic antibiotic before surgery or dental procedures for patients with histories of rheumatic fever.

Therapeutic Outcome

The primary therapeutic outcome expected from penicillin therapy is elimination of bacterial infection.

❖ Nursing Implications for Penicillins

◆ Premedication assessment

1. Obtain baseline assessments of presenting symptoms.
2. Record temperature, pulse, respirations, blood pressure, and hydration status.
3. Assess for and record any allergies, symptoms of diarrhea, and abnormal liver or renal function test results. If present, withhold drug and report findings to the healthcare provider.
4. Obtain baseline laboratory studies ordered and review results (e.g., CBC with differential, culture and sensitivity).

◆ *Availability, dosage, and administration.* See Table 45.6.

Admixture compatibilities. *Do not* mix with other drugs in the same syringe with penicillins or infuse with other drugs. See the Drug Interactions later in this section for incompatibilities.

◆ *Common adverse effects*
Gastrointestinal

Diarrhea. Penicillins cause diarrhea by altering the bacterial flora of the GI tract. The diarrhea is usually not severe enough to warrant discontinuation. Encourage the patient not to discontinue therapy without first consulting the healthcare provider. If diarrhea persists, monitor the patient for signs of dehydration.

◆ *Severe adverse effects*
Gastrointestinal

Hepatotoxicity. Transient elevations of liver function test results (e.g., AST, ALT, alkaline phosphatase levels) have been reported. Monitor returning laboratory data and report abnormal findings to the healthcare provider.
Renal

Nephrotoxicity. Transient elevations of renal test results (e.g., BUN, serum creatinine levels) have been reported. Renal toxicity, as evidenced by proteinuria, hematuria, casts, decreased creatinine clearance, and decreased urine output, also has been reported. Monitor returning laboratory data and report abnormal findings to the healthcare provider.
Hematologic

Electrolyte imbalance. The electrolyte content of the antibiotics may cause hyperkalemia or hypernatremia. Some of the penicillins (e.g., penicillin G intravenously, piperacillin, ticarcillin) have a high electrolyte content.
Vascular

Thrombophlebitis. Carefully assess patients receiving IV penicillins for the development of thrombophlebitis. Inspect the IV infusion area frequently when providing care; inspect during dressing changes and when the infusion is changed to a new site. Always investigate pain at the IV site. Report redness, warmth, tenderness to touch, and edema in the affected part.

◆ *Drug interactions*
Probenecid. Patients receiving probenecid in combination with penicillins are more susceptible to toxicity because probenecid inhibits renal excretion of the penicillins. Monitor closely for adverse effects.

This combination may be used advantageously when treating infections in which high serum levels of penicillin are required.

Ampicillin, amoxicillin, and allopurinol. When ampicillin or amoxicillin is used concurrently with allopurinol, there is a higher incidence of a skin rash. Do not label the patient as allergic to penicillins until further skin testing has verified that there is a true hypersensitivity to penicillins.

Antacids. Excessive use of antacids may diminish the absorption of oral penicillins.

Oral contraceptives. Penicillins may interfere with the activity of oral contraceptives. Oral contraceptives should not be discontinued, but counseling regarding use of additional methods of contraception (e.g., condoms and foam) should be planned.

Table 45.6 Penicillins

GENERIC NAME	BRAND NAME	AVAILABILITY	ADULT DOSAGE RANGE
amoxicillin	—	Tablets: 500, 875 mg Tablets, extended release (24 hr): 775 mg Tablets, chewable: 125, 250 mg Capsules: 250, 500 mg Suspension: 125, 200, 250, 400 mg/5 mL	PO: 250-875 mg q8-12h
ampicillin	—	Capsules: 500 mg Suspension: 125, 250 mg/5 mL Injection: 0.125-, 0.25-, 0.5-, 1-, 2-, 10-g vials	IM, IV: 0.5-1 g q4-6h PO: 250-500 mg q6h
dicloxacillin ⇄ *Do not confuse dicloxacillin with doxycycline.*	—	Capsules: 250, 500 mg	PO: 250-500 mg q6h
nafcillin	—	IV: 1-, 2-, 10-g powder; 1-, 2-g premixed containers	IV: 500-1000 mg q4h
oxacillin	—	Injection: 1-, 2-, 10-g vials	IM, IV: 0.5-1 g q4-6h
penicillin G, potassium or sodium	Pfizerpen-G	Injection: vials of 0.2, 0.4, 0.6, 5, 20 million units	IM, IV: 600,000 to 30 million units daily
penicillin V potassium	—	Tablets: 250, 500 mg Suspension: 125, 250 mg/5 mL	PO: 125-500 mg q6h
Combination Products			
amoxicillin and potassium clavulanate (co-amoxiclav)	Augmentin Clavulin ✚	Tablets, chewable: 200, 400 mg Tablets: 250, 500, 875 mg Tablets, extended release (12 hr): 1000 mg Suspension: 125, 250, 400, 600 mg/5 mL	PO: 250 mg q8h or 500-875 mg q12h Extended release: 2000 mg q12h Extra-strength suspension: 600 mg q12h
ampicillin and sulbactam sodium	Unasyn	Injection: 1.5-, 3-, 15-g bottles and vials	IM, IV: 1.5-3 g q6h
piperacillin and tazobactam	Zosyn	IV: 2.25-, 3.375-, 4.5-, 13.5-, 40.5-g vials	3.375-4.5 g q6h; Maximum dose: 18 g/day

✚ Available in Canada.

DRUG CLASS: QUINOLONES

Actions

Quinolone antibiotics are an important class of therapeutic agents. The subclass known as the fluoroquinolones is effective against a wide range of gram-positive and gram-negative bacteria, including some anaerobes. The fluoroquinolones act by inhibiting the activity of DNA gyrase, an enzyme essential for the replication of bacterial DNA.

Uses

- Ciprofloxacin was the first well-tolerated, broad-spectrum oral antibiotic in the quinolone series. It is used for the treatment of UTIs, infectious diarrhea, and chronic bacterial prostatitis caused by *E. coli* or *Proteus mirabilis*. Although ciprofloxacin is indicated in adult patients for treatment of lower respiratory tract infections caused by *E. coli, K. pneumoniae, Proteus mirabilis, Pseudomonas aeruginosa, Haemophilus influenzae, Haemophilus parainfluenzae,* or *Strep. pneumoniae*, it is not the first choice in the treatment of pneumonia secondary to *Strep. pneumoniae*. Because

fluoroquinolones have been associated with serious adverse reactions, reserve fluoroquinolones for treatment of uncomplicated UTIs and acute exacerbations of chronic bronchitis in patients who have no alternative treatment options.

- Delafloxacin is specifically indicated in adults with acute bacterial skin and skin structure infections caused by certain gram-positive and gram-negative pathogens, including MRSA. It is the only fluoroquinolone active against MRSA.
- Gemifloxacin is similar in spectrum of activity and use to levofloxacin and moxifloxacin. It also has an advantage of once-daily oral dosing.
- Levofloxacin has broad-spectrum activity against gram-negative, gram-positive, and anaerobic bacteria. It is used to treat maxillary sinusitis, acute bacterial exacerbations of chronic bronchitis, community-acquired pneumonia, skin and soft tissue infections, chronic bacterial prostatitis, UTIs, acute pyelonephritis, and inhalational anthrax. It has an advantage of once-daily oral dosing. Levofloxacin should be used with caution in older patients who may be susceptible to prolongation of the Q–T interval and

the development of potentially life-threatening dysrhythmias. Levofloxacin is contraindicated in patients with hypokalemia or those receiving amiodarone, sotalol, and other antiarrhythmic agents.

- Moxifloxacin is active against gram-positive microorganisms such as *Strep. pneumoniae* and *Staph. aureus*, gram-negative organisms such as *H. influenzae*, and atypical causes of pneumonia such as *Chlamydia pneumoniae* and *Mycoplasma pneumoniae*. It is approved for use in patients with acute bacterial sinusitis, acute bacterial exacerbation of chronic bronchitis, and community-acquired pneumonia caused by susceptible organisms. Moxifloxacin should be used with caution in older patients who may be susceptible to prolongation of the Q–T interval and the development of potentially life-threatening dysrhythmias. Moxifloxacin is contraindicated in patients with hypokalemia or those receiving amiodarone, sotalol, or other antiarrhythmic agents.
- Ofloxacin has broad-spectrum activity against gram-negative, gram-positive, and anaerobic bacteria. It differs from ciprofloxacin in that it has greater activity against STIs such as *Chlamydia trachomatis* and genital ureaplasma. Ofloxacin is also less susceptible to drug interactions than are other fluoroquinolones. Ofloxacin is used to treat UTIs, prostatitis, skin infections (e.g., cellulitis and impetigo), lower respiratory pneumonia, and STIs other than syphilis and gonorrhea.

Therapeutic Outcome

The primary therapeutic outcome expected from quinolone therapy is elimination of bacterial infection.

❖ Nursing Implications for Quinolones

◆ Premedication assessment

1. Obtain baseline assessments of presenting symptoms.
2. Record temperature, pulse, respirations, blood pressure, and hydration status.
3. Assess for and record any gastric symptoms before initiation of therapy.
4. Assess for any allergies.
5. Obtain baseline laboratory studies ordered and review results (e.g., CBC with differential, culture and sensitivity).
6. Ensure that the patient is not pregnant.
7. Warn patients of possible phototoxicity (see Serious Adverse Effects later in this section).

◆ Availability, dosage, and administration. See Table 45.7.
Children and older adults, patients taking corticosteroids, transplant patients. Fluoroquinolones should not be prescribed for patients younger than 18 years. Use in pediatric patients has resulted in an increased incidence of musculoskeletal disorders such as arthralgia, tendinopathy, and gait abnormality. This risk is further increased in older patients (usually older than 60 years of age), in patients taking corticosteroids (e.g.,

prednisone, dexamethasone), and in patients with organ transplants.

Pregnant women. Quinolone therapy is not recommended during pregnancy unless the benefit of therapy outweighs the risk. No studies have been completed in human patients, but animal studies have demonstrated various teratogenic effects.

◆ Common adverse effects
Gastrointestinal
Nausea, vomiting, diarrhea, abdominal discomfort. These adverse effects are usually mild and tend to resolve with continued therapy. Encourage the patient not to discontinue therapy without first consulting the healthcare provider. If the patient becomes debilitated, contact the healthcare provider.

Neurologic
Dizziness, lightheadedness. Although uncommon, ciprofloxacin may cause these disturbances. They tend to be self-limiting, and therapy should not be discontinued until the patient consults the healthcare provider. Caution the patient against driving or performing hazardous tasks until adjusted to the effects of the medication.

◆ Serious adverse effects
Metabolic
Hypoglycemia. Fluoroquinolones have been associated with the development of serious, and sometimes fatal, hypoglycemia. These events have occurred most often in elderly patients with diabetes but have also been reported in patients without a prior history of diabetes. Prompt identification and treatment of hypoglycemia is essential. Individual quinolones may differ in their potential to cause this effect.

Integumentary
Phototoxicity. Phototoxic reactions have been reported in patients treated with fluoroquinolones. Exposure to direct and indirect sunlight and the use of sun lamps should be avoided. These reactions have occurred with and without the use of sunblocks and sunscreens and with single doses of fluoroquinolones. The patient should not take additional doses and should contact the healthcare provider if a sensation of skin burning, redness, swelling, blisters, rash, itching, or dermatitis develops. Suggest wearing long-sleeved clothing, a hat, and sunglasses when exposed to sunlight.

Rash. Report a rash or pruritus immediately and withhold additional doses pending approval by the healthcare provider.

Gastrointestinal
Hepatotoxicity. Transient elevations of liver function test results (e.g., AST, ALT, alkaline phosphatase levels) have been reported. Monitor returning laboratory data and report abnormal findings to the healthcare provider.

Renal
Nephrotoxicity. Transient elevations of renal test results (e.g., BUN, serum creatinine levels) have been reported.

Table 45.7 Fluoroquinolones

GENERIC NAME	BRAND NAME	AVAILABILITY	DOSAGE RANGE
ciprofloxacin ⇄ *Do not confuse ciprofloxacin with cephalexin.*	Cipro	Tablets: 100, 250, 500, 750 mg Tablets, extended release (24 hr): 500, 1000 mg Suspension: 250, 500 mg/5 mL Injection: 200-, 400-mg vials	PO: 0.2-1.5 g daily in two divided doses 2 hr after meals IV: 400-800 mg daily in two divided doses q12h
delafloxacin	Baxdela	Injection: 300-mg vial Tablets: 450 mg	IV: 300 mg; infuse over 60 min q12h PO: 450 mg q12h
gemifloxacin	Factive	Tablets: 320 mg	PO: 320 mg once daily; may be taken with or without food
levofloxacin		Tablets: 250, 500, 750 mg Solution: 25 mg/mL Injection: 250-, 500-, 750-mg containers	PO: 250-750 mg once daily IV: 250-750 mg infused slowly over at least 60 min
moxifloxacin	Avelox ⇄ *Do not confuse Avelox with Avandia, Avapro, or Cerebyx.*	Tablets: 400 mg Injection: 400 mg/250 mL	IV, PO: 400 mg once daily; may be taken with or without food
ofloxacin		Tablets: 300, 400 mg	PO: 400-800 mg daily in two divided doses q12h, 1 hr before or 2 hr after meals, with a large glass of fluid

Renal toxicity, as evidenced by proteinuria, hematuria, casts, decreased creatinine clearance, and decreased urine output, also has been reported. Monitor returning laboratory data and report abnormal findings to the healthcare provider.

Neurologic

Tinnitus, headache, dizziness, mental depression, drowsiness, confusion. Quinolone therapy may cause these disturbances. Consult with the healthcare provider when these effects occur. Caution the patient against driving or performing hazardous tasks until adjusted to the effects of the medication.

Worsening symptoms for those with myasthenia gravis. Quinolones may exacerbate muscle weakness in patients with myasthenia gravis. Avoid in patients with known history of myasthenia gravis.

Irreversible peripheral neuropathy (serious nerve damage). Fluoroquinolones have been associated with an increased risk of peripheral neuropathy. Discontinue immediately if the patient experiences symptoms of peripheral neuropathy (including pain, burning, tingling, numbness, and/or weakness) or other alterations in sensations (including light touch, pain, temperature, position sense and vibratory sensation, and/or motor strength) to minimize the development of an irreversible condition. Avoid fluoroquinolones in patients who have previously experienced peripheral neuropathy.

◆ *Drug interactions*

Iron, antacids, sucralfate. Iron salts, zinc salts, sucralfate, and antacids containing magnesium hydroxide or aluminum hydroxide decrease the absorption of quinolones. Administer at least 2 hours before or 6 hours after ingestion of antacids, sucralfate, or iron-containing products, depending on the quinolone.

Nonsteroidal antiinflammatory drugs. The concurrent administration of nonsteroidal antiinflammatory drugs with fluoroquinolones (e.g., levofloxacin, ofloxacin) may increase the risk of central nervous system stimulation with seizures. Use with extreme caution. Consider the use of other analgesics or antiinflammatory agents.

Theophylline. The fluoroquinolones (e.g., ciprofloxacin, moxifloxacin, ofloxacin), when given with theophylline, may produce theophylline toxicity. Observe for vomiting, dizziness, restlessness, and cardiac dysrhythmias. Monitor theophylline serum levels. The dosage of theophylline may need to be reduced.

DRUG CLASS: STREPTOGRAMINS

quinupristin-dalfopristin (kwĭ-nyū-PRĬS-tĭn dăl-fō-PRĬS-tĭn) **Synercid** (SĬN-ŭr-sĭd)

Actions

Quinupristin-dalfopristin is the first of a new class of antimicrobial agents known as *streptogramins*. These two agents were developed from pristinamycin. When used in combination, they are synergistic and act by inhibiting protein synthesis in bacterial cells.

Uses

Quinupristin and dalfopristin are agents that can be used in the treatment of serious or life-threatening infections that are associated with VRE bacteria and cSSSIs caused by methicillin-susceptible *Staph. aureus* or *Strep. pyogenes.* The use of quinupristin-dalfopristin, a representative of a new class of antibiotics, should be reserved for those cases in which other antibiotics such as vancomycin are ineffective, so that resistant strains of bacteria do not rapidly develop.

Therapeutic Outcome

The primary therapeutic outcome expected from quinupristin-dalfopristin therapy is elimination of bacterial infection.

❖ **Nursing Implications for Streptogramins**
◆ *Premedication assessment*
1. Obtain baseline assessments of presenting symptoms.
2. Record temperature, pulse, respirations, blood pressure, and hydration status.
3. Assess for and record any gastric symptoms before initiating therapy.
4. Assess for any allergies.
5. Obtain baseline laboratory studies ordered and review results (e.g., CBC with differential, platelets, blood glucose, electrolytes, creatine kinase, liver function tests, culture and sensitivity).

◆ *Availability.* *IV:* 500 mg (150 mg quinupristin and 350 mg dalfopristin) in 10-mL vial. All dosage recommendations are based on total quinupristin and dalfopristin, in milligrams.

◆ *Dosage and administration.* **Adult:** *IV:* 7.5 mg/kg every 8 hours for the treatment of VRE bacteremia or every 12 hours for treatment of cSSSIs. Infuse the dose over 60 minutes.

Admixture compatibility. Reconstitute only with 5% dextrose or sterile water for injection and then dilute with 5% dextrose to a final concentration of 100 mg/mL. A precipitate will form if reconstituted with other standard diluents. If infused in an IV line being used for other medicines, flush the line with 5% dextrose. Do not flush with heparin or sodium chloride.

◆ *Serious adverse effects*
Vascular
Pain, infusion site inflammation. The most frequent adverse venous events include pain at the administration site, edema, infusion site reaction, and thrombophlebitis.
Gastrointestinal
Nausea, vomiting, anorexia, abdominal cramps, diarrhea. These adverse effects are usually mild and tend to resolve with continued therapy.
Hepatotoxicity. The symptoms of hepatotoxicity are anorexia, nausea, vomiting, jaundice, hepatomegaly, splenomegaly, and abnormal liver function tests (e.g., elevated bilirubin, AST, ALT, GGT, and alkaline phosphatase levels; increased INR).

Musculoskeletal
Arthralgia, myalgia. Arthralgias and myalgias may occur during therapy. Decreasing the frequency of administration to every 12 hours may minimize recurrence.

◆ *Drug interactions*
Toxicity induced by quinupristin-dalfopristin. Quinupristin-dalfopristin may decrease the metabolism of HMG-CoA reductase inhibitors (e.g., atorvastatin, lovastatin, pravastatin, fluvastatin, simvastatin), cyclosporine, ritonavir, vincristine, paclitaxel, docetaxel, tamoxifen, diazepam, midazolam, methylprednisolone, carbamazepine, nifedipine, verapamil, diltiazem, lidocaine, and other potent CYP3A enzyme system inhibitors. Serum concentrations of these agents should be monitored closely if used concurrently with quinupristin-dalfopristin.

DRUG CLASS: SULFONAMIDES

Actions

The sulfonamides are not true antibiotics because they are not synthesized by microorganisms. However, they are highly effective antibacterial agents. Sulfonamides act by inhibiting bacterial biosynthesis of folic acid, which eventually results in bacterial cell death. Human cells do not synthesize folic acid and therefore are not affected.

Uses

Sulfonamides are used primarily to treat UTIs and otitis media. They may also be used to prevent streptococcal infection or rheumatic fever in those allergic to penicillin.

Because of an increasing incidence of organisms resistant to sulfonamide therapy and the unreliability of in vitro sulfonamide sensitivity tests, patients should be monitored closely for continued therapeutic response to treatment. This is particularly important for patients being treated for chronic and recurrent UTIs.

The sulfonamide most commonly used today is actually a combination of trimethoprim (TMP) and sulfamethoxazole (SMX) (e.g., co-trimoxazole, TMP-SMX). This combination blocks two steps in the pathway of folic acid production; therefore fewer resistant strains of microorganisms have developed. Co-trimoxazole is often used for treatment of UTIs, otitis media in children, traveler's diarrhea, acute exacerbations of chronic bronchitis in adults, and prophylaxis and treatment of *Pneumocystis jiroveci* pneumonia in immunocompromised patients.

Therapeutic Outcome

The primary therapeutic outcome expected from sulfonamide therapy is elimination of bacterial infection.

❖ **Nursing Implications for Sulfonamides**
◆ *Premedication assessment*
1. Obtain baseline assessments of presenting symptoms.
2. Record temperature, pulse, respirations, blood pressure, and hydration status.

3. Assess for and record any gastric symptoms before beginning therapy.
4. Assess for any allergies.
5. Obtain baseline laboratory studies ordered and review results (e.g., CBC with differential, culture and sensitivity).

◆ *Availability, dosage, and administration.* See Table 45.8.

 Medication Safety Alert

Patients should be encouraged to drink water several times daily while receiving sulfonamide therapy. In rare situations, crystals form in the urinary tract if the patient becomes too dehydrated.

◆ **Common adverse effects**
Gastrointestinal
Nausea, vomiting, anorexia, diarrhea. These adverse effects are usually mild and tend to resolve with continued therapy. Encourage the patient not to discontinue therapy without first consulting the healthcare provider. If the patient becomes debilitated, contact the healthcare provider.

Integumentary
Dermatologic reactions. Report a rash or pruritus immediately and withhold additional doses pending approval by the healthcare provider.

Photosensitivity. The patient should be cautioned to avoid exposure to sunlight and ultraviolet light. Suggest wearing long-sleeved clothing, a hat, and sunglasses when outdoors. Discourage the use of tanning lamps.

Hematologic
Hematologic reactions. Routine laboratory studies (e.g., CBC with differential) are scheduled for patients taking sulfonamides for 14 days or longer. Stress the importance of returning for this laboratory work. Monitor for the development of a sore throat, fever, purpura, jaundice, or excessive and progressive weakness.

Neurologic
Neurologic effects. Report the development of tinnitus, headache, dizziness, mental depression, drowsiness, or confusion.

◆ **Drug interactions**
Oral hypoglycemic agents. Sulfonamides may displace sulfonylurea oral hypoglycemic agents (e.g., glipizide, glimepiride, glyburide) and meglitinide oral hypoglycemic agents (repaglinide, nateglinide) from protein-binding sites, resulting in hypoglycemia. Monitor for hypoglycemia, headache, weakness, decreased coordination, general apprehension, diaphoresis, hunger, and blurred or double vision. The dosage of the hypoglycemic agent may need to be reduced. Notify the healthcare provider if any of these symptoms appear.

Warfarin. Sulfonamides may enhance the anticoagulant effects of warfarin. Observe for petechiae; ecchymoses; nosebleeds; bleeding gums; dark, tarry stools; and bright red or coffee-ground emesis. Monitor INR and reduce dosage of warfarin if necessary.

Methotrexate. Sulfonamides may produce methotrexate toxicity when given simultaneously. Monitor patients on concurrent therapy for oral stomatitis and for signs of nephrotoxicity (e.g., oliguria, hematuria, proteinuria, casts).

Phenytoin. Sulfisoxazole may displace phenytoin from protein-binding sites, resulting in phenytoin toxicity. Monitor patients on concurrent therapy for signs of phenytoin toxicity (e.g., nystagmus, sedation, lethargy); serum levels may be ordered. A reduced dosage of phenytoin may be required.

Angiotensin-converting enzyme inhibitors, angiotensin receptor blockers, eplerenone, spironolactone. With concurrent use of these agents and TMP-SMX, trimethoprim may act additively to suppress aldosterone, resulting in hyperkalemia that may lead to cardiac arrhythmias. Monitor serum potassium levels.

DRUG CLASS: TETRACYCLINES

Actions
Tetracyclines are a class of antibiotics that are effective against gram-negative and gram-positive bacteria. They act by inhibiting protein synthesis by bacterial cells.

Uses
The tetracyclines are often used in patients allergic to penicillins for the treatment of certain STIs, UTIs, upper respiratory tract infections, pneumonia, and meningitis. They are particularly effective against skin (acne), rickettsial, and mycoplasmic infections. The newest tetracycline, eravacycline, is approved for the treatment of complicated intraabdominal infections caused by *E. coli, E. cloacae, K. oxytoca, E. faecalis, S. aureus, S. anginosus, C. perfringens,* and *Bacteroides* species in patients 18 years or older.

Tetracyclines administered during the ages of tooth development (last half of pregnancy through 8 years of age) may cause enamel hypoplasia and permanent yellow, gray, or brown staining of teeth. Tetracyclines are secreted in breast milk, so nursing mothers on tetracycline therapy are advised to feed their infants formula or cow's milk, as appropriate.

Therapeutic Outcome
The primary therapeutic outcome expected from tetracycline therapy is elimination of bacterial infection.

❖ **Nursing Implications for Tetracyclines**
◆ *Premedication assessment*
1. Obtain baseline assessments of presenting symptoms.
2. Record temperature, pulse, respirations, blood pressure, and hydration status.
3. Assess for and record any gastric symptoms present before beginning therapy.
4. Assess for any allergies.

Table 45.8　Sulfonamides

GENERIC NAME	BRAND NAME	AVAILABILITY	ADULT DOSAGE RANGE
sulfadiazine		Tablets: 500 mg	PO: Initial dose: 2-4 g, then 2-4 g/day in three to six divided doses
sulfasalazine	Azulfidine	Tablets: 500 mg Tablets, delayed release: 500 mg	PO: Initial therapy: 3-4 g daily in three to four divided doses; maintenance dosage: 2 g daily
co-trimoxazole	Bactrim, Bactrim DS ⇄ Do not confuse Bactrim with Biaxin.	Tablets: 400/80-, 800/160-mg sulfamethoxazole/trimethoprim Suspension: 200/40-, 400/80-mg sulfamethoxazole/ trimethoprim IV: 80/16 mg/mL sulfamethoxazole, trimethoprim	PO: 2-4 tablets daily, depending on strength, disease being treated IV: 8-10 mg/kg/day (based on trimethoprim) in two to four divided doses *Pneumocystis* pneumonia: 15-20 mg/kg/24 hr (based on trimethoprim) in three or four divided doses for up to 14 days

5. Obtain baseline laboratory studies ordered and review results (e.g., CBC with differential, culture and sensitivity).

◆ **Availability, dosage, and administration.** See Table 45.9. **PO:** Emphasize the importance of taking medication 1 hour before or 2 hours after ingesting antacids, milk, or other dairy products, or products containing calcium, aluminum, magnesium, or iron (e.g., vitamins). *Exception:* Food and milk do not interfere with the absorption of doxycycline.

◆ **Common adverse effects**
Gastrointestinal
Nausea, vomiting, anorexia, abdominal cramps, diarrhea. These adverse effects are usually mild and tend to resolve with continued therapy. Encourage the patient not to discontinue therapy without first consulting the healthcare provider.
Integumentary
Photosensitivity. Photosensitivity resulting in an exaggerated sunburn after short exposure has been reported. The patient should be cautioned to avoid exposure to sunlight and ultraviolet light. Suggest wearing long-sleeved clothing, a hat, and sunglasses when outdoors. Discourage the use of tanning lamps. Consult the healthcare provider about the advisability of discontinuing therapy.

◆ **Drug and other interactions**
Warfarin. Tetracyclines may enhance the anticoagulant effects of warfarin. Observe for petechiae; ecchymoses; nosebleeds; bleeding gums; dark, tarry stools; and bright red or coffee-ground emesis. Monitor the INR and reduce the dosage of warfarin if necessary.
Impaired absorption. Iron, calcium-containing foods (milk and dairy products), and calcium, aluminum, or magnesium preparations (antacids) decrease absorption of tetracyclines. Administer all tetracycline products 1 hour before or 2 hours after ingestion of these foods or products. *Exceptions:* Food and milk do not interfere with the absorption of doxycycline.

Phenytoin, carbamazepine. These agents reduce the half-life of doxycycline. Monitor patients for lack of clinical improvement from the infection.

Tooth development. Do not administer tetracyclines to pregnant patients or to children younger than 8 years. The infant's or child's tooth enamel may be permanently stained yellow, gray, or brown.

Lactation. Nursing mothers must switch their babies to formula while taking tetracyclines because tetracyclines are present in breast milk.

Oral contraceptives. Tetracyclines may interfere with the activity of oral contraceptives. Oral contraceptives should not be discontinued, but counseling regarding use of additional methods of contraception (e.g., condoms and foam) should be planned.

DRUG CLASS: ANTITUBERCULAR AGENTS

ethambutol (ĕth-ĂM-byū-tŏl)

Actions
Ethambutol inhibits tuberculosis bacterial growth by altering cellular RNA synthesis and phosphate metabolism.

Uses
Ethambutol is an antitubercular agent. It must be used in combination with other antitubercular agents to prevent the development of resistant organisms.

Therapeutic Outcome
The primary therapeutic outcome expected from ethambutol therapy is elimination of tuberculosis.

❖ **Nursing Implications for Ethambutol**
◆ **Premedication assessment**
1. Obtain baseline assessments of presenting symptoms.

Table **45.9**   **Tetracyclines**

GENERIC NAME	BRAND NAME	AVAILABILITY	ADULT DOSAGE RANGE
doxycycline ⇄ *Do not confuse doxycycline with dicloxacillin or dicyclomine.*	Vibramycin ⇄ *Do not confuse Vibramycin with vancomycin.* Adoxa, Doryx	Tablets: 20, 50, 75, 100, 150 mg Tablets, delayed release: 50, 75, 100, 120, 150, 200 mg Capsules: 50, 75, 100, 150 mg Capsules delayed release: 40 mg Suspension: 25 mg/5 mL Syrup: 50 mg/5 mL IV: 100-mg vials	PO: 100 mg twice daily IV: 100 mg twice daily or 200 mg once daily
eravacycline	Xerava	Injection: 50-mg vials	IV: 1 mg/kg over 60 min every 12 hr for 4 to 14 days
minocycline	Minocin	Capsules: 50, 75, 100 mg Tablets: 50, 75, 100 mg Tablets, extended release (24 hr): 45, 55, 65, 80, 90, 105, 115, 135 mg Capsules, extended release (24 hr): 90, 135 mg Extended-release powder in dental base: 1 mg IV: 100-mg vial	PO, IV: 200 mg, followed by 100 mg q12h
tetracycline		Capsules: 250, 500 mg	PO: 250-500 mg four times daily

2. Record temperature, pulse, respirations, blood pressure, and hydration status.
3. Assess for and record any gastric symptoms before initiating therapy.
4. Assess for any allergies.
5. Perform baseline mental status assessment (e.g., orientation and alertness), assess for GI symptoms, and test color vision (e.g., red-green discrimination) before initiating therapy.
6. Review laboratory data of tuberculin testing and cultures in the patient's chart.

◆ *Availability. PO:* 100- and 400-mg tablets.

◆ *Dosage and administration.* **Adult:** *PO:* Initial treatment: 15 mg/kg administered as a single dose every 24 hours. Re-treatment: 25 mg/kg as a single daily dose. After 60 days, reduce the dosage to 15 mg/kg and administer as a single dose every 24 hours. Administer once daily with food or milk to minimize gastric irritation.

[!] Medication Safety Alert

The patient should be warned that omission of doses or interrupted intake of ethambutol may result in bacterial drug resistance, reversal of clinical improvement, and increased susceptibility of family members and others to tuberculosis.

◆ **Common adverse effects**
Gastrointestinal
Nausea, vomiting, anorexia, abdominal cramps. These adverse effects are usually mild and tend to resolve with continued therapy. Encourage the patient not to discontinue therapy without first consulting the

healthcare provider. Administer the daily dosage with food to minimize nausea and vomiting.

◆ **Serious adverse effects**
Neurologic
Confusion, hallucinations. Perform a baseline assessment of the patient's degree of alertness and orientation to name, place, and time before initiating therapy. Make regularly scheduled subsequent mental status evaluations and compare findings. Report development of alterations. Provide for patient safety during episodes of altered behavior or periods of dizziness.
Sensory
Blurred vision, red-green vision changes. Before initiating therapy, check for any visual alterations using a color vision chart. Schedule subsequent evaluations on a regular basis. Report the development of visual disturbances for the healthcare provider's evaluation. These adverse effects disappear within a few weeks after therapy has been discontinued.

◆ **Drug interactions**
Antacids. Aluminum salts may delay and reduce absorption of ethambutol. Separate administration by at least 2 hours.

---

isoniazid (ī-sō-NĪ-ă-zĭd)
   INH

Actions
Isoniazid has been a mainstay for many years in the prevention and treatment of tuberculosis. Despite this, its mechanism of action is still not fully known. It

appears to disrupt the *Mycobacterium tuberculosis* cell wall and inhibit replication.

Uses

Isoniazid is used for both prophylaxis and treatment of tuberculosis. It should be used in combination with other antitubercular agents for therapy of active disease.

Therapeutic Outcomes

The primary therapeutic outcomes expected from isoniazid therapy are as follows:

- Prevention of tuberculosis in people with a positive skin test
- Elimination of tuberculosis in people with active disease

❖ Nursing Implications for Isoniazid

◆ *Premedication assessment*

1. Obtain baseline assessments of presenting symptoms.
2. Record temperature, pulse, respirations, blood pressure, and hydration status.
3. Assess for and record any gastric symptoms, abnormal liver function test results, or paresthesias present before initiation of therapy.
4. Assess for any allergies.
5. Check medication orders for concurrent administration of other antitubercular drugs and for an order for pyridoxine.

◆ *Availability.* *PO:* 100- and 300-mg tablets; 50-mg/5-mL syrup. *IM:* 100 mg/mL in 10-mL vials.

◆ *Dosage and administration.* **Adult:** *PO:* *Treatment of active tuberculosis:* 5 mg/kg to a maximum of 300 mg daily, or 15 mg/kg/day (900 mg maximum per dose) two or three times per week. Isoniazid should be used in conjunction with other effective antitubercular agents. *Prophylactic therapy:* 300 mg daily in a single dose. Administer on an empty stomach for maximum effectiveness. Pyridoxine, 25 to 50 mg daily, is often given concurrently with isoniazid to diminish peripheral neuropathies, dizziness, and ataxia. *IM:* Same as for PO administration.

Pediatric: *PO:* 10 to 15 mg/kg/day (maximum dose of 300 mg daily) in single dose, or 20 to 40 mg/kg/day (900 mg maximum per dose) two or three times weekly. Infants and children tolerate larger dosages than adults.

◆ *Common and serious adverse effects*

Gastrointestinal

Nausea, vomiting. Nausea and vomiting are relatively common adverse effects of isoniazid and are dose related. Concurrent use of pyridoxine, 25 to 50 mg daily, will usually prevent these symptoms.

Hepatotoxicity. The incidence of hepatotoxicity increases with age and with the consumption of alcohol. This reaction usually occurs within the first 3 months of therapy and is thought to be an allergic reaction. The symptoms of hepatotoxicity are anorexia, nausea, vomiting, jaundice, hepatomegaly, splenomegaly, and abnormal liver function test results (e.g., elevated bilirubin, AST, ALT, GGT, and alkaline phosphatase levels; increased INR).

Neurologic

Tingling, numbness. Tingling and numbness of the hands and feet are relatively common adverse effects of isoniazid and are dosage related. Concurrent use of pyridoxine, 25 to 50 mg daily, will usually prevent these symptoms. When paresthesias are present, the patient must be cautioned to inspect the extremities for any skin breakdown because of the diminished sensation. Caution patients not to immerse feet or hands in water without first testing the temperature. Monitor patients with paresthesias for adequate nutrition.

Dizziness, ataxia. Provide for patient safety and assistance in ambulation until either a dosage adjustment or addition of pyridoxine provides symptomatic relief.

◆ *Drug interactions*

Disulfiram. Patients receiving concurrent therapy may experience changes in physical coordination and mental affect and behavior. Provide for patient safety and monitor the patient's mental status before and during therapy. If possible, avoid concomitant therapy.

Carbamazepine. Isoniazid may inhibit the metabolism of carbamazepine. Monitor patients receiving concurrent therapy for signs of carbamazepine toxicity (e.g., ataxia, headache, vomiting, blurred vision, drowsiness, confusion).

Theophylline. Isoniazid may inhibit the metabolism of theophylline. Monitor patients receiving concurrent therapy for signs of theophylline toxicity (e.g., anxiety, tachycardia, nausea, headache, vomiting).

Phenytoin. Isoniazid may inhibit the metabolism of phenytoin. Monitor patients receiving concurrent therapy for signs of phenytoin toxicity (e.g., nystagmus, sedation, lethargy). Serum levels may be ordered and the dosage of phenytoin reduced.

---

pyrazinamide (pī-rah-ZIN-a-mīd)
 Tebrazid ♦ (teb RAH zid)

Actions

Pyrazinamide is converted to pyrazinoic acid in the mycobacterium organism, which lowers the pH of the environment, although the exact mechanism of action is not known.

Uses

Pyrazinamide is used in the treatment of tuberculosis. It must be used in combination with other antitubercular agents to prevent the development of resistant organisms. Pyrazinamide may inhibit uric acid excretion; acute gouty attacks have been reported. Use with caution in patients with chronic gout. Its use is contraindicated with acute gout.

Therapeutic Outcome

The primary therapeutic outcome expected from pyrazinamide therapy is elimination of tuberculosis.

❖ Nursing Implications for Pyrazinamide
◆ Premedication assessment
1. Obtain baseline assessments of presenting symptoms.
2. Record temperature, pulse, respirations, blood pressure, and hydration status.
3. Assess for and record any gastric symptoms before initiating therapy.
4. Assess for any allergies.
5. Perform baseline mental status assessment (e.g., orientation and alertness).
6. Review laboratory data of tuberculin testing and cultures in the patient's chart.

◆ Availability. *PO:* 500-mg tablets.

◆ Dosage and administration. **Adult:** *PO: dosage by weight:* 40 to 55 kg: 1000 mg once daily; 56 to 75 kg: 1500 mg once daily; 76 to 90 kg: 2000 mg once daily.
NOTE: The preferred frequency of administration is once daily.

> **⚠ Medication Safety Alert**
>
> The patient should be warned that omission of doses or interrupted intake of pyrazinamide may result in bacterial drug resistance, reversal of clinical improvement, and increased susceptibility of family members and others to tuberculosis.

◆ Common adverse effects
Gastrointestinal
Nausea, vomiting, anorexia. These adverse effects are usually mild and tend to resolve with continued therapy. Encourage the patient not to discontinue therapy without first consulting the healthcare provider. Administer the daily dosage with food to minimize nausea and vomiting.

Skeletal and neuromuscular effects
Arthralgia, myalgia. These adverse effects are usually mild and tend to resolve with continued therapy. Encourage the patient not to discontinue therapy without first consulting the healthcare provider.

◆ Serious adverse effects
Hepatotoxicity. Monitor liver function tests periodically.

◆ Drug interactions
Cyclosporine. Pyrazinamide may decrease the serum concentration of cyclosporine.

---

rifampin (rĭf-ĂM-pĭn)
 Do not confuse rifampin with ramipril or rifabutin.
Rifadin (RĬF-ă-dĭn)
 Do not confuse Rifadin with Rifater.

Actions

Rifampin prevents RNA synthesis in mycobacteria by inhibiting DNA-dependent RNA polymerase. This action blocks key metabolic pathways needed for mycobacterium cells to grow and replicate.

Uses

Rifampin is used in combination with other agents for the treatment of tuberculosis. Rifampin is also used to eliminate meningococci from the nasopharynx of asymptomatic *N. meningitidis* carriers and to eliminate *H. influenzae* type b from the nasopharynx of asymptomatic carriers.

Therapeutic Outcomes

The primary therapeutic outcomes expected from rifampin therapy are as follows:
1. Elimination of tuberculosis
2. Eradication of meningococci or *H. influenzae* type b from asymptomatic carriers of these diseases

❖ Nursing Implications for Rifampin
◆ Premedication assessment
1. Obtain baseline assessments of presenting symptoms.
2. Record temperature, pulse, respirations, blood pressure, and hydration status.
3. Assess for and record any gastric symptoms present before beginning therapy.
4. Assess for any allergies.
5. Obtain baseline laboratory studies ordered and review results (e.g., CBC with differential, tuberculin tests, chest radiography).

◆ Availability. *PO:* 150- and 300-mg capsules. 25 mg/mL per 120 mL bottle suspension. *IV:* 600-mg vials.

◆ Dosage and administration. **Adult:** *PO:* 10 mg/kg (maximum 600 mg) once daily, either 1 hour before or 2 hours after a meal. *IV:* same as for PO.
Pediatric: *PO:* 10 mg/kg/day, with a maximum daily dose of 600 mg. *IV:* same as for PO.

> **⚠ Medication Safety Alert**
>
> Patients should be warned that omission of doses or interrupted intake of rifampin may result in bacterial drug resistance, reversal of clinical improvement, and increased susceptibility of family members to tuberculosis.

◆ Common adverse effects
Excretory
Reddish orange secretions. Urine, feces, saliva, sputum, sweat, and tears may be tinged reddish orange. This effect is harmless and will disappear after discontinuing therapy. However, rifampin may permanently discolor soft contact lenses.

◆ *Serious adverse effects*
Gastrointestinal
Nausea, vomiting, anorexia, abdominal cramps. These adverse effects are usually mild and tend to resolve with continued therapy. Encourage the patient not to discontinue therapy without first consulting the healthcare provider. If these symptoms are accompanied by fever, chills, or muscle and bone pain, or if unusual bruising or a yellowish discoloration of the skin or eyes appears, contact the healthcare provider.

◆ *Drug interactions*
Warfarin. Rifampin may diminish the anticoagulant effects of warfarin. Monitor the INR and increase the dosage of warfarin if necessary.

Isoniazid. Concurrent therapy may rarely result in hepatotoxicity. Patients on combined therapy should have liver function tests monitored periodically.

Decreased therapeutic effects induced by rifampin. Rifampin stimulates the metabolism of benzodiazepines (e.g., diazepam, midazolam, triazolam), quinidine, amiodarone, verapamil, nifedipine, mexiletine, enalapril, theophylline, beta-blocking agents (e.g., bisoprolol, metoprolol, propranolol), phenobarbital, fluoroquinolones, ondansetron, haloperidol, losartan, protease inhibitors, sulfonylureas, and many other drugs. Long-term combined therapy may require an increase in dosages for therapeutic effect.

Ketoconazole. Administration of rifampin and ketoconazole decreases serum levels of both drugs. Avoid concurrent use if possible.

Oral contraceptives. Rifampin interferes with the activity of oral contraceptives. Counseling regarding alternative methods of birth control should be planned.

DRUG CLASS: MISCELLANEOUS ANTIBIOTICS

aztreonam (ăz-TRĒ-ō-năm)
⇄ *Do not confuse aztreonam with azithromycin.*
Azactam (ăz-ĂK-tăm)

Actions
Aztreonam is a monobactam antibiotic, acting by inhibition of cell wall synthesis.

Uses
The monobactams have a high degree of activity against beta-lactamase–producing aerobic gram-negative bacteria, including *P. aeruginosa*. Aztreonam has essentially no activity against anaerobes or gram-positive microorganisms. It is used to treat urinary tract, lower respiratory tract, skin, intraabdominal, gynecologic, and bacteremic infections and meningitides caused by *P. aeruginosa, Salmonella, Shigella, N. gonorrhoeae,* and ampicillin-resistant *H. influenzae.* It is recommended that aztreonam be combined with a broad-spectrum antibiotic in the initial treatment of an infection of unknown cause to treat susceptible anaerobes or gram-positive organisms.

Therapeutic Outcome
The primary therapeutic outcome expected from aztreonam therapy is elimination of bacterial infection.

❖ **Nursing Implications for Aztreonam**
◆ *Premedication assessment*
1. Obtain baseline assessments of presenting symptoms.
2. Record temperature, pulse, respirations, blood pressure, and hydration status.
3. Assess for and record any gastric symptoms before initiating therapy.
4. Assess for any allergies.
5. Obtain baseline laboratory studies ordered and review results (e.g., CBC with differential, culture and sensitivity).

◆ *Availability.* **IM, IV:** 1- and 2-g/vial. *Inhalation:* 75 mg/vial for reconstitution.

◆ *Dosage and administration.* **Adult: IM or IV:** *Urinary tract infections:* 0.5 to 1 g every 8 to 12 hours. *Moderately severe systemic infections:* 1 to 2 g every 8 to 12 hours. *Life-threatening infections:* 2 g every 6 to 8 hours.

Inhalation: Usual dosage: 75 mg three times daily using an Altera Nebulizer System (PARI Respiratory Equipment, Midlothian, VA). Reconstitute the powder using the supplied diluent just prior to inhalation. Patients should use a short- or long-acting bronchodilator prior to administration of aztreonam.

◆ *Common adverse effects*
Gastrointestinal
Nausea, vomiting, diarrhea. These adverse effects are usually mild and tend to resolve with continued therapy.

◆ *Serious adverse effects*
Gastrointestinal
Severe diarrhea. Severe diarrhea may develop from the use of aztreonam. Report diarrhea of five or more stools daily to the healthcare provider. This may be an indication of drug-induced pseudomembranous colitis. Blood or mucus in the stool also should be reported to the healthcare provider. **Warn patients not to treat diarrhea themselves when taking this drug.** The use of paregoric, diphenoxylate, or loperamide may prolong or worsen the condition.
Vascular
Phlebitis. Avoid IV infusion in the lower extremities or in areas with varicosities. Use proper technique in starting the IV solution.

Carefully assess at regularly scheduled intervals for signs of developing phlebitis. Inspect for redness, warmth, tenderness to touch, edema, or pain. Always assess complaints of pain at the infusion site. If signs of inflammation accompany complaints, discontinue and restart elsewhere.

Immune system (opportunistic infections)

Secondary infections. Oral thrush, genital and anal pruritus, vaginitis, and vaginal discharge may occur. Report promptly because these infections are resistant to the original antibiotic used. Teach the importance of meticulous oral and perineal hygiene measures.

◆ *Drug interactions*

Beta-lactamase antibiotics. These antibiotics (e.g., cefoxitin, imipenem) induce the production of beta-lactamase in some gram-negative organisms, resulting in possible antagonism with a beta-lactam antibiotic such as aztreonam. It is recommended that beta-lactamase–stimulating antibiotics not be used concurrently with aztreonam.

---

clindamycin (klĭn-dă-MĬ-sĭn)
Cleocin (klē-Ō-sĭn)

Actions
Clindamycin is an antibiotic that acts by inhibiting protein synthesis.

Uses
Clindamycin is useful against infections caused by gram-negative aerobic organisms and a variety of gram-positive and gram-negative anaerobes.

Therapeutic Outcome
The primary therapeutic outcome expected from clindamycin therapy is elimination of bacterial infection.

❖ **Nursing Implications for Clindamycin**
◆ *Premedication assessment*
1. Obtain baseline assessments of presenting symptoms.
2. Record temperature, pulse, respirations, blood pressure, and hydration status.
3. Record pattern of bowel elimination before initiating drug therapy.
4. Assess for any allergies.
5. Obtain baseline laboratory studies ordered and review results (e.g., CBC with differential, culture and sensitivity).

◆ *Availability.* **PO:** 75-, 150-, and 300-mg capsules; 75-mg/5-mL suspension. **IV:** 150 mg/mL in 2-, 4-, and 6-mL ampules.

◆ *Dosage and administration.* **Adult:** *PO:* 150 to 450 mg every 6 hours. *Do not* refrigerate the suspension. It is stable at room temperature for 14 days. *IM:* 600 to 2700 mg/24 hr. *Do not* exceed 600 mg per injection. Pain, induration, and sterile abscesses have been reported. Deep IM injection is recommended to help minimize this reaction. *IV:* 600 to 2700 mg/24 hr. Dilute to less

than 6 mg/mL and administer at a rate less than 30 mg/min. Administration by IV push is not recommended.

Pediatric: *PO:* Suspension: 8 to 25 mg/kg/24 hr in three or four divided doses. Capsules: 8 to 20 mg/kg/24 hr in three or four divided doses. Capsules should be taken with a full glass of water to prevent esophageal irritation. *IM:* 15 to 40 mg/kg/24 hr in four divided doses. *IV:* same as for IM use. Dilute to less than 6 mg/mL and administer at a rate less than 30 mg/min.

◆ *Common adverse effects*
Gastrointestinal
Diarrhea. This adverse effect is usually mild and tends to resolve with continued therapy. Encourage the patient not to discontinue therapy without first consulting the healthcare provider.

◆ *Serious adverse effects*
Gastrointestinal
Severe diarrhea. Severe diarrhea may develop from the use of clindamycin. Report diarrhea of five or more stools daily to the healthcare provider. This may be an indication of drug-induced pseudomembranous colitis. Blood or mucus in the stool should also be reported to the healthcare provider. **Warn patients not to treat diarrhea themselves when taking this drug.** The use of paregoric, diphenoxylate, or loperamide may prolong or worsen the condition.

◆ *Drug interactions*
Neuromuscular blockade. Label charts of patients scheduled for surgery who are taking clindamycin. When combined with surgical muscle relaxants or aminoglycosides, neuromuscular blockade may result.

These combinations also may potentiate respiratory depression. Check the anesthesia record of surgical patients. Monitor postoperative patients for respiratory depression for a prolonged period. This can occur 48 hours or more after the drug administration.

Erythromycin. Therapeutic antagonism has been reported between clindamycin and erythromycin. Do not administer concurrently.

---

daptomycin (dăp-tō-MĬ-sĭn)
Cubicin (KYŪ-bĭ-sĭn)

Actions
Daptomycin is in the class of antibiotics known as *cyclic lipopeptide antibiotics*. It has a unique mechanism of action among the antibiotics. It binds to bacterial membranes and causes a rapid depolarization of membrane potential, leading to inhibition of protein, RNA, and DNA synthesis, which leads to cell death. Because of its unique mechanism of action, daptomycin is effective against microorganisms that have developed resistance to other commonly used antibiotics.

Uses

Daptomycin has been approved for the treatment of cSSSIs caused by *Staph. aureus, Strep. pyogenes, Strep. agalactiae,* and *Enterococcus faecalis.* It is particularly valuable in cases of gram-positive organisms becoming resistant to the beta-lactam antibiotics (penicillins and cephalosporins) and vancomycin. In an effort to slow the development of strains of bacteria resistant to daptomycin, it should be used only when the pathogen is resistant to other available antibiotics.

Therapeutic Outcome

The primary therapeutic outcome expected from daptomycin therapy is elimination of bacterial infection.

❖ Nursing Implications for Daptomycin
◆ Premedication assessment
1. Obtain baseline assessments of presenting symptoms.
2. Record temperature, pulse, respirations, blood pressure, and hydration status.
3. Assess for any allergies.
4. Assess the bowel elimination patterns and record before initiating therapy.
5. Ensure that blood for a baseline creatine phosphokinase (CPK) and creatinine kinase study has been drawn and sent to the laboratory before daptomycin is started. Also, inquire and record whether the patient has any particular muscle weakness or pains, particularly in the extremities.
6. Obtain other baseline laboratory studies ordered and review results (e.g., CBC with differential, culture and sensitivity).

◆ Availability. *IV:* 500-mg vials.

◆ Dosage and administration. *IV:* Complicated skin and skin structure infections: 4 mg/kg once every 24 hours for 7 to 14 days.

Endocarditis: 6 mg/kg infused over 30 minutes every 24 hours for 2 to 6 weeks.

Patients who have reduced renal function with a creatinine clearance of less than 30 mL/min should have the same doses administered every 48 hours.

Admixture compatibility. Daptomycin is not compatible with dextrose-containing diluents, and additives or other medications should not be added to daptomycin or infused simultaneously through the same IV line. If the same IV line is used for sequential infusion of several different drugs, the line should be flushed with a compatible infusion solution before and after infusions with daptomycin.

◆ Common adverse effects
Gastrointestinal
Gastric irritation. The most common adverse effects of daptomycin therapy are diarrhea, constipation, nausea, and vomiting. These adverse effects are usually mild and tend to resolve with continued therapy.

◆ Serious adverse effects
Gastrointestinal
Severe diarrhea. Severe diarrhea may develop from the use of daptomycin. Blood and mucus in the stool also may be present. This may be an indication of drug-induced pseudomembranous colitis and should be reported immediately. Withhold the next dose of antibiotic until the healthcare provider gives approval for administration.

Musculoskeletal
Skeletal muscle weakness and pain. Patients should be monitored for the development of muscle pain or weakness, particularly in the distal extremities. It is recommended that CPK concentrations be monitored weekly in patients treated with daptomycin and more frequently in those who develop unexplained elevations of CPK levels during therapy.

◆ Drug interactions
HMG-CoA reductase inhibitors. The statins (e.g., atorvastatin, lovastatin, simvastatin, others) may infrequently cause skeletal muscle myopathy and potentially rhabdomyolysis when administered with daptomycin. It is therefore suggested that statin therapy be discontinued in patients being treated with daptomycin. Statin therapy may be reinitiated after daptomycin therapy has been completed.

---

metronidazole (mĕt-rō-NĪ-dă-zŏl)
⇄ *Do not confuse metronidazole with metoclopramide, metoprolol, miconazole, or methazolamide.*
Flagyl (FLĂ-jĭl)

Actions

Metronidazole is a nitroimidazole. It is a somewhat unusual medication in that it has bactericidal, trichomonacidal, and protozoacidal activity. Its mechanism of action is unknown.

Uses

Metronidazole is used to treat trichomoniasis, giardiasis, amebic dysentery, amebic liver abscess, and anaerobic bacterial infections.

Therapeutic Outcome

The primary therapeutic outcome expected from metronidazole therapy is elimination of infection.

❖ Nursing Implications for Metronidazole
◆ Premedication assessment
1. Obtain baseline assessments of the presenting symptoms.
2. Record temperature, pulse, respirations, blood pressure, and hydration status.
3. Assess for and record any gastric symptoms, peripheral neuropathy, or seizure disorders before initiating therapy.

4. Assess for any allergies.

5. Perform a baseline assessment of the patient's degree of alertness and orientation to name, place, and time before initiating therapy.

6. Obtain baseline laboratory studies ordered and review results (e.g., CBC with differential, culture and sensitivity).

◆ *Availability. PO:* 250- and 500-mg tablets; 375-mg capsules; 750-mg extended-release tablets (24 hr). *Suspension:* 50, 100 mg/mL in 150 mL bottles. *Injection:* 500-mg powder/vial.

◆ *Dosage and administration.* **Adult:** *PO:*

- *Trichomoniasis:* Men and women: 500 mg twice daily for 7 days (CDC) *or* 250 mg three times daily or 375 mg twice daily for 7 days (manufacturer). Sexual partners must be treated concurrently to prevent reinfection. Single doses of 2 g or two doses of 1 g each administered the same day appear to provide adequate treatment for trichomoniasis in men and women.
- *Giardiasis:* 250 mg three times daily for 5 to 7 days.
- *Amebic dysentery:* 750 mg three times daily for 5 to 10 days.
- *Amebic liver abscess:* 7.5 mg/kg every 6 hours for 7 to 10 days.
- *Anaerobic bacterial infections:* Administer with parenteral therapy initially. The usual oral dosage is 7.5 mg/kg every 6 hours. Do not exceed 4 g/24 hr. The usual duration is 7 to 10 days. Infections of the bones and joints, lower respiratory tract, and endocardium may require longer treatment.

Adult: *IV: Anaerobic bacterial infections:* Loading dose: 15 mg/kg infused over 1 hour. Maintenance dosage: 7.5 mg/kg infused over 1 hour every 6 hours. Do not exceed 4 g/24 hr. Convert to oral dosages when clinical condition is stable. Dosage reduction is necessary in patients with hepatic impairment but not renal impairment.

Pediatric: *PO: Trichomoniasis:* 15 mg/kg/24 hr in three divided doses for 7 days. *Amebiasis:* 35 to 50 mg/kg/24 hr in three divided doses for 7 to 10 days. *Giardiasis:* 15 mg/kg/24 hr in three divided doses (maximum of 250 mg/dose) for 5 days.

◆ *Common adverse effects*

Gastrointestinal

Nausea, vomiting, diarrhea, metallic taste. These adverse effects are usually mild and tend to resolve with continued therapy.

◆ *Serious adverse effects*

Neurologic

Dizziness. Provide for patient safety during episodes of dizziness; report to the healthcare provider for further evaluation.

Confusion, seizures. Patients receiving high doses of metronidazole, those with histories of seizure activity,

and those with significant hepatic impairment are at greater risk of confusion and seizures. Perform a baseline assessment of the patient's degree of alertness and orientation to name, place, and time before initiating therapy. Make regularly scheduled subsequent mental status evaluations and compare findings. Report the development of alterations.

Implement seizure precautions (padded side rails, available oxygen, and suction sets). Make sure that the patient continues with anticonvulsant therapy. If seizures develop, provide for patient safety and then record the exact time of seizure onset and duration of each phase, a description of the specific body parts involved, and any progression in the affected parts. Describe the automatic responses seen during the clonic phase—altered, jerky respirations; frothy salivation; dilated pupils and eye movements; cyanosis; diaphoresis; or incontinence.

Vascular

Thrombophlebitis. Carefully assess patients receiving IV metronidazole for the development of thrombophlebitis. Inspect the IV infusion area frequently when providing care; visually inspect during dressing changes and whenever the infusion is changed to a new site. Always investigate pain at the IV site. Report redness, warmth, tenderness to touch, and edema in the affected part.

◆ *Drug interactions*

Alcohol. Use of alcohol and alcohol-containing preparations, such as OTC cough medications and mouthwashes (e.g., Listerine, Cēpacol), should be avoided during and up to 48 hours after discontinuation of metronidazole therapy. Metronidazole inhibits enzymes required to metabolize alcohol, resulting in mild symptoms of abdominal cramping, flushing, headache, nausea, vomiting, and sweating.

Warfarin. Metronidazole may enhance the anticoagulant effects of warfarin. Observe for the development of petechiae; ecchymoses; nosebleeds; bleeding gums; dark, tarry stools; and bright red or coffee-ground emesis. Monitor the INR and reduce the dosage of warfarin if necessary.

Disulfiram. Combined use of disulfiram and metronidazole may result in mental confusion and psychoses. Concurrent therapy is not recommended.

Lithium. Patients receiving higher dosages of lithium are more susceptible to lithium toxicity and potential renal damage. Metronidazole should be initiated only if absolutely necessary. Frequently monitor serum lithium and creatinine concentrations when metronidazole and lithium are administered concurrently.

Phenytoin, fosphenytoin. Metronidazole inhibits phenytoin metabolism. Monitor patients with concurrent therapy for signs of phenytoin toxicity: nystagmus, sedation, and lethargy. Serum levels may be ordered and the dosage of phenytoin reduced.

tinidazole (tĭn-Ĭ-dă-zōl)
Tindamax (TĬN-dă-măks)

Actions

Tinidazole is a nitroimidazole similar to metronidazole. Its mechanism of action is unknown.

Uses

Tinidazole is used to treat parasitic infections such as trichomoniasis caused by *Trichomonas vaginalis* in female and male patients, giardiasis caused by *Giardia lamblia*, and intestinal amebiasis and amebic liver abscess caused by *Entamoeba histolytica*.

Therapeutic Outcome

The primary therapeutic outcome expected from tinidazole therapy is elimination of parasitic infection.

❖ Nursing Implications for Tinidazole

◆ *Premedication assessment*

1. Obtain baseline assessments of the presenting symptoms.
2. Record temperature, pulse, respirations, blood pressure, and hydration status.
3. Assess for and record any gastric symptoms, peripheral neuropathy, or seizure disorders before initiating therapy.
4. Assess for any allergies.
5. Perform a baseline assessment of the patient's degree of alertness and orientation to name, place, and time before initiating therapy.
6. Obtain baseline laboratory studies ordered and review results (e.g., CBC with differential, culture and sensitivity).

◆ *Availability.* PO: 250- and 500-mg tablets.

◆ *Dosage and administration.* PO: *Trichomoniasis:* Men and women: 2 g once. Sexual partners must be treated concurrently to prevent reinfection. *Amebic dysentery and amebic liver abscess:* 2 g once daily for 3 days. *Giardiasis:* 2 g once.

Note: Tinidazole should be administered with food to reduce the incidence of GI effects.

◆ *Common adverse effects*

Gastrointestinal

Nausea, vomiting, diarrhea. These adverse effects are usually mild and tend to resolve with continued therapy.

◆ *Serious adverse effects*

Neurologic

Dizziness. Provide for patient safety during episodes of dizziness; report for further evaluation.

Confusion, seizures. Patients receiving high doses of tinidazole, those with histories of seizure activity, and those with significant hepatic impairment are at greater risk of confusion and seizures. Perform a baseline assessment of the patient's degree of alertness and orientation to name, place, and time before initiating therapy. Make regularly scheduled subsequent mental status evaluations and compare findings. Report the development of alterations.

Implement seizure precautions (padded side rails, available oxygen, and suction sets). Make sure that the patient continues with anticonvulsant therapy. If seizures develop, provide for patient safety and then record the exact time of seizure onset and duration of each phase, a description of the specific body parts involved, and any progression in the affected parts. Describe the automatic responses seen during the clonic phase—altered, jerky respirations; frothy salivation; dilated pupils and eye movements; cyanosis; diaphoresis; or incontinence.

◆ *Drug interactions*

Alcohol. Use of alcohol and alcohol-containing preparations, such as OTC cough medications and mouthwashes (e.g., Listerine, Cēpacol), should be avoided during therapy and for 72 hours after discontinuation of tinidazole therapy. Tinidazole inhibits enzymes required to metabolize alcohol, resulting in mild symptoms of abdominal cramping, flushing, headache, nausea, vomiting, and sweating.

Warfarin. Tinidazole may enhance the anticoagulant effects of warfarin during and up to 8 days after taking tinidazole. Observe for the development of petechiae; ecchymoses; nosebleeds; bleeding gums; dark, tarry stools; and bright red or coffee-ground emesis. Monitor the INR and reduce the dosage of warfarin if necessary.

Lithium. Patients receiving higher dosages of lithium are more susceptible to lithium toxicity and potential renal damage. Tinidazole should be initiated only if absolutely necessary. Frequently monitor serum lithium and creatinine concentrations when tinidazole and lithium are administered concurrently.

Phenytoin, fosphenytoin. Tinidazole inhibits phenytoin metabolism. Monitor patients with concurrent therapy for signs of phenytoin toxicity: nystagmus, sedation, and lethargy. Serum levels may be ordered and the dosage of phenytoin reduced.

DRUG CLASS: TOPICAL ANTIFUNGAL AGENTS

Actions

The exact mechanisms whereby antifungal agents act are unknown. However, it is known that cell membranes are altered, resulting in increased permeability, leakage of amino acids and electrolytes, and impaired uptake of essential nutrients needed for cell growth.

Uses

The common topical fungal infections caused by several different dermatophytes are tinea pedis (athlete's foot), tinea cruris (jock itch), tinea corporis (ringworm), and tinea versicolor. *Candida albicans* is the most common cause of oral candidiasis (thrush), cutaneous candidiasis (e.g., diaper rash), and vaginal candidiasis (moniliasis [yeast infection]).

Therapeutic Outcome

The primary therapeutic outcome expected from topical antifungal therapy is elimination of fungal infection.

❖ Nursing Implications for Topical Antifungals
◆ Premedication assessment
1. Obtain baseline assessments of presenting symptoms.
2. Assess for any allergies.

◆ Availability, dosage, and administration. See Table 45.10.
Topical. Apply clean gloves. Wash hands thoroughly before and immediately after application. Cleanse skin with soap and water and dry thoroughly.

For athlete's foot, the powder is most effective in intertriginous areas and in patients for whom a dry environment may enhance the therapeutic response. Instruct patients to wear cotton socks (avoid nylon) if possible and change them two or three times daily. Treatments may be required for 6 weeks or longer with long-standing infections and in areas of thickened skin.

For jock itch or ringworm, wear well-fitting, non-constricting, ventilated clothing.

For all fungal infections, instruct patients to avoid tight-fitting clothing and occlusive dressings unless otherwise instructed by the healthcare provider.

Eye contact. Instruct patients to avoid contact with the eyes and to wash their eyes immediately if contact occurs.

Intravaginal. Give the patient the following instructions:
1. Wash the applicator in warm soapy water after each use so that it does not become a vehicle for reinfection.
2. Consider using a pad to protect clothing.
3. Use the number of doses prescribed even if symptoms disappear or menstruation begins.
4. Refrain from sexual intercourse during therapy (or the male should wear a condom to avoid reinfection).
5. When being treated with vaginal ointment (e.g., Vagistat-1), use contraception other than a diaphragm or condom. Prolonged contact with petrolatum-based products may cause the diaphragm and condom to deteriorate.

◆ Common and serious adverse effects
Integumentary

Irritation. Some patients experience vulvar or vaginal burning, vulvar itching, discharge, soreness, or swelling from the intravaginal products. These adverse effects are usually mild and tend to resolve with continued therapy. Encourage the patient not to discontinue therapy without first consulting the healthcare provider.

Redness, swelling, blistering, oozing. These signs may be an indication of hypersensitivity. Inform the healthcare provider.

◆ Drug interactions. No clinically significant drug interactions have been reported.

DRUG CLASS: SYSTEMIC ANTIFUNGAL AGENTS

amphotericin B (ăm-fō-TĔR-ĭ-sĭn)
amphotericin B sodium desoxycholate ("conventional")
amphotericin B lipid complex
   Abelcet
amphotericin B liposome
   AmBisome

Actions

Amphotericin B is a fungistatic agent that disrupts the cell membrane of fungal cells, resulting in a loss of cellular contents.

Uses

Amphotericin B is used primarily in treating systemic life-threatening fungal infections. It should not be used to treat noninvasive fungal infections such as oral thrush, vaginal candidiasis, and esophageal candidiasis in immunocompetent patients with normal neutrophil counts. There are three dosage forms of amphotericin B, each with different brand names and somewhat different approval for use. Each has different requirements for reconstitution, dilution, filtration, and administration rate. Work closely with the pharmacy department to ensure that the correct dosage form is being reconstituted and diluted properly, and that proper administration technique, including the use of appropriate inline filters and rate of infusion, is being used.

Therapeutic Outcome

The primary therapeutic outcome expected from amphotericin B therapy is elimination of fungal infection.

❖ Nursing Implications for Amphotericin B
◆ Premedication assessment
1. Obtain baseline assessments of presenting symptoms.
2. Record temperature, pulse, respirations, blood pressure, and hydration status.
3. Assess for normal renal function and normal electrolytes before initiating therapy.
4. Assess for any allergies.
5. Gather baseline data about the patient's mental status (e.g., alertness, orientation, confusion), muscle strength, presence of muscle cramps, tremors, nausea, and general appearance (e.g., drowsy, anxious, lethargic).
6. Obtain baseline laboratory studies ordered and review results (e.g., CBC with differential, culture and sensitivity).

◆ Availability
IV:
- Amphotericin B sodium desoxycholate ("conventional" amphotericin B): 50 mg/vial

Table 45.10 Topical Antifungal Agents

GENERIC NAME	BRAND NAME	AVAILABILITY	ADULT DOSAGE RANGE
butenafine	Lotrimin Ultra, Mentax	Cream: 1%	For ringworm, jock itch, athlete's foot: Apply topically to affected area one or two times daily for 1-4 wk
butoconazole	Gynazole-1	Vaginal cream: 2%	For vaginal candidiasis: Insert 1 applicatorful intravaginally at bedtime once
ciclopirox	Loprox	Cream: 0.77% Gel: 0.77% Shampoo: 1% Solution for nails: 8% Topical suspension: 0.77%	For ringworm, jock itch, athlete's foot, cutaneous candidiasis, and tinea versicolor: Massage product into affected skin twice daily for at least 4 wk; shampoo: twice weekly for 4 wk
clotrimazole	Gyne-Lotrimin 3	Vaginal cream: 2%	For vaginal candidiasis: Insert 1 applicatorful at bedtime for 3-7 nights
	Desenex, Alevazol Lotrimin AF	Cream and ointment: 1% Solution: 1% Oral lozenges: 10 mg (troches)	For ringworm, jock itch, athlete's foot: Apply topically to affected skin morning and evening; gently rub in For oral candidiasis: Allow 1 lozenge to dissolve slowly in mouth five times daily for 14 consecutive days
econazole	Ecoza	Cream: 1% Foam: 1%	For ringworm, jock itch, athlete's foot, tinea versicolor: Apply over affected area once daily For cutaneous candidiasis: Apply twice daily (morning and evening)
efinaconazole	Jublia	Solution: 10%	For fungal infections of the toes: Apply to affected toenails once daily for 48 wk
ketoconazole	Nizoral	Cream: 2% Foam: 2% Gel: 2% Shampoo: 1%, 2%	For ringworm, jock itch, athlete's foot, cutaneous candidiasis, tinea versicolor: Massage cream into affected and surrounding tissue once daily; may require 2-4 wk of treatment For seborrheic dermatitis: Cream and foam: Massage into affected area twice daily for 4 wk Gel: Massage into affected area once daily for 2 wk For dandruff: Moisten hair and scalp with water; apply shampoo and lather gently for 1 min; rinse and reapply, leaving lather on scalp for 3 min; rinse thoroughly and dry hair; apply shampoo twice weekly for 4 wk with at least 3 days between shampooing
luliconazole	Luzu	Cream, external 1%	For jock itch, truncal lesions: Apply once daily for 1 wk For athlete's foot: Apply once daily for 2 wk
miconazole	Monistat 3	Vaginal suppositories: 200 mg Vaginal cream: 2%	For vaginal candidiasis: Monistat 3: Insert 1 suppository intravaginally at bedtime for 3 days
	Monistat 7	Vaginal suppositories: 100 mg Vaginal cream: 2%	Monistat 7: Insert 1 applicatorful or 1 suppository intravaginally at bedtime for 7 days
	Micatin	Cream: 2% Powder: 2% Solution: 2% Spray: 2% Ointment: 2%	For ringworm, jock itch, athlete's foot, cutaneous candidiasis, tinea versicolor: Cover affected areas twice daily (morning and evening); treatment may require 2-4 wk
naftifine	Naftin	Cream: 1, 2% Gel: 1, 2%	For ringworm, jock itch, athlete's foot: Cream: massage into affected area once daily Gel: massage into affected area twice daily

Table 45.10 Topical Antifungal Agents—cont'd

GENERIC NAME	BRAND NAME	AVAILABILITY	ADULT DOSAGE RANGE
nystatin		Vaginal tablets: 100,000 units	For vaginal candidiasis: Insert 1 tablet intravaginally daily for 2 wk
		Oral suspension: 100,000 units/mL	For oral candidiasis: Sip 4-6 mL four times daily; retain in mouth as long as possible before swallowing
		Oral tablets: 500,000 units	For nonesophageal mucous membrane GI candidiasis: 1 or 2 tablets to three times a day
		Cream, ointment, powder	For cutaneous candidiasis: Apply to affected area two or three times daily
oxiconazole nitrate	Oxistat	Cream: 1% Lotion: 1%	For ringworm, jock itch, athlete's foot: Massage into affected areas once to twice daily at bedtime
sertaconazole	Ertaczo	Cream: 2%	For athlete's foot: Apply twice daily for 4 wk
sulconazole	Exelderm	Cream: 1% Solution: 1%	For ringworm, jock itch, athlete's foot: Massage into affected area once or twice daily
tavaborole	Kerydin	Solution: 5%	For onychomycosis of the toenail: Apply to affected toenail(s) once daily for 48 wk
terbinafine	Lamisil AT	Cream: 1% Spray: 1% Gel: 1%	For tinea versicolor, athlete's foot, jock rash, ringworm: Massage into affected area once or twice daily; treatment may require 2-4 wk
terconazole	Terazol 7 Terazol 3 Zazole	Vaginal cream: 0.4% Vaginal cream: 0.8% Vaginal suppository: 80 mg	For vaginal candidiasis: Insert 1 applicatorful intravaginally daily at bedtime for 3 (0.8% cream) or 7 (0.4% cream) consecutive days Insert 1 suppository intravaginally once daily at bedtime for 3 consecutive days
tioconazole	Vagistat-1	Vaginal ointment: 6.5%	For vaginal candidiasis: Insert 1 applicatorful intravaginally at bedtime once
tolnaftate	Tinactin	Cream: 1% Solution: 1% Spray: 1% Powder: 1%	For ringworm, jock itch, athlete's foot, cutaneous candidiasis, tinea versicolor: Cover affected areas twice daily (morning and evening); treatment may require 2-4 wk

- Amphotericin B lipid complex (Abelcet): 5 mg/mL in 20-mL vial
- Amphotericin B liposome (AmBisome): 50 mg/vial

◆ *Dosage and administration.* Dosage varies depending on the dosage form and the organism for which the medicine is being used. Consult the healthcare provider, laboratory results, and the pharmacist to provide checks on the appropriate dose and administration of the antifungal agent.

◆ *Common and serious adverse effects*
General
Malaise, fever, chills, headache, nausea, vomiting. These adverse effects tend to be dose related and may be minimized by slow infusion, reduction of dosage, and alternate-day administration. Check PRN and standing orders for drugs (e.g., antihistamines, aspirin, antiemetics) that may alleviate these symptoms.
Urinary
Nephrotoxicity. Nephrotoxicity may be manifested by increases in excretion of uric acid, potassium, and magnesium; oliguria; granular casts in the urine; proteinuria; and increased BUN and serum creatinine levels.

Monitor urinalysis and kidney function tests for abnormal results. Report increasing BUN and creatinine levels, decreasing urine output or decreasing urine specific gravity (despite amount of fluid intake), casts or protein in the urine, frank blood or smoky-colored urine, or RBCs in excess of 0 to 3 RBCs/HPF (see Table 41.1) on the urinalysis report. Report input and output, as well as a progressive decrease in daily urine volume or changes in visual characteristics.
Hematologic
Electrolyte imbalance. The electrolytes most commonly altered are potassium (K^+) and magnesium (Mg^{2+}). Hypokalemia is most likely to occur. Many symptoms associated with altered fluid and electrolyte balance are subtle and resemble general symptoms of drug toxicity or the disease process itself. Gather data about changes in the patient's mental status (e.g., alertness, orientation, confusion), muscle strength, muscle cramps, tremors, nausea, and general appearance (e.g., drowsy, anxious, lethargic). Always check the electrolyte reports for early

indications of electrolyte imbalance. Keep accurate records of input and output, daily weights, and vital signs.

Vascular

Thrombophlebitis. Carefully assess patients receiving IV amphotericin B for the development of thrombophlebitis. Inspect the IV infusion area often when providing care; inspect during dressing changes and whenever the infusion is changed to a new site. Always investigate pain at the IV site. Report redness, warmth, tenderness to touch, and edema in the affected part.

◆ *Drug interactions*

Corticosteroids. The concurrent use of amphotericin B and corticosteroids (e.g., prednisone) may enhance the loss of potassium. Check potassium levels and monitor more closely for hypokalemia.

Nephrotoxic potential. Combining amphotericin B with other nephrotoxic agents such as aminoglycosides, diuretics, or cisplatin should be done with extreme caution. Monitor closely for signs of nephrotoxicity.

Digoxin. Because amphotericin B may induce hypokalemia, use cautiously in patients receiving digoxin. Hypokalemia may induce digoxin toxicity. Monitor patients for dysrhythmias, nausea, and bradycardia.

Diuretics. Thiazide and loop diuretics may induce hypokalemia. Monitor patients receiving amphotericin B and diuretic therapy very closely for hypokalemia.

---

fluconazole (flū-KŎN-ă-zōl)
Diflucan (DĪ-flū-kăn)
⇄ *Do not confuse Diflucan with Dilantin or Diprivan.*

Actions

Fluconazole is an antifungal agent chemically related to ketoconazole and itraconazole. It acts by inhibiting certain metabolic pathways in fungi, thus interfering with cell wall synthesis.

Uses

Fluconazole is used for oral and IV treatment of cryptococcal meningitis and oropharyngeal, esophageal, vulvovaginal, or systemic candidiasis. Fluconazole therapy is usually reserved for patients in whom other antifungal therapy was not tolerated or was ineffective. Fluconazole is also used prophylactically to prevent candidiasis in bone marrow transplant patients who are receiving radiation or chemotherapy treatment and in patients with human immunodeficiency virus (HIV) infection. Fluconazole is also approved as a single-dose treatment of vaginal candidiasis in immunocompetent patients.

Therapeutic Outcomes

The primary therapeutic outcomes expected from fluconazole therapy are as follows:

1. Prevention of systemic fungal infections
2. Elimination of fungal infection

❖ **Nursing Implications for Fluconazole**

◆ *Premedication assessment*

1. Obtain baseline assessments of presenting symptoms.
2. Record temperature, pulse, respirations, blood pressure, and hydration status.
3. Assess for and record any gastric symptoms and abnormal liver and renal function before initiating therapy.
4. Assess for any allergies.
5. Obtain baseline laboratory studies ordered and review results (e.g., CBC with differential, culture and sensitivity).

◆ *Availability.* **PO:** 50-, 100-, 150-, and 200-mg tablets; 10 and 40 mg/mL in 35-mL bottle. **IV:** 100-, 200- and 400-mg vials.

◆ *Dosage and administration.* **PO:** 100 to 400 mg daily; dosage must be individualized to type of infection being treated. **IV:** same as for PO.

◆ *Common adverse effects*

Gastrointestinal

Nausea, vomiting, diarrhea. These adverse effects are usually mild and tend to resolve with continued therapy. Encourage the patient not to discontinue therapy without first consulting the healthcare provider.

◆ *Serious adverse effects*

Integumentary

Rash. Report symptoms for further evaluation by the healthcare provider. Do not administer any further doses until so ordered by the healthcare provider.

Gastrointestinal

Hepatotoxicity. The symptoms of hepatotoxicity are anorexia, nausea, vomiting, jaundice, hepatomegaly, splenomegaly, and abnormal liver function test results (e.g., elevated bilirubin, AST, ALT, GGT, and alkaline phosphatase levels; increased INR).

◆ *Drug interactions*

Cimetidine. Cimetidine inhibits the absorption of fluconazole. Concurrent use is not recommended.

Diuretics. Diuretics inhibit the excretion of fluconazole. Monitor patients for an increase in frequency of adverse effects. The dosage of fluconazole may need to be decreased if concurrent therapy with diuretics is required.

Toxicity induced by fluconazole. Fluconazole can increase serum concentrations of alfentanil, benzodiazepines, buspirone, cyclosporine, losartan, phenytoin, vincristine, zidovudine, zolpidem, tricyclic antidepressants, HMG-CoA reductase inhibitors (e.g., simvastatin, atorvastatin), protease inhibitors (e.g., ritonavir, indinavir), and oral sulfonylurea hypoglycemic agents (e.g., glipizide, glyburide). Fluconazole can also potentiate the anticoagulant effects of warfarin. Read individual drug monographs for monitoring parameters of toxicity from these agents.

griseofulvin microsize (grĭz-ē-ō-FŬL-vĭn)
griseofulvin ultramicrosize

Actions

Griseofulvin is a fungistatic agent that acts by stopping cell division and new cell growth.

Uses

Griseofulvin is used to treat ringworm of the scalp, body, nails, and feet. After griseofulvin is absorbed, it is incorporated into the keratin of the nails, skin, and hair in therapeutic amounts. The infecting fungus is not killed, but its growth into new cells is prevented. Once the cells are shed or removed, they are replaced by new cells that are free from the infection. Because of slow nail growth, treatment is often required for several months.

Therapeutic Outcome

The primary therapeutic outcome expected from griseofulvin therapy is elimination of fungal infection.

❖ **Nursing Implications for Griseofulvin**

◆ *Premedication assessment*

1. Obtain baseline assessments of presenting symptoms.
2. Record temperature, pulse, respirations, blood pressure, and hydration status.
3. Assess for and record any gastric symptoms or abnormal hematologic, liver, or renal function tests before initiating therapy.
4. Assess for any allergies.
5. Obtain baseline laboratory studies ordered and review results (e.g., CBC with differential, culture and sensitivity, liver and renal function tests).
6. Record results of baseline mental status examination.

◆ *Availability.* **PO:** *Microsize:* 500-mg tablets; 125-mg/5-mL oral suspension in 120-mL bottle. *Ultramicrosize:* 125- and 250-mg tablets.

◆ *Dosage and administration.* **Adult:** *PO: Microsize:* depending on the specific organism and the location of the infection, 500 mg to 1 g in single or divided doses daily. Absorption from the GI tract may be increased by administering griseofulvin with a high-fat meal.

Adult: PO: *Ultramicrosize:* depending on the specific organism and the location of the infection, 375 to 750 mg daily in divided doses. Absorption from the GI tract may be increased by administering griseofulvin with a high-fat meal.

◆ *Common adverse effects*
Gastrointestinal

Nausea, vomiting, anorexia, abdominal cramps. These adverse effects are usually mild and tend to resolve with continued therapy. Encourage the patient not to discontinue therapy without first consulting the healthcare provider.

◆ *Serious adverse effects*
Integumentary, hypersensitivity

Urticaria, rash, pruritus. Hypersensitivity reactions, manifested by itching, urticaria, and rash, are relatively common. Report symptoms for further evaluation by the healthcare provider. Pruritus may be relieved by adding baking soda to the bath water.

Photosensitivity. The patient should be cautioned to avoid exposure to sunlight and ultraviolet light. Suggest wearing long-sleeved clothing, hat, and sunglasses when outdoors. Discourage the use of tanning lamps. Consult the healthcare provider about the advisability of continuing therapy.

Neurologic

Confusion. Perform a baseline assessment of the patient's degree of alertness and orientation to name, place, and time before initiating therapy. Make regularly scheduled subsequent mental status evaluations, and compare findings. Report the development of alterations.

Dizziness. Provide for patient safety during episodes of dizziness; report to the healthcare provider for further evaluation.

Immune system (opportunistic infections)

Secondary infections. With griseofulvin, oral thrush, genital and anal pruritus, vaginitis, and vaginal discharge may occur. Report promptly to the healthcare provider because these infections are resistant to the original antimicrobial agent. Teach the importance of meticulous oral and perineal personal hygiene.

Hematologic. Routine laboratory studies (e.g., RBC, white blood cell, and differential counts) are scheduled for patients taking griseofulvin for 30 days or longer. Stress the importance of returning for this laboratory work. Monitor for sore throat, fever, purpura, jaundice, or excessive and progressive weakness.

Renal

Nephrotoxicity. Monitor urinalysis and kidney function tests for abnormal results. Report increasing BUN and creatinine levels, decreasing urine output or decreasing urine specific gravity (despite amount of fluid intake), casts or protein in the urine, frank blood or smoky-colored urine, or RBCs in excess of 0 to 3 RBCs/HPF (see Table 41.1) on the urinalysis report.

Gastrointestinal

Hepatotoxicity. The symptoms of hepatotoxicity are anorexia, nausea, vomiting, jaundice, hepatomegaly, splenomegaly, and abnormal liver function test results (e.g., elevated bilirubin, AST, ALT, GGT, and alkaline phosphatase levels; increased INR).

◆ *Drug interactions*

Warfarin. Griseofulvin may diminish the anticoagulant effects of warfarin. Monitor the INR and increase the dosage of warfarin if necessary.

Phenobarbital. The absorption of griseofulvin is impaired when combined with phenobarbital. If concurrent therapy cannot be avoided, administer the griseofulvin in divided doses three times daily.

Oral contraceptives. Griseofulvin may cause amenorrhea, increased breakthrough bleeding, and possibly decreased contraceptive efficacy when used concomitantly with oral contraceptives. Other methods of contraception (e.g., condoms and foam) should be considered during griseofulvin therapy.

---

itraconazole (ĭt-ră-KŎN-ă-zōl)
    Sporanox (SPŌR-ă-nŏks)

Actions

Itraconazole is an antifungal agent chemically related to fluconazole and ketoconazole. It acts by interfering with cell wall synthesis, causing leakage of cellular contents.

Uses

Itraconazole is used orally to treat candidiasis, chronic mucocutaneous candidiasis, oral thrush, onychomycosis, candiduria, coccidioidomycosis, histoplasmosis, chromomycosis, blastomycosis, and paracoccidioidomycosis. It is also effective against *Aspergillus* spp.

> **! Medication Safety Alert**
>
> Do not administer itraconazole to patients with a history of heart failure. Itraconazole is a negative inotropic agent and may seriously aggravate heart failure.
>
> Itraconazole has many drug interactions because it is a potent inhibitor of CYP3A4-metabolizing enzymes in the liver (see Drug Interactions later in this section). Coadministration of itraconazole with pimozide, dofetilide, or quinidine is *contraindicated*. Fatal reactions may result.

Therapeutic Outcome

The primary therapeutic outcome expected from itraconazole therapy is elimination of fungal infection.

 Nursing Implications for Itraconazole

◆ *Premedication assessment*

1. Obtain baseline assessments of presenting symptoms.
2. Record temperature, pulse, respirations, blood pressure, and hydration status.
3. Assess for and record any gastric symptoms, abnormal liver function tests, or heart failure before beginning therapy.
4. Assess for any allergies.
5. Obtain baseline laboratory studies ordered and review results (e.g., liver function tests).

◆ *Availability.* **PO:** 100-mg capsules; 200-mg tablets; 10 mg/mL oral solution in 150-mL containers.

◆ *Dosage and administration.* **Adult:** *PO:* 100 to 400 mg daily. Dosages of more than 200 mg should be given in two divided doses. Instruct the patient to take with a full meal to ensure maximum absorption.

> **! Medication Safety Alert**
>
> Do not use itraconazole capsules and itraconazole oral solution interchangeably. Capsules are used to treat systemic fungal infections. The oral solution should only be used to treat oral or esophageal candidiasis in adult HIV-positive or other immunocompromised patients.

◆ *Common adverse effects*

Gastrointestinal

Nausea, vomiting. These adverse effects are usually mild and tend to resolve with continued therapy. Encourage the patient not to discontinue therapy without first consulting the healthcare provider. Administer with a full meal for maximum absorption.

◆ *Serious adverse effects*

Gastrointestinal

Hepatotoxicity. Liver function tests are recommended before initiating therapy, with follow-up tests biweekly to monthly. The symptoms of hepatotoxicity are anorexia, nausea, vomiting, jaundice, hepatomegaly, splenomegaly, and abnormal liver function tests (e.g., elevated bilirubin, AST, ALT, GGT, and alkaline phosphatase levels; increased INR).

Cardiovascular

Heart failure. Monitor the six cardinal signs of heart disease—dyspnea, chest pain, fatigue, edema, syncope, and palpitations—and individualize care to deal with the degree of impairment (see also Chapter 27).

Integumentary

Pruritus, rash. Report symptoms to the healthcare provider for further evaluation. Pruritus may be relieved by adding baking soda to the bath water.

◆ *Drug interactions*

Histamine-2 antagonists, antacids, protease inhibitors. Histamine-2 antagonists (e.g., cimetidine, famotidine, ranitidine, nizatidine), antacids, indinavir, and ritonavir inhibit the absorption of itraconazole. Concurrent use is not recommended.

Carbamazepine, phenytoin, rifampin. Concurrent administration of itraconazole and these agents has resulted in a significant decrease in itraconazole activity and clinical failure. The mechanism is unknown, but it is suspected that these agents stimulate the metabolism of itraconazole. If these agents are to be used concurrently, itraconazole levels must be monitored to ensure therapeutic effect.

Toxicity induced by itraconazole. Itraconazole can increase serum concentrations of alfentanil, benzodiazepines (e.g., triazolam, midazolam, alprazolam), buspirone, calcium channel blockers (e.g., felodipine, nisoldipine, nifedipine, verapamil), carbamazepine, cyclosporine, digoxin, dofetilide, haloperidol, HMG-CoA reductase inhibitors (e.g., atorvastatin, lovastatin), isoniazid, pimozide, tacrolimus, tolterodine, vincristine, zolpidem, and oral sulfonylurea hypoglycemic agents (e.g., glipizide, glyburide) and other drugs metabolized by the CYP3A4-metabolizing enzymes. Itraconazole can also potentiate the anticoagulant effects of warfarin. Read individual drug monographs for monitoring parameters of toxicity from these agents.

---

terbinafine (tŭr-BĬN-ă-fēn)

Actions

Terbinafine is an allylamine derivative that acts by inhibiting squalene epoxidase, a key enzyme required in sterol biosynthesis in fungi. This action causes accumulation of squalene and a deficiency of ergosterol, resulting in fungal cell death.

Uses

Terbinafine is used in the treatment of onychomycosis of the toenail or fingernail caused by dermatophytes. Maximum clinical effect is observed months after the fungus has been eradicated when a new nail has grown. The granules are used to treat tinea capitis in children 4 years of age and older.

Therapeutic Outcome

The primary therapeutic outcome expected from terbinafine therapy is elimination of fungal infection in toenails and fingernails.

❖ **Nursing Implications for Terbinafine**
◆ *Premedication assessment*
   1. Obtain baseline assessments of presenting symptoms.
   2. Record temperature, pulse, respirations, blood pressure, and hydration status.
   3. Assess for and record any gastric symptoms before initiating therapy.
   4. Assess for any allergies.
   5. Obtain baseline laboratory studies ordered and review results (e.g., CBC with differential, culture, liver function tests, and electrolyte levels).

◆ *Availability.* **PO:** 250-mg tablets.

◆ *Dosage and administration.* **Adult:** *PO:* 250 mg daily for 6 weeks to treat fungal infections of the fingernail and 12 weeks for treatment of infections of the toenail.
   Pediatric: *PO: dosage by weight:* less than 25 kg, 125 mg/day; 25 to 35 kg, 187.5 mg/day; more than 35 kg, 250 mg/day.

◆ *Serious adverse effects*
   Integumentary, immune system
   Pruritus, rash, fever, chills. Report symptoms to the healthcare provider for further evaluation. Pruritus may be relieved by adding baking soda to the bath water.
   Renal
   Nephrotoxicity. Assess for increasing BUN and creatinine levels, decreasing urine output, decreasing urine specific gravity, casts or protein in the urine, frank blood

or smoky-colored urine, or RBCs in excess of 0 to 3 RBCs/HPF (see Table 41.1) on the urinalysis report.
   Gastrointestinal
   Hepatotoxicity. Review laboratory studies (e.g., bilirubin, AST, ALT, GGT, alkaline phosphatase levels; increased INR) and report abnormal findings to the healthcare provider.
   Hematologic
   Neutropenia, lymphopenia. Neutropenia (neutrophil count <1000 cells/mm^3) and lymphopenia have been observed in patients receiving terbinafine. Monitor the CBC with differential in patients receiving treatment for longer than 6 weeks.

◆ *Drug interactions*
   Selective serotonin reuptake inhibitors and tricyclic antidepressants. Terbinafine can increase serum concentrations of selective serotonin reuptake inhibitors and tricyclic antidepressants. Monitor patients for signs of toxicity such as central nervous system stimulation, seizure activity, and arrhythmias.
   Cyclosporine. Terbinafine can decrease serum concentrations of cyclosporine. Monitor patients for signs of transplant rejection. Check trough cyclosporine levels.
   Caffeine. Terbinafine can increase serum concentrations of caffeine. Monitor patients for excitability, agitation, irritability, and tachycardia.
   Dextromethorphan. Terbinafine can increase serum concentrations of dextromethorphan. Monitor patients for dizziness, drowsiness, GI disturbances, altered sensory perception, ataxia, slurred speech, and dysphoria.
   Rifampin. Rifampin reduces serum levels of terbinafine. Use of another antifungal agent whose metabolism is not induced by rifampin may be necessary.
   Cimetidine. Cimetidine may inhibit the metabolism of terbinafine, increasing the potential for toxicity from terbinafine. Switching to another H$_2$ antagonist, such as famotidine, that is not likely to inhibit metabolism may resolve the interaction. Continue to monitor for terbinafine toxicity.

DRUG CLASS: ANTIVIRAL AGENTS

---

acyclovir (ă-SĬK-lō-vĭr)
Zovirax (ZŌ-vĭr-ăks)
⇄ *Do not confuse Zovirax with Zyvox.*

Actions

Acyclovir is an antiviral agent that acts by inhibiting viral cell replication.

Uses

Acyclovir is used topically to treat initial infections of herpes genitalis and non–life-threatening cases of mucocutaneous herpes simplex virus infections in patients with suppressed immune systems. The oral form is used to treat initial episodes and for management of recurrent episodes of genital herpes in certain patients. The IV form is used to treat initial and recurrent mucosal and cutaneous herpes simplex virus types 1 and 2 infections in immunosuppressed adults and children and to treat severe initial clinical episodes of herpes genitalis in patients who are not immunosuppressed.

Therapeutic Outcome

The primary therapeutic outcome expected from acyclovir therapy is elimination of symptoms of viral infection.

❖ Nursing Implications for Acyclovir

◆ Premedication assessment

1. Obtain baseline assessments of presenting symptoms.
2. Record temperature, pulse, respirations, blood pressure, and hydration status.
3. Assess for and record any abnormal renal function before beginning therapy.
4. Assess for any allergies.
5. Obtain baseline laboratory studies ordered and review results (e.g., renal function tests).
6. Perform baseline mental status examination (e.g., orientation).

◆ Availability. *Topical:* 5% ointment and cream. *PO:* 200-mg capsules; 400- and 800-mg tablets; 200-mg/5-mL suspension. *IV:* 50 mg/mL in 10- and 20-mL vials.

◆ Dosage and administration. **Adult:** *Topical:* Apply to each lesion every 3 hours, six times daily for 7 days. A finger cot or rubber gloves should be used to avoid the spread of virus to other tissues and people. Use meticulous hand hygiene technique before and after applying the ointment. *Do not* apply to the eyes. It is not an ophthalmic ointment.

IV: Dosage for patients with normal renal function: 5 to 10 mg/kg every 8 hours for 5 to 7 days. Acyclovir is reconstituted with 10 mL of preservative-free sterile water for injection to provide a solution concentration of 50 mg/mL. The solution is stable for 12 hours. This solution should be further diluted by a glucose and electrolyte IV fluid to a concentration of 1 to 7 mg/mL before administration (stable for 24 hours). Infuse over at least 1 hour to well-hydrated patients to prevent renal damage. Observe for phlebitis at the infusion site. Bolus or rapid IV infusions may result in renal tubular damage.

PO: Initial treatment of genital herpes: 200 mg every 4 hours while the patient is awake, for a total of 1000 mg daily for 10 days. *Chronic suppressive therapy for recurrent disease:* 400 mg twice daily for up to 12 months. Some patients require 200 mg five times daily. *Intermittent therapy:* 200 mg every 4 hours while the patient is awake, for a total of 1000 mg for 5 days. Therapy should be initiated at the earliest sign or symptom (prodrome) of recurrence.

Pediatric: *Topical:* same as for adult patients. *IV:* patients older than 12 years: same as for adult patients.

◆ Serious adverse effects

Integumentary

Pruritus, rash, burning. Report symptoms to the healthcare provider for further evaluation. Pruritus may be relieved by adding baking soda to the bath water.

Rash, hives. Assess, describe, and chart the location and extent of these presenting symptoms. Report to the healthcare provider for further evaluation.

Diaphoresis. Diaphoresis can be serious if the patient is not well hydrated. Assess hydration state, monitor electrolytes, and provide nursing interventions (e.g., clean, dry linens; adequate fluid intake).

Vascular

Intravenous therapy. Avoid IV infusion in the lower extremities and areas with varicosities. Use proper technique when starting the IV solution. Carefully assess at regularly scheduled intervals for signs of developing phlebitis. Inspect for redness, warmth, tenderness to touch, edema, or pain.

Renal

Nephrotoxicity. Monitor urinalysis and kidney function tests for abnormal results. Report increasing BUN and creatinine levels, decreasing urine output or decreasing urine specific gravity (despite amount of fluid intake), casts or protein in the urine, frank blood or smoky-colored urine, or RBCs in excess of 0 to 3 RBCs/HPF (see Table 41.1) on the urinalysis report.

Cardiovascular

Hypotension. Record the blood pressure in both supine and sitting positions before and during administration of this drug. Caution the patient to rise slowly from a supine or sitting position.

Neurologic

Confusion. Perform a baseline assessment of the patient's degree of alertness and orientation to name, place, and time *before* initiating therapy. Make regularly scheduled subsequent mental status evaluations and compare findings. Report development of alterations in consciousness.

◆ Drug interactions

Probenecid. Probenecid may reduce urinary excretion of acyclovir. Monitor closely for signs of toxicity from acyclovir.

Theophylline. Acyclovir may increase theophylline levels. Monitor theophylline serum levels.

Phenytoin, fosphenytoin, valproic acid. Acyclovir may decrease phenytoin, fosphenytoin, and valproic acid levels. Monitor serum levels and observe for increased frequency of seizure activity.

Zidovudine. Patients may complain of severe drowsiness and lethargy when acyclovir and zidovudine are used concurrently. Observe for patient safety.

---

famciclovir (făm-SĬK-lō-vĭr)

Actions

Famciclovir is a prodrug of penciclovir, an antiviral agent that acts by inhibiting viral cell replication.

Uses

Famciclovir is used orally to treat recurrent infections of genital herpes and for the management of acute herpes zoster (shingles). In patients with genital herpes, famciclovir reduces the time of viral shedding, the duration of symptoms, and the time of healing if started within 6 hours of the onset of symptoms and continued for 5 days. In patients with shingles, if therapy is begun within 72 hours and continued for 7 days, famciclovir reduces the times to full crusting, loss of vesicles, loss of ulcers, and loss of crusts more effectively than placebo treatment. Early treatment with famciclovir can also reduce the duration of postherpetic neuralgia.

Therapeutic Outcome

The primary therapeutic outcome expected from famciclovir therapy is elimination of symptoms of viral infection.

❖ Nursing Implications for Famciclovir
◆ *Premedication assessment*
1. Obtain baseline assessments of presenting symptoms.
2. Record temperature, pulse, respirations, blood pressure, and hydration status.
3. Assess for and record any abnormal renal function before initiating therapy.
4. Assess for any allergies.
5. Perform baseline mental status examination (e.g., orientation).
6. Obtain baseline laboratory studies ordered and review results (e.g., renal function tests).

◆ *Availability. PO:* 125-, 250-, and 500-mg tablets.

◆ *Dosage and administration.* **Adult:** *PO: Treatment of genital herpes:* Recurrent episodes: 1000 mg twice daily for 1 day. Therapy should be started within 6 hours of the first sign or symptom of herpes breakout. *Treatment of herpes zoster (shingles):* 500 mg every 8 hours for 7 days. To be effective, therapy must be started within 72 hours of the onset of symptoms.

◆ *Common adverse effects*
Gastrointestinal
Nausea, vomiting. These adverse effects are usually mild and tend to resolve with continued therapy. Encourage the patient not to discontinue therapy without first consulting the healthcare provider. Administer with food or milk to reduce irritation.
Neurologic
Headache. This adverse effect is usually mild and tends to resolve with continued therapy. Encourage the patient not to discontinue therapy without first consulting the healthcare provider.

◆ *Serious adverse effects*
Neurologic
Confusion. Perform a baseline assessment of the patient's degree of alertness and orientation to name, place, and time before initiating therapy. Make regularly scheduled subsequent mental status evaluations and compare findings. Report the development of alterations in consciousness.

◆ *Drug interactions*
Probenecid. Probenecid may reduce urinary excretion of famciclovir. Monitor closely for signs of toxicity from famciclovir.

oseltamivir (ō-sĕl-TĂM-ĭ-vĭr)
Tamiflu (TĂM-ĭ-flū)
⇄ *Do not confuse Tamiflu with tamoxifen or Theraflu.*

Actions

Oseltamivir is an antiviral agent that acts by inhibiting neuraminidase, an enzyme on the viral cell coat necessary for reproduction and spread of viral cell particles.

Uses

Oseltamivir was the first neuraminidase inhibitor approved for oral use in treating uncomplicated acute illness caused by influenza. Studies show that the duration of symptoms of influenza infection (e.g., nasal congestion, sore throat, cough, myalgia, fatigue, headache, chills, sweats) will be reduced by about 1 day (4 days versus 5 days) if the patient has been symptomatic for no more than 2 days when treatment is started. The severity of symptoms and potential for complications from secondary infection are also significantly reduced. It is not known whether oseltamivir is effective in preventing influenza infection, and it should not be used as a substitute for annual influenza vaccination. Oseltamivir has not been shown to reduce the risk of transmission of influenza to others.

Therapeutic Outcomes

The primary therapeutic outcome expected from oseltamivir therapy is reduced symptomatology caused by influenza virus infection. It may also reduce the incidence of opportunistic secondary infections such as pneumonia.

❖ Nursing Implications for Oseltamivir
◆ *Premedication assessment*
1. Obtain baseline assessments of presenting symptoms.
2. Record temperature, pulse, respirations, blood pressure, and hydration status.
3. Assess for and record any gastric symptoms before initiating therapy.
4. Assess for any allergies.
5. Obtain baseline laboratory studies ordered and review results.

◆ *Availability. PO:* 30-, 45-, and 75-mg capsules; 6 mg/mL oral suspension in 60-mL container.

◆ *Dosage and administration.* **Adult:** *PO:* 75 mg twice daily for 5 days. Treatment should begin within 2 days after the onset of symptoms of influenza. Patients may also take decongestants, analgesics, and antipyretic agents to reduce symptomatology.

◆ *Common adverse effects*
Gastrointestinal
Nausea, vomiting. Patients receiving oseltamivir may develop nausea and vomiting within the first 2 days of treatment. Administering with food or milk will minimize the incidence of nausea and vomiting. If these symptoms continue, report to the healthcare provider for evaluation of other potential complications.

Immune system
Cough, sore throat, fever, continuing symptoms. If the patient starts coughing up yellow or green sputum, if a sore throat worsens and becomes severe, if fever returns after going away, or if symptoms last longer than 1 or 2 weeks, report to the healthcare provider for evaluation of other potential complications.

◆ *Drug interactions.* No clinically significant drug interactions have been reported.

---

ribavirin (rī-bă-VĪ-rĭn)
  Virazole (VĪ-ră-zōl) (aerosol)
  Rebetol (rĕ-bĕt-ōl) (oral capsules and suspension)
  Ribasphere (RĪ-bă-sfēr) (oral tablets and capsules)

Actions
The mechanism of action of ribavirin is unknown.

Uses
Ribavirin has been shown to have inhibitory activity against members of the DNA-type viral families of Adenoviridae, Herpesviridae, and Poxviridae. The RNA viruses for which ribavirin exerts inhibitory activity are the influenza and parainfluenza viruses and respiratory syncytial virus (RSV).

Ribavirin has been given US Food and Drug Administration (FDA) approval to be used by aerosol administration to treat severe lower respiratory tract infections caused by RSV in infants and young children. Ribavirin aerosol (Virazole) should not be used in adults.

Ribavirin has also been given FDA approval to be used in oral capsular form (Rebetol) in combination with interferon alfa-2b, recombinant (Intron A) injection for the treatment of chronic hepatitis C in patients with compensated liver disease previously untreated with interferon alfa or in those who have relapsed following interferon alfa therapy. Because of the potential for hemolytic anemia, patients with a history of heart disease should not be treated with ribavirin.

Ribavirin has also been given FDA approval to be used in oral tablet form (Ribasphere) in combination with peginterferon alfa-2a injection for the treatment of chronic hepatitis C in patients with compensated liver disease previously untreated with interferon alfa.

Therapeutic Outcome
The primary therapeutic outcome expected from ribavirin therapy is elimination of viral infection—RSV in infants and children and chronic hepatitis C in adults.

❖ **Nursing Implications for Ribavirin**
◆ *Premedication assessment*
1. Obtain baseline assessments of presenting symptoms.
2. Record temperature, pulse, respirations, blood pressure, and hydration status.
3. Assess for and record any gastric symptoms before initiating therapy.
4. Assess for any allergies.
5. Obtain baseline laboratory studies ordered and review results (e.g., pulmonary function tests, hemoglobin, hematocrit, CBC with differential, platelets, liver function tests [GGT, AST, and ALT levels]).
6. Determine if the patient is pregnant; if pregnancy is suspected, check with the healthcare provider before administering the drug.

◆ *Availability. PO:* 200-, 400-, 600-mg tablets; 200-mg capsules; 40 mg/mL oral solution in 100-mL containers.
  Inhalation: aerosol powder: 6-g vials of powder for reconstitution.

◆ *Dosage and administration.* **PO:** *Capsules (dosage by weight):* less than 75 kg: 400 mg in the morning, 600 mg in the evening daily; more than 75 kg: 600 mg in the morning; 600 mg in the evening daily. *Tablets:* 800 to 1200 mg administered orally in two divided doses with food. The dose should be individualized to the patient, depending on baseline disease genotype, response to therapy, and tolerability of the regimen.

  Inhalation: *Aerosol powder:* Ribavirin must be administered through a specific, small-particle aerosol generator (SPAG-2):
1. Using aseptic technique, reconstitute 6 g of drug by adding at least 75 mL of sterile water for injection to the 100-mL vial. Shake well.
2. When dissolved, transfer the contents to a clean, sterilized, 500-mL, wide-mouth Erlenmeyer flask (SPAG-2 reservoir) and further dilute with sterile water for injection to a final volume of 300 mL. The final concentration is 20 mg/mL.
3. Administer ribavirin at an initial concentration of 20 mg/mL through the SPAG-2 reservoir. Treatment is carried out for 12 to 18 hours daily for at least 3 and no more than 7 days. The aerosol is delivered from the generator to the patient via an oxygen hood or face mask. It should not be

administered concurrently with any other aerosolized medication.

4. The liquid in the reservoir should not have any other substances (e.g., antibiotics) added to it. Discard and replace ribavirin solution in the SPAG-2 at least every 24 hours.

Pregnant women. Ribavirin is contraindicated for women who are or may become pregnant during exposure to the drug. It is also contraindicated in the male partners of women who are pregnant or who may become pregnant. Ribavirin has been reported to cause birth defects in several animal species. It is not completely eliminated from human blood for at least 4 weeks after administration. It is recommended that at least two reliable forms of effective contraception be used during treatment and during the 6-month posttreatment follow-up to prevent pregnancy.

Patients on respirators. Ribavirin is not recommended for patients requiring assisted ventilation because precipitation of the drug in the respiratory equipment may interfere with safe and effective use of the ventilator by these patients. If it is deemed necessary to treat a patient with ribavirin who is also receiving ventilatory support, prefilters must be placed in the equipment to prevent precipitation in the endotracheal tube or on the valves and tubing.

◆ *Common adverse effects.* Rash and conjunctivitis tend to occur because of local irritation from poorly placed inhalation equipment. Work with the patient for optimal fit. Methylcellulose eyedrops may be applied to reduce conjunctival irritation.

◆ *Serious adverse effects*

Respiratory

Diminishing pulmonary function. Perform baseline pulmonary function tests to assess whether the patient shows deterioration after therapy is initiated. If initiation of treatment appears to produce sudden deterioration of respiratory function, treatment should be discontinued immediately and reinstituted only with extreme caution and continuous monitoring. Immediately report complaints of chest soreness, shortness of breath, or other adverse effects.

Hematologic

Anemia. The primary toxicity of ribavirin capsules is hemolytic anemia, which develops in about 10% of patients treated with ribavirin–Intron A after 1 to 2 weeks of therapy. It is recommended that a baseline hemoglobin or hematocrit level be obtained and at weeks 2 and 4 of therapy. Fatal and nonfatal myocardial infarctions have been reported in patients who develop anemia secondary to ribavirin therapy.

◆ *Drug interactions*

Stavudine, zidovudine, peginterferon alfa-2a. Ribavirin may antagonize the in vitro antiviral activity of stavudine and zidovudine against HIV. Combination therapy with zidovudine, ribavirin, and peginterferon alfa-2a has resulted in severe neutropenia and severe anemia. Monitor closely for treatment-associated toxicities. Consider dose reduction or discontinuation of ribavirin, peginterferon alfa-2a, or both if worsening toxicities occur.

---

valacyclovir (văl-ă-SĬK-lō-vĭr)
Valtrex (VĂL-trĕks)
⇌ *Do not confuse Valtrex with Valcyte.*

Actions

Valacyclovir is a prodrug of acyclovir, an antiviral agent that acts by inhibiting viral cell replication.

Uses

Valacyclovir is used orally in adults to treat acute herpes zoster (shingles) and herpes labialis (cold sores and genital herpes) in immunocompetent patients. It is also approved to treat varicella virus (chickenpox) in children ages 2 through 18 years.

Therapeutic Outcome

The primary therapeutic outcome expected from valacyclovir therapy is elimination of symptoms of viral infection.

❖ **Nursing Implications for Valacyclovir**
◆ *Premedication assessment*

1. Obtain baseline assessments of presenting symptoms.
2. Record temperature, pulse, respirations, blood pressure, and hydration status.
3. Assess for and record any abnormal renal function before initiating therapy.
4. Assess for any allergies.
5. Perform baseline mental status examination (e.g., orientation).
6. Obtain baseline laboratory studies ordered and review results.

◆ *Availability.* *PO:* 500-mg and 1-g tablets.

◆ *Dosage and administration.* **Adult:** *PO:*
Treatment of herpes zoster (shingles): 1 g three times daily for 7 days. To be effective, therapy must be started within 48 hours of the onset of the zoster rash.
Treatment of genital herpes—initial episode: 1 gm twice daily for 10 days. Treatment is most effective if started within 48 hours of first symptoms. *For recurrent episodes:* 500 mg twice daily for 3 days, initiating treatment at the first sign of symptoms of an episode.
Pediatric: *PO: Treatment of Varicella virus (chickenpox):* 20 mg/kg administered 3 times daily for 5 days. Start at the earliest sign of symptoms. Do not exceed 1 gm 3 times daily.

◆ *Serious adverse effects and drug interactions.* See earlier section on Acyclovir.

zanamivir (zăn-ĂM-ĭ-vĭr)
Relenza (rĕl-ĔN-ză)

Actions

Zanamivir is an antiviral agent that acts by inhibiting neuraminidase, an enzyme on the viral cell coat necessary for replication and spread of viral cell particles.

Uses

Zanamivir was the first neuraminidase inhibitor marketed for use for the treatment of uncomplicated acute illness caused by influenza. Studies show that the duration of symptoms (nasal congestion, sore throat, cough, myalgia, fatigue, headache, chills, and sweats) of influenza infection will be reduced by about 1 day (4 days versus 5 days) if the patient has been symptomatic for no more than 2 days when treatment is started. The severity of symptoms and potential for complications from secondary infection are also significantly reduced. It is not known whether zanamivir is effective in preventing influenza infection, and it should not be used as a substitute for annual influenza vaccination. Zanamivir has not been shown to reduce the risk of transmission of influenza to others.

Therapeutic Outcomes

The primary therapeutic outcome expected from zanamivir therapy is reduced symptomatology caused by influenza virus infection. It may also reduce the incidence of opportunistic secondary infections such as pneumonia.

❖ Nursing Implications for Zanamivir

◆ *Premedication assessment*
1. Obtain baseline assessments of presenting symptoms.
2. Record temperature, pulse, respirations, blood pressure, and hydration status.
3. Assess for any allergies.

4. Obtain baseline laboratory studies ordered and review results (e.g., pulmonary function tests).

◆ *Availability.* **Inhaler:** 5-mg blisters of powder for inhalation through a Diskhaler.

◆ *Dosage and administration.* **Adult:** *Inhalation:* Two inhalations (one 5-mg blister per inhalation for a total of 10 mg) twice daily (approximately 12 hours apart) for 5 days. Treatment should begin within 2 days after the onset of symptoms of influenza. On the first day of treatment, two doses should be taken, provided there are at least 2 hours between doses. On subsequent days, doses should be approximately 12 hours apart at approximately the same time each day.

Patients who are scheduled to use an inhaled bronchodilator should use the bronchodilator before taking zanamivir. Patients may also take decongestants, analgesics, and antipyretic agents to reduce symptomatology.

◆ *Serious adverse effects*
Respiratory
Asthma, bronchospasm, diminishing pulmonary function. Perform baseline pulmonary function tests to assess whether the patient shows deterioration after therapy is started. If starting inhalation treatment appears to produce sudden bronchospasm or deterioration of respiratory function, treatment should be discontinued immediately and the healthcare provider contacted. Immediately report complaints of chest soreness, shortness of breath, or other adverse effects.
Immune system
Cough, sore throat, fever, continuing symptoms. If the patient starts coughing up yellow or green sputum, if a sore throat worsens and becomes severe, if fever returns after going away, or if symptoms last longer than 1 or 2 weeks, report to the healthcare provider for evaluation of other potential complications.

◆ *Drug interactions.* No clinically significant drug interactions have been reported.

Get Ready for the NCLEX® Examination!

Key Points

- Antimicrobial agents are chemicals that eliminate living microorganisms that are pathogenic to the patient.
- If at all possible, the infecting organisms should first be isolated and identified. The antimicrobial therapy is then started based on the sensitivity results and the clinical judgment of the healthcare provider.
- Nurses must consider the entire patient when administering and monitoring antimicrobial therapy.
- It is essential that the nurse be knowledgeable about the drugs, including physiologic parameters for monitoring expected therapeutic activity and potential adverse effects.

- Beginning nursing students need to focus on the commonality of the premedication assessments and adverse effects that may occur with the various drugs prescribed for infectious disease. Because of the numerous drug interactions listed in the drug monographs, it is essential to consult a drug reference before administering a prescribed antimicrobial.
- It is important to teach the individual with an infection basic principles of self-care that will enhance the recovery process and measures to prevent the spread of the infection. In the case of communicable diseases, exposed individuals must be contacted for follow-up testing and appropriate treatment.

Additional Learning Resources

SG Go to your Study Guide for additional Review Questions for the NCLEX® Examination, Critical Thinking Clinical Situations, and other learning activities to help you master this chapter content.

Go to your Evolve website (https://evolve.elsevier.com/Clayton) for additional online resources.

Review Questions for the NCLEX® Examination

1. The nurse is administering tobramycin, an aminoglycoside, to a patient with a wound infected with *Klebsiella* and is alert for which adverse effects? *(Select all that apply.)*
   1. Ototoxicity
   2. Nystagmus
   3. Nephrotoxicity
   4. Photosensitivity
   5. Dizziness

2. Prophylactic antibiotics are prescribed prior to dental procedures for patients at risk for developing infective endocarditis with which of the following medical conditions? *(Select all that apply.)*
   1. Hypertension
   2. Previous heart transplantation
   3. History of infective endocarditis
   4. Congestive heart failure
   5. Congenital heart defects

3. A patient was complaining of nausea and vomiting after taking ampicillin. After reassuring the patient, the nurse responded with which appropriate statement?
   1. "I would not worry about feeling this way; these symptoms will go away in a couple of hours."
   2. "Since the symptoms of nausea and vomiting are common responses to antibiotics, it may be helpful to take ampicillin with food."
   3. "This is a sign that you are allergic to the drug. I will notify your physician."
   4. "The drug needs to be discontinued, and you will need to be started on another drug."

4. A patient presented with the symptoms of white patches over the tongue while taking ceftriaxone for pneumonia. The nurse recognized this reaction as what?
   1. Ototoxicity
   2. An allergic reaction
   3. A secondary infection
   4. Photosensitivity

5. A nurse knows that patients receiving amphotericin B may develop nephrotoxicity. The nurse knows which of the following laboratory values need to be monitored for this adverse effect?
   1. Elevated AST and ALT levels
   2. Increased BUN and creatinine levels
   3. Decreased BUN and creatinine levels
   4. Decreased AST and ALT levels

6. While talking with a patient, the nurse noticed that the patient frequently asked the nurse to repeat what was said. After reviewing the chart, the nurse found there was no prior mention of hearing loss. The nurse became concerned about possible ototoxicity when the patient was also receiving which drug?
   1. ciprofloxacin (Cipro)
   2. linezolid (Zyvox)
   3. azithromycin (Zithromax)
   4. tobramycin (Tobrex)

7. Ertapenem (Invanz) was prescribed for a patient who came in to the hospital with cellulitis. The nurse performs which of the following assessments before administration? *(Select all that apply.)*
   1. Assess for any allergies.
   2. Record the patient's temperature, pulse, respirations, and blood pressure.
   3. Obtain baseline assessments of presenting symptoms.
   4. Assess for any respiratory symptoms before initiating therapy.
   5. Obtain baseline height and weight.

8. When an antibiotic is prescribed for use before culture and sensitivity results are available, this refers to what type of treatment?
   1. Empirical treatment
   2. Prediagnosis treatment
   3. Definitive treatment
   4. Primary treatment

9. The nurse was instructing a patient who was diagnosed with tuberculosis on the medications that will be used to treat the disease. The nurse knows further education is needed when the patient makes which statement?
   1. "The drugs that I need to take for tuberculosis are the isoniazid (INH) and the rifampin (Rifadin)."
   2. "One of the common effects that I should be aware of is the potential for nausea and vomiting."
   3. "My urine and tears may turn bright yellow with these drugs."
   4. "I understand I need to take these drugs consistently or the organism develops a resistance to the drugs."

10. The antiviral agent ribavirin (Virazole) is used for treatment for which of the following infections? *(Select all that apply.)*
    1. HIV-1
    2. Herpes zoster (shingles)
    3. Influenza
    4. Chronic hepatitis C
    5. Respiratory syncytial virus

46

Nutrition

https://evolve.elsevier.com/Clayton

Objectives

1. Identify sources of dietary fiber and dietary fats.
2. Differentiate between fat-soluble and water-soluble vitamins and discuss their functions.
3. Discuss the functions of minerals in the body.
4. Describe physical changes associated with a malnourished state.

5. Discuss nursing assessments and interventions required during the administration of enteral nutrition.
6. Describe the advantages and disadvantages of providing nutrition by peripheral parenteral nutrition (PPN) and central parenteral nutrition (CPN).

Key Terms

macronutrients (măk-rō-NŪ-trē-ĕnts) (p. 736)
Dietary Reference Intakes (DRIs) (DĪ-ĕ-tār-ē RĚF-rĕns ĬN-tāks) (p. 741)
Estimated Average Requirement (EAR) (ĔS-tǐ-mā-tĕd ĂV-ĕ-rĕj rē-KWĪ-ŭr-mĕnt) (p. 741)
Recommended Dietary Allowances (RDAs) (rĕk-ō-MĚN-dĕd DĪ-ĕ-tār-ē ă-LŌ-ĕn-sĕz) (p. 741)
Adequate Intake (AI) (ĂD-ĕ-kwĕt ĬN-tāk) (p. 742)
Tolerable Upper Intake Level (UL) (TŎL-ŭr-ă-bŭl ŬP-ŭr ĬN-tāk LĚ-vŭl) (p. 742)
kilocalories (kǐl-ō-KĂL-ŏ-rēz) (p. 742)
Estimated Energy Requirement (EER) (ĔS-tǐm-ă-tĕd ĔN-ŭr-jē rē-KWĪ-ŭr-mĕnt) (p. 742)
carbohydrates (kăr-bō-HĪ-drāts) (p. 742)
monosaccharides (mŏn-ō-SĂK-ă-rīdz) (p. 742)
disaccharides (dī-SĂK-ă-rīdz) (p. 742)
polysaccharides (pŏ-lē-SĂK-ă-rīdz) (p. 742)

fiber (FĪ-bĕr) (p. 742)
lipids (LĬ-pĭdz) (p. 743)
essential fatty acids (ĂS-ĭdz) (p. 743)
gluconeogenesis (glū-kō-nē-ō-JĚN-ĕ-sĭs) (p. 743)
vitamins (VĪ-tă-mĭnz) (p. 743)
minerals (MĬN-ĭ-rŭlz) (p. 745)
physical exercise (FĬZ-ĭ-kŭl ĔKS-ŭr-sīz) (p. 745)
marasmus (mă-RĂZ-mŭs) (p. 746)
kwashiorkor (kwăsh-ē-ŌR-kōr) (p. 746)
mixed kwashiorkor-marasmus (p. 746)
enteral nutrition (ĔN-tĕr-ăl nū-TRĬ-shŭn) (p. 746)
tube feedings (p. 746)
parenteral nutrition (pă-RĔN-tĕr-ŭl nū-TRĬ-shŭn) (p. 746)
total parenteral nutrition (TPN) (TŌ-tăl) (p. 747)
peripheral parenteral nutrition (PPN) (pĕ-RĬF-ĕr-ăl) (p. 747)
central parenteral nutrition (CPN) (SĚN-trŭl) (p. 747)

 Clinical Goldmine

"For the two out of three adult Americans who do not smoke and do not drink excessively, one personal choice seems to influence long-term health prospects more than any other: what we eat" (*The Surgeon General's Report on Nutrition and Health*, 1988; retrieved from https://profiles.nlm.nih.gov/NN/B/C/Q/G).

PRINCIPLES OF NUTRITION

It is no coincidence that eating is one of life's greatest pleasures. The body needs a regular source of energy to sustain its various functions, including respiration, nerve transmission, circulation, physical work, and maintenance of core temperature. There are many environmental, cultural, and behavioral reasons for what and how people eat, but the most basic is to sustain life. Because the body cannot make most of the needed nutrients, these chemicals must be supplied from external sources. For the most part, they are supplied from the food people eat. Other chemicals are supplied by air, such as oxygen; by water; and by sunlight, which helps the body manufacture vitamin D. The energy derived from external sources is converted to chemical energy by the body, which sustains the body's functions. The heat produced during these chemical reactions maintains body temperature. Energy sources required for balanced metabolism are the macronutrients—fats, carbohydrates, fiber, and proteins—which are measured in calories (see

Macronutrients section later in this chapter). Other essential nutrients include vitamins, minerals, and water. Imbalances between energy intake (food) and energy expenditure result in gain or loss of body composition, primarily in the form of fat, which determines changes in weight.

Nutritional requirements vary based on level of activity, age of the individual (e.g., infant, preschool child, adolescent, adult, and older adult), and gender. For example, there are differences in nutritional requirements for a pregnant teenager, an adult woman, and a lactating mother. The presence of disease, wound healing, and the degree of catabolism also can influence nutritional needs. Therefore the reader should consult a reliable nutrition textbook for current detailed information.

Nutritional needs are met primarily from foods. Foods in nutrient-dense forms contain essential vitamins and minerals and also dietary fiber. In some cases, fortified foods and dietary supplements may be useful in providing one or more nutrients if necessary. No one food source can meet all of the body's basic nutritional requirements. Foods from a variety of groups are required to provide an optimal nutrient balance and to minimize naturally occurring toxic substances from a single food source.

METHODS FOR ASSESSING NUTRITION

Governmental Guidelines

Two federal agencies, the US Department of Agriculture (USDA) and the US Food and Drug Administration, collaborate to publish *Dietary Guidelines for Americans* every 5 years. The latest edition is the *2015-2020 Dietary Guidelines for Americans* (8th edition). These guidelines are based on research of nutrients in foods and recommend how to make the best food choices to promote good health (Box 46.1). These guidelines encourage a healthy eating pattern as described in the USDA Food Patterns (with vegetarian adaptations) and the DASH (*D*ietary *A*pproaches to *S*top *H*ypertension) Eating Plan. The USDA's website (https://www.choosemyplate.gov) contains a wealth of information on how people can become more informed and more calorie conscious and plan nutrient-rich meals with suggested proportions (Fig. 46.1).

The key recommendations in the 2015-2020 *Dietary Guidelines* are to develop a healthy eating pattern and to develop healthy eating pattern limits. Healthy eating patterns can help reduce the risk of chronic disease throughout periods of growth, development, and aging as well as during pregnancy. An eating pattern represents the totality of all foods and beverages consumed. All foods consumed as part of a healthy eating pattern fit together like a puzzle to meet nutritional needs without exceeding limits, such as those for saturated fats, added sugars, sodium, and total calories. All forms of foods, including fresh, canned, dried, and frozen, can be included in healthy eating patterns.

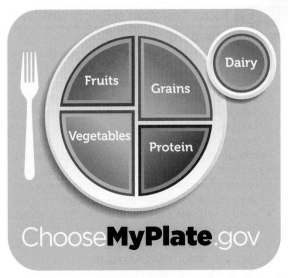

Fig. 46.1 MyPlate Food Guide. (From US Department of Health and Human Services/US Department of Agriculture, 2011.)

With obesity, metabolic syndrome, and type 2 diabetes mellitus reaching epidemic proportions over the past decade in the United States and recent research findings raising concerns, the *Dietary Guidelines* have undergone substantial scrutiny. The 2015-2020 version was revised and updated extensively to address issues and trends related to nutrition and overall health. The 2015-2020 *Dietary Guidelines* encourage the intake of whole grains and suggest that people limit sugar intake. Another concern in the average American diet is the consumption of *trans*-fatty acids (also called *hydrogenated fats*) and saturated fats, which have no known nutritional benefit but increase cholesterol levels and the frequency of heart disease. The guidelines now emphasize that intake of *trans* fats should be as low as possible. As of January 2006, food labels are required to list *trans* fat content to help consumers become aware of and reduce their intake. The primary sources of *trans* fats are commercially fried foods, stick margarine, processed and ready-to-eat foods, and snack foods. Research indicates that monounsaturated and polyunsaturated fats have some health benefits, so the guidelines also recommend obtaining between 20% and 35% of daily calories from these types of fats. Saturated fats should continue to be limited. Primary sources of saturated fats are red meats, butter, and high-fat dairy products (e.g., whole milk) (Box 46.2; see Fig. 46.2).

The *2015-2020 Dietary Guidelines for Americans* are recommending two variations of the Healthy U.S.-Style Eating Pattern as examples of additional healthy eating patterns—the Healthy Mediterranean-Style Eating Pattern and the Healthy Vegetarian Eating Pattern. Both of these patterns align with the 2015-2020 *Dietary Guidelines*. A healthy eating pattern made under these guidelines includes:

- A variety of vegetables from all of the subgroups—dark green, red and orange, legumes (beans and peas), starchy, and other

Box **46.1**   **Recommendations of Dietary Guidelines for Americans, 2015-2020**

FIVE DIETARY GUIDELINES:

1. Follow a healthy eating pattern across the life span.
- All food and beverage choices matter.
- Choose a healthy eating pattern at an appropriate calorie level to help achieve and maintain a healthy body weight, support nutrient adequacy, and reduce the risk of chronic disease.

2. Focus on variety, nutrient density, and amount.
- To meet nutrient needs within calorie limits, choose a variety of nutrient-dense foods across and within all food groups in recommended amounts.
- Shifts are needed within the protein foods group to increase seafood intake, but the foods to be replaced depend on the individual's current intake from the other protein subgroups.
- Strategies to increase the variety of protein foods include incorporating seafood as the protein foods choice in meals twice per week in place of meat, poultry, or eggs, and using legumes or nuts and seeds in mixed dishes instead of some meat or poultry.
- For example, choosing a salmon steak, a tuna sandwich, bean chili, or almonds on a main-dish salad could all increase protein variety.

3. Limit calories from added sugars and saturated fats and reduce sodium intake.
- Consume an eating pattern low in added sugars, saturated fats, and sodium.
- Cut back on foods and beverages higher in these components to amounts that fit within healthy eating patterns.
- The most commonly used oil in the United States is soybean oil. Other commonly used oils include canola, corn, olive, cottonseed, sunflower, and peanut oil. Oils also are found in nuts, avocados, and seafood.
- Coconut, palm, and palm kernel oils (tropical oils) are solid at room temperature because they have high amounts of saturated fatty acids and are therefore classified as a solid fat rather than as an oil.

4. Shift to healthier food and beverage choices.
- Choose nutrient-dense foods and beverages across and within all food groups in place of less healthy choices.
- Consider cultural and personal preferences to make these shifts easier to accomplish and maintain.
- Shift to eating more vegetables.
- One strategy to do that would mean choosing a green salad or a vegetable as a side dish and incorporating vegetables into most meals and snacks.
- Shift to eating more fruits, by choosing more fruits as snacks, in salads, as side dishes, and as desserts in place of foods with added sugars, such as cakes, pies, cookies, doughnuts, ice cream, and candies.
- Shift to make half of all grains consumed be whole grains.
- Strategies to increase dairy intake include drinking fat-free or low-fat milk (or a fortified soy beverage) with meals, choosing yogurt as a snack, or using yogurt as an ingredient in prepared dishes such as salad dressings or spreads.
- Strategies for choosing dairy products in nutrient-dense forms include choosing lower fat versions of milk, yogurt, and cheese in place of whole milk products and regular cheese.

5. Support healthy eating patterns for all.
- Everyone has a role in helping to create and support healthy eating patterns in multiple settings nationwide, from home to school to work to communities.
- In order to improve individual and population lifestyle choices, strategies need to be implemented such as expanding access to healthy, safe, and affordable food choices that align with the *Dietary Guidelines*.
- Adopt organizational changes and practices, including those that increase the availability, accessibility, and consumption of foods that align with the *Dietary Guidelines*.
- Provide nutrition assistance programs that support education and promotional activities tailored to the needs of the community.

Adapted from U.S. Department of Agriculture and U.S. Department of Health and Human Services. *Dietary Guidelines for Americans, 2015-2020.* 8th ed. Washington, DC: U.S. Government Printing Office; 2015.

- Fruits, especially whole fruits
- Grains, at least half of which are whole grains
- Fat-free or low-fat dairy, including milk, yogurt, cheese, and/or fortified soy beverages
- A variety of protein foods, including seafood, lean meats and poultry, eggs, legumes (beans and peas), and nuts, seeds, and soy products
- Oils

The guidelines also make recommendations for healthy eating pattern limits, which include:
- Limiting saturated fats and *trans* fats, added sugars, and sodium
- Consuming less than 10% of calories per day from added sugars

- Consuming less than 10% of calories per day from saturated fats
- Consuming less than 2300 mg per day of sodium
- If alcohol is consumed, it should be consumed in moderation and only by adults of legal drinking age

Several nutrients are considered as being underconsumed: vitamins A, D, E, and C; folate; calcium; magnesium; fiber; and potassium. These shortfalls are identified as low intakes of vegetables, fruits, whole grains, and dairy. The 2015-2020 *Dietary Guidelines* encourage dietary patterns that are rich in vegetables, fruit, whole grains, seafood, legumes, and nuts; moderate in low- and nonfat dairy products and alcohol (among adults); lower in red

| Box **46.2** | **Dietary Fat Sources** |

MONOUNSATURATED FATS
- Olives
- Olive oil
- Canola oil
- Peanut oil
- Cashews
- Peanuts
- Avocados

POLYUNSATURATED FATS
- Corn oil
- Soybean oil
- Safflower oil
- Cottonseed oil
- Fish

SATURATED FATS
- Whole milk
- Cheese
- Ice cream
- Red meat
- Chocolate
- Coconut
- Coconut oil

***TRANS* FATS**
- Stick margarines
- Vegetable shortening
- Deep-fried chips
- French fries
- Many fast foods
- Most commercial baked goods

and processed meat; and low in sugar-sweetened foods and beverages and refined grains (https://health.gov/dietaryguidelines/2015/guidelines/).

Alternatives to Governmental Guidelines

Nutrition experts at the Harvard University School of Public Health have proposed the Healthy Eating Plate (Fig. 46.3), the Kid's Healthy Eating Plate (Fig. 46.4), and the Healthy Eating Pyramid (Fig. 46.5) to address deficiencies in the USDA's MyPlate Food Guide (https://www.hsph.harvard.edu/nutritionsource/healthy-eating-plate/). Some of the highlights of the Healthy Eating Pyramid are as follows:

- Daily activity and weight control serve as the foundation for the pyramid.
- Whole-grain foods, fruits, and vegetables (sources of fiber, vitamins, and minerals) are emphasized.
- Vegetable oils and nuts (sources of unsaturated fats) and legumes receive greater emphasis as sources of protein, fiber, vitamins, and minerals. Good sources of healthy unsaturated fats include olive, canola, soy, corn, sunflower, and peanut oils.
- Red meat should be consumed sparingly because of saturated fat content. Switching to fish or chicken several times a week can improve cholesterol levels.
- Food sources high in refined carbohydrates (e.g., white rice, white bread, potatoes, pasta, sweets) should be consumed only sparingly. They can cause rapid increases in blood sugar levels that can lead to weight gain, diabetes, and heart disease.

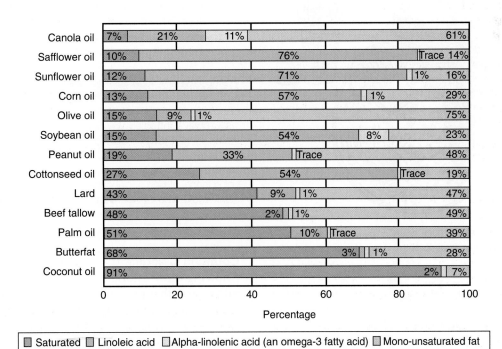

Fig. 46.2 All plant oils used in food preparation contain saturated, monounsaturated, and polyunsaturated fatty acids. It is recommended that the use of those oils higher in saturated fatty acids be minimized. (From Thomas DQ, Kotecki JE. *Physical Activity and Health: An Interactive Approach.* 2nd ed. Sudbury, MA: Jones and Bartlett; 2007. Reprinted with permission.)

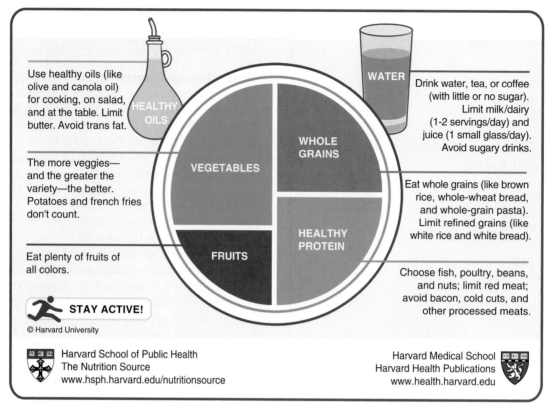

Fig. 46.3 The Healthy Eating Plate. (As print in image and © Harvard University. For more information, visit https://www.health.harvard.edu.)

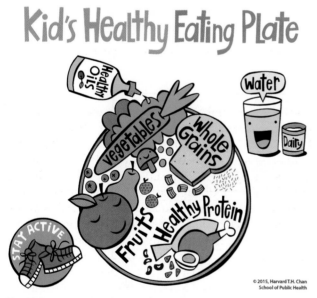

Fig. 46.4 Kids Healthy Eating Plate. (As print in image and © Harvard University. For more information, visit https://www.health.harvard.edu.)

Whole-grain carbohydrates cause slower, steadier increases in blood sugar that do not overwhelm the body's ability to metabolize sugars.

• Dairy products are deemphasized and placed in their own category; it is believed that dairy products being consumed as a calcium source could be replaced with a calcium supplement to avoid unneeded calories and saturated fats.

• A daily multivitamin is recommended for most people.
• Moderate daily alcohol may be a healthy option unless contraindicated for specific people. A good balance for men is one or two drinks daily. Women should limit alcohol consumption to no more than one drink per day. (See https://www.cdc.gov/alcohol/fact-sheets.htm.)

Cultural Considerations

Another excellent source of healthy nutritional information is Oldways (https://www.oldwayspt.org), a nutritional food think tank. Oldways develops education programs to help consumers make informed choices about eating, drinking, and lifestyle. Their principles are grounded in a combination of science, strong social conscience, and culinary excellence. Oldways promotes Asian, Latin, Mediterranean, and vegetarian evidence-based food pyramids for healthy eating.

Counting Calories

Knowing daily calorie needs may be useful for determining whether the number *consumed* is appropriate in relation to the number *needed* each day. The best way to assess the appropriate number of calories is to monitor body weight and adjust calorie intake and participation in physical activity based on changes in weight over time. A reduction of 500 calories or more per day is a common initial goal for weight loss for adults. However, maintaining a smaller deficit can have a meaningful influence on

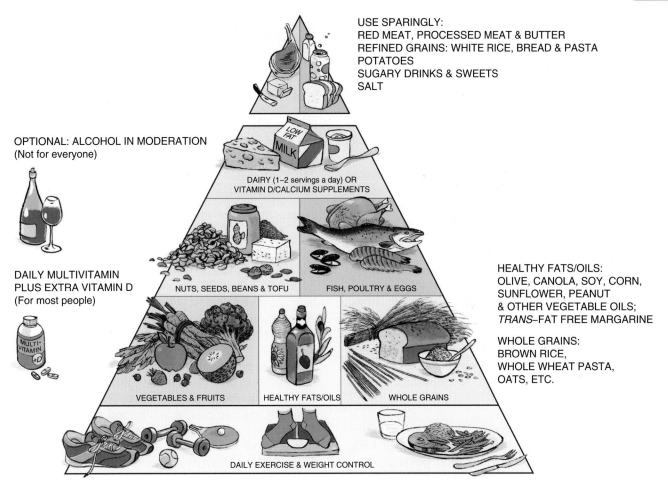

USE SPARINGLY:
RED MEAT, PROCESSED MEAT & BUTTER
REFINED GRAINS: WHITE RICE, BREAD & PASTA
POTATOES
SUGARY DRINKS & SWEETS
SALT

OPTIONAL: ALCOHOL IN MODERATION
(Not for everyone)

DAIRY (1–2 servings a day) OR
VITAMIN D/CALCIUM SUPPLEMENTS

DAILY MULTIVITAMIN
PLUS EXTRA VITAMIN D
(For most people)

NUTS, SEEDS, BEANS & TOFU

FISH, POULTRY & EGGS

HEALTHY FATS/OILS:
OLIVE, CANOLA, SOY, CORN,
SUNFLOWER, PEANUT
& OTHER VEGETABLE OILS;
TRANS–FAT FREE MARGARINE

WHOLE GRAINS:
BROWN RICE,
WHOLE WHEAT PASTA,
OATS, ETC.

VEGETABLES & FRUITS

HEALTHY FATS/OILS

WHOLE GRAINS

DAILY EXERCISE & WEIGHT CONTROL

Fig. 46.5 The Healthy Eating Pyramid. (As print in image and © Harvard University. For more information, visit https://www.health.harvard.edu.)

body weight over time. The effect of calorie reduction on weight does not depend on how the reduction is produced—by reducing calorie intake, increasing caloric expenditure (more exercise), or both—yet, in research studies, a greater proportion of the calorie reduction is often due to decreasing calorie intake, with a relatively smaller fraction due to increased physical activity.

Life Span Considerations
Food for Thought

Because a pound of stored fat represents about 3500 excess kilocalories (kcal):
- An average excess of only 10 kcal/day in energy intake over energy expenditure can result in about a 1-pound weight gain in 1 year (10 kcal/day × 365 days = 3650 kcal).
- Cutting back on only 100 kcal/day (e.g., 1 soft drink) results in approximately a 10-pound weight loss in 1 year (100 kcal/day × 365 days = 36,500 kcal), or consuming an extra 100 kcal/day will result in a 10-pound gain.
  - For weight gain, add 500 cal/day to gain approximately 1 pound/wk.
  - For weight loss, subtract 500 cal/day for a loss of approximately 1 pound/wk.

DIETARY REFERENCE INTAKES

The National Academies of Sciences, Engineering, and Medicine collect data and publish a series of tables known as **Dietary Reference Intakes (DRIs)**, which provide quantitative estimates of nutrient intakes for planning and assessing diets for healthy people. The DRIs are actually a set of four reference values: Estimated Average Requirement, Recommended Dietary Allowances, Adequate Intake, and Tolerable Upper Intake Level. Links to the DRIs updated in 2017 may be retrieved at http://www.nationalacademies.org/hmd/Activities/Nutrition/SummaryDRIs/DRI-Tables.aspx.

The **Estimated Average Requirement (EAR)** is a nutrient intake value that is estimated to meet the requirement of half of the healthy individuals in a group. The most widely known component of the DRIs is the **Recommended Dietary Allowances (RDAs)** table. It lists the average daily dietary intake level that is sufficient to meet the nutrient requirements of almost all (97% to 98%) healthy individuals in a group. (Groups are based on gender, age, and, if applicable, pregnancy or lactation.) Recommended Dietary Allowances are goals in meeting nutritional needs. They do not meet the nutritional needs of ill patients and do not account for nutritional value that may be lost in cooking.

The RDA is based on the EAR plus twice the standard deviation: the RDA for a nutrient is a value to be used as a goal for dietary intake by healthy individuals. There is no established benefit for healthy persons if they consume nutrient intakes greater than the RDA or Adequate Intake.

Adequate Intake (AI) is a value based on observed or experimentally determined approximations of nutrient intake by a group of healthy people. The AI is used when the RDA cannot be determined.

Another category in the DRI tables is the **Tolerable Upper Intake Level (UL)**. This level is defined as the highest level of daily nutrient intake that is likely to pose no risk of adverse health effects to almost all those in the general population. As intake increases above the UL, the risk of adverse effects increases. The UL is not intended to be a recommended level of intake. For many nutrients, there are insufficient data on which to develop a UL. This does not mean that there is no potential for adverse effects resulting from high intake. Over time, these data will help establish the value of megadoses of vitamins and nutrients and provide information about whether there are therapeutic and toxic effects to ingestion of large doses of these chemicals.

MACRONUTRIENTS

The metabolism of the macronutrients—carbohydrates, fiber, fats, and proteins—provides energy for the body to maintain life (respiration, circulation, physical work, nerve transmission, core body temperature) and to repair damage induced by illness or injury. Energy is measured in **kilocalories** (kcal). The heat generated during these processes is reflected as body temperature. Energy balance in an individual depends on dietary energy intake and energy expenditure. An excess of energy (food) intake over that which is burned results in weight gain. Body weight is lost through burning more kilocalories than are consumed. A pound of body weight is approximately 3500 kcal.

The **Estimated Energy Requirement (EER)** is defined as the average dietary energy intake that is predicted to maintain energy balance in a healthy adult of a defined age, gender, weight, height, and level of physical activity consistent with good health (Table 46.1).

The National Academy of Sciences published the *Dietary Reference Intakes for Energy, Carbohydrate, Fiber, Fat, Fatty Acids, Cholesterol, Protein and Amino Acids* in 2005. This report on macronutrients was sponsored for both the United States and Canada by several government agencies, including Health Canada, the US Department of Health and Human Services, the US Food and Drug Administration, the National Institutes of Health, the Centers for Disease Control and Prevention, the USDA, and private sources. These guidelines are based on research of nutrients in foods and how the body uses energy from foods. The report recommends that to meet the body's energy and nutritional needs while *minimizing risk for chronic disease,* adults

Table **46.1**	Calculation of Estimated Energy Requirements (EERs)	
LIFESTYLE	**MEN**[a]	**WOMEN**[b]
Sedentary	1.00	1.00
Low active	1.11	1.12
Active	1.25	1.27
Very active	1.48	1.45

[a]Men ages 19 years and older: EER = 662 − (9.53 × age [yr]) + PA × (15.91 × weight [kg] + 539.6 × height [m])
[b]Women ages 19 years and older: EER = 354 − (6.91 × age [yr]) + PA × (9.36 × weight [kg] + 726 × height [m])
PA, Physical activity coefficient.
Data from Institute of Medicine, Food and Nutrition Board. *Dietary Reference Intakes for Energy, Carbohydrate, Fiber, Fat, Fatty Acids, Cholesterol, Protein, and Amino Acids.* Washington, DC: National Academies Press; 2005:185. Retrieved from http://www.nap.edu/catalog.php?record_id=10490.

should obtain 45% to 65% of their calories from carbohydrates, 20% to 35% from fat, and 10% to 35% from protein. (See Chapter 35 for the American Diabetes Association recommendations for intake of carbohydrates, fats, and proteins for a patient with diabetes mellitus.)

Carbohydrates, often referred to as *sugars* because many of them taste sweet, are the major source of energy for body activities and metabolism. They occur in nature as simple and complex molecules and are water soluble. The simple carbohydrates are also known as *monosaccharides* and *disaccharides*. **Monosaccharides** such as glucose (also known as *dextrose*), fructose, and galactose are the only sugars that can be absorbed directly from the gastrointestinal (GI) tract into the blood. They are the most rapidly available sources of energy and are the only sugars capable of being used directly to produce energy for the body. **Disaccharides** such as sucrose (common table sugar), maltose, and lactose are the most common sugars in foods, but they must be metabolized to monosaccharides before being absorbed into the bloodstream. For example, a molecule of lactose is metabolized by the enzyme lactase into a molecule each of glucose and galactose, which are then absorbed through the gut wall into the blood. Complex carbohydrates such as starch, dextrin, and fiber are also known as *polysaccharides*. Complex carbohydrates must also be metabolized into simple sugars in the intestine before being absorbed. The carbohydrates provide about 4 kcal of energy per gram. Daily caloric needs from carbohydrates range from 3 to 5.5 g/kg/day, depending on energy requirements for daily living, stress, and wound healing. Fruits, grains, and vegetables are excellent sources of carbohydrates. Candies and carbonated beverages are commonly used sources of calories but contain no other nutrients. End products of carbohydrate metabolism are carbon dioxide (excreted primarily through the lungs) and water.

A by-product of some complex carbohydrate metabolism is **fiber.** Until recently, fiber was thought to be only a by-product of carbohydrate metabolism that needed to be eliminated from the body. It is recognized now as a macronutrient, a separate factor necessary for complete nutrition and wellness. *Dietary fiber* is derived from plant sources and consists of undigestible carbohydrates and lignin and digestible macronutrients (carbohydrates, proteins) such as cereal brans, sweet potatoes, and legumes that contribute to overall nutrition. Another category of fiber is *functional fiber,* which consists of undigestible carbohydrates that have a beneficial physiologic effect on humans. An excellent example of a functional fiber is psyllium, an undigestible fiber that adds bulk to fecal content, which helps timely passage of fecal contents in the GI tract, preventing constipation. Functional fiber content may delay gastric emptying, giving a sense of fullness, which may contribute to weight control. Delayed gastric emptying may also reduce postprandial blood glucose concentrations, potentially preventing excessive insulin secretion and insulin sensitivity. Fibers can reduce the absorption of dietary fat and cholesterol, as well as enterohepatic recirculation of cholesterol and bile acids, which may also reduce blood cholesterol concentrations. *Total fiber* is the sum of dietary fiber and functional fiber.

Fats, also known as **lipids**, serve as the body's major form of stored energy and are key components of membranes, prostaglandins, and many hormones. They are not water soluble. Examples of lipids are cholesterol, fatty acids, triglycerides, and phospholipids. Excess dietary carbohydrates and proteins are converted to fat for storage. When used as an energy source, fats generate 9 kcal of energy per gram. Fat intake usually constitutes 25% to 40% of total caloric intake, although the DRIs recommend limits of 20% to 35% from fat. Healthy adults require 1 to 1.5 g/kg/day. Even when patients severely restrict intake for dieting purposes, 4% to 10% of total calories must be supplied in the form of fats to prevent essential fatty acid deficiency.

Essential fatty acids are not produced by the body and must be obtained from dietary sources. The most prominent essential fatty acids are omega-3 and omega-6 fatty acids. They are polyunsaturated fatty acids, also known as *alpha-linolenic acid* and *linoleic acid,* respectively. Both fatty acids are required for eicosanoid and prostaglandin production and cell membrane structure.

Dietary fats can be subdivided into four categories: monounsaturated, polyunsaturated, saturated, and *trans* fats (see Box 46.2 for sources of dietary fats). Monounsaturated fats decrease low-density lipoproteins (LDLs) and increase high-density lipoproteins (HDLs) and are considered to be cardioprotective. Polyunsaturated fats also lower LDL and raise HDL levels. Saturated fats raise both LDL and HDL and are thought to increase atherosclerotic plaque formation in the arteries. Only recently has it been recognized that *trans* fats may induce more heart disease than saturated fats because, in addition to raising LDL cholesterol, *trans* fats *decrease* HDL cholesterol and increase triglycerides, as well as another undesirable blood fat, lipoprotein. Saturated fats and *trans* fats have no known beneficial nutritional effect

and should be eliminated as much as possible from the diet. Note in Fig. 46.2 how all plant oils used in food preparation contain saturated, monounsaturated, and polyunsaturated fatty acids. It is recommended that we minimize the use of those oils higher in saturated fatty acids. (See also Chapter 21 for further discussion of lipoproteins and cholesterol.) End products of fat metabolism are water and carbon dioxide and insoluble substances excreted in sweat, bile, and feces.

Proteins are complex molecules composed of amino acid chains. Amino acids can be subclassified as essential and nonessential. The essential amino acids must be provided from external sources to sustain life; nonessential amino acids can be synthesized to meet metabolic requirements. Before absorption, proteins must be metabolized in the gut to the individual amino acids. Once absorbed, the amino acids are used to build new proteins, such as muscle and other vital tissues, or are used as an energy source if other energy sources are depleted. Amino acids generate 4 kcal of energy per gram, similar to carbohydrates. Sources of highest protein value are dairy products (e.g., milk, eggs, cheese), fish, and meat. Grains and beans have less protein value. End products of amino acid metabolism are nitrogenous products such as urea, uric acid and ammonium, carbon dioxide, and water. Protein requirements for healthy people are 0.5 to 1 g/kg/day. Depending on the amount of stress that a patient is experiencing and the amount of tissue building and wound healing required, protein requirements may range from 1.5 to 2.5 g/kg/day. Calories from proteins generally constitute 12% to 20% of total calorie intake, but the National Academy of Sciences recommends 10% to 35% for healthy nutrition.

It is crucial that calorie intake be balanced among carbohydrates, proteins, and fats. If there is an inadequate amount of carbohydrates to provide energy to break down the proteins, fats, and carbohydrates, the body will actually metabolize body proteins and fats through a process called **gluconeogenesis** to provide glucose energy to use the incoming proteins and fats. Even though patients are receiving adequate total calories, they may develop a protein-wasting condition.

VITAMINS

Vitamins, whose name derives from the term *vital amines*, are a specific set of chemical molecules that regulate human metabolism necessary to maintain health. To be classified as a vitamin, a chemical must be ingested, because the human body does not make sufficient quantities to maintain health, and the lack of a vitamin in the diet produces a specific vitamin deficiency disease (e.g., beriberi is a thiamine deficiency, and scurvy is an ascorbic acid deficiency). To date, 13 compounds have been identified as vitamins, 9 of which are classified as water soluble and 4 as fat soluble (Table 46.2). Vitamins were originally named according to letters of the alphabet, but as a result of the diversity of actions of different vitamins, they are commonly referred to by

Table 46.2   **Vitamins**

TYPE OF VITAMIN	ACTIONS	SOURCES
Fat-Soluble Vitamins		
Vitamin A (retinol)	Essential for proper vision, growth, cellular differentiation, healthy skin and mucous membranes, reproduction, and immune system integrity; needed to maintain healthy skin and mucous membranes *Deficiency:* Night blindness, conjunctival xerosis	Liver, fish liver oils, eggs, whole milk, sweet potatoes, cantaloupe, carrots, spinach, broccoli, raw apricots
Vitamin D (ergocalciferol, D_2; cholecalciferol, D_3)	Regulates calcium and phosphorus metabolism *Deficiency:* Rickets	Liver, cod liver oil, egg yolks, butter, and oily fish; produced in skin by exposure to sunlight
Vitamin E (alpha-tocopherol)	Acts as antioxidant; protects essential cellular components from oxidation	Wheat germ oil, sunflower oil, cottonseed oil, safflower oil, corn oil, soybean oil, almonds, peanuts, green leafy vegetables
Vitamin K (phytonadione)	Used for synthesis of prothrombin and coagulation factors VII, IX, and X needed for blood coagulation	Kale, collard greens, spinach, broccoli, asparagus, lettuce, soybeans, pickles, pine nuts, blueberries; needs bile salts to be adequately absorbed in the intestines; malabsorptive disease processes can lead to decreased vitamin K absorption; vitamin K synthesized by intestinal flora; severe diarrhea or use of antibiotics that kill intestinal flora may result in deficiency; deficiency exists in newborn infants
Water-Soluble Vitamins		
Vitamin C (ascorbic acid)	Antioxidant; aids in formation and maintenance of intracellular cement substances *Deficiency:* Scurvy	Citrus fruits and juices, fruits, and vegetables such as broccoli, cabbage
Niacin (nicotinic acid, vitamin B_3)	Used to decrease cholesterol levels; regulates energy metabolism; helps maintain health of skin, tongue, and digestive system *Deficiency:* Pellagra	Organ meats, poultry, fish, meats, yeast, bran cereal, peanuts, brewer's yeast
Riboflavin (vitamin B_2)	Affects fetal growth and development; coenzyme for production of mitochondrial energy	Green leafy vegetables, fruit, eggs and dairy products, enriched cereal products, organ meats, peanuts and peanut butter
Thiamine (vitamin B_1)	Coenzyme for carbohydrate metabolism; used for nerve conduction and energy production *Deficiency:* Beriberi	Pork products, whole grains, wheat germ, meats, peas, cereal, dry beans, peanuts
Pyridoxine (vitamin B_6)	Metabolism of amino acids and proteins; may be important in red blood cell regeneration and normal nervous system functioning *Deficiency:* Anemia, spotty hair loss, paresthesias	Milk, meats, whole-grain cereals, fish, vegetables
Cyanocobalamin (vitamin B_{12})	Needed as coenzyme for red blood cell synthesis *Deficiency:* Megaloblastic anemia	Seafood, egg yolks, organ meats, milk, most cheeses
Folic acid (folacin)	Essential for cell growth and reproduction, synthesis of DNA in red blood cells *Deficiency:* Impaired development of central nervous system; anencephaly, spina bifida	Liver, beans, green vegetables, yeast, nuts, fruit
Biotin	Essential for gluconeogenesis, fatty acid synthesis, metabolism of branched-chain amino acids	Soy flour, cereals, egg yolk, liver; also synthesized in lower gastrointestinal tract by bacteria and fungi
Pantothenic acid (vitamin B_5)	Essential for fat, carbohydrate, protein metabolism	Organ meats, beef, and egg yolk

their generic names (e.g., phytonadione is vitamin K, and thiamine is vitamin B$_1$).

MINERALS

Minerals (Table 46.3) are inorganic chemicals found in nature. Minerals are essential to life, serving as components of enzymes, hormones, and bone and tooth structure. They help regulate acid-base and water balance, osmotic pressure and cell membrane permeability, nerve conduction, muscle contractility, metabolism of nutrients in foods, oxygen transport, and blood clotting, to name a few.

WATER

Water is another nutrient essential for life. As noted in Table 3.2 (p. 25), water accounts for 60% to 83% of total body weight and plays a crucial role in transport of nutrients, temperature regulation, and metabolic reactions. Normal water losses occur through urination, perspiration, defecation, and vaporization through the lungs. Normal daily intake is highly variable, depending on climate, activity level, and presence of a fever, but ranges from 1.5 to 3 L/day for the average adult. Intake should slightly exceed losses so that the person maintains adequate urine output to help flush waste products through the kidneys and minimize constipation.

PHYSICAL ACTIVITY

Balanced nutrition plays a key role in health and wellness, but another equally important component is **physical exercise** and activity. Throughout history, it was known that the intake of food was necessary to

Table 46.3 Essential Minerals

MINERAL	ACTIONS	SOURCES
Calcium	Nerve transmission, bone and tooth formation, blood clotting; most abundant mineral in body	Milk, cheese, vegetables
Chlorine	Acid-base balance, gastric acid	Table salt
Chromium	Glucose and energy metabolism	Vegetables, oils, meats, fats, brewer's yeast, cheddar cheese, wheat germ
Cobalt	Component of cyanocobalamin (vitamin B$_{12}$)	Meats, milk
Copper	Component of enzymes needed for iron metabolism	Meats, drinking water
Fluorine	Bone and tooth structure	Drinking water, seafood, tea
Iodine	Component of thyroid hormones	Seafood, vegetables, dairy products, iodized salt
Iron	Component of hemoglobin for oxygen transport, enzymes for energy metabolism	Meats, legumes, grains, leafy vegetables, eggs, clams, prunes, raisins
Magnesium	Component of bones, enzymes; protein synthesis, nerve transmission	Grains, green leafy vegetables, nuts, legumes, oysters, crab, cornmeal
Manganese	Component of enzymes; fat synthesis, bone and connective tissue synthesis	Whole grains, cereals, green vegetables, tea, ginger, cloves
Molybdenum	Component of enzymes; metabolize iron and uric acid	Cereals, legumes, meat, sunflower seeds, wheat germ
Phosphorus	Acid-base balance, bone and tooth structure, energy production	Milk, cheese, grains, meats, green leafy vegetables, fish
Potassium	Acid-base balance, nerve conduction, body water balance, muscle contractions	Citrus fruits, meat, milk, bananas, liver
Selenium	Antioxidant	Seafood, meat, grains, liver, kidney
Sodium	Water balance, membrane transport, muscle contraction, acid-base balance	Table salt, soy sauce, cured meats
Sulfur	Component of many tissue types such as tendons and cartilage, metabolic pathways, blood clotting	Sulfur-containing amino acids (e.g., methionine, cystine), garlic, onion, seafood, asparagus
Ultratrace Minerals		
Nickel	Cofactor in enzyme reactions	Chocolate, nuts, fruits
Silicon	Bone calcification, collagen	Chicken skin, whole grains
Tin	Exact functions unknown	General diet
Vanadium	Cofactor in enzyme reactions	Olives, shellfish, mushrooms
Zinc	Component of enzymes required for digestion, wound healing, vision, sexual development	Oysters, liver, milk, fish, meats, carrots, oatmeal, peas

meet the physical energy needs to sustain life. The balance of dietary energy intake and energy expenditure was accomplished almost subconsciously by most individuals because of the need for manual labor in everyday life. Since the beginning of the Industrial Revolution in the mid-1800s, the invention of many labor-saving devices (e.g., manufacturing assembly lines, telegraph, telephone, e-mail, cell phones, automobile, remote control) and new forms of entertainment (e.g., radio, television, the Internet) has reduced energy expenditure for most people. Today, despite common knowledge that regular exercise is healthful, more than 60% of Americans are not regularly physically active and 25% are not active at all. In the past 50 years, society has welcomed an immense variety of new types of foods made from basic food sources (animals, plants). Ease and convenience of food preparation (e.g., fast food restaurants, drive-throughs, use of a microwave versus a convection oven) and increases in portion sizes to increase commercial market share have placed too many easily consumed calories on the tables of the American public. Consequently, reduced physical activity and increased caloric intake have resulted in a national epidemic of obesity, causing metabolic syndrome (see Chapter 20) and premature death.

The latest reports from the National Academies of Sciences, Engineering, and Medicine (2017) focus on combating obesity with food literacy and physical exercise. The Academies have stressed the importance of balancing diet with physical activity for years and make recommendations about daily maximum caloric intake of food to be consumed based on height, weight, and gender for four different levels of physical activity (sedentary, low active, active, and very active). The reports illustrate how difficult it is to lose weight based on reduction of calories alone and how important it is to maintain a level of physical activity to prevent reduction in lean body mass (muscle or protein wasting). The reports now recommend moderate physical activity of at least 30 minutes daily, such as brisk walking, to reduce risk of heart attack, stroke, colon cancer, high blood pressure, diabetes, and other medical problems. To manage weight and prevent gradual, unhealthy weight gain, 60 to 90 minutes of moderate-intensity physical activity (e.g., walking at a rate of 4 to 5 miles/hr) or high-intensity activity (e.g., jogging at a rate of 4 to 5 miles for 20 to 30 minutes) four to seven times weekly, in addition to the activities of daily living, is recommended to maintain body weight (in adults) in the recommended body mass index range (18 to 25 kg/m^2).

MALNUTRITION

Nutrition plays a vital role in helping a patient recover from illness. Adequate intake of nutrients is critical to restoring normal homeostasis and rebuilding damaged tissue. If nutritional needs are not adequately addressed, malnutrition results. Malnutrition is a major source of morbidity and mortality in patients who suffer from disease because they are much more susceptible to infections and organ failure. Malnutrition generally results from inadequate intake of protein and calories or from a deficiency of one or more vitamins and minerals.

Malnutrition resulting from inadequate ingestion of proteins and calories may be subdivided into three types—marasmus, kwashiorkor, and mixed kwashiorkor-marasmus. **Marasmus**, the most common form of malnutrition in hospitalized patients, results from a lack of both total energy calories and protein. Marasmus occurs most commonly in patients who suffer from chronic disease and who do not ingest or use adequate amounts of proteins and calories. These patients, in essence, are starving, and they have a cachectic appearance. Laboratory tests indicate normal serum albumin and transferrin concentrations but delayed cutaneous hypersensitivity. In severe cases, muscle function is diminished. **Kwashiorkor** is a protein deficiency that develops when the patient receives adequate fats and carbohydrates in the diet but little or no protein. These patients are often difficult to recognize because they appear well nourished. They are often edematous, and laboratory tests may show hypoalbuminemia. **Mixed kwashiorkor-marasmus** results from inadequate protein building combined with a wasting of fat stores and skeletal muscle. This most often results in a patient with marasmus who is suddenly stressed with a new insult, such as infection. The additional stress causes a greater energy need, leading to a greater loss of fat stores, muscle mass, and serum proteins. These patients often have lower immunocompetence, are hypoalbuminemic, and have wounds that heal very slowly.

A patient's nutritional status must be assessed to diagnose a nutritional deficiency. Nutrition assessment requires completion of a medical history, dietary history, physical examination, and anthropometric measurements (height, weight, skinfold thickness, limb size, and wrist circumference) and collection of laboratory data. Laboratory tests used to assess lean body mass include albumin, prealbumin, retinol binding protein, and transferrin levels. Tests commonly used to assess immune function are total lymphocyte count and delayed cutaneous hypersensitivity reactions.

THERAPY FOR MALNUTRITION

During illness, patients may require partial or full supplementation of their nutritional needs to prevent metabolic imbalances and starvation. One of two forms of supplementation is often used, depending on the patient's requirements. **Enteral nutrition** is administered orally, either by drinking or by instillation into the stomach through a feeding tube (**tube feedings**—nasogastric, nasoduodenal, or nasojejunal tube) or feeding gastrostomy tube (see Chapter 8). Administration of nutrients directly into veins is known as *parenteral* *nutrition.* **Total parenteral nutrition (TPN)** may be subdivided into **peripheral parenteral nutrition (PPN)** and **central parenteral nutrition (CPN)**. The PPN refers to solutions that are administered using the peripheral veins, and the CPN refers to solutions administered using a central vein (see Chapter 11 for a discussion of central venous access and implantable vascular access devices that may be used to administer parenteral nutrition).

 Clinical Pitfall

Total parenteral nutrition orders are formulated daily based on the patient's status, weight, and fluid and electrolyte balance. It is essential to check all aspects of the healthcare provider's order against the actual container of TPN solution with a second qualified nurse and initiate the flow rate specified using an infusion pump. Follow clinical practice guidelines for changing the TPN container and tubing, generally every 24 hours.

❖ NURSING IMPLICATIONS FOR NUTRITIONAL SUPPORT

The purpose of enteral or parenteral nutrition is to supply the patient with an adequate intake of nutrients to meet the body's metabolic needs. Enteral and parenteral forms of nutritional support are undertaken for individuals who are unable to eat, have altered absorptive processes, or are unable to meet the body's required nutritional demands resulting from coexisting disease.

◆ Assessment

History of nutritional deficit. Review the patient's history to identify the rationale for use of nutritional support (e.g., protein-calorie malnutrition [kwashiorkor and marasmus], burn, surgery, cancer, acquired immunodeficiency syndrome, hyperemesis gravidarum, infection, radiation therapy, chemotherapy, malabsorptive disorders, anorexia).

Nutritional history
- Are socioeconomic factors influencing the individual's dietary practices?
- Are cultural or religious practices affecting the individual's food intake pattern? What are the patient's food preferences and food customs?
- Ask the patient to describe the pattern of the developing nutritional problem (e.g., amount of weight loss and period of time over which it has occurred; any concurrent symptoms).
- Ask the patient to do a 24-hour recall of foods eaten and fluids ingested, including an estimate of serving sizes.
- As time permits and condition of the patient warrants, have the person keep a record of all foods eaten and fluids ingested over a specific time, usually 3 days. It may be useful to have the patient record the times of meals and any activities that coincide with the food intake. This will help establish a pattern of the daily eating cycle.
- Are there any physical conditions that alter the patient's ability to ingest food? Examine the oral cavity for dentition or chewing problems, observe swallowing, and check history regarding any incidence of aspiration.
- Ask whether patient has any food or drug allergies.
- Is the patient taking any prescription or nonprescription medicines, especially corticosteroids or anabolic steroids; medicines for diabetes, hypertension, or heart disease; tetracycline; or vitamins?
- Is the patient pregnant or planning to become pregnant in the next several months? Is the patient breast feeding?

Physical changes related to a malnourished state
- Obtain height, weight, arm muscle circumference, and triceps skinfold thickness.
- Check the skin integrity, skeletal muscle mass, and subcutaneous fat distribution. When performing an examination, take into consideration normal alterations in fat distribution throughout the life cycle.
- *Skin integrity, muscle mass, and fat distribution:* Starvation may be manifested by depletion of skeletal muscle mass; however, it may also be caused by muscle atrophy from disease or lack of use. Another indication of starvation is fat depletion in the waist, arms, and legs. Dry, dull hair that can be easily pulled from the scalp is associated with protein deficiency. With advanced protein deficiency, known as *kwashiorkor*, the skin may become dry and flaky. Observe for edema in the abdomen and subcutaneous tissues, another sign of possible protein deficiency.
- *Cardiovascular alterations:* Caloric deficiencies over a long period may cause hypotension, generalized weakness, and low energy levels. A thiamine deficiency can increase heart rate and heart size and may be recognized by a widened pulse pressure.
- *Respiratory alterations:* Obese patients may have an increase in fat sufficient to restrict expansion and contraction of the chest, thereby compromising pulmonary function. Patients need to have lung sounds assessed to detect crackling sounds (crackles), an indication of overhydration and excessive fluid intake.
- *Neurologic alterations:* Vitamin B deficiencies may be related to abnormal findings with accompanying symptoms, such as decreased position sense and diminished vibratory sense, decreased tendon reflexes, weakness, paresthesias, or decreased tactile sensations; therefore these patients require a more thorough neurologic evaluation. Thiamine deficiency may result in neurologic deficit.
- *Abdominal alterations:* Perform an examination of the abdomen by inspection, auscultation, percussion, light palpation, and deep palpation as dictated by the nurse's level of knowledge and assessment skills.

- Obtain a history of GI symptoms such as diarrhea, vomiting, constipation, and abdominal pain and their relationship to food consumption; ask specifically for details on how any of these conditions have been self-treated or treated by a healthcare provider.
- *Thyroid function:* The thyroid gland and its hormones influence all body cells. Be aware of the signs and symptoms of hypothyroidism (e.g., weight gain, dry brittle hair, facial edema, enlarged breasts, slowed pulse, coarse dry skin, deepening of the voice, lethargy, slowed speech and impaired memory, muscle weakness, altered reflexes). Conversely, be aware of the signs and symptoms of hyperthyroidism (e.g., goiter, hyperactive reflexes, weight loss, increased pulse rate, dysrhythmias, elevated blood pressure, emotional lability, heat intolerance).

◆ Implementation

- Implement orders for diet, nutritional supplements, vitamins, minerals, tube feedings, intravenous (IV) therapy, or TPN.
- Perform assessments for nutritional and fluid deficits and excess.
- Implement proper administration and monitoring for complications associated with enteral, parenteral, or total parenteral administration.
- Perform verification of tube placement, including pH testing, in accordance with clinical site policies.
- Implement institutional policies for flushing and administration of medications via feeding tubes.
- Document all aspects of patient care relating to nutritional therapy and the patient's response to therapy.
- If the patient is to continue special feedings after discharge, assure that the patient understands proper storage of nutritional products or parenteral solutions.

Monitoring tube feedings

- Check tube placement and gastric pH according to clinical practice guidelines or healthcare provider orders.
- In general, check tube placement and residual volumes before the administration of each bolus tube feeding, or every 4 or 8 hours for continuous feedings. When residual volumes exceed 100 mL or another limit is specified by the healthcare provider's order, hold further tube feeding and recheck residual volume in 1 hour. Most clinical settings then resume the prescribed ordered volume if the repeat residual volume is less than 100 mL. Because higher residual volumes may indicate obstruction, the healthcare provider should be notified if the residual amount has not diminished to less than 100 mL.
- Follow the healthcare provider's orders for the amount, type, strength of solution, and rate of administration, as well as the method of administration prescribed (e.g., continuous, intermittent, bolus, cyclic). Enteral feedings are often initiated at half strength to determine how well the patient's GI tract tolerates the solution. If abdominal distention, nausea, vomiting, diarrhea, or cramping starts, discontinue administration and notify the healthcare provider for further orders.
- Initiate enteral feeding at a lower rate of about 20 mL/hr. Every 12 to 24 hours, increase the rate by about 10 mL/hr until the appropriate hourly volume has been attained.
- Perform daily weights and monitor for signs of dehydration or overhydration. Monitor blood glucose and other laboratory or diagnostic test results (notify healthcare provider of abnormal results).
- Change tube feeding apparatus in accordance with clinical facility policy, usually every 24 hours.
- Handle enteral feedings carefully to prevent bacterial contamination. Store in a clean, cool place and wash lids before opening the ready-to-use preparations. Check manufacturer's recommendations for the length of time that a formula is considered safe at room temperature (usually 12 hours). Many clinical sites suggest placing only enough formula for 4 or 8 hours in the delivery apparatus; check individual clinical site guidelines.

Monitoring peripheral parenteral nutrition

- Observe IV site for signs of infiltration, phlebitis, or local reaction.
- Monitor actual IV infusion rate and all aspects of the IV order (type and strength of solution, rate of administration). Check date on IV container and tubing for need to be changed, usually every 24 hours.
- Monitor the patient for signs and symptoms of fluid overload (e.g., bounding pulse rate, hoarseness, dyspnea, cough, venous distention).
- Monitor for pyrogenic reaction (e.g., fever, chills, general malaise, vomiting), usually within 30 minutes of initiating therapy.
- Monitor for anaphylactic reaction to proteins (e.g., wheezing, itching, hypotension, tightness in chest).

Monitoring central parenteral nutrition

- Monitor daily weights and laboratory or diagnostic test results (notify healthcare provider of abnormal results).
- Check all aspects of the healthcare provider's order against the actual container of CPN solution with a second qualified nurse, and initiate the flow rate specified using an infusion pump. Follow clinical practice guidelines for changing of CPN container and tubing, generally every 24 hours.
- Provide site care for central venous access in accordance with clinical site policy. Assess site for redness, swelling or drainage, elevated temperature, or fatigue (signs of infection).
- Perform glucose and urine ketone tests as specified by the healthcare provider's orders, and administer regular insulin according to orders. Check patient

for signs of hypoglycemia (e.g., nausea, weakness, thirst, rapid respirations, headache).

- Assess for signs of refeeding syndrome during the first 24 to 48 hours after initiation of CPN or tube feeding (e.g., changes in electrolytes, respiratory depression, confusion, weakness, irritability, generalized lethargy).
- Observe for fluid and electrolyte imbalances and hyperglycemia resulting from high glucose content of solution. Do not speed up CPN solution to catch up if the amount delivered is behind schedule. This practice may overload the individual's system with glucose.
- Individuals are tapered from CPN by gradually slowing the infusion rate of the CPN while simultaneously increasing oral intake over a few days. This procedure ensures that the patient's GI system can tolerate adequate oral feedings without diarrhea developing.

 Clinical Pitfall

Do not speed up CPN solution infusion to "catch up" if the amount delivered is "behind schedule." This practice may cause significant hyperglycemia and metabolic imbalance.

◆ Patient Education

- Patients being discharged with enteral nutrition for home use require considerable education for themselves and family or significant others.
- Give specific written instructions on the administration procedures, type, rate and frequency, storage, and handling of tube feedings ordered. Include in the description signs that indicate a need to call the healthcare provider (e.g., diarrhea, nausea, vomiting, signs of infection).
- Teach the patient or primary caregiver the procedure used in the hospital to administer the enteral or parenteral solutions.
- Ask the appropriate individual(s) to demonstrate competency in performing the procedures before discharge. As appropriate, request a referral to a community agency, such as visiting nurses, for assistance in the home with the feedings.
- Give specific instructions on changing tubing and apparatus used and the importance of adhering to the techniques taught in the hospital to prevent infection.
- Have the patient role-play the resolution of common problems associated with the prescribed nutritional therapy (e.g., tube obstruction, cramping, diarrhea, nausea).
- Teach the person with a central IV line the proper care of the line and dressing changes, as permitted by the employing institution.
- Teach the individual to perform daily weights at the same time of day in similar clothing on the same scale.

- Teach appropriate oral hygiene measures and include ways to alleviate thirst and mouth dryness (e.g., rinsing the mouth frequently, use of hard candy or sugarless gum).
- Give written instructions of what to do if the patient aspirates or the tube comes out.
- Explain techniques that can be used to self-administer tube feedings ordered for intermittent administration.
- Explain the importance of having the prescribed laboratory tests done as scheduled to evaluate the response to the nutritional therapy.
- Teach the patient to maintain a record of temperature, pulse, respirations, blood pressure, and defined monitoring parameters.

Fostering health maintenance

- Provide the patient and significant others with important information for the specific medications prescribed. For example, when an iron preparation is prescribed, the patient should understand it is best taken between meals; however, as a result of stomach irritation, it may be best to take it with food or immediately after meals. Liquid iron should be taken with a straw placed well back on the tongue, and the mouth should be rinsed immediately after administration to prevent staining of the teeth. When vitamins and minerals are prescribed, it is necessary to continue their use for the period specified by the healthcare provider and to adhere to the prescribed dosage.
- Ensure that the patient understands the care, handling, and storage of all enteral, supplemental, or parenteral solutions, and the need to prevent infection through use of the proper administration techniques.
- Discuss ways that the individual who is to be maintained on enteral nutrition or TPN for a long time can be involved, as appropriate, with other household members during mealtimes.
- Seek cooperation and understanding of the following points so that medication compliance is increased: name of medication; dosage, route, and time of administration; and common and serious adverse effects. For all supplemental, enteral, or TPN solutions, the individual must understand all components of the healthcare provider's orders.

Patient self-assessment. Enlist the patient's help in developing and maintaining a written record of monitoring parameters. See the Patient Self-Assessment Form for Nutritional Therapy on the Evolve website. Complete the Premedication Data column for use as a baseline to track response to drug therapy. Ensure that the patient understands how to use the form, and instruct the patient to take the completed form to follow-up visits. During follow-up visits, focus on issues that will foster adherence with the therapeutic interventions prescribed.

ENTERAL NUTRITION

Actions

Enteral nutrition is the provision of nutrients through the GI tract. Formulas may be administered orally or by nasogastric, nasoduodenal, or nasojejunal tube; feeding gastrostomy tube; or needle-catheter jejunostomy.

Uses

There is an adage often used in medicine: "When the gut works, and can be safely used, use it." Supplementation with enteral food formulas is indicated when oral consumption is inadequate. Examples of when tube feedings might be necessary are head and neck surgery, esophageal obstruction, stroke resulting in inability to chew or swallow food, and dementia. Advantages to enteral nutrition, when compared with parenteral nutrition, are that it avoids risks associated with IV therapy, provides GI stimulation, and is physiologic; protocols for administration are much less stringent because there is less risk of infection; and enteral feeding is less expensive. Enteral feedings are contraindicated when there is intractable vomiting, a paralyzed ileum, and/or the presence of certain types of fistulas. See Table 46.4 for examples of oral supplements, standard feeding tube formulas, pediatric formulas, and formulas for special cases such as hepatic, renal, or pulmonary failure or malabsorption syndrome.

Therapeutic Outcomes

The primary therapeutic outcomes expected from enteral nutrition are the following:

1. Stabilization of the patient's weight within identified parameters
2. Sufficient intake of nutrients to maintain age-appropriate growth and development
3. Improved results seen in laboratory assessments of nutrition

❖ Nursing Implications for Enteral Nutrition

◆ Premedication assessment

1. Assess for underlying diseases such as heart disease or renal or liver impairment that may limit the rate of administration and type of enteral formula to be used.
2. Assess for food allergies and lactose intolerance.
3. Review and record daily weights, changes in gastric motility, and stool characteristics.
4. Review enteral formula for type ordered and expiration date of formula.
5. Monitor for signs and symptoms of aspiration (e.g., respiratory rate and depth, lung sounds) and elevation in body temperature.
6. Check tube placement and residual volume present according to policy (see Chapter 8).
7. Check all aspects of the healthcare provider's order for a tube feeding—type, amount, rate of administration, method of administration (bolus or continuous)—and for specific orders regarding additional water intake.

8. Check to ensure that laboratory tests have been completed before starting enteral therapy (e.g., serum prealbumin, albumin, urea nitrogen, creatinine, electrolytes, hemoglobin, hematocrit, lipids, liver function studies, glucose, total lymphocyte count, ferritin, transferrin, urine specific gravity, and urine ketones).
9. Be prepared to monitor for potential signs and symptoms of enteral nutrition complications throughout the shift (e.g., tube obstruction, skin and mucous membrane breakdown, nausea, diarrhea, constipation, pulmonary complications, hyperglycemia, hypercapnia, fluid volume excess or deficits).

◆ *Availability.* See Table 46.4.

◆ *Dosage and administration.* Tube feedings, especially those that have an osmolality of 300 mOsm/L water or higher, need to be started with a quarter- or half-strength formula to prevent diarrhea from a hypertonic solution. The patient is positioned in the high Fowler's position during administration and for a period of 30 to 60 minutes after feeding.

Tube feedings are administered by one of the following methods:

1. *Intermittent or bolus feedings:* Administer 200 mL or more of formula over 20 to 30 minutes using a reservoir bottle or bag. Formula is advanced by gravity.
2. *Continuous drip:* Formula is slowly administered continuously over 12 to 24 hours using an infusion pump. This method is recommended when feeding is infused into the jejunum.

Administration of medicines to the tube-fed patient

- Administer each drug separately; do not combine.
- Stop formula and flush tubing with 15 to 30 mL water.
- Administer prescribed medication, one crushed tablet at a time, suspended in tepid water, followed by 5 to 10 mL of water.
- Flush tube with 15 to 30 mL of water.
- Reinitiate tube feeding and record total amount of water used for flushes.

[!] Medication Safety Alert

- Do not add prescribed medications directly to the formula being administered.
- Do not crush and administer any enteric-coated, chewable, or sublingual tablets via the feeding tube. Obtain a liquid form of the medication when possible.
- Do not crush slow-release tablets and give via the tube. If the size of the tube is sufficient, the slow-release capsules may be opened, added to water, and given via the tube with adequate water to clear the tubing completely following administration.

◆ *Common adverse effects*

Metabolic

Hyperglycemia. Hyperglycemia may develop easily, especially when feeding is started for a malnourished

Table 46.4   Enteral Formulas[a]

BRAND NAMES	CALORIES (kcal/mL)	PROTEIN CONTENT (g/L)	OSMOLALITY (mOsm/kg water)	COMMENTS
Oral Supplements				
Ensure Liquid	0.93	38	500	These products are dietary supplements and are available in a variety of flavors for oral use. They require full digestive capability by gut. At recommended dosages, these formulas provide 100% of the RDA for vitamins and minerals.
Ensure HN	0.5	60	610	
Ensure Plus	1.50	54.2	680	
Boost	1.01	42	610-670	
Standard Isotonic Formulas				
Isocal	1.06	34.0	300	These products are standard formulas used for tube feeding. They are lactose free to prevent bloating and flatulence, and are of low residue and low viscosity. At recommended dosages, these formulas provide 100% of the RDA for vitamins and minerals.
Osmolite 1	1.06	44	300	
Osmolite 1.2	1.2	55.5	360	
Nutren 1.0	1.00	40.0	315	
Isosource HN	1.20	53.6	—	
Pediatric Formulas				
Similac Soy Isomil	0.67	15.7	200	Soy-based infant formula; for infants with allergy to cow's milk or those with lactose intolerance or galactosemia.
Similac Alimentum	0.67	19.0	320	For patients with severe food allergies, protein maldigestion, and fat malabsorption.
Pregestimil	0.67	18.7	290	Predigested; for patients with severe malabsorption.
Phenex-1	Dependent on prepared; 480 cal/100 g of powder	15.0 g per 100 g of powder	370 per 100 g of powder	Phenylalanine free; for patients with phenylketonuria.
Specialized Formulas				
Glucerna 1.0 Cal	1.00	41.8	355	High-fat, low-carbohydrate formula for patients with glucose intolerance.
Nutren Pulmonary	1.50	68	330 unflavored; 450 vanilla	High-fat, low-carbohydrate formula for patients with pulmonary disorders; reduced CO_2 production
Peptamen	1.00	40.0	—	Predigested; for patients with protein maldigestion.
NovaSource Renal	2.0	90	800	Essential amino acids for patients with renal failure.
NutriHep	1.5	40.0	790	High in branched-chain and low in aromatic amino acids; for patients with hepatic encephalopathy.

[a]Formulas listed are representative examples and are not intended to be a complete list.
RDA, Recommended Dietary Allowance.

person. Check healthcare provider's orders for frequency of blood glucose monitoring and whether insulin has been ordered for elevated glucose levels.

◆ *Serious adverse effects*

Respiratory

Pulmonary complications. Assess for symptoms of aspiration.

Gastrointestinal

Diarrhea or constipation. Changes in bowel pattern and consistency often develop when enteral nutrition is initiated. If diarrhea starts, discontinue feedings immediately and report findings to the healthcare provider for further orders.

Nausea, vomiting, increased residual volumes. These signs are an indication of bowel obstruction. Discontinue feedings and report findings to the healthcare provider for further orders.

Hypersensitivity, immune system

Rash, chills, fever, respiratory difficulty. These signs are an indication of allergy to the formula. Provide emergency care as needed. Immediately discontinue feedings and report findings to the healthcare provider for further orders.

◆ *Drug interactions.* Food can affect medicines by altering absorption, metabolism, and excretion; conversely, medicines can affect nutrition by similar pathways. Interactions between drugs and nutrients are particularly significant in older adult patients who often have several chronic diseases requiring long-term multiple drug therapy and who may often have poor nutrition. The following entries provide a synopsis of the more common potential food-drug interactions.

Alcohol and disulfiram, metronidazole, and tinidazole. Alcohol interacts with these three medicines, causing nausea, vomiting, abdominal cramps, headache, sweating, and flushing of the face. Use of alcohol and alcohol-containing preparations, such as over-the-counter cough medications and mouthwashes (e.g., Listerine, Cēpacol), should be avoided during therapy and for 72 hours after discontinuation of metronidazole or tinidazole therapy. The interaction with disulfiram may last several weeks.

Tetracycline, doxycycline, ciprofloxacin, levofloxacin. The patient should avoid taking these antibiotics within 2 hours before or after antacids, iron, zinc, and dairy products (e.g., milk, ice cream, cheese, yogurt). If taken close together, the absorption of the antibiotic is inhibited.

Itraconazole (capsules), ganciclovir, ritonavir. These medicines should be taken with food to increase absorption and therapeutic effect.

Itraconazole (suspension), didanosine, indinavir. These medicines should be taken at least 1 hour before or 2 hours after meals. They need to be taken on an empty stomach to increase absorption and therapeutic effect.

Alendronate, risedronate, ibandronate. Alendronate should be taken at least 30 minutes before the first food, beverage, or medication of the day (for risedronate and ibandronate, at least 2 hours). The patient should take the drug with a full glass of plain water and not lie down for at least 30 minutes with alendronate or risedronate or 60 minutes with ibandronate.

Monoamine oxidase inhibitors (tranylcypromine, phenelzine, isocarboxazid). A major potential complication with monoamine oxidase inhibitor (MAOI) therapy is hypertensive crisis, particularly with tranylcypromine. Because MAOIs block amine metabolism in tissues outside the brain, patients who consume foods or medications containing indirect sympathomimetic amines are at considerable risk for a hypertensive crisis. Foods containing significant quantities of tyramine include well-ripened cheeses (e.g., Camembert, Edam, Roquefort, Parmesan, mozzarella, cheddar), yeast extract, red wines, pickled herring, sauerkraut, overripe bananas, figs, avocados, chicken livers, and beer. Other foods containing vasopressors include fava beans, chocolate, coffee, tea, and colas. Common prodromal symptoms of hypertensive crisis include severe occipital headache, stiff neck, sweating, nausea, vomiting, and sharply elevated blood pressure. This drug-food interaction may occur for up to 2 weeks after discontinuation of the MAOI.

Warfarin. Patients receiving warfarin should avoid extreme changes in diet and daily consumption of large amounts of dark green vegetables. Herbal medicines (e.g., ginseng, ginkgo biloba, garlic) inhibit platelet aggregation. Monitor patients for signs of bleeding.

Grapefruit juice. Fresh or frozen grapefruit juice inhibits the metabolism of several drugs. The severity of the interaction varies among people, among drugs, and with the quantity of grapefruit juice consumed.

Potentially serious interactions between grapefruit juice and other medicines

Calcium channel blockers. These include members of the dihydropyridine class (e.g., felodipine, nifedipine, nimodipine, amlodipine, isradipine, nicardipine). Monitor for signs of toxicity such as flushing, headache, tachycardia, and hypotension.

Carbamazepine. Monitor for signs of toxicity such as dizziness, drowsiness, sedation, nausea, vomiting, blurred vision, and hepatotoxicity.

Antidepressant and antianxiety medicines. Serum concentrations of buspirone, diazepam, triazolam, nefazodone, and trazodone may be increased by concurrent administration with grapefruit juice. Avoid multiday administration of grapefruit juice with any of these agents. Monitor for increased sedation.

Cyclosporine. Monitor for signs of toxicity such as nephrotoxicity, hepatotoxicity, and increased immunosuppression.

Caffeine. Monitor for signs of toxicity such as nervousness and overstimulation.

 Herbal Interactions

Patients receiving warfarin should avoid herbal medicines (e.g., ginseng, ginkgo biloba, garlic) that inhibit platelet aggregation.

PARENTERAL NUTRITION

Actions
Parenteral nutrition is the administration of nutrients by IV infusion. Parenteral nutrient solutions provide a balanced combination of carbohydrates, amino acids, and essential fats, along with appropriate minerals, vitamins, and electrolytes.

Uses
Parenteral nutrition is used for patients who are unable to take nutrition enterally for more than 7 days. It is generally used for intractable vomiting and diarrhea, malabsorption syndromes, bowel surgery, coma, and bowel rest and for conditions requiring additional nutrition, such as massive wound healing secondary to trauma or major infection.

The type of parenteral nutrition prescribed depends on the patient's status, metabolic needs, and disease process and how long the individual will not be able to meet metabolic demands through normal oral intake.

Peripheral parenteral nutrition is used for patients requiring support for a limited time, usually lasting less than 3 to 4 weeks. It is appropriate for the patient who is anticipated to have normal GI functioning reestablished within a short time. Peripheral parenteral nutrition administration generally requires a relatively high fluid volume of approximately 2000 mL/day and therefore may not be tolerated well or indicated for some coexisting disease processes such as heart failure. Peripheral parenteral nutrition solutions consist of 2% to 5% crystalline amino acid preparations with 5% or 10% dextrose and added electrolytes and vitamins.

Central parenteral nutrition consists of glucose (15% to 25%); amino acids (3.5% to 15%); fat emulsion (10% to 20%); and electrolytes, vitamins, and minerals. The Harris-Benedict equation may be used to estimate caloric and nutritional requirements. Special hepatic, renal, and stress formulations are also available.

Therapeutic Outcomes

The primary therapeutic outcomes expected from parenteral nutrition are as follows:
1. Stabilization of the patient's weight within identified parameters
2. Sufficient intake of nutrients to maintain age-appropriate growth and development
3. Improved results seen in laboratory assessments of nutrition

❖ **Nursing Implications for Parenteral Nutrition**
◆ *Premedication assessment*
1. Assess for underlying disorders such as heart disease or renal or liver impairment, which may limit the rate of administration and type of parenteral formula to be used.
2. Review and record daily weight; note hydration of mucous membranes.
3. Check to ensure that laboratory tests have been completed before starting parenteral therapy (e.g., serum prealbumin, albumin, urea nitrogen, creatinine, electrolytes, hemoglobin, hematocrit, lipids, liver function studies, glucose, total lymphocyte count, ferritin, transferrin, urine specific gravity, and urine ketones).
4. Compare the entire healthcare provider's order with the actual contents of the TPN container before initiating or adding it to the running access site.
5. Check the patient's identification and the expiration date and time on the TPN to be hung.
6. Discard any TPN solution that remains at the end of 24 hours. Have the next container of TPN ready. If it is not ready, hang a solution of 10% dextrose. Do *not* simply shut off the infusion.
7. Take vital signs at least every 4 hours while TPN is being administered.
8. Be prepared to monitor for potential signs and symptoms of parenteral nutrition complications throughout the shift (e.g., pulmonary complications, hyperglycemia, hypercapnia, and fluid volume excess or deficits).

◆ *Availability*
• Check at least 1 to 2 hours in advance of needing the next container of TPN to be certain that it will be ready.
• Always use an infusion pump for administration of TPN.
• Do not speed up TPN if it gets behind schedule. Speeding it up could result in hyperglycemia, seizures, coma, or death.
• Schedule blood glucose monitoring as prescribed by the healthcare provider, generally every 4 hours during initiation or every 6 hours thereafter.
• Schedule daily electrolyte studies as prescribed.

◆ *Dosage and administration.* Do not use TPN IV lines or central venous catheters for delivery of any other medications or solutions.

◆ *Common adverse effects*
   Metabolic
   Hyperglycemia. Hyperglycemia may develop easily, especially when CPN is initiated for a malnourished person. Symptoms include headache, nausea and vomiting, abdominal pain, dizziness, rapid pulse, rapid shallow respirations, and a fruity odor to the breath from acetone. Check the healthcare provider's orders for frequency of blood glucose monitoring and whether insulin has been ordered for elevated glucose levels.

◆ *Serious adverse effects*
   Metabolic
   Hypoglycemia. Signs of hypoglycemia include nervousness, tremors, headache, apprehension, sweating, cold clammy skin, and hunger. This may progress to blurred vision, lack of coordination, incoherence, coma, and death.
   Fluid imbalance. Overhydration may be recognized by weight gain, neck vein distention, change in mental status, edema, dyspnea, crackles and rhonchi, tachycardia, and bounding pulses. Dehydration may be noted by loss of skin turgor, sticky oral mucous membranes, a shrunken or deeply furrowed tongue, crusted lips, weight loss, deteriorating vital signs, soft or sunken eyeballs, weak pedal pulses, delayed capillary refill, excessive thirst, and mental confusion.
   Electrolyte imbalances. Check for indications of electrolyte imbalance (e.g., mental status [alertness, orientation, confusion], muscle strength, muscle cramps, tremors, nausea, decline in general appearance). Check laboratory values and report abnormal values to the healthcare provider.
   Vitamin deficiencies. Deficiencies of fat-soluble vitamins:
• *Vitamin A:* Diarrhea; dry, scaly, rough, cracked skin; alterations in adaptation to light and dark

- *Vitamin D:* Involuntary spasms and twitching, decreased calcium and phosphorus, demineralization of bones
- *Vitamin E:* Hemolysis of red blood cells; in older children, neurologic syndrome of vitamin E deficiency
- *Vitamin K:* Symptoms of bleeding and/or delayed clotting

  Deficiencies of water-soluble vitamins:
- *Cyanocobalamin:* Anorexia, ataxia, diarrhea, constipation, irritability, paresthesia, delirium, hallucinations
- *Folic acid:* Diarrhea, glossitis, macrocytic anemia, low serum levels
- *Niacin:* Glossitis, diarrhea, rashes, weakness, anorexia, indigestion; as deficiency progresses, central nervous system involvement is manifested by confusion, disorientation, neuritis
- *Pyridoxine:* Anemia, dyspnea, cheilosis (cracks in the corner of the mouth), glossitis (inflammation of the tongue), convulsions
- *Riboflavin:* Cheilosis, glossitis, seborrheic dermatitis, photophobia, poor wound healing

- *Thiamine:* Anorexia (poor to no appetite), constipation, indigestion, confusion, edema, muscle weakness, cardiomegaly, heart failure
- *Vitamin C:* Anemia, petechiae, depression, delayed wound healing

  Gastrointestinal

  Hepatotoxicity. Fatty liver may develop. Check liver function tests (elevated bilirubin, aspartate aminotransferase, alanine aminotransferase, gamma-glutamyltransferase, and alkaline phosphatase levels; increased prothrombin time) and report abnormal laboratory values to the healthcare provider.

  Hypersensitivity, immune system

  Rash, chills, fever, respiratory difficulty. These signs are an indication of allergy to the formula. Provide emergency care as needed. Immediately discontinue feedings and report findings to the healthcare provider for further orders.

◆ *Drug Interactions.* No other drugs should be administered concurrently with TPN. Consult a pharmacist for parenteral nutrition solutions and compatibility with specific medicines.

Get Ready for the NCLEX® Examination!

Key Points

- Energy sources required for balanced metabolism are the macronutrients—fats, carbohydrates, and proteins. Other essential nutrients include vitamins, minerals, fiber, and water. Nutritional requirements vary based not only on the age of the individual but also on the gender and level of activity.
- No one food source can meet all of the basic nutritional requirements. Healthful diets provide a balance of carbohydrates, fiber, fat, protein, and essential nutrients to reduce the risks of chronic diseases and support a full and productive lifestyle. Healthful nutrition must be accompanied by regular mild-to-moderate physical activity to help maintain muscle tone and agility.
- Nutrition plays a vital role in helping a patient recover from illness. Adequate intake of nutrients is critical to restoring normal homeostasis and rebuilding damaged tissue. If nutritional needs are not adequately addressed, malnutrition results. Malnutrition is a major source of morbidity and mortality in patients who are suffering from disease because they are much more susceptible to infections and organ failure than are healthy individuals.
- During illness, patients may require partial or full supplementation of their nutritional needs. One of two forms of supplementation is often used. Enteral nutrition is administered orally, either by the patient drinking the liquid or by administration into the GI tract by a feeding tube. Administration of nutrients directly into veins is known as *parenteral nutrition.*

- Nurses need to understand the importance of cultural beliefs whenever special diets are prescribed. Because the nurse may not have knowledge of the cultural aspects of dietary adaptations, it is essential to involve a nutritionist in the dietary planning process.

Additional Learning Resources

SG Go to your Study Guide for additional Review Questions for the NCLEX® Examination, Critical Thinking Clinical Situations, and other learning activities to help you master this chapter content.

Go to your Evolve website (https://evolve.elsevier.com/Clayton) for additional online resources.

Review Questions for the NCLEX® Examination

1. The nurse asked the patient to pick out good food sources of dietary fiber from the menu. Which selection indicates adequate patient understanding?
   1. Lettuce salad with dressing
   2. Potatoes, pasta, and white bread
   3. Beef, chicken, fish, and tofu
   4. Cereal brans, sweet potatoes, vegetables, and fruits

2. After discussing sources of dietary fats that have health benefits with the patient, the nurse expects that the patient will identify which sources? *(Select all that apply.)*
   1. Whole milk
   2. Olive oil
   3. Coconut oil
   4. Ice cream
   5. Avocados

3. A patient who has a diet high in fruits and vegetables may be getting which vitamins? *(Select all that apply.)*
   1. Vitamin A
   2. Vitamin B_3
   3. Vitamin C
   4. Vitamin E
   5. Vitamin K

4. A patient who had been instructed by the healthcare provider to increase the amount of calcium in the diet asked the nurse what would be recommended. Which would be an appropriate response by the nurse?
   1. "Cook with ginger and cloves, and eat more whole grains."
   2. "Be sure to eat more chicken, beans, and green leafy vegetables."
   3. "I think that you can have more oysters and liver, as well as oatmeal."
   4. "Milk, cheese, and vegetables should be part of your diet."

5. The nurse was assessing the patient's nutritional status and became concerned about which findings that point to possible malnutrition? *(Select all that apply.)*
   1. Reports of increased physical activity
   2. Dry, dull hair that falls out easily
   3. Generalized weakness and lethargy
   4. Recent intended weight loss
   5. Laboratory tests that indicate hypoalbuminemia

6. Which assessment finding that the nurse discovered during a gastrostomy feeding requires the prescriber to be notified?
   1. A gastric residual of 120 mL after the tube feeding was held for 1 hour.
   2. The tube-feeding formula was kept at room temperature in a cabinet.
   3. The patient's abdomen was soft and nausea was absent.
   4. The feeding tube was kinked, and only half of the formula was administered during that hour.

7. The nurse reviewing an order for PPN notifies the healthcare provider after checking the formula and finding the dextrose amount to be which value?
   1. 5%
   2. 7%
   3. 10%
   4. 15%

8. The nurse discussing the difference between PPN and CPN with the patient used which accurate statement?
   1. "You will be getting nutrition through the tube in your nose to help you meet your daily requirements of calories and nutrients."
   2. "This solution of PPN will be given in your vein in your arm to provide you with your daily requirements of calories and nutrients."
   3. "This solution of CPN will be given in your vein in your arm to provide you with your daily requirements of calories and nutrients."
   4. "When you get home, you will need to give yourself nutrition through your feeding tube in your abdomen."

Objectives

1. Summarize the primary actions and potential uses of the herbal and dietary supplement products cited.

2. Describe the interactions between commonly used herbal and dietary supplement products and prescription medications.

Key Terms

dietary supplements (DĬ-ĕ-tār-ē SŬP-lĕ-mĕnts) (p. 756)
herbal medicines (ĔR-băl MĔD-ĭ-sĭnz) (p. 758)
botanicals (bō-TĂN-ĭ-kălz) (p. 758)

phytomedicine (fī-tō-MĔD-ĭ-sĭn) (p. 758)
phytotherapy (fī-tō-THĔR-ă-pē) (p. 758)

HERBAL MEDICINES, DIETARY SUPPLEMENTS, AND RATIONAL THERAPY

Over the past two decades, there has been a tremendous resurgence in the popularity of self-care and alternative therapies, including acupuncture, aromatherapy, homeopathy, vitamin and other supplement therapy, and herbal medicine. When herbal preparations are labeled "all natural," these products become attractive to the general public because the common perception is that "all natural" is synonymous with "better" and not harmful.

There also has been a greater emphasis on health, wellness, and disease prevention, which contributes to the perception that herbal preparations are harmless. Some of the more than 250 herbal medicines and hundreds of combinations of other supplements may be beneficial, but unfortunately the whole field of complementary medicine is fraught with false claims, lack of standardization, and adulteration and misbranding of products.

REGULATORY LEGISLATION

In the early 1990s, the US Food and Drug Administration (FDA) threatened to ban from the US market herbal medicines and other types of supplements that were being touted as good for health until appropriate scientific studies were completed to prove that these products were safe and effective. Such an uproar was created by this threat that Congress passed the Dietary Supplement Health and Education Act of 1994. Under this act, almost all herbal medicines, vitamins, minerals, amino acids, and other supplemental chemicals used for health were reclassified legally as dietary supplements, a food category. The legislation also allows manufacturers to include information on the label and through advertisements about how these products affect the human body. These labels and advertisements also must contain a statement that the product has not yet been evaluated by the FDA for treating, curing, or preventing any disease. The law does not prevent other people (e.g., nutritionists, health food store clerks, herbalists, strength coaches, or other unlicensed individuals) from making claims (founded or unfounded) about the therapeutic effects of supplement ingredients.

The result of the new law is that dietary supplements are not required to be safe and effective, and unfounded claims of therapeutic benefit abound. Hundreds of herbal medicines and other dietary supplements are marketed in the United States as single- and multiple-ingredient products for an extremely wide variety of uses, all implying that they will improve one's health.

INDEPENDENT PRODUCT TESTING

The vast majority of the popular claims made for herbal medicines and dietary supplements are unproven. The FDA issued Good Manufacturing Practices, which became mandatory for the dietary supplement industry as of June 2010 (https://www.fda.gov/Drugs/DevelopmentApprovalProcess/Manufacturing/ucm090016.htm).

Since 1999, ConsumerLab.com has been testing dietary supplements, and the United States Pharmacopeial Convention launched the Dietary Supplement Verification Program in 2001 and began testing products that year. The United States Pharmacopeial Convention is a scientific nonprofit standards-setting organization that establishes federally recognized standards for the quality of drugs and dietary supplements. It is the only such organization recognized in US federal law that also offers voluntary verification services to help ensure dietary supplement quality, purity, and potency. Its standards for prescription drugs and over-the-counter (OTC) medicines are FDA enforceable per the Federal Food, Drug, and Cosmetic Act of 1938. In 2003 the NSF (National Sanitation Foundation) International began testing dietary supplements. Products that pass testing are eligible to bear the mark of approval from the testing agency (Fig. 47.1).

It is important to remember that the products are tested for labeled potency, good manufacturing practices, and lack of contamination, but they are not tested for safety and efficacy or for manufacturer's claims on the label. Dietary supplement therapy, under current legal standards, creates an ethical dilemma for nurses and other healthcare professionals. Licensed healthcare professionals have a moral and ethical responsibility to recommend only medicines that are proven to be safe and effective. They should be aware of a medicine's legal use versus its popular use, its potential for toxicity, and its potential for interactions with other medicines. Box 47.1 lists the factors to consider when discussing dietary supplements.

Studies have shown that 40% to 78% of patients fail to disclose the use of complementary and herbal therapy to their healthcare provider, resulting in a lack of guidance for these products (Chong, 2006). It is important for the nurse to inquire about the use of these products when obtaining a history from the patient. The nurse can direct the patient and family toward reliable web resources, such as the National Institutes of Health website, that provide sound scientific data on supplements.

❖ NURSING IMPLICATIONS FOR HERBAL AND DIETARY SUPPLEMENT THERAPY

◆ Assessment
- Discuss specific dietary supplement products and the patient's reasons for using these products.
- Obtain a list of the specific symptoms that the patient is treating with the supplement products and details of whether the symptoms have improved (or worsened) since beginning therapy. Ask whether the patient has informed his or her healthcare provider of this use of supplement products.
- Did anyone in particular recommend herbal products? If yes, what was the basis of the recommendations?
- Obtain a detailed list of all prescribed, OTC, and supplemental products in use. Have any prescribed medications been discontinued in lieu of initiating supplements?
- What cultural or ethnic beliefs does the individual espouse?

History of symptoms. Examine data to determine the individual's understanding of the symptoms or the disease process for which the individual began taking supplements.

Medication history
- Check the history and physical assessment by the healthcare provider to determine whether any supplement products are listed.
- Research dietary supplements being taken and identify drug interactions, actions, and adverse effects that may occur.
- Check the hospital policy regarding the administration and recording of the products. Because they are not medications, but rather are classified legally as dietary supplements (a food category), how are the orders

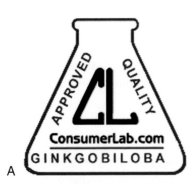 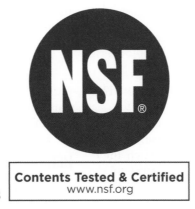 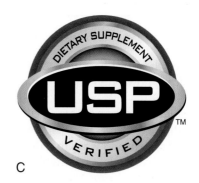

A   B   C

Fig. 47.1 These certification marks signify that the dietary supplements to which the mark is affixed contain ingredients as listed on the label and that they were manufactured using good manufacturing practices, but they do not certify whether the products are safe and effective for the labeled use. (*A,* Used with permission from ConsumerLab.com, White Plains, NY. *B,* Used with permission from NSF International, Ann Arbor, MI. *C,* Used with permission from the United States Pharmacopeial Convention, Rockville, MD.)

Box 47.1	Factors to Consider When Recommending Herbal Medicines and Other Dietary Supplements

1. Dietary supplements are not miraculous cure-alls. Most of those intended for therapeutic use are technically unapproved drugs. They may have been used for centuries, but substantial data on safety and efficacy of long-term use are often lacking.
2. Prospective consumers may be seriously misinformed about the value of certain dietary supplements as a result of false advertising and unsubstantiated claims made by advocacy literature.
3. Dietary supplements are generally mild medications and should not be endorsed for the treatment of human immunodeficiency virus (HIV) infection, cancer, self-diagnosed heart disease, or other serious conditions.
4. Quality control of dietary supplements is often deficient in the United States. Patients should purchase them only from the most reliable producers and purchase standardized products when possible.
5. Do not recommend dietary supplement use for pregnant women, lactating mothers, infants, or young children without approval from the patient's healthcare provider.
6. Advise patients to cease taking a dietary supplement immediately if adverse effects (e.g., allergy, stomach upset, skin rashes, headache) occur.
7. Products containing many different ingredients, such as herbs, should be carefully examined to determine whether the ingredients are present in therapeutic amounts. Some contain only a few milligrams of each ingredient in quantities insufficient for any beneficial effect.
8. Be cautious in recommending any product that does not indicate, or permit calculation of, the quantity of individual ingredients contained in it.
9. The labels of dietary supplement products should also show the scientific name of the ingredients, the name and address of the actual manufacturer, a batch or lot number, the date of manufacture, and the expiration date.
10. Do not confuse herbal medicine, which uses therapeutic doses of drugs of botanical origin, with homeopathy, which uses products containing few or no active ingredients.

Adapted from Tyler VE. What pharmacists should know about herbal remedies. *J Am Pharm Assoc.* 1996;NS36(1):29.

for their use handled? Are they self-administered? If so, how often and in what quantity?

Cultural and ethnic beliefs. If cultural issues are involved in the use of the supplement products, research the belief system and ways that the nurse can appropriately be involved in supporting the individual.

◆ **Implementation**
• Perform detailed nursing assessments of the symptoms for which the products are being taken, including any adverse effects.

• Record data in the nursing notes regarding the use, response, or lack of response to the products.
• Label the front of the chart with a listing of supplement products being used in case the healthcare provider does not have knowledge of their use.
• Discuss cultural and ethnic beliefs with the individual patient and consult other members of the healthcare team regarding appropriate approaches for patient care and education.

◆ **Patient Education**
Expectations of therapy. Discuss the expectations of therapy with the patient and why self-treatment needs to be discussed with other members of the healthcare team. Emphasize to the patient that dietary supplements can and do interact with other medications.

Fostering health maintenance
• Discuss medication information and how it will benefit the course of treatment to produce an optimal response. Have the healthcare provider or pharmacist discuss implications of medications and products being used.
• Seek cooperation and understanding of the following points so that medication compliance is increased: name of medication; dosage, route, and times of administration; and common and serious adverse effects. The patient must understand not only prescribed medication data, but that of the dietary supplements as well. The individual must believe in the prescribed regimen in order for compliance to be enhanced.

Patient self-assessment. Enlist the patient's help in developing and maintaining a written record of monitoring parameters (e.g., blood pressure, pulse, daily weight, degree of pain relief). See Appendix B: Template for Developing a Written Record for Patients to Monitor Their Own Therapy. Complete the Premedication Data column for use as a baseline to track response to drug therapy. Ensure that the patient understands how to use the form, and instruct the patient to take the completed form to follow-up visits. During follow-up visits, focus on issues that will foster adherence with the therapeutic interventions prescribed. The healthcare team members must understand that simply telling the patient not to take supplements may result in the patient's hiding the use of these products, creating additional problems.

HERBAL THERAPY

Herbal medicine is perhaps as old as the human race. For thousands of years, civilizations have depended on substances found in nature to treat illnesses. **Herbal medicines** are defined as natural substances of botanical or plant origin. Other names for herbal medicines are *botanicals*, *phytomedicine*, and *phytotherapy*.

> **Common name: aloe** (ĂL-ō)
> Other names: aloe vera, salvia, burn plant
> Botanical source: **Aloe barbadensis**
> Parts used: **aloe gel:** clear, jellylike secretion obtained from the thin-walled, sticky cells of the inner portion of the leaf; **aloe latex:** cells just below the outer skin of the aloe plant

Actions

Two products derived from aloe plant leaves are aloe gel and aloe latex. Aloe gel (commonly known as *aloe vera*) is a gelatinous extract from the sticky cells lining the inner portion of the leaf. Aloe gel is composed of polysaccharides and lignin, salicylic acid, saponin, sterols, triterpenoids, and a variety of enzymes. Aloe gel may possibly inhibit bradykinin and histamine, reducing pain and itching. Aloe latex (resin), also known as an *aloin*, contains pharmacologically active anthraquinone derivatives that, when taken orally, act as a laxative by irritating the intestinal lining, increasing peristalsis and fluid and electrolyte secretions.

Uses

Aloe has been used as a medicinal agent for more than 5000 years for a vast array of internal and external illnesses, including arthritis, colitis, the common cold, ulcers, hemorrhoids, seizures, and glaucoma. Aloe gel is the form most commonly used in the cosmetic and health food industries. Most recently, aloe gel has been marketed for topical use to treat pain, inflammation, and itching and as a healing agent for sunburn, skin ulcers, psoriasis, and frostbite. The FDA has reviewed clinical studies of aloe gel and has not found adequate scientific evidence to support these claims. Therefore aloe gel is not classified as a drug but is allowed to remain on the market as a cosmetic for topical use. It is frequently used as a co-ingredient in skin care products; however, the product labeling should not make therapeutic claims regarding the aloe gel because none has been substantiated through scientific studies.

Aloe latex contains anthraquinone derivatives that, when taken orally, act as a laxative. There is a concern, however, about carcinogenicity, so aloe latex has been removed from the pharmaceutical market because it is not proven to be safe and effective. Historically, aloe has been known as a fragrant wood used as incense, unrelated to aloe vera.

❖ Nursing Implications for Aloe

◆ *Availability.* *Aloe gel:* Moisturizing lotion, shampoo, hair conditioner, gels, toothpaste, aloe juice for topical application. Capsules and tinctures are also available for oral use. There are no proven therapeutic effects from these products.

Aloe latex: Aloe juice drinks for catharsis; whole-leaf aloe vera: juice.

◆ *Adverse effects.* When applied to the skin, no adverse effects have been reported. When taken orally, aloe products may cause diarrhea due to anthraquinone content.

◆ *Drug interactions*

Diabetic therapy. Monitor blood glucose levels closely because of claims that, when taken orally, aloe may have hypoglycemic effects.

> **Common name: black cohosh** (KŌ-hŏsh)
> Other names: squawroot, black snakeroot, bugbane, bugwort
> Botanical source: **Cimicifuga racemosa**
> Parts used: fresh and dried root

Actions

The active ingredients in black cohosh are complex triterpenes and flavonoids. It is thought that these agents have estrogenlike effects by suppressing release of luteinizing hormone and by binding to estrogen receptors in peripheral tissue.

Uses

Black cohosh is used to reduce symptoms of premenstrual syndrome, dysmenorrhea, and menopause. Therapy is not recommended for longer than 6 months. Black cohosh should not be used in the first two trimesters of pregnancy because of its uterine-relaxing effects.

Avoid use in the following situations:
- Hypotension: may cause low blood pressure; avoid concurrent use with antihypertensive agents.
- People with a history of hormone-sensitive conditions (e.g., breast cancer, uterine cancer, or endometriosis).
- People with known seizure disorders, liver disease, or a history of stroke or blood clots.

❖ Nursing Implications for Black Cohosh

◆ *Availability.* *PO:* Elixirs, tablets, capsules.

◆ *Adverse effect.* Upset stomach is rare.

◆ *Comments.* Do not confuse black cohosh with blue cohosh. Blue cohosh is used as an antispasmodic and uterine stimulant to promote menstruation or labor, but it is different and potentially more toxic than black cohosh. Beware of commercial products that contain both black and blue cohosh when only black cohosh is sought.

Actions

Two herbs are known as chamomile: German chamomile and Roman chamomile. The therapeutic effects of chamomile derive from a complex mixture of different compounds. The antiinflammatory and antispasmodic effects come from a volatile oil containing matricin,

Herbal Interactions

Black Cohosh

HORMONE REPLACEMENT THERAPY
Women already receiving hormone replacement therapy (usually estrogen and progestin) to treat symptoms associated with menopause and to prevent osteoporosis should be cautious about receiving additional estrogenic effects from concurrent use of black cohosh.

ANTIHYPERTENSIVE THERAPY
Black cohosh may cause added antihypertensive effects when taken with other antihypertensive agents. If black cohosh is being taken, monitor the blood pressure response to the cumulative effects. Take blood pressures in the supine and erect positions.

Common name: chamomile (KĂM-ō-mē-ŭl)
Other names: German or Hungarian chamomile: pinheads, chamomilla, genuine chamomile; Roman or English chamomile: ground apple, whig plant, common chamomile
Botanical source: **Matricaria recutita** (German or Hungarian chamomile); **Chamaemelum nobile** (Roman or English chamomile)
Parts used: predominantly flower heads, but other above-ground parts also contain the volatile oils

bisabolol, bisabolol oxides A and B, and flavonoids such as apigenin and luteolin. Coumarins, herniarin, and umbelliferone exhibit antispasmodic properties. Chamazulene has also been shown to possess antiinflammatory and antibacterial properties.

Uses

Both chamomiles are used in herbalism and medicine; however, German chamomile is the species most commonly used in the United States and Europe, whereas Roman chamomile is favored in Great Britain. Chamomile is used as a digestive aid for bloating, an antispasmodic and antiinflammatory in the gastrointestinal (GI) tract, an antispasmodic for menstrual cramps, an antiinflammatory for skin irritation, and a mouthwash for minor mouth irritation or gum infections. Plant extracts are used in cosmetic and hygiene products in the form of ointments, lotions, and vapor baths for topical application. For internal use, chamomile is taken in the form of a strong tea.

❖ Nursing Implications for Chamomile

◆ *Availability, dosage, and administration.* German chamomile is available as ointment and gel in strengths of 3% to 10%. As a bath additive, 50 g is added to 1 L of water. For internal use as a tea, pour 150 mL of boiling water over 3 g of chamomile (1 teaspoon = 1 g of chamomile), cover for 5 to 10 minutes, and then strain.

◆ *Adverse effects.* Rare hypersensitivity reactions may occur in patients who are allergic to ragweed, asters, chrysanthemums, or daisies.

◆ *Drug interactions.* No clinically significant drug interactions have been reported with chamomile.

Common name: echinacea (ĕk-ĭn-Ā-shĕ)
Other names: purple coneflower, coneflower, black sampson
Botanical source: **Echinacea angustifolia, E. purpurea,** and other related species
Parts used: roots, rhizomes, above-ground parts

Actions

Echinacea is a nonspecific stimulator of the innate (nonspecific) immune system. It stimulates phagocytosis and effector cell activity. There is an increased release of tumor necrosis factors and interferons from macrophages and T lymphocytes, which increases the body's resistance to bacterial and viral infection. It may have antiinflammatory effects by inhibiting hyaluronidase, a potent inflammatory agent. Echinacea has no direct bactericidal or bacteriostatic effects.

Uses

As a nonspecific immunostimulant, echinacea may prevent or treat viral respiratory tract infections such as the common cold or flu. Well-designed clinical studies have shown equivocal results. Symptoms of the common cold may be reduced if echinacea is taken during the early, acute phase. Echinacea has also been used to treat urinary tract infections and may be applied externally to difficult-to-heal superficial wounds. Because of its immunomodulating effects, it is recommended that it not be used for more than 8 weeks at a time.

Avoid use in the following situations:
- People with heart disease; echinacea may cause abnormal or irregular heartbeat.
- People taking anticoagulants or who are at increased risk of bleeding.
- People with skin disorders; echinacea may cause burning sensations, hives, itching, rashes, and skin redness.
- People who are taking agents that may be toxic to the liver, including anabolic steroids, amiodarone, methotrexate, and ketoconazole; echinacea may cause hepatotoxicity.

❖ Nursing Implications for Echinacea

◆ *Availability. PO:* Echinacea is available as dried roots, teas, tinctures, and dry powder extracts.

◆ *Adverse effects.* Rare hypersensitivity reactions may occur in patients who are allergic to ragweed, asters, chrysanthemums, or daisies.

◆ *Comments.* Because echinacea appears to be an immunomodulator, it is not recommended for patients with autoimmune diseases, such as multiple sclerosis or lupus erythematosus, or diseases affecting the immune system, such as acquired immunodeficiency syndrome (AIDS).

Herbal Interactions

Echinacea

Echinacea may interfere with immunosuppressive therapy. Concurrent use with immunosuppressants (e.g., azathioprine, cyclosporine) is not recommended.

Common name: ephedra (ē-FĔ-dră)
Other names: ma huang, desert herb, ephedrine
Botanical source: ***Ephedra sinica***
Parts used: stems, rhizomes with roots

Action

The active ingredient in ephedra is the alkaloid ephedrine.

Uses

Ephedra was perhaps the first Chinese herbal medicine to be used in Western medicine. It is used as a bronchodilator for asthma, as a nasal decongestant, and as a central nervous system (CNS) stimulant. It is contraindicated in patients with heart conditions, hypertension, diabetes, and thyroid disease. The FDA first banned the sale of all dietary supplements containing ephedra in April 2004 based on a lack of evidence to support efficacy claims and more than 16,000 reported cases of adverse reactions. The ban was later overturned by a federal judge in April 2005 for products containing ephedra 10 mg or less. However, in May 2007, the ban was upheld by the US Supreme Court based on a final FDA regulation declaring dietary supplements containing adulterated ephedrine alkaloids as presenting an unreasonable risk of illness or injury.

❖ Nursing Implications for Ephedra

◆ *Adverse effects.* Ephedra elevates systolic and diastolic blood pressures and heart rate, causing palpitations. It also causes nervousness, headache, insomnia, and dizziness.

◆ *Comments*
- In recent years, popular culture has touted ephedra as a weight loss product, an energy booster, an aphrodisiac, and a mental stimulant. There is no substantial evidence that supports these claims. It is commonly found in OTC weight loss products. Deaths have been reported from its overuse and in those patients who may have underlying cardiovascular disease.
- Because ephedrine can serve as a precursor to the synthesis of illegal methamphetamine (speed), several states have passed laws regulating the sale of products containing ephedrine.
- Ephedrine is a medicine approved as safe and effective by the FDA and is readily available commercially. There are several other medicines that are safer, with fewer adverse effects (e.g., pseudoephedrine). There

is really no need to use herbal ephedra for rational medical therapy.

Herbal Interactions

Ephedra

DRUGS THAT ENHANCE TOXIC EFFECTS
Beta-adrenergic stimulants (e.g., pseudoephedrine, phenylpropanolamine) and monoamine oxidase inhibitors (MAOIs) (e.g., isocarboxazid, tranylcypromine, phenelzine):
- Excessive use may result in significant hypertension.
- Patients already receiving antihypertensive therapy should not use decongestants such as ephedrine because they raise blood pressure.

METHYLDOPA, RESERPINE
Frequent use of decongestants inhibits the antihypertensive activity of these agents. Concurrent therapy is not recommended.

Common name: feverfew (FĒ-vĕr-fyū)
Other names: featherfoil, flirtwort, bachelor's buttons
Botanical source: ***Tanacetum parthenium***
Parts used: leaves

Actions

There is significant controversy as to which ingredients in feverfew are therapeutic. Several sesquiterpene lactones are smooth muscle relaxants in the walls of the cerebral blood vessels and may be the source of antimigraine activity. Feverfew has also been shown to inhibit the release of arachidonic acid, which serves as a substrate for production of prostaglandins and leukotrienes. It also inhibits release of serotonin and histamine from platelets and white cells, which helps prevent or control migraine headaches. Parthenolide, long thought to be the primary active ingredient, has been shown by one well-controlled study to be of minimal therapeutic effect. Perhaps additional compounds work synergistically with parthenolide to prevent migraine headaches.

Uses

Feverfew is used to reduce the frequency and severity of migraine headaches. Its antiinflammatory effects have also been used to treat rheumatoid arthritis. Feverfew is contraindicated in women who are pregnant. It may cause uterine contractions, increasing the risk of miscarriage or premature delivery.

❖ Nursing Implications for Feverfew

◆ *Availability.* *PO:* Leaf powder for making tea; tablets.

◆ *Adverse effects.* Fresh feverfew leaves appear to be most effective in reducing the frequency and pain associated with migraine headaches. Ulcerations of the oral mucosa and swelling of the lips and tongue have been reported by 7% to 12% of patients. Feverfew therapy should be discontinued if these lesions develop.

Rare hypersensitivity reactions may occur in patients who are allergic to ragweed, asters, chrysanthemums, or daisies.

◆ *Comments*
• The sesquiterpene lactone content is higher in the flowering tops than in the leaves, stalks, and roots. This diminishes with time and with exposure to light. Because the active ingredients are not known, there are no standards established for purity. Many products sold in the United States have been found to have low, variable quantities of sesquiterpene lactones.
• People who take feverfew for a long time and then stop taking it may have difficulty sleeping, headaches, joint pain, nervousness, and stiff muscles.

 Herbal Interactions

Feverfew

NONSTEROIDAL ANTIINFLAMMATORY DRUGS
Even though feverfew has antiinflammatory properties, concurrent use with nonsteroidal antiinflammatory drugs may reduce the effectiveness of feverfew.

ANTICOAGULANTS
Because feverfew reduces platelet aggregation, it should be used with extreme caution in patients who are also receiving platelet inhibitors (e.g., aspirin, ticlopidine, dipyridamole, clopidogrel), anticoagulants (e.g., warfarin), and herbal medicines (e.g., ginkgo, garlic, ginger, ginseng). Monitor patients for signs of bleeding.

Common name: garlic (GĂR-lĭk)
   Other names: none
   Botanical source: ***Allium sativum***
   Parts used: bulb

Actions

Garlic contains a large variety of chemicals, making it difficult to determine which ingredients are responsible for its biologic effects. Alliin is a major component of garlic that, when crushed, is acted on by the enzyme alliinase to produce allicin. Allicin is thought to have the greatest pharmacologic activity but is also responsible for garlic's characteristic odor. A metabolite of allicin, ajoene (Ă-hō-wĕn), is also thought to have biologic activity.

Uses

Garlic has been one of the most widely used herbal medicines for centuries. At various times, claims have been made for it curing almost all diseases, as well as being an excellent aphrodisiac. It also has been widely used in folklore to ward off vampires, demons, and witches. Its most frequent use supported by scientific literature is in reducing cholesterol and triglyceride levels. Garlic has been shown to lower levels of serum cholesterol by 9% to 12% and triglycerides by as much as 17%. It also demonstrates antiplatelet activity similar to aspirin and may also modestly lower high blood pressure.

❖ **Nursing Implications for Garlic**
◆ *Availability. PO:* Cloves, oil, enteric-coated tablets, capsules, elixirs.

◆ *Adverse effects.* The most common adverse effect of garlic is its characteristic taste and odor, frequently resulting in halitosis. Enteric-coated oral preparations minimize this problem. There are rare reports of patients developing nausea and vomiting and burning of the mouth and stomach after ingesting various commercial preparations.

◆ *Comments.* Fresh garlic is the most potent from a biologic standpoint, releasing the active ingredients in the mouth when chewed. The enzyme alliinase, necessary for conversion of alliin to the active principles of allicin and ajoene, is inactivated in stomach acid. The active ingredients of garlic are easily destroyed by freeze drying or heat drying and commercial products are of variable potency. Dried garlic preparations are most effective if they are enteric coated, allowing them to pass into the intestine before dissolution. These products tend to have less of the characteristic odor associated with garlic because the allicin is released in the intestine. One fresh clove daily or a daily dose of 8 mg of alliin from a product standardized for alliin content is the current dosage recommendation to treat hypercholesterolemia. Diet and exercise will aid the garlic in reducing high blood pressure and cholesterol levels.

 Herbal Interactions

Garlic

ANTICOAGULANTS
Because garlic reduces platelet aggregation, it should be used with extreme caution in patients who are also receiving platelet inhibitors (e.g., aspirin, ticlopidine, dipyridamole, clopidogrel), anticoagulants (e.g., warfarin), and herbal medicines (e.g., ginkgo, ginger, feverfew, ginseng). Monitor patients for signs of bleeding.

Common name: ginger (JĬN-jĕr)
   Other names: African ginger, Jamaica ginger, race ginger
   Botanical source: ***Zingiber officinale***
   Parts used: roots and rhizomes

Actions

The active ingredients in ginger roots and rhizomes are known as *gingerols*. They increase the rate of GI motility, act as serotonin antagonists, and inhibit cyclooxygenase pathways.

Uses

Ginger has been used for centuries to alleviate nausea and vomiting from a variety of causes. It is thought to act as an antiemetic by increasing gastroduodenal motility and by blocking serotonin receptors that, when stimulated, may trigger nausea and vomiting. Ginger is possibly safe when used in pregnancy, and a few controlled studies indicate that it may reduce the frequency of morning sickness. The use of ginger in pregnancy is controversial, however, because it has never been studied thoroughly for safety in this patient population.

Ginger has also been shown to be modestly effective in reducing inflammation and pain in patients with rheumatoid arthritis, osteoarthritis, and muscle discomfort because it is a cyclooxygenase-2 inhibitor.

The rhizome is used as the source for the dried powder used in food preparation.

❖ Nursing Implications for Ginger
◆ *Availability and dosage. PO:* Powdered ginger root; ginger tea made from ginger root; tinctures. The dosages are quite variable, but it is recommended that the dosage not exceed 4 g daily.

◆ *Adverse effects.* Generally, ginger is well tolerated. There have been reports of heartburn, diarrhea, and irritation to the mouth and throat.

◆ *Comments.* Ginger is generally recognized as safe when used in food preparation. The dosages used for nausea, vomiting, and analgesia are substantially higher and have not been proven to be safe or effective.

Herbal Interactions

Ginger

ANTICOAGULANTS

Because ginger reduces platelet aggregation, it should be used with extreme caution in patients who are also receiving platelet inhibitors (e.g., aspirin, ticlopidine, dipyridamole, clopidogrel), anticoagulants (e.g., warfarin), and herbal medicines (e.g., garlic, ginkgo, ginseng, feverfew). Monitor for signs of bleeding.

Common name: ginkgo (GĬNK-ō)
  Other names: maidenhair tree
  Botanical source: ***Ginkgo biloba***
  Parts used: green-picked leaves

Actions
The active ingredients in ginkgo leaves are flavonoids and terpenes. Because higher concentrations of these chemicals are necessary for biologic activity, the green-picked leaves are processed to form a concentrated ginkgo biloba extract (GBE). Ginkgo biloba extract is standardized to a potency of 24% flavonoids (primarily flavonoid glycosides and quercetin) and 6% terpenes (primarily composed of ginkgolides A, B, C, and J and bilobalide). Ginkgo biloba extract is a smooth muscle relaxant and vasodilator that improves blood flow in arteries and capillaries. It may also be a free radical scavenger, preventing endothelial cell damage. Ginkgolides inhibit platelet-activating factor, inhibiting platelet aggregation.

Uses
Ginkgo biloba extract is used primarily for increasing cerebral blood flow, particularly in geriatric patients. Conditions treated are short-term memory loss, headache, dizziness, tinnitus, and emotional instability with anxiety. Patients with Alzheimer's disease may show modest improvement in cognitive performance and social functioning. Other uses include improved walking distance in patients with intermittent claudication, improvement in erectile dysfunction secondary to antidepressant therapy, improved peripheral blood flow in patients with diabetes mellitus, and improved hearing in patients whose hearing is impaired secondary to poor circulation to the ears. Therapy must be continued for up to 6 months to assess optimal response.

❖ Nursing Implications for Ginkgo
◆ *Availability and dosage. PO:* 40 mg GBE in liquid, tablets, and capsules. Dosages range from 120 to 240 mg of GBE twice daily.

◆ *Adverse effects.* Large doses of GBE may cause mild restlessness, diarrhea, nausea, vomiting, and dizziness. Adverse effects may be minimized by slowly titrating the dose upward as tolerated.

Herbal Interactions

Ginkgo

ANTICOAGULANTS

Because ginkgo reduces platelet aggregation, it should be used with extreme caution in patients who are also receiving platelet inhibitors (e.g., aspirin, ticlopidine, dipyridamole, clopidogrel, prasugrel, ticagrelor), anticoagulants (e.g., warfarin), and herbal medicines (e.g., ginger, garlic, feverfew, ginseng). Monitor patients for signs of bleeding.

Common name: ginseng (JĬN-sĕng)
  Other names: ***Aralia quinquefolia,*** five fingers, tartar root, red berry
  Botanical source: ***Panax ginseng*** (Chinese or Korean ginseng)
  Parts used: root

Actions
Ginseng contains a large variety of chemicals, making it difficult to determine which components are responsible for its biologic effects. The ingredients believed to be responsible are triterpenoid saponins, classified into panaxosides, ginsenosides, and chikusetsusaponins. Unfortunately, the literature is extremely difficult to interpret because of differences in composition between Asian and American ginseng species, different scientific

terms for active ingredients, and the lack of well-controlled scientific studies.

Uses

Ginseng is not used to cure a disease but is an "adaptogen" in maintaining health. Current claims for ginseng are that it increases the body's resistance to stress, overcomes disease by building up defenses, and strengthens general vitality. It has also been used for centuries as an aphrodisiac. There is no scientific basis for its claims as an aphrodisiac and little scientific evidence as an adaptogen.

❖ Nursing Implications for Ginseng

◆ *Availability.* *PO:* Teas, powders, capsules, tablets, liquids. There are no standardized methods of purity. Commercial ginseng extract products range from 100 to 600 mg standardized to a percentage of ginsenosides.

◆ *Adverse effects.* Many adverse effects have been reported with the use of ginseng, but most are single case reports and may be the pharmacologic effect of adulterants added to ginseng. Adverse effects most commonly attributed to ginseng are insomnia, diarrhea, and skin eruptions.

◆ *Comments.* Even though thousands of articles have been written lauding its praises, ginseng has not undergone much scientific study. Most of the literature is based on superstition and anecdotal reports. Many of the reports have been written by governments and companies making claims for financial gain. Ginseng is an herbal medicine that is commonly adulterated, so it is difficult to know whether the results of studies are because of the ginseng content or the added ingredients.

Siberian ginseng (*Eleutherococcus senticosus;* also known as *eleuthero*) is different from American or Asian ginseng and should not be substituted. It has been marketed as a cheaper form of ginseng but is known to have many adulterants, and there are no scientific studies to support its claims as an immune system stimulant and enhancer of endurance.

 Herbal Interactions

Ginseng

ANTICOAGULANTS

Ginseng may affect platelet aggregation and blood coagulation. It should be used with extreme caution in patients who are also receiving platelet inhibitors (e.g., aspirin, ticlopidine, dipyridamole, clopidogrel, prasugrel, ticagrelor), anticoagulants (e.g., warfarin), and herbal medicines (e.g., garlic, feverfew, ginger, ginkgo). Monitor for signs of bleeding.

INSULIN

Ginseng has been shown to raise insulin levels in laboratory animals. It may have the potential to induce hypoglycemia. Blood glucose levels of patients with type 1 or type 2 diabetes mellitus should be monitored closely if the patient insists on taking ginseng.

Common name: goldenseal (GŌL-děn-sē-ăl)
Other names: yellow root, Indian dye, Indian paint, jaundice root
Botanical source: **Hydrastis canadensis**
Parts used: rhizomes with root fibers

Actions

The active ingredients in goldenseal are contained in a group of plant alkaloids, the most active of which are hydrastine and berberine. Berberine gives the herb its characteristic golden color.

Uses

Goldenseal is popular in herbal medicine as an antiseptic and astringent, reducing inflammation of mucous membranes. It is used topically as a tea for treatment of canker sores, sore mouth, and cracked and bleeding lips. Goldenseal may have weak antibacterial properties and may stimulate the immune system to help fight viral upper respiratory infections such as a cold or flu. Goldenseal is sometimes marketed in combination with echinacea to ward off bouts of the common cold. No controlled studies have been completed to validate this combined therapy. In high doses, goldenseal may have uterine stimulant effects and should not be taken during pregnancy. In recent years, there has been a common myth that goldenseal, when taken as tea or put into urine, will mask assays for street drugs (see Comments later in this section).

❖ Nursing Implications for Goldenseal

◆ *Availability.* *PO:* Powder for tea, tincture, fluid extract, freeze-dried root.

◆ *Adverse effects.* The alkaloids in goldenseal are not absorbed to any extent when swallowed, producing no systemic effects. High doses may cause nausea, vomiting, diarrhea, and CNS stimulation.

◆ *Comments.* One of the more recent popular uses for goldenseal is to mask the presence of illicit drugs in urine samples. Contrary to popular belief, goldenseal does not prevent detection of drugs by urine tests, nor does it flush illicit drugs from the body. When goldenseal is present, the urine takes on a distinctive dark amber or brown color.

Common name: green tea
Other names: Chinese tea, teagreen
Botanical source: **Camellia sinensis,** evergreen shrub
Parts used: leaf, leaf bud, and stem

Actions

When steamed, green tea leaves and stems yield high concentrations of polyphenols, such as gallic acid, and catechins and caffeine, which are thought to be the active ingredients of green tea. Mechanisms of action are unknown. Green tea also contains B vitamins and ascorbic acid.

Uses

Green tea has been used as a very common beverage in Asian cultures for centuries. The caffeine produces CNS stimulation and is thought to improve cognitive performance. It raises blood pressure, heart rate, and contractility and acts as a diuretic. Green tea has been shown to lower cholesterol, triglyceride, and low-density lipoprotein (LDL) levels and raise high-density lipoprotein (HDL) level. There is some evidence that green tea might reduce the risk of bladder, esophageal, and pancreatic cancers and reduce or prevent the onset of parkinsonism. Green tea is also used to treat diarrhea.

❖ Nursing Implications for Green Tea

◆ *Availability and dosage. PO:* Green tea is readily available in premade tea bags and in bulk form for brewing. Moderate consumption of one to four cups daily appears to provide therapeutic benefits. Consumption of five or more cups daily has significantly more adverse effects that are associated with excessive caffeine.

◆ *Adverse effects.* Many of the adverse effects of green tea are an extension of the pharmacologic effects of caffeine: anxiety, nervousness, headache, diuresis, insomnia, tremor, irritability, palpitations, and dysrhythmias. The chronic use and consumption of high quantities can produce tolerance, habituation, and psychological dependence. The abrupt discontinuation may cause withdrawal headaches, irritation, and nervousness.

 Herbal Interactions

Green Tea

INCREASED THERAPEUTIC AND TOXIC EFFECTS

The following drugs, when used concurrently with green tea, may significantly increase the stimulant effects and the adverse effects of the caffeine in green tea by inhibiting its metabolism: ephedrine, cimetidine, disulfiram, grapefruit juice, MAOIs (e.g., tranylcypromine, phenelzine, isocarboxazid), mexiletine, oral contraceptives, quinolones (e.g., ciprofloxacin, norfloxacin), theophylline, and verapamil.

BETA-ADRENERGIC AGENTS (ALBUTEROL, METAPROTERENOL, TERBUTALINE)

Concurrent consumption of green tea (caffeine) with beta agonists can increase the heart rate and the potential for dysrhythmias. Use with caution. Discontinue green tea consumption if palpitations develop.

EPHEDRA

Concurrent consumption of ephedra and the caffeine in green tea results in significantly more stimulant effects with greater possibility of adverse effects.

WARFARIN

Concurrent consumption of large quantities of green tea with warfarin may antagonize the anticoagulant effects of warfarin. Monitor the patient's international normalized ratio (INR) for the therapeutic effect of warfarin.

Common name: St. John's wort (SĀNT JŎNZ WŌRT)
Other names: Klamath weed, hardhay, amber
Botanical source: ***Hypericum perforatum***
Parts used: fresh buds and flowers

Actions

The active ingredients of St. John's wort are unknown. Studies indicate that it behaves as a reuptake inhibitor, prolonging the effect of serotonin, dopamine, and norepinephrine.

Uses

St. John's wort is used orally to treat mild depression and to heal wounds.

❖ Nursing Implications for St. John's Wort

◆ *Availability and dosage.* St. John's wort is available as powder, tablets, capsules, and liquid. It is also found in semisolid preparations for topical use. It is commonly standardized to hypericin content, but it has been shown that hypericin content is not related to antidepressant effect, so this standard is of little value. Therapeutic effects are variable between various products and different batches of the same product. Because the therapeutic ingredients are unknown, there is no effective standardization for St. John's wort products. The average daily dosage for internal use is 2 to 4 g of herb or 0.2 to 1 mg of total hypericin.

◆ *Adverse effects.* St. John's wort may cause photosensitivity. Patients should discontinue the herbal medicine and report excessive sunburn, pruritus, and edema immediately.

There is concern about St. John's wort contributing to the development of serotonin syndrome. The seriousness of this adverse effect warrants that patients be informed of this complication of therapy. Serotonin syndrome may result from taking two or more drugs that affect serotonin levels. Symptoms associated with the syndrome are confusion, agitation, shivering, fever, diaphoresis, nausea, diarrhea, muscle spasms, and tremor. These symptoms have a sudden onset, somewhat like a panic attack, and may progress to a coma. The syndrome is life threatening. When switching between serotonergic agents and St. John's wort, a 5- to 7-day washout period is recommended (see Chapter 16).

◆ *Comments*
- Folklore tells us that St. John's wort received its name because its golden flower is particularly abundant on June 24, the day celebrated as the birthday of John the Baptist.
- St. John's wort products are light and heat sensitive. Exposure to light and excessive heat for 2 weeks will alter the content of the chemical constituents.
- Depression is a serious, potentially fatal illness. It is important that patients discuss their symptoms and the use of St. John's wort before starting self-treatment.

Herbal Interactions

St. John's Wort

SEROTONIN STIMULANTS

Selective serotonin reuptake inhibitors (SSRIs) (e.g., paroxetine, sertraline, fluoxetine), tricyclic antidepressants (e.g., amitriptyline, imipramine, doxepin), MAOIs (e.g., isocarboxazid, phenelzine, tranylcypromine), and dopamine agonists (e.g., bromocriptine) may induce a serotonin syndrome when taken concurrently with St. John's wort. Patients should contact their healthcare provider immediately if they start noticing symptoms of this syndrome (see Adverse Effects earlier in this section).

Common name: valerian (văl-ĀR-ē-ăn)
  Other names: Amantilla, setwall, heliotrope, vandal root
  Botanical source: *Valeriana officinalis*
  Parts used: dried roots and rhizomes
  ⇄ *Do not confuse valerian with Valium.*

Actions

The chemical constituents that are responsible for the therapeutic effects of valerian have not been fully identified.

Uses

Valerian has been used for more than 1000 years as a mild tranquilizer. It is used for restlessness and may promote sleep.

❖ Nursing Implications for Valerian

◆ *Availability. PO:* Valerian may be administered in the form of a tea, tincture, extract, tablets, or capsules. Some preparations are standardized for valepotriate content, but it is not known whether these compounds are the active ingredients.

◆ *Adverse effects.* Adverse effects are rare; chronic users may experience excitability, uneasiness, and headache.

◆ *Comments.* Because of similarity in names, valerian and Valium have sometimes been confused. Valerian is a mild tranquilizer, whereas Valium is the brand name of a much more potent tranquilizer (generic name: diazepam). Diazepam is a member of the benzodiazepines (see Chapter 15).

◆ *Drug interactions.* No clinically significant drug interactions have been reported, but concurrent use of other medicines with sedative properties, such as antihistamines, benzodiazepines, alcohol, and phenobarbital, should be avoided.

OTHER DIETARY SUPPLEMENTS

Common name: coenzyme Q10 (kō-ĔN-zīm)
  Other names: CoQ10, ubiquinone
  Sources: commercial sources—fermentation of cane sugar and beets using special strains of yeast; natural sources—beef, soy oil, sardines, peanuts

---

Description and Actions

Coenzyme Q10 is a provitamin found in every living cell and is essential for energy production in the mitochondria. Organs with high energy requirements contain the highest levels of CoQ10; these organs are the heart muscle, liver, kidneys, and pancreas. Human cells synthesize CoQ10 from the amino acid tyrosine in a series of chemical reactions that also require folic acid, niacin, riboflavin, and pyridoxine. A deficiency of any of these vitamins may result in a deficiency in CoQ10. Deficiency of CoQ10 also results from diminished dietary intake, impairment of biosynthesis, and increased usage of CoQ10 by the body.

Uses

CoQ10 has been used to treat a variety of disorders. Its primary use is as an adjunctive therapy for chronic heart failure. It has also been tested with varying degrees of success in other cardiovascular diseases (e.g., ischemic heart disease [angina], hypertension, dysrhythmias, toxin-induced cardiomyopathy, surgery for heart valve replacement), cancer (breast, lung, prostate, pancreatic, colon), muscular dystrophy, periodontal disease, and AIDS. Additional studies are required to determine the degree of therapeutic benefit for these diseases.

❖ Nursing Implications for CoQ10

◆ *Availability. PO:* Powder-filled capsules, tablets, liquid-filled gel capsules, chewable wafers, intraoral spray.

◆ *Dosage and administration*
  • Usual dosage 10 to 300 mg/day in 1 or in divided dose(s) up to 3 times per day. Up to 3000 mg/day have been used.
  • Coenzyme Q10 deficiency: 150-2400 mg daily in up to three divided doses.
  • Administer with meals that contain some fat to enhance absorption.
  • Dosages of more than 100 mg daily should be divided into two or three doses.
  • The safety of CoQ10 in pregnancy and lactation has not been established, and its use is not recommended.

◆ *Adverse effects.* No serious adverse effects have been reported. Less than 1% of patients describe symptoms of nausea, upset stomach, diarrhea, and appetite suppression. Doses of 100 mg or more taken at bedtime may cause mild insomnia. Patients taking 300 mg daily for extended periods demonstrate mild elevations of liver enzyme levels, but no cases of hepatotoxicity have been reported.

 Herbal Interactions

Coenzyme Q10

ANTILIPEMIC AGENTS
Several antilipemic agents—3-hydroxy-3-methylglutaryl coenzyme A reductase inhibitors ("statins") and gemfibrozil—appear to reduce total body levels of CoQ10 by inhibiting its synthesis by the body. The clinical significance of this interaction is not known at this time.

BETA-ADRENERGIC BLOCKING AGENTS
Beta-adrenergic blocking agents appear to reduce total body levels of CoQ10 by inhibiting its synthesis. The clinical significance of this interaction is not known at this time.

INSULIN, ORAL HYPOGLYCEMIC AGENTS
CoQ10 supplementation has been reported to reduce insulin requirements in diabetes mellitus. Oral hypoglycemic agents (e.g., tolazamide, glyburide) have also been reported to reduce total body levels of CoQ10; therefore patients with diabetes who are taking CoQ10 require close monitoring of blood glucose levels with adjustment in dosages of antidiabetic medicines as needed.

WARFARIN
The chemical structures of CoQ10 and vitamin K are similar. There are reports that administration of CoQ10 to patients receiving warfarin causes a decrease in the INR. Monitor the INR closely for therapeutic effect.

Common name: creatine (KRĒ-ă-tēn)
Other names: creatine monohydrate
Sources: natural: meat and fish (muscle)

Description and Actions
Creatine is a naturally occurring, energy-producing substance in the human body synthesized from amino acids. It plays a key role in providing energy to muscles for short-duration, high-intensity exercise. About 95% of the body's creatine is in skeletal muscle, of which 60% is in the form of creatine phosphate. Muscle adenosine triphosphate (ATP) provides immediate energy for muscle contraction, after which it is replenished by creatine phosphate. The rapidity with which creatine phosphate is replenished depends on the amount of free creatine available.

Uses
Creatine is used as a performance-enhancing substance. Creatine supplementation is thought to enhance muscle performance for short bouts of repeated, intense exercise such as sprinting, jumping, and power lifting. Increasing creatine phosphate stores enhances rapid replenishment of ATP, and increased supplies of free creatine shorten muscle recovery time by rebuilding depleted creatine phosphate stores faster. Many small studies have attempted to document the benefits of creatine supplementation but with mixed results. At best, some studies indicate a 1% to 3% improvement in performance for brief periods.

Small clinical studies also indicate that patients with heart failure and muscular dystrophy might benefit from creatine supplementation by preserving energy stores in the myocardium and skeletal muscle, respectively. Additional studies are needed to assess long-term benefits of creatine therapy in these and other conditions.

❖ **Nursing Implications for Creatine**

◆ *Availability. PO:* Powder, candy, gum, and liquid. It is often combined with other supplements for energy.

◆ *Dosage.*
- Dosage regimens in clinical trials vary from 2 to 20 g daily and from 1 week up to 4 years.
- Skeletal muscle enhancement regimens include "high dose, short term" of 20 g daily for 7 days and a "lower dose, longer term" regimen of 2 to 5 g for 4 to 6 weeks.

◆ *Adverse effects.* No serious adverse effects have been reported, but long-term studies that might document adverse effects have not been completed. Creatine causes weight gain of 3 to 6 pounds because of water retention. Other adverse effects of creatine may include muscle cramping, dehydration, and GI bloating and diarrhea.

◆ *Comments*
- It is recommended that at least eight 8-ounce glasses of water be consumed daily while taking creatine supplements.
- Creatine supplementation should be avoided by people who have impaired renal function or are taking potentially nephrotoxic medicines.
- The safety of creatine in pregnancy and lactation has not been established, and its use is not recommended.

Common name: gamma-hydroxybutyrate (GHB) (GĂ-mă hī-drŏk-sē-BYŪ-tĭr-āt)
Other names: Georgia home boy (GHB), liquid ecstasy, salty water, many others

---

Description and Actions
Gamma-hydroxybutyrate occurs naturally in the brain, kidneys, heart, and skeletal muscle. It is a metabolite of gamma-aminobutyric acid, an inhibitory neurotransmitter. A wide variety of physiologic responses occur when GHB receptors are stimulated, including dopamine release, growth hormone release, and induction of sleep.

Uses
In the late 1980s GHB was marketed and sold in the health food industry as a growth hormone stimulator to help bodybuilders promote muscle mass and maintain weight, and as an OTC sedative. The drug was banned by the FDA in 1990 after several reports of adverse

reactions in individuals using nutritional and weight loss supplements containing GHB. Despite the FDA ban, GHB continues to be marketed as a dietary supplement. Home manufacturing kits can be purchased, and recipes are readily available on the Internet.

Gamma-hydroxybutyrate is usually abused for its intoxicating, sedative, and euphoric properties. It is an increasingly popular drug of abuse, particularly at rave parties where it is used as a euphoriant, and as a date rape drug that is added to alcoholic drinks. Like alcohol, GHB's intoxicating effects begin 10 to 20 minutes after ingestion. The effects typically last up to 4 hours, depending on the dose. In progressively higher doses, the sedative effects may progress from sleep to coma to death. As with other commonly abused substances, repeated exposure leads to reinforcement, tolerance, and dependence. Dependence may be manifested by withdrawal symptoms, such as the need to continue to take the drug, anxiety, insomnia, and abnormal thinking.

❖ Nursing Implications for GHB
◆ *Availability.* Gamma-hydroxybutyrate is available as a prescription product (sodium oxybate [Xyrem]) for treating a small population of patients with narcolepsy who experience episodes of cataplexy, a condition characterized by weak or paralyzed muscles. Because of safety concerns associated with the use of the drug, sodium oxybate is a Schedule III controlled substance and the distribution of Xyrem is tightly restricted. The medicine is to be used only at bedtime because it induces sleep very quickly.

◆ *Adverse effects.* Adverse effects related to GHB ingestion are highly variable among individuals, possibly relating to contaminating chemicals from home manufacturing kits. A wide range of effects have been reported, including impairment of judgment, aggression, and hallucinations, but those that are potentially life threatening are vomiting (with aspiration into the lungs), respiratory depression, bradycardia, and hypotension.

Herbal Interactions

Gamma-Hydroxybutyrate

DRUGS THAT INCREASE TOXIC EFFECTS
Alcohol, antihistamines, analgesics, anesthetics, tranquilizers, antidepressants, valproic acid, phenytoin, and sleep aids will increase the sedative-hypnotic effects of GHB.

Common name: lycopene (LĪ-kō-pēn)
Sources: natural: tomatoes, watermelon, pink grapefruit

Description and Actions
Lycopene is a carotenoid, a family of more than 50 nutrients from yellow, red, and orange plant pigments that act as antioxidants to protect the body against free radicals (unstable molecules released when the body uses oxygen).

Uses
There is some evidence to suggest that diets high in lycopene may reduce the risk of prostate cancer and possibly lung, colon, and breast cancer. Small studies also indicate that the antioxidant properties have a lowering effect on LDL cholesterol and can protect against heart attack and stroke. Lycopene may also help prevent ophthalmic conditions such as macular degeneration and cataracts.

❖ Nursing Implications for Lycopene
◆ *Availability.* Research indicates that lycopene in tomatoes can be absorbed more efficiently by the body if processed into tomato juice, sauce, paste, and ketchup. Most products are sold as a carotenoid complex containing natural tomato powder and tomato extract.

◆ *Dosage.* Optimal dosages of lycopene have not been established. Analysis of major studies indicates that 5 to 10 servings per week of tomato-based sauces and other products (juices, extracts) may have a protective effect against developing prostate cancer. Dosage guidelines from manufacturers range from 10 to 30 mg taken twice daily with meals. Lycopene is also incorporated in multivitamin and multimineral products.

◆ *Adverse effects.* No serious adverse effects have been reported.

Common name: melatonin (mĕl-ă-TŌ-nĭn)
Other names: sleep hormone, MEL, MLT

Description and Actions
Melatonin is a human hormone synthesized from serotonin and secreted by the pineal gland. Its secretion is increased by dark and suppressed by light through the retina.

Uses
Melatonin is best known as a sleep aid and treatment for jet lag. It may also be helpful in patients withdrawing from benzodiazepine therapy. Melatonin has also been recommended as an antiaging medicine, but good clinical studies do not support this claim.

❖ Nursing Implications for Melatonin
◆ *Availability. PO:*
Tablets: 0.3, 1, 3, 5, 10 mg
Chewable tablets: 2.5 mg
Oral disintegrating tablets: 3, 5, 10 mg
Extended-release tablets: 10 mg
Capsules: 1, 2.5, 3, 5, 10 mg
Oral liquid: 0.25, 1 mg/mL

◆ *Dosage.* **PO:** *Insomnia:* Melatonin 3 to 5 mg given orally 3 to 4 hours before an imposed sleep period over 4 weeks.

PO: *Jet lag prevention:* There is little information on the best dose or formulation because studies have used different dosage regimens. In general, lower oral doses (0.5 to 2 mg) preflight and higher oral doses (5 mg) postflight over a period of up to 4 days appear to be adequate.

◆ *Comments.* The safety of melatonin in children and during pregnancy and lactation has not been established, and its use is not recommended.

◆ *Adverse effects*
Neurologic
Drowsiness, sedation, lethargy. Because melatonin causes drowsiness, people who work around machinery, drive a car, administer medicines, or perform other duties in which they must remain mentally alert should not take melatonin while working.

Paradoxical response. Occasionally, melatonin causes a paradoxical reaction such as agitation and insomnia. Provide supportive care and safety during these responses. Assess the level of excitement and deal calmly with the individual. During periods of excitement, protect the patient from harm and provide for physical channeling of energy (e.g., walking). Seek a change in the medication order.

Herbal Interactions

Melatonin

CENTRAL NERVOUS SYSTEM DEPRESSANTS
Melatonin may add to CNS depression caused by alcohol, benzodiazepines, sleep aids, and other sedative-hypnotics. Do not administer melatonin to patients already receiving any of these medications without healthcare provider approval.

Common name: policosanol (pŏl-ē-KŌ-săn-ŏl)
Other names: policosanol, **N**-octacosanol, octacosyl alcohol, octacosanol, wheat germ oil

Description and Actions

Policosanol is a plant sterol that contains a mixture of waxy-type alcohols derived from plant sources, including sugarcane and wheat germ oil. The alcohols that comprise policosanol are primarily octacosanol, tetracosanol, hexacosanol, heptacosanol, nonacosanol, triacontanol, dotriacontanol, and tetratriacontanol. Policosanol appears to lower cholesterol levels by inhibiting hepatic cholesterol synthesis and by increasing the degradation of LDL cholesterol. Policosanol also reduces platelet aggregation but does not seem to significantly affect coagulation time.

Uses

Plant sterols are included in the National Cholesterol Education Program guidelines as part of the Therapeutic Lifestyle Changes program. Orally, policosanol is used to treat dyslipidemia, lowering LDL cholesterol 17% to 27% and increasing HDL 7% to 10%. It has no effect on triglyceride levels. Clinical studies indicate that policosanol has similar efficacy in treating dyslipidemias as do lower doses of the statins. As a platelet inhibitor, policosanol is used to treat intermittent claudication in patients with peripheral artery disease and myocardial ischemia in patients with coronary heart disease.

❖ **Nursing Implications for Policosanol**
◆ *Availability.* **PO:** 10- and 20 mg tablets.

◆ *Dosage.* The dosage is 5 to 10 mg twice daily of a product containing at least 60% octacosanol. Two months of therapy may be required to see significant changes in cholesterol levels. Doses of 40 mg daily do not appear to have added benefit.

◆ *Adverse effects.* No serious adverse effects have been reported. Only mild adverse effects such as nervousness, headache, diarrhea, and insomnia have been reported. In long-term studies of 2 to 4 years, adverse effects occurred in less than 1% of patients. Weight loss, excessive urination, and insomnia were reported.

◆ *Drug interactions*
Aspirin, warfarin, heparin, clopidogrel, ticlopidine, pentoxifylline. The blood-thinning properties of policosanol may enhance the anticoagulant effects of these agents. Use with extreme caution and monitor closely for bruising and bleeding.

Garlic, ginkgo, high-dose vitamin E. The blood-thinning properties of policosanol may enhance the blood-thinning effects of these agents. Use with extreme caution and monitor the patient closely for bruising and bleeding.

Common name: omega-3 fatty acids (ō-MĔG-ă)
Other names: fish oils, omega-3 (ω-3) polyunsaturated fatty acids (PUFAs)

Description and Actions

Omega-3 polyunsaturated fatty acids (ω-3 fatty acids) are found in a variety of plant (flaxseed, soybean, walnut, canola) and fish (tuna, salmon, herring, mackerel, sardine) oils. However, it is now recognized that the cardioprotective benefits of omega-3 fatty acids are primarily caused by eicosapentaenoic acid (EPA) and docosahexaenoic acid (DHA), which are found primarily in fish oils. Omega-3 fish oil supplements may modestly lower the risk of death from a recent heart attack or from heart failure but do not prevent heart disease. Most recent studies indicate that omega-3 fish oils reduce deaths from myocardial infarction by about 10% and deaths and hospitalizations from heart failure by 9%.

Uses

Omega-3 fatty acids are used for reduction of risk of death from myocardial infarction or heart failure.

❖ Nursing Implications for Omega-3 Fatty Acids

◆ *Availability.* Omega-3 fatty acid content is highly variable in OTC supplements, ranging from 300 to 2700 mg of EPA-DHA per teaspoonful or capsule. It is also available as a prescription-only product (Lovaza capsules) containing 840 mg of EPA-DHA, which is a highly purified product with a low incidence of adverse effects.

◆ *Dosage.* The American Heart Association recommends a daily intake of omega-3 fatty acids (Table 47.1).

◆ *Adverse effects.* Dyspepsia and eructation (burping or belching) with a fishy aftertaste are the most common problems reported. These adverse effects can be minimized by using a more purified product (more EPA-DHA per serving), taking smaller doses with meals throughout the day, gradually building up the dosage over several weeks, taking enteric-coated tablets, and freezing non–enteric-coated tablets prior to administration.

◆ *Comments.* Factors to consider in product selection are purity, strength, calories, cholesterol count, and other ingredients, such as vitamins. Different products may need to be tried for optimal benefit to the consumer. More purified products generally have fewer adverse effects, such as a fishy aftertaste, but are usually more expensive. Some products are available with an enteric coating that reduces aftertaste.

Table 47.1	American Heart Association Recommended Daily Intake of Omega-3 Fatty Acids	
PATIENT POPULATION	**RECOMMENDATIONS**
No CHD	Consume a variety of preferably oily fish at least twice weekly[a]
CHD present	1 g EPA-DHA daily, preferably from fatty fish (tuna, salmon, herring, mackerel, sardines); use supplements under physician supervision
Reduced left ventricular function	Use supplement under physician supervision
Elevated triglyceride levels	2-4 g EPA-DHA daily from a supplement under physician supervision

[a]Pregnant and nursing women and young children should avoid swordfish, shark, king mackerel, and tilefish and limit their consumption of other fish to 12 ounces per week (recommendation of the U.S. Food and Drug Administration). Oily fish: salmon, mackerel, herring, lake trout, sardines, albacore tuna.
CHD, Coronary heart disease; *DHA,* docosahexaenoic acid; *EPA,* eicosapentaenoic acid.
Data from Siscovick DS, Barringer TA, Fretts AM. Omega-3 polyunsaturated fatty acid (fish oil) supplementation and the prevention of clinical cardiovascular disease: a science advisory from the American Heart Association. *Circulation.* 2017;135:e867–e884. doi: 10.1161/CIR.

Labels of supplement products should be read carefully because it is routine to report fish oil content per serving as much higher (e.g., 1000 mg) than it actually is because of including other fish oils (impurities), whereas the actual content of EPA-DHA is only 300 mg (EPA, 180 mg, plus DHA, 120 mg). Carbohydrates are often added as sweetening agents, making the product more palatable, but some products, when used in therapeutic doses, may be a hidden source of over 100 calories daily. Some products also contain cholesterol (an impurity) that can be significant for patients on a reduced cholesterol diet. Vitamin content (sometimes an impurity) can also be a potential for toxicity if the product is being taken in higher doses to treat hypertriglyceridemia.

Common name: *S-adenosylmethionine* (SAM-e)
Other names: Sammy, SAM

Description and Actions

S-adenosylmethionine (SAM-e) is a naturally occurring substance found in all cells of the human body, particularly in the brain and liver. It is produced from ATP, an energy-producing compound, and methionine, an amino acid. SAM-e is involved in a wide range of essential biochemical reactions, including synthesis, activation, and metabolism of hormones, neurotransmitters, proteins, and phospholipids and deactivation of toxic substances.

Uses

As a supplement, SAM-e has been proposed for treating depression, osteoarthritis, and fibromyalgia. It is thought that SAM-e may have a dopaminergic effect in treating depression, but study results have been highly variable and inconclusive. In small studies for the treatment of osteoarthritis, SAM-e has been compared with nonsteroidal antiinflammatory drugs (e.g., ibuprofen, naproxen, indomethacin) and placebo, and produced mild symptomatic improvement after 2 weeks. Other small studies suggest a possible benefit in relieving symptoms associated with liver disease (e.g., chronic fatigue) and fibromyalgia (e.g., pain, depression, morning stiffness). SAM-e is relatively expensive, so other, more conventional treatments for osteoarthritis and depression are warranted for several weeks before considering courses of SAM-e treatment.

❖ Nursing Implications for *S*-Adenosylmethionine

◆ *Availability.* A variety of tablet and capsule dosage forms are available, but the enteric forms that dissolve in the intestines (not the stomach) are recommended as more effective. There are two forms of SAM-e: the preferred form is *S*-adenosylmethionine 1,4-butanedisulfonate (sulfate form) rather than the toluene sulfonate (tosylate) form. There are cases of misleading labeling; for example, 400 mg SAM-e disulfate tosylate actually contains only 200 mg or less of the preferred sulfate form.

◆ *Dosage. PO:* 400 mg three or four times daily is recommended. Patients should start with lower dosages and gradually increase to a higher dosage to avoid mild stomach distress.

◆ *Comments*
- Do not administer to patients diagnosed with manic depression. SAM-e has been reported to trigger manic episodes in patients with bipolar disease.
- The safety of SAM-e in pregnancy and lactation and in children has not been established, and its use is not recommended.

◆ *Adverse effects.* No serious adverse effects have been reported. Mild stomach distress has been reported at starting doses of 400 mg three or four times daily.

Herbal Interactions
S-Adenosylmethionine

ANTIDEPRESSANTS
S-adenosylmethionine (SAM-e) may interfere with the actions of several antidepressants (tricyclic antidepressants, SSRIs, MAOIs) or magnify their adverse effects. Combined use of antidepressants and SAM-e should be recommended only by a healthcare provider.

LEVODOPA
It is reported that SAM-e may reduce some of the adverse effects of levodopa used to treat parkinsonism, but it is also thought that SAM-e may reduce the beneficial effects of levodopa in the treatment of parkinsonism over time.

Get Ready for the NCLEX® Examination!

Key Points

- Herbal therapies are as old as the human race. Herbal medicines are defined as those natural substances derived from botanical or plant origin.
- Over the past two decades, there has been a tremendous resurgence in the popularity of self-care and alternative therapies, including acupuncture, aromatherapy, homeopathy, vitamin therapy, and herbal therapy. Some of the more than 250 herbal medicines may be beneficial, but unfortunately the whole field of herbal therapy is fraught with false claims, lack of standardization, and adulteration and misbranding of products.
- Dietary supplement therapy under the current legal standards creates an ethical dilemma for nurses and other healthcare professionals. Licensed healthcare professionals have a moral and ethical responsibility to recommend only medicines that are proven to be safe and effective. Regarding dietary supplements, including herbal medicines, the healthcare professional should be aware of their legal uses versus their popular uses, their potential for toxicity, and their potential for interaction with other medicines.

Additional Learning Resources

SG Go to your Study Guide for additional Review Questions for the NCLEX® Examination, Critical Thinking Clinical Situations, and other learning activities to help you master this chapter content.

Go to your Evolve website (https://evolve.elsevier.com/Clayton) for additional online resources.

Review Questions for the NCLEX® Examination

1. After reviewing the medication history with the patient, the nurse noted that the herbal therapy St. John's wort was on the list. The nurse then made which appropriate statement?
   1. "I see you are taking St. John's wort. Please tell me if you think it is working for you."
   2. "I see you are taking St. John's wort. I would advise you to stop immediately because it is not safe to take."
   3. "I take St. John's wort, too. It works great for me. Tell me, how do you like it?"
   4. "I believe this St. John's wort is available in premade tea bags and also in bulk form."

2. Coenzyme Q10 is used primarily as an adjunctive therapy for which of the following disorders?
   1. Chronic heart failure
   2. Insomnia
   3. Depression
   4. Migraine headaches

3. A patient was discussing with the nurse the dietary supplement melatonin and stated that he intended to take it to help his recent insomnia. Which statement by the nurse would be appropriate?
   1. "It should be okay to take it with other sleeping pills."
   2. "I don't believe these dietary supplements work."
   3. "I believe it can be used for treatment of jet lag because it can help you adjust to changes in time zones."
   4. "I would recommend that you take it if you wake up after falling asleep because it will help you get back to sleep."

4. A pregnant patient came into the clinic and was discussing with the nurse some options for her persistent nausea. She asked the nurse which herbal supplement might help. What would be an appropriate response by the nurse?
   1. "I think that the herbal supplement ginger is helpful for nausea."
   2. "I think that the herbal supplement garlic is helpful for nausea."
   3. "I think that the herbal supplement feverfew is helpful for nausea."
   4. "I think that the herbal supplement ephedra is helpful for nausea."

5. While teaching a patient about home-going medications, the nurse asked about the use of any dietary supplements or herbal medications. The nurse knows that further education is needed after the patient made which statement?
   1. "I do not take any supplements or over-the-counter medications anymore."
   2. "I heard that there is a new law requiring herbal medicines and supplements to be standardized."
   3. "From what I understand, the herbal medications and dietary supplements have been unproven to work."
   4. "Herbal therapy has been around a long time and involves the use of plant leaves and such to make teas and salves."

6. The nurse reviewing the medications the patient indicated were taken at home and noticed feverfew was listed. Which symptom would the patient possibly use feverfew for?
   1. Poor circulation
   2. Nasal decongestion
   3. Menopausal hot flashes
   4. Migraine headaches

Substance Abuse

Objectives

1. Identify the differences between mild, moderate, and severe substance abuse disorder.
2. Differentiate between the screening instruments for substance use disorders.
3. Cite the responsibilities of professionals who suspect substance abuse by a colleague.
4. Explain the primary long-term goals in the treatment of substance abuse.
5. Identify the withdrawal symptoms for major substances that are commonly abused.

Key Terms

substance use disorder (SŬB-stăns ăb-YŪS) (p. 773)
impairment (ĭm-PĀR-měnt) (p. 773)
dependence (dē-PĚN-děns) (p. 773)

illicit substance (ĭl-LĬS-ĭt) (p. 774)
intoxication (ĭn-tŏks-ĭ-KĀ-shŭn) (p. 781)

CLASSIFICATION OF SUBSTANCE ABUSE

The new *Diagnostic and Statistical Manual of Mental Disorders, 5th edition (DSM-5)*, redefines substance abuse under a new category termed *Substance Use Disorders*, with the specific substance used defining the specific disorder (e.g., alcohol use disorder, cannabis use disorder, inhalant use disorder), each with its own diagnostic criteria. The *DSM-5* groups substances of abuse into 12 categories (Box 48.1). Many other medications taken for therapeutic purposes can induce substance-related disorders as an adverse effect (Box 48.2), especially when large doses of the medications are taken for longer periods. Symptoms usually disappear when the dosage is lowered or the medication is stopped.

SUBSTANCE USE DISORDERS

The diagnosis of a substance use disorder is based on a pathologic pattern of behaviors related to the use of the substance. Over time, an important characteristic of substance use disorders is an underlying change in brain chemistry. The criteria for diagnosis can be subdivided into groupings of impaired control, social impairment, risky use, and pharmacologic criteria (Table 48.1). Substance use disorders occur in a broad range of severity, from mild to severe, based on the number of symptom criteria present. As a general rule, a *mild* substance use disorder has the presence of two or three symptoms, *moderate* has four to five symptoms, and *severe* has six or more symptoms. Severity can fluctuate over time based on changes in frequency and/or dose of substance use.

A term no longer used in the *DSM-5* diagnostic criteria for substance use disorder is *addiction*, although it is often used in medical and common terminology. There is no true definition of the term *addiction*, and its use often has negative connotations. The more neutral term *substance use disorder* is used to describe the wide range of the disorder, from a mild form to a severe state of chronically relapsing, compulsive drug taking.

Substance abuse is the periodic, purposeful use of a substance that leads to clinically significant impairment. The impairment results in failure to fulfill major obligations at work, school, or home (e.g., absenteeism, poor work performance, neglect of responsibilities); places the person in physically hazardous situations (e.g., operating a vehicle or machinery when impaired); and creates legal problems (e.g., arrests for intoxication, disorderly conduct) or social problems that are aggravated by the substance (e.g., physical fights, spousal arguments). If the substance use disorder is not stopped, substance abuse may lead to more serious medical conditions known as *tolerance* and *withdrawal*, which are normal physiologic responses to long-term use of substances (see Table 48.1). Symptoms of severe abuse include overwhelming compulsive use, tolerance of higher amounts of the substance, and withdrawal symptoms on discontinuation. A phrase that characterizes chemical dependency is "using a substance to live and living to use." The amount of drug exposure and the frequency of use necessary to develop dependence are unknown and highly individual, based on the

| Box 48.1 | Substances of Abuse |

- Alcohol (ethanol)
- Caffeine
- Cannabis (marijuana)
- Hallucinogens
- Inhalants
- Opioids
- Phencyclidine (PCP) or similarly acting arylcyclohexylamines
- Sedatives, hypnotics, and anxiolytics
- Stimulants (including amphetamines, cocaine)
- Tobacco
- Other (or unknown) substance-related disorders
- Nonsubstance-related disorder: gambling disorder

Data from the National Institute of Drug Abuse. Commonly abused prescription drugs chart; 2015. https://www.drugabuse.gov/drugs-abuse/commonly-abused-drugs-charts; *American Psychiatric Association: Diagnostic and Statistical Manual of Mental Disorders.* 5th ed. Washington, DC: American Psychiatric Publishing; 2013.

| Box 48.2 | Medications Whose Adverse Effects May Induce Substance Abuse |

- Analgesics
- Anesthetics
- Anticholinergic agents
- Anticonvulsants
- Antidepressants
- Antihistamines
- Antihypertensive and cardiovascular medications
- Antimicrobial medications
- Antiparkinsonian medications
- Chemotherapeutic agents
- Corticosteroids
- Gastrointestinal medications
- Muscle relaxants
- Nonsteroidal antiinflammatory drugs

Data from the National Institute of Drug Abuse. Commonly abused prescription drugs chart; 2015. https://www.drugabuse.gov/drugs-abuse/commonly-abused-drugs-charts.

pharmacology of the drug, the emotional condition of the person, heredity, and environmental factors. A term frequently associated with substance abuse is *illicit substance*—any chemical or mixture of chemicals that alters biologic function and is not required to maintain health. The term applies primarily to illegal substances. Any chemical that can produce a pleasurable state of mind has potential for abuse. Commonly abused substances, their pharmacologic effects, their street names, and their potential long-term consequences are listed in Table 48.2.

Substance abuse is a societal issue that plagues many cultures and all races throughout the world. In the United States, according to the 2014 National Survey on Drug Use and Health, an estimated 17 million (6.4% of the population) individuals age 12 or older had an alcohol use disorder in 2014. This percentage has remained steady between 2011 and 2014. There were 679,000 adolescents ages 12 to 17 in 2014 with alcohol use disorder (2.7% of adolescents). This was a lower percentage of alcohol use

| Table 48.1 | Measures of Substance Use Disorders |
GROUPING	DESCRIPTION
Impaired Control	Intake of substance in larger quantities or over a longer time period than originally planned or prescribed. The desire to cut down substance use may exist along with multiple unsuccessful attempts to reduce or discontinue use. Substantial time spent in obtaining, using, or recovering from the effects of the substance. Craving exhibited by a powerful urge for the substance; more common in circumstances in which the substance was used before.
Social Impairment	Failure to meet responsibilities at work, school, or home because of recurrent substance use. Substance use continues despite repeated social or interpersonal problems caused by the effects of the substance. Reduction or cessation of important social, occupational, or recreational pursuits because of substance use. Withdrawal from family activities and hobbies to use the substance.
Risky Use	Repeated substance use even when in settings or circumstances where doing so may be physically risky. Continued substance use regardless of known recurrent physical or psychological problems caused by or worsened by the substance. (Failure to abstain despite the problems it is causing.)
Pharmacologic	Development of tolerance manifested by the necessity to consume larger quantities to reach the desired effect, or a reduced effect achieved when the usual dose is consumed. Development of withdrawal symptoms occurs when blood levels decline. Symptoms vary widely across the classes of substances.

Data from American Psychiatric Association. *Diagnostic and Statistical Manual of Mental Disorders.* 5th ed. Washington, DC: American Psychiatric Publishing; 2013:483-484.

disorder in adolescents in 2014 than the percentages in 2002 to 2012. During this same time period, 7.1 million people (2.7% of US population) age 12 or older had an illicit drug disorder. This percentage has remained steady between 2005 and 2014.

SIGNS OF IMPAIRMENT

When signs of impairment start showing, it is usually not one sign alone but a cluster that raises questions of an impairment problem. The disease is usually first manifested in family life (e.g., domestic violence, separation, financial problems, problem behavior in children) and then in social life (e.g., overt public intoxication; isolation from friends, peers, church). Physical and mental changes may be manifested by excessive tiredness, multiple illnesses, frequent injuries or accidents, and emotional crises. Deterioration in physical status is an important sign but occurs late in the disease. Flagrant evidence of impairment at the worksite is relatively rare and usually occurs after the disease is advanced. In many cases the workplace is the source of the drug of choice, so the impaired person will strive to protect the source with appropriate behavior.

SCREENING FOR ALCOHOL AND SUBSTANCE ABUSE

Because of the large number of health problems associated with alcohol and substance abuse, *Healthy People 2020,* the US Preventive Services Task Force, the American Medical Association, and the American Nurses Association support and encourage screening patients for alcohol and other substance abuse. Screening instruments for substance abuse can be divided into the following four categories: (1) comprehensive drug abuse screening and assessment, (2) brief drug abuse screening, (3) alcohol abuse screening, and (4) drug and alcohol abuse screening for use with adolescents (Table 48.3). All the screening instruments listed in Table 48.3 have been validated for accuracy for specific purposes (e.g., differentiating between early detection of excessive drinking versus alcoholism; the potential for a substance use disorder). Another example of assessment for specific purposes is the Drug Abuse Screening Test, which can be used to differentiate among alcohol problems only, drug problems only, and both drug and alcohol problems. Some instruments are designed to be administered through an interview by a trained health professional, whereas others are designed for self-assessment by the patient using pencil and paper or computer entry. It is crucial that the proper assessment instrument be selected for use with a specific patient to attain meaningful results for an appropriate diagnosis. A disadvantage of some of the comprehensive screening instruments is the length of time required to administer the assessment and the availability of a qualified data interpreter. Many of the comprehensive instruments have been modified to be used as quick-screening instruments. A four-question assessment for alcohol abuse commonly used in the primary care setting because of its ease of administration is the CAGE questionnaire. CAGE (*c*ut down, *a*nnoyed, *g*uilty, and *e*ye opener) is an acronym that provides the interviewer with a quick reminder of questions to be asked about the patient's feelings toward his or her intake of substances (Ewing, 1984). A disadvantage of many of the instruments is that they were developed using adult male patients and have not been validated in other populations (e.g., women, older adults, and adolescents).

HEALTH PROFESSIONALS AND SUBSTANCE ABUSE

Although the prevalence of substance abuse among physicians, nurses, pharmacists, and other health professionals is not precisely known, it is probably similar to that of the general population. There is thought to be more prescription drug use and less street drug use because of easier access to prescription drugs. It is a misperception that education somehow protects healthcare professions from substance use disorders because "they know better." An individual's inability to manage stress brought on by intense patient care practice, managing more patients with the same resources, zero tolerance for making a mistake in association with the expectation of 100% perfection, and financial debt are thought to be major contributing factors to substance abuse among healthcare professionals.

Healthcare professionals are responsible for maintaining a code of ethics and standards of care, and the inappropriate use of substances puts these principles in jeopardy. Signs that raise suspicion of substance abuse include behavioral changes (e.g., wearing long-sleeved garments all the time, diminished alertness, lack of attention to hygiene, mood swings) and performance deterioration (e.g., requests for frequent schedule changes, errors in clinical judgment, excessive absenteeism, frank odor of alcohol on the breath and attempts to camouflage it with breath fresheners, frequent or long breaks, or deterioration in professional practice and patient care).

If a healthcare professional suspects that a colleague is impaired, a confidential report should be made to an appropriate supervisor familiar with institutional policy. An investigation should be initiated; observation and documentation are crucial to building a record of repeat instances over time to support the suspicion of impairment. Because of faulty memory on the part of the impaired individual, examples of inappropriate actions need to be well documented over time. An accurate record can also be useful in helping the impaired individual recognize the problem and submit voluntarily to treatment.

When considering whether to report a colleague for suspected drug abuse, remember the following:
- Clinical practice is a privilege, not a right.
- Good-faith reporting should not be considered unfair or disloyal to a colleague; protecting patients and the profession from harm should be paramount.
- It is very unlikely that an individual making a confidential report to a supervisor will be sued if a reasonable effort is made to establish that the concerns are legitimate and it is clear that patient safety is the primary concern.

Table 48.2 | **Substances of Abuse: Psychoactive Drugs Identification Chart**

DRUGS	MEDICAL USES	MEDICAL NAMES	SLANG NAMES	FORMS	USUAL METHOD OF ADMINISTRATION
Stimulants					
Nicotine	None	nicotine	Butt, chew, smoke, cig	Pipe, tobacco, cigarettes, snuff	Sniff, chew, smoke
Caffeine	Hyperkinesis, stimulant	caffeine	Java, cup of joe, morning thunder	Chocolates, tea, soft drinks, coffee	Swallow
Amphetamines	Hyperkinesis, narcolepsy, weight control, mental disorders	dexedrine, benzedrine	Speed, bennies, dexies, pep pills; doll, black beauties, crystal meth	Capsules, liquid, tablets, powder	Inject, swallow; inhale
Cocaine	Local anesthetic	cocaine	Coke, rock, Big C, blow, tool, white, blast, snow, flake	Powder, rock	Inject, smoke, inhale
Depressants					
Alcohol	None	ethyl alcohol	Booze	Liquid	Swallow
Sedatives	Anesthetic, sedative-hypnotic, anticonvulsant	secobarbital, phenobarbital, Seconal	Barbs, reds, downers, spoors	Capsules, tablets, powder	Inject, swallow
Tranquilizers	Antianxiety, sedative-hypnotic	Valium, Librium, meprobamate	Downers	Capsules, tablets	Swallow
Opioids					
Opium	Analgesic, antidiarrheal	paregoric	Midnight oil, Auntie	Powder, liquid	Smoke, swallow
Morphine	Analgesic, antitussive	morphine	None	Powder, tablet, liquid	Inject, smoke, swallow
Heroin	Research	diacetylmorphine	China white, smack, junk, H, horse	Powder	Inject, swallow
Fentanyl derivatives	Analgesic	fentanyl	Apache, China girl, dragon	Powder, liquid	Inject, snort, swallow
Codeine	Analgesic, antitussive	codeine, Empirin compound with codeine, Robitussin AC	None	Capsules, tablets, liquid	Inject, swallow

EFFECTS SOUGHT	POSSIBLE EFFECTS	OVERDOSAGE	LONG-TERM EFFECTS
Relaxation	Respiratory difficulties, fatigue, high blood pressure	None	Dependency, lung cancer, heart attacks, respiratory ailments
Alertness	Increased alertness, pulse rate, blood pressure; excitation, insomnia, loss of appetite	Irritability	Dependency may aggravate organic actions
Alertness, activeness	Increased alertness, pulse rate, and blood pressure; excitation, insomnia, loss of appetite	Agitation, increase in body temperature, hallucinations, convulsions, possible death	Severe withdrawal, possible convulsions, toxic psychosis; periodontitis, advanced tooth decay; dermatitis
Excitation, euphoria	Increased alertness, pulse rate, and blood pressure; excitation, insomnia, loss of appetite	Agitation, increase in body temperature, hallucinations, convulsions, possible death	Dependency, depression, paranoia, convulsions
Sense alteration, anxiety reduction	Loss of coordination, sluggishness, slurred speech, disorientation, depression	Total loss of coordination, nausea, unconsciousness, possible death	Dependency, toxic psychosis, neurologic damage
Anxiety reduction, euphoria, sleep	Loss of coordination, sluggishness, slurred speech, disorientation, depression	Cold clammy skin, dilated pupils, shallow respiration, weak and rapid pulse, coma, possible death	Dependency, severe withdrawal, possible convulsions, toxic psychosis
Anxiety reduction, euphoria, sleep	Loss of coordination, sluggishness, slurred speech, disorientation, depression	Cold clammy skin, dilated pupils, shallow respiration, weak and rapid pulse, coma, possible death	Dependency, severe withdrawal, possible convulsions, toxic psychosis
Euphoria, prevent withdrawal, sleep	Euphoria, drowsiness, respiratory depression, constricted pupils, sleep, nausea	Clammy skin, slow and shallow breathing, convulsions, coma, possible death	Dependency, constipation, loss of appetite, severe withdrawal
Euphoria, prevent withdrawal, sleep	Euphoria, drowsiness, respiratory depression, constricted pupils, sleep, nausea	Clammy skin, slow and shallow breathing, convulsions, coma, possible death	Dependency, constipation, loss of appetite, severe withdrawal
Euphoria, prevent withdrawal, sleep	Euphoria, drowsiness, respiratory depression, constricted pupils, sleep, nausea	Clammy skin, slow and shallow breathing, convulsions, coma, possible death	Dependency, constipation, loss of appetite, severe withdrawal
Euphoria, prevent withdrawal, sleep	Euphoria, drowsiness, respiratory depression, constricted pupils, sleep, nausea	Clammy skin, slow and shallow breathing, convulsions, coma, possible death	Dependency, constipation, loss of appetite, severe withdrawal
Euphoria, prevent withdrawal, sleep	Euphoria, drowsiness, respiratory depression, constricted pupils, sleep, nausea	Clammy skin, slow and shallow breathing, convulsions, coma, possible death	Dependency, constipation, loss of appetite, severe withdrawal

Continued

Table 48.2   **Substances of Abuse: Psychoactive Drugs Identification Chart—cont'd**

DRUGS	MEDICAL USES	MEDICAL NAMES	SLANG NAMES	FORMS	USUAL METHOD OF ADMINISTRATION
Cannabis					
THC	Research, cancer chemotherapy antinauseant	tetrahydrocannabinol	THC	Tablets, liquid	Swallow
Hashish	None	tetrahydrocannabinol	Hash	Solid resin	Smoke
Marijuana	Research	tetrahydrocannabinol	Pot, grass, doobie, ganja, dope, gold, herb, weed, reefer	Plant particles	Smoke, swallow
Hallucinogens					
PCP	None	phencyclidine	Angel dust, zombie peace pill, hog	Tablets, powder	Smoke, swallow
LSD	Research	lysergic acid diethylamide	Acid, sugar, cubes	Capsules, tablets, liquid	Swallow
Organics	None	mescaline, psilocybin	Mescal, mushroom	Crude preparations, tablets, powder	Swallow
Inhalants					
Aerosols and solvents	None	None	Glue, benzene, toluene, Freon	Solvents, aerosols	Inhale

For more information, contact the Florida Alcohol and Drug Abuse Association Resource Center, 2868 Mahan Dr. Tallahassee, FL, 32308.
National Institute on Drug Abuse: Commonly Abused Drugs Charts: https://www.drugabuse.gov/drugs-abuse/commonly-abused-drugs-charts.

- An unreported colleague is more likely than a reported one to die as a result of the impairment (from suicide, accidental overdose, other accident, disease, or violence).
- Colleagues who are reported to licensing authorities (especially those who self-report) have a very good chance of retaining their license and salvaging their careers.
- If a healthcare professional has knowledge of suspected impairment of another healthcare professional but fails to report it, that healthcare professional may potentially be named in a civil lawsuit or be named as a contributor in a malpractice suit against the impaired healthcare provider.
- In some states, if impairment of a colleague is suspected, filing a report with the licensing authority is mandatory. Failure to do so may result in a reprimand or probation from the licensing authority.

LEGAL CONSIDERATIONS OF SUBSTANCE ABUSE AND DEPENDENCE

All states have laws pertaining to the reporting of impairment of healthcare workers. Some require that suspected impairment be reported to the healthcare professional's licensure or disciplinary board. Other states allow referral to a professional society's impairment committee, which then contracts with the impaired individual to participate in a recovery program. As long as the healthcare professional continues to participate, the committee can refrain from notifying the licensure board.

The healthcare professional who makes a conscious effort to be treated for a substance use disorder has a

EFFECTS SOUGHT	POSSIBLE EFFECTS	OVERDOSAGE	LONG-TERM EFFECTS
Relaxation, euphoria, increased perception	Relaxed inhibitions, euphoria, increased appetite, distorted perceptions, disoriented behavior	Fatigue, paranoia, possible psychosis	Amotivational syndrome, respiratory difficulties, lung cancer, interference with physical and emotional development
Relaxation, euphoria, increased perception	Relaxed inhibitions, euphoria, increased appetite, distorted perceptions, disoriented behavior	Fatigue, paranoia, possible psychosis	Amotivational syndrome, respiratory difficulties, lung cancer, interference with physical and emotional development
Relaxation, euphoria, increased perception	Relaxed inhibitions, euphoria, increased appetite, distorted perceptions, disoriented behavior	Fatigue, paranoia, possible psychosis	Amotivational syndrome, respiratory difficulties, lung cancer, interference with physical and emotional development
Distortion of sense, insight, exhilaration	Illusions and hallucinations, distorted perception of time and distance	Longer and more intense "trips" or episodes, psychosis, convulsions, possible death	May intensify existing psychosis, flashbacks, panic reactions
Distortion of sense, insight, exhilaration	Illusions and hallucinations, distorted perception of time and distance	Longer and more intense "trips" or episodes, psychosis, convulsions, possible death	May intensify existing psychosis, flashbacks, panic reactions
Distortion of sense, insight, exhilaration	Illusions and hallucinations, distorted perception of time and distance	Longer and more intense "trips" or episodes, psychosis, convulsions, possible death	May intensify existing psychosis, flashbacks, panic reactions
Intoxication	Exhilaration, confusion, poor concentration	Heart failure, unconsciousness, asphyxiation, possible death	Impaired perception, coordination, and judgment; neurologic damage

variety of legal protections that can be helpful to reestablishing a career. The Americans with Disabilities Act (ADA) came into effect in 1992 and defines a disabled person as one "with a physical or mental impairment seriously limiting one or more major life activities." People who were dependent on drugs but who are no longer using drugs illegally and are receiving treatment for chemical dependence, or who have been rehabilitated successfully, are protected by the ADA from discrimination on the basis of past drug addiction. However, a substance abuser whose current use of chemicals impairs job performance or conduct may be disciplined, discharged, or denied employment to the extent that this person is not a "qualified individual with a disability." An individual who is currently engaging in the illegal use of drugs is not an "individual with a disability" under the ADA. State and federal handicap laws also mandate that every employer, including healthcare institutions, ensure that each recovering chemically impaired individual who applies for employment or reinstatement be afforded the same protection received by anyone with a handicap.

Once a chemically dependent person has been through treatment, an ongoing monitoring program is routinely established to help ensure that the person is free of the abused substance. Urinalysis for drugs is the most common form of drug testing. The Drug-Free Workplace Act of 1988 encourages (but does not require) drug screening in an effort to provide drug-free workplaces. The Drug-Free Schools and Communities Act Amendments of 1989 extend this act to all educational institutions.

The Supreme Court has ruled that drug screening does not violate one's constitutional right to privacy or

Table 48.3	Screening Instruments for Substance Abuse

NAME OF INSTRUMENT	ACRONYM	NAME OF INSTRUMENT	ACRONYM
Comprehensive Drug Abuse Screening and Assessment Instruments		**Alcohol Abuse Screening Instruments**	
Addiction Severity Index	ASI	CAGE	CAGE
Alcohol, Smoking and Substance Involvement Screening Test	ASSIST	Michigan Alcoholism Screening Test	MAST
		Millon Clinical Multiaxial Inventory	MCMI
Alcohol Use Disorders Identification Test	AUDIT	Millon Clinical Multiaxial Inventory, Scale B– Alcohol Dependence	MCMI (I-III)
Composite International Diagnostic Interview– Substance Abuse Module	CIDI-SAM	Short Michigan Alcohol Screening Test	SMAST
Drug Abuse Screening Test	DAST	**Drug and Alcohol Abuse Screening Instruments for Adolescents**	
Drug Use Screening Inventory-Revised	DUSI-R	Adolescent Alcohol Involvement Scale	AAIS
Individual Assessment Profile	IAP	Adolescent Drug Abuse Diagnosis	ADAD
MacAndrew Alcoholism Scale	MAC	Adolescent Drinking Index	ADI
Millon Clinical Multiaxial Inventory	MCMI	Adolescent Drug Involvement Scale	ADIS
Minnesota Multiphasic Personality Inventory	MMPI	Comprehensive Adolescent Severity Inventory	CASI
Minnesota Multiphasic Personality Inventory–2	MMPI-2	Drug and Alcohol Problem Quick Screen	DAP Quick Screen
Brief Drug Abuse Screening Instruments		Home, Education/Employment, Activities, Drugs, Sexuality, Suicide/Depression	HEADSS
CAGE Questionnaire Adapted to Include Drugs	CAGE-AID	Home, Education, Abuse, Drugs, Safety, Friends, Image, Recreation, Sexuality, and Threats	HEADS FIRST
Millon Clinical Multiaxial Inventory	MCMI		
Millon Clinical Multiaxial Inventory, Scale T–Drug Dependence	MCMI (I-III)	Problem-Oriented Screening Instrument for Teenagers	POSIT
Minnesota Multiphasic Personality Inventory–2	MMPI-2		
Addiction Potential Scale	APS		
Addiction Acknowledgment Scale	AAS		
Screening Instrument for Substance Abuse Potential	SISAP		
Short Michigan Alcoholism Screening Test—Adapted to Include Drugs	SMAST-AID		

Modified from McPherson TL, Hersch PK. Brief substance use screening instruments for primary care settings: A review. *J Subst Abuse Treat.* 2000;18:193-202.

represent unreasonable search. Drug screening may be required for employment and can be requested for cause (e.g., suspicious behavior, arrest, after an accident), or a random test can be requested as a part of a return-to-work agreement for people in recovery. A positive drug test means that the reported drug is present in the specimen. It does not establish that the person is dependent on the drug, and it does not, by itself, prove the drug was the cause of an impaired performance.

EDUCATING HEALTHCARE PROFESSIONALS ABOUT SUBSTANCE ABUSE

The curricula of healthcare profession educational programs should ensure that all students have multiple opportunities during their development of professional attitudes and behaviors to consider and formulate values about self-medication and substance abuse consistent with professional and legal standards. Employers should make available drug abuse resources, such as information about employee assistance programs and policies,

professional recovery assistance (e.g., recovery networks), and educational opportunities. Prevention of drug misuse, whether it is illegal or inappropriate use or drug abuse, is an important priority in the practice of every healthcare profession.

PRINCIPLES OF TREATMENT FOR SUBSTANCE ABUSE

It is important to recognize that substance-related disorders as described in *DSM-5* cover 10 separate classes of drugs and are considered treatable disorders. This focus is essential to successful treatment. The American Psychiatric Association lists long-term goals in treating substance abuse as follows:

- Reduction or abstinence in the use and effects of substances
- Reduction in the frequency and severity of relapse
- Improvement in psychological and social functioning

By the time a person seeks treatment for substance abuse or is ordered into a treatment program by the courts, the illness has become very complex, affecting almost every aspect of the person's life. Treatment requires lifelong effort, with a combination of psychosocial support and sometimes pharmacologic treatment. Key factors associated with long-term recovery are negative consequences of substance use (e.g., deteriorating health, divorce, loss of job, problems with family and friends) and social and community support, particularly with participation by self-help organizations whose goals include total abstinence of substances being abused (e.g., Alcoholics Anonymous, Narcotics Anonymous, Women for Sobriety, Rational Recovery). The types of social support given by the 12-step programs (e.g., Alcoholics Anonymous, Narcotics Anonymous), such as 24-hour availability when cravings arise, networking, role modeling, and advice on abstinence based on direct personal experiences, appear to be primary characteristics for success in maintaining recovery (Box 48.3).

Diagnostic criteria for assessment of substance use disorders are defined in the *DSM-5*. A combination of interviews, screening tools (see Table 48.3), information from colleagues, and laboratory tests will determine whether there is a single diagnosis of abuse of one or more substances or if there are multiple diagnoses. Other psychiatric conditions (e.g., depression, psychosis, delirium, dementia) and medical conditions (e.g., anemia, cirrhosis, hepatic encephalopathy, nutrition deficiencies, cardiomyopathy) may be induced by substance abuse. Based on the findings, priorities must be assigned. Immediate medical needs must be addressed first (e.g., thiamine deficiency, withdrawal and detoxification, safety). Detoxification programs are an important first step in substance abuse treatment. Detoxification initiates abstinence, reduces the severity of withdrawal symptoms, and retains the person in treatment to forestall relapse. During detoxification, behavioral interventions (e.g., contingency management, motivational enhancement, and cognitive therapies) can also be started.

ALCOHOL

In the United States, the 2015 National Survey on Drug Use and Health reports that binge drinking, defined as five or more drinks on one or more occasions in the past month, occurred in approximately 27% of people age 18 or older. Data from 2014 indicated that binge drinking appeared to be declining among individuals 18 to 25 years of age. Despite this decrease, more than one-third of young adults still binge drink.

A common characteristic of alcohol abusers is denial of a problem. Individuals who abuse alcohol may continue to consume alcohol despite the knowledge that continued consumption poses a significant social and health hazard to themselves.

Research over the past 25 years indicates that with *acute* ingestion of alcohol, the central nervous system (CNS) depressant effects of alcohol come from release of the major inhibitory neurotransmitter gamma-aminobutyric acid (GABA) and suppression of the major excitatory neurotransmitter glutamate, a byproduct of the N-methyl-D-aspartate (NMDA) receptors. With long-term *chronic* ingestion, the reverse occurs: tolerance to alcohol leads to reduced GABAergic activity and higher levels of NMDA activity. There are also inconsistent effects on the serotonin, dopamine, and opioid receptors of the CNS that may account for some of the acute and chronic effects of alcohol ingestion. Stimulation of opioid and dopamine receptors appears to be related to the alcohol "high," or the rewarding aspects of drinking alcohol.

Intoxication

Alcohol abuse, or more appropriately ethanol abuse, is commonly called *alcohol intoxication*. **Intoxication** is defined as the ingestion of ethanol to the point of clinically significant maladaptive behavioral or psychological changes (e.g., inappropriate sexual or aggressive behavior, mood lability, impaired judgment, impaired social or occupational functioning). These changes are

---

Box 48.3	**The 12 Steps of Alcoholics Anonymous**

1. We admitted we were powerless over alcohol—that our lives had become unmanageable.
2. Came to believe that a Power greater than ourselves could restore us to sanity.
3. Made a decision to turn our will and our lives over to the care of God as we understood Him.
4. Made a searching and fearless moral inventory of ourselves.
5. Admitted to God, to ourselves, and to another human being the exact nature of our wrongs.
6. Were entirely ready to have God remove all these defects of character.
7. Humbly asked Him to remove our shortcomings.
8. Made a list of all people we had harmed, and became willing to make amends to them all.
9. Made direct amends to such people wherever possible, except when to do so would injure them or others.
10. Continued to take personal inventory and when we were wrong promptly admitted it.
11. Sought through prayer and meditation to improve our conscious contact with God as we understood Him, praying only for knowledge of His will for us and the power to carry that out.
12. Having had a spiritual awakening as the result of these steps, we tried to carry this message to alcoholics and to practice these principles in all our affairs.

From Alcoholics Anonymous World Services, Inc. The Twelve Steps are reprinted with permission of Alcoholics Anonymous World Services, Inc. (AAWS). Permission to reprint the Twelve Steps does not mean that AAWS has reviewed or approved the contents of this publication, or that AAWS necessarily agrees with the views expressed herein. Alcoholics Anonymous (AA) is a program of recovery from alcoholism only; use of the Twelve Steps in connection with programs and activities patterned after AA but which address other problems, or in any other non-AA context, does not imply otherwise.

accompanied by evidence of slurred speech, incoordination, unsteady gait, nystagmus, impairment in attention or memory, or stupor or coma (American Psychiatric Association, 2013).

Withdrawal

When alcohol is ingested in quantities leading to intoxication, symptoms of overindulgence (e.g., hangover, queasy stomach, headache) are common over the next several hours because of direct toxic effects on body cells. If a person frequently drinks to intoxication over long periods (i.e., months to years), a physical dependence develops and a decrease in the blood alcohol level over 4 to 12 hours may cause symptoms of alcohol withdrawal. Development of withdrawal symptoms and craving often induces the person to continue to abuse alcohol (see Fig. 48.1 for symptoms and a time sequence of alcohol withdrawal). The person may no longer get much effect from the alcohol other than its ability to prevent withdrawal.

Alcohol withdrawal symptoms can begin within a few hours of discontinuation of drinking and may continue for 3 to 10 days. Withdrawal can progress to more severe symptoms, including visual and auditory hallucinations and seizures (usually of the tonic-clonic type). Less than 10% of patients develop delirium tremens (the DTs), the worst of the withdrawal symptoms. This syndrome is manifested by hyperactivity, delirium, and severe hyperthermia. The mortality rate of patients who progress to delirium tremens is 20%, most commonly as a result of stroke or cardiovascular collapse. Because it is difficult to predict who may have severe withdrawal, anyone experiencing alcohol withdrawal should be observed closely and treated if necessary.

Treatment

Patients who appear to be developing withdrawal symptoms should be quickly assessed for hydration and electrolyte and nutritional status. Excessive loss of fluids and electrolytes may occur through vomiting, sweating, and hyperthermia. Dehydration also may be caused by inadequate fluid intake and diuresis during prolonged and heavy alcohol consumption. Thiamine and multiple vitamins should be administered routinely to patients in alcohol withdrawal. Intravenous (IV) fluid therapy for rehydration may be necessary, but thiamine must be administered before glucose infusion to prevent Wernicke's encephalopathy.

If a person with an alcohol-related disorder seeks treatment for withdrawal symptoms, benzodiazepines (e.g., diazepam, chlordiazepoxide, clorazepate, oxazepam, lorazepam) are commonly used for detoxification because they enhance GABA activity that has been suppressed by chronic alcohol ingestion. The benzodiazepines are effective in sedating and controlling autonomic hyperactivity and reducing seizure risk in patients experiencing alcohol withdrawal. They are not effective in treating or controlling delirium.

There are two approaches for benzodiazepine dosing in treating withdrawal symptoms. The fixed-dose schedule uses a set dose of benzodiazepine administered at specific intervals. Usually, at about the second day, smaller tapering doses of benzodiazepines are administered on a fixed schedule. The symptom-triggered schedule depends on the use of a rating scale such as the Clinical Institute Withdrawal Assessment for Alcohol–Revised (CIWA-Ar). The CIWA-Ar protocol calls for administration of a benzodiazepine when the patient shows certain symptoms (symptom-triggered

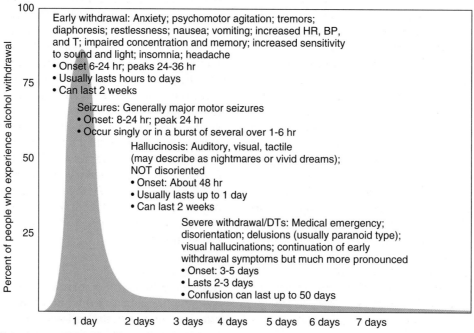

Fig. **48.1** Alcohol withdrawal syndrome. *BP*, Blood pressure; *DTs*, delirium tremens; *HR*, heart rate; *T*, temperature. (From Stuart GW. Principles and Practice of Psychiatric Nursing. 10th ed. St. Louis: Mosby; 2013.)

regimen) rather than a fixed-schedule regimen. It is hypothesized that the symptom-triggered medication regimen significantly reduces the amount of medication given and may shorten the length of treatment necessary.

The longer-acting benzodiazepines (e.g., chlordiazepoxide, diazepam, clorazepate) offer advantages of less fluctuation in blood levels and appear to be associated with fewer rebound effects and fewer withdrawal seizures on discontinuation. Because of the longer half-lives and active metabolites, patients taper themselves off just by discontinuing the dosage. The short-acting benzodiazepines (e.g., oxazepam, lorazepam) have the advantage of having no active metabolites that may produce additional adverse effects in older adults or those with concurrent liver disease. They do, however, have to be administered more often and tapering may be required. Carbamazepine is also effective in decreasing seizure frequency and some of the psychiatric symptoms associated with withdrawal (e.g., anxiety, agitation). Beta blockers (e.g., atenolol, propranolol) and an alpha agonist such as clonidine may reduce craving and decrease the severity of withdrawal symptoms.

Relapse Prevention

Lifelong effort with a combination of psychosocial support and sometimes pharmacologic treatment is necessary to prevent relapse. Key factors associated with long-term recovery are social and community support through participation with self-help organizations and negative consequences of substance use (e.g., job loss, divorce, loss of child custody). Current treatments are effective for about 50% of patients and significantly reduce the cost of healthcare, morbidity, and mortality associated with alcoholism.

Three medicines have been approved for use in helping to promote abstinence. Disulfiram (Antabuse) (see Drugs Used to Treat Alcoholism section later in this chapter) helps reduce the desire for alcohol by inducing nausea and vomiting (disulfiram reaction) if alcohol is ingested while disulfiram is being taken. Reactions can be severe, so it is essential that the patient understands the consequences of drinking alcohol while taking the medicine. It also means that the patient must avoid alcohol taken in the form of medicines (e.g., cough and cold elixirs, nighttime sedatives, mouthwashes), soups and sauces containing cooking sherry, and aftershave lotions or perfumes that contain alcohol that can be absorbed through the skin. Success with disulfiram very much depends on adherence to the medication regimen, and many alcoholics become lax in taking their medication as prescribed.

Naltrexone (see Chapter 19) is an opioid antagonist prescribed to block the pharmacologic effects of the high associated with alcohol. Studies report less alcohol craving and fewer drinking days, especially when naltrexone is combined with psychosocial treatment. Success is somewhat limited with naltrexone, because although it blocks the high from drinking, it provides no relief or promise of reward against the emotions that trigger the desire to drink in the first place.

Acamprosate (Campral) (see Drugs Used to Treat Alcoholism section later in this chapter) helps individuals maintain abstinence from alcohol. It enhances abstinence and reduces drinking rates in alcohol-dependent patients who are abstinent at the beginning of treatment. It is neither a sedative nor an anxiolytic, and it is not habit forming. Unlike naltrexone, it does not reduce the rewarding effects of alcohol, and unlike disulfiram, it does not cause nausea and vomiting when alcohol is consumed. Studies indicate similar rates of success with naltrexone and acamprosate and a slightly higher success rate when used together.

OPIOIDS

Commonly abused opiates (i.e., derived from opium) are heroin, morphine, hydromorphone (Dilaudid), codeine, oxycodone, and hydrocodone, as well as the synthetic opiatelike (opioid) substances such as methadone, meperidine, fentanyl, pentazocine, buprenorphine, and butorphanol. Heroin is a street drug derived from opium; there are no approved medicinal uses for heroin. Heroin use has been growing in recent years because it is now available in a purer form. Improved purity means a heroin user can get high from smoking or sniffing heroin and can avoid injecting it. There is also a misconception that inhaling heroin does not lead to dependence. As many as 40% of individuals who initially sniff heroin become IV users of it. The other opiates and opioids are made by legitimate manufacturers in specific concentrations for prescription use as anesthetics, analgesics, antidiarrheal agents, and cough suppressants but have been diverted from medicinal use into the illicit drug market for pleasure and profit. Obtaining prescriptions from one or more healthcare providers simultaneously for fake or exaggerated medical conditions (e.g., "severe" pain, back injury) is another mechanism of acquisition for illicit use by abusers. Healthcare providers who abuse opioids may write prescriptions for self-use or steal medicines intended for other patients or from pharmacy or floor stock.

The National Center for Health Statistics has shown that drug overdose deaths increased every year from 2002 to 2015. In 2015 there were 52,404 overdose deaths. Prescription opioids and benzodiazepines were responsible for 22,598 and 8791 overdose deaths, respectively, in 2015. More people are dying annually now from prescription drug overdoses than from illicit street drug abuse (heroin, cocaine, amphetamines).

Intoxication

Indications of opioid intoxication are the presence of inappropriate behaviors after administration, such as initial euphoria ("high") followed by apathy, dysphoria, agitation, impaired judgment, and/or impaired social and occupational functioning. Additional signs are pupillary constriction (miosis) and one or more of the following: drowsiness, slurred speech, and impairment of attention and memory. Intoxicated people also may show an indifference to placing themselves in potentially hazardous situations. The extent to which an intoxicated person shows these signs and symptoms depends on the dosage taken, route of administration, frequency of use, and acquired tolerance. Intoxication will usually last for several hours but depends on the half-life of the drug taken and the frequency of readministration of the opioid. Overdosage, especially with street drugs in which the concentration of drug is not known, can lead to severe intoxication manifested by coma, respiratory depression, pupillary dilation (mydriasis), and death.

Withdrawal

All opioids produce similar signs and symptoms of withdrawal. Onset of withdrawal symptoms in opioid-dependent people is somewhat predictable based on the half-life of the drug being abused; the symptoms begin two or three half-lives after the last dose has been taken. Onset of withdrawal symptoms from heroin or morphine is usually within 6 to 12 hours after the last dose, whereas it may take 2 to 4 days following discontinuation of longer-acting drugs such as methadone. Onset of withdrawal for people who abuse a variety of drugs and alcohol is extremely variable. Physical signs and symptoms associated with withdrawal are anxiety and restlessness, increased blood pressure and pulse, pupillary dilation, rhinorrhea, sweating, nausea, vomiting, and diarrhea. In severe cases, piloerection and fever may be present. Subjectively, the person may complain of an achy feeling, often located in the back and legs, an increased sensitivity to pain, and drug-seeking behavior (craving). Acute withdrawal symptoms from short-acting opiates (e.g., heroin) usually peak in 1 to 3 days and dissipate over the next 5 to 7 days. Chronic withdrawal symptoms (e.g., insomnia, anxiety, drug craving, apathy toward the pleasures in life [anhedonia]) may require weeks to months to dissipate.

Treatment

Withdrawal from opioids is uncomfortable but usually not life threatening unless there are coexisting medical conditions. Treatment is focused on relieving the acute symptoms. Clonidine (see Drug Class: Central-Acting Alpha-2 Agonists section in Chapter 22) is useful for decreasing tremors, sweating, and agitation; cyclobenzaprine (see Table 44.1) reduces skeletal muscle spasms; and loperamide (see Table 34.2) reduces gastrointestinal cramping and diarrhea. A protocol such as the Clinical Institute Narcotic Assessment rating scale is helpful for assessing and monitoring a patient undergoing opioid withdrawal.

Another approach to treatment of opioid dependence is the substitution of another opioid, usually long-acting methadone, to reduce the severity of withdrawal symptoms. Once the person has been detoxified from the abused opiate substance, the methadone can be tapered gradually to allow the person to be drug free. The long half-life of the methadone requires that the taper be prolonged over several weeks.

Another treatment alternative is an opioid maintenance program. The patient is started on methadone to minimize withdrawal symptoms. Instead of being tapered off the methadone, however, the person is maintained on a daily dose to prevent the development of withdrawal symptoms. The benefits to this approach are that the person can be maintained on a stable dosage without the development of tolerance and substantial craving and can function more normally in the work and home environment, although still addicted to an opiate. Opioid maintenance programs have been shown to reduce opioid use, criminal activity, and the transmission of human immunodeficiency virus (HIV) and hepatitis in opioid-dependent people.

Relapse Prevention

As with alcoholism, a lifelong effort with a combination of psychosocial support and sometimes pharmacologic treatment is necessary to prevent relapse. Key factors associated with long-term recovery are social and community support through participation with self-help organizations (e.g., Narcotics Anonymous) and the negative consequences of substance use. Current treatments are effective for maintaining abstinence for some patients and significantly reduce the cost of health care, morbidity, and mortality associated with opioid addiction.

Naltrexone (see Chapter 19) is an opioid antagonist prescribed to block the pharmacologic effects of the high associated with opioids. Studies report less drug craving and a reduced use of illicit drugs, especially when naltrexone is combined with psychosocial treatment. Success is somewhat limited with naltrexone, however, because although it blocks the high from opioid use, it provides no relief or promise of reward against the emotions that triggered the desire to get high in the first place.

Another approach to reducing the abuse of opioids is the methadone long-term maintenance program described as a treatment option. A disadvantage of this program is that the drug is available only through specially registered clinics and patients often have to travel long distances to the clinics, sometimes as often as six times per week. The Drug Addiction Treatment Act of 2000 opened up the possibility of physician office–based management of addicted patients who meet certain criteria by legalizing the prescribing of Schedule III, IV, and V medications for the treatment of opioid dependence. A drug that has been well studied in office practice is buprenorphine (see Chapter 19), a partial opioid agonist. Because it has opioid agonist and antagonist properties, it has a ceiling effect on analgesia and respiratory depression, giving it a much greater safety profile. Two dosage forms of buprenorphine have been approved for maintenance opioid programs: buprenorphine only, as a sublingual tablet; and buprenorphine-naloxone (Suboxone), as a sublingual film. The naloxone in the Suboxone product is to prevent abuse of the buprenorphine as a narcotic antagonist. Specifically trained prescribers administer the buprenorphine-only sublingual tablets directly to the patient in their offices, usually for 2 days. After dosage adjustment, the patient is switched to Suboxone for maintenance therapy.

AMPHETAMINE-TYPE STIMULANTS

Amphetamine-type stimulants are a group of chemically related compounds that are manufactured synthetically as CNS stimulants. Amphetamine, levoamphetamine, dextroamphetamine, and methamphetamine are all members of the amphetamine-type stimulants class. The amphetamines have been used medically over the years to treat schizophrenia, depression, opiate and nicotine addiction, and radiation sickness and have been used as bronchodilators in treating asthma. Dextroamphetamine and amphetamine are combined in the product Adderall, which is approved for the treatment of attention-deficit/hyperactivity disorder. The amphetamines have been commonly used for those persons in occupations that require mental stimulation during long hours of monotony, such as interstate truck drivers and assembly line workers.

The amphetamines have a high potential for abuse and dependence with prolonged use. Methamphetamine is most commonly used for nontherapeutic purposes.

The amphetamines became popular in the 1960s because of the perception of enhanced performance and communication, embodying a modern and fashionable lifestyle. Recreational use was not thought to be harmful and was perceived as easily controlled compared with cocaine or heroin. Methamphetamine ("meth" or "crystal meth"), in particular, is cheaper than cocaine and has a longer half-life (10 to 12 hours) than cocaine (1.5 to 2 hours) for longer duration of effect. Although it is most commonly smoked for its quick onset (euphoric rush), methamphetamine can also be taken orally or rectally, injected, or snorted through the nostrils. In some social circles, it is perceived as being acceptable to take methamphetamine orally rather than by injection or smoking, which carries negative connotations.

From a manufacturing standpoint, methamphetamine is not dependent on climate or geographic location like heroin (poppy plants) and cocaine (coca trees). Manufacture does not require advanced knowledge of chemistry and recipes are readily available on the Internet. Some recipes use ephedrine or pseudoephedrine, easily purchased over the counter (OTC) in some states as nasal decongestants. (Most states now require that these products be kept behind the prescription counter and sold only by a pharmacist in limited quantities.) Other ingredients are available for legitimate purposes in hardware and convenience stores. Although most methamphetamine is smuggled into the United States, "meth labs" are very easily assembled in the trunk of a car, the back of a van, or a rural farmhouse. A "cooker" can set up a lab, cook a batch, and then move on to another location. There is also a high margin of profit when the product is sold.

Intoxication

The intensity of physiologic response to methamphetamine intake depends on how it is ingested. If smoked, snorted, or injected, it produces a rapid, pleasurable "rush" within a few minutes because of the release of dopamine, norepinephrine, and serotonin neurotransmitters in the CNS. If taken orally, onset starts in about 20 minutes and peaks in 2 to 3 hours. Low doses tend to produce a sense of heightened alertness, attentiveness, self-confidence, powerfulness, and energy, whereas high doses produce a sense of well-being, euphoria, and enhanced self-esteem. Hypomania and grandiosity are more common with prolonged use. There is an increased libido and enhanced sense of sexual pleasure that is often associated with high-risk sexual behavior during a high. A methamphetamine high may last for 12 hours, but a user "on a run" taking additional doses may stay awake for 7 to 10 days, often with little food or water intake. As the drug starts to wear off, users may experience anxiety, depression, mental confusion, fatigue, and headaches. Prolonged sleep often follows.

Tolerance can occur with repeated use, requiring larger and more frequent doses to get high. The most common adverse effects are weight loss, insomnia, paranoia, hallucinations, and psychosis with violent behavior. Poor oral hygiene, in combination with the effects of methamphetamine use, such as dry mouth, teeth grinding, and jaw clenching, can lead to periodontitis and advanced tooth decay known as *meth mouth*. Other physiologic effects of methamphetamine are hypertension and tachycardia. Overdoses may induce myocardial infarction, stroke, and seizures.

Withdrawal

Abrupt discontinuation of methamphetamine after long-term use may result in withdrawal symptoms of severe depression, fatigue, lack of energy, loss of memory, and inability to manipulate information. These symptoms are frequently accompanied by drug craving. Because of its longer half-life and affinity for lipid tissues, methamphetamine withdrawal is substantially more prolonged than that of cocaine, and patients should be monitored closely for suicidal ideation.

Treatment

There are no antidotes to reverse methamphetamine intoxication, so treatment is largely supportive. If methamphetamine has been taken orally, activated charcoal may be administered. Rehydration is often necessary. Patients should be placed in a quiet area to reduce environmental stimuli. Patients demonstrating severe agitation may be sedated with a benzodiazepine such as diazepam. Antipsychotic agents such as haloperidol, a dopamine antagonist, may be necessary, but haloperidol may lower the seizure threshold in patients already at higher risk for seizures.

After withdrawal symptoms have subsided, the patient should be encouraged to undergo a psychiatric evaluation because methamphetamine is a neurotoxin that damages dopaminergic and serotonergic neurons in the brain. Damage to the dopaminergic centers may result in symptoms of parkinsonism and serotonergic damage may result in depression, anxiety, and impulsive behavior that may be treatable with appropriate medication. Ongoing outpatient behavior therapies such as cognitive behavior therapy, contingency management programs, and support groups or 12-step drug treatment programs may also be beneficial.

COCAINE

Cocaine is obtained from the leaves of trees indigenous to Bolivia, Colombia, Peru, Indonesia, and other parts of the world. For centuries, workers who traveled in mountainous South American countries have chewed coca leaves to improve stamina and suppress hunger. It has been used in Western medicine as a topically applied local anesthetic, particularly in ophthalmic, nasal, oral, and laryngeal procedures, for more than 100 years. Pharmacologically, cocaine blocks the transmission of nerve impulses when applied to tissues in these areas. When injected intravenously, inhaled as smoke, or sniffed onto the mucous membranes of the nose (snorted using a straw), it blocks the reuptake of catecholamines in the brain, causing sudden CNS stimulation with euphoria (the rush).

Popular as a recreational drug for its euphoric effects, cocaine soared in use in the United States through the 1970s and 1980s. When treated with hydrochloric acid, cocaine becomes cocaine hydrochloride, which can be dried to a powder for sniffing or dissolved in water for IV injection for an immediate rush. Another method of extraction of cocaine led to the creation of the more potent "freebase" and "crack" cocaine. Freebase is formed when cocaine hydrochloride is mixed with ammonia to form a base, which then is dissolved in ether. The ether evaporates, leaving a powder residue. The powder is then smoked for the rush, but ether vapors remaining are extremely flammable and can ignite, causing a small explosion with severe burns to the face and airways if inhaled. Crack cocaine is formed when the cocaine hydrochloride is mixed with baking soda and then heated. The resulting mass that forms is left to harden into slabs of cocaine. Chunks of the slab are sold as "rocks" of cocaine. This form of cocaine is the cheapest and most potent. When smoked, it makes a crackling sound, hence its name. Other drugs (e.g., nicotine, alcohol, heroin) are frequently used at the same time to enhance and prolong the euphoria. Cocaine smoking and IV use tend to be particularly associated with a rapid progression from use to abuse to dependence, often occurring over weeks to months. Intranasal use is associated with a more gradual progression, usually occurring over months to years. With continued use, tolerance and dependence develop, leading to increases in dosage and a reduction in the pleasurable effects of the euphoria.

Intoxication

Acute cocaine intoxication usually begins with a euphoric feeling and can then lead to a variety of other behaviors, including enhanced vigor, hyperactivity, restlessness, hypervigilance, talkativeness, anxiety, tension, alertness, grandiosity, anger, and impaired judgment. Signs and symptoms that develop are tachycardia or bradycardia, pupillary dilation, hyper- or hypotension, sweating or chills, and nausea and vomiting. With chronic use, fatigue, sadness, social withdrawal, respiratory depression, chest pain, cardiac dysrhythmias, and confusion may manifest. Severe intoxication can lead to hyperpyrexia, seizures (primarily tonic-clonic), respiratory depression, coma, and death.

Withdrawal

Because cocaine has a short half-life, withdrawal symptoms (a "crash") may begin within a few hours of a reduction in dosage or frequency of administration, or discontinuation. Acute withdrawal symptoms are more likely to be seen after periods of repetitive high-dose use ("runs" or "binges"). People often complain of fatigue, vivid and unpleasant dreams, extreme depression, insomnia or hypersomnia, and increased appetite. There is often an intense craving and drug-seeking behavior. These symptoms cause significant distress and social withdrawal, with the inability to continue work. Several days of rest and recuperation are required for symptoms to resolve. Depression with suicidal ideation is generally the most serious problem associated with cocaine withdrawal.

Treatment

There are no medicines approved to treat cocaine dependence. Many classes of drugs (e.g., dopamine agonists, antidepressants, anticonvulsants, calcium channel blockers, serotonin reuptake inhibitors) have been tested in controlled studies, with minimal effect. Studies are ongoing with GABA, the inhibitory neurotransmitter. Two additional areas of investigation are vaccines and maintenance drugs. Animal studies have shown that vaccines trigger the formation of antibodies that might increase the metabolism of cocaine. Long-acting maintenance medicines similar to methadone or buprenorphine for opioid addiction are also under investigation. Unfortunately, the rate of relapse for patients who develop a cocaine dependency is very high.

❖ NURSING IMPLICATIONS FOR SUBSTANCE ABUSE

◆ Assessment

Despite early detection of an overdose of a substance, the adverse effects of the ingested substance on multiple body systems may result in death. Assess the ABCs—*a*irway, *b*reathing, and *c*irculation—immediately on admission. A thorough physical and neurologic examination must be undertaken to detect life-threatening symptoms. Care must be prioritized, based on the individual patient's care needs.

Refer to Table 48.2 for a listing of substances abused and symptoms associated with each substance. Table 48.3 can serve as a reference for screening instruments for substance abuse, and the CAGE questionnaire (https://psychology-tools.com/cage-alcohol-questionnaire/) can be used as an index for individuals suspected of alcoholism. Screening instruments will have to be administered in a manner appropriate to circumstances and the overall condition of the patient.

History of the event, accident, or behavior. For the person who appears to be intoxicated, ask simple, direct questions about whether the person has been drinking or using drugs. "Do you drink alcohol?" If the answer is "yes," ask, "When was your last drink (time)?" "How much have you had to drink?" "Approximately how much alcohol have you consumed over the past week or month?" This would be an appropriate time to administer the CAGE questionnaire if other, more urgent care is not needed. If the answer to the question regarding drug and alcohol use is "no," ask whether the individual has a history of drinking alcohol or treatment for alcohol abuse, or has lost a driver's license, been fined, or ordered to a treatment program as a result of alcohol or drug abuse. Ask specific questions regarding the use of any "street drugs" or prescription drugs. Be direct and name examples, such as cocaine, marijuana, amphetamines, crack cocaine, tranquilizers, opioids, phencyclidine (PCP), and lysergic acid diethylamide (LSD). It is essential to try to identify the abused substance so that reversal agents may be used to minimize respiratory depression.

People with symptoms of bizarre or inappropriate behavior and who are combative, violent, and possibly hallucinating should be screened not only for substance abuse but also for possible psychiatric disorders that may be the primary cause of the presenting symptoms, a result of substance abuse, or a combination of both (see also Chapters 15, 16, and 17 for further information). Know how to summon security personnel or have them present to provide for patient and personnel safety. It is important to include past medical history in the nursing assessment. For example, a history of stroke may include slurred speech as a residual deficit that will not improve with an overdose treatment regimen.

If the patient has been injured, follow emergency department policies regarding forms and legal documents that need to be completed (e.g., screening toxicology, rape kit procedures) to meet the medicolegal requirements.

Vital signs. Persistent abnormal vital signs during routine testing should raise suspicion of substance abuse. Vital signs should be taken as often as necessary to monitor the patient's status.

- *Blood pressure:* Blood pressure may be elevated from the use of stimulants and other coexisting conditions. Blood pressure should be determined at least twice daily and more often if indicated by the patient's symptoms or the healthcare provider's orders.
- Record the blood pressure in both arms. A systolic pressure variance of 5 to 10 mm Hg is normal; readings reflecting a variance of more than 10 mm Hg should be reported for further evaluation. **Always report a narrowing pulse pressure** (difference between systolic and diastolic readings).
- *Pulse:* Assess bilaterally the rhythm, quality, equality, and strength of peripheral pulses. Note if any pulse is diminished or absent. **Report irregular rate, rhythm, and palpitations.**
- *Respirations:* Table 48.2 notes that respirations are affected by narcotics and depressants; however, because the patient may have coexisting medical conditions, respiratory rate cannot be relied on as a definitive observation for substance abuse. Lungs also may have substantial damage from smoking or prolonged inhalations of drugs, aerosols, and solvents, making the patient susceptible to respiratory abnormalities. Check breath sounds for abnormal breath sounds (e.g., crackles, wheezes). Observe the degree of dyspnea that occurs and whether it happens with or without exertion.
- *Temperature:* Record the temperature.

Basic mental status. Be alert for fluctuating levels of consciousness; lack of awareness or attention; paranoid thoughts; visual, auditory, or tactile hallucinations; and confusion about the immediate surroundings.

Note the patient's level of consciousness and clarity of thought; both are indicators of cerebral perfusion. Assess level of consciousness for improvement or deterioration. Report declining mental status to the healthcare provider.

Appearance. Describe the individual's gait, coordination, and physical appearance.

Neurologic assessment. Determine the Glasgow Coma Scale score if appropriate (Table 48.4).

Heart assessment. Heart palpitations and irregularity may occur during withdrawal. Cocaine is associated with causing cardiotoxicity that can be fatal to a first-time user or to an individual who has cardiovascular disease. (See Chapters 22, 23, and 24 for further details relating to heart assessments.)

Table 48.4	Determination of Glasgow Coma Scale Score[a]		
EYE OPENING (E)	**VERBAL RESPONSE (V)**	**MOTOR RESPONSE (M)**
4 = Spontaneous	5 = Normal conversation	6 = Normal
3 = To voice	4 = Disoriented conversation	5 = Localizes to pain
2 = To pain	3 = Words, but not coherent	4 = Withdraws to pain
1 = None	2 = No words, only sounds	3 = Decorticate posture
	1 = None	2 = Decerebrate posture
		1 = None

[a]Total score = E + V + M.

Eyes. Check pupil size, equality, light reaction, and accommodation. Note ptosis, nystagmus, or other abnormal eye movements. Abnormal pupil changes include either enlarged dilated pupils (mydriasis); very small, pinpoint pupils (miosis); or nonreactive pupils (do not respond to light).

Dry eyes may be a problem in a person with alcoholism. Blurred vision is common with alcoholism, and the condition may resolve after approximately 3 to 4 months of sobriety, but if the condition persists or increases, an eye examination should be scheduled.

Ears, oral cavity, nose, and throat. The range of symptoms associated with substance abuse is extensive in these tissues. Ringing, buzzing, and roaring in the ears are most common among benzodiazepine users.

The oral cavity, which is often ignored by people who abuse drugs, may have bleeding gums, canker sores, cold sores, dental caries, and infections. During withdrawal, the mouth may be very dry. The long-term use of alcohol, especially when combined with smoking, increases the risk of oral cancer, so a thorough examination of the mouth and throat should be completed.

Snorting of cocaine and heroin can seriously damage tissues in the nose, showing evidence of inflammation, ulceration, and perforation of the nasal septum. Nosebleeds are common.

Skin assessment. Check skin color; jaundice may indicate hepatitis, which is common in drug abusers who share needles and in alcoholics with advanced disease. Check skin for rashes, abscesses, and evidence of "tracking" along veins on the forearm, wrist, dorsum of hand, antecubital area, ankle, scrotal area, between the toes, and under the tongue. Is the skin dry, moist, or clammy? Sweating may be observed during withdrawal.

Musculoskeletal assessment. Alcohol depletes calcium from the bones, making them more susceptible to fractures. Osteoporosis also may be prevalent in alcoholics. Muscle pains (myalgia) and weakness in the muscles may be associated with withdrawal. Fine hand tremors may be observed with alcohol withdrawal.

Medication history. Ask specific questions relating to the use of prescription, OTC, and street or illicit drugs. Does the individual also use any herbal products?

Coexisting diseases and disorders. Is the individual currently under treatment for other diseases? Is there a history of any cardiac, respiratory, renal, endocrine, or neurologic disorders? Is there a history of head trauma or seizures?

Sexually transmitted infections. The individual will need examination and testing for the entire scope of sexually transmitted infections. Sexual activity is common during drug and alcohol intoxication. Prostitution is commonly used to support a substance abuse habit.

Pregnancy. Ask female patients if they are pregnant. Use of drugs and alcohol while pregnant has a strong likelihood of harming not only the mother but also the baby before and after birth. Alcohol and drug use during pregnancy may cause preterm birth, low birth weight, birth defects, fatal bleeding disorders, and behavioral problems later in life. Intravenous drug abusers who share needles may expose the fetus to hepatitis B virus, HIV, or acquired immunodeficiency syndrome. Sexually transmitted infections also place both the mother and fetus at risk. Infants of drug addicts must be monitored closely for symptoms of withdrawal after delivery.

Laboratory tests. Urine and/or blood toxicology screening; complete blood cell count; electrolyte studies; renal and liver function tests; thyroid levels; serologic tests for hepatitis B virus, venereal disease, and HIV; chest x-ray; tuberculosis skin test; and electrocardiography constitute a routine panel for most individuals suspected of substance abuse.

The sensitivity of the blood and urine testing for drugs depends on the amount, frequency of use, and time of last use. The presence of any drug depends on the drug's half-life and metabolites. Hallucinogens may be detected in urine for up to 28 days after last use in regular users, whereas opiates may be detectable for only 12 to 36 hours after the last use.

Emergency treatment. The nurse should be aware of the policy for calling codes, location of the emergency cart, and procedures used to check the emergency cart supplies and understand the procedure for defibrillation and cardioversion. The nurse should also be familiar with the medicolegal components of providing care to injured or impaired patients.

Safety. Provide for patient safety during and following detoxification until the individual is able to assume self-responsibility.

Goal setting for the patient. Establish goals and outcomes for the immediate needs of an individual who has had an injury or has inflicted injury on others.

Plan for the patient's immediate care needs and arrange for follow-up in an inpatient or outpatient detoxification and rehabilitation program designed to help the individual reach the goal of long-term abstinence. Involve the patient in goal setting as the ability to assume responsibility for his or her own actions evolves.

In a rehabilitation program, the individual will be given factual information regarding the harmful use of drugs and/or alcohol. The individual will often not acknowledge that he or she has a problem (denial); when the problem is recognized, the person does not have insight into how to overcome the problem. Throughout the program, the patient will need to explore positive and negative aspects of his or her behavior to develop new behaviors that do not include the use of drugs and alcohol.

Family and support involvement. Integrate family and others within the patient's support network into the interdisciplinary team for long-term planning for treatment and support. Encourage them to become involved in the rehabilitation program. Family members and friends need guidance in appropriate ways to be involved in the recovery of an individual who exhibits symptoms of a dysfunctional family relationship. Enrollment in community groups (e.g., Al-Anon, Nar-Anon) designed to provide support for family and friends will assist them in understanding the addiction problem and provide guidance in coping with potential problems.

◆ Implementation

- In an emergency department setting, the immediate care needs of the individual must be met to stabilize the person and provide for patient safety. Deliver physical care and provide psychological support of the individual and significant others. Orient the patient to date, time, place, person, and situation. Once stabilized, the patient may be admitted to an intensive care, acute care, psychiatric, or rehabilitation facility designed to provide treatment of the presenting problems.
- The nurse needs to be familiar with the protocol and healthcare provider orders used during detoxification. Refer to the earlier section on Principles of Treatment for Substance Abuse, and to other textbooks with more extensive coverage of substance abuse, for details regarding detoxification for specific agents being abused.
- During withdrawal, patients need a quiet, safe care environment with staff experienced in detoxification methods.

- Provide for patient and staff safety. Have emergency equipment available at all times, and be particularly vigilant for seizure activity.
- Perform physical assessments of the patient in accordance with clinical policies (e.g., every 2, 4, or 8 hours or as indicated by the patient's status).
- Have medications listed in the protocol or healthcare provider's orders readily available for administration (e.g., benzodiazepines, clonidine, beta blockers for treatment of withdrawal; carbamazepine for seizures; cyclobenzaprine for muscle spasms; naltrexone to reduce craving).
- Implement measures to reduce anxiety, including administering prescribed medications that can best alleviate the patient's symptoms and provide maximum level of comfort. Support the patient in a calm manner, even if the patient responds in a hostile or confrontational way. React appropriately to the patient's expressions of resistance (e.g., arguing, denying, ignoring).
- As the patient progresses, encourage the patient to make choices and take responsibility for those decisions. See discussions earlier in the chapter for intoxication, withdrawal, treatment, and relapse prevention for various substances.

◆ Patient Education

Design an individualized approach to help the patient modify factors that are in the patient's control.

Nutrition status

- Encourage a well-balanced diet. Consultation with a dietitian may be necessary. The B vitamins, especially thiamine, are vital to the repair of the nervous system; calcium may be needed for weakened bones; and excessive amounts of vitamins A and D may be harmful.
- If the patient is anemic, an iron preparation may also be prescribed. Consult with the healthcare provider or a pharmacist about an appropriate vitamin supplement.
- Have the patient drink 8 to 10 eight-ounce glasses of water daily, unless coexisting medical problems prohibit it.
- Sugars may affect the mood of some individuals. If mood swings are a problem, it may be wise to limit the patient's sugar intake.

Stress management. Identify stress-producing situations in the patient's life and seek means to reduce these factors significantly. In some cases, referral for training in stress management, relaxation techniques, mediation, or biofeedback may be necessary. If stress is produced in the work setting, it may be appropriate to involve the nurse at the patient's place of employment.

Fostering health maintenance. Seek the patient's cooperation and understanding of the following points so that medication adherence is increased: name of medication; dosage, route, and times of administration; and common and serious adverse effects. The person who has an alcohol or drug abuse problem needs to reveal his or her history to all healthcare providers so that the prescriber can take this into account when selecting agents for use. At the supermarket, pharmacy, or nutrition center, the patient should always read labels thoroughly to avoid food and medicinal products that contain alcohol.

Patient self-assessment. Enlist the patient's help in developing and maintaining a written record of monitoring parameters for coexisting medical problems (e.g., pulse rate, blood pressure, degree of dyspnea and what precipitates it, chest pain, edema). See Appendix B: Template for Developing a Written Record for Patients to Monitor Their Own Therapy. Complete the Premedication Data column for use as a baseline to track response to drug therapy. Ensure that the patient understands how to use the form, and instruct the patient to take the completed form to follow-up visits. During follow-up visits, focus on issues that will foster adherence with the therapeutic interventions prescribed.

DRUGS USED TO TREAT ALCOHOLISM

acamprosate (ā-KĂM-prō-sāt)
Campral (KĂM-prăl) ✦

Actions
Acamprosate is classified as a weak NMDA receptor antagonist. It is a synthetic compound structurally related to GABA. A variety of mechanisms have been proposed, but none has been well proven.

Uses
Acamprosate is used in alcohol rehabilitation programs for chronic alcoholic patients who want to maintain sobriety. It should be used only in conjunction with other rehabilitative therapy. It enhances abstinence and reduces drinking rates in alcohol-dependent patients who are abstinent at the beginning of treatment. It is neither a sedative nor an anxiolytic, and it is not habit forming. It does not reduce the rewarding effects of alcohol as does naltrexone, and it does not cause nausea and vomiting when alcohol is consumed, as does disulfiram. Studies indicate similar rates of success with naltrexone and acamprosate and a slightly higher success rate when used together. Acamprosate may also be used in cases when naltrexone is contraindicated, such as for patients with liver disease or those receiving concurrent opioid therapy or methadone maintenance therapy. Acamprosate does not treat withdrawal symptoms.

Therapeutic Outcome
The primary therapeutic outcome expected from acamprosate is improved adherence with an alcohol treatment program by abstinence from alcohol.

❖ **Nursing Implications for Acamprosate**
◆ *Premedication assessment*
1. Perform baseline neurologic assessment (e.g., orientation to date, time, and place; mental alertness; bilateral hand grip; motor functioning).
2. Take vital signs (temperature, blood pressure, pulse, respirations).
3. Check laboratory values for urine screen for alcohol use and blood urea nitrogen and serum creatinine levels for renal function.
4. Monitor for gastrointestinal symptoms before and during therapy.

◆ *Availability.* **PO:** 333-mg delayed-release tablets.

◆ *Dosage and administration.* **Adult: PO:** Two 333-mg tablets (666 mg) three times daily. Tablets may be taken without regard to meals. Acamprosate should be started as soon as possible after the period of alcohol withdrawal, when the patient has become abstinent.

Patients with moderate renal function as indicated by a creatinine clearance of 30 to 50 mL/min should take one 333-mg tablet three times daily.

Behavior modification. Acamprosate therapy in combination with behavior therapy has been shown to be more effective than acamprosate or behavior therapy alone in prolonging alcohol cessation in patients who were formerly physically dependent on alcohol.

> [!] **Medication Safety Alert**
> Acamprosate is contraindicated in patients with severe renal failure as indicated by a creatinine clearance lower than 30 mL/min.

◆ *Common adverse effects*
Gastrointestinal
Diarrhea. Diarrhea may occur in 10% to 20% of patients taking acamprosate but rarely is it a cause for discontinuing therapy. Symptoms are usually mild and tend to resolve with continued therapy. Encourage the patient not to discontinue therapy without first consulting with the healthcare provider and treatment program.

◆ *Serious adverse effects*
Psychological
Suicidal actions. In clinical studies with acamprosate, suicidal ideation, suicide attempts, and completed suicides were infrequent but were more common in acamprosate-treated patients than in patients treated with placebo (2.4% vs. 0.8%). The interrelationship of alcohol dependence, depression, and suicide is well recognized and complex. Monitor alcohol-dependent patients, including those patients being treated with acamprosate, for symptoms of negative thoughts, feelings, behaviors, depression, or suicidal thinking. Alert families and caregivers of patients being treated with acamprosate of the need to monitor patients for the

emergence of these symptoms and ask them to report such symptoms to the patient's healthcare provider.

◆ *Drug interactions.* No clinically significant drug interactions have been reported.

---

disulfiram (dī-SŬL-fĭr-ăm)
Antabuse (ĂN-tĕ-byūs)

Actions

Disulfiram is an agent that, when ingested before any form of alcohol is consumed, produces a very unpleasant reaction to the alcohol. Disulfiram blocks the metabolism of acetaldehyde, a metabolite of alcohol. Elevated levels of acetaldehyde produce the disulfiram-alcohol reaction, which is manifested by nausea, severe vomiting, sweating, throbbing headache, dizziness, blurred vision, and confusion. The intensity of the reaction depends somewhat on the sensitivity of the individual and the amount of alcohol consumed. The duration of the reaction depends on the presence of alcohol in the blood. Mild reactions may last from 30 to 60 minutes, whereas more severe reactions may last for several hours. Prolonged administration of disulfiram does not produce tolerance; indeed, the longer a patient remains on therapy, the more exquisitely sensitive the person becomes to alcohol.

Uses

Disulfiram is used in alcohol rehabilitation programs for chronic alcoholic patients who want to maintain sobriety. It should be used only in conjunction with other rehabilitative therapy. Patients must be fully informed of the consequences of drinking alcohol while receiving disulfiram therapy. As little as 10 to 15 mL of alcohol may produce a reaction. Patients must not drink or apply alcohol in any form, including OTC products such as sleep aids, cough and cold products, aftershave lotions, mouthwashes, and rubbing alcohol. Dietary sources, such as sauces and vinegars containing alcohol, are prohibited. A disulfiram-alcohol reaction may occur with the ingestion of any alcohol for 1 to 2 weeks after discontinuing disulfiram therapy. Disulfiram must never be administered to a patient who is intoxicated. Because of the consequences of a disulfiram-alcohol reaction on other disease states, disulfiram therapy must be used very cautiously in patients with diabetes mellitus, hypothyroidism, epilepsy, cerebral damage, chronic or acute nephritis, hepatic cirrhosis, or hepatic failure.

Therapeutic Outcome

The primary therapeutic outcome expected from disulfiram is improved adherence to an alcohol treatment program by abstinence from alcohol.

❖ Nursing Implications for Disulfiram

◆ *Premedication assessment*

1. Perform baseline neurologic assessment (e.g., orientation to date, time, and place; mental alertness; bilateral hand grip; motor functioning).

2. Take vital signs (i.e., temperature, blood pressure, pulse, respirations).
3. Check laboratory values for hepatotoxicity; screen urine for alcohol use.
4. Monitor for gastrointestinal symptoms before and during therapy.
5. The manufacturer recommends that baseline determinations of liver function should be performed in all patients before initiation of therapy and repeated in 10 to 14 days. A baseline complete blood cell count and serum chemistries are recommended and should also be repeated every 6 months, along with the liver function tests.

◆ *Availability.* *PO:* 250- and 500-mg tablets.

◆ *Dosage and administration.* **Adult:** *PO:* Initially a maximum of 500 mg once daily for 1 to 2 weeks. The maintenance dosage is usually 250 mg daily (range 125 to 500 mg). Do not exceed 500 mg daily. Administer at bedtime to avoid the complications of sedative effects.

Behavior modification. Disulfiram therapy, in combination with behavior therapy, has been shown to be more effective than disulfiram or behavior therapy alone in prolonging alcohol cessation in patients who were formerly physically dependent on alcohol.

- Disulfiram must never be administered to patients when they are in a state of intoxication or when they are unaware that they are receiving therapy. Family members should be told about the treatment so that they can provide motivation and support and help the patient avoid accidental disulfiram-alcohol reactions.
- Do not administer disulfiram until the patient has abstained from alcohol for a period of at least 12 hours.
- It is recommended that all patients who are receiving disulfiram carry a patient identification card stating the use of disulfiram and describing the symptoms that are most likely to occur as a result of the disulfiram-alcohol reaction. This card also should indicate the healthcare provider or institution that should be contacted in an emergency.

◆ *Common adverse effects.* These adverse effects are usually mild and tend to resolve with continued therapy. Encourage the patient not to discontinue therapy without first consulting with the healthcare provider and treatment program.

Neurologic. Drowsiness, fatigue, headache.
Reproductive. Impotence.
Gastrointestinal. Metallic taste.

◆ *Serious adverse effects*
Gastrointestinal
Hepatotoxicity. The symptoms of hepatotoxicity are jaundice, nausea, vomiting, anorexia, hepatomegaly, splenomegaly, and abnormal liver function tests (e.g., elevated bilirubin, aspartate aminotransferase, alanine aminotransferase, and alkaline phosphatase levels;

increased prothrombin time). Because many of these patients do not develop clinical symptoms but do develop abnormal liver function test results, strongly encourage patients to report for blood tests as scheduled. Report abnormal values to the appropriate healthcare provider.

Hypersensitivity, immune system

Hives, pruritus, rash. Report symptoms of hives, pruritus, or rash for further evaluation by the healthcare provider. Pruritus may be relieved by taking antihistamines and adding baking soda to the bath water.

◆Drug interactions

Warfarin. Disulfiram may enhance the anticoagulant effects of warfarin. Observe for the development of petechiae; ecchymoses; nosebleeds; bleeding gums; dark, tarry stools; and bright red or coffee-ground emesis. Monitor the prothrombin time (international normalized ratio) and reduce the dosage of warfarin if necessary.

Phenytoin. Disulfiram inhibits the metabolism of phenytoin. Monitor patients with concurrent use for signs of phenytoin toxicity (i.e., nystagmus, sedation, lethargy). Serum levels may be monitored, and the dosage of phenytoin may need to be reduced.

Isoniazid. Disulfiram alters the metabolism of isoniazid. Perform a baseline assessment of the patient's degree of alertness (e.g., orientation to name, place, time) and coordination before initiating therapy. Make regularly scheduled subsequent mental status evaluations and compare findings. Report to the healthcare provider any development of alterations in mental status.

Metronidazole. Concurrent administration of disulfiram and metronidazole may result in psychotic episodes and confusional states. Concurrent therapy is not recommended.

Benzodiazepines. Disulfiram inhibits the metabolism of specific benzodiazepines (e.g., chlordiazepoxide, diazepam, clorazepate, flurazepam, quazepam, estazolam). When benzodiazepine therapy is indicated, use oxazepam, alprazolam, temazepam, or lorazepam because of a different metabolic pathway not inhibited by disulfiram.

Caffeine. The cardiovascular and CNS stimulant effects of caffeine may be increased by disulfiram. If tachycardia or nervousness is noted, cut back on the consumption of caffeine-containing products such as coffee.

Get Ready for the NCLEX® Examination!

Key Points

- Substance abuse is defined as the periodic, purposeful use of a substance that leads to clinically significant impairment.
- Table 48.3 summarizes several screening instruments used for substance abuse.
- Frequency of substance abuse among healthcare providers is probably similar to that of the general population.
- Healthcare professionals suspecting a colleague of substance abuse need to observe, document, and report relevant data to the supervisor and to the licensing agency or disciplinary board in states in which mandatory reporting is required. Many states have licensee assistance programs and procedures for reporting or seeking counseling from this resource.
- The *DSM-5* has redefined substance use disorders and recognizes that they are treatable disorders. Treatment needs to be individualized to the person's needs.
- Professionals providing healthcare to people with a substance abuse problem need to be vigilant for coexisting medical or psychiatric problems.
- People with a substance use disorder must be encouraged to assume responsibility for their own actions and to focus not only on the need for a change in behavior, but also on strategies for managing their lives and approaches to coping more effectively with life situations.

- Group support for the individual and for family and significant others needs to be established. Many rehabilitation programs involve family as part of the treatment regimen. Others suggest community resources such as Alcoholics Anonymous or Narcotics Anonymous for the person in recovery and Al-Anon or Nar-Anon for family members.

Additional Learning Resources

SG Go to your Study Guide for additional Review Questions for the NCLEX® Examination, Critical Thinking Clinical Situations, and other learning activities to help you master this chapter content.

Go to your Evolve website (https://evolve.elsevier.com/Clayton) for additional online resources.

Review Questions for the NCLEX® Examination

1. A patient reported to the clinic in a state of intoxication. The nurse questioned the patient about alcohol use and determined that the patient may be considered under the classification of moderate alcohol use disorder with the finding of how many symptoms?
   1. Two
   2. Four
   3. Six
   4. Eight

2. The screening instrument used commonly in acute care settings to determine alcohol abuse is referred to by which acronym?
   1. DAST
   2. CASI
   3. CAGE
   4. MMPI

3. Which signs and symptoms raise the suspicion of substance use disorder by a healthcare professional? *(Select all that apply.)*
   1. Infrequent breaks
   2. Diminished alertness
   3. Rarely being absent from work
   4. Requests for frequent schedule changes
   5. Wearing long-sleeved garments all the time

4. The nurse recognizes that the amphetamine-type stimulants can have which of the following effects? *(Select all that apply.)*
   1. They produce excitation and insomnia.
   2. They may cause sluggishness and increased appetite.
   3. They produce hypotension and bradycardia.
   4. They may produce parkinsonism symptoms as a result of long-term use.
   5. They cause prolonged withdrawal due to their affinity for lipid tissues.

5. Which symptoms are associated with alcohol withdrawal? *(Select all that apply.)*
   1. Nausea
   2. Vomiting
   3. Hypotension
   4. Diaphoresis
   5. Psychomotor agitation

6. The nurse realizes that the patient who is being treated for cocaine dependence has insight about cocaine use after making which statement?
   1. "When getting clean, I sometimes have thoughts of ending it all."
   2. "Cocaine withdrawal is relatively easy."
   3. "The only form of cocaine that is dangerous is freebase."
   4. "There are several approved treatment medications for cocaine dependence."

7. The nurse was instructing a patient taking disulfiram (Antabuse) on which of the following precautions while on the medication? *(Select all that apply.)*
   1. Avoid foods high in purines.
   2. Avoid all alcoholic beverages.
   3. Avoid foods high in tyramine.
   4. Avoid topical products and lotions with alcohol.
   5. Review all drug labels for ingredients, particularly alcohol.

8. The nurse educating a patient being treated for substance abuse reviewed the list of medications that have the adverse effect of inducing substance abuse. Which class of medications would the nurse caution the patient on? *(Select all that apply.)*
   1. Analgesics
   2. Corticosteroids
   3. Diuretics
   4. Antihistamines
   5. Antidiabetic agents

Nomogram for Calculating the Body Surface Area of Adults, Children, and Infants

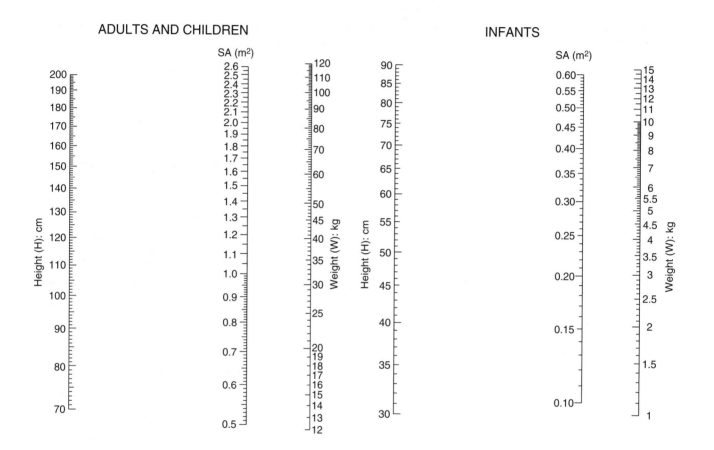

ADULTS AND CHILDREN

INFANTS

Template for Developing a Written Record for Patients to Monitor Their Own Therapy

---

PATIENT SELF-ASSESSMENT FORM   Self-Monitoring Drug Therapy Record

MEDICATIONS	COLOR	TO BE TAKEN

Patient _____

Health Care Provider _____

Health Care Provider's phone _____

Next appt.* _____

What I Should Monitor	Premedication Data	Date	Date	Date	Date	Date	Date	Comments

Complete the premedication data column for use as a baseline to track response to drug therapy.
Instruct patient to bring this record to the next appointment.
Use the back of this sheet for additional information.

Bibliography

ONLINE RESOURCES

https://beckinstitute.org/tag/beck-depression-inventory/.

http://consumer.healthday.com/encyclopedia/pain-management-30/pain-health-news-520/pain-care-bill-of-rights-646163.html [Pain Care Bill of Rights, American Pain Foundation].

http://health.gov/dietaryguidelines/2015-scientific-report/pdfs/scientific-report-of-the-2015-dietary-guidelines-advisory-committee.pdf.

http://naturaldatabase.therapeuticresearch.mancom. [Therapeutic Research Faculty; Natural Medicines database].

http://www.miccsi.org/wp-content/uploads/2016/01/CMAG2.pdf [Case Management Adherence Guidelines].

http://www.nationalacademies.org/hmd/Activities/Nutrition/SummaryDRIs/DRI-Tables.aspx [Institute of Medicine: Dietary Reference Intakes Tables and Application. 2017].

http://www8.nationalacademies.org/onpinews/newsitem.aspx?recordid=10490.

http://www.nlm.nih.gov/medlineplus/ency/article/004024.htm [Drugs that may cause impotence, 10/07/17].

http://www.samhsa.gov/data/: Center for Behavioral Health Statistics and Quality.(2015). [Behavioral health trends in the United States: Results from the 2014 National Survey on Drug Use and Health (HHS Publication No. SMA 15-4927, NSDUH Series H-50)].

https://www.diabeteseducator.org/docs/default-source/legacy-docs/_resources/pdf/general/Insulin_Injection_How_To_AADE.pdf.

https://www.drugabuse.gov/drugs-abuse/commonly-abused-drugs-charts [Commonly abused drugs chart}.

https://ginasthma.org [Global Initiative for Asthma (GINA): Global strategy for asthma management and prevention Revised 2017].

https://goldcopd.org/gold-2017-global-strategy-diagnosis-management-prevention-copd/ [GOLD 2017 Global Strategy for the Diagnosis, Management and Prevention of COPD].

https://health.gov/dietaryguidelines/2015/guidelines/ [U.S. Department of Health and Human Services and U.S. Department of Agriculture. *2015–2020 Dietary Guidelines for Americans.* 8th Edition. December 2015].

https://rarediseases.info.nih.gov/ [National Institutes of Health, Office of Rare Diseases Research: Rare diseases information, 2017].

https://www.cancer.org/research/cancer-facts-statistics.html [American Cancer Society: Cancer facts and figures, 2017, Atlanta, 2017, American Cancer Society].

https://www.cdc.gov/brfss [Centers for Disease Control and Prevention: National Center for Chronic Disease Prevention and Health Promotion: Behavioral risk factor surveillance system: Survey data and downloads, Atlanta, 2017, U.S. Department of Health and Human Services].

https://www.cdc.gov/diabetes/pdfs/data/statistics/national-diabetes-statistics-report.pdf [National Diabetes Statistics Report 2017].

https://www.cdc.gov/nchs/data/databriefs/db282.pdf [Drug Overdose Deaths Among Adolescents Aged 15–19 in the United States: 1999–2015].

https://www.columbia.edu/ [Columbia University: Partnership for Gender-Specific Medicine, New York, Columbia University].

https://www.fda.gov/Drugs/ResourcesForYou/Consumers/BuyingUsingMedicineSafely/EnsuringSafeUseofMedicine/SafeDisposalofMedicines/ucm186187.htm [U.S. Food and Drug Administration: Disposal of unused medicines: What you should know. Rockville, MD, 2013, U.S. Food and Drug Administration].

www.cdc.gov/diabetes/home/index.html [Centers for Disease Control and Prevention: National diabetes fact sheet: General information and national estimates on diabetes in the U.S., Atlanta, 2017, U.S. Department of Health and Human Services].

www.cdc.gov/nchs/fastats/deaths.htm [Centers for Disease Control and Prevention; National Center for Health Statistics: Deaths and mortality, Atlanta, 2014, U.S. Department of Health and Human Services].

www.cdc.gov/obesity/data/adult.html [Centers for Disease Control and Prevention: Prevalence of obesity, 2016, U.S. Department of Health and Human Services].

www.drugabuse.gov/publications/drugfacts/methamphetamine [National Institute on Drug Abuse—Methamphetamine—2017].

www.fda.gov/downloads/Drugs/DrugSafety/UCM353335.pdf [Magnesium Sulfate Drug Safety Communication—Recommendation against prolonged use in pre-term labor; U.S. Food and Drug Administration].

www.fda.gov/downloads/Drugs/DrugSafety/PostmarketDrugSafetyInformationforPatientsandProviders/UCM192556.pdf [Statistical Review And Evaluation Antiepileptic Drugs And Suicidality].

www.fda.gov/drugs/scienceresearch/ucm572698 [Center for Drug Evaluation and Research: Table of valid genomic biomarkers in the context of approved drug labels, Rockville, MD, 2017, U.S. Food and Drug Administration].

www.idf.org/ [The IDF consensus worldwide definition of the metabolic syndrome, Metabolic Syndrome 2006, Brussels, Belgium. International Diabetes Federation].

www.ins1.org [Infusion Nurses Society: Infusion nursing. The Infusion Nurses Society promotes excellence in infusion nursing through standards, education, advocacy, and outcomes research].

www.ismp.org/Tools/highalertmedications.pdf [Institute for Safe Medication Practices: ISMP's list of high-alert medications, Horsham, PA].

www.jointcommission.org/SentinelEvents/SentinelEventAlert/sea_35.htm [The Joint Commission: Sentinel event alert: Using medication reconciliation to prevent errors, Oakbrook Terrace, IL, 2017, The Joint Commission].

www.nap.edu/openbook.php?isbn=0309085373 [Food and Nutrition Board; Institute of Medicine of the National Academies: Dietary reference intakes for energy, carbohydrate, fiber, fat, fatty acids, cholesterol, protein, and amino acids, Washington DC, 2005, National Academies Press].

www.nccn.org/professionals/physician_gls/PDF/antiemesis.pdf [NCCN Guidelines Version 2.2017. Antiemesis; National Comprehensive Cancer Network, 2017].

www.nhlbi.nih.gov/guidelines/asthma/asthgdln.htm [National Heart Lung and Blood Institute: Expert Panel Report 3 (EPR3): Guidelines for the diagnosis and management of asthma, Bethesda, MD, 2007, National Institutes of Health, U.S. Department of Health and Human Services].

www.nhlbi.nih.gov/health/public/heart/obesity/phy_active.pdf [U.S. Department of Health and Human Services; National Institutes of Health; National Heart, Lung, and Blood Institute: Your guide to physical activity and your heart. NIH Publication No. 06–5714, Bethesda, MD, 2006, U.S. Department of Health and Human Services].

www.oldwayspt.org [Food issues think tank. Oldways, 2017].

www.painfoundation.org. [Pain care bill of rights, Baltimore, MD, American Pain Foundation].

www.surgeongeneral.gov/library/mentalhealth/home.html [U.S. Department of Health and Human Services: Mental health: A report of the Surgeon General, Rockville, MD, 1999, U.S. Department of Health and Human Services].

PUBLICATIONS

Abramowicz M. *Treatment Guidelines, Medical Letter.* New Rochelle, NY: The Medical Letter; 2015.

Abrams P, et al. The standardisation of terminology of lower urinary tract function: report from the Standardisation Subcommittee of the International Continence Society. *Neurourol Urodyn.* 2002;21:167.

Alberti KG, et al. Harmonizing the metabolic syndrome: a joint interim statement of the International Diabetes Federation Task Force on Epidemiology and Prevention; National Heart, Lung, and Blood Institute; American Heart Association; World Heart Federation; International Atherosclerosis Society; and International Association for the Study of Obesity. *Circulation.* 2009;120(16):1640–1645.

Alden K, Lowdermilk DL, et al. *Maternity and Women's Health Care.* 11th ed. St. Louis: Mosby; 2016.

American Association of Clinical Endocrinologists. Clinical practice guidelines for developing a diabetes mellitus comprehensive care plan – 2015. *Endocr Pract.* 2015;21(suppl 1):1–87.

American College of Obstetricians and Gynecologists' Committee on Practice Bulletins—Obstetrics. Practice Bulletin No. 171: management of preterm labor. *Obstet Gynecol.* 2016;128(4):e155–e164.

American Diabetes Association. Standards of medical care in diabetes—2017. *Diabetes Care.* 2017;40(suppl 1):S1–S135.

American Diabetes Association. Standards of medical care in diabetes – 2018. *Diabetes Care.* 2018;41(suppl 1):S1–S153. http://care.diabetesjournals.org/content/diacare/suppl/2017/12/08/41.Supplement_1.DC1/DC_41_S1_Combined.pdf.

American Geriatrics Society. 2015 Updated Beers Criteria for potentially inappropriate medication use in older adults. *J Am Geriatr Soc.* 2015;63(11):2227–2246.

American Pain Society. *Principles of Analgesic Use in the Treatment of Acute Pain and Cancer pain.* 6th ed. Chicago, IL: American Pain Society; 2008.

American Psychiatric Association. *Diagnostic and Statistical Manual of Mental Disorders.* 5th ed. Washington DC: American Psychiatric Publishing; 2013.

Baldwin JN, Thibault ED. Substance abuse by pharmacists: stopping the insanity. *J Am Pharm Assoc.* 2001;41:373.

Beck AT, Steer RA, Brown GK. *Beck Depression Inventory II (BDI-II) Manual.* 2nd ed. Indianapolis: Pearson Education; 1996.

Benjamin EJ, et al. Heart disease and stroke statistics-2017 update: a report from the American Heart Association. *Circulation.* 2017;135(10):e146–e603.

Berger MJ, et al. National comprehensive cancer network guidelines insights: antiemesis, version 2.2017. *J Natl Compr Canc Netw.* 2017;15:883–893.

Bickley LS. *Bates' Guide to Physical Examination and History Taking.* 10th ed. Philadelphia: Wolters Kluwer Health/Lippincott Williams & Wilkins; 2009.

Billups NF, Billups SM, eds. *American Drug Index 2014.* 58th ed. Philadelphia: Lippincott, Williams & Wilkins; 2014.

Brown LM, Isetts BJ. Patient assessment and consultation. In: *Handbook of Non-Prescription Drugs.* 17th ed. Washington, DC: American Pharmacists Association; 2012:27.

Brunton L, et al. *Goodman and Gilman's the Pharmacological Basis of Therapeutics.* 13th ed. New York: McGraw-Hill; 2018.

Busse JW, Craigie S, Juurlink DN, et al. Guideline for opioid therapy and chronic noncancer pain. *CMAJ.* 2017;189(18):E659–E666.

Camacho LH, Frost CP, Abella E, Morrow PK, Whittaker S. Biosimilars 101: considerations for U.S. oncologists in clinical practice. *Cancer Med.* 2014;3(4):889–899.

Camacho PM, Petak SM, Binkley N, et al. American Association of Clinical Endorinologists and American College of Endocrinology Clinical Practice Guidelines for the diagnosis and treatment of postmenopausal osteoporosis-2016. *Endocr Pract.* 2016;22(suppl 4):1–42.

Canadian Pharmacists Association, ed. *Compendium of Pharmaceuticals and Specialties 2014.* Ottawa, Canada: Canadian Pharmacists Association; 2014.

Canadian Pharmacists Association, ed. *Compendium of Self-Care Products 2010.* Ottawa, Canada: Canadian Pharmacists Association; 2010.

Carpenito LJ. *Nursing Diagnosis: Application to Clinical Practice.* 14th ed. Philadelphia: Wolters Kluwer Health/Lippincott Williams & Wilkins; 2013.

Centers for Disease Control and Prevention. *National Diabetes Statistics Report: Estimates of Diabetes and Its Burden in the United States, 2014.* Atlanta, GA: U.S. Department of Health and Human Services; 2014.

Centers for Disease Control and Prevention. *National Diabetes Statistics Report, 2017.* Atlanta, GA: Centers for Disease Control and Prevention, U.S. Dept of Health and Human Services; 2017.

Centers for Disease Control and Prevention. Sexually transmitted diseases treatment guidelines. 2015. *MMWR Recomm Rep.* 2015;64(RR–03):1–137.

Chabner BA. Clinical strategies for cancer treatment. The role of drugs. In: Chabner BA, Longo DL, eds. *Cancer Chemotherapy and Biotherapy: Principles and Practice.* 5th ed. Philadelphia: Lippincott Williams & Wilkins; 2010.

Chandola T, Brunner E, Marmot M. Chronic stress at work and the metabolic syndrome: prospective study. *BMJ.* 2006;332:521.

Chen JJ, Dashtipour K. Parkinson's disease. In: DiPiro JT, et al, eds. *Pharmacotherapy: A Pathophysiologic Approach.* 10th ed. New York: McGraw-Hill; 2017.

Chong OT. An integrative approach to addressing clinical issues in complementary and alternative medicine in an outpatient oncology center. *Clin J Oncol Nurs.* 2006;10:83.

Clayton BD, Brown BK. Nausea and vomiting. In: Helms RA, et al, eds. *Textbook of Therapeutics, Drug and Disease Management.* 8th ed. Philadelphia: Lippincott Williams & Wilkins; 2006.

Clinical guidelines on the identification, evaluation, and treatment of overweight and obesity in adults: executive summary. Expert Panel on the Identification, Evaluation, and Treatment of Overweight in Adults. *Am J Clin Nutr.* 1998;68(4):899–917.

Cohen H. Be on the alert for high-alert drugs. *Nursing Made Incredibly Easy.* 2008;6(2):7–11.

Criteria Committee of the New York Heart Association. *Nomenclature and Criteria for Diagnosis of Diseases of the Heart and Great Vessels.* 9th ed. Boston: Little, Brown; 1994.

Curtis KM, Tepper NK, Jatlaoui TC, et al. U.S. medical eligibility criteria for contraceptive use, 2016. *MMWR Recomm Rep.* 2016;65(RR–3):1–104.

DiPiro JT, et al. *Pharmacotherapy: A Pathophysiologic Approach.* 10th ed. New York: McGraw-Hill; 2017.

Dopheide JA, Stimmel GL. Sleep disorders. In: Koda-Kimble MA, Young LY, eds. *Applied Therapeutics.* 10th ed. Philadelphia: Lippincott Williams & Wilkins; 2013.

Dowell D, Haegerich TM, Chou R. CDC guideline for prescribing opioids for chronic pain—United States, 2016. *JAMA.* 2016;315(15):1624–1645.

Eckel RH, Jakcic JM, Ard JD, et al. 2013 AHA/ACC Guideline on lifestyle management to reduce cardiovascular risk: a report of the American College of Cardiology/American

Heart Association Task Force on Practice Guidelines. *Circulation*. 2014;129(25 suppl 2):S76–S99. doi:10.1161/01.cir.0000437740.48606.d1.

Ewing JA. Detecting alcoholism: the CAGE questionnaire. *JAMA*. 1905;252:1984.

Facts and comparisons. *Drug Facts and Comparisons, 2015*. St. Louis: Wolters Kluwer; 2015.

Ferrell B, Argoff CE, Epplin J, et al. Pharmacological management of persistent pain in older persons. *J Am Geriatr Soc*. 2009;57(8):1331–1346.

Ford A, et al. American College of gastroenterology monograph on the management of irritable bowel syndrome and chronic idiopathic constipation. *Am J Gastroenterol*. 2014;109:S2–S26.

French JA, Pedley TA. Clinical practice. Initial management of epilepsy. *N Engl J Med*. 2008;359:166.

Garber AJ, et al. Consensus statement by the American Association of Clinical Endocrinologists and American College of endocrinology on comprehensive type 2 diabetes management algorithm-2018. *Endocr Pract*. 2018;24(1):91–120.

Garvey WT, Mechanick JI, Brett EM, et al. American Association of Clinical Endocrinologists and American College of Endocrinology Comprehensive Clinical Practice Guidelines for medical care of patients with obesity. *Endocr Pract*. 2016;22(7):842–884.

Gerhard-Herman MD, Gornik HL, Barrett C, et al. 2016 AHA/ACC Guideline on the management of patients with lower extremity peripheral artery disease: executive summary: a report of the American College of Cardiology/American Heart Association Task Force on Clinical Practice Guidelines. *Circulation*. 2017;135(12):e686–e725.

Gilbert DN, et al. *The Sanford Guide to Antimicrobial Therapy 2014*. 44th ed. Sperryville, VA: Antimicrobial Therapy, Inc; 2014.

Go AS, Mozaffarian D, Roger VL, et al. Heart disease and stroke statistics—2014 update: a report from the American Heart Association. *Circulation*. 2014;129:e28–e292.

Goldman L, et al, eds. *Cecil Textbook of Medicine*. 24th ed. Philadelphia: Saunders; 2012.

Gordon DB, Dahl JL, Miaskowski C, et al. American pain society recommendations for improving the quality of acute and cancer pain management: American Pain Society Quality of Care Task Force. *Arch Intern Med*. 2005;165(14):1574–1580.

Guyton AC, Hall J. *Textbook of Medical Physiology*. 12th ed. Philadelphia: Saunders; 2011.

Haas DM, Caldwell DM, Kirkpatrick P, et al. Tocolytic therapy for preterm delivery: systematic review and network meta-analysis. *BMJ*. 2012;345:e6226. doi:10.1136/bmj.e6226.

Hatcher RA, et al. *Contraceptive Technology*. 20th ed. New York: Ardent Media; 2008.

Helms RA, ed. *Textbook of Therapeutics, Drug and Disease Management*. 8th ed. Philadelphia: Lippincott Williams & Wilkins; 2006.

Henderson ML. Self-care and nonprescription pharmacotherapy. In: Krinsky DL, et al, eds. *Handbook of Non-Prescription Drugs*. 17th ed. Washington, DC: American Pharmacists Association; 2012.

Hesketh PJ, et al. Antiemetics: American Society of Clinical Oncology clinical practice guideline update. *J Clin Oncol*. 2017;35(28):3240–3261.

Hockenberry M, Wilson D. *Wong's Nursing Care of Infants and Children*. 9th ed. St. Louis: Mosby; 2011.

Ignatavicius DD, Workman ML. *Medical-Surgical Nursing: Patient-Centered Collaborative Care*. 7th ed. Philadelphia: Saunders; 2013.

Infusion Nurses Society. *Infusion nursing standards of practice (2011), Store.untreedreads.com Institute of Medicine, Food and Nutrition Board: dietary reference intakes: a risk assessment model for establishing upper intake levels for nutrients*. Washington, DC: National Academy Press; 1998.

International Association for the Study of Pain, Subcommittee on Taxonomy. Classification of chronic pain. Descriptions of chronic pain syndromes and definitions of pain terms. *Pain Suppl*. 1986;3:S1.

Jarvis C. *Physical Examination and Health Assessment*. 6th ed. St. Louis: Saunders; 2011.

Joint National Committee on Detection, Evaluation and Treatment of High Blood Pressure. *The seventh report of the National Committee on Detection, Evaluation and Treatment of High Blood Pressure (JNC 7), NIH Publication 03–5233*. Bethesda, MD: National Institutes of Health; 2003.

Jones CM, Mack KA, Paulozzi LJ. Pharmaceutical overdose deaths, United States, 2010. *JAMA*. 2013;309(7):657–659.

Kaskutas LA, Bond J, Humphreys K. Social networks as mediators of the effects of Alcoholics Anonymous. *Addiction*. 2002;97:891.

Keltner NL, Steele D. *Psychiatric Nursing*. 7th ed. St. Louis: Mosby; 2014.

Koda-Kimble MA, Young LY, eds. *Applied Therapeutics*. 10th ed. Philadelphia: Wolters Kluwer/Lippincott, Williams and Wilkins; 2013.

Kotecki JE. *Physical Activity and Health: An Interactive Approach*. 4th ed. Boston: Jones & Bartlett Learning, Inc; 2013.

Lasser KE, et al. Timing of new black box warnings and withdrawal for prescription medications. *JAMA*. 2002;287:2215.

László KD, et al. Job strain predicts recurrent events after a first acute myocardial infarction: the Stockholm Heart Epidemiology Program. *J Intern Med*. 2010;267(6):599–611.

Laudet AB, Savage R, Mahmood D. Pathways to long-term recovery: a preliminary investigation. *J Psychoactive Drugs*. 2002;34:305.

Lazarou J, Pomeranz B, Corey P. Incidence of adverse drug reactions in hospitalized patients: a meta-analysis of prospective studies. *JAMA*. 1998;279:1200.

Leininger M. *Transcultural Nursing: Concepts, Theories, and Practices*. 3rd ed. New York: McGraw-Hill; 2002.

LeMone P, Burke K. *Medical-Surgical Nursing: Critical Thinking in Client Care*. 6th ed. Upper Saddle River, NJ: Pearson; 2015.

Lewis S, et al. *Medical-Surgical Nursing: Assessment and Management of Clinical Problems*. St. Louis: Mosby; 2014.

Lineberry TW, Bostwick JM. Methamphetamine abuse: a perfect storm of complications. *Mayo Clin Proc*. 2006;81:77.

Lloyd-Jones DM, Morris PB, Ballantyne CM, et al. 2017 focused update of the 2016 ACC expert consensus decision pathway on the role of non-statin therapies for LDL-cholesterol lowering in the management of atherosclerotic cardiovascular disease risk: a report of the American College of Cardiology Task Force on Expert Consensus Decision Pathways. *J Am Coll Cardiol*. 2017;70(14):1785–1822.

Longo DL, ed. *Cancer Chemotherapy and Biotherapy: Principles and Practice*. 5th ed. Philadelphia: Lippincott Williams & Wilkins; 2010.

McCance KL, Huether SE. *Pathophysiology: The Biologic Basis for Disease in Adults and Children*. 7th ed. St. Louis: Mosby; 2013.

McEvoy G, ed. *AHFS Drug Information 2015*. Bethesda, MD: American Society of Health-System Pharmacists; 2015.

McPherson TL, Hersch RK. Brief substance use screening instruments for primary care settings: a review. *J Subst Abuse Treat*. 2000;18:193.

McVary KT. Clinical practice. Erectile dysfunction. *N Engl J Med*. 2007;357:2472.

Meiner S, Lueckenotte AG. *Gerontologic Nursing*. 4th ed. St. Louis: Mosby; 2011.

Melzack R. The McGill pain questionnaire: major properties and scoring methods. *Pain*. 1975;1:277.

Moore N, et al. Frequency and cost of serious adverse drug reactions in a department of general medicine. *Br J Clin Pharmacol*. 1998;45:301.

Moore TJ, Cohen MR, Furberg CD. Serious adverse drug events reported to the Food and Drug Administration, 1998-2005. *Arch Intern Med*. 2007;167(16):1752–1759.

Mulhall A. Nursing, research, and the evidence. *Evid Based Nurs*. 1998;1:4.

National Academies of Sciences, Engineering, and Medicine. *The Challenge of Treating Obesity and Overweight: Proceedings of a Workshop-in Brief.* Washington, DC: The National Academies Press; 2017. doi:10.17226/24830.

National Research Council. *To Err Is Human: Building a Safer Health System.* Washington, DC: The National Academies Press; 2000.

Nguyen Viet-Huong V, Baca CB, Chen JJ, Rogers SJ. Epilepsy. In: DiPiro JT, et al, eds. *Pharmacotherapy.* 10th ed. New York: McGraw-Hill; 2017 [chapter 56].

Niebyl JR. Nausea and vomiting in pregnancy. *N Engl J Med.* 2010;363:1544–1550.

Nishimura RA, Otto CM, Bonow RO, et al. 2017 AHA/ACC focused update of the 2014 AHA/ACC Guideline for the management of patients with valvular heart disease: a report of the American College of Cardiology/American Heart Association Task Force on Clinical Practice Guidelines. *Circulation.* 2017;135:e1159–e1195.

Nix S. *Williams' Basic Nutrition and Diet Therapy.* 14th ed. St. Louis: Mosby; 2012.

O'Gara PT, Kushner FG, Aschei DD, et al. 2013 ACCF/AHA Guideline for the management of ST-elevation myocardial infarction. *Circulation.* 2013;127:e362–e425. doi:10.1161/CIR.Ob013e3182742cf6.

Pagana KD, Pagana TJ. *Mosby's Manual of Diagnostic and Laboratory Tests.* 5th ed. St. Louis: Mosby; 2013.

Parker RB, Nappi JM, Cavallari LH. Chronic heart failure. In: DiPiro JP, et al, eds. *Pharmacotherapy: A Pathophysiologic Approach.* 10th ed. New York: McGraw-Hill; 2017 [chapter 14].

Physicians' Desk Reference. 69th ed. Montvale, NJ: PDR Network, LLC; 2015.

Potter PA, Perry AG. *Fundamentals of Nursing.* 8th ed. St. Louis: Mosby; 2012.

Prochaska J, DiClemente C. Towards a comprehensive model of change. In: Miller W, Heather N, eds. *Treating Addictive Behaviors: A Process of Change.* New York: Plenum Press; 1986.

Qaseem A, Forciea MA, McLean RM. Treatment of low bone density or osteoporosis to prevent fractures in men and women: a clinical practice guideline update from the American College of Physicians. *Ann Intern Med.* 2017;166(11):818–839.

Reid WH. Recognizing and dealing with impaired clinicians, part I: recognition and reporting. *J Med Pract Manage.* 2001;17:97.

Reid WH. Recognizing and dealing with impaired clinicians, part II: treatment options. *J Med Pract Manage.* 2001;17:145.

Repchinsky C, ed. *Patient Self-Care: Helping Patients Make Therapeutic Choices.* 2nd ed. Ottawa, Canada: Canadian Pharmacists Association; 2010.

Romanelli F, Smith KM. Clinical effects and management of methamphetamine abuse. *Pharmacotherapy.* 2006;26:1148.

Rossouw JE, et al. Lessons learned from the women's health initiative trials of menopausal hormone therapy. *Obstet Gynecol.* 2013;121:172–176.

Rossouw JE, et al. Risks and benefits of estrogen plus progestin in healthy postmenopausal women: principal results from the Women's Health Initiative randomized controlled trial. *JAMA.* 2002;288:321.

Sateia MJ, et al. Clinical practice guideline for the pharmacologic treatment of chronic insomnia in adults: an American Academy of Sleep Medicine clinical practice guideline. *J Clin Sleep Med.* 2017;13(2):307–349.

Scheffer IE, et al. ILAE classification of the epilepsies: position paper of the ILAE Commission for Classification and Terminology. *Epilepsia.* 2017;58(4):512–521.

Siscovick DS, Barringer TA, Fretts AM. Omega-3 polyunsaturated fatty acid (fish oil) supplementation and the prevention of clinical cardiovascular disease: a science advisory from the American Heart Association. *Circulation.* 2017;135:e867–e884. doi: 10.1161/CIR.

Skidmore-Roth L. *Mosby's Handbook of Herbs and Natural Supplements.* 4th ed. St. Louis: Mosby; 2009.

Smith SC, Grundy SM. 2013 ACC/AHA Guideline recommends fixed-dose strategies instead of targeted-dose strategies instead of targeted goals to lower blood cholesterol. *J Am Coll Cardiol.* 2014;64:601–612.

Sprague RL, Kalachnik JE. Reliability, validity and a total score cutoff for the Dyskinesia Identification System: Condensed User Scale (DISCUS) with mentally ill and mentally retarded populations. *Psychopharmacol Bull.* 1991;27:51.

Stone NJ, Robinson JG, Lichtenstein AH, et al. 2013 ACC/AHA Guideline on the treatment of blood cholesterol to reduce atherosclerotic cardiovascular risk in adults: a report of the American College of Cardiology/American Heart Association Task Force on Practice Guidelines. *J Am Coll Cardiol.* 2014;63:2889–2934.

Substance Abuse and Mental Health Services Administration. *Behavioral Health Barometer: United States, 2014.* HHS Publication No. SMA–15–4895. Rockville, MD: Substance Abuse and Mental Health Services Administration; 2015.

Sweetman SC, ed. *Martindale: The Complete Drug Reference.* 37th ed. London: Pharmaceutical Press; 2011.

Taylor D, Stuart G. Chemically mediated responses and substance-related disorders. In: Stuart GW, eds. *Principles and Practice of Psychiatric Nursing.* 10th ed. St. Louis: Mosby; 2010.

Therapeutic Research Faculty. *Natural Medicines Comprehensive Database.* 11th ed. Stockton, CA: Therapeutic Research Faculty; 2009.

Tice SA, Parry D. Medications that require hepatic monitoring. *Hosp Pharm.* 2001;38:456. 39:595–606, 2004.

Trissel LA. *Handbook on Injectable Drugs.* 18th ed. Bethesda, MD: American Society of Health-System Pharmacists; 2015.

Tyler VE. What pharmacists should know about herbal remedies. *J Am Pharm Assoc NS.* 1996;36:29.

US Department of Health and Human Services and US Department of Agriculture. *2015–2020 Dietary Guidelines for Americans.* 8th ed. December 2015. https://health.gov/dietaryguidelines/2015/guidelines/.

US Pharmacopeia 39/National Formulary 33. Rockville, MD: U.S. Pharmacopeial Convention; 2015.

USP Dictionary of USAN and International Drug Names. Rockville, MD: U.S. Pharmacopeial Convention; 2015.

Vasilakou D, Karagiannis T, et al. Sodium-glucose cotransporter 2 inhibitors for type 2 diabetes. *Ann Intern Med.* 2013;159:262–274.

Vlasnik JJ, Aliotta SL, DeLor B. Evidence-based assessment and intervention strategies to increase adherence to prescribed medication plans. *Case Manager.* 2005;16:55.

Vlasnik JJ, Aliotta SL, DeLor B. Medication adherence: factors influencing compliance with prescribed medication plans. *Case Manager.* 2005;16:47.

Wein AJ, Rovner ES. Definition and epidemiology of overactive bladder. *Urology.* 2002;60(5 suppl 1):7–12.

Whelton PK, Carey RM, Aronow WS, et al. 2017 ACC/AHA/AAPA/ABC/ACPM/AGS/APhA/ASH/ASPC/NMA/PCNA Guideline for the prevention, detection, evaluation, and management of high blood pressure in adults: a report of the American College of Cardiology/American Heart Association Task Force on Clinical Practice Guidelines. *J Am Coll Cardiol.* 2017; http://www.onlinejacc.org/content/early/2017/11/04/j.jacc.2017.11.005. Published online November 13.

Willett WC. *Eat, Drink, and Be Healthy: The Harvard Medical School Guide to Healthy Eating.* Florence, MA: Free Press/Simon & Schuster; 2005.

Wilson W, Taubert KA, Gewitz M, et al. Prevention of infective endocarditis: guidelines from the American Heart Association: a guideline from the American Heart Association Rheumatic Fever, Endocarditis, and Kawasaki Disease Committee, Council on Cardiovascular Disease in the Young, and the Council on Clinical Cardiology, Council on Cardiovascular Surgery and Anesthesia, and the Quality of Care and Outcomes

Research Interdisciplinary Working Group. *J Am Dent Assoc.* 2007;*139*(suppl):3S–24S.

Workowski KA, Bolan GA, Centers for Disease Control and Prevention. Sexually transmitted diseases treatment guidelines, 2015. *MMWR Recomm Rep.* 2015;*64*(RR–3):1–137.

Yancy CW, Jessup M, Bozkurt B, et al. 2013 ACCF/AHA Guideline for the management of heart failure: a report of the American Colleges of Cardiology Foundation/American Heart Association Task Force on Practice Guidelines. *Circulation.* 2013;*128*:e240–e327. doi:10.1161/CIR.0b013e31829e8776.

Yancy CW, Jessup M, Bozkurt BJ, et al. 2017 ACC/AHA/HFSA focused update of the 2013 ACCF/AHA Guideline for the management of heart failure: a report of the American College of Cardiology/American Heart Association Task Force on Clinical Practice Guidelines and the Heart Failure Society of America. *J Card Fail.* 2017;*23*(8):628–651. doi:10.1016/j.cardfail.2017.04.014.

Yu DT, et al. Impact of implementing alerts about medication black-box warnings in electronic health records. *Pharmacoepidemiol Drug Saf.* 2011;*20*(2):192–202.

Index